Postgraduate Haematology

Postgraduate Haematology

Third Edition

Edited by

A. V. Hoffbrand

MA, DM, FRCP, FRCPath, FRCP (Edin), DSc

Professor of Haematology, Royal Free Hospital School of Medicine, Honorary Consultant Haematologist, The Royal Free Hospital, London

S. M. Lewis

BSc, MD, FRCPath, DCP

Reader in Haematology, Royal Postgraduate Medical School and Consultant Haematologist, Hammersmith Hospital, London

HEINEMANN PROFESSIONAL PUBLISHING

Heinemann Medical Books
An imprint of Heinemann Professional Publishing Ltd
Halley Court, Jordan Hill, Oxford OX2 8EJ

OXFORD LONDON SINGAPORE NAIROBI IBADAN KINGSTON

First published 1972
Reprinted 1975
Second edition 1981
Reprinted 1983, 1986
Third edition 1989
(The first edition was published under the title of
Haematology in the series *Tutorials in Postgraduate
Haematology*)

British Library Cataloguing in Publication Data

Postgraduate haematology.—3rd ed.
  I. Man. Blood. Diseases
  I. Hoffbrand, A. V. (Allan Victor)
  II. Lewis, S. M. (Shirley Mitchell)
  616.1′5

  ISBN 0-433-15054-8

Typeset by Macmillan (India) Ltd, Bangalore 560 025 and
printed in Great Britain by Butler and Tanner Limited, Frome

CONTENTS

PREFACE TO THE FIRST EDITION

In this book the authors combine an account of the physiological and biochemical basis of haematological processes, with descriptions of the clinical and laboratory features and management of blood disorders. Within this framework, each author has dealt with the individual subjects as he or she thought appropriate. Because this book is intended to provide a foundation for the study of haematology and is not intended to be a reference book, it reflects, to some extent, the views of the individual authors rather than providing comprehensive detail and a full bibliography. For these the reader is referred to the selected reading given at the end of each chapter. It is hoped that the book will prove of particular value to students taking either the Primary or Final Part of the examination for Membership of the Royal College of Pathologists and the Diplomas of Clinical Pathology. It should also prove useful to physicians wishing to gain special knowledge of haematology, and to technicians taking the Advanced Diploma in Haematology of the Institute of Medical Laboratory Technology, or the Higher National Certificate in Medical Laboratory subjects.

We wish to acknowledge kind permission from the Editors and Publishers of the British Journal of Haematology, the Journal of the Royal College of Physicians of London and the Quarterly Journal of Medicine for permission to reproduce figures 4.1, 4.5, 4.10, 4.11, 4.12, 9.4 and 9.10, also the publishers of "Progress in Haematology" for figure 7.2, and many other publishers who, together with the authors, have been acknowledged in the text. We are particularly grateful to Professor J. V. Dacie for providing material which formed the basis of many of the original illustrations in Chapters 4–8. We are greatly indebted to Mrs. T. Charalambos, Mrs. J. Cope and Mrs. D. Haysome for secretarial assistance, to Mrs. P. Schilling and the Department of Medical Illustration for photomicrography, art work and general photography.

Finally, we are grateful for the invaluable help and forbearance we have received from Mr. R Emory and William Heinemann Medical Books.

London, 1972

A.V.H.
S.M.L.

PREFACE TO THE THIRD EDITION

The first edition of this book was published in 1972; when the second edition appeared in 1981, its considerable expansion was an indication of the advances which had taken place in the science and practice of haematology. Since then there has been an even more dramatic growth in understanding of the functions of blood in health and its abnormalities in disease. These advances are mainly due to the application of new techniques in biochemistry, molecular biology, molecular genetics and monoclonal antibody technology. The editors were faced with the formidable task of retaining the essential substance of the previous edition and adding important new aspects whilst endeavouring to keep the book to a reasonable size and maintaining the original intent. It is intended to provide a foundation to the study of haematology for postgraduate students specializing in haematology, especially those taking the examination for Membership of the Royal College of Pathologists, for physicians with an interest in haematology and also for scientists and technologists working in this area.

An increasing amount of clinical work and responsibility for the clinical management of patients is being undertaken by haematologists. In this edition this is recognized in the detailed descriptions which are given of the clinical aspects of blood diseases and the range of treatments which are now available. The book will, we hope, serve as a bridge between scientists carrying out experimental research, and laboratory-based and clinically-based haematologists.

The first edition was written exclusively by the members of the Department of Haematology of the Royal Postgraduate Medical School. Some of those original authors have moved to other institutions where they have established their own centres of excellence; these and other authors were invited to contribute to the new edition which now reflects British haematology more broadly. The book is not intended as a reference book, but gives the viewpoint of the individual authors who are all eminent teachers and workers in their specialized fields. However, each chapter includes selected key references, especially to important reviews, and where there may be differing and controversial opinions the authors have in general tried to give a balanced critical view. The book does not include technical material, but where necessary the reader is referred to appropriate texts on laboratory practice.

We are grateful to all our authors for their excellent contributions despite many other demands on their time and to Caroline Creed and Richard Barling, our publishers, for their enthusiastic support and help at all stages in the preparation of this new edition.

London, 1988

A.V.H.
S.M.L.

LIST OF CONTRIBUTORS

M K Brenner MA MB MRCP MRCPath PhD
Senior Lecturer in Haematology
Honorary Royal Free Hospital School of Medicine
    Consultant Haematologist
The Royal Free Hospital
Pond Street
London NW3 2QG

D Catovsky MD MRCP FRCPath DSc
Professor of Haematology
Honorary Consultant Haematologist
Royal Marsden Hospital
Fulham Road
London Sw3 6JJ

Marcela Contreras BSc MD MRCPath
Director
National Blood Transfusion Unit
North London Blood Transfusion Centre
Deansbrook Road
Edgware
Middlesex
HA8 8BD

D A G Galton MA MD FRCP FRCPath
Formerly Honorary Director
MRC Leukaemia Unit
Royal Postgraduate Medical School
Hammersmith Hospital
Ducane Road
London W12 OHS

J M Goldman DM FRCP FRCPath
Professor of Leukaemia Biology
Royal Postgraduate Medical School
Honorary Consultant Physician
Hammersmith Hospital
Ducane Road
London W12 OHS

E C Gordon-Smith MA MSc BM FRCP FRCPath
Professor of Haematology
St George's Hospital Medical School
Honorary Consultant Haematologist
St George's Hospital
Cranmer Terrace
Blackshaw Road
Tooting
London SW17 OQT

R M Hardisty MD FRCP FRCPath
Emeritus Professor of Haematology
Katherine Dormandy Haemophilia Centre and
    Haemostasis Unit
The Royal Free Hospital
Pond Street
London NW3 2QG

Patricia Hewitt MB MRCP MRCPath
Deputy Director
Edgware Blood Transfusion Centre
Deansbrook Road
Edgware
Middlesex
HA8 9BD

A V Hoffbrand MA DM FRCP FRCPath FRCP
    (Edin) DSc
Professor of Haematology
Royal Free Hospital
School of Medicine
Honorary Consultant Haematologist
The Royal Free Hospital
Pond Street
London NW3 2QG

J M Hows MD, MSc, MRCP, MRCPath
Senior Lecturer in Immunohaematology
Royal Postgraduate Medical School
Consultant Haematologist
Royal Postgraduate Medical School
Hammersmith Hospital
Ducane Road
London W12 OHS

R A Hutton PhD FIMLS
Principal Biochemist
Katherine Dormandy Haemophilia Centre and
    Haemostasis Unit
The Royal Free Hospital
Pond Street
London NW3 2QG

P B A Kernoff MD FRCP MRCPath
Director
Katherine Dormandy Haemophilia Centre and
    Haemostasis Unit
Consultant Haematologist
The Royal Free Hospital
Pond Street
London NW3 2QG

S M Lewis Bsc MD FRCPath DCP
Reader in Haematology
Royal Postgraduate Medical School
Consultant Haematologist
Hammersmith Hospital
Ducane Road
London W12 OHS

Anatole Lubenko BA PhD
Head of Department of Immunology
National Blood Transfusion Unit
North London Blood Transfusion Centre
Deansbrook Road
Edgware, Middlesex, HA8 9BD

L Luzzatto MD FRCP FRCPath
Professor of Haematology
Royal Postgraduate Medical School
Honorary Director MRC and LRS Leukaemia Unit
Honorary Consultant Haematologist
Hammersmith Hospital
Ducane Road
London W12 OHS

S J Machin MB MRCPath
Reader in Haematology
Middlesex Hospital Medical School
Consultant Haematologist
The Middlesex Hospital
Mortimer Street
London W1N 8AA

T C Pearson MD MRCPath
Reader in Haematology
Consultant Haematologist
United Medical and Dental Schools of Guy's
    Hospital and St. Thomas's Hospital
Lambeth Palace Road
London SE1 7EH

M J Pippard BSc MB MRCP MRCPath
Consultant Haematologist
Northwick Park Hospital and Clinical Research
    Centre
Harrow
Middlesex

Lorna M Secker-Walker MA PhD
Senior Lecturer in Haematology
Royal Free Hospital School of Medicine
Pond Street
London NW3 2QG

E G D Tuddenham MD FRCP FRCPath
Consultant Haematologist
Clinical Research Centre
Watford Road
Harrow
Middlesex
HA1 3UJ

J S Wainscoat MSc MB MRCP MRCPath
Consultant Haematologist
John Radcliffe Hospital
Headington
Oxford
OX3 9DU

Chapter 1

ERYTHROPOIESIS

S. M. LEWIS

The essential purpose of erythropoiesis is to provide a vehicle for the transport of haemoglobin. Normal erythropoiesis requires the production of an adequate number of erythrocytes at a rate determined by the body's demand. They enter circulation at a correct state of maturity, and contain an adequate content of normal adult haemoglobin for oxygen uptake, transport and exchange. This process requires an intact and integrated system of enzymes and other factors for multiplication, maturation and release of erythrocytes; it also requires an effective enzyme-controlled metabolic system to enable the cells to survive in circulation for the duration of a normal lifespan. If the controls are deranged for one or other reason, or if an essential factor is lacking, erythropoiesis will be disturbed. This will result in diminished production (i.e. marrow hypoplasia), defective production (i.e. dyserythropoiesis), or the production of erythrocytes which have intrinsic defects and are liable to premature death and to haemolysis by a normally harmless environment. These abnormalities are frequently interrelated; thus, for example, dyserythropoiesis will almost invariably result in the production of abnormal erythrocytes with shortened survival. The defects of erythropoiesis and of the erythrocyte which give rise to various types of anaemia will be described in subsequent chapters. This chapter will be devoted mainly to the process of normal erythropoiesis.

THE ORIGIN AND SITES OF ERYTHRO-POIESIS (Fig. 1.1)

In common with granulocytes and megakaryocytes, erythroid cells are derived from a mesenchymal stem cell which appears in the yolk sac in two-week-old embryos. At six weeks the liver becomes a haemopoietic organ and the mesenchymal cell differentiates into reticulum cells and colony-forming cells.

The liver becomes the main site of haemopoiesis by the 12th to 16th week and remains active until a few weeks before birth. The spleen is a relatively minor organ of erythropoiesis, beginning to function in this role at about the same time as the liver and continuing until gestation. The bone marrow becomes a site of erythropoiesis from about 20 weeks, increasing rapidly in its activity during the last trimester of pregnancy. Meanwhile, during the developmental process, the cells have further differentiated into primitive erythroblasts and then into the definitive pronormoblasts and normoblasts which characterize normal postnatal erythropoiesis and which differentiate into the mature erythrocytes. In the postnatal marrow all three cell lines—erythroid, granulocytic and megakaryocyte—are derived from a common 'pluripotent' progenitor stem cell, or 'colony-forming unit', known as a CFU. This has the ability to reproduce itself, but, also, its progeny become progressively more committed to one of the lines of blood cell production: the progenitor stem cells of erythropoiesis are known as burst-forming units (BFU–E); these give rise to the erythroid colony-forming units (CFU–E). CFU–GM give rise to granulocyte-macrophages, and CFU–Mk are the progenitor cells for megakaryocyte production. The haemopoietic stem cell appears also to differentiate into precursors of T-lymphocytes and B-lymphocytes (see Chapter 11). Erythropoiesis is regulated by the interaction of BFU–E with auxiliary cells which regulate their growth and differentiation; these auxiliary cells are

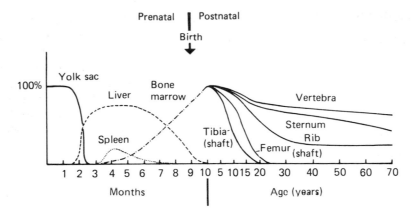

Fig. 1.1. *Sites of erythropoietic tissue in fetus and throughout life.*

thought to be macrophages, T-lymphocytes and cells of the haemopoietic microenvironment (see below). T-cells are an important source of interleukin 3 (a burst-promoting activity) which stimulates BFU–E formation from the earlier, pluripotent precursor. Another factor which is essential for erythropoiesis is erythropoietin (p. 7). Acting as a 'colony-stimulating factor' (CSF), it stimulates the proliferation and differentiation of CFU–E; it also induces proliferation of late BFU–E.

At birth, haemopoietic (red) marrow occupies the entire capacity of the bones. From childhood there is a gradual replacement of the red marrow by fatty (yellow) marrow until, in the adult, red marrow is confined to the sternum, ribs and vertebrae, cranium, and pelvis. In old age these sites, too, become increasingly replaced with fatty marrow. This is important when assessing the cellularity of the bone marrow from an aspirated sample or trephine biopsy at any one site. In an iliac crest trephine section in the normal adult there is usually a cellular:fat ratio of about 1:1 to 2:1 (Fig. 1.2). It must, however, be remembered that the marrow spaces do not have uniform cellularity, and a solitary sampling cannot be assumed to represent the overall pattern.

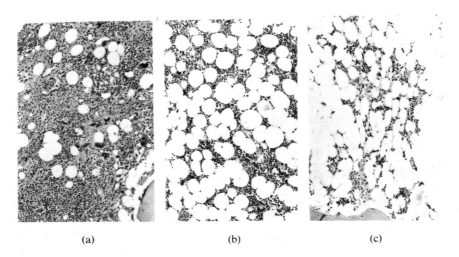

(a)   (b)   (c)

Fig. 1.2. *Range of cellularity of marrow in normal subjects (iliac crest trephine biopsies). (H & E × 100.)*

Haemopoietic Microenvironment

Bone marrow consists of fat cells, reticulum cells, mast cells, plasma cells, fibroblasts and the endothelial cells which line the vascular structures (Fig. 1.3). The stroma, together with the vascular channels, provides the microenvironment necessary for supporting the viability of the haemopoietic cells. Precisely how the microenvironment influences haemopoiesis is not known. Some aspects have been elucidated by in-vitro culture studies and the functions of the various stromal cells are described on p. 297. In addition to these specific cellular functions the stroma itself provides the structural framework which allows the haemopoietic cells to retain their place between the fat cells, and adjacent to the vessels and sinusoids. The extracellular glycoprotein fibronectin is important for adhesion of early erythroid precursors. The cells of the microenvironment also produce collagen, proteoglycans and laminin.

Another cell with important influence on haemopoiesis is the bone marrow macrophage. The macrophage has a number of different functions. Apart from being a haemopoietic cell, it has a role in the regulation of haemopoiesis by its capacity to synthesize and/or transport haemopoietic growth factors and also inhibitory factors which affect both granulocytic and erythroid cell lines. Macrophages are found at the centre of erythropoietic islands in the marrow. The marrow is an active site of phagocytosis of normal red cells at the end of their lifespan

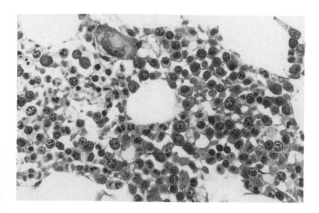

Fig. 1.3. *Section of normal bone marrow; methacrylate embedding (× 300).*

and it may become a major site of erythrophagocytosis when there is intramedullary cell destruction or severe haemolysis. Macrophages contain iron, set free from phagocytosed erythrocytes, and which in turn attaches to transferrin. T-lymphocytes which are present in the marrow also appear to have a controlling influence on haemopoiesis by producing GM-CSF and IL-3.

ERYTHROCYTE CELL PROLIFERATION AND MATURATION

Cells of the erythroid series have the same mechanism for synthesis as any cell, but with the unique capacity for haemoglobin synthesis. The earliest morphologically distinct erythroid precursor is the pro-erythroblast (or pronormoblast). It can synthesize DNA, RNA and protein together with carbohydrate and enzymes. It is characterized by a large nucleus with a clear and delicate chromatin pattern and nucleoli. The cytoplasm contains abundant RNA, ribosomes mainly in the form of polyribosomes, endoplasmic reticulum, together with a few microtubules and fibrils, a large number of mitochondria and a centrosome composed of centrioles and a well-formed Golgi body. There may be ferritin molecules scattered throughout the cytoplasm; this ferritin comes from iron which has been brought to the cell membrane bound to transferrin (see p. 28) and then passes across the membrane into the cell. Some of the iron is taken up in the mitochondria, where protoporphyrin rings are synthesized from succinate and glycine, into which the iron is incorporated to form the haem which will be used subsequently to produce haemoglobin.

As the cell matures, the nucleus loses its nucleolus and the chromatin begins to condense to form coalescent clumps. The residual ferritin becomes grouped in small (siderotic) clusters. In the polychromatic normoblasts, ferritin clusters are still present and there are abundant ribosomes, mainly in the form of polyribosomes but also in scattered solitary units. At this stage DNA and RNA synthesis ceases so that all subsequent protein synthesis (mainly haemoglobin) must utilize preformed mRNA. Haemoglobin is manufactured within the cytoplasm by the combination of two alpha and two beta polypeptide globin chains and four haem groups (see p. 121).

The penultimate stage of maturation is the reticulocyte; this cell contains no nucleus but RNA, ribosomes and some mitochondria are still present so that the cell is still capable of (limited) haemoglobin production. In the last stages of maturation the mitochondria, RNA and ribosomes disappear. The mature erythrocyte has no synthetic capability but is able to metabolize glucose by means of the enzyme systems of the glycolytic pathways.

The features of erythroid cells during their maturation, as demonstrated by electron microscopy, are illustrated in Fig. 1.4.

DNA provides the genetic control for cell synthesis. The way in which genetic information stored in the DNA of the cell nucleus is transferred to the cytoplasm and provides the blueprint for protein synthesis within the cell is described at the molecular level in Chapter 5. The process of cell proliferation at the cellular level will be described below.

In the erythropoietic system there are always some cells in a resting stage and some in a proliferative cycle (Fig. 1.5). There are three mitotic divisions during the evolution of the pronormoblasts to the late (pyknotic) normoblast (Fig. 1.6): the interphase (intermitotic interval) lasts 16 hours, so that maturation to the late normoblasts takes 2 days. Haemoglobinization takes 2–4 days.

Cell Division

Mitosis commences at prophase when the nuclear membrane disintegrates and the nuclear chromatin becomes rearranged into individual chromosomes, which then duplicate (Fig. 1.7). The dissolution of the nuclear membrane gives rise to vesicles and cisternae of endoplasmic reticulum. The chromosome-pairs are joined at their midpoints (centromeres). At metaphase the paired chromosomes begin to separate, and mitotic spindles, which form from microtubules, connect the centromeres to the centrioles which are situated at the two poles of the cell. At anaphase the spindles contract and one half of each of the duplicated chromosomes is drawn towards each of the centrioles. At telophase the chromatin becomes rearranged into a nucleus, the

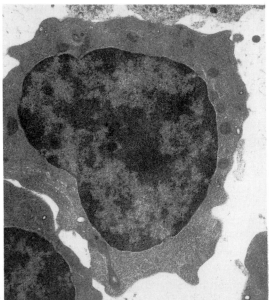
(a)

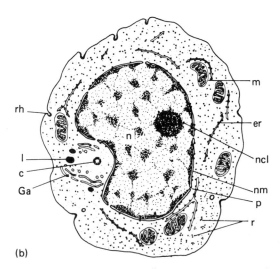
(b)

Fig. 1.4. *Transmission electron microscope appearance of section of an erythroid cell (a) (× 15 000). A schematic drawing (b) identifies the constituents of the cell. (n, nucleus; ncl, nucleolus; nm, nuclear membrane; p, pore; m, mitochondria; er, endoplasmic reticulum; Ga, Golgi apparatus; c, centriole; r, ribosomes; lysosome; rh, rhopheocytosis.)*

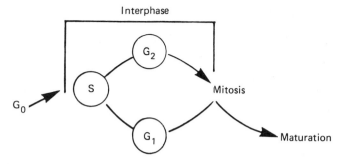

Fig. 1.5. *Model of cell cycle. (G_0, resting phase; S, DNA synthetic stage; G_1 and G_2 are postmitotic and postsynthetic gaps; at G_0 the resting cell is not yet committed.)*

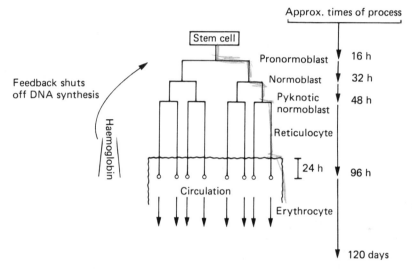

Fig. 1.6. *Model of erythroid cell proliferation and maturation.*

cytoplasmic membrane invaginates around each nucleus and the cell separates as interphase begins.

The nuclear membrane plays an important part in mitosis. It appears to control the ordered process by which chromatin is arranged during interphase and rearranged in prophase as a prerequisite for division. There are a number of situations which cause a variation in the normal sequence of erythropoiesis.

(a) *Shortening of intermitotic time with normal maturation time* will result in the production of an increased number of cells in a given time; it is the usual response to anaemia caused by haemorrhage or haemolysis. In studies with radioactive iron (^{59}Fe) this is demonstrated by a shortened marrow transit time with an unusually rapid reappearance of radioactivity in the circulation. In severe anaemia there may also be an accelerated maturation time which will result in premature release into circulation of cells which still contain residual material from their development, i.e. nuclear remnants and basophilic reticulocytes (see p. 6). These cells are also macrocytic ('shift reticulocytes').

(b) *Additional mitotic division* may occur if the control mechanism which determines cessation of division becomes disordered, as, for example, in iron deficiency anaemia, when the reduced content of haemoglobin is responsible (see p. 6). In this event the ultimate cells are microcytic.

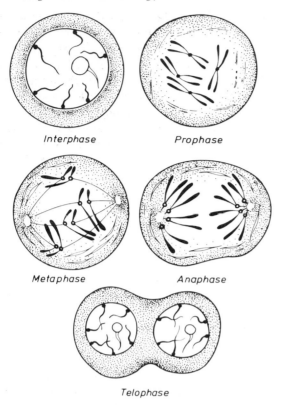

Fig. 1.7. *The different phases of mitotic cell division.*

(c) *Omission of one or more mitotic divisions* produces a converse effect, and the cells are left as macrocytes.

Cell proliferation is thought to be regulated by tissue-specific substances called chalones, which interact with DNA. Inhibition of erythroblast proliferation is caused by a chalone derived from erythrocytes. In addition, in the erythrocyte there is another specific control mechanism; when a critical haemoglobin concentration is reached, a feedback mechanism is triggered which shuts off further nucleic acid synthesis and cell division, Thus, the number of divisions in a fixed interphase time is determined by the rate of haemoglobin synthesis: when haemoglobin synthesis is accelerated, critical haemoglobin concentration is reached more rapidly—in haemoglobin deficiency the shut-off fails and this results in an increased number of divisions with the production of microcytes (see Fig. 1.6).

Disappearance of Nucleus

The erythroid cell is unique in that it loses its nucleus whilst retaining its functional capacity. As the cell matures, its DNA activity becomes suppressed. This leads to chromosome condensation with cessation of differentiation. The pyknotic nucleus is then extruded by a process of cytoplasm cleavage for which active cell movement is required. Thus, this depends on the functional integrity of both the nuclear envelope and the cell membrane. Residual remnants of the nucleus which are retained during the cleavage will be removed subsequently when the cells pass through the spleen (p. 18).

Erythrocytes

Reticulocytes mature in 2–3 days, 24 hours of which are spent in the circulation. However, if the reticulocyte is released into circulation prematurely, its maturation time in circulation will be prolonged for up to 3 days. This is an important point to remember when using the reticulocyte count as a measurement of erythropoietic activity; it is usually said that marrow activity can be deduced from reticulocyte numbers, on the assumption that reticulocytes remain in circulation for one day. However, as this is not necessarily true, especially in situations of increased demand, it would be more informative to relate the reticulocyte count to the stage of their development as indicated by the amount of reticulum in stained preparations or their RNA content, or by calculating a corrected reticulocyte count per day from an estimated maturation time.

$$\frac{\text{Corrected}}{\text{reticulocyte count}} = \frac{\text{Absolute reticulocyte count}}{\text{Maturation time (days)}}$$

After the erythrocytes have matured, they survive in circulation for about 120 days (S.D. $\pm$ 15 days). There are two methods for measuring the lifespan and rate of destruction of red cells using radionuclide markers, namely cohort and random labelling. In cohort labelling a population of red cells is labelled during the production in the bone marrow. Peripheral blood radioactivity is then monitored over a period of time to detect the release of these cells into the circulation and their subsequent removal. Labelled amino acids such as glycine and radioactive iron (^{59}Fe) are generally used for cohort labelling. Random labelling, in which a sample of the circulating blood is labelled with radioactive sodium chromate (^{51}Cr), is simpler and is the method of choice in most clinical situations. Technical details and interpretation of the results of red cell survival studies are outside the scope of this book; they can be found in Dacie and Lewis (1984).

Supplementary information about the mechanism of haemolysis can be obtained from in-vivo surface counting carried out during the red cell survival study. The destruction of the red cells at the end of their lifespan is by phagocytosis in the reticuloendothelial (RE) system. This occurs partly in the spleen, but RE cells throughout the body, notably in the bone marrow, also take part in the process. With phagocytosis the constituents of the erythrocyte are disassembled: amino acids are returned to the body protein pool; iron is freed from haem and is transported, bound to a beta-globulin protein (transferrin), back to the marrow for re-use in a new cycle of erythropoiesis; the breakdown of the protoporphyrin ring releases carbon which escapes through the lungs as carbon monoxide, whilst the remaining pyrrole ring is carried as bilirubin to the liver where it is conjugated to glucuronide and excreted. During the phase of excretion in the gut, bacterial action converts the conjugated bilirubin to urobilinogen—it is in this form that it appears in the stool, whilst a small proportion is reabsorbed and excreted in the urine.

BONE MARROW CONTROL OF BLOOD CELL DELIVERY

Each day some 2×10^{11} erythrocytes enter the circulation. To do so the mature blood cells must pass the vascular barrier, at a rate determined by the porosity of the sinusoidal wall and/or the ability of the cells to squeeze through a narrow gap. When haemopoietic cells proliferate, they exert pressure on the membrane of endothelial cells lining the sinusoids. These endothelial cells normally overlap, but when the lumen of the sinus expands, the overlapping cells separate, thus opening intercellular pores through which the migrating cells can pass. Control of the mechanism of erythroid cell

release appears to be mediated by erythropoietin and it may also be influenced by other hormonal and humoral factors. Porosity is especially increased when the marrow is infiltrated by malignant cells or fibrosis, and this leads to the release into circulation of immature cells. Cell deformability is a feature of the mature erythrocyte; nucleated erythroid cells do not have the pliability to pass through the normal sinus wall. Fibronectin adhesion, present on the immature cells, is lost on mature erythrocytes.

REGULATION OF ERYTHROPOIESIS

The maintenance of a relatively constant circulating red cell mass requires an erythropoietic stimulus which ensures that under physiological conditions the rate of production of new erythrocytes equals the rate of destruction, and that there is an increased production rate in response to anoxia, high altitude, haemorrhage or haemolysis. The most important factors are erythropoietin and, as nutrients, iron, vitamin B_{12} and folate. Other essential factors are vitamin B_6 (pyridoxine), riboflavin, vitamin E (alpha tocopherol), and copper, as well as proteins and carbohydrates. Several hormones (e.g. androgens, thyroxine) also play a part, either directly or by stimulating erythropoietic activity. Interleukin 3 is necessary in vitro to induce the formation of the earliest detectable red cell progenitor, the BFU–E.

ERYTHROPOIETIN

Erythropoietin is a heat-stable glycoprotein. The gene on chromosome 7q11–q22 has been characterized and a purified erythropoietin has been produced by recombinant DNA methods. It contains a protein backbone consisting of 166 amino acids with a 27-amino-acid leader peptide. It has a molecular weight of 18 398; in its native form erythropoietin is heavily glycosylated and has a molecular weight of about 34 000. It has a terminal sialic acid residue which is necessary for its in-vivo biological activity.

Erythropoietin is produced mainly in the kidney (about 90%) but also in the liver and possibly to a slight extent in the spleen. In the renal tissue it is located in the light mitochondrial and microsomal subcellular fractions. It is thought to be generated in the microsomes and then transported to the mitochondria. Erythropoietin can be demonstrated in plasma or urine: (a) by biological assay based on the measurement of ^{59}Fe uptake by a laboratory animal following injection of test material, (b) by in-vitro assay of incorporation of ^{59}Fe into haem in fetal liver cells, and (c) by radioimmunoassay. Estimates by the different methods do not give identical results as they reflect different functional and structural characteristics of erythropoietin and its degradation products. However, they show comparable trends in various conditions. Radioimmunoassay is a sensitive and convenient method; it gives a range of 13–37 mi.u./ml in the serum of normal individuals (Chapter 20, Fig. 20.2).

Erythropoietin stimulation affects erythrocyte production at several levels. Primarily it stimulates proliferation of late BFU–E and controls the rate at which the erythropoietin-sensitive marrow progenitor cells (CFU–E) give rise to pronormoblasts. It also influences the rate of maturation, haemoglobin synthesis and release of the cell from the marrow into circulation. In a subject in whom the marrow is capable of normal response, erythropoietic stimulus of severe anaemia (Hb < 80 g/l) can cause a six- to ninefold increase in erythroid marrow. This results in expansion of the marrow into the long bones and sometimes into extramedullary sites. The place of erythropoietin in the regulation of erythropoiesis is illustrated in Fig. 1.8. Conditions associated with increased or decreased erythropoietin are listed in Table 1.1. The role of erythropoietin in the anaemia which occurs in chronic renal failure has been shown by a remarkable rise in haemoglobin after administration of recombinant human erythropoietin to patients with end-stage renal disease undergoing regular haemodialysis.

For erythropoietin to have its predictable effect, an adequate iron supply is necessary for haemoglobin synthesis: in the normal adult this means 20–30 mg/day. The bulk of this iron will be derived from normal erythrocyte breakdown, with direct transfer of the iron from RE cells to erythroid marrow. Only 1 mg is obtained daily from the absorption of dietary iron and 3–4 mg are available from labile stores. The normal adult man has about 1000 mg of stored iron and can temporarily mobilize 10–30 mg per day. Conversely, without adequate stores blood production will be limited by the small amount of iron derived from diet. In extravascular haemolytic anaemia there is an adequate and readily available iron supply of up to several hundred milligrams per day derived from the destroyed erythrocytes. It is in this group of diseases that the marrow is best able to respond to the anaemia over long periods of time.

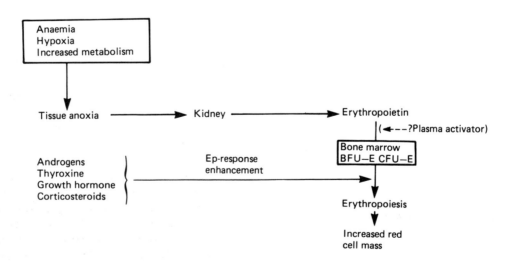

Fig. 1.8. *Schematic diagram of erythropoietin production and its role in erythropoiesis (see text).*

Table 1.1
Erythropoietin production

Erythropoietin increased
Physiologically appropriate (compensatory)
Hypoxia*
  High altitude
  Cardiovascular shunt
  Chronic pulmonary disease
  Massive obesity
  High O_2 affinity haemoglobinopathies
  Congenital low red cell DPG
Anaemias
  Haemolytic
  Haemorrhagic
  Megaloblastic, iron deficiency etc.
  Aplastic and red cell aplasia (but inhibitor may be present)

Physiologically inappropriate
Renal disease*
  Cysts
  Hydronephrosis
  Carcinoma
  Renal transplant
Tumours*
  Renal carcinoma
  Cerebellar haemangioblastoma
  Hepatoma
  Uterine fibroma
  Ovarian carcinoma
  Adrenocortical adenoma
Endocrine disease*
  Adrenal cortical hyperplasia/tumour
Drugs
  Androgens†
  Corticosteroids
  Thyroxine
  Growth hormone
  Cobalt

Erythropoietin decreased
Renal failure
Oestrogen
Secondary anaemia of chronic disease (?)

Erythropoietin normal or low
Polycythaemia vera

---

*Likely to result in polycythaemia.
†Also causes increased erythropoietic response to normal amounts of erythropoietin.

HORMONES

An association of sex hormones with the regulation of erythropoiesis is suggested by the relationship of haemoglobin to age and sex. Testosterone is known to cause a rise in haemoglobin, and androgens have been shown to be beneficial in at least some patients with aplastic anaemia. Conversely, patients with hypofunction of the anterior lobe of the pituitary, the thyroid, testes or adrenal gland may suffer from anaemia which responds to therapy with the deficient hormone.

Corticosteroids, androgens, growth hormones and thyroxine are thought to enhance erythropoietin response by the red cell precursors. Thyroid hormones stimulate erythropoietin production indirectly by increasing the general metabolism, resulting in increased oxygen requirement. Corticosteroids also have a direct stimulatory effect on erythropoiesis. Oestrogen inhibits erythropoiesis both by reducing erythropoietin production and by antagonizing its effect.

BLOOD VOLUME

Total blood volume comprises the red cell mass (RCM) and plasma volume (PV), with an almost negligible contribution, as a rule, from platelets and leucocytes. The ratio of RCM to PV differs in the venous system, the capillaries and the splenic blood pool (p. 18).

The venous haematocrit (PCV) is about 10% higher than the overall body haematocrit. The RCM does not fluctuate to any significant extent provided that the circulation and erythropoiesis are in a steady state. It is influenced by age and sex, by compensation for increased oxygen needs and by other factors which affect erythropoietin production (see p. 8). The PV is more labile and is influenced by bedrest, exercise, change in posture, food, and ambient temperature. Short-term regulation of PV is designed to maintain a constant circulating blood volume; as a rule, rapid adjustments take place, immediately in the case of shock or haemolysis or a few hours after blood transfusion or intravenous infusion. Fluctuation in PV is responsible for haemodilution, when PV expands, and haemoconcentration, when PV is reduced. The effects of

PV changes on the blood count in pathological conditions are illustrated in Table 1.2.

In pregnancy, both PV and RCM increase: PV increases especially in the first trimester, RCM later, and by full term PV has increased by about 40% and the total blood volume by 32% or more. The blood volume returns to normal within a few weeks postpartum.

Plasma Volume Control

Changes in plasma volume are achieved by alteration in the distribution of water between the intravascular and extracellular fluid compartments across the capillary wall. The capillary has a semipermeable membrane which allows water, electrolytes and protein molecules (but not red cells) to diffuse through its pores which increase in size as a result of hydrostatic pressure and distension of the capillaries. Capillary permeability is influenced by pH, PO_2 and PCO_2, changes in oncotic and intravascular pressure, hormones, enzymes and toxic agents.

Fluid balance is thought to be regulated by 'stretch receptors' situated in the vena cava and right atrium. With low PV, a decrease in stretch triggers neurovascular signals which stimulate pituitary secretion of antidiuretic hormone and adrenal cortex secretion of aldosterone. The antidiuretic hormone causes reduced water excretion; aldosterone causes sodium retention and water reabsorption. Both effects result in increased PV.

Other stretch receptors, present in the renal glomerular arterioles, react to distension caused by increased PV by depressing the release of renin and angiotensin; this in turn inhibits aldosterone, resulting in water loss and reduced PV. Conversely, decreased stretch leads to renin activation, aldosterone secretion and increased PV (Fig. 1.9).

MEASUREMENT OF BLOOD VOLUME

The principle of measurement of blood volume is dilution analysis. A small amount of a readily identifiable radionuclide is injected intravenously either bound to the red cells or to a plasma protein and its dilution is measured after complete mixing within the circulating red cell volume or plasma volume respectively. Previously ^{51}Cr was the usual red cell label for measuring red cell volume. It is not ideal but is still used, especially when this measure-

Table 1.2
Influence of red cell volume and plasma volume on blood count

Red cell volume	Plasma volume	Cause	Effect
Normal	High	Pregnancy	Pseudoanaemia
Normal	Low	Stress; Peripheral circulatory failure; Diuretics; Dehydration; Prolonged bedrest	Pseudopolycythaemia
Normal or low	High	Cirrhosis; Nephritis; Myelomatosis; Marked splenomegaly	Pseudoanaemia or anaemia less severe than indicated by PCV and RBC
High	Normal or low	Polycythaemia	Accurate reflection of polycythaemia or polycythaemia less severe than apparent

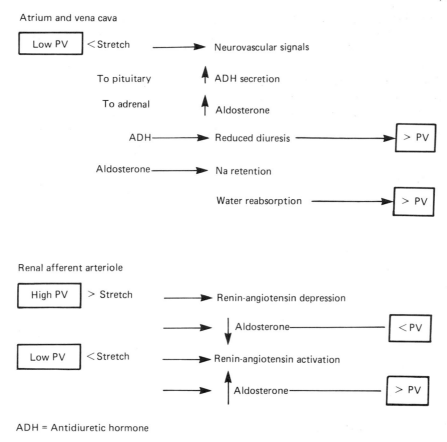

Atrium and vena cava

Low PV < Stretch ⟶ Neurovascular signals

To pituitary ↑ ADH secretion

To adrenal ↑ Aldosterone

ADH ⟶ Reduced diuresis ⟶ > PV

Aldosterone ⟶ Na retention

Water reabsorption ⟶ > PV

Renal afferent arteriole

High PV > Stretch ⟶ Renin-angiotensin depression

⟶ ↓ Aldosterone ⟶ < PV

Low PV < Stretch ⟶ Renin-angiotensin activation

⟶ ↑ Aldosterone ⟶ > PV

ADH = Antidiuretic hormone

Fig. 1.9. *Role of stretch receptors in control of plasma volume.*

ment is combined with a red cell survival study (p. 14). Currently the most practical labels for red cell volume are technetium (^{99m}Tc) and indium (^{111}In or ^{113m}In). Plasma volume is measured with human serum albumin labelled with ^{125}I or ^{131}I. Details of the labelling procedures are described in Dacie and Lewis (1984).

Normal Range of Blood Volume

Red cell mass in men is 30 ml/kg (2S.D. range ±5 ml). In women, RCM is 25 ml/kg; (2S.D. range ±5 ml. Plasma volume is 40–50 ml/kg in both men and women. As PV is labile, confidence limits for normal values are less reliable than for RCM. Total blood volume is 60–80 ml/kg in men and women. In children the RCM and PV are the same, relative to body weight, as in adults.

These values are likely to be overestimates in obese subjects as fatty tissue is relatively avascular and blood volume is more closely correlated with lean body mass or an ideal weight based on height, age, sex and build. Formulae exist for predicting normal RCM and PV related to surface area; in normal subjects the RCM should be no more than 125% of the predicted value and the PV not less than 80% of the predicted value.

QUANTITATIVE MEASUREMENT OF ERYTHROPOIESIS

Ferrokinetics

The rate and effectiveness of erythropoiesis can be analysed by studying the disposal by the body of an injected dose of radioactive iron (^{59}Fe) bound to the circulating plasma transferrin. It is possible to measure the rate of clearance of the iron from plasma and to calculate iron turnover from this measurement and plasma iron content. The half-time of plasma clearance is normally 60–140 minutes (Fig. 1.10), and the turnover rate of iron (PIT) is 70–140 μmol/1 (4–8 mg/l) of blood per day. Non-erythroid iron turnover accounts for a small but significant proportion of the total PIT; it occurs as extramedullary and tissue iron.

Reappearance of the radio-iron in circulating erythrocytes is an indication of effective erythropoiesis. Normally, about 70%–80% of the

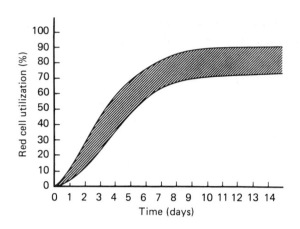

Fig. 1.11. *Normal pattern of erythrocyte iron utilization. After intravenous injection of radioactive iron (^{59}Fe), 70–80% of the dose will appear in circulating erythrocytes.*

administered iron is thus utilized (Fig. 1.11); the rest is involved in ineffective erythropoiesis (i.e. intramedullary cell destruction after synthesis has commenced), or enters non-erythroid tissues and thus fails to enter the circulating blood. If there is rapid haemolysis, the utilization curve will be distorted by destruction of some of the labelled cells. This will be recognized if daily samples are measured. Effective and ineffective iron turnover together constitute the total marrow iron turnover (MIT). Erythrocyte iron turnover (EIT) is the product of red cell utilization and PIT. Typical results in various conditions are shown in Table 1.3.

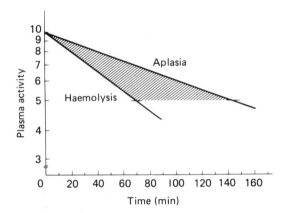

Fig. 1.10. *Normal range of plasma clearance of radioactive iron (^{59}Fe). Data are plotted on logarithmic graph paper, from which half-time clearance is read.*

Table 1.3
Typical ferrokinetic data in various conditions

	Plasma clearance T1/2 (min)	Plasma turnover (μmol/l per day)	Red cell utilization (%)
Normal	60–140	70–10	70–80
Aplastic anaemia	250	96	20
Red cell aplasia	330	110	0
Myelosclerosis	50	270	53
Infection	54	120	75
Iron deficiency	20	145	90
Thalassaemia major	25	915	17
Dyserythropoietic anaemias*	60	460	35

* Dyserythropoiesis also occurs frequently to a greater or lesser extent in the other disorders which are listed.

Marrow transit time is the time taken to reach one-half of the maximum red cell utilization. It is normally about 80 hours. It provides a fairly reliable reflection of marrow response to erythropoietin.

The sites of erythropoiesis can be demonstrated by counting radioactivity over various parts of the body. This method of surface counting will also indicate whether there is ineffective erythropoiesis and the extent to which the administered iron might be diverted for storage because of failure of cell synthesis. Surface counts in normal and some abnormal states are illustrated in Fig. 1.12. In the normal individual, plasma iron clearance is paralleled by a rise in marrow radioactivity. Within the marrow, the iron is rapidly incorporated into haemoglobin and the marrow radioactivity then gradually falls over a period of 10–14 days as newly formed erythrocytes are released into circulation and, after a delay, some of the radioactivity builds up in the spleen and to a lesser extent in the liver (i.e. the iron accumulates in the RE system). When the marrow is non-functioning, as in aplastic anaemia, there is a slow plasma clearance, little or no uptake of iron in the marrow but, instead, rapid accumulation of radioactivity in the liver as the iron is stored in the parenchymal cells of that organ; there is negligible re-entry of radioactivity in circulation. In contrast to the continuing build-up of radioactivity when the liver or the spleen is the site of storage, in cases of extramedullary haemopoiesis, after the initial accumulation, the activity in these organs subsequently decreases, corresponding to the appearance of radioactivity in circulating erythrocytes.

The pattern seen in haemolysis is one of rapid clearance, rapid increase in marrow and then rapid release of newly formed isotope-containing cells into circulation; however, there will also be considerable activity over the spleen or liver, or over both organs, indicating sequestration or increased destruction of circulating erythrocytes, and this will correspond to a decline in the circulating radioactivity. It should be remembered, however, that these 'characteristic' patterns, as described, may be confused by combination of circumstances, e.g. a degree of ineffective erythropoiesis is often associated with hypoplastic marrow, or in myelosclerosis there may be extramedullary erythropoiesis at the

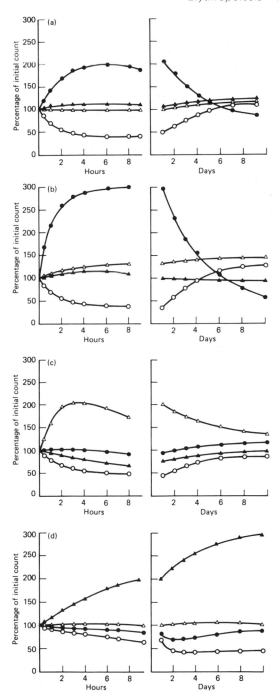

Fig. 1.12. *Surface-counting patterns following an intravenous injection of ^{59}Fe: (a) normal, (b) iron deficiency, (c) myelosclerosis with extramedullary erythropoiesis in spleen, (d) aplastic anaemia. Radioactivity measured over sacrum (●), spleen (▲), liver (x) and heart (o).*

same time as haemolysis. Moreover, surface counting is usually performed at circumscribed sites, e.g. the sacrum is taken to represent the bone marrow, and no account is taken of marrow variability. For this reason, whole body scans with ^{52}Fe provide a more reliable method for gauging the extent and distribution of erythropoietic tissue, both intramedullary and extramedullary (Fig. 1.13). Unfortunately, this radionuclide, which has a very short half-life (8.2 hours), is only available in a few centres. It has been suggested that as ^{111}In chloride binds to transferrin, it might be used instead. However, results with this radionuclide are inconsistent and its distribution in the body does not always parallel that of iron.

Reticulocyte Count

The reticulocyte count is commonly used as a measure of marrow production. As described in a previous section, this is valid only if the circulating reticulocyte maturation time is known, so that a corrected reticulocyte count and reticulocyte production index per day can be calculated. If the reticulocyte count is expressed in absolute numbers per litre, a constant number might be expected to be produced by a normally functioning marrow, irrespective of the severity of anaemia. In fact, there will be an increase with expanded marrow. In normal subjects there is considerable individual variation; the mean is about $50–75 \times 10^9/l$.

Blood Volume

The total erythrocyte count and packed cell volume do not invariably reflect the total red cell volume. There is a roughly exponential relationship between PCV and red cell volume, but with wide dispersion so that the PCV is a poor guide in any individual case, especially when the PCV is greater than 0.5 or less than 0.15, when the plasma volume tends also to become disproportionately reduced or increased. Moreover, a disproportionate increase in plasma volume occurs, irrespective of PCV, in cirrhosis, nephritis and splenomegaly, and this results in an anaemia more apparent than real. Conversely, when the red cell volume is normal but the plasma volume is decreased, the peripheral count will suggest a polycythaemia where none exists (see p. 531).

It is thus obvious that measurement of blood volume has a place in the elucidation of obscure anaemias and in evaluating the effectiveness of erythropoietic response to an apparent anaemia.

Erythrocyte Lifespan

Measurement of the mean cell life (MCL) of the erythrocytes is useful to distinguish between an anaemia due to failure of the marrow to respond to a demand for increased activity which is within the ability of a normally functioning marrow, and anaemia which occurs because of an excessive demand. There are two ways in which red cells can be labelled with radionuclides for measuring their lifespan—*cohort labelling*, in which red cells produced over a restricted period of time are labelled, and *random labelling*, in which a population of circulating red cells of all ages is labelled . ^{59}Fe is a suitable radionuclide for cohort labelling. It is incorporated into haemoglobin during its synthesis in erythroblasts. The MCL can be deduced fairly reliably from the rate of red cell production, as described above. For random labelling, either ^{51}Cr or DF^{32}P (di-isosopropyl phosphofluoridate) can be used; the former can only be used to label the red cells in vitro, whereas the latter is normally used as an in-vivo label.

The normal marrow can expand about six- to ninefold. Thus, haemolysis in which the MCL is more than 20 days should not lead to anaemia (i.e. there is a compensated haemolysis), whereas a more intense haemolysis will lead to anaemia. When the MCL is 15 days of less, anaemia is inevitable, but a disproportionate anaemia suggests a degree of marrow incapacity. These measurements can only be used as a rough guide as there are limitations of accuracy in the measurement of erythrocyte survival, and the usual methods of random labelling do not measure the destruction of erythroid cells occurring in the marrow.

Other Methods

Indirect assessment of erythropoiesis can be obtained from the daily faecal urobilinogen excretion or from the endogenous production of bilirubin or

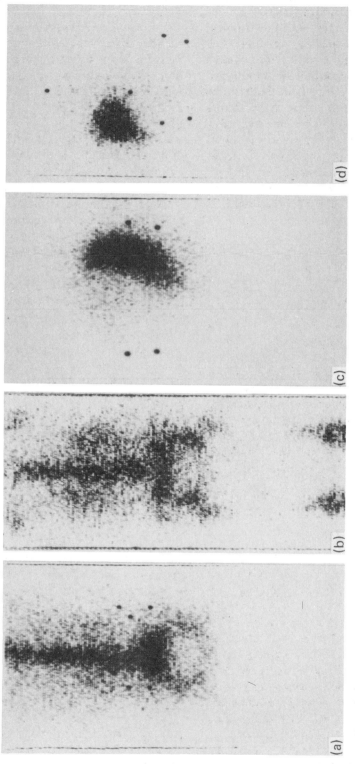

Fig. 1.13. ^{52}Fe *scans: (a) normal, (b) polycythaemia, (c) myelofibrosis with extramedullary erythropoiesis in spleen, (d) aplastic anaemia.*

carbon monoxide. These are a measure of haemo-globin catabolism and are, thus, an indication of the efficiency of haemoglobinopoiesis rather than of erythropoiesis.

Erythropoietin assay (see p. 8) provides a method for assessing the function of the erythro-poietic system. A high level occurs in the serum in most anaemias in inverse proportion to the haemo-globin concentration, except in patients with renal failure, when a low erythropoietin level is found. There are conflicting reports as to whether pro-duction of erythropoietin is reduced in patients with anaemia of rheumatoid arthritis and other systemic chronic disorders, but recent studies show a re-sponse to recombinant erythropoietin in rheuma-toid arthritis.

THE SPLEEN

The normal spleen weighs about 150–250 g, but there is considerable variation between normal individuals and at various times in the same indiv-idual. At puberty, it weighs about 200–300 g, and after the age of 65 its weight decreases to 100–150 g or less. In the adult its length is 8–13 cm, width 4.5–7 cm, surface area 45–80 cm^2 and its volume less than 275 cm^3. A spleen greater than 14 cm long is usually palpable. It enlarges in a wide range of diseases (Table 1.4), up to a massive 2 kg in weight in some blood diseases.

The spleen has a complicated structure and sev-eral different functions. Essentially, it consists of a connective tissue framework, vascular channels,

Table 1.4
Causes of splenomegaly

Haematological
Acute leukaemia
Chronic granulocytic leukaemia*
Chronic lymphocytic leukaemia
Malignant lymphomas
Chronic (primary) myelofibrosis*
Polycythaemia vera
Hairy cell leukaemia*
Gaucher's disease, Niemann–Pick disease and histiocytosis X*
Non-tropical primary splenomegaly (? malignant lymphoma)
Thalassaemia
Sickle cell disease and other haemoglobinopathies
Haemolytic anaemias

Minor
Iron deficiency anaemia
Megaloblastic anaemia
Thrombocytopenic purpura

Systemic
Acute infections: septicaemia, subacute bacterial endocarditis, typhoid, infectious mono-
  nucleosis
Chronic infections: tuberculosis, syphilis, brucellosis
Tropical parasitic infections (tropical splenomegaly)*: malaria, leishmaniasis, schisto-
  somiasis
Collagen diseases: systemic lupus erythematosus, rheumatoid arthritis (Felty)
Sarcoidosis
Amyloidosis
Portal hypertension and congestive splenomegaly
  Cirrhosis
  Splenic/portal/hepatic venous thrombosis

---

* Often associated with massive splenomegaly.

lymphatic tissue, lymph drainage channels and cellular components of the haemopoietic and reticuloendothelial systems. The circulation within the spleen is illustrated in Fig. 1.14. Blood is brought to the spleen via the splenic artery, and then, through its branches (the trabecular arteries), into the central arteries which are sited in the white pulp. These central arteries run in the central axis of periarteriolar lymphatic sheaths; they give off many arterioles and capillaries, some of which terminate in the white pulp whilst others go on to enter the red pulp. In the red pulp there are endothelial-lined sinuses, 20–40 μm in diameter, and also cords (Bilroth cords) which are spaces lined by adventitial cells and macrophages. The arterial capillaries either connect directly with the sinuses and thence, via the collecting vein, to the trabecular vein (closed system), or they first pass into the cord spaces before joining up with the sinuses (open system). There is

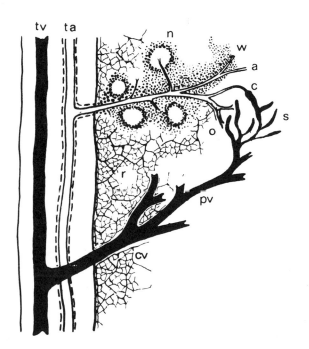

Fig. 1.14. *Schematic diagram of the circulation of the spleen. (tv, trabecular vein; ta, trabecular artery; n, nodular white pulp; w, white pulp; a, artery of the pulp; c, direct vascular connection between arterial capillary and splenic sinus; o, 'open' vascular pathway from arterial capillary to splenic sinus; s, splenic sinuses; r, reticulum; pv, pulp vein; cv, collecting vein.) (Reproduced from Bowdler (1982), with permission.)*

thus both a rapid and a slow transit component in the splenic circulation. The rapid transit is of the order of 1–2 minutes; the slow mixing which occurs notably when there is splenomegaly (see later) has a circulation time of 30–60 minutes or even longer. In normal subjects, the open system has a minor role and the blood flows through the spleen as rapidly as through other organs, at a rate of about 5% of the blood volume per minute, so that each day the blood has repeated passages through the spleen. During the flow, by a process of plasma skimming, the plasma and the leucocytes pass preferentially to white pulp whilst the red cells remain in the axial stream of the central artery. Some of this blood flows directly through the sinusoids to the venous system, whilst the remainder passes into the cords of the red pulp. The red cells are normally flexible enough to squeeze through the endothelial slits into the sinuses, whereas cells with abnormal membranes or with inclusions which render them relatively inflexible remain in the cords where they either become conditioned for later transit or are destroyed.

The various functions of the spleen are determined by the organ's anatomical and histological structures. Some of these functions are interrelated.

Phagocytosis and Sequestration

It is important to distinguish that three mechanisms are involved in the action of the spleen: sequestration, phagocytosis and pooling. Sequestration is a reversible process whereby cells are held up temporarily before returning to the circulation. Phagocytosis is the irreversible uptake of nonviable cells by macrophages or the destruction of viable cells which have been damaged by prolonged sequestration or by antibody coating. Pooling is the presence of an increased amount of blood in the spleen in continuous exchange with the circulation (see p. 18).

As the red and white blood cells, platelets and other discrete matter in the bloodstream pass through the cords, effete or damaged cells or foreign matter are readily phagocytosed by the macrophages and reticulum cells. The red cells are subject to a further hazard: as the blood passes through the spleen, plasma skimming causes a high haematocrit and increased viscosity, resulting in slow flow almost to the point of stasis. In the presence of metabolically active macrophages, the densely packed red cells are deprived of oxygen and glucose. This stress increases membrane rigidity and reduces the natural deformability of the biconcave cell. The red cell needs to be able to deform to pass between adjacent sinus endothelial cells and so enter the splenic sinus lumen. Cells which have become too inflexible will fail to do so. This occurs especially as a result of excessive reaction to stress, e.g. because of an underlying abnormality of the red cell metabolic system, or because the cells are already spherical or antibody coated or are fragmented or misshapen in other ways; they will remain trapped in the cord space and will there undergo phagocytosis.

Siderotic granules, Howell–Jolly bodies, nuclear remnants and Heinz bodies are removed (culling or pitting) during temporary sequestration; after removal of the inclusions the red cells return to the circulation. Sequestration of reticulocytes has been shown to occur both in humans and in experimental animals. In humans, reticulocytes may be retained in the splenic cords for a considerable proportion of their 2–3 days maturation time, while they lose their intracellular inclusions, alter the lipid composition of their surface and become smaller in size. It is not clear whether the spleen has any special role at the other end of the life of the red cell in the normal process of elimination of senescent cells; it seems more likely that such cells are removed by the general reticuloendothelial system, including the spleen to some extent, and especially in the marrow.

Blood Pooling

The normal red cell content of the spleen is 30–70 ml, or less than about 5% of the total red cell mass. When the spleen is enlarged it is capable of developing a considerable pool with high haematocrit and only slow exchange of red cells with the general circulation. In myelofibrosis, hairy cell leukaemia and prolymphocytic leukaemia, especially, as much as 40% of the red cell mass may be pooled in the spleen. This pooling will functionally exclude a relatively large volume of red cells from the main arteriovenous circulation, and thus cause anaemia. In such cases, it should be noted that the red cell mass, measured by a radionuclide-labelling technique, may give a misleadingly normal result whereas the peripheral blood packed cell volume will give a more reliable measurement of the effectively circulating red cell mass.

As far as granulocytes are concerned, no pool is demonstrable in the normal spleen, but splenic sequestration of granulocytes is thought to be responsible for the neutropenia which often occurs in patients with splenomegaly. Platelets, on the other hand, have been shown to have a significant reservoir in the spleen, rapidly interchangeable with the circulation. In normal subjects, 20%–40% of the total platelet mass is pooled in the spleen and the platelets spend up to one-third of their lifespan there. The pool increases when the spleen is enlarged. This pooling and temporary sequestration must be distinguished from destruction of platelets in the spleen which occurs in many cases of thrombocytopenia.

Immunological Function

The spleen has the largest single accumulation of lymphoid tissue in the body. It contains 25% of the T-lymphocyte pool and 10%–15% of the B-lymphocyte pool. T cells are found predominantly in periarteriolar lymphatic sheaths, and B cells in germinal centres in the white pulp. There is a constant flow of both T and B cells through the spleen; T cells stay in the spleen for 4–6 hours, or longer when they are activated by antigen, while B cells stay for up to 24 hours. T-cell interaction with the corresponding B cells takes place mainly when they are juxtaposed in the periarteriolar sheath.

During a primary immune response, antigenic material such as blood-borne organisms which are taken up by the splenic cord macrophages are then delivered to immunocompetent lymphoid cells. This results in production of humoral antibody and an increase in lymphoid germinal centres in the spleen. Secondary stimulation with the antigen enhances antibody production, usually IgG. Red cells sensitized by IgG antibodies do not, as a rule, agglutinate in the peripheral blood, but the environment of the spleen promotes agglutination of such cells with consequent sequestration. The antibody-coated cells in contact with macrophages which have Fc receptors lose pieces of their membrane, becoming more spherical and less flexible each time they traverse the endothelial pores and thus are trapped. Apart from the type of antibody, several other factors also influence the role of the spleen in immune red cell destruction, e.g. the number of macrophages present and the rate of splenic blood flow. Increased haemolysis results in an increased number of phagocytes accumulating in the splenic cords, with consequent increasing lysis, in a spiralling system. Conversely, however, phagocytic action may be reduced, at least temporarily, as the damaged red cell load blockades the RE cells.

Extramedullary Haemopoiesis

Experimental studies in mice have shown that there are haemopoietic stem cells (CFU–S) as well as crythroid progenitors (BFU–E) in the spleen, but whilst the spleen is a minor organ of haemopoiesis in fetal life, normally no erythropoietic activity is demonstrable in the spleen after birth. In myelosclerosis, and occasionally in patients with secondary carcinomatosis and leukaemia when there is myeloid metaplasia, the spleen reverts to its embryonic function, and foci of haemopoietic tissue become established. Extramedullary erythropoiesis may also occur by way of a compensatory erythroblastic hyperplasia in chronic haemolytic anaemias, megaloblastic anaemia and in thalassaemia.

Although in the past, because of its large volume of lymphoid tissue, the spleen was considered an important lymphopoietic organ, it now seems more likely that most of the lymphocytes have migrated from other sites of origin such as bone marrow and thymus.

Regulation of Erythropoiesis

The spleen is a site of limited production or storage of erythropoietin, but there is no convincing evidence that it exerts a direct humoral effect on the marrow, whether suppressive or stimulating. It may, however, play an important indirect role. Splenomegaly is often associated with an increased plasma volume (see below). This results in a pseudoanaemia ('dilutional anaemia'), whilst an increasing splenic red cell pool may cause true anaemia in the peripheral circulation. This anaemia, whether absolute or only apparent, will result in erythropoietic stimulation.

Control of Plasma Volume

The neurohumoral mechanism which controls the plasma volume is described on p. 10. Under physiological conditions, the red cell volume is fairly constant while the plasma volume undergoes continual transient variations which trigger off the necessary adjustments which ensure that the total blood volume remains constant. There is no evidence that the normal spleen is involved in this mechanism. When the spleen is enlarged, it does play a role, and splenomegaly is frequently associated with an increased plasma volume which may lead to a dilutional pseudoanaemia. Possible mechanisms which have been suggested to explain expanded plasma volume in splenomegaly include the following.

(a) The enlarged organ, acting as a large arteriovenous fistula, requires an expansion of blood volume to fill the additional intravascular space; in conditions where marrow erythropoietic activity is reduced, as in myelosclerosis, it may not be possible to maintain the normal red cell : plasma ratio and the additional volume is provided by plasma alone.

(b) Protein alterations, especially increased globulin levels with reduced albumin, result in an alteration in colloid oncotic pressure. This has been suggested as a factor in tropical splenomegaly and in cirrhosis.

In blood dyscrasias, the increase in plasma volume is directly proportional to the size of the spleen, less so in cirrhosis.

CAUSES OF SPLENOMEGALY

Splenomegaly is a frequent and important clinical sign (see Table 1.4). In some of the diseases listed, splenic enlargement is only found occasionally and, when it occurs, it is seldom marked, e.g. in acute septicaemias, the megaloblastic and iron deficiency anaemias, idiopathic thrombocytopenic purpura, most collagen disorders, amyloidosis and hyperthyroidism. In other conditions the spleen may become grossly enlarged and be the dominant clinical feature.

The relative incidence of the cause of splenomegaly is subject to enormous geographical variation. In Europe the leukaemias, malignant lymphomas, myeloproliferative disorders, haemolytic anaemias and portal hypertension account for most cases. Infective endocarditis is also relatively frequent. In tropical countries, however, the incidence of these haematological causes of splenomegaly is swamped by the great preponderance of splenic enlargement caused by the parasitic tropical infections: malaria, leishmaniasis and schistosomiasis. Portal hypertension is an important cause of splenomegaly in most tropical countries but it is especially prevalent in North-Eastern India and Southern China. The 'tropical splenomegaly syndrome' is seen in large numbers of patients in New Guinea and Central Africa. Splenomegaly is also associated with haemoglobin C disease in West Africa, haemoglobin E disease in the Far East, and with thalassaemia syndromes which have a wide distribution throughout the Tropics. Because of the multiplicity of factors responsible for splenomegaly in such countries, more than one pathology may contribute to an increase in splenic size in a particular patient. The prevalence of malaria is thought to explain the anomaly of splenic enlargement in surviving African adults with homozygous sickle-cell disease.

Hypersplenism

Hypersplenism is a clinical syndrome; it does not imply a specific causal mechanism. It has the following characteristic features.

1. Enlargement of the spleen.
2. Reduction in one or more of the cell lines in the peripheral blood.
3. Normal or hyperplastic cellularity of the bone marrow, often with orderly maturation of earlier stages but paucity of more mature cells.
4. Premature release of cells into peripheral blood, resulting in reticulocytosis and/or large immature platelets.
5. Increased splenic red cell pool, decreased red cell survival and increased splenic pooling of platelets with shortening of their lifespan.

The diagnosis of hypersplenism is ultimately confirmed by response to splenectomy, although an immediate remission may be followed in the longer term by partial relapse with some cytopenia.

Most of the diseases listed in Table 1.4 can give rise to secondary hypersplenism. In these conditions the haematological features of hypersplenism may be obscured or dominated by the primary disease, especially if it involves the marrow. Hypersplenism also occurs as a primary event due to an unknown pathogenetic stimulus. It is sometimes termed primary splenic hyperplasia, splenic neutropenia or splenic anaemia, and it includes those cases of non-tropical primary splenomegaly in which there is no firm evidence for an underlying lymphoma.

HAEMATOLOGICAL EFFECTS OF SPLENECTOMY OR SPLENIC ATROPHY

Characteristic blood changes occur following splenectomy. Similar changes are seen with atrophy of the spleen to less than 20% of normal size and when there is functional asplenia with or without reduction in size of the organ. Hypofunction may occur in sickle cell disease, dermatitis herpetiformis, amyloidosis, adult coeliac disease and, less frequently, in Crohn's disease and ulcerative colitis, and in essential thrombocythaemia.

Red Cell Changes

The changes in red cell morphology include the presence of Howell–Jolly bodies and siderotic granules in some of the cells and the appearance of target cells. In a proportion of subjects, irregularly contracted or crenated, acanthocytic forms are also a feature (Fig. 1.15). There is usually an increase in the number of reticulocytes in the circulation and occasionally isolated erythroblasts are seen. There is, however, no alteration in red cell survival.

Under normal circumstances, some of the red cells leaving the marrow contain siderotic granules and Howell–Jolly bodies. As the number of cells containing siderotic granules is related to the sideroblastic percentage in the bone marrow, the siderocyte count in the peripheral blood is low in the absence of marrow pathology. In patients suffering from haemolytic anaemias, thalassaemia and the sideroblastic anaemias, a major proportion of the red cells may contain siderotic granules. The

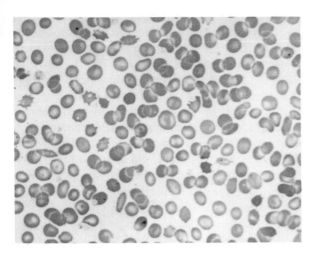

Fig. 1.15. *Red cell appearances after splenectomy; Howell–Jolly bodies, target cells and contracted cells can be seen.*

number of Howell–Jolly bodies is also variable and is most marked in conditions characterized by dyserythropoiesis. Other red cell inclusions may be prominent in the post-splenectomy state: Heinz bodies are found following oxidative injury by drugs and in patients who have glucose-6-phosphate dehydrogenase (G6PD) deficiency or an unstable haemoglobin; precipitated alpha chains are found in beta-thalassaemia; and crystalline deposits of haemoglobin C in Hb-C disease. The presence of red cell inclusions will, to some extent, reflect the absence of the splenic 'pitting' function. Demonstration of the presence of pits is a more reliable indication of splenic dysfunction. They are readily identified in unstained blood films by means of interference-contrast (Nomarski) microscopy. They appear as crater-like indentations on the surfaces of red cells. When the spleen is functioning normally, less than 2% of the red cells will be pitted.

If the output from the bone marrow remains constant, lack of a temporary sequestration in the spleen results in an increased number of reticulocytes in the circulation. Erythroblasts are only prominent during times of erythropoietic stress.

Leucocyte Changes

After splenectomy there is a rise in total leucocyte count. A neutrophil leucocytosis in the immediate postoperative period is, in the majority of subjects, later replaced by a significant and permanent increase in both lymphocytes and monocytes. After a few weeks the neutrophil count returns to normal or near-normal levels. Minor increases in blood eosinophils and basophils have been noted after splenectomy but this is not a regular feature.

In response to infection, splenectomized subjects produce a much greater leucocytosis than persons with intact spleens, and often there is a marked left shift in the differential leucocyte count with myelocytes and occasionally more primitive cells.

Platelet Changes

In the immediate postoperative period in uncomplicated splenectomy patients, the platelet count rises steeply to a maximum of usually $600–1000 \times 10^9/l$, with a peak at 7–12 days. The thrombocytosis is usually transitory, and a fall to near-normal values over the following 1–2 months is the rule. However, even if the platelet count has returned to normal values, occasional large and bizarre platelets can be seen in the blood films of many splenectomized subjects; their presence suggests that these particular platelets are normally removed by the spleen.

In a number of patients, the thrombocytosis persists indefinitely after splenectomy and this usually appears to be a consequence of continuing anaemia with a hyperplastic marrow—an inverse relationship exists between the severity of the anaemia and the height of the platelet counts. Although a reactive thrombocytosis is not usually associated with thromboembolic problems, the high platelet counts may have contributed to the serious and sometimes fatal episodes of pulmonary embolism that have occurred following splenectomy. It is advisable to give antiplatelet therapy (e.g. aspirin 100 mg daily) as long as thombocytosis is present.

Immunological Effects

The spleen plays an important role in immunoglobin synthesis, and a fall in the IgM fraction of the serum immunoglobulins is commonly found post-splenectomy. Removal of an organ with a unique ability to recognize and phagocytose circulating particulate antigen would be expected to have serious consequences. Despite these facts, splenectomy in adults without complicating disease is not usually associated with a substantially increased incidence of infection. It must be assumed, therefore, that an increase in activity of other lymphoreticular organs compensates for any defects in the immunological defence mechanisms that result from this operation.

In the young, however, splenectomy is associated with a significant increase in overwhelming bacterial infections. This is particularly noticeable during the first five years of life. Septicaemia and meningitis are the usual documented causes of death, and there is an overwhelming predominance of the pneumococcus in most reports. The vulnerability of young children and their dependence on the spleen to deal with blood-borne infection during this time would appear to be explained by the general immaturity of their lymphoreticular systems. In the absence of the spleen, the defective reticuloendothelial clearance of an encapsulated, rapidly growing organism such as the pneumococcus may lead to dangerous bloodsteam concentration in too short a time for an adequate immunological defence to be mounted. Splenectomy is therefore usually postponed until after the age of 6–7 years wherever possible, and in all splenectomized subjects prophylactic penicillin (250 mg twice daily) is advocated postoperatively, continuing in young subjects until the age of 18. Polyvalent pneumococcal vaccine is also given preoperatively.

INVESTIGATION OF SPLENIC FUNCTION USING RADIONUCLIDES

The role of the spleen in the pathogenesis of anaemia has been widely investigated. Surface counting following the injection of ^{51}Cr-labelled erythrocytes provides a qualitative guide to splenic red cell destruction. The factors which require elucidation are *red cell pooling*, the *relative amounts of functioning tissue and non-functioning tissue* within the spleen, and the presence of *extramedullary erythropoiesis*. In cases of splenomegaly, especially, it is important to distinguish increased reticuloendothelial activity causing cell destruction

from increased red cell content due to a large splenic pool, and from enlargement of the organ due to tumour infiltration. In practice, all three mechanisms may act at the same time and it may be of value to assess the relative importance of each in the individual patient in relation to the haematological parameters. It is important to clarify the changes produced by treatment and to correlate the observations in patients who undergo splenectomy. Imaging techniques, especially when used in quantitative methods, allow a more extensive assessment of the various splenic mechanisms responsible for the production of anaemia. In hypersplenism there may be thrombocytopenia and neutropenia as well as anaemia. Thus, there have been a number of studies of the role of the spleen using labelled platelets and white cells as well as in-vivo studies with red cells.

Visualization of the Spleen

The spleen can be visualized by means of a scintillation camera following injection of labelled red cells after they have been manipulated by a procedure which ensures that they are removed from the circulation by the spleen. The most effective method is by exposing the red cells, which have been labelled with ^{51}Cr, ^{111}In or ^{99m}Tc, to a temperature of 49.5°C for precisely 20 minutes. This demonstrates the functional size of the spleen; it is more reliable than radiological or clinical examination in detecting minor degrees of splenic enlargement, in diagnosing space-occupying lesions such as splenic cysts and tumour deposits, in determining whether an upper abdominal mass is of splenic origin, and in identifying abnormally positioned and accessory splenic tissue. Conversely, functional asplenia or atrophy is well demonstrated by this procedure.

Ultrasonic imaging provides similar information on spleen size, while computerized tomography gives an accurate representation of the anatomy of the spleen and its position in relation to adjacent organs.

From the radionuclide image, the area (A) of the spleen can be obtained from the linear measurements. Several formulae have been proposed for estimating the volume of the spleen from these measurements. The following appears to be fairly reliable:

Spleen volume (ml) $= 9.9A - 540$

Splenic Red Cell Volume

A similar procedure to that for visualizing the spleen, but with undamaged, labelled red cells, provides a relatively simple method for measuring the splenic red cell volume. By quantitative imaging, the fraction of the administered radionuclide present in the spleen 20–30 minutes after injection is measured. Normally the spleen contains 5% or less of the red cell volume and there is general correlation between splenic red cell volume and physical size of the spleen. There is a proportionately greater pool in certain disorders (see p. 18), and in these the pool may be a major cause of splenomegaly. Discrepancies between the volume of the spleen (see above) and of the red cell pool suggest that the splenomegaly is due, at least in part, to cell or tumour infiltration. The extent of the splenic red cell pool should be taken into account when assessing the significance of anaemia; also it makes it possible to predict the degree to which anaemia will improve following splenectomy.

Sites of Red Cell Destruction

In-vivo surface counting during survival studies with ^{51}Cr-labelled red cells provides a means for determining the sites of red cell destruction. The principle is that the destruction of red cells in an organ is manifested by an increase in radioactive counts over that organ relative to the count rate over other organs and in the blood. By this means it is possible to identify the principal site of red cell sequestration and destruction, and to determine the relative activities of the spleen and liver in a haemolytic process. Four patterns of surface counting occur: (a) excess accumulation in spleen alone, (b) excess accumulation in liver alone, (c) no excess accumulation in either organ, and (d) excess accumulation in both organs. Some congenital haemolytic anaemias (hereditary spherocytosis and hereditary elliptocytosis) generally fall into group (a), autoimmune haemolytic anaemias into group (a) or (d), hereditary non-spherocytic haemolytic anaemia

into group (c), PNH and cases of intravascular haemolysis into group (c) or (d). In patients with haemolytic disease, the results taken in conjunction with the clinical details of the patients have value in deciding whether splenectomy should be undertaken. A good response can be expected only in patients who show the first pattern.

The surface-counting method will demonstrate a trend but does not provide the quantitative information which should be more reliable in predicting the value of splenectomy, especially in those patients in whom the spleen is not the only organ of red cell destruction. A quantitative method has been devised and it is possible to provide measurements of the fractions of red cell destruction in spleen, liver and other RE tissue. By this technique, it has been shown that normally the spleen accounts for 20% of the total red cell destruction, the main part of which is in the general reticuloendothelial system.

Measurement of Splenic Phagocytic Function

Irreversible trapping of particulate matter is a function of the reticuloendothelial system. Colloid particles 1 μm in size or less will be taken up by the liver, larger particles by the spleen. There is a well-established relationship between splenic reticuloendothelial function and the rate at which heat-damaged red cells are removed from the circulation. The half-clearance time in normal subjects is about 5–15 minutes. Significantly increased times occur in thrombocythaemia, sickle cell disease, coeliac disease, Crohn's disease, ulcerative colitis, dermatitis herpetiformis, amyloidosis and malignant histiocytosis. In these conditions, a slow clearance rate may identify splenic hypofunction before the blood film shows Howell–Jolly bodies and other morphological features. Faster than normal clearance times have been observed in patients with haemolytic anaemia and in some patients with splenomegaly. The curve of the clearance time is complex, as it comprises three overlapping components, namely, intrasplenic cell transit, sequestration and phagocytosis or irreversible extraction (Fig. 1.16). There is also a rapid uptake of some of the labelled material by the liver. When the spleen is functioning normally, the transit time is 5–10% per minute, with extraction of 20–50% of the labelled cells.

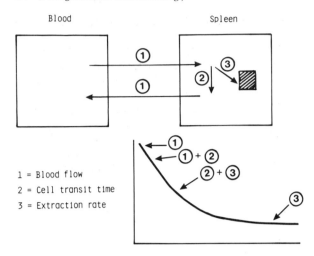

Blood   Spleen

1 = Blood flow
2 = Cell transit time
3 = Extraction rate

Fig. 1.16. *Curve of disappearance from circulation of heat-damaged red cells. The components of the curve reflect transit, pooling, sequestration and irreversible trapping of cells.*

Identification of Platelet Sequestration

When ^{51}Cr-labelled platelets are administered, combined measurements of radioactivity in the liver and spleen and in the blood show that normally about one-third of the platelets are promptly extracted from circulation by the spleen and are released later, with a subsequent mono-exponential equilibration with the circulating platelets. A small fraction of the labelled platelets is taken up rapidly and irreversibly by the liver; this is assumed to be due to their being damaged by the labelling process. Splenomegaly is associated with a marked increase in splenic pooling; by contrast, in asplenia, nearly 100% of the labelled platelets are recovered in the circulating blood. Surface counting and quantitative scanning have been used to identify the role of the spleen in thrombocytopenia. The clinical usefulness of such data in predicting the results of splenectomy in such patients is, however, debatable, as there is both sequestration and destruction of platelets in the spleen; sequestration is, as a rule, a temporary phase, which does not necessarily mean subsequent destruction, as with red cells.

Plasma Volume

As described on p. 19, splenomegaly is often associated with an increased plasma volume and splenectomy is usually followed by a reduction in plasma volume. This means that in splenomegaly the blood count may give an exaggerated impression of anaemia so that measurement of red cell and plasma volume must be included in clarifying the cause of anaemia in conditions associated with splenomegaly.

Assessment of Splenic Erythropoiesis

As described on p. 11, ferrokinetic studies provide useful information in patients with myelosclerosis, dyserythropoiesis and other obscure anaemias. The normal spleen is unable to remove iron from transferrin. Uptake of iron in the spleen, demonstrable by surface counts shortly after administration of ^{59}Fe or by scan after [52]Fe, thus indicate that erythropoiesis is occurring in that organ. The degree of ineffective erythropoiesis can be assessed by surface counts on subsequent days and by measurement of red cell utilization. In myeloproliferative disorders, radionuclide studies will distinguish splenic enlargement due to myeloid metaplasia from that caused by red cell pooling. Also, they will indicate when splenic red cell destruction exceeds that organ's contribution to total erythropoiesis— an aspect which must be taken into account when deciding on splenectomy.

SELECTED BIBLIOGRAPHY

Barrett A. J., Gordon M. Y. (1985). *Bone marrow disorders: the biological basis of clinical problems.* Oxford: Blackwell Scientific Publications.

Bentley S. A. (1982). Bone marrow connective tissue and the haemopoietic microenvironment. *British Journal of Haematology*, **50**, 1–6.

Berlin N. I., Berk P. D. (1981). Quantitative aspects of bilirubin metabolism for hematologists. *Blood*, **57**, 983–999.

Bessis M. (1973). *Living blood cells and their ultrastructure.* Berlin, New York: Springer-Verlag.

Bowdler A. J. (1982). The spleen in disorders of the blood. In *Blood and its disorders*, pp. 751–797 (Eds. R. M. Hardisty and D. J. Weatherall). Oxford: Blackwell Scientific Publications.

Cavill I., Ricketts C., Napier J. A. F., Jacobs A. (1977). Ferrokinetics and erythropoiesis in man; red cell production and destruction in normal and anaemic subjects. *British Journal of Haematology*, **35**, 33–40.

Cotes P. M. (1982). Immunoreactive erythropoietin in serum. I. Evidence for the validity of the assay method and the physiological relevance of estimates. *British Journal of Haematology*, **50**, 427–438.

Cotes P. M. (1983). Erythropoietin. In *Hormones in blood*, 3rd edn, Vol. 4, pp. 195–218 (Eds. C. H. Gracy and V. H. T. James). London, New York: Academic Press.

Crane C. G. (1981). Tropical splenomegaly. Part 2; Oceania. *Clinics in Haematology*, **10**, 976–982.

Dacie J. M., Lewis S. M. (1984). *Practical haematology* 6th edn. Edinburgh: Churchill Livingstone.

Dacie J. V., White J. M. (1949). Erythropoiesis with particular reference to its study by biopsy of human bone marrow: a review. *Journal of Clinical Pathology*, **2**, 1–32.

Dunn C. D. R. (Ed.) (1983). *Current concepts in erythropoiesis*. Chichester: Wiley.

Fakunle Y. M. (1981). Tropical splenomegaly. Part 1; Tropical Africa. *Clinics in Haematology*, **10**, 963–975.

Ferrant A., Cauwe F., Michaux J. L., Beckers C., Verwilghen R. L. (1982). Assessment of the sites of red cell destruction using quantitative measurements of splenic and hepatic red cell destruction. *British Journal of Haematology*, **50**, 591–598.

Finch C. A. (1982). Erythropoiesis, erythropoietin and iron. *Blood*, **60**, 1241–1246.

Giblett E. R., Coleman D. H., Pirzio-Biroli G., Donohue D. M., Motulsky A. G., Finch C. A. (1956). Erythrokinetics; quantitative measurements of red cell production and destruction in normal subjects and patients with anemia, *Blood*, **11**, 291–309.

Golde D. W. (Ed.) (1984). Hematopoietic stem cells. *Methods in Hematology*, **11**.

Goldwasser E., Sherwood J. B. (1981). Annotation: Radioimmunoassay of erythropoietin. *British Journal of Haematology*, **48**, 359–363.

Heier H. E. (1980). Splenectomy and serious infection. *Scandinavian Journal of Haematology*, **24**, 5–12.

Hillman R. S. (1969). Characteristics of marrow production and reticulocyte maturation in normal man in response to anemia. *Journal of Clinical Investigation*, **48**, 443–453.

Hoffbrand A. V., Pettit J. E. (1988). *Sandoz atlas of clinical haematology*. London: Gower Medical.

Izak G. (1977). Erythroid cell differentiation and maturation. *Progress in Hematology*, **10**, 1–41.

Jacobs K. *et al.* (1985). Isolation and characterization of genomic and cDNA clones of human erythropoietin. *Nature*, **313**, 806–810.

Lai P-H. *et al.* (1986). Structural characterisation of human erythropoietin. *Journal of Biological Chemistry*, **261**, 3116–3121.

Lewis S. M. (Ed.) (1983). The spleen. *Clinics in Haematology*, **12**(2), 361–608.

Lewis S. M., Bayly R. J. (Eds.) (1985). Radionuclides in haematology. *Methods in Hematology*, **12**, 1–262.

Lichtman M. A. (1981). The ultrastructure of the hemopoietic environment of the marrow: a review. *Experimental Haematology*, **9**, 391–410.

Najean Y., Cacchione R. (1977). Blood volume in health and disease. *Clinics in Haematology*, **6**, 543–566.

Ricketts C., Cavill I., Napier J. A. F., Jacobs A. (1977). Ferrokinetics and erythopoiesis in man: an evaluation of ferrokinetic measurements. *British Journal of Haematology*, **35**, 41–47.

Testa N. G. (1979). Erythroid progenitor cells; their relevance for the study of haematological disease. *Clinics in Haematology*, **8**, 311–333.

Videbaek A., Christensen B. E., Jønsson V. (1982). *The spleen in health and disease*. Copenhagen: FADL's Farlag.

Wickramasinghe S. M. (1986). *Blood and bone marrow*. Edinburgh: Churchill Livingstone.

Winearls C. G., Oliver D. O., Pippard M. J., Reid C., Downing M. R., Cotes P. M. (1986). Effect of human erythropoietin derived from recombinant DNA on the anaemia of patients maintained by chronic haemodialysis. *Lancet*, **2**, 1175–1177.

Zucker-Franklin D., Greaves M. F., Grossi C. E., Marmont A. M. (1988). *Atlas of blood cells*, 2nd edn. Philadelphia: Lea & Febiger.

Chapter 2

IRON

M. J. PIPPARD AND A. V. HOFFBRAND

Iron is essential for many metabolic processes. Its ability to exist in both ferric and ferrous states underlies its importance in the oxygen and electron transport systems concerned with cellular energy production. Many of the physiologically active iron compounds in the body are haem proteins, but there are also specialized proteins of iron transport and storage. The latter are necessary to enable iron to remain in solution at neutral pH, where ferric iron is virtually completely insoluble, and to limit the potential toxicity of this reactive metal. The insolubility of ferric iron also means that although the earth's crust consists of approximately 4% of iron, and iron may be plentiful in the diet, much of this is unavailable. As a result, the body is limited in the adjustments it can make to excessive loss of iron which frequently occurs due to haemorrhage, and iron deficiency is the commonest cause of anaemia throughout the world. The general need to conserve the metal is reflected in the absence of any physiological mechanism for excretion of iron, with control of iron balance being at the level of iron absorption. This is important in the rarer but potentially fatal disorders of iron overload.

BODY IRON

The distribution of body iron is shown in Fig. 2.1. The largest component is circulating haemoglobin, 450 ml (1 unit) of whole blood containing about 200 mg of iron. Most of the remaining iron is contained in the storage proteins, haemosiderin and ferritin. These are found mainly in the reticuloendothelial cells of the liver, spleen and bone marrow (which gain iron from breaking down

red cells) and in parenchymal liver cells (which gain most of their iron from the plasma iron-transporting protein, transferrin).

Functional Iron-Containing Proteins

Haemoglobin (mol. wt 64 500) contains four haem groups linked to four globin chains, and can bind four molecules of oxygen. Myoglobin (mol. wt. 17 000) contains 4–5% of body iron as a single haem group attached to its one polypeptide chain. It has a higher affinity for oxygen than haemoglobin and behaves as an oxygen reserve in muscles. The mitochondria contain a series of haem and non-haem iron-proteins (including the cytochromes a, b and c, succinate dehydrogenase and cytochrome oxidase) which form an electron-transport pathway responsible for the oxidation of intracellular substrates and the simultaneous production of ATP. Cytochrome P_{450} is found in the endoplasmic reticulum and is involved in hydroxylation reactions, including drug detoxification by the liver. Other haemoproteins include the enzymes catalase and lactoperoxidase, concerned in peroxide breakdown, and tryptophan pyrrolase, concerned in the oxidation of tryptophan to formyl-kynurenine. There is a smaller group of iron sulphur proteins, e.g. xanthine oxidase, aconitase and NADH dehydrogenase, and iron is also necessary for the function of ribonucleotide reductase, a key enzyme in DNA synthesis.

Ferritin and Haemosiderin

Ferritin is the primary iron storage protein and provides a reserve of iron which may be used for

Iron-donating tissues and iron stores

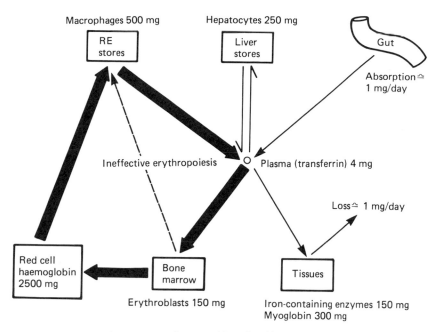

Fig. 2.1. *The major compartments of iron in a 70-kg male. Iron supply for erythropoiesis and turnover of iron from senescent red cells (heavy arrows) dominate internal iron exchange.*

haem synthesis if required. It consists of an approximately spherical apoprotein shell (mol. wt 480 000) enclosing a core of ferric hydroxyphosphate (up to 4000 iron atoms). The internal cavity communicates with the exterior via six channels through which iron may enter (after oxidation) or leave (after reduction, e.g. by dihydroflavins or ascorbic acid). However, the mechanisms by which ferritin iron is mobilized are poorly understood, and a process by which the entire ferritin molecule is degraded within lysosomes prior to iron release has also been suggested. Human ferritin is made up from 24 subunits of two immunologically distinct types, H subunits (mol. wt 21 000) and L subunits (mol. wt 19 000). These are coded for by genes on chromosomes 11 and 19, respectively. However, there are multiple gene copies, many of which are presumably pseudogenes, on 12 different chromosomes. Variation in the proportion of H to L subunits explains the heterogeneity of ferritin from different tissues on isoelectric focusing: L-rich ferritins (from spleen,

liver and placenta) are more basic than H-rich ferritins (from heart and red cells). There may be functional differences between different isoferritins (e.g. in iron storage or intracellular iron transport) but this is not established. The small amount of ferritin normally present in serum contains little iron and consists almost exclusively of L subunits. However, it also is heterogeneous due to it being around 60% glycosylated. This glycosylation and the direct relationship of serum ferritin concentration to body iron stores (p. 35) suggest that serum ferritin may be secreted by macrophages and/or hepatocytes which have been stimulated by iron to synthesize ferritin.

Haemosiderin, unlike ferritin, is water insoluble, and is a non-crystalline, protein–iron complex visible by light microscopy when stained by the Prussian-blue (Perls') reaction. It has an amorphous structure, with a higher iron to protein ratio (up to 37%) than ferritin (up to 20%), and is probably formed by the partial digestion of ferritin aggregates by lysosomal enzymes. In normal subjects, storage iron is about two-thirds ferritin and one-third haemosiderin, but in iron overload the proportion as haemosiderin increases considerably.

Transferrin

This contains only about 4 mg of body iron but is vital to iron transport (Fig. 2.1). It is a β-globulin glycoprotein (6% carbohydrate) of molecular weight 79 500, which is present in plasma and extravascular spaces, with a plasma half-life of 8–11 days. The transferrin gene is on chromosome 3 and the protein is synthesized in the liver, synthesis being inversely related to iron stores. Normal plasma contains 1.8–2.6 g/l. Two atoms of ferric iron may be attached to each molecule, the binding sites (N-terminal and C-terminal) being thought to contain three tyrosine and two histidine residues and an arginine group. Binding of iron involves simultaneous attachment of an anion, usually bicarbonate.

Lactoferrin is a related glycoprotein, of molecular weight approximately 77 000, which also binds two atoms of iron per molecule. It is found in milk and other secretions and in neutrophils and is thought to have a bacteriostatic action by depriving micro-organisms of the iron needed for their growth.

Intracellular Transit Iron

It is thought that in all cells there is a transit pool of 'metabolically active' iron which receives iron from degraded haem or ferritin, is in exchange with circulating transferrin, and is utilized for newly synthesized iron-proteins. The chemical nature of this iron is not known, though low molecular weight chelates may be involved. It is likely to be the main stimulus to ferritin protein synthesis, and also a major source of iron chelated by desferrioxamine (p. 52).

NORMAL IRON BALANCE

The amount of iron in the body at birth depends on the blood volume and haemoglobin concentration, the birth weight which determines blood volume, being particularly important. Delay in clamping the cord leads to an increased red cell mass by placental transfusion. The amount of maternal iron stores has little effect on the fetal iron endowment. On average, the newborn contains about 80 mg/kg at full term. Neonatal iron reserves are utilized for growth in early infancy, and between 6 months and 2 years virtually no iron stores are present. Thereafter, iron stores gradually accumulate during childhood to around 5 mg/kg. In men there is a further increase between 15 and 30 years to about 15 mg/kg (total approximately 1 g), whereas iron stores remain lower in women (average 300 mg) until the menopause.

Table 2.1 lists the normal daily losses of iron and hence the requirements to compensate for this as well as for growth. The main loss in males is in the stools as a result of shedding of intestinal cells and iron-laden macrophages. The urine contains less than 0.1 mg daily in red cells and renal cells. Losses also occur in nails, hair and desquamated skin cells. Requirements are higher in menstruating women, and during periods of rapid growth in infancy, and adolescence. Menstrual loss has a median value of 30 ml, but a proportion of women have losses of 80 ml a month (equivalent to 1.4 mg iron a day) or more, which has been found to be significantly associated with iron deficiency. Requirements are highest of all in pregnancy, when the overall net loss may be 500 mg or more.

Losses are reduced as body iron stores fall, and it has been estimated that it would take 6–8 years for an adult male to deplete the body iron stores and develop iron deficiency anaemia solely due to lack of dietary intake or malabsorption.

IRON ABSORPTION

Iron absorption depends not only on the amount of iron in the diet but also, and more importantly, on the bioavailability of that iron, as well as the body's needs for iron. A normal Western diet provides approximately 15 mg iron daily (6 mg/kcal). Of that iron, digestion within the gut lumen solubilizes about one-half, from which about 3 mg may be taken up by mucosal cells and only about 1 mg (or 5–10% of dietary iron) transferred to the portal blood in a healthy adult male. Iron absorption can thus be influenced at several different stages.

Table 2.1

Daily iron losses and requirements (WHO Technical Reports Series No. 452)

	Daily loss (mg)		Requirement for growth (mg)	Total loss (= requirement) (mg)
	Urine, skin, faeces, etc.	Menses		
Infant (0–4 months)	0.5			0.5
(5–12 months)	0.5		0.5	1.0
Child	0.5		0.5	1.0
Adolescent male	0.9		0.9	1.8
Adolescent female	0.9	1.0	0.5	2.4
Menstruating female	0.9	1.9		2.8
Adult male	0.9			0.9
Post-menopausal female	0.9			0.9

N.B. Average daily requirement during pregnancy is 3.0–4.0 mg.

Dietary Factors

Much of the dietary iron is non-haem iron derived from cereals (commonly fortified with additional iron in the UK), with a lesser component of haem iron derived from haemoglobin or myoglobin in red or organ meats. Haem iron is more readily absorbed than non-haem iron, being less subject to influence by other dietary constituents which can produce wide variations in the ionization, solubility and thus availability of non-haem iron (Table 2.2). Nevertheless, even in iron deficiency, the maximum iron absorption from a mixed Western diet is no more than 3–4 mg daily, and this figure is much less with the predominantly vegetarian, cereal-based diets of most of the world's population. Even when animal foods form only a small part of the diet, they contribute a relatively larger fraction to the total iron absorbed. This is because of the direct availability of haem iron, and also because an unidentified ligand present in meat promotes an enhanced availability of the non-haem iron in the rest of the diet.

Luminal Factors

Iron is released from protein complexes by acid and proteolytic enzymes in the stomach and small intestine, and haem is liberated from haemoglobin and myoglobin. Iron is maximally absorbed from the duodenum and less well from the jejunum, probably because the increasingly alkaline environment leads to the formation of insoluble ferric hydroxide complexes. Low molecular weight substances such as sugars and ascorbic acid (Table 2.2) form highly soluble iron chelates and facilitate attachment of iron to the intestinal mucosa. Ascorbic acid also helps to keep iron in the ferrous form which remains more soluble than ferric iron as the pH increases. By contrast, absorption of non-haem iron is inhibited by binding to phosphates and phytates in the diet. Alkalis and tea also reduce iron absorption. Therapeutic ferrous iron salts are well absorbed on an empty stomach, but when taken with meals, absorption is reduced due to the same ligand-binding processes that affect dietary non-haem iron. Absorption of haem iron is much less dependent on the luminal environment.

Mucosal Factors

Iron uptake by mucosal cells appears to involve binding to specific receptors on the brush borders followed by an energy-dependent transfer across the cell membrane. At higher doses of iron, passive diffusion may also occur. Haem enters the small intestinal mucosal cell intact and is then broken down within the cell, possibly by the enzyme haem oxygenase, to release its iron into a common intra-

Table 2.2
Iron absorption

Favoured by	Reduced by
Dietary factors	
Increased haem iron	Decreased haem iron
Increased animal foods	Decreased animal foods
Ferrous iron salts	Ferric iron salts
Luminal factors	
Acid pH (e.g. gastric HCl)	Alkalis (e.g. pancreatic secretions)
Low molecular weight soluble chelates (e.g. vitamin C, sugars, amino acids)	Insoluble iron complexes (e.g. phytates, phosphates, tea (tannates), bran)
Ligand in meat (unidentified)	
Mucosal factors	
Iron deficiency	Iron overload
Increased erythropoiesis (e.g. after haemorrhage)	Decreased erythropoiesis
Ineffective erythropoiesis	Acute or chronic inflammation
Pregnancy	
Anoxia	

cellular transit iron pool. From there, iron may either be transferred to the portal circulation, or may enter ferritin to be eventually lost with the exfoliation of the mucosal cell. The relative proportions following these alternative pathways vary with the body's iron needs. The nature of the transit iron pool remains uncertain. The suggestion that a transferrin-like protein is involved in mucosal iron uptake and/or subsequent transport through the cell has not been generally accepted.

Regulation of Iron Absorption

Iron absorption may be regulated both at the stage of mucosal uptake (possibly by varying the number of brush border iron receptors) and at the stage of transfer to the blood. Factors favouring increased iron absorption include iron deficiency, pregnancy, anoxia and increased erythropoiesis. Iron absorption is usually decreased when the body is overloaded with iron, and in acute and chronic infection. How each of these factors influences the intestine and informs the mucosal cells how much iron to take up or to transfer to the plasma is not clear. The

plasma iron and transferrin saturation do not seem to be involved (indeed, in the very rare condition of congenital atransferrinaemia, iron absorption is increased, with the development of liver iron overload in association with a hypochromic anaemia). Attempts to demonstrate a possible humoral factor have been unsuccessful. One hypothesis concerning the transfer stage suggests that each of the iron-donating tissues (macrophages, liver and gut, see Fig. 2.1) may supply iron to plasma transferrin in proportion to the amount of available iron in those tissues, the iron being transported to satisfy the needs of the main receptor tissue, the erythroid marrow. Within this framework, the amount of iron to be supplied by the intestinal cells would be dependent on the output from other donor tissues being increased when there is tissue iron deficiency. Furthermore, where there is a rise in plasma iron turnover due to increased erythron demands for iron, output from all the donor tissues, including the gut, might be expected to increase. However, the nature of the mechanism which ensures that iron supply is closely matched to tissue demands for iron is not known. It breaks down in some conditions where iron absorption remains normal or even raised despite the presence of increased iron stores. This occurs in idiopathic haemochromatosis and also where there is an increase in plasma iron turnover associated with massive ineffective erythropoiesis, particularly in thalassaemia and sideroblastic anaemia. If absorption occurs despite a high serum iron concentration, free iron may be present in plasma and is rapidly deposited in parenchymal cells, particularly those of the liver.

INTERNAL IRON EXCHANGE

After phagocytosis by macrophages, haem from senescent red cells is broken down by haem oxygenase to release iron. As ferrous iron, it can then either enter ferritin (where it is oxidized to ferric iron by the ferritin protein) or be released into plasma, where its binding to transferrin (also as the ferric form) may be facilitated by a plasma ferrous oxidase (e.g. caeruloplasmin). The mechanisms of iron donation to transferrin are poorly understood, but binding of apotransferrin to the macrophage cell membrane does not appear to be essential. There is still dispute as to whether the two iron-binding sites of the transferrin molecule are loaded randomly with iron, or whether there may be preferential loading of the N- rather than the C-terminal site. Changes in release of iron from macrophages are thought to account for the diurnal rhythm of serum iron concentration, which is highest in the morning and lowest in the evening.

Uptake of iron from transferrin requires that the protein is attached to specific receptor sites on the surface of developing red cells and reticulocytes, hepatocyes, placenta, and to a lesser extent on all other tissues of the body. The number of receptors in any given cell type increases with an increase in proliferation. It has recently been shown that some of the receptors are shed into the plasma, where their concentration, measured by immunoassay, correlates particularly with the overall activity of the erythron; the measurement may therefore provide a novel alternative to ferrokinetic techniques for assessing erythroid activity. The transferrin receptor is a transmembrane protein consisting of two monomers linked by a disulphide bridge, each subunit being able to bind one transferrin molecule.

The human transferrin receptor is identified by the monoclonal antibody OKT 9. It has a much higher affinity for fully saturated, diferric transferrin than for monoferric transferrin, and a very low affinity for apotransferrin at neutral, but not acid, pH. Although some workers believe that the transferrin–receptor complex remains on the cell surface during iron removal, there is good evidence in both reticulocytes and hepatocytes of a process of receptor-mediated endocytosis (Fig. 2.2). The iron is released, perhaps by a fall of pH in an acidic endosome, before the apotransferrin and receptor are recycled to plasma and cell membrane, respectively. There is no evidence that, in vivo, the two iron-binding sites of transferrin differ in their iron-donating properties. Whether or not a specific intracellular carrier, either a protein or low molecular weight chelate, is then involved in transport of iron to the mitochondria or to ferritin remains uncertain. The suggestion that developing red cells might also gain a small amount of iron directly from macrophage cells by micropinocytosis of ferritin molecules (rhopheocytosis) is now thought to be of no physiological significance.

After intravenous injection, about 80–90% of a trace dose of ^{59}Fe bound to transferrin normally enters developing red cells, the rest going to other tissues (especially liver, but also to skeletal muscle and intestinal epithelium). It should be noted (see Fig. 2.1) that the liver hepatocytes have a central position in iron metabolism, acting as a buffer capable both of taking up extra iron when the transferrin saturation (and thus the proportion of diferric transferrin) is increased, and of releasing iron from stores when there is an increased need in other tissues for iron. An increased percentage iron saturation of the plasma transferrin (iron-binding capacity) is thus the earliest indication of a risk of parenchymal iron overload in idiopathic haemochromatosis and the iron-loading anaemias. Other variations in plasma iron and transferrin levels in disease states are illustrated in Fig. 2.3.

About 90% of the iron used by the marrow each day derives from breaking down red cells; the remainder is derived from the slow turnover of the storage pool and from absorption from the gut. Some 5–10% of haemoglobin broken down is released intravascularly and attached to haptoglobin prior to its removal by hepatocytes. An increase in

Mitochondria
Ribosomes
Haem
Globin
α β
Ferritin
Haemoglobin
Fe
Endosome (Acidic)
Transferrin receptor
Diferric transferrin
Transferrin receptor
Apotransferrin

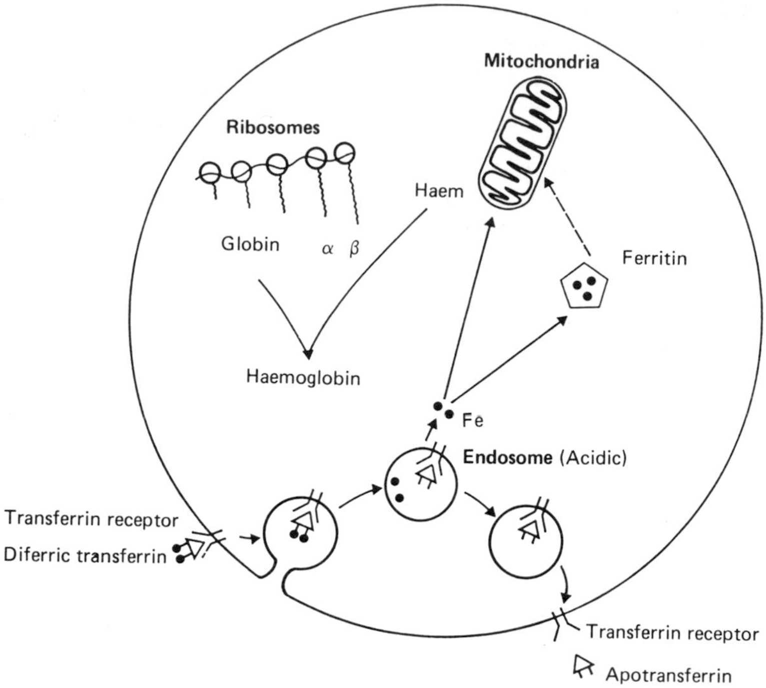

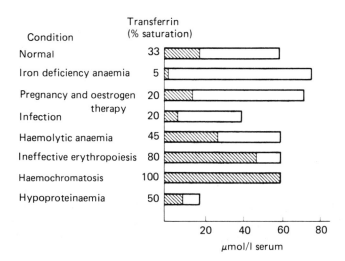

Fig. 2.2. *Incorporation of iron from plasma transferrin into haemoglobin in developing red cells. Uptake of transferrin iron is by receptor-mediated endocytosis.*

Condition
Transferrin (% saturation)
Normal 33
Iron deficiency anaemia 5
Pregnancy and oestrogen therapy 20
Infection 20
Haemolytic anaemia 45
Ineffective erythropoiesis 80
Haemochromatosis 100
Hypoproteinaemia 50
20
40
60
80
μmol/l serum

Fig. 2.3. *Typical values of the serum iron (▧) and unsaturated iron-binding capacity (□) in various conditions (1 μmol/l = 18 μg/100 ml).*

this pathway is seen in haemolytic and dyserythro-poietic anaemias, and may provide a further route by which hepatocytes accumulate excess iron in disorders such as thalassaemia, in addition to the uptake of transferrin iron and any free iron in the plasma. By contrast, large particles of colloidal iron, including therapeutic parenteral iron preparations, are removed from circulation by macrophages of the reticuloendothelial system.

Fate of Iron in the Erythroid Cell

Some 80–90% of iron taken into developing erythroblasts is converted to haem within 1 hour. The main non-haem protein present is ferritin, which is actively synthesized in proportion to the amount of iron entering the cells. Iron uptake is greatest in early erythroblasts, prior to the peak in haem synthesis, a pattern which would be consist-ent with a possible role for ferritin as an obligatory intermediate in the movement of iron from plasma to haemoglobin (Fig. 2.2). Any iron taken up in excess of the requirement for haem synthesis re-mains in ferritin, and the red cell ferritin content is therefore increased when the plasma transferrin is fully saturated with iron, or when haemoglobin synthesis is impaired, as in thalassaemia syndromes or sideroblastic anaemia. Excess iron may also be seen in mature red cells as one or more siderotic granules. These are composed of haemosiderin, and stain blue with Perls' reaction and purplish blue with Romanowsky stains, when they are called 'Pappenheimer bodies'. The spleen removes these granules by its pitting action (see p. 18), but it is also possible that they are actively extruded from the cells into the circulation. The bulk of iron entering red cells is, however, converted to haem, and this process is discussed next.

HAEM SYNTHESIS

Haem consists of a protoporphyrin ring with an iron atom at its centre. The porphyrin ring consists of four pyrrole groups which are united by methene ($=C-$) bridges (Fig. 2.4). The hydrogen atoms in the pyrrole groups are replaced by four methyl (CH_3-), two vinyl ($-C=CH_2$) and two proprionic acid ($-CH_2-CH_2-COOH$) groups.

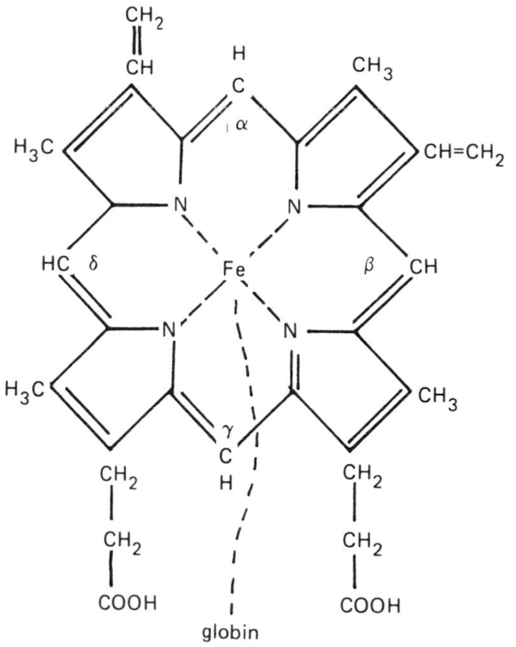

Fig. 2.4. *Haem. (Adapted from Wintrobe, et al. 1981.)*

Haem is synthesized from the precursors succinic acid and glycine (Fig. 2.5). Succinate (derived from α-ketoglutarate in the Krebs' tricarboxylic acid cycle, and from proprionate via the intermediate methylmalonate) is converted to its coenzyme A derivative in the presence of magnesium ions and ATP. Succinyl CoA condenses with glycine to form delta amino-laevulinic acid (ALA) under the action of ALA synthase (ALA-S), with pyridoxal-5'-phosphate as coenzyme. Iron has also been impli-cated as a cofactor in the reaction. It is possible that an intermediate α-amino-β-ketoadipic acid is form-ed from glycine and succinate which is then decarboxylated to ALA. ALA can be utilized for the formation of both purines and haem. Under the action of the enzyme ALA dehydrase, two mole-cules of ALA due to be made into haem condense to form a monopyrrole, porphobilinogen (PBG). Glu-tathione is needed as coenzyme in this reaction. Four molecules of porphobilinogen then condense to form the tetrapyrrole ring compound uropor-phyrinogen III. Uroporphyrinogen III is decarbox-ylated to form coproporphyrinogen III, which is then oxidized to protoporphyrin IX. Iron in the

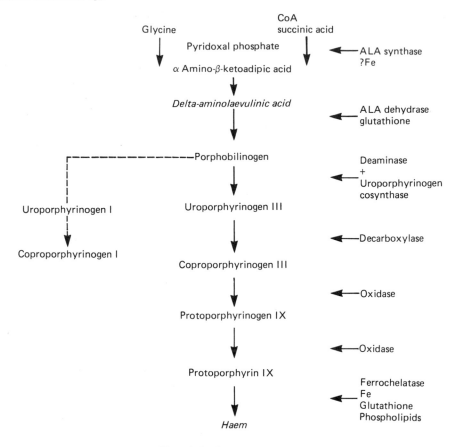

Fig. 2.5 *Synthesis of haem.*

ferrous form is then incorporated (either before or after globin has been attached) under the influence of the enzyme ferrochelatase and glutathione. This reaction has also been shown to be stimulated by phospholipids. Iron in haem has six co-ordinating valencies: four (in one plane) link the iron to nitrogen atoms in each of the pyrrole rings, while the remaining two link haem to histidine residues in the globin chain, the distal bond being unstable and easily replaced by oxygen to form oxyhaemoglobin.

The mitochondria are the main subcellular sites of haem synthesis since ALA-S, coproporphyrinogen oxidase and ferrochelatase are all present in them, and only the enzyme sequence from ALA to coproporphyrinogen is situated in the cytoplasm. The mitochondria are also the sites of the citric acid cycle which supplies succinate. The mature red cell,

which lacks mitochondria, is therefore unable to synthesize haem.

A number of porphyrins are formed by side reactions during the synthesis of protoporphyrin. Uroporphyrinogen III and coproporphyrinogen III are relatively easily oxidized to uroporphyrin III and coproporphyrin III respectively. Oxygen tension and reducing or oxidizing agents may therefore have a significant influence on the regulation of haem synthesis. Uroporphyrinogen I (as well as uroporphyrinogen III) is formed from porphobilinogen when there is a deficiency of uroporphyrinogen cosynthase, and this leads to a series of compounds of the porphyrin I structure in which the substituent groups in the porphyrin ring alternate regularly (in Type III, one pair is asymmetrical). In the porphyrias (Table 2.5), many of these compounds accumulate in the major sites of haem synthesis, the liver and red cells.

Control Mechanisms in Haem Synthesis

It is necessary to switch on haem formation in the developing red cell and to inhibit haem synthesis in the mature cell. Synthesis of haem and globin must also be co-ordinated so that there is no significant excess of either. Moreover, the entry of iron into the cell and to the mitochondria and its incorporation into haem must be regulated so that the normal cell gets sufficient iron for its needs, but not a vast excess.

The accepted view has been that the enzyme ALA-synthase is a major site of control for haem synthesis. The activity of ALA-S rises in the basophilic normoblast to reach a peak in the polychromatic normoblast, and then diminishes so that no activity is present in the mature cell. The appearance of the enzyme in the early cells may partly depend on hormonal control since certain steroid hormones derived from testosterone and progesterone have been found to stimulate formation of ALA-S in the chick embryo. The rate of haem synthesis is thought to be regulated through the inhibition by haem of both ALA-S enzyme activity (end-product inhibition) and enzyme synthesis (end-product repression). However, in erythroid cells there is some evidence that the availability of iron from transferrin may be rate limiting for the incorporation of glycine into haem and that haem may in turn inhibit the cellular uptake of iron from transferrin. This has raised the possibility that haem may regulate its own synthesis at the level of iron uptake rather than by direct inhibition of ALA-S.

Haem formation enhances globin, and lack of haem reduces globin formation, having a more marked effect on production of the α than of the β chain. Exactly how haem has this effect is unknown. It may also be that globin enhances haem synthesis. Certainly, removal of haem into haemoglobin would lead to reduced feedback inhibition on ALA-S, and this is one likely mechanism. A direct stimulatory effect of globin on haem synthesis has also been suggested but not confirmed experimentally.

DIAGNOSTIC METHODS FOR IRON STATUS

In order to assess body iron status the three main compartments of iron shown in Fig. 2.1 (storage iron, transport iron, and functional iron compounds, particularly haemoglobin in red cells) should be considered. Ferrokinetic measurements using radio-iron (see Chapter 1) may also be used to quantify the major pathways of internal iron exchange, iron absorption and blood loss, though this is rarely necessary clinically.

Storage Iron

Serum Ferritin

In normal people, the serum ferritin concentration is well correlated with hepatic and macrophage iron stores, as assessed by quantitative phlebotomy or tissue biopsy (see below). This has led to the widespread use of immunoassays for serum ferritin as a convenient, non-invasive measure of iron stores. Serum ferritin is usually of low iron content, even in conditions of iron overload, is rich in L subunits and is partially glycosylated. It has a much slower clearance from plasma (half-life approximately 30 hours) than non-glycosylated tissue ferritins (half-life approximately 10 minutes), and is probably cleared via specific ferritin receptors on hepatocytes. Normal concentrations of serum ferritin range from about 15 μg/l to 300 μg/l, and are higher in adult males (mean 100 μg/l) than in premenopausal women (mean 30 μg/l). In neonates, the concentration in cord blood (approximately 200 μg/l) rises further over the first 2 months of life as fetal haemoglobin is broken down, and thereafter falls to low levels (20–30 μg/l) during growth through childhood.

Values for serum ferritin concentration which are below 15 μg/l are virtually specific for storage-iron depletion, but values above 300 μg/l do not necessarily, or even usually, indicate iron overload. This is because ferritin synthesis is influenced by factors other than iron (in particular, it acts as an acute phase reactant in many inflammatory diseases), and because damage to ferritin-rich tissues can release large amounts of tissue ferritins into the plasma (Table 2.3). Increased serum ferritin concen-

Table 2.3
Changes in serum ferritin

Rise with	Fall with
Increased body iron stores Idiopathic haemochromatosis Iron-loading anaemas (e.g. thalassaemia)	*Decreased body iron stores* Iron deficiency Pregnancy
Redistribution of body iron Anaemia not due to iron deficiency or blood loss (e.g. megaloblastic or hypoplastic anaemias)	*Decreased ferritin synthesis (rare)* Ascorbate deficiency Hypothyroidism
Increased ferritin synthesis Inflammation/infection Malignancy: acute leukaemias, carcinoma and lymphoma, hepatoma Hyperthyroidism	
Release of tissue ferritins Cell necrosis: hepatic necrosis,* chronic liver disease, spleen or bone marrow infarction (e.g. sickle cell disease)	

*May be massive increase.

trations in malignancy may be due to associated anaemia (in which redistribution of iron from hae-moglobin to macrophage stores is to be expected), tissue necrosis, or changes in liver function leading to accumulation of ferritin in plasma. The presence of somewhat more acidic (H-subunit-rich) ferritins in some tumours has suggested that they may produce their own, qualitatively different, ferritin, but this is not proven, and is not of any diagnostic significance. Although, in the absence of additional pathology, serum ferritin generally gives a reliable guide to the severity of iron overload, it has been found to give false normal results in occasional cases of early idiopathic haemochromatosis and where there is associated ascorbate deficiency which lowers the serum ferritin. It may also be normal in the early stages of iron loading due to excessive iron absorption in dyserythropoietic anaemias (e.g. β-thalassaemia intermedia, HEMPAS). Conversely, very high serum ferritin concentrations (>4000 μg/l) in transfusion-dependent anaemias may reflect liver dysfunction in addition to increased iron stores.

Tissue Biopsy

Liver biopsy (in the diagnosis of iron overload) or bone marrow biopsy (in the differential diagnosis of iron deficiency) allows direct examination of iron stores by histological staining for iron or chemical measurement of iron. Liver iron is normally found mainly in hepatocytes rather than macrophages and is higher in men (on average 400 mg) than in women (average 130 mg in menstruating women and 245 mg in post-menopausal women) in Western communities. Chemical determination of marrow non-haem iron is not usually carried out. Research studies have shown that it correlates well with the more usual microscopical grading, though there is some overlap between different grades. It can be particularly difficult to determine with certainty from marrow iron stains, that iron stores are completely absent.

Chelating Methods

The measurement of urine iron excretion following a single intramuscular injection of 0.5 g desferrioxamine is still occasionally useful in the assessment of possible iron overload, particularly when clinical considerations make the more definitive liver biopsy impossible. Urine excretion of greater than 8 mg in 24 hours (normal < 1.5 mg) can be expected in established idiopathic haemochromatosis, though much lower values are sometimes seen in precirrhotic disease. A number of other factors influence iron chelation by desferrioxamine (p. 52), and although the hepatocyte is a major site of action of the drug, these limit the value of the test as a measure of parenchymal iron overload.

Mobilization by Phlebotomy

This is carried out by repeated venesections at frequent intervals so that iron absorption is negligible during the period. The amount of iron removed (as blood) before anaemia develops is calculated. However, anaemia may sometimes occur in subjects with increased iron stores even though some haemosiderin remains, presumably because of slow iron release from this insoluble compound. The amount of storage iron measured by the technique in normal adults has been about 750 mg in males and 250 mg in females.

Other Techniques

Computerized tomographic (CT) scanning and magnetic resonance imaging (MRI) have been used as non-invasive methods to measure liver iron.

Transport Iron

Serum Iron and Iron-binding Capacity

The serum iron and, more particularly, the saturation of the iron-binding capacity, give a measure of the iron supply to the tissues at the time of sampling. In normal subjects the serum iron is labile, showing marked fluctuations from hour to hour. However, in iron deficiency and iron overload, values stabilize at low or high levels, respectively. A serum transferrin saturation which is persistently less than 15% is insufficient to support normal erythropoiesis, which becomes iron deficient. A sustained increase (more than 60%) in transferrin saturation is the first change in the development of parenchymal iron loading, and its

measurement is thus an essential part of screening for iron overload. Both measures can be affected by factors other than iron status (see Fig. 2.3), and both are considerably lower in children than adults.

Red Cell Iron

Red Cell Protoporphyrin

Where iron supply to the erythron is limited, iron incorporation into haem is restricted, leading to accumulation of the immediate precursor, protoporphyrin. This is lost only slowly from circulating red cells, and concentrations greater than the normal 40 µg/100 ml red cells therefore indicate that a reduction in iron supply has been present over the previous few weeks. However, protoporphyrin may be increased by other defects of haem synthesis, including sideroblastic anaemia and lead poisoning.

Red Cell Ferritin

The ferritin content of red cells is directly related to the iron supply to the erythron, and is increased where the plasma transferrin saturation is raised. It has therefore been suggested as a measure of parenchymal iron stores, less subject to those many factors which can elevate the serum ferritin independently of iron status. However, it is also increased in disorders of haemoglobin synthesis (including iron-loading anaemias such as the thalassaemia disorders), limiting its use for this purpose, and it remains a research tool.

Haemoglobin

Reduced amounts of haemoglobin accompany an overall reduction in body iron in iron deficiency anaemia or acute blood loss. In other anaemias, such as megaloblastic anaemias, iron is redistributed from red cells to macrophage iron stores, and a corresponding increase in marrow stainable iron and serum ferritin should be expected.

Clinical Use of Measures of Iron Status

The large amount of iron present as haemoglobin means that the degree of any anaemia must always be considered in assessing iron status. It should be remembered that iron stores should be sufficient to replenish any deficit in the haemoglobin compartment, and that in anaemic patients, values for measures of iron stores that are within the 'normal' range may in fact indicate inadequate reserves. No single measurement of iron status is ideal for all clinical circumstances since changes may develop sequentially (as in progressive negative iron balance) or may affect particular body iron compartments. In an uncomplicated microcytic anaemia with an obvious cause for iron deficiency, either a reduced serum iron in the presence of an increased total iron-binding capacity (TIBC), or a low serum ferritin concentration will be sufficient to confirm the diagnosis. In a mild normocytic anaemia the situation may be less clear cut, and measures of both iron supply and iron stores may be necessary. Estimation of the serum ferritin can make a bone marrow biopsy for assessment of iron stores unnecessary in many cases. However, in hospital patients, the behaviour of ferritin as an acute phase protein means that, on occasion, marrow examination may be the quickest way of being certain of whether storage iron depletion is complicating an inflammatory disorder. In assessing iron overload, screening measures must include estimation of the saturation of the serum TIBC and serum ferritin, where these are abnormal liver biopsy is likely to be necessary in order to quantitate the iron overload and assess possible iron-induced tissue damage.

IRON DEFICIENCY ANAEMIA

Sequence of Events

Depletion of Iron Stores

When the body is in a state of negative iron balance, the first event is depletion of body stores which are mobilized for haemoglobin production. Iron absorption is increased when stores are reduced, before anaemia develops and even when the serum iron level is still normal although the serum ferritin will have already fallen. When the stores are entirely depleted there is no stainable iron present in the bone marrow, and the serum ferritin is less than 15 μg/l unless there is accompanying inflammatory disease.

Iron-deficient Erythropoiesis

With further iron depletion, the serum transferrin saturation falls to less than 15%, leading to the development of iron-deficient erythropoiesis and increasing concentrations of red cell protoporphyrin. At this stage, the haemoglobin, mean corpuscular volume (MCV) and mean corpuscular haemoglobin (MCH) may still be within the normal range, though they may rise significantly when iron therapy is given. There has been recent concern that a reduced tissue iron supply, even in the absence of anaemia, may lead to impaired exercise tolerance and reduced learning and mental performance in children. In addition, tissue changes attributable to iron deficiency may occasionally be present without overt anaemia.

Iron Deficiency Anaemia

If the negative iron balance continues, frank iron deficiency anaemia develops. The patient may show breathlessness, pallor and tachycardia. The red cells become more obviously microcytic and hypochromic, and poikilocytosis becomes more marked in the blood film (Fig. 2.6a). The MCV, mean corpuscular haemoglobin concentration (MCHC) and MCH are all reduced, and target cells may be present. The reticulocyte count is low for the degree of anaemia. The serum total iron-binding capacity (TIBC) rises (due to increased hepatic transferrin synthesis) and the serum iron falls, so that when anaemia is present the percentage saturation of the total iron-binding capacity of serum is usually less than 10% (see Fig. 2.3).

The number of erythroblasts containing iron (sideroblasts) is reduced at an early stage in the development of deficiency, and siderotic granules are entirely absent from these cells when iron deficiency anaemia is established. The erythroblasts have a ragged, vacuolated cytoplasm and relatively pyknotic nuclei (Fig. 2.6b). The bone marrow macrophages show a total absence of iron except where very rapid blood loss outstrips the ability to mobilize the storage iron; parenteral iron dextran may also result in poorly available macrophage iron. The survival of iron-deficient erythrocytes is moderately reduced due to an intracorpuscular defect. The white cell series is usually normal, though there is some evidence that hypersegmentation of neutrophil nuclei and large metamyelocytes may occur rarely in iron deficiency uncomplicated by either folate or vitamin B$_{12}$ deficiencies.

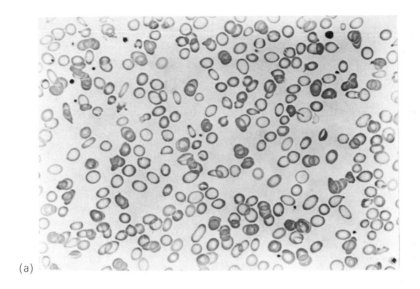

(a)

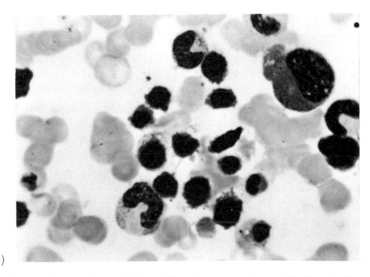

(b)

Fig. 2.6. *(a) The peripheral blood film from a patient with chronic iron deficiency anaemia (haemoglobin 64 g/l), (May-Grünwald Giemsa × 650). (b) The bone marrow of a patient with severe iron deficiency anaemia. The normoblasts show ragged cytoplasm and pyknotic nuclei (May-Grünwald Giemsa × 1300).*

When these changes are obvious, however, folate or vitamin B_{12} deficiency is usually present, probably because the underlying condition (poor nutrition, malabsorption or excess demands) affects both nutrients. Platelets are frequently increased, possibly as a result of stimulation of megakaryocyte, and hence platelet, formation by erythropoietin. There have also been occasional reports of associated thrombocytopenia responding to iron therapy.

When iron deficiency is severe and chronic, widespread tissue changes may be present including koilonychia, angular stomatitis (especially in those with badly fitting dentures), glossitis, pharyngeal and oesophageal webs (Kelly–Paterson syndrome) and atrophic gastritis (p. 41). Partial villous atrophy, with minor degrees of malabsorption of xylose and fat reversible by iron therapy, has been described in infants suffering from iron deficiency, but not in adults. Pica is sometimes present in iron-deficient subjects; in some who eat clay or chalk, this may cause rather than be the result of iron deficiency. Iron-containing enzymes such as the cytochromes, catalase and tryptophan pyrrolase are usually better preserved in the tissues than other iron-containing compounds. In severe iron deficiency, however, these enzymes are not inviolate and their levels may fall. This may be partly responsible for the general tissue changes, with mitochondrial swelling in many different cells (including, in the experimental animal, hepatic and myocardial cells), poor lymphocyte transformation and diminished cell-mediated immunity, and impaired intracellular killing of bacteria by neutrophils.

CAUSES OF IRON DEFICIENCY
(Table 2.4)

Diet

Defective intake of iron is rarely the sole or major cause of iron deficiency in adults in Western communities since it takes many years for the deficiency to develop solely on the basis of poor nutrition. It occurs when the diet is lacking in meat, liver, vegetables and other foods containing iron. This

may arise through poverty, religious tenets, food faddism or because of gastrointestinal disorders. Iron deficiency is more likely to develop in subjects taking a largely vegetarian diet who also have increased physiological demands for iron.

Increased Physiological Iron Requirements

Iron deficiency is common in infancy when demands for growth may be greater than dietary supplies. It is aggravated by prematurity, by infections, and by delay in mixed feeding. It is also frequent in adolescence when demands are again increased, particularly at the menarche in girls. Menstrual blood loss is extremely variable, being of clinical importance when it exceeds 80 ml each month. Iron requirements are even higher in the second and third trimester of pregnancy, when they usually are 3.0–4.0 mg but may reach figures of up to 7.5 mg daily. The fetus acquires about 280 mg of iron and a further 400–500 mg is required for the temporary expansion of the maternal red cell mass. Though iron absorption increases throughout pregnancy and increased requirements are partly offset by amenorrhoea, this may not be sufficient to meet the resultant net maternal outlay of over 500 mg iron.

Table 2.4
Causes of iron deficiency

Blood loss	
Uterine	Menorrhagia, post-menopausal bleeding, parturition
Gastrointestinal	Oesophageal varices, hiatus hernia, peptic ulcer, aspirin ingestion, hookworm, hereditary telangiectasia, carcinoma of stomach, caecum or colon, ulcerative colitis, angiodysplasia, Meckel's diverticulum, diverticulosis, piles etc.
Renal tract	Haematuria (e.g. renal or bladder lesion), haemoglobinuria (e.g. paroxysmal nocturnal haemoglobinuria)
Pulmonary tract Widespread bleeding disorders Self-inflicted	Overt haemoptyses, idiopathic pulmonary haemosiderosis
Malabsorption	Gluten-induced enteropathy (child or adult), gastrectomy, atrophic gastritis, chronic inflammation, clay eating etc.
Dietary	Especially vegetable diet

Blood Loss

Blood loss is the most common cause of iron deficiency. A loss of more than about 8 ml of blood (4 mg iron) daily becomes of importance since this equals the maximum amount of iron that can be absorbed from a normal diet. The loss is usually from the genital tract in women or from the gastro-intestinal tract in either sex. The most common cause on a world basis is infestation with hook-worm, in which anaemia is related to the degree of infestation. In the UK, menorrhagia, haemorrhoids and peptic ulceration are common, as well as salicylates or other non-steroidal anti-inflammatory drugs, hiatus hernia, diverticulosis and bowel tumours. Some of the other causes are listed in Table 2.4.

Some unusual causes of blood loss deserve mentioning. Cows' milk intolerance in infants may lead to gastrointestinal haemorrhage. Self-induced haemorrhage may occur as an unusual form of Munchausen's syndrome. Chronic intravascular haemolysis, such as that in paroxysmal nocturnal haemoglobinuria or mechanical haemolytic anaemia, may be a serious source of iron loss, while haemorrhage into the lungs in pulmonary haemosiderosis and into the joints in rheumatoid arthritis may cause a general body iron deficiency in the face of local iron overload.

Malabsorption

Malabsorption may sometimes be the primary cause of iron deficiency. In other cases it prevents the body adjusting to iron deficiency from other causes by increasing iron absorption. Dietary iron is poorly absorbed in coeliac disease both in children and adults, though often patients with this disease show a response, albeit sluggish, to oral therapy with inorganic iron. Excess loss of iron from exfoliating small intestinal cells may also contribute to the iron deficiency since turnover of intestinal cells may be increased up to several times normal in untreated coeliac disease. After partial gastrectomy, up to 65% of patients become iron deficient. The cause is multifactorial—haemorrhage (before and after the operation), poor diet, and malabsorption of food iron due to reduced gastric acid and loss of the stomach's 'hopper' function, are probably all important.

Atrophic Gastritis

There is a higher incidence of atrophic gastritis and histamine-fast achlorhydria in iron-deficient patients than in controls. In addition, many iron-deficient patients show parietal cell antibody in the serum and atrophic gastritis on gastric biopsy. Acid secretion has been shown to increase in some of these patients with iron therapy, particularly in younger subjects, and this suggests that the deficiency may be causing the gastric atrophy.

The reverse situation may also occur in some patients. Gastric acid is known to favour absorption of inorganic and other non-haem iron derived from food, and some degree of malabsorption of iron occurs in achlorhydric patients. In addition, atrophic gastritis may be a source of iron loss from local haemorrhage.

The known association between iron deficiency anaemia and pernicious anaemia (PA) could be explained by either theory. It may be that chronic iron deficiency predisposes to the gastritis of PA. More probably, autoimmune gastritis leads both to PA and to iron deficiency.

TREATMENT OF IRON DEFICIENCY

This entails (a) treatment of the underlying cause, and (b) correction of the deficiency by therapy with inorganic iron. Iron deficiency is commonly due to blood loss and, wherever possible, the site of this must be identified and the lesion treated.

Oral Therapy

In most patients, body stores of iron can be repleted by oral iron therapy, and several simple iron salts are satisfactory for this purpose. Iron is equally well absorbed from ferrous sulphate, gluconate, succinate, fumarate, lactate and glutamate, and since ferrous sulphate is the cheapest, this is the drug of choice; 200 mg ferrous sulphate contains 60 mg iron, 300 mg ferrous gluconate 36 mg, 300 mg ferrous succinate 70 mg, and 200 mg ferrous fumarate 65 mg. It is usual to give from 100 mg to 200 mg of elemental iron each day to adults and about 3 mg/kg per day as a liquid iron preparation to infants and children. The side-effects of oral iron, such as nausea, epigastric pain, diarrhoea, and constipation, are related to the amount of available iron which they contain; if iron does cause gastrointestinal symptoms, these can usually be obviated by reducing the dosage. Doses may be taken with food to reduce gastrointestinal intolerance, but this also reduces the amount absorbed. Enteric-coated and sustained-release preparations should not be used since much of the iron is released past the duodenum at sites of poor absorption and their effect of reducing symptoms can be achieved far more cheaply by using ordinary iron preparations at reduced dosage or with food.

A reticulocytosis begins on the third or fourth day after starting iron therapy and lasts from 12 to 21 days. The reticulocytosis does not reach the heights seen during treatment of megaloblastic anaemia and shows a more sustained plateau. The minimum rate of response should be 20 g/l rise in haemoglobin every 3 weeks, and the usual rate is 1.5–2 g/l daily. It will be slower where the dose of oral iron which is tolerated is less than 100 mg/day, but this is seldom of clinical importance. It is usually necessary to give iron for 3–6 months to correct the deficit of iron in circulating haemoglobin and in stores (shown by a rise in serum ferritin to normal).

Failure to respond to oral iron may be due to continued haemorrhage, malabsorption, or because the patient is not taking the drug. It is of course to be expected if the diagnosis is incorrect. For instance, many patients with thalassaemia or sideroblastic anaemia or other anaemias have been treated with iron before haemoglobin studies, bone marrow examination, or other tests have revealed the correct diagnosis. A poor response may also be obtained if the patient has an infection, renal or hepatic failure or an underlying malignant disease, or any other cause of anaemia additional to iron deficiency.

Parenteral Therapy

This is usually unnecessary but may be given if subjects genuinely cannot tolerate oral iron, particularly if a gastrointestinal disease such as ulcerative colitis or Crohn's disease is present. It is also occasionally necessary in coeliac disease and when it is essential to replete body stores rapidly (e.g. where severe iron deficiency anaemia is first diagnosed in late pregnancy) or when oral iron cannot keep pace with continuing haemorrhage (e.g. in patients with hereditary telangiectasia).

From all parenteral preparations, the iron complex is taken up by macrophages of the reticuloendothelial system, from where iron is released to circulating transferrin which then takes it to the marrow. Parenteral therapy does not lead to a more rapid rise in haemoglobin than that obtained with adequate oral iron therapy.

Parenteral preparations include iron dextran (Imferon) and iron-sorbitol (Jectofer) for intramuscular injection (50–100 mg iron/day). Local skin staining may occur with both preparations, which should be given by deep intramuscular injection. Iron dextran may also be given as a 'total dose' intravenous infusion over 6 hours. Whichever route is chosen, the deficit in body iron should be calculated from the degree of anaemia, and is usually 1–2 g. Total dose infusion of iron dextran should not be used if there is a history of allergy, since anaphylaxis occasionally occurs. A test dose should therefore be given slowly, followed by close medical supervision of the rest of the infusion. Flushing, nausea, urticaria, shivering, general aches and pains, dyspnoea and syncope are possible immediate adverse effects. Delayed reactions, including arthralgia, fever and lymphadenopathy, are well described and can persist for several days. An exacerbation of rheumatoid arthritis may also be precipitated. With iron sorbitol, some low molecular weight iron is released into circulation and excreted in the urine, and this may exacerbate urinary tract infection.

ANAEMIA OF CHRONIC DISORDERS

One of the commonest types of anaemia, particularly in hospital patients, is that due to chronic infections such as tuberculosis, to malignant diseases such as carcinoma and lymphoma, to chronic inflammatory diseases such as connective tissue diseases and rheumatoid arthritis, or to renal failure. In each of these conditions, iron deficiency, folate deficiency, and other causes of anaemia may also be present but there is an underlying, usually mild (PCV 0.3–0.4) anaemia, the degree being related to the activity of the disease. The peripheral blood characteristically shows normocytic and normochromic red cells, but where the illness results in a prolonged low saturation of plasma transferrin, the anaemia may be microcytic. Here the question of possible coexistent iron deficiency anaemia frequently arises. Diagnosis depends upon the demonstration of normal or increased iron stores (e.g. normal or raised serum ferritin) accompanying a reduced serum iron and TIBC (see Figs. 2.2 and 2.3). The bone marrow shows adequate iron in the macrophages but reduced amounts of iron in developing erythroblasts. Although the serum ferritin is an acute phase reactant, and may therefore be in the normal range despite coexistent iron deficiency, values below 50 μg/l are usually associated with absent iron stores in rheumatoid arthritis, renal disease and inflammatory bowel disease. All these are disorders in which chronic blood loss, due to disease or therapy, is common, and in which a fall in serum ferritin concentration below this level may be a useful guide to the need for iron therapy.

The pathogenesis of the anaemia is still incompletely defined. A mild shortening of red cell lifespan is sometimes present, together with a failure of the marrow to mount an appropriate increase in red cell production. There are conflicting data on whether erythropoietin production and/or erythroblast response to this hormone may be reduced, though the former is clearly important in chronic renal failure where a response to recombinant erythropoietin has been described. There is some evidence that serum from patients with rheumatoid arthritis may contain a factor which inhibits in-vitro erythroid colony growth. Although the changes in iron metabolism are striking and consistent with a block in the release of macrophage iron, their contribution in limiting erythropoiesis is not fully established. Increased lactoferrin production from granulocytes, with subsequent uptake of lactoferrin iron by macrophages, and increased apoferritin synthesis by macrophages, have both been suggested as possible explanations for the hypoferraemia. It seems likely that the anaemia is multifactorial in origin, with several different effects being mediated by inflammatory mediators such an interleukin-1. However, some of the more severe red cell changes may be explained by an imbalance between plasma iron supply and the erythroid marrow requirements.

PATHOLOGICAL ALTERATIONS IN HAEM SYNTHESIS

Porphyrias

These are a group of inherited or acquired diseases each characterized by a partial defect in one of the enzymes of haem synthesis. Increased amounts of intermediates of haem synthesis accumulate, the disorders being classified by whether the effects are predominantly in the liver or the erythron (Table 2.5). A full discussion of these disorders is beyond the scope of this chapter, but those with a particular haematological overlap will be mentioned briefly.

Congenital Erythropoietic Porphyria

This is a very rare autosomal recessive disorder which is due to reduced uroporphyrinogen cosynthase activity. Large amounts of porphyrinogens accumulate, and their conversion by spontaneous oxidation to photoactive porphyrins leads to severe, and disfiguring, cutaneous photosensitivity and dermatitis, as well as a haemolytic anaemia with splenomegaly. Increased amounts of uroporphyrin and coproporphyrin, mainly Type I, are found in bone marrow, red cells, plasma, urine and faeces. The disease is present from infancy and treatments, including avoidance of sunlight and splenectomy to improve red cell survival, are only partially effective. High level blood transfusions to suppress erythropoiesis completely (combined with iron chelation therapy to deal with the inevitable transfusional iron overload) have been reported to reduce porphyrin production sufficiently to abolish the clinical symptoms.

Erythropoietic Protoporphyria

This is caused by an autosomal dominant inherited deficiency of ferrochelatase, which results in increased free protoporphyrin concentrations in bone marrow, red cells, plasma and bile. Onset of the disease is usually in childhood. Expression of the gene is variable and photosensitivity and dermatitis vary from mild or absent to moderate in degree. There is no haemolysis, but accumulation of protoporphyrins in the liver can lead to rapidly progressive cirrhosis and hepatic failure. Treatment is by

Table 2.5
Human porphyrias

Form	Inheritance	Enzyme defect	Clinical features
Hepatic			
Acute intermittent porphyria	Autosomal dominant	Porphobilinogen deaminase	Acute attacks of gastrointestinal and/or nervous system involvement
Hereditary coproporphyria	Autosomal dominant	Coproporphyrinogen oxidase	
Porphyria variegata	Autosomal dominant	Protoporphyrinogen oxidase	
Porphyria cutanea tarda	Acquired or (rare) autosomal dominant	Uroporphyrinogen decarboxylase	Photosensitive dermatitis
Erythropoietic			
Congenital erythropoietic porphyria	Autosomal recessive	Uroporphyrinogen cosynthase	
Erythropoietic protoporphyria	Autosomal dominant	Ferrochelatase	

Photosensitive skin lesions are seen when the level of the enzyme defect in the haem synthetic pathway (Fig. 2.5) leads to the accumulation of formed porphyrins, while acute attacks are related to the accumulation of porphyrin precursors (ALA and PBG). For further details see Kappas *et al.*(1983).

avoidance of sunlight, and β-carotene may also diminish photosensitivity. Iron deficiency should be avoided since this may increase the amount of free protoporphyrin.

Porphyria Cutanea Tarda

The commonest of the hepatic porphyrias, this is usually due to an acquired defect affecting liver uroporphyrinogen decarboxylase, though there is a rarer genetic defect of this enzyme. There is increased excretion of urinary uroporphyrin I and coproporphyrin III, and the disease is characterized by photosensitivity and dermatitis. It appears to be precipitated in middle or later life, more often in men than women, by factors such as liver disease, alcohol excess, or oestrogen therapy. Hepatic siderosis is a common feature. Iron is known to inhibit uroporphyrinogen decarboxylase, and removal of the moderate iron overload by repeated phlebotomy is standard treatment, usually leading to remission.

Lead Poisoning

Chronic ingestion of lead in humans causes an anaemia which is usually normochromic or slightly hypochromic. Red cell lifespan is shortened and there is a mild rise in reticulocytes, but jaundice is rare. Basophilic stippling is a characteristic, though not universal, finding and it is thought to be due to precipitation of RNA, resulting from inhibition of the enzyme pyrimidine 5′-nucleotidase. Siderotic granules, and occasionally Cabot rings, are found in circulating red cells. The bone marrow shows increased sideroblast formation, in some cases with ring sideroblasts present. Red cell protoporphyrin and coproporphyrin are raised, as are urinary excretion of ALA, coproporphyrin III and uroporphyrin I.

The cause of the anaemia appears to be multifactorial. Haemolysis, probably due to the blocking of sulphydryl groups with consequent denaturation of structural proteins, enzymes and damage to mitochondria, and defective haemoglobin synthesis due to inhibition of enzymes in haem synthesis, are the major factors.

Sideroblastic Anaemia

The sideroblastic anaemias comprise a group of refractory dyserythropoietic disorders in which there are a variable number of hypochromic cells in

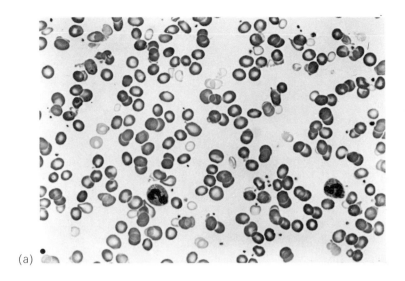

(a)

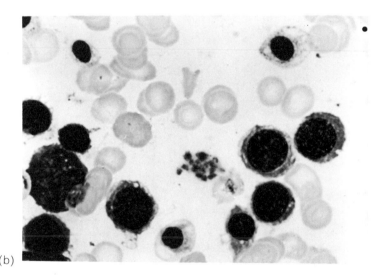

(b)

Fig. 2.7. *(a) The peripheral blood film of a patient with primary acquired sideroblastic anaemia (May-Grünwald Giemsa × 650). (b) The bone marrow of a patient with primary acquired sideroblastic anaemia. The normoblasts show a vacuolated appearance (May-Grünwald Giemsa × 1300).*

the peripheral blood (Fig. 2.7a) and an excess of iron in the bone marrow, many of the developing erythroblasts containing iron granules arranged in a ring around the nucleus (Fig. 2.8). These ring sideroblasts (more than six perinuclear granules/cell) are the diagnostic feature of the anaemia, and though they may form a small percentage of the erythroblasts in a wide variety of clinical disorders, are only present in large numbers in sideroblastic anaemia. The various types of sideroblast that may be

seen in the marrow are classified in Table 2.6 and illustrated in Fig. 2.9.

Classification (Table 2.7)

Congenital Sideroblastic Anaemia

This is a rare disorder manifesting mainly in males, usually in childhood or adolescence. In most reported families inheritance has followed an

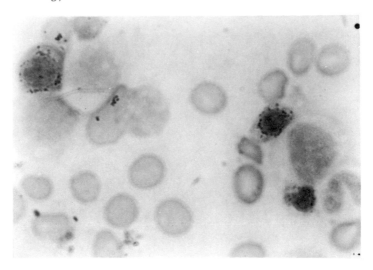

Fig. 2.8. *The bone marrow of a patient with primary acquired sideroblastic anaemia stained for iron (Perls' stain). Three ring sideroblasts are present (× 1300).*

Table 2.6
Siderocytes and sideroblasts

Siderocyte
Mature red cell containing one or more siderotic granules (Pappenheimer bodies)

Normal sideroblast
Nucleated red cell containing one or more siderotic granules; granules few, difficult to see, randomly distributed in the cytoplasm. Reduced proportion of sideroblasts in iron deficiency and anaemia of chronic disorders

Abnormal sideroblasts
(a) *Cytoplasmic iron deposits (ferritin aggregates)*
    Increased granulation; granules larger and more numerous than normal, easily visible and randomly distributed; proportion of sideroblasts usually parallels the percentage saturation of transferrin (e.g. haemolytic anaemia, megaloblastic anaemia, iron overload, thalassaemia disorders)
(b) *Mitochondrial iron deposits (non-ferritin iron)*
    Ring sideroblasts in inherited and acquired sideroblastic anaemias

---

X-linked pattern; females may show partial expression, usually with only mild or no anaemia, though, rarely, severe dimorphic anaemia has been described. This may depend on variation in the severity of the defect, as well as the degree of Lyonization of the affected X-chromosome. The latter is presumably responsible for the demonstration of a true dual population of normal and microcytic cells. Autosomal inheritance may also occur. The patients show a hypochromic, often microcytic, anaemia with reduced MCV, MCH and MCHC. There may be a few circulating siderocytes, normoblasts and cells with punctate basophilia, but these features become pronounced only if the spleen

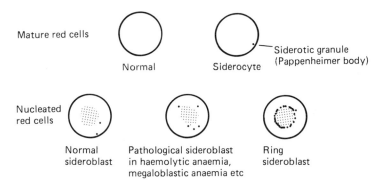

Fig. 2.9. *Siderocytes and sideroblasts.*

Table 2.7

Classification of causes of ring sideroblasts

Hereditary	X-linked
	Autosomal (rare)
Acquired	
(1) Primary	Refractory anaemia with ring sideroblasts in FAB classification of myelodysplastic syndromes
(2) Associated with myeloproliferative and other myelodysplastic diseases	Acute myeloid leukaemia, myelosclerosis, polycythaemia rubra vera, erythroleukaemia, other myelodysplastic syndromes (including chronic myelomonocytic leukaemia, and refractory anaemia with excess blasts)
Also reported in association with myeloma, chronic lymphocytic leukaemia	
(3) Secondary	
(a) Conditions with abnormalities of vitamin B_6 metabolism	Antituberculous chemotherapy, coeliac disease, haemolytic anaemia, alcoholism
(b) Conditions with a known disturbance of haem synthesis or mitochondrial function	Lead poisoning, alcohol, chloramphenicol
(c) Other conditions (? by chance)	Rheumatoid arthritis, carcinoma, megaloblastic anaemia, phenacetin

has been removed. The bone marrow shows erythroid hyperplasia: the erythroblasts tend to be microcytic with ragged, vacuolated cytoplasm, resembling severely iron-deficient cells. When the anaemia is severe there is usually an increased proportion of early cells with some later cells appearing non-viable. The iron stain shows increased iron in the fragments and macrophages, and excessive siderotic granulation in the developing erythroblasts. There are usually many ringed sideroblasts, the most obviously affected cells being the late forms, though in mildly affected females only a small proportion of erythroblasts may be affected. The spleen may be enlarged, presumably due to the excess pitting function in removing iron from circulating red cells; a mild decrease in platelet and leucocyte counts may result from hypersplenism. The serum iron is usually raised, the total iron-binding capacity saturated, and the reticulocytes inappropriately low at between 1% and 4%. Patients may present with severe iron overload despite a relatively mild anaemia and absence of previous iron therapy or blood transfusions, though the rate of iron loading is accelerated if the latter are needed.

Primary Acquired Sideroblastic Anaemia (see also Chapter 17)

This is a disease predominantly of middle-aged and elderly subjects and is one type of myelodysplasia. The sexes are affected equally and there is no family history. The disease may be present for many years before the diagnosis is made and, rarely, the patient may show the clinical features of haemochromatosis on presentation.

The peripheral blood film is characteristically dimorphic (see Fig. 2.7a). The proportion of hypochromic cells is usually lower than in the inherited disease, and the MCH and MCHC tend to be higher. The serum iron is usually raised but is normal more often than in the inherited disease. Macrocytosis is often present and the MCV raised. The white cells are usually normal but occasionally show myelodysplastic features, e.g. Pelger phenomenon, low alkaline phosphatase, agranular forms, an increased monocyte count, a few myelocytes or even occasional myeloblasts. When these features are present acute myeloblastic leukaemia is more likely to develop. However, the overall risk of this (approximately 10%) is lower in sideroblastic anaemia, particularly in those with marked erythroid hyperplasia, than in the other myelodysplastic syndromes (p. 470). Thrombocytopenia may also occur, and occasionally there may be a striking thrombocytosis.

The bone marrow, as in the inherited disease, is usually hypercellular, though the erythroblasts in the acquired disease tend to show more macronormoblastic or megaloblastic changes. They have a characteristic vacuolated appearance (see Fig. 2.7b). Bone marrow iron is increased to a variable degree, and at least 15% of erythroblasts should have rings to make the diagnosis; these are found in both early and late erythroblasts in the acquired disease.

Ring Sideroblasts in Association with Other Marrow Disorders

Ring sideroblasts may be present in patients with other myelodysplastic and myeloproliferative diseases (Table 2.7). In some patients the two may present simultaneously. In other cases, ring sideroblasts develop in a patient known to have had a previous marrow disorder. Yet other patients present with apparently primary sideroblastic anaemia and subsequently develop acute myeloblastic leukaemia after a variable period of follow-up.

Secondary Ring Sideroblasts

Pure nutritional vitamin B_6 deficiency in experimental animals produces a hypochromic anaemia in which ring sideroblasts may be seen. It is likely that abnormalities of vitamin B_6 metabolism may predispose to sideroblastic anaemia in several clinical situations but are not established to be the sole cause.

Vitamin B_6 deficiency. Sideroblastic anaemia associated with vitamin B_6 deficiency has been described, though not completely documented, in a few patients with coeliac disease and pregnancy, and with haemolytic anaemias such as sickle-cell anaemia, mechanical haemolytic anaemia and autoimmune haemolytic anaemia. It is possible that associated folate deficiency in some way exaggerates the tendency to form ring sideroblasts in these diseases.

Vitamin B_6 antagonists. Sideroblastic anaemia may be found as a complication of antituberculous chemotherapy, particularly with the vitamin B_6 antagonists isoniazid and cycloserine. The exact frequency is unknown but it probably requires at least 6 months of chemotherapy for the anaemia to manifest. Only a small proportion of tuberculous patients appear to be susceptible to this complication and it may be that these particular patients have an underlying genetic tendency to form ring sideroblasts.

Lead poisoning. Lead inhibits several enzymes concerned in haem and probably in globin synthesis. The anaemia of lead poisoning is discussed on p. 44; in some cases, ring sideroblasts are visible in the marrow.

Chloramphenicol. This drug inhibits mitochondrial protein synthesis and in some patients causes ring sideroblast formation, presumably as a result of impaired haem formation in the mitochondria.

Alcoholism. Sideroblastic anaemia is associated with the 'Skid-Row' type of alcoholism in which there is associated malnutrition and folate deficiency. Suggested mechanisms include direct interference with haem formation and interference with pyridoxal kinase, an enzyme involved in vitamin B_6 metabolism. The anaemia rapidly reverses with abstinence from alcohol, a normal diet, and pyridoxine therapy.

Other drugs. Ring sideroblasts have been found in the bone marrow of patients receiving phenacetin and paracetamol, but the exact association is still obscure.

Other diseases. Occasional patients with rheumatoid arthritis, carcinomatosis, myxoedema and other chronic disorders have been reported to show ring sideroblasts. Whether these are significant associations is still uncertain.

Pathogenesis

A common end-point in the sideroblastic anaemias appears to be defective haem synthesis. Reduced levels of ALA-synthase are common in both inherited and primary acquired disease. Other enzymes may also be affected, e.g. ferrochelatase is impaired by chloramphenicol. ALA-synthase requires pyridoxal-phosphate as coenzyme, and reduced affinity of apoenzyme for coenzyme might explain responses to pyridoxine therapy (see below). No case of primary sideroblastic anaemia has been shown to be due to a defect of vitamin B_6 metabolism. In some cases of secondary sideroblastic anaemia, however, vitamin B_6 deficiency or faults in its metabolism may play a role.

It remains unclear, however, whether deficient synthesis of haem is the cause of ring sideroblast formation. Primary defects of haem synthetic enzymes alone do not seem to be sufficient explanation for sideroblastic changes as these are not characteristic of any of the porphyrias. An alternative possibility is that a primary defect in erythroblast iron metabolism (e.g. of transport or maintenance of iron in the reduced ferrous state in which it is incorporated into haem) may produce mito-

chondrial iron overload and damage, resulting in secondarily impaired haem synthesis. In primary acquired sideroblastic anaemia, multiple mitochondrial enzyme defects have been shown to occur. Whatever the primary mechanism, impaired mitochondrial function is likely to contribute to the defect of erythroblast maturation, where arrest in G_2 phase is typical.

In the inherited sideroblastic anaemias an inborn error is likely to be the fault, whereas in primary acquired disease a clonal mutation is likely to be responsible. Indeed, G6PD isoenzyme and cytogenetic studies confirm a clonal abnormality affecting all haemopoietic cell lines but not fibroblasts. Chromosome analysis is normal in the hereditary disease, but a small minority of patients with primary acquired disease have cytogenetic abnormalities (e.g. monosomy); their presence is usually associated with a more rapid clinical progression and increased risk of leukaemic change. Mutations in ras oncogenes have also been described in 15% of patients in most studies.

Treatment of Sideroblastic Anaemia

Often the patient is refractory to all forms of therapy and the treatment resolves itself to management of a patient with chronic refractory anaemia. In many patients the anaemia may remain stable and asymptomatic for years, but in others it may progress, possibly due to an increasing accumulation of iron in mitochondria and consequent increasing inhibition of haem synthesis. Because of the problems of iron overload, transfusions should be used sparingly and iron therapy must be avoided.

Pyridoxine

About a third of patients with sideroblastic anaemia, whether acquired or inherited, show some response to pyridoxine. However, the minority of patients who respond well have an inherited form of the disease, and in most of the others the response is only partial, with a reticulocytosis but suboptimal rise in haemoglobin. In some, the rise in haemoglobin may occur slowly over several months without any definite reticulocytosis. It is usually necessary to give pharmacological doses of 50–100 mg or even 500 mg of pyridoxine daily to obtain these responses.

A few patients have been reported who had secondary sideroblastic anaemia completely reversed by pyridoxine therapy. This has been described in alcoholism, in haemolytic anaemia and in coeliac disease. Completely reversible sideroblastic anaemia has also been reported in patients receiving antituberculous chemotherapy in whom the drugs have been stopped and pyridoxine administered. However, no patient with either inherited or primary acquired sideroblastic anaemia has shown complete reversal of the condition.

Folic Acid

Folate deficiency is particularly common in secondary sideroblastic anaemias but occurs in all forms of the disease, presumably due to increased marrow cell turnover. Some of the patients show an improvement in haemoglobin when given folic acid, and surprisingly this may occur both in patients with and without megaloblastic erythropoiesis. In addition to pyridoxine, folic acid therapy may therefore be tried. In patients with primary acquired disease, megaloblastic erythropoiesis is often not converted to normoblastic by folic acid (or vitamin B_{12}), even in large doses.

Other Forms of Treatment

In younger patients with iron overload, attempts to prevent tissue damage by iron chelation and/or phlebotomy therapy should be considered. Indeed, in a few cases, improvement in the anaemia has followed iron removal by phlebotomy. Androgens do not seem to have any beneficial effect. A single case has responded to injections of pyridoxal-phosphate after not responding to pyridoxine. Responses to immunosuppressive therapy have been described in a few patients with other evidence of an immune aetiology for the anaemia. Splenectomy should not be carried out as it does not benefit the anaemia and leads to persistently high platelet counts postoperatively with a high incidence of thromboembolism.

IRON OVERLOAD

The association of excessive parenchymal iron stores with tissue damage, particularly of the liver, is conventionally called haemochromatosis. By contrast, increased amounts of iron which are situated mainly in macrophages of the reticuloendothelial system appear relatively harmless. Parenchymal iron overload commonly arises when excess iron enters the body from the intestine, whereas iron administered parenterally, e.g. as multiple transfusions, is first taken up in senescent red cells by macrophages. However, there is no absolute distinction between the two sites, and iron from macrophages is slowly released to transferrin and then enters parenchymal cells. A classification of the conditions of iron overload is shown in Table 2.8.

Table 2.8
Causes of iron overload

(a) Excess iron absorption	Idiopathic haemochromatosis
	Massive ineffective erythropoiesis (thalassaemia intermedia, sideroblastic anaemia, congenital dyserythropoietic anaemias)
(b) Blood transfusion	Refractory anaemias (β thalassaemia major, red cell aplasia, etc.)
(c) Increased iron intake	Excess oral iron (patients in (a) at particular risk) or parenteral iron
	Bantu siderosis (high iron diet and beverages)
(d) Liver disease	Alcoholic cirrhosis
	Post-portocaval anastomosis
(e) Local: Pulmonary	Idiopathic pulmonary haemosiderosis
Renal	Paroxysmal nocturnal haemoglobinuria
Joints	Rheumatoid arthritis

For a detailed discussion of these syndromes the reader is referred elsewhere, but some features relating to haematological conditions are mentioned below.

Idiopathic Haemochromatosis

This manifests the features of cirrhosis, endocrine disorders, skin pigmentation and cardiac failure. It is usually a disease of middle and later life and is thought to arise after many years of increased iron absorption due to an unknown genetic defect of iron metabolism. At least one determinant of the disease is closely linked with the HLA locus on chromosome 6, particularly with HLA-A3. The disease is inherited as an autosomal recessive, the haemochromatosis allele having a frequency as high as 1 in 20 in some populations. The amount of iron in the body revealed by therapeutic phlebotomy may be 20 g or more in symptomatic disease. The disease is commoner in males than females, presumably because of the protective effect of regular menstruation in premenopausal women. Other factors such as dietary iron intake and alcoholism probably also contribute to the rate of development of the disease. First-degree relatives, particularly siblings, are also at risk of the disease, and should be regularly screened for evidence of iron loading. It has been suggested that the occasional occurrence of iron overload in haematological disorders such as congenital spherocytosis, where it is otherwise uncommon, might be due to the coincidental inheritance of the heterozygous state for idiopathic haemochromatosis.

Liver Disease

Idiopathic haemochromatosis must be distinguished from cirrhosis with increased liver iron, which most frequently arises in alcoholics. These patients usually show lower amounts of iron in the body, with rapid development of iron deficiency on repeated venesection, and more features of hepatocellular insufficiency and portal hypertension than patients with primary haemochromatosis.

Increased Iron Intake

Excess iron ingestion from food and beer prepared in iron pots is probably the major factor in Bantu siderosis, where there is iron overload of both parenchymal and reticuloendothelial cells. Alcoholism, malnutrition and infections may also contribute to the iron overload and determine its distribution in individual cases. Haemochromatosis has also been described in subjects given therapeutic oral iron for many years and, in Brescia in Italy, in subjects drinking the local red wine of high iron content.

IRON-LOADING ANAEMIAS

Iron overload in patients with chronic anaemias is the most difficult of all to treat and can arise from (a) increased iron absorption, (b) repeated blood transfusion, or (c) prolonged administration of therapeutic iron. Iron loading from regular blood transfusions occurs at 20–30 mg/day in adults and, in patients with β-thalassaemia major, leads to endocrine damage, increasing hepatic fibrosis, and death by the end of the second decade from cardiac failure or arrhythmias. The endocrine damage is manifest by failure of pubertal growth and development (due to variable damage to the hypothalamus, pituitary and gonads), and sometimes diabetes mellitus, hypoparathyroidism and hypothyroidism. Increased iron absorption appears to occur only in those patients with a hypercellular marrow (and not, for instance, in aplastic anaemia) and to be particularly important in conditions of ineffective erythropoiesis (Table 2.8), rather than chronic haemolytic anaemias. The risk of iron loading from the gut is variable and may be concealed in some patients since a mild and asymptomatic anaemia can sometimes coexist with a marked expansion of dyserythropoietic marrow. Such patients are also particularly vulnerable to the inappropriate administration of oral iron therapy.

Mechanism of Iron Damage

Adults who have received 50–100 units of blood usually develop tissue damage. In infants even 10 units may cause liver damage. Resting rather than proliferating cells are affected. Peroxidation of lipids of cell membranes, due to iron-catalysed hydroxyl radical formation, and oxidation of intracellular proteins have been suggested.

Damage to lysosomal membranes by haemosiderin has also been shown to occur, with release of lysosomal enzymes into other cell compartments. However, the degree of damage in various organs shows poor correlation with the amount of iron in the organ. The heart in particular often seems to show functional damage in excess of that expected. The length of time the iron has been present may also be relevant, although damage to the liver, assessed by electron microscopy, has been found in children with thalassaemia major in the first or second year of life. Liver damage in multiply transfused patients is, however, frequently due to hepatitis B virus or non-A, non-B hepatitis.

IRON CHELATION THERAPY

The improved survival in idiopathic haemochromatosis after iron removal by phlebotomy has encouraged the use of iron-chelating agents in the iron-loading anaemias. Desferrioxamine mesylate (DF, mol. wt 657) is the main agent in current clinical use. It is not absorbed orally, and after parenteral injection it is rapidly cleared from the plasma, with a half-life of 5–10 minutes, being excreted in the urine, taken up by hepatocytes, or metabolized in the tissues. This probably accounts for the much greater mobilization of iron by continuous intravenous or subcutaneous infusions, which allow a more prolonged exposure of the drug to the chelatable iron. As a result, subcutaneous infusions (self-administered, usually over 12 hours every night, using a small battery-driven pump and a fine needle inserted over the anterior abdominal wall) have, over the last few years, become the standard way of using the drug. DF is a trihydroxamic acid, one molecule binding one ferric ion to form the red chelate, ferrioxamine. This is excreted in urine and bile (appearing in the faeces). Faecal iron is derived from hepatocytes, probably from an intracellular transit iron pool in exchange with ferritin iron stores. Urine iron, which has received the most attention, being more easily measured, also derives, at least in part, from hepatocytes, though other body sources, including iron released from macrophages, may also contribute. Urinary iron excretion tends to level off at higher doses, but this does not occur with bile iron excretion, which increases linearly with the dose: bile iron may

therefore predominate at high doses and this is also the major route of excretion when total body iron has been reduced to relatively low levels. Urine iron excretion also tends to be less immediately after blood transfusions, but this is accompanied by a reciprocal increase in faecal iron excretion so that total iron mobilized may be little changed. On the other hand, increased erythropoiesis, as in haemolytic anaemias, is associated with an increase in urine iron excretion in relation to body iron stores.

Planning Treatment

Therapy with DF is expensive and inconvenient. Its use should therefore be restricted to those patients, e.g. with congenital anaemias, in whom iron overload is the main threat to life. In elderly patients with acquired, transfusion-dependent, refractory anaemias, the prognosis of the underlying haematological disease may not justify therapy designed to prevent iron-overload complications several years hence. In children, tissue damage from iron may be present from very early life, and regular iron chelation should begin by 2 to 3 years. The dose should be 'tailored' for each individual to give optimum urinary iron excretion, and is usually around 40 mg/kg as a 12-hour subcutaneous infusion. Careful planning has become even more important, with reports of auditory and visual neurotoxicity and growth defects with large doses, particularly in young patients with relatively low body iron stores. The hearing loss is characterized by a high frequency sensorineural deficit, while the eye changes consist of an optic neuropathy with decreased acuity, loss of colour vision and pigment changes in the retina. It is, however, well worthwhile using larger doses (e.g. 150 mg/kg over 12–24 hours) by intravenous infusion at the time of each blood transfusion, in order to take advantage of the increased bile iron excretion at high doses: as much as 200 mg of iron can be mobilized by a single such infusion in some older patients. Repletion of the ascorbic acid deficiency which sometimes accompanies iron overload, or ascorbic therapy even in those with normal tissue levels of ascorbate, increases urinary iron excretion, but has no effect on bile iron excretion. Worries about a possible increase in iron toxicity due to mobilization of storage iron by ascorbate mean that supplements of vitamin

C should not exceed 100–200 mg/day. The effect of ascorbate may disappear as iron stores decline. In some less severely anaemic patients with chronic ineffective erythropoiesis and iron loading from the gut, e.g. with thalassaemia intermedia or sideroblastic anaemia, cautious phlebotomy may be added to regular subcutaneous DF to produce a rate of iron mobilization comparable to that achieved in the treatment of idiopathic haemochromatosis.

Effect of Iron Chelation

Even relatively inadequate therapy with intramuscular DF (0.5–2.0 g/day) was found to prevent progress of hepatic fibrosis, possibly by interfering with the action of an enzyme requiring iron as a cofactor in collagen synthesis. Nevertheless, tissue iron and serum ferritin levels remained well above normal with this therapy. By contrast, regular subcutaneous infusions offer the hope of preventing iron accumulation, since they can mobilize sufficient iron to produce negative iron balance even in young children with low iron loads. There is increasing evidence of improved hepatic and cardiac function, and hepatic iron removal, in patients who comply with the rigorous therapy. Growth and pubertal development are improved in many but not all patients, but diabetes and other endocrine abnormalities still occur frequently. Serum ferritin levels in well-chelated thalassaemia major patients usually plateau between 500 μg/l and 1500 μg/l. Possible adverse effects of DF, in addition to the largely reversible neurotoxicity and growth defects described above, include sensitivity reactions, local soreness related to the site of injection (usually due to the needle being inserted too superficially), and exacerbation of some infections, notably of the urinary tract and Yersinia enterocolitis. Cataracts have been described in experimental animals, but not in humans. Regular eye and auditory examinations are advisable.

Other Iron Chelators

Although DF is relatively safe and highly specific for iron, its expense and inconvenient route of administration mean that it is unavailable in many parts of the world where thalassaemia is common. Diethylene triamine penta-acetic acid (DTPA) is cheaper but must also be given parenterally and has the disadvantage that it chelates substantial amounts of zinc. With repeated frequent use, DTPA produces severe toxic effects as a result of zinc depletion, though it may be possible to ameliorate these with oral zinc supplements. There is now some prospect for the clinical development of a cheap oral iron-chelating drug. A variety of compounds are active by mouth in animals (including pyridoxal isonicotinoyl hydrazone and pyridine derivatives, and some phenolic chelators), and early clinical studies with 1,2 dimethyl-3-hydroxypyrid-4-one raise the hope that one or other drug may eventually prove non-toxic and suitable for long-term clinical use.

Endocrine Replacement Therapy

Patients with chronic iron overload, particularly from childhood, may develop a variety of endocrine abnormalities requiring treatment, e.g. with insulin, gonadotrophin-releasing hormone (GnRH), gonadotrophins, sex hormones, vitamin D and calcium supplements, or thyroxine.

Therapy of Acute Iron Poisoning

In this case, DF is given both orally and parenterally. Instillation of 5 g into the stomach after a 1% sodium bicarbonate gastric lavage and an injection of 1–2 g intramuscularly may be tried. If more severe poisoning has occurred, an intravenous DF infusion up to a maximum dose of 80 mg/kg in 24 hours should be set up.

SELECTED BIBLIOGRAPHY

Bothwell T. H., Charlton R. W., Cook J. D., Finch C. A. (1979). *Iron metabolism in man.* Oxford: Blackwell Scientific Publications.

Cartwright G. E., Deiss A. (1975). Sideroblasts, siderocytes and sideroblastic anemia. *New England Journal of Medicine*, **29**, 185–193.

Cazzola M., Huebers H. A., Sayers M. H., MacPhail P., Eng M., Finch C. A. (1985). Transferrin saturation, plasma iron turnover and transferrin uptake in normal humans. *Blood*, **66**, 935–939.

Charlton R. W., Bothwell T. H. (1983). Iron absorption. *Annual Review of Medicine*, **34**, 55–68.

Cook J. D. (1982). Clinical evaluation of iron deficiency. *Seminars in Hematology*, **19**, 6–18.

Hershko C., Weatherall D. J. (1988). Iron chelating therapy. *C.R.C. Critical Reviews in Medicine* (in press).

Hoffbrand A. V., Gorman A., Laulicht M. *et al.* (1979). Improvement in iron status and liver function in patients with transfusional iron overload with long-term subcutaneous desferrioxamine. *Lancet*, **i**, 947–949.

Jacobs A. (Ed.) (1982). *Disorders of iron metabolism. Clinics in Haematology*, **11**, 241–486.

Jacobs A. (1985). Iron deficiency and iron overload. *CRC Critical Reviews in Oncology/Hematology*, **3**, 143–186.

Jacobs A. (1986). Primary acquired sideroblastic anaemia. *British Journal of Haematology*, **64**, 415–418.

Kappas A., Sassa S., Andreou K. E. (1983). The porphyrias. In *The metabolic basis of inherited disease*, 5th edn, pp. 1301–1384. (Eds. J. B. Stanbury, J. B. Wyngaarden, D. S. Fredrickson, J. L. Goldstein, M. S. Brown). New York: McGraw Hill.

Kontoghiorghes G. J., Aldouri M. A., Hoffbrand A. V., Barr J., Wonke B., Kourouclaris T., Sheppard L. (1987). Effective chelation of iron in beta-thalassaemia with the oral chelator 1,2-dimethyl-3-hydroxypyrid-4-one. *British Medical Journal*, **295**, 1509–1512.

Kontoghiorghes G. J., Hoffbrand A. V. (1988). Transfusional iron overload: prospects for effective oral iron chelation. In *Recent advances in haematology*, Vol. 5, pp. 75–98. (Ed. A. V. Hoffbrand). Edinburgh: Churchill Livingstone.

Lee G. R. (1983). The anemia of chronic disease. *Seminars in Hematology*, **20**, 61–80.

Marcus R. E., Huehns E. R. (1985). Transfusional iron overload. *Clinical and Laboratory Haematology*, **7**, 195–212.

Olivieri N. F., Buncic J. R., Chew E. *et al.* (1986). Visual and auditory toxicity in patients receiving subcutaneous deferoxamine infusions. *New England Journal of Medicine*, **314**, 869–873.

Oski F. A., Honig A. S., Helu B., Howanitz P. (1983). Effect of iron therapy on behaviour performance in non-anemic, iron deficient infants. *Pediatrics*, **71**, 877–880.

Peto T. E. A., Pippard M. J., Weatherall D. J. (1983). Iron overload in mild sideroblastic anaemias. *Lancet*, **1**, 375–378.

Pippard M. J., Callender S. T. (1983). The management of iron chelation therapy. *British Journal of Haematology*, **54**, 503–507.

Wolfe L., Olivieri W., Sallan D. *et al.* (1985). Prevention of cardiac disease by subcutaneous deferoxamine in patients with thalassemia major. *New England Journal of Medicine*, **312**, 1600–1603.

Worwood M. (1986) Serum ferritin. *Clinical Science*, **70**, 215–220.

Wintrobe M. N., Lee G. R., Bogg D. R. *et al.* (1981). *Clinical haematology*, 8th edn, p. 199. Philadephia: Lea & Febiger.

Chapter 3

MEGALOBLASTIC ANAEMIA

A. V. HOFFBRAND

The megaloblastic anaemias are a group of disorders characterized by the presence of distinctive morphological appearances of the developing red cells in the bone marrow. The cause is usually deficiency of either vitamin B_{12} or folate but megaloblastic anaemia may arise because of abnormal metabolism of these vitamins or because of faults in DNA synthesis not related to vitamin B_{12} or folate (Table 3.1).

CLINICAL FEATURES

Many patients are detected by routine blood counts, often because of a raised MCV before any symptoms are present. The main clinical features in more severe cases are those of anaemia such as weakness, tiredness, shortness of breath and occasionally angina of effort or heart failure. Anorexia is usually marked and there may be weight loss, diarrhoea or constipation. Other particular features of megaloblastic anaemia include glossitis ('beefy red'), angular cheilosis, a mild fever in the more severely anaemic patients, jaundice of the unconjugated type, and reversible melanin skin pigmentation which may occasionally be marked and occurs with both B_{12} and folate deficiencies. The low platelet count sometimes leads to bleeding manifestations and this may be exaggerated by vitamin C deficiency in a few patients, and the anaemia and low leucocyte count may predispose to infections, particularly of the respiratory or urogenital tracts. Aphthous ulceration has been suggested but not proven to be a sign of the deficiencies. Sterility may occur in both sexes. The spleen may be palpable in the more anaemic cases.

Neurological Manifestations

Vitamin B_{12} deficiency may cause bilateral peripheral neuropathy or degeneration of the posterior and pyramidal tracts of the spinal cord, optic atrophy or mental abnormalities. The patient with vitamin B_{12} neuropathy usually presents with paraesthesiae, muscle weakness, difficulty in walking or psychotic disturbances. Visual impairment may be due to a retrobulbar neuritis with optic atrophy or, in severely anaemic patients, to retinal haemorrhages. Folate deficiency may cause mental changes such as slowness and even mild dementia and has been suggested to cause organic nervous disease but this is uncertain. Methotrexate injected into the cerebrospinal fluid may, however, cause brain or spinal cord damage.

HAEMATOLOGICAL FINDINGS

Peripheral Blood

The presence of oval macrocytes, usually with considerable anisocytosis and poikilocytosis, is the main feature (Fig. 3.1a). The MCV is usually raised above 100 fl unless a cause of microcytosis, e.g. iron deficiency or thalassaemia trait, is present when the film is dimorphic and the MCV may be normal. In some cases, the MCV may be normal due to excess fragmentation of red cells. Some of the neutrophils are hypersegmented (more than five nuclear lobes). Both macrocytosis and hypersegmented neutrophils may occur in other situations (Table 3.2). Together, however, they strongly suggest megaloblastic haemopoiesis. The total white cell count tends to fall due to reduction of granulocytes and

Table 3.1
Causes of megaloblastic anaemia

Vitamin B_{12} deficiency or abnormalities of vitamin B_{12} metabolism (see Table 3.4)

Folate deficiency or abnormalities of folate metabolism (see Table 3.8)
Therapy with antifolate drugs, e.g. methotrexate

Independent of either vitamin B_{12} or folate deficiency and refractory to vitamin B_{12} and folate therapy

(a) Some cases of erythroleukaemia,* other leukaemias,* myelodysplasia*
(b) Orotic aciduria (responds to uridine)
(c) Therapy with drugs interfering with synthesis of DNA, e.g. cytosine arabinoside, hydroxyurea, 6-mercaptopurine, azidothymidine (AZT)
(d) Alcohol ingestion
(e) Thiamine responsive (one documented case)

Suggested but poorly documented causes of megaloblastic anaemia not due to vitamin B_{12} or folate deficiency or metabolic abnormality:
Vitamin E deficiency
Lesch–Nyhan syndrome (? responds to adenine)

---

* Folate deficiency also occurs frequently in these diseases.

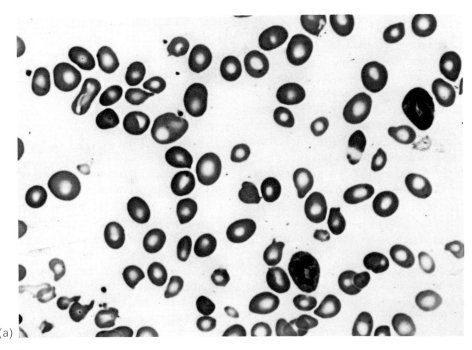

(a)

Fig. 3.1a. *The peripheral blood in severe megaloblastic anaemia (May–Grünwald Giemsa × 650).*

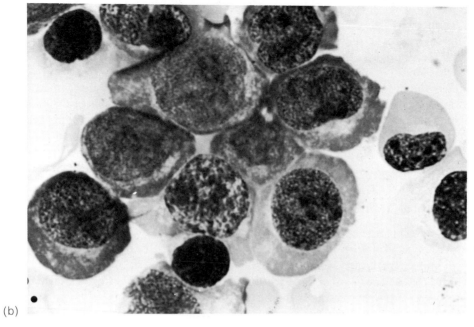

(b)

Fig. 3.1b. *The bone marrow in severe megaloblastic anaemia (May–Grünwald Giemsa × 1300)*

Table 3.2

Conditions in which macrocytosis or hypersegmented neutrophils may occur in the absence of megaloblastic anaemia

Macrocytosis	Alcoholism
	Liver disease (especially alcoholic)
	Reticulocytosis (haemolysis or haemorrhage)
	Aplastic anaemia or red cell aplasia
	Hypothyroidism
	Myelodysplasia including primary acquired sidero-blastic anaemia
	Myeloma and macroglobulinaemia
	Leucoerythroblastic anaemia
	Myeloproliferative disease and leukaemia
	Chronic respiratory failure
	Pregnancy
	Newborn
Hypersegmented neutrophils	Renal failure
	Congenital (familial) abnormality
	? Iron deficiency

Note: High MCV recorded when cold agglutinins or paraproteins are present.

lymphocytes but is not usually less than $1.5 \times 10^9/1$; the platelet count may be moderately reduced, though in extreme cases it falls to levels of $40 \times 10^9/1$ or less. Occasionally a leucoerythroblastic blood picture is seen. The severity of all these changes parallels the degree of anaemia (provided no other cause of anaemia is present); in the non-anaemic patient, the presence of a few macrocytes and hypersegmented polymorphs in the peripheral blood may be the only indication of the underlying disorder.

Bone Marrow

In the severely anaemic patient, the marrow is hypercellular; the myeloid:erythroid ratio is normal or reduced and there is an accumulation of primitive cells due to selective death of more mature forms. The most characteristic finding is dissociation between nuclear and cytoplasmic development in the erythroblasts, the nucleus maintaining a primitive appearance despite maturation and haemoglobinization of the cytoplasm; fully haemoglobinized (orthochromatic) cells may be seen which retain nuclei. The nucleus of the megaloblast also has an open, fine, lacey appearance, the cells are larger than normoblasts and an increased number of cells with eccentric lobulated nuclei or nuclear fragments may be present (Fig. 3.1b). Mitoses and dying cells are more frequent than normal. The leucocyte series shows the presence of giant and abnormally shaped metamyelocytes, while the megakaryocytes may be enlarged and show increased numbers of nuclei (hyperpolyploidy). Rarely, red cell precursors are lost almost completely from the marrow and a mistaken diagnosis of myeloid leukaemia may be made. Iron staining shows increase in both RE stores and in the developing megaloblasts.

In less anaemic cases, the changes in the marrow may be difficult to recognize. The terms 'intermediate', 'moderate', 'mild' or 'early' are used to describe megaloblastic changes not so florid as those seen in the severely anaemic, uncomplicated case. The changes may be mild and difficult to recognize, even in a severely anaemic patient if the anaemia is largely due to other factors, e.g. iron deficiency, infection, malignant disease, haemolysis, etc., and the megaloblastosis is an incidental phe-

nomenon. The term 'megaloblastoid' has several different connotations and is best avoided.

Chromosomes

Bone marrow cells, transformed lymphocytes and other proliferating cells in the body show a variety of changes, including random breaks, reduced contraction, spreading of the centromere and exaggeration of secondary chromosomal constrictions and overprominent satellites. Similar abnormalities may be produced by antimetabolite drugs, e.g. cytosine arabinoside, hydroxyurea and methotrexate, which also cause megaloblastic appearances.

INEFFECTIVE HAEMOPOIESIS

There is an accumulation of unconjugated bilirubin in plasma partly due to the decreased survival of circulating red cells but mainly due to death of nucleated red cells in the marrow, so called ineffective erythropoiesis. Other evidence for this includes raised urine urobilinogen and faecal stercobilinogen excretion, reduced haptoglobins, a positive Schumm's test, positive urine haemosiderin, raised serum lactate dehydrogenase (LDH) to values between 1000 and 10 000 i.u./dl, and a raised serum iron level with rapid clearance of injected radio-iron and poor incorporation of the isotope into circulating red cells. Radio-labelled glycine studies have shown an increase in the later (erythropoietic) phase rather than in the earlier (hepatic) phase of the early (1–4 day) appearance of the isotope in bilirubin and stercobilinogen. Carbon monoxide production is also increased. The serum lysozyme is also raised in some cases, suggesting ineffective granulopoiesis.

GENERAL TISSUE EFFECTS OF VITAMIN B_{12} AND FOLATE DEFICIENCIES

The deficiencies, when severe, affect all rapidly growing (DNA synthesizing) tissues. After the marrow, the next most affected tissues are the epithelial cell surfaces of the mouth, stomach, small intestine, respiratory, urinary, and female genital tracts. The cells show macrocytosis with increased numbers of multinucleate and dying cells. The gonads are also affected and sterility is common in patients with either deficiency.

Less well-established effects include a number of complications of pregnancy (recurrent abortions, antepartum haemorrhage, abruptio placentae, congenital malformations, stillbirth and prematurity), inhibition of osteoblast activity (a low serum alkaline phosphatase has been recorded in untreated pernicious anaemia) and reduced regeneration of the cirrhotic liver. Patients with coeliac disease and with sickle-cell anaemia have also been reported to show stunted growth, which has been improved coincidentally with commencement of folic acid therapy, but it is not certain how much the growth improvement in these children was due to folic acid and how much to other, simultaneously administered, therapy. Vitamin B_{12} deficiency, but not folate deficiency, has been associated with defective intracellular killing by neutrophils of ingested bacteria. In the fragile X syndrome, sister chromatid exchange and DNA breaks are increased in vitro in folate-deficient medium, apparently at the X q28 site. No in-vivo abnormality of folate metabolism can be detected.

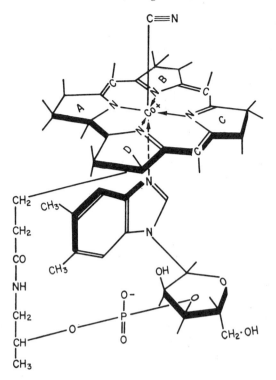

Fig. 3.2. *The structure of vitamin B_{12} (cyanocobalamin).*

VITAMIN B_{12}

Vitamin B_{12} exists in a number of different chemical forms, called the cobalamins. It was first crystallized as cyanocobalamin which is a stable form, has a molecular weight of 1355 in the unhydrated state and forms dark-red prisms. The molecule consists of two halves, a 'planar group' and 'nucleotide' set at right angles to it (Fig. 3.2). The planar group is a corrin ring and the nucleotide consists of the base, 5,6-dimethylbenziminazole, and a phosphorylated sugar, ribose-3-phosphate. In nature, the vitamin is mainly in the 5′-deoxyadenosylcobalamin form in which the –CN group is replaced by the 5′-deoxyadenosyl group. This is the main form in human liver and most other tissues. Minor constituents of natural cobalamins are methylcobalamin, the major form in human plasma, and hydroxocobalamin, which is the form to which methyl-and 5′-deoxyadenosylcobalamin are rapidly converted by

exposure to light, hydroxocobalamin having its cobalt atom in the fully oxidized, Cob III state, whereas the cobalt exists as the reduced Cob I in the methyl- and deoxyadenosyl-coenzyme forms (Fig. 3.3).

Dietary Sources and Requirements

Vitamin B_{12} is synthesized solely by microorganisms. Ruminants obtain vitamin B_{12} from the foregut but the only source for humans is food of animal origin. The highest amounts are found in liver and kidney (up to 100 μg/100 g) but it is also present in shellfish, organ and muscle meats, fish, chicken and dairy products—eggs, cheese and milk, which contain small amounts (6 μg/l). On the other hand, vegetables, fruits and all other foods of non-animal origin are free from vitamin B_{12} unless they are contaminated by bacteria. Cooking does not usually destroy vitamin B_{12} but in alkaline conditions some loss may occur.

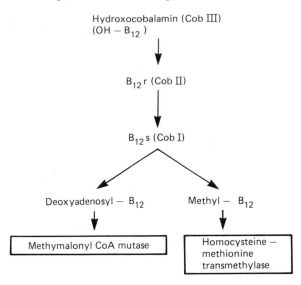

Hydroxocobalamin (Cob III)
(OH − B$_{12}$)

↓

B$_{12}$ r (Cob II)

↓

B$_{12}$ s (Cob I)

Deoxyadenosyl − B$_{12}$ Methyl − B$_{12}$

↓   ↓

| Methymalonyl CoA mutase |

| Homocysteine − methionine transmethylase |

Fig. 3.3. *The reduction of hydroxocobalamin to the two active cobalamin coenzymes.*

A normal Western diet contains between 5 μg and 30 μg vitamin B$_{12}$ daily. Adult daily losses (mainly in urine and faeces) are between 1 μg and 3 μg (about 0.1% of body stores) and, since the body does not seem to have the ability to degrade vitamin B$_{12}$, daily requirements are also about 1–3 μg. Stores are of the order of 2–3 mg, sufficient for 3–4 years if supplies are completely cut off.

ABSORPTION OF VITAMIN B$_{12}$

Two mechanisms exist for vitamin B$_{12}$ absorption. One is passive, occurs equally through the jejunum and the ileum, is rapid but extremely inefficient since less than 1% of an oral dose of vitamin B$_{12}$ can be absorbed by this process. The other mechanism is active, occurs through the ileum in humans and is efficient for small oral doses of vitamin B$_{12}$. This is the normal mechansim by which the body acquires vitamin B$_{12}$ and is mediated by *gastric intrinsic factor.*

Dietary vitamin B$_{12}$ is released from protein complexes by enzymes in the stomach, duodenum and jejunum and combines rapidly, one molecule to one molecule, with intrinsic factor. All forms of vitamin B$_{12}$ are absorbed by the same intrinsic factor mechanism and it has been suggested that the nucleotide portion of the molecule fits into a pit on the surface of the protein, while the -CN, -OH, -CH$_3$ or deoxyadenosyl group are opposite the site of attachment (Fig. 3.4). Pseudovitamin B$_{12}$ compounds in which the 5,6-dimethylbenziminazole nucleotide is replaced by other nucleotides usually do not attach to intrinsic factor and therefore remain unabsorbed.

Intrinsic factor (IF) is a glycoprotein of molecular weight 45 000. The gene has been cloned. It is produced in the microsomes or endoplasmic reticulum of the gastric parietal cells in the fundus and body of the stomach of humans. The IF–B$_{12}$ complex, in contrast to free IF, is resistant to enzyme digestion. It appears that IF–B$_{12}$ has a smaller molecular radius than free intrinsic factor and that some enzyme bonds which are open to attack by proteolytic enzymes when intrinsic factor is free are protected in the complex (Fig. 3.4). Pancreatic trypsin is necessary to free vitamin B$_{12}$

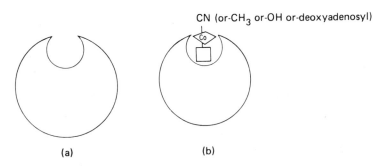

CN (or-CH$_3$ or-OH or-deoxyadenosyl)

(a)   (b)

Fig. 3.4. *(a) Intrinsic factor and (b) intrinsic factor–vitamin B$_{12}$ complex. Intrinsic factor has been estimated to have a molecular radius of 3.6 nm, vitamin B$_{12}$ 0.8 nm, and the complex 3.2 nm.*

that becomes attached to the non-intrinsic factor, R binder (see below) present in gastric juice.

The IF–B_{12} complex passes to the ileum where the intrinsic factor attaches to specific receptor sites on the microvillus membrane of the brush border surface of the ileal absorptive cells. The attachment requires calcium ions and a pH around neutral, and is probably a physical process, not requiring energy. The receptor consists of an α subunit facing out which binds IF, and a β subunit which faces into the cell. Vitamin B_{12} then enters the ileal cell but the exact fate of the intrinsic factor is unknown. Intrinsic factor does not enter the bloodstream as such, since after a delay of about 6 hours absorbed vitamin B_{12} appears in portal blood attached to the B_{12} transport protein, transcobalamin II, probably synthesized in the ileum. During the period of mucosal delay, vitamin B_{12} may be concentrated in the lysosomes of the ileal cells, where IF is probably digested away. There may also be partial conversion of cyano- to deoxyadenosylcobalamin.

The ileum has a limited capacity to absorb vitamin B_{12} at any one time because of limited receptor sites, and though 50% or more of a single dose of 1 μg vitamin B_{12} may be absorbed, with doses above 2 μg the proportion absorbed falls rapidly. Moreover, after one dose of IF–B_{12} complex has been presented, the ileal cells become refractory to further doses for about 6 hours.

Enterohepatic Circulation

Between 0.5 μg and 5.0 μg of vitamin B_{12} enter the bile every day. This is normally reabsorbed together with vitamin B_{12} derived from sloughed intestinal cells.

TRANSPORT OF VITAMIN B_{12}

Two main vitamin B_{12} transport proteins exist in human plasma which both bind vitamin B_{12} one molecule for one molecule (Fig. 3.5). One, transcobalamin I (TCI), a glycoprotein, electrophoreses as an alpha globulin and has a molecular weight of 56 000–58 000. It is closely related to other so-called 'R' B_{12}-binding proteins in milk, gastric juice, bile, saliva, and other fluids. These glycoproteins differ from each other only in the carbohydrate moiety of the molecule. Transcobalamin III is a name used to

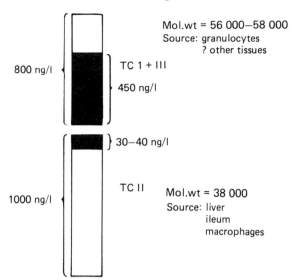

Fig. 3.5. *The serum vitamin B_{12}-binding proteins. (Closed rectangles = endogenous serum vitamin B_{12}, open rectangles = vitamin B_{12}-binding protein.)*

describe an isoprotein of TCI in plasma which differs from TCI by its composition of sugars and B_{12} content. TCI is normally about two-thirds saturated with B_{12}, which it binds tightly. It gives up B_{12} to tissues less readily than free B_{12} enters tissues. Glycoprotein receptors on liver cells are concerned in the removal of R proteins from plasma.

Transcobalamin II is a beta-globulin, (mol. wt 38 000), synthesized by liver, and by other tissues including macrophages and probably ileum. It normally carries only 20–60 ng of B_{12}/l of plasma and readily gives up B_{12} to marrow, placenta, and other tissues, which it enters by endocytosis. The protein itself is not reutilized. Alterations may occur in the transcobalamin levels in a variety of disease states (Table 3.3). In general, an increase in TCI causes an increase in serum vitamin B_{12}, whereas an increase in TCII does not. Five different inherited isoproteins of TCII, separated by polyacrylamide gel electrophoresis, have been described. All are functionally active.

VITAMIN B_{12} ANALOGUES

Vitamin B_{12} analogues are corrinoids which may be cobamides (which contain substitutions in the

Table 3.3

Alterations in plasma vitamin B_{12}-binding proteins in disease

TCI (and/or TCIII)	Increased (usually with elevated serum B_{12}) 1. Myeloproliferative diseases, especially chronic granulocytic leukaemia, myelosclerosis, polycythaemia vera 2. Hepatoma 3. Increased granulocyte production, e.g. inflammatory bowel disease, liver abscess 4. Eosinophilia due to hypereosinophilic syndrome

Congenital absence: low serum vitamin B_{12}; no clinical abnormality

TCII	Increased (sometimes with no elevation of serum B_{12}) 1. Liver disease 2. Gaucher's disease 3. Autoimmune diseases 4. Long-continued hydroxocobalamin therapy

Congenital absence: normal serum B_{12}; megaloblastic anaemia within a few weeks of birth; impaired B_{12} absorption

place of ribose, e.g. adenosine) or cobinamides (which have no nucleotide at all). The analogues are relatively inert for the microbiological assay organisms *Euglena gracilis* or *Lactobacillus leichmannii*. In radioisotope dilution assays that use R-binder but not pure intrinsic factor they may, after extraction from proteins with the cobalamins, lead to false high serum B_{12} levels. TCI may carry them to the liver for excretion in bile. It is unclear whether they are inert, or inhibit vitamin B_{12}-dependent reactions, or are active as co-enzymes in these reactions. The proportion derived from diet, gut bacteria or endogenous breakdown of B_{12} is unknown.

CAUSES OF VITAMIN B_{12} DEFICIENCY

Vitamin B_{12} deficiency is usually due to malabsorption. The only other cause is inadequate dietary intake. Vitamin B_{12} deficiency due to excess degradation, utilization or loss has not been adequately documented.

Inadequate Dietary Intake

Adult

Dietary vitamin B_{12} deficiency arises in vegans who for religious reasons omit meat, fish, eggs, cheese and other animal produce from their diet. The largest group in the world comprises Hindus and it is likely that many millions of Indians are deficient in vitamin B_{12} on a nutritional basis. Not all vegans, however, develop vitamin B_{12} deficiency of sufficient severity to cause anaemia or neuropathy, even though subnormal serum vitamin B_{12} levels have been found in up to 50% of randomly selected young adult Indian vegans. Explanations as to why nutritional vitamin B_{12} deficiency may not progress to megaloblastic anaemia include the following.

(a) The diet of most vegans is probably not totally lacking in vitamin B_{12}. The serum B_{12} level may not be an accurate measure of their body stores—red cell B_{12} levels have been found to be generally much closer to those of subjects on a normal diet.

(b) The enterohepatic circulation of vitamin B_{12} is still intact in vegans and thus losses are less than in conditions of malabsorption.

(c) Daily losses of vitamin B_{12} are thought to be related to body stores; therefore, as the body stores become depleted, daily losses become smaller and the amount of vitamin B_{12} needed to maintain the *status quo* may also become smaller.

Dietary vitamin B_{12} deficiency may rarely arise in non-vegetarian subjects who exist on grossly inadequate diets because of poverty or psychiatric disturbance.

Infancy

Vitamin B_{12} deficiency has been described in infants born to severely vitamin B_{12}-deficient mothers. These infants develop megaloblastic anaemia at about 3–6 months of age, presumably because they are born with low stores of vitamin B_{12} and because they are fed breast-milk of low vitamin B_{12} content. They have been shown to respond satisfactorily to as little as 0.1 μg vitamin B_{12} daily by mouth. The condition occurs most commonly in India but a similar condition has also been described elsewhere where the mother had unrecognized pernicious anaemia.

MALABSORPTION OF VITAMIN B_{12}

Table 3.4 lists the conditions which may cause malabsorption of vitamin B_{12} sufficiently severe and prolonged to cause vitamin B_{12} deficiency with megaloblastic anaemia or neuropathy. The conditions giving rise to less severe malabsorption of vitamin B_{12} are listed in Table 3.5.

Table 3.4
Causes of vitamin B_{12} deficiency

Nutritional	Vegans
Malabsorption	
Gastric causes	Pernicious anaemia (congenital, acquired)
	Total and partial gastrectomy
Intestinal causes	Intestinal stagnant-loop syndrome
	Jejunal diverticulosis
	Ileocolic fistula
	Anatomical blind-loop
	Intestinal stricture, etc.
	Tropical sprue
	Ileal resection and Crohn's disease
	Selective malabsorption with proteinuria
	Fish tapeworm

Table 3.5
Causes of malabsorption of vitamin B_{12} usually without severe vitamin B_{12} deficiency

Malabsorption of vitamin B_{12} may occur in the following conditions but is not usually sufficiently prolonged to cause clinically significant vitamin B_{12} deficiency

Simple atrophic gastritis
Coeliac disease
Severe pancreatitis
Total body irradiation
Zollinger–Ellison syndrome
Deficiencies of vitamin B_{12}, folate, protein, ?riboflavin, ?nicotinic acid
Therapy with colchicine, PAS, neomycin, slow-release potassium chloride, anticonvulsant drugs, metformin, phenformin, cytotoxic drugs
Alcohol

Gastric Causes of Vitamin B$_{12}$ Deficiency: Pernicious Anaemia

Adult pernicious anaemia may be defined as severe lack of intrinsic factor due to gastric atrophy. It is a common disease in North Europeans and is rare in Asia and Africa. The overall incidence is about 120 per 100 000 population in Great Britain, but there is a wide variation between one area and the next. The incidence in men and women is approximately 1:1.6 and the peak age incidence is 60, only 10% of cases presenting under 40 years of age. The disease occurs more commonly than by chance in close relatives, and in subjects with autoimmune diseases (see below) and those with premature greying, blue eyes, vitiligo, and in persons of blood group A. An association with HLA-3 has been reported in some but not all series.

Prognosis

The life expectancy in females once regular treatment has begun is normal. Males have a slightly subnormal life expectancy due to a higher incidence of carcinoma of the stomach than in controls.

Diagnosis

This is usually suspected from the clinical picture and the finding of megaloblastic anaemia due to vitamin B$_{12}$ deficiency. Lack of intrinsic factor may be demonstrated directly or by vitamin B$_{12}$ absorption studies. Tests for gastric autoantibodies are also important.

Gastric Secretion Studies

Intrinsic Factor

This is measured by its vitamin B$_{12}$ binding, one unit binding 1 ng vitamin B$_{12}$. Normal adult males secrete more than 2000 units in an hour after maximal stimulation, females about half this amount. Patients with PA usually secrete no measurable IF, but a few secrete up to 250 units in an hour. Greater amounts of IF can be detected if steps are taken to dissociate local IF antibody from IF. It has been estimated that 500 units or more are needed to maintain normal vitamin B$_{12}$ absorption.

Hydrochloric Acid

The resting juice usually has a pH more than 7 and does not fall more than 1 pH unit with maximal stimulation. The volumes of gastric secretion and pepsin secretion are also markedly low. The serum gastrin level is usually raised, the hormone coming from endocrine cells in the gastric fundus.

Gastric Biopsy

This usually shows gastric atrophy with loss of glandular elements and replacement by mucous cells, a mixed inflammatory cell infiltrate and perhaps intestinal metaplasia. In some cases, glandular elements remain.

Immune Phenomenon

In addition to the appearance of the gastric mucosa, there is a large body of evidence which suggests that immune mechanisms play an important role in the pathogenesis of pernicious anaemia and this aspect of the disease is discussed next under four main headings.

Antibodies to Gastric Antigens

Intrinsic Factor Antibodies

Two types of intrinsic factor antibody may be found in the serum of patients with pernicious anaemia; both are IgG. One, the 'blocking' or 'Type I' antibody, prevents the combination of intrinsic factor and vitamin B$_{12}$, whereas the other, the 'binding', 'Type II' or 'precipitating' antibody, which attaches to intrinsic factor whether attached to vitamin B$_{12}$ or not, prevents attachment of intrinsic factor to ileal mucosa. The blocking antibody occurs in the serum of about 55% of the patients and the binding antibody in 35%. The sera of 45% of patients show neither antibody.

Intrinsic factor antibodies are rarely found in conditions other than pernicious anaemia, but Type I antibody has been detected in the sera of rare patients without pernicious anaemia with thyrotoxicosis, myxoedema, Hashimoto's disease, diabetes and in relatives of the pernicious anaemia patients.

Intrinsic factor antibodies have also been detected in *gastric juice* in about 80% of pernicious anaemia patients. These antibodies may well reduce absorption of dietary vitamin B_{12} by combining with small amounts of remaining intrinsic factor in the gastric juice. Achlorhydria favours the formation of this antigen–antibody complex whereas acid secretion (with a consequent low pH) dissociates intrinsic factor from its antibodies and favours its combination with vitamin B_{12}, and therefore vitamin B_{12} absorption.

Parietal Cell Antibody

This is detected by immunofluorescent or complement fixation techniques. It is present in the sera of nearly 90% of adult patients with pernicious anaemia but it is by no means diagnostic since it is frequently present in other subjects. Thus, it occurs in as many as 16% of randomly selected female subjects aged over 60 and in a smaller proportion of younger controls and is found more frequently than in controls in relatives of PA patients, in patients with simple atrophic gastritis, chronic active hepatitis, thyroid disorders and their relatives, Addison's disease, diabetes, rheumatoid arthritis, chronic active hepatitis, iron deficiency anaemia and other conditions. The parietal cell antibody has also been found in gastric juice in PA.

Association with Other 'Autoimmune' Diseases

There is also a clinical association between PA and thyroid diseases, hypoparathyroidism and Addison's disease but not with systemic lupus erythematosus. These diseases occur together more than by chance and they are often found in close relatives of patients with one or other overt disease. The serum of PA patients may also contain an autoantibody to the gastrin receptor.

Response to Steroid Therapy

Steroid therapy improves the gastric lesion, at least temporarily, in a proportion of patients with PA. There may be regeneration of the mucosa, with a return of secretion of acid and intrinsic factor, and an improvement in vitamin B_{12} absorption. When steroid therapy is withdrawn, there is a relapse

within a few weeks. These findings suggest that an 'autoimmune' process is continuously damaging the gastric mucosa in PA and preventing regeneration.

Hypogammaglobulinaemia

Pernicious anaemia is found more often than by chance in patients with deficiency of IgA or with complete hypogammaglobulinaemia. These subjects resemble other subjects with PA except they often present relatively young (before the age of 40), they have a lower incidence of serum intrinsic factor and parietal cell antibodies than other PA patients and they may show intestinal malabsorption. They may also have a history of recurrent infections. The gastric lesion is similar to that in other cases except plasma cells are absent from the inflammatory cell infiltrate.

Lymphocyte Subpopulations

An increased CD4 (helper) to C8 (suppressor) cell population in peripheral blood has been described in patients showing intrinsic factor antibodies.

Conclusion

Adult pernicious anaemia seems to consist of a local 'autoimmune' gastritis, partly congenitally determined and possibly partly due to acquired factors. The unique event is the appearance of intrinsic factor antibodies in the gastric juice which inhibit any remaining intrinsic factor. The exact relation between the antibodies and the gastric lesion and the reason why intrinsic factor antibodies virtually only occur in PA remain obscure.

Childhood Pernicious Anaemia

Two types exist. One, usually in older children, resembles PA of adults. Gastric atrophy, achlorhydria and serum intrinsic factor antibody are all present, though parietal cell antibody is usually absent. About half of these patients show an associated endocrinopathy such as myxoedema, Addison's disease or hypoparathyroidism.

In the second, more common type, the child usually shows no demonstrable intrinsic factor but has a normal gastric mucosa and normal secretion of acid. These patients usually present with megaloblastic anaemia in the first, second, or third year of life when stores of vitamin B_{12}, accumulated from the mother *in utero*, are used up; a few have presented as late as the second decade. Parietal cell and intrinsic factor antibodies are absent. The inheritance of this condition follows a recessive, autosomal pattern. A variant of this type has been described in which the child is born with intrinsic factor present which is functionally inactive.

Gastrectomy

Following *total gastrectomy*, vitamin B_{12} deficiency is inevitable and prophylactic vitamin B_{12} therapy should be commenced immediately following the operation. After partial gastrectomy, 10–15% of patients also develop the deficiency. This usually manifests 4 years or more following the operation. The exact incidence may depend partly on the type of operation and the site of the ulcer but is most influenced by the size of the resection. The vitamin B_{12} deficiency may cause uncomplicated megaloblastic anaemia in about 4% of cases, but more frequently occurs in patients with associated iron deficiency anaemia (about 7% of all cases).

The explanation of the vitamin B_{12} deficiency is usually lack of intrinsic factor. This is due to resection of intrinsic-factor-secreting tissue, atrophy of remaining stomach and possibly inhibition of secreted intrinsic factor by bile. Secretion of intrinsic factor in post-gastrectomy patients is stimulated by food, and tests of absorption in the fasting state may therefore be misleading. In a few patients, the deficiency is due solely to the creation of a bacterially contaminated intestinal stagnant loop, and in other patients an abnormal jejunal flora may be a partial cause of vitamin B_{12} malabsorption.

Intestinal Causes of Vitamin B_{12} Deficiency

Intestinal Stagnant-Loop Syndrome

Malabsorption of vitamin B_{12} occurs in a variety of intestinal lesions in which there is colonization of the upper small intestine by faecal organisms. This may occur in patients with jejunal diverticulosis, entero-anastomosis, intestinal stricture or fistula, or with an anatomical blind-loop due to Crohn's disease, tuberculosis or created at operation. It is not known with certainty which organism is responsible for the malabsorption of vitamin B_{12}.

Ileal Resection

Removal of 1.2 metres or more of terminal ileum causes malabsorption of vitamin B_{12}. In some patients following ileal resection, particularly if the ileocaecal valve is incompetent, colonic bacteria may contribute to the malabsorption.

Selective Malabsorption of Vitamin B_{12} with Proteinuria (Imerslund's syndrome: Imerslund–Gräsbeck syndrome; congenital vitamin B_{12} malabsorption)

The patients, who usually present with megaloblastic anaemia between the ages of 6 months and 3 years, secrete normal amounts of intrinsic factor and gastric acid but are unable to absorb vitamin B_{12} due to a congenital defect of the ileum. In some cases, ileal brush border receptors for intrinsic factor are absent. Other tests of intestinal absorption are normal. Over 90% of the patients show non-specific proteinuria but renal function is otherwise normal and renal biopsy has not shown any consistent renal defect; a few of the patients have shown aminoaciduria and congenital renal abnormalities such as duplication of the renal pelvis. The inheritance is autosomal recessive.

Tropical Sprue

Nearly all patients with acute and subacute tropical sprue show malabsorption of vitamin B_{12} and this may persist as the principal abnormality in the chronic form of the disease when the patient may present with megaloblastic anaemia or neuropathy due to vitamin B_{12} deficiency. Absorption of vitamin B_{12} usually improves after antibiotic therapy and, in the early stages, may also improve considerably after folic acid.

Fish Tapeworm (*Diphyllobothrium latum*) Infestation

This tapeworm lives in the small intestine of humans and accumulates vitamin B_{12} from food, rendering this unavailable for absorption. People acquire the worm by eating raw or partly cooked fish and infestation is common around the lakes of Scandinavia, Germany, Japan, North America and Russia. Megaloblastic anaemia or vitamin B_{12} neuropathy occurs only in those with a heavy infestation, with the worm high in the small intestine, and many carriers have no vitamin B_{12} deficiency.

MALABSORPTION OF VITAMIN B_{12} USUALLY WITHOUT SEVERE VITAMIN B_{12} DEFICIENCY (Table 3.5)

Simple Atrophic Gastritis

About a third of these patients show malabsorption of vitamin B_{12} and some show borderline serum B_{12} levels, but none shows clinically important vitamin B_{12} deficiency; otherwise, they are, by definition, cases of pernicious anaemia.

Adult Coeliac Disease

Malabsorption of vitamin B_{12} occurs in about 30% of untreated patients (presumably those in whom the disease extends to the ileum) and correlates with the degree of steatorrhoea. Vitamin B_{12} deficiency is not usually severe in these patients and is probably never the cause of megaloblastic anaemia. The absorption improves when the patients are treated with a gluten-free diet.

Severe Chronic Pancreatitis

In this condition, lack of trypsin is thought to cause dietary vitamin B_{12} attached to gastric non-IF(R) binder to be unavailable for absorption. In pancreatitis, it may also be that the concentration of calcium ions in the ileum falls below the level needed to maintain normal vitamin B_{12} absorption.

Alteration in pH of the Ileum

Malabsorption of vitamin B_{12} has been reported in the Zollinger–Ellison syndrome and during treatment with slow-release potassium chloride. It is thought that in these situations the pH of the ileum may fall below 6 and reduce ileal uptake of IF–B_{12} complex.

Drugs

Neomycin, colchicine, phenytoin (diphenylhydantoin), para-aminosalicylate(PAS), phenformin, metformin and alcohol have all been reported to cause malabsorption of vitamin B_{12}.

Vitamin B_{12}, Folate Deficiencies

Both vitamin B_{12} and folate deficiencies affect the function of the small intestine, and malabsorption of vitamin B_{12} due to ileal dysfunction may be found in patients with either deficiency. Surprisingly, it may take several weeks of vitamin B_{12} therapy to correct the ileal absorptive defect in patients with pernicious anaemia.

Deficiency of protein, riboflavin and pyridoxine have also been reported to cause malabsorption of vitamin B_{12}.

ABNORMALITIES OF VITAMIN B_{12} METABOLISM

Congenital TCII Deficiency or Abnormality

These infants present with megaloblastic anaemia within a few weeks of birth. Serum vitamin B_{12} and folate levels are normal but the anaemia responds to massive (e.g. 1 mg three times weekly) injections of vitamin B_{12} which cause free vitamin B_{12} to enter marrow cells by passive diffusion in the absence of the specific transport protein. In some cases, the protein is present in normal amounts but is unable to bind B_{12} or to attach to the cell surface and so is functionally dead. The infants do not show methylmalonic aciduria, but malabsorption of vitamin B_{12} has been described in all and reduced immunoglobulins in some cases. Failure to institute vitamin B_{12} therapy may allow neurological damage to occur.

Congenital Methylmalonic Aciduria (Fig. 3.6)

The infants with this abnormality are ill from birth, with vomiting, failure to thrive, ketosis and mental

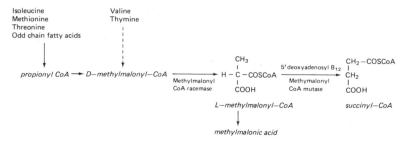

Fig. 3.6. *The role of deoxyadenosyl-cobalamin in methylmalonyl CoA metabolism.*

retardation. Anaemia, if present, is normocytic and normoblastic. A proportion of the infants respond to vitamin B_{12} in large doses whereas the others are unresponsive. In the patients who do respond, it is likely that there is failure of conversion of vitamin B_{12} to its deoxyadenosyl coenzyme form; in those who do not, the enzyme methylmalonyl CoA mutase is probably lacking or defective. Some children have combined methylmalonic aciduria and homocystinuria due to defective formation of both vitamin B_{12} coenzymes. Surprisingly, only two of five such children showed megaloblastic haemopoiesis.

Acquired Abnormality of Vitamin B_{12} Metabolism

Nitrous Oxide Inhalation

Nitrous oxide has been found to oxidize methylcobalamin from its active, fully reduced, Cob I state to an inactive precursor with the Cob II state (see Fig. 3.3). This has been shown to lead to failure of thymidylate synthesis in both humans and experimental animals and to be of importance in the megaloblastic anaemia that occurs in patients undergoing prolonged N_2O anaesthesia, e.g. in intensive care units. A neuropathy resembling vitamin B_{12} neuropathy has been described in dentists repeatedly exposed to N_2O and in monkeys exposed to the gas for many months. Under more usual circumstances, the nitrous oxide effect presumably reverses with no clinical abnormality resulting.

Cyanide Inactivation of Vitamin B_{12}

The theory that certain foods and smoking inactivate vitamin B_{12} as cyano B_{12} in sufficient amounts to cause vitamin B_{12} neuropathy is no longer thought true, although hydroxocobalamin is still used in the treatment of tobacco amblyopia and Leber's optic atrophy.

DIAGNOSIS OF VITAMIN B_{12} DEFICIENCY

There are four methods used clinically to diagnose the deficiency.

Therapeutic Trial

The first step in the diagnosis of either vitamin B_{12} or folate deficiency is recognition of the relevant abnormalities in the peripheral blood and/or bone marrow. The diagnosis of vitamin B_{12} or folate deficiency as the cause of megaloblastic anaemia can be accomplished by a therapeutic trial. This is performed by: (1) placing the patient on a diet of low vitamin B_{12} and folate content, (2) allowing a period of 7–10 days after admission to exclude a 'spontaneous' response or response to a haematinic given before admission, and then (3) treatment with a physiological dose of vitamin B_{12} (e.g. 1 μg intramuscularly daily) or of folic acid (100 μg daily).

An optimal haematological response is shown by a reticulocytosis beginning on the third day and reaching a peak on the sixth or seventh day of therapy, with considerable conversion of erythropoiesis to normoblastic after 48 hours and leucopoiesis to normal by the 12th to 14th day. There is a rise in haemoglobin of about 10 g/l per week. The leucocyte and platelet counts become normal after about 7 days.

In a non-anaemic patient or a patient with iron deficiency or other complicating cause of anaemia, or with an infection, the therapeutic trial cannot be carried out. It is also unwarranted in an extremely ill patient when it is necessary to treat quickly with large doses of vitamin B_{12} and folic acid.

Deoxyuridine Suppression Test

In normal bone marrow, deoxyuridine (dU) considerably suppresses uptake of radioactive thymidine into DNA. This is thought to be due to conversion of dU to thymidine triphosphate (dTTP) which inhibits thymidine kinase, on which thymidine uptake depends (Fig. 3.7). The dU suppresses radioactive thymidine incorporation less effectively in megaloblastic anaemia due to folate or B_{12} deficiency because of the block in dUMP conversion to dTMP (Fig. 3.7). In B_{12} deficiency, the test can be corrected with B_{12} or 5-formyl tetrahydrofolate (folinic acid) but not by methyltetrahydrofolate, whereas in folate deficiency, both the folate analogues but not B_{12} correct the test. In refractory megaloblastic anaemia (e.g. of sideroblastic anaemia or erythroleukaemia or due to antimetabolite drugs which inhibit DNA synthesis at a separate point

from thymidylate synthesis) the test gives results as in a normoblastic marrow. The test can also be performed on stimulated peripheral lymphocytes.

Measurement of the Serum Vitamin B_{12} Level

This is the most satisfactory routine method of diagnosing the deficiency and may be accomplished by microbiological assay, using *Lactobacillus leichmannii*, *Euglena gracilis* (or, less commonly, *Escherichia coli* or *Ochromonas malhamensis*) as test organism. Serum vitamin B_{12} can also be measured by one of a number of radioisotope dilution assays. Normal (*E. gracilis*) serum vitamin B_{12} levels range from about 160 ng/l to 925 ng/l while in patients with megaloblastic anaemia due to vitamin B_{12} deficiency, the level is usually less than 100 ng/l. The more severe the deficiency, the lower the serum vitamin B_{12} level, and in patients with spinal cord damage due to the deficiency, levels are 50 ng/l or less even in the absence of anaemia. Values between 100 ng/l and 160 ng/l are regarded as borderline and may be found in patients with mild vitamin B_{12} deficiency, and, in the absence of vitamin B_{12} deficiency, in pregnancy and in patients with

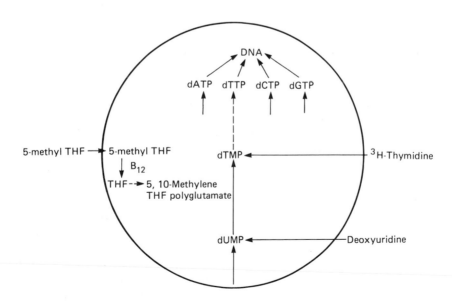

Fig. 3.7. *Deoxyuridine suppression test. The circle represents a bone marrow or other haemopoietic cell. (THF, tetrahydrofolate; MP, monophosphate; TP, triphosphate; d, deoxyribose; A, adenine, T, thymine; C, cytosine; G, guanine.)*

megaloblastic anaemia due to folate deficiency. The isotope assays should use pure intrinsic factor or R protein already blocked by analogue as binding protein, otherwise B_{12} analogues in serum are measured and falsely high results obtained (see above). This may be because vitamin B_{12} analogues may be circulating which do not support the growth of the micro-organisms used in assay but do compete with vitamin B_{12} for non-IF binding proteins used in the isotope assays. Raised serum vitamin B_{12} levels (if not due to recent therapy or bacteriological contamination of the specimen) are usually due to a rise in transcobalamin I (see Table 3.3) or to liver or renal disease with increased saturation of transcobalamins I and II.

Methylmalonic Acid Excretion

Deoxyadenosyl cobalamin is required as coenzyme in the isomerization of methylmalonyl CoA to succinyl CoA, and in patients with vitamin B_{12} deficiency sufficient to cause anaemia or neuropathy, methylmalonic acid excretion is usually raised. Normal excretion ranges from 0 to 4 mg in 24 hours. The test can be made more sensitive by loading the patient with 10 g L-valine. The test is almost specific since rare congenital abnormalities of metabolism are the only causes, other than vitamin B_{12} deficiency, of raised methylmalonic acid excretion.

TESTS FOR THE CAUSE OF VITAMIN B_{12} DEFICIENCY

The principal methods used in diagnosing the cause of vitamin B_{12} deficiency are listed in Table 3.6. Many of these tests are mentioned elsewhere in this chapter, and others are described in texts of gastroenterology. Studies of vitamin B_{12} absorption are of particular importance, however.

Vitamin B_{12} Absorption

This may be assessed by five different techniques: faecal excretion, whole-body counting, urinary excretion (Schilling test), hepatic uptake and plasma radioactivity. Four isotopes of cobalt, ^{56}Co, ^{57}Co, ^{58}Co and ^{60}Co, are available but vitamin B_{12} labelled with ^{57}Co or ^{58}Co is used clinically. The test is performed giving radioactive vitamin B_{12} (a dose of 1 μg) alone, and then if this shows malabsorption, the dose is given with a commercial preparation of intrinsic factor. The results distinguish between gastric and intestinal causes of vitamin B_{12} deficiency. If intestinal malabsorption is present, the test may be repeated after antibiotic therapy to reduce possible bacterial interference with vitamin B_{12} absorption. The Schilling test involves injection of 1 mg of non-radioactive B_{12} and this will also treat the patient. A combined test has been introduced in which two isotopes of

---

Table 3.6

Tests for the cause of vitamin B_{12} deficiency

Clinical history—diet, drugs, operations, etc.
Vitamin B_{12} absorption using radioactive B_{12}:
    (a) alone
    (b) with food
    (c) with intrinsic factor (IF)
    (d) after a course of antibiotics
Measurement of IF in gastric juice after maximal stimulation, e.g. with pentagastrin
Tests for tissue-specific antibodies in serum, e.g. IF, parietal cell, thyroid antibodies
Barium meal (or endoscopy with gastric biopsy) and follow-through examination
Faecal fat excretion, xylose absorption, jejunal biopsy, etc.
Examination of urine for proteinuria; stools for fish tapeworm ova

Table 3.7

Biochemical reactions of folate coenzyme

Reaction	Coenzyme form of folate involved (THF = tetrahydrofolate)	Single carbon unit transferred	Importance
Formate activation	THF	$-CHO$	Generation of 10-formyl THF
Purine synthesis			
1. Formylation of glycine amidoribotide	5,10-methenyl THF	$-CHO$	Formation of purines needed for DNA, RNA synthesis but reactions probably not rate limiting
2. Formylation of amino-imidazole-carboxamide-ribotide (AICAR)	10-formyl THF	$-CHO$	
Pyrimidine synthesis			
Methylation of deoxyuridylate* to thymidylate[+]	5,10-methenyl THF	$-CH_3$	1. Rate-limiting step in DNA synthesis 2. Oxidizes THF to DHF
Amino acid interconversion			
1. Serine–glycine interconversion	THF	$=CH_2$	Entry of single carbon units into active pool
2. Homocysteine to methionine	5-methyl THF	$-CH_3$	Demethylation of 5-methyl THF; also requires vitamin B_{12}, FAD, ATP and adenosylmethionine
3. Formiminoglutamic acid to glutamic acid	THF	$-HN-CH=$	Basis of the Figlu test (now obsolete)

*Deoxyuridylate = deoxyuridine 5'-monophosphate.
[+]Thymidylate = thymidine 5'-monophosphate.

vitamin B_{12} are given simultaneously, one alone and one attached to intrinsic factor; the excretion of the two isotopes in the same 24-hour urine is compared. The results are less clear-cut than when the two tests are performed separately.

The standard test is performed using crystalline B_{12}. Tests using food-bound (e.g. egg ova albumin) radioactive B_{12} have been devised to parallel normal dietary B_{12} more closely. Such tests may detect malabsorption of B_{12} in some patients, e.g. with atrophic gastritis and low serum B_{12} levels but with normal absorption of crystalline B_{12}.

FOLATE

Dietary Folate

Folic acid (pteroylglutamic acid) is a yellow, crystalline, water-soluble substance of molecular weight 441. It is the parent compound of a large family of compounds, now termed folates but previously called the Wills' factor, vitamin B_c, vitamin M and the 'Norite eluate' factor. The molecule of folic acid consists of three parts: pteridine, para-amino-benzoate and L-glutamic acid (Fig. 3.8). Folic acid itself is only a minor component of normal food (probably less than 1%) and the naturally occurring compounds differ from it in three respects (Fig. 3.8): first, they are partly or completely reduced at positions 5,6,7,8, in the pteridine portion to di- or tetrahydrofolate derivatives; second, they usually contain a single carbon unit of varying degrees of reduction such as a methyl group at N_5 or a formyl group at N_5 or N_{10}; third, 70–90% of natural folates contain a chain of three or more glutamate residues linked to each other by the unusual γ-

peptide bond and are called pteroyl- or folate-polyglutamates. In human cells, 4,5 or 6 glutamate residues are usually present.

Most articles of food contain some folate and highest concentrations are found in liver and yeast ($>200\ \mu g/100g$), spinach, other greens and nuts ($>100\ \mu g/100g$). The total folate content of an average Western diet is about 650 μg daily, but the amount varies widely according to the type of food eaten and the method of cooking. Folate is easily destroyed by heating, particularly in large volumes of water, and over 90% may be lost.

Body Stores and Requirements

Total body folate in the adult is about 10 mg, the liver containing the largest store. Daily adult requirements are about 100 μg. Up to 13 μg of folate is lost as such in the urine each day, but breakdown products of folate are also lost in urine. Losses of folate also occur in sweat and skin; faecal folate is largely derived from colonic bacteria. Stores are only sufficient for about 4 months in normal adults, so severe folate deficiency may develop extremely rapidly.

Absorption

The principal site of folate absorption is the upper small intestine and there is a steep fall-off in absorptive capacity in the lower jejunum and ileum. Absorption of all forms tested is rapid, a rise in blood level occurring within 15–20 minutes of ingestion.

The small intestine has a tremendous capacity to absorb folic acid (pteroylglutamic acid) or other folate monoglutamates, since about 90% of a single

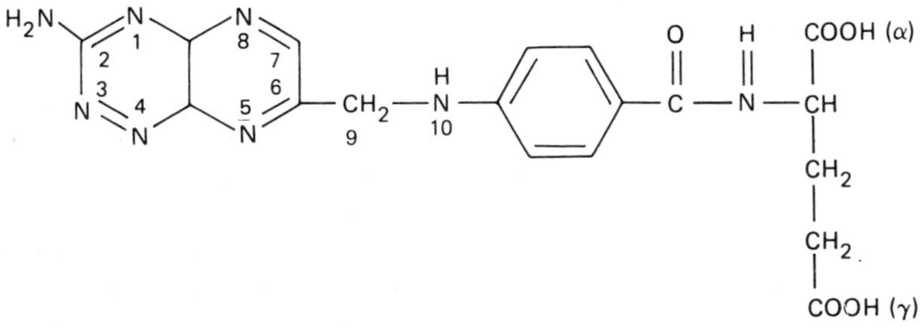

Fig. 3.8. *The structure of folic acid (pteroylglutamic acid).*

dose is absorbed whether this is small (100 μg) or large (15 mg). Absorption of pteroylglutamic acid occurs by a saturable process both in humans and experimental animals, though whether an active mechanism or facilitated diffusion is involved is not known. The existence of patients with a specific defect in absorption of folates, including pteroylglutamic acid itself, however, does suggest that a special mechanism exists.

Absorption of folate polyglutamates with higher numbers of glutamate residues is more limited than absorption of folate monoglutamates. This may be due to limited capacity of the small intestine to hydrolyse these compounds or to limited transfer of these compounds into the mucosal cell. On average, about 50% of food folates are probably absorbed.

Polyglutamate forms are hydrolysed to the monoglutamate derivatives, either in the lumen of the intestine or within the mucosa, and they do not enter portal blood intact. The enzyme which carries out the hydrolysis is called pteroylpolyglutamate hydrolase (PPH) or folate conjugase or gamma-glutamyl carboxypeptidase. The exact intracellular site of hydrolysis of dietary pteroylpolyglutamates in the jejunal mucosa is unknown though PPH has been shown to be concentrated in the lysosomes of the cells. Mono- or polyglutamate forms of dietary folate, which are already mainly partly or completely reduced, are converted to 5-methyltetrahydrofolate within the small intestinal mucosa before entering portal plasma (Fig. 3.9). Pteroyl-

glutamic acid is largely absorbed unchanged and converted to 5-methyltetrahydrofolate by the liver.

Enterohepatic Circulation

About 60–90 μg of folate enters the bile each day and is excreted into the small intestine. Loss of this folate, together with the folate of sloughed intestinal cells, accelerates the speed with which folate deficiency develops in malabsorptive conditions.

Biochemical Functions

Folates (as the intracellular polyglutamate derivatives) act as coenzymes in the transfer of single carbon units from one compound to another (Table 3.7). Two of these reactions are involved in DNA and RNA synthesis, a third is a rate-limiting step in DNA synthesis, and, in another reaction, methionine synthesis, vitamin B_{12} is also involved.

CAUSES OF FOLATE DEFICIENCY
(Table 3.8)

Nutritional

Dietary folate deficiency is common. Indeed, in most patients with folate deficiency, a nutritional element is present. Certain individuals are particularly prone to have diets containing inadequate amounts of folate—the old, edentulous, poor, alcoholics, psychiatrically disturbed and patients following gastric operations such as partial gastrectomy. Nutritional folate deficiency occurs in kwashiorkor and scurvy and in infants with repeated infections, or fed solely on goats' milk which has a very low folate content.

Malabsorption

Malabsorption of dietary folate occurs in tropical sprue, coeliac disease in children and adults, coeliac disease associated with dermatitis herpetiformis, and in the rare congenital condition of selective malabsorption of folate (only three cases of this syndrome have been reported and two of them showed megaloblastic anaemia, mental retardation, and fits.) Minor degrees of malabsorption may also

Role of vitamin B_{12} in folate metabolism

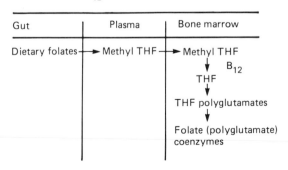

Fig. 3.9. *The absorption of dietary folates and role of vitamin B_{12} in intracellular folate coenzyme synthesis. (THF = tetrahydrofolate (monoglutamate).)*

Table 3.8
Causes of folate deficiency

Dietary
Particularly in old age, infancy, poverty, alcoholic, chronic invalids, psychiatrically disturbed; may be associated with scurvy or kwashiorkor

Malabsorption
Major cause of deficiency: tropical sprue, coeliac disease in child and adult and in association with dermatitis herpetiformis, specific malabsorption of folate
Minor cause of deficiency: extensive jejunal resection, Crohn's disease, partial gastrectomy, congestive heart failure, Whipple's disease, scleroderma, amyloid, diabetic enteropathy, systemic bacterial infection, lymphoma, salazopyrine
Disputed cause of deficiency: anticonvulsant drug, folate deficiency, alcohol, oral contraceptives

Excess utilization or loss
(a) Physiological: pregnancy and lactation, prematurity
(b) Pathological
    Haematological diseases: chronic haemolytic anaemias, myelosclerosis, sideroblastic anaemia
    Malignant diseases: carcinoma, lymphoma, leukaemia, myeloma
    Inflammatory diseases: tuberculosis, Crohn's disease, psoriasis, exfoliative dermatitis, malaria
    Metabolic disease: homocystinuria
    Excess urinary loss: congestive heart failure, active liver disease
    Haemodialysis, peritoneal dialysis

Antifolate drugs
Anticonvulsant drugs (diphenylhydantoin, primidone and barbiturates)
Nitrofurantoin, tetracycline, antituberculosis (less well documented)

Mixed causes
Liver diseases, alcoholism, intensive care units

N.B. In severely folate-deficient patients with causes other than those listed under 'Dietary', poor dietary intake is usually present.

---

occur following jejunal resection, partial gastrectomy, in Crohn's disease and in systemic infections, but in these conditions, if severe deficiency occurs, it is usually largely due to poor nutrition.

Malabsorption of folate has also been described in patients receiving salazopyrine, cholestyramine and triamterene. It has also been associated with anticonvulsant drug therapy, the contraceptive pill, alcohol and folate deficiency but these are less well established. Indeed, in the intestinal stagnant-loop syndrome, the predominant effect of the small intestinal bacteria is to cause a rise in serum folate by synthesizing folate which is then absorbed.

Excess Utilization or Loss

Pregnancy

Folate requirements are increased by 100 μg to 300 μg daily in a normal pregnancy because of transfer of the vitamin to the fetus. Megaloblastic anaemia due to the deficiency is now largely prevented by prophylactic folic acid therapy. It occurs in about 0.5% of pregnancies in England and other Western countries but the incidence is much higher in countries where the general nutritional status is poor, e.g. megaloblastic haemopoiesis occurs in over 50% of pregnant women in South India. The anaemia is more common in twin pregnancies, is most likely to occur in the last trimester and the late winter and early spring months (in Britain) and may also present in the early post-partum period during lactation. The deficiency is more common in pregnant women who also suffer from iron deficiency, probably because these patients take a poor diet. The usual presentation of the anaemia is similar to that of other megaloblastic anaemias but occasionally, when there is an associated infection, acute arrest of haemopoiesis with pancytopenia may occur which resembles aplastic anaemia, except that the marrow shows obvious megaloblastic changes.

Prematurity

The newborn infant, whether full-term or premature, has higher serum and red cell folate concentrations than the adult, but the newborn infant's demands for folate have been estimated to be up to ten times those of adults on a weight basis and the neonatal folate levels fall rapidly to lowest values at about 6 weeks of age. The falls are steepest, and are liable to reach subnormal levels in premature babies, a number of whom develop megaloblastic anaemia responsive to folic acid at about 4–6 weeks of age. This occurs particularly in the smallest babies, and in those who have feeding difficulties, infections or multiple exchange transfusions.

Haematological Disorders

Folate deficiency frequently occurs in chronic haemolytic anaemia, particularly in thalassaemia major, sickle cell disease, autoimmune haemolytic anaemia and congenital spherocytosis. It is not immediately obvious why patients with these and other conditions of increased cell turnover should develop folate deficiency (they do not develop iron or vitamin B_{12} deficiencies). Urinary excretion of folate as such in these diseases is normal. It seems more likely that folate is not completely reutilized after performing coenzyme functions and is partly

lost at pteridines due to cleavage at the C_9–N_{10} bond. The incidence of folate deficiency is much lower in pyruvate kinase deficiency and other red cell enzyme deficiencies, unstable haemoglobin states and in PNH where cell turnover is not so high.

Myelosclerosis

Patients with chronic myelosclerosis may develop folate deficiency at some stage of the illness and in about 10–30% of patients in Britain, this is severe. The deficiency may easily be overlooked because marrow is difficult to aspirate and because the natural course of the disease includes increasing anaemia. Thrombocytopenia may in some cases be the principal sign. Megaloblastic anaemia may supervene in the transition period between polycythaemia vera and myelosclerosis, when total nucleic acid turnover seems to be considerably increased and when gout may also be a feature. Severe folate deficiency is more common in myelosclerosis following polycythaemia than in primary myelosclerosis but does not occur in uncomplicated polycythaemia vera unless some other cause, such as poor diet, is present.

Leukaemia, Carcinoma, Lymphoma, Myeloma

There is a high incidence of mild deficiency in all these diseases, though it is unusual for this to progress to gross megaloblastic anaemia.

Inflammatory Conditions

Chronic inflammatory diseases such as tuberculosis, rheumatoid arthritis, Crohn's disease, psoriasis, exfoliative dermatitis, bacterial endocarditis and chronic bacterial infections cause deficiency by reducing appetite and by increasing demands for folate. Systemic infections may also cause malabsorption of folate. Severe deficiency is virtually confined to the patients with the most active disease. Fever per se has also been suggested to interfere with folate metabolism by inhibiting certain temperature-dependent folate enzymes. In patients with subclinical folate deficiency from causes other than infection, intercurrent infections often precipitate severe megaloblastic anaemia.

Homocystinuria

This is a rare metabolic defect in conversion of homocysteine to cystathione. Folate deficiency occurs in most of the patients and is thought to be due to excessive utilization due to compensatory increased conversion of homocysteine to methionine.

Long-term Dialysis

Since folate is only loosely bound to plasma proteins, it is easily removed from plasma by haemodialysis or peritoneal dialysis. (Vitamin B_{12}, in contrast, is not removed from plasma by dialysis since it is firmly protein bound.) The amount of body folate that can be removed in this way is relatively small. Nevertheless, in patients with anorexia, vomiting, infections and haemolysis, folate stores may become depleted and megaloblastic anaemia supervene.

Congestive Heart Failure, Liver Disease

Excess urinary folate losses of more than 100 μg a day may occur in some of these patients. The explanation appears to be release of folate from damaged liver cells.

Antifolate Drugs

Anticonvulsants

A large number of epileptics receiving long-term therapy with diphenylhydantoin (Phenytoin, Dilantin) or primidone (Mysoline) with or without barbiturates develop low serum and red cell folate levels, and in some of the patients, megaloblastic anaemia supervenes. A number of mechanisms have been suggested—inhibition of absorption of pteroylglutamic acid or specifically of pteroylpolyglutamates, inhibition of the action of or synthesis of folate-dependent enzymes, displacement of folate from its plasma transport protein and induction of folate-utilizing enzymes; none of these theories has been established. A dietary element is present in the patients with the severest deficiency.

Alcohol

Alcohol may also be a folate antagonist since patients drinking spirits may develop megaloblastic anaemia which will respond to normal quantities of dietary folate or to physiological doses of pteroylglutamic acid only if the alcohol is withdrawn. Resumption of alcohol intake rapidly inhibits the haematological response to small doses of folate. The mechanism is unknown, though inhibition of folate absorption and of the folate-requiring enzymes has been suggested. Inadequate folate intake is the major factor in the development of deficiency in spirit-drinking alcoholics. Beer is relatively folate rich.

The drugs which inhibit dihydrofolate reductase (methotrexate, pyrimethamine and trimethoprim) are discussed later (p. 79).

Congenital Abnormalities of Folate Metabolism

A number of babies have been described, mainly in Japan, with congenital defects of folate enzymes, e.g. cyclohydrase, methylfolate transferase, dihydrofolate reductase. Some had megaloblastic anaemia.

DIAGNOSIS OF FOLATE DEFICIENCY

Therapeutic Trial

If the patient has uncomplicated megaloblastic anaemia due to folate deficiency, there will be a satisfactory haematological response to physiological doses of folic acid (e.g. 100–200 μg daily). Response to a larger dose is not diagnostic, since patients with vitamin B_{12} deficiency may respond haematologically to 400 μg or more of folic acid daily. If malabsorption of folate is suspected, physiological doses of folic acid should be given *parenterally* while performing the therapeutic trial.

A poor response may be due to an associated deficiency, e.g. of vitamin B_{12} or iron, to infection or to another cause for anaemia being present. It may also occur in diseases of increased folate utilization, e.g. haemolytic anaemia or myelosclerosis, where demands for folate may be as much as ten times normal.

Deoxyuridine Suppression Test (see page 69)

Serum Folate

This may be measured microbiologically with *Lactobacillus casei* or by radioassay. The serum folate level is low in all folate-deficient patients. In most laboratories the normal range is quoted as from 3.0 μg/l to about 15 μg/l, though levels between 3.0 μg/l and 6.0 μg/l are regarded as borderline. The serum folate is markedly affected by recent diet, and inadequate intake for as little as a week may cause the level of a healthy adult to become subnormal. Because of this, the serum folate assay is a very sensitive test and may be low before there is haematological or other biochemical evidence of the deficiency.

The serum folate level rises in severe vitamin B_{12} deficiency, and raised levels have also been reported in the intestinal stagnant-loop syndrome, acute renal failure, and in active liver damage. (High levels are also obtained when the patient is receiving folic acid therapy or when the serum for assay is contaminated with folate or folate-producing bacteria or if a sample is haemolysed.) 'False' low levels of serum folate are obtained in patients receiving drugs which inhibit the growth of *L. casei* (e.g. methotrexate, trimethoprim or antibiotics in large doses). Otherwise the serum folate assay is a specific test for the deficiency.

Red Cell Folate

This can also be measured microbiologically or by radioassay. Most of the folate in blood is contained in the red cells and the red cell folate assay is a valuable test of body folate stores. It is less affected by recent diet and traces of haemolysis than the serum assay. In normal adults, concentrations range from 160 μg/l to 640 μg/l of packed red cells. Subnormal levels occur in patients with megaloblastic anaemia due to folate deficiency but also occur in nearly two-thirds of patients with megaloblastic anaemia due to vitamin B_{12} deficiency. If vitamin B_{12} deficiency is excluded, however, a low red cell folate can be used as an indication that severe folate deficiency is present and warrants full investigation and treatment. False normal results may occur if the folate-deficient patient has received a recent blood transfusion (since the folate content of the transfused red cells will be measured), or if the patient has a raised reticulocyte count for any reason (e.g. haemorrhage or haemolytic anaemia).

GENERAL MANAGEMENT OF MEGALOBLASTIC ANAEMIA

It is usually possible to establish which of the two deficiencies is the cause of the anaemia and to treat only with the appropriate vitamin. In patients who enter hospital severely ill, however, it may be necessary to treat immediately with both vitamins in large doses. Transfusion is usually unnecessary and inadvisable. If it is essential, packed cells should be given slowly and one or two units are ample. Exchange transfusion as well as usual treatment of heart failure should be considered in patients with extreme anaemia and congestive heart failure. Platelet concentrates are of value in reducing spontaneous bleeding in the rare patients with severe thrombocytopenia. Potassium supplements have been recommended to obviate the danger of hypokalaemia that has been recorded in some patients during the initial haematological response.

TREATMENT OF VITAMIN B_{12} DEFICIENCY

Indications

It is usually necessary to treat patients who have developed vitamin B_{12} deficiency with life-long regular vitamin B_{12} therapy. In a few instances the underlying cause of vitamin B_{12} deficiency can be permanently corrected; for instance, the fish tapeworm, tropical sprue or an intestinal stagnant-loop which is amenable to surgery.

The indications for starting vitamin B_{12} therapy are a well-documented megaloblastic anaemia or neuropathy due to the deficiency. It is also necessary to treat any patient with haematological abnormalities due to vitamin B_{12} deficiency even in the absence of anaemia, e.g. hypersegmented neutrophils or megaloblastic erythropoiesis, as a case of pernicious anaemia. Patients with borderline serum vitamin B_{12} levels but no haematological or other abnormality should either be followed at, for example, yearly intervals to make sure the vitamin B_{12} deficiency does not progress, or if malabsorption of vitamin B_{12} has also been demonstrated, should also be given regular maintenance vitamin B_{12} therapy. Vitamin B_{12} should also be given routinely to all patients who have had a total gastrectomy or ileal resection.

Parenteral Vitamin B_{12} Therapy

Replenishment of body stores should be complete with six 1000-μg, intramuscular injections of *hydroxocobalamin* at 3–7-day intervals. Larger and more frequent doses are usually used in patients with vitamin B_{12} neuropathy but there is no evidence that these produce a better response. For maintenance therapy, 1000 μg hydroxocobalamin intramuscularly once every 3 months is satisfactory. Cyanocobalamin should no longer be used for treating vitamin B_{12} deficiency since this is less well retained in the body than hydroxocobalamin. Toxic reactions are extremely rare and are usually due to contamination in the preparation, rather than to vitamin B_{12} itself.

Oral Vitamin B_{12} Therapy

This is only satisfactory in patients with nutritional deficiency of vitamin B_{12}, but even so, regular daily doses are needed because of the normal body's limited ability to absorb vitamin B_{12}. In patients with malabsorption of the vitamin, oral doses of at least 500–1000 μg daily are needed to supply the body's daily requirements by passive diffusion through the jejunum. Oral therapy with vitamin B_{12} combined with hog intrinsic factor soon leads to resistance to the intrinsic factor preparation.

TREATMENT OF FOLATE DEFICIENCY

There is probably never any need to give folic acid parenterally except in parenteral nutrition when patients cannot swallow tablets. Oral doses of 5–15 mg folic acid daily are satisfactory since sufficient folate is absorbed from these extremely large doses even in patients with severe malabsorption. The length of time therapy must be continued is uncertain. It is customary to continue therapy for about 4 months, when all folate-deficient red cells will have been eliminated and replaced by a new folate-replete population.

Before large doses of folic acid are given, vitamin B_{12} deficiency must be excluded and, if present, corrected, otherwise vitamin B_{12} neuropathy may be precipitated.

Long-term folic acid therapy is required when the underlying cause of the deficiency cannot be corrected and the deficiency is likely to recur, for instance in chronic haemolytic anaemias such as thalassaemia and sickle-cell anaemia and in chronic myelosclerosis. It may also be necessary in coeliac disease if this does not respond to a gluten-free diet. Where mild but chronic folate deficiency occurs, it is preferable to encourage an improvement in the diet after correcting the deficiency with a short course of folic acid. In any patient receiving long-term folic acid therapy it is important to measure the serum vitamin B_{12} level at regular (e.g. once yearly) intervals to exclude the coincidental development of vitamin B_{12} deficiency.

Folinic Acid (5-Formyltetrahydrofolate)

This is given orally or parenterally to overcome the toxic effects of methotrexate or other dihydrofolate reductase inhibitors.

Prophylactic Folic Acid

Pregnancy

Most workers now give about 300–400 μg folic acid daily throughout pregnancy, i.e. the amount by which folate requirements are thought to be increased. Combined iron and folic acid preparations are generally satisfactory, except they are usually expensive and if the patient cannot tolerate the iron and stops taking the tablets, folic acid therapy will also be discontinued.

Prematurity

The incidence of folate deficiency is so high in the smallest premature babies during the first 6 weeks of life that folic acid should be given routinely to babies weighing less than 1500 g at birth and to larger premature babies who require exchange transfusions or develop feeding difficulties, infections, or vomiting and diarrhoea.

Haemolytic Anaemia and Dialysis

Prophylactic folic acid is also usually given to patients with chronic haemolytic anaemia or undergoing long-term haemodialysis.

BIOCHEMICAL BASIS OF MEGALOBLASTIC ANAEMIA

Vitamin B_{12}–Folate Relations

The anaemia is due to impaired synthesis of DNA and this is due to reduced supply of one or other of the four immediate precursors of DNA, the deoxyribonucleoside triphosphates dATP and dGTP (purines) and dTTP and dCTP (pyrimidines) (Fig. 3.10). Folate deficiency principally impairs synthesis of dTTP since folate is needed, as 5,10-methylene tetrahydrofolate polyglutamate, as coenzyme in thymidylate synthesis, a rate-limiting reaction in DNA synthesis. The integrity of this reaction is tested in the dU suppression test (p. 69, Fig. 3.7). During this reaction, the folate coenzyme is oxidized to the dihydrofolate state and the enzyme dihydrofolate reductase (DHFR) is required to return the folate to its active tetra-hydro state. DHFR is inhibited by methotrexate, pyrimethamine, and in bacteria, but only very weakly in human tissues, by trimethoprim. Folate is required for many other reactions in mammalian tissues, including two in purine synthesis (Table 3.7), but impairment of these seems to be far less important clinically.

Only two reactions in the body are known to require vitamin B_{12} (see Fig. 3.3); methylmalonyl CoA isomerization which requires deoxyadenosyl cobalamin has been discussed earlier (p. 70). The methylation of homocysteine to methionine requires both methyltetrahydrofolate (methyl THF) as methyl-donor and methylcobalamin as coenzyme. This reaction, which is almost completely irreversible, is the first step in the pathway by which methyl THF which enters bone marrow and other cells from plasma is converted into all the intracellular folate enzymes (see Fig. 3.9). Reduced folates other than methyl THF are the correct substrates for polyglutamate addition needed to keep folate inside the cells and to form the various polyglutamate derivatives, including the 5,10-methylene coenzyme needed for thymidylate synthesis as well as the coenzymes needed in purine synthesis and for Figlu breakdown. Thus, in vitamin B_{12} deficiency, methyl THF formed by the small intestinal cells from dietary folates cannot be metabolized by cells at a normal rate and piles up in plasma, while intracellular folate concentrations fall due to failure of formation of intracellular folate polyglutamates since methyl THF is not the correct folate substrate. The exact substrate for folate polyglutamate formation may be THF or formyl THF.

This theory explains the abnormalities of folate metabolism which occur in vitamin B_{12} deficiency (high serum folate, low cell folate, positive purine precursor, AICAR, excretion), and also why the anaemia will respond to folic acid in large doses. The explanation as to why the serum vitamin B_{12} falls in folate deficiency may also be related to impairment of the homocysteine–methionine reaction with reduced formation of methylcobalamin, the main form of vitamin B_{12} in plasma, but other mechanisms may occur. The biochemical basis for vitamin B_{12} neuropathy, however, remains obscure, although its occurrence in the absence of methylmalonic aciduria in TC II deficiency and in monkeys given nitrous oxide suggests that the neuropathy is related to the defect in homocysteine–methionine conversion, possibly due to lack of methylation reactions in lipid synthesis mediated by S-adenosyl methionine. Measurements of methylation of arginine in myelin basic protein in fruit bats with vitamin B_{12} neuropathy or in rats exposed to N_2O, however, show no defect of methylation.

DNA Replication

Synthesis of new strands of DNA during the 'S' phase of the cell cycle commences with separation of the two parent strands from each other at many points along the chromosome. At a number of points or origins, RNA primers are synthesized first and new DNA strands are then synthesized bidirectionally, using the parent strands as templates, adenine pairing with thymine, guanine with cytosine. The RNA primer is ultimately hydrolysed and the gap filled with DNA. The small pieces of DNA are then joined up to make complete new chromosomal DNA. During this process it is likely that the chromosomal proteins are concerned in allowing separation and unwinding of the two chromosomes and their subsequent contraction. A DNA polymerase is concerned with synthesis of new DNA, while DNA ligases link up shorter pieces to each other and take part with DNA-ases in repair processes.

Reduced supply of dTTP in megaloblastic anaemia due to folate or vitamin B_{12} deficiency, or to antifolate drug therapy, appears to slow elongation of newly orginated replicating segments. Thus, small fragments accumulate, single-stranded areas become points of weakness where mechanical or enzymatic breakage may occur, and the failure to form bulk DNA may impair contraction of newly replicated lengths of DNA, thus leaving the chromosomes elongated, despirillated and with random breaks. There is evidence that late replicating DNA may be particularly A-T rich and that a special DNA polymerase may be concerned with late replication. This may also be the time when supplies of dTTP become particularly reduced, and many of the gross defects in DNA appear in late replication. Indeed, some cells become arrested and die at this stage.

Reduced supply of one of the other three deoxyribonucleoside triphosphates due to a metabolic error or drug therapy may cause a similar fault in DNA replication, and thus a megaloblastic appearance of the cells (Fig. 3.10).

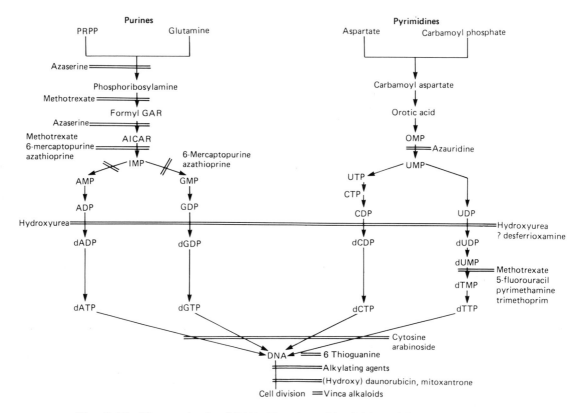

Fig. 3.10. *The synthesis of DNA. The sites of inhibition of DNA synthesis and replication by drugs are shown. (PRPP, phosphoribosylpyrophosphate; GAR, glycinamide ribotide; AICAR, amino imidazole carboxamide ribotide; MP, monophosphate; DP, diphosphate; TP, triphosphate; A, adenine; G, guanine; C, cytosine; T, thymine; I, inosine; U, uridine; d, deoxyribose; O, orotidine.)*

OTHER NUTRITIONAL ANAEMIAS

Protein Deficiency

Anaemia is usual in children and adults with severe protein deficiency (kwashiorkor). The anaemia, which may be partly masked by haemoconcentration, is usually orthochromic, normocytic and normoblastic but megaloblastic changes have been described in from 10% to 60% of cases in different series. Hypoplasia, or even aplasia, of the marrow has also been recorded. The mechanism by which protein deficiency causes anaemia is not completely understood. Lack of protein does not seem to reduce haemoglobin synthesis directly. Studies on experimental animals suggest that the major factor is diminution of erythropoietin secretion. This is probably due to reduction of general tissue metabolism and therefore oxygen consumption, with consequent reduced stimulus for erythropoietin secretion.

In most patients, other factors contribute to the anaemia. These include infections, deficiencies of folate and iron and also possibly deficiencies of vitamins C, E, B_{12} and other trace substances. Riboflavin deficiency may also contribute to the anaemia and become apparent only during the response to protein.

Scurvy

There is usually a moderate or severe normocytic, normochromic anaemia arising because of external haemorrhage, haemorrhage into tissues and from impaired erythropoiesis. In some cases the anaemia is megaloblastic, which appears to be partly due to associated nutritional folate deficiency and partly due to impairment of folate metabolism caused by vitamin C deficiency. Vitamin C is not established, however, to play a role in normal folate metabolism.

Other Deficiencies

Deficiencies of nicotinic acid and pantothenic acid cause anaemia in experimental animals but have not been shown to do so in humans. On the other hand, riboflavin deficiency may cause anaemia in humans resembling the anaemia of protein deficiency. Copper is essential for haemopoiesis and normal iron metabolism, and deficiency of copper causes an anaemia resembling iron deficiency in experimental animals. Anaemia due to copper deficiency however, has never been documented in humans. Copper excess (as in Wilson's disease) causes a haemolytic anaemia.

SELECTED BIBLIOGRAPHY

Babior B. M. (Ed.) (1975). *Cobalamin. Biochemistry and pathophysiology*. New York: John Wiley.

Blakely R. L. (1969). *The biochemistry of folic acid and related pteridines*. Amsterdam: North-Holland.

Blakely R. L., Whitehead V. M. (1986). *Folates and pterins*. Vol. 3: *Nutritional, pharmacological and physiological aspects*. New York: John Wiley.

Botez M. I., Reynolds E. H. (Eds.) (1979). *Folic acid in neurology, psychiatry and internal medicine*. New York: Raven Press.

Chanarin I. (1979). *The megaloblastic anaemias*, 2nd edn. Oxford: Blackwell Scientific Publications.

Chanarin I. (1982). The effects of nitrous oxide on cobalamins, folate and on related events. *CRC Critical Reviews in Toxicology*, 179–213.

Chanarin I., Deacon R., Lumb M., Muir M., Perry J. (1985). Cobalamin–folate interrelations: a critical review. *Blood*, **66**, 479–489.

Cooper B. A., Rosenblatt D. S. (1987). Inherited defects of vitamin B_{12} metabolism. *Annual Review of Nutrition*, **1**, 291–320.

Cooper B. A., Zittoun J. (Eds.) (1987). *Cobalamin and folate. Progress en hematologie*. Paris: Doin.

Food and Nutrition Board (1977). *Folic acid. Biochemistry and physiology in relation to the human nutrition requirement*. Washington, DC: Food and Nutrition Board, National Research Council. National Academy of Sciences.

Hall C. A. (Ed.) (1983) *Methods in haematology, 10. The cobalamins*. Edinburgh: Churchill.

Hoffbrand A. V. (Ed.) (1976). *Megaloblastic anaemia. Clinics in haematology*, Vol. 5, No. 3, pp. 471–769. London: W. B. Saunders.

Hoffbrand A. V. (1983). Pernicious anaemia. *Scottish Medical Journal*, **28**, 218–227.

Hoffbrand A. V., Wickremasinghe R. G. (1982). Megaloblastic anaemia. In *Recent advances in haematology*, Vol. 3, pp. 25–44. (Ed. A. V. Hoffbrand). Edinburgh: Churchill Livingstone.

Kapadia C. R., Donaldson R. M. Jr (1985). Disorders of cobalamin (vitamin B_{12}) absorption and transport.

Annual Review of Medicine, **36**, 93–110.

Kass L. (1976). *Pernicious anaemia*, Vol. VII: *Major problems in internal medicine*. Philadelphia: W. B. Saunders.

Smyth E. L. (1965). *Vitamin B$_{12}$*, 3rd edn. London: Methuen.

Zagalak B., Friedrich W. (Eds.) (1979). *Vitamin B$_{12}$*. Berlin: Walter de Gruyter.

Other Nutritional Anaemias

Adams E. B. (1970). Anaemia associated with protein deficiency. *Seminars in Haematology*, **7**, 55–66.

Cox E. V. (1960). The anaemia of scurvy. *Vitamins and Hormones*, **26**, 635–652.

Darby W. J. (1968). Tocopherol-responsive anaemias in man. *Vitamins and Hormones*, **26**, 685–699.

Chapter 4

APLASTIC ANAEMIA AND OTHER TYPES OF BONE MARROW FAILURE

E.C. GORDON-SMITH AND S.M. LEWIS

Bone marrow failure implies that peripheral blood cytopenia has arisen primarily as a result of a specific failure of bone marrow precursor cells to produce mature cells rather than the production of abnormal cells which have a shortened survival or the production of normal cells which are subjected to an abnormal environment. In the bone marrow failures the remaining cells in the marrow appear morphologically normal, or near normal, reflecting only minor changes produced by 'marrow stress' including a mild increase in dyserythropoietic forms, often with some macrocytosis. The stroma of the marrow does not appear to be disturbed. These observations distinguish the true marrow failures from the myelodysplastic and myeloproliferative syndromes.

There are two major groups of bone marrow failure: the aplastic anaemias, where the failure lies in the pluripotent stem cell, and the single cell cytopenias, where the failure lies in one or other of the committed cell lines. There is overlap between these groups for single cell failure may occasionally progress to total marrow failure and, following partial recovery, aplastic anaemia may continue with a prolonged period of single cell deficiency. It is convenient to consider the two groups separately.

APLASTIC ANAEMIA

Aplastic anaemia is defined by the presence of pancytopenia in the peripheral blood and a hypocellular marrow in which normal haemopoietic marrow is replaced by fat cells. Abnormal cells are not found in either the peripheral blood or bone marrow. The diagnosis is based on the absence of cells, not the presence of any characteristic feature.

There are a variety of ways in which this haematological pattern can be produced, as indicated in Table 4.1. Distinguishing between these forms of aplastic anaemia is a matter of awareness, careful observation of haematological material, particularly the granulocyte and megakaryocyte morphology, history and physical examination.

Inevitable Aplastic Anaemia

Most cytotoxic drugs, penetrating ionizing radiation and radioactive substances concentrated in the marrow are capable of producing aplastic anaemia through their effects on actively dividing cells. The timing and duration of the aplasia and the order in which cell lines recover depend to some extent on the nature of the cytotoxic agent and the dose. Recovery is usual, with the exception of marrow rendered aplastic by whole body irradiation given in a critical dose which destroys the haemopoietic system without killing the patient from additional toxicity. Although in general the development and recovery of aplasia following exposure to cytotoxic drugs are predictable, there are exceptions. Repeated or prolonged exposure to small doses of alkylating agents, particularly busulphan, may lead to a prolonged and unpredictable aplasia, even when given for myeloproliferative disorders such as chronic granulocytic leukaemia, essential thrombocythaemia or myelofibrosis.

Table 4.1
The aplastic anaemias

Aetiology	Examples	Clinical course
Inevitable	Ionizing radiation Cytotoxic drugs	Predictable Recovery usual
Idiosyncratic	Idiopathic Drug induced Viral Commercial solvents	Prolonged Unpredictable recovery
Inherited	Fanconi's anaemia Dyskeratosis congenita Others	Usually progressive Increased malignancy
Industrial	Benzene	Dose dependent Proliferative disorders more common
Immune	Drug induced Viruses, e.g. EBV Systemic lupus erythematosus	Usually recovers spontaneously
Malignant	Acute lymphoblastic leukaemia Hypoplastic acute myeloid leukaemia Hypoplastic myelodysplastic syndrome	Usually but not exclusively in children

Idiosyncratic Aplastic Anaemia

Idiosyncratic aplastic anaemia may occur spontaneously or appear following exposure to drugs or viruses which do not produce marrow failure in the great majority of persons exposed to these agents. The disease is characterized by its unpredictable onset and prolonged course, death usually occurring as a result of deficiency of granulocytes or platelets with a failure in support measures.

Aetiology

In about one-third of the patients with aplastic anaemia, suspicion may be directed to a particular agent, usually a drug or virus.

Drugs

The list of drugs which have been recorded as 'causing' aplastic anaemia is long, but mostly only single or a few cases have been reported for each drug and it is not profitable to detail them in lists because the evidence against them is slim. Some of the more definitely implicated drugs are listed in Table 4.2. Perhaps most attention has been given to chloramphenicol. This antibiotic was introduced into general use in 1948 and it was predicted, on the basis of its similarity of chemical structure to amidopyrine (a drug notorious for producing blood dyscrasias), that it would cause haematological toxicity. In fact amidopyrine most commonly produces an immune agranulocytosis, though aplastic anaemia has been reported, and it was suggested that chloramphenicol would also produce agranulocytosis. In the event the first case of blood dyscrasia following chloramphenicol was described in 1950 and was fatal aplastic anaemia. It is estimated that somewhere between $1:25\,000$ and $1:40\,000$ people exposed to oral chloramphenicol will develop aplastic anaemia. The evidence is purely epidemiological, there being no tests to demonstrate that chloramphenicol is responsible for aplastic anaemia in any particular case.

Chloramphenicol also causes a dose-dependent suppression of haemopoiesis, particularly affecting erythropoiesis, through its action on mitochondrial DNA, but this suppression is not related to the

Table 4.2
Drugs with a strong link with aplastic anaemia

Antibiotics	Chloramphenicol
	Sulphonamides—including co-trimoxazole
Anti-inflammatory drugs	Phenylbutazone—pyrazolones
	Oxyphenbutazone
	Gold salts
	Indomethacin—indole derivatives
	Benoxaprofen*—propionic acid derivative
	Piroxicam
	Amidopyrine*
Antithyroid drugs	Thiouracils
	Carbimazole†
Antimalarials	Amodiaquine
	Mepacrine
	Pyrimethamine
Anticonvulsants	Phenytoin‡
Antidepressants	Prothiaden
	Chlorpromazine

*Withdrawn from the market. Included to warn of possible danger of similarly structured drugs.
†More commonly neutropenia.
‡May produce an immune recoverable aplasia.

development of prolonged aplastic anaemia. Some six cases of aplastic anaemia have been reported in people using chloramphenicol eye-drops or ointment, in most cases for a prolonged period of time. Much of the dose of these preparations is absorbed through the mucous membranes, though the total amount is small. This has given rise to the idea that the development of aplastic anaemia following chloramphenicol is not dose related, but from the literature it would appear that aplastic anaemia is more common in patients given large or repeated doses of oral chloramphenicol and that the incidence of aplasia in patients given eye preparations approaches the background incidence. In Western countries the incidence of aplastic anaemia is of the order of 4–5 per million per year. It has been estimated that the incidence following chloramphenicol exposure is 30 per million per year, while the incidence in people with no known exposure to any drug or virus is of the order of 4 per million per

year. All these figures are very approximate, but do emphasize that drugs which are suspected of causing aplasia should be used only with the proper indications and with a knowledge of the risks.

Non-steroidal anti-inflammatory agents have been incriminated in causing aplastic anaemia. The pyrazalone derivatives phenylbutazone and oxyphenbutazone have the highest incidence of aplasia in this group but the indole derivatives indomethacin and sulindac have both been reported in association with aplastic anaemia. Benoxaprofen (Opren) was associated with a number of cases, as has been piroxicam. These are propionic acid derivatives which seem in general to cause a low but definite incidence of blood dyscrasias. This group of drugs illustrates well the difficulties in establishing causal relationships with aplastic anaemia. They are widely used by patients with an underlying disease which may have an autoimmune basis (rheumatoid arthritis) and who might have an increased risk of developing blood dyscrasias anyway. The incidence of aplastic anaemia may not be higher than the spontaneous background.

Gold salts deserve a special mention. Neutropenia and eosinophilia are common. Persistence with gold injections in the face of a falling neutrophil count may lead to aplasia or aplasia may appear without warning. Gold salts are one of the few drugs for which careful monitoring of blood counts may prevent the development of aplasia. Gold may be removed from the body by chelation with dimercaprol (British anti-Lewisite, BAL). BAL is usually given by intramuscular injection which makes it difficult to administer to patients with aplastic anaemia. There is no evidence that removal of gold in this way accelerates recovery and it is possible to detect gold in the marrow of patients who have recovered from gold-induced aplasia over a year after recovery.

Sulphonamides have also been thought to cause aplastic anaemia and there are several reports of aplasia following co-trimoxazole administration. Again it is difficult to be sure of the strength of the association, especially as the antibiotics may be given for an infection which is the first marker of an undetected marrow dyscrasia.

Viruses

Virus infections have been associated with aplasia. Hepatitis viruses, mainly hepatitis A or the non A, non B diseases, are the most common. About 15% of patients with aplasia have a history of hepatitis or biochemical tests suggestive of recent hepatitis. The delay between the clinical hepatitis and the onset of pancytopenia is of the order of 6–12 weeks, a similar period to that between drug exposure and aplasia. There is some suggestion that chloramphenicol administration followed by hepatitis is particularly likely to be associated with aplastic anaemia. Parvovirus infection in non-immune individuals may lead to a transient pure red cell aplasia of clinical importance to people with haemolytic anaemia (see below). The virus specifically infects the erythroid burst-forming units (BFU-E) and does not normally produce true aplastic anaemia. One particular strain, parvovirus 19, has been detected in the marrow of a patient with anaemia and neutropenia. In cats, certain combinations of infection by the feline leukaemia virus group may cause aplastic anaemia rather than proliferative diseases. The role of viruses in human aplastic anaemia is thus intriguing but uncertain.

Pathogenesis

The way in which these agents produce aplastic anaemia is unknown. Genetic factors may play a role but the evidence for this is not strong. There is debate as to whether the primary defect is in the haemopoietic stem cell itself or is the result of environmental factors, particularly immunological attack, on the cell. The answer might have come from observing identical twin bone marrow transplants. Unfortunately about half of syngeneic transplants have been successful without prior immunosuppression of the recipient, suggesting a pure stem cell deficit, while the other half have required immunosuppression before a successful graft has been obtained, suggesting that immune mechanisms may play a part, at least in prolonging the aplasia.

Various cell populations in the lymphocytes, including activated T cells of the cytotoxic suppressor phenotype $CD8^+$, Tac^+ of normal people, may be shown to be cytotoxic to normal marrow, but so far an increase in these cell types or their direct implication in marrow suppression has not been demonstrated in untransfused patients.

In a small minority of patients with aplastic anaemia who have been studied in detail, a humoral inhibitor of haemopoiesis has been detected but this does not seem to be a general phenomenon. One of the difficulties in determining the role of either cellular or humoral immunity in the production or prolongation of aplastic anaemia is the effect of repeated exposure to blood products in the patients. Transfusions produce allogeneic effects which give rise to lymphocyte populations which are cytotoxic to allogeneic marrow either specifically (HLA antibodies or restricted cell killing) or nonspecifically (natural killer cells). The nature of aplastic anaemia means that the appropriate target marrow is not available for study. Recent work has concentrated on the possible role of cytokines, particularly the interferons (IFN) in the pathogenesis of the disease. IFN-γ, and to a lesser extent IFN-α, are inhibitors of haemopoiesis whereas interleukins 1 and 3 will stimulate haemopoiesis, as will other growth factors produced by lymphocytes or monocytes. Whilst increased levels of IFN-γ have been detected in the blood and marrow of patients with aplastic anaemia by some workers, this has not been confirmed by others. Once again the interpretation of data is difficult because of the repeated transfusion effects and the effects of infection in these neutropenic patients.

Clinical Features

Haematology

The peripheral blood film shows pancytopenia without gross morphological abnormalities in the remaining cells. There may be some macrocytosis of remaining red cells, usually with an absolute reticulocytopenia. A relative reticulocytosis should always raise the possibility of associated paroxysmal nocturnal haemoglobinuria (PNH). Granulocytes often show increased staining of granules, the so-called toxic granulation of neutropenia. The neutrophil alkaline phosphatase score is increased (it falls if PNH develops). Monocytes are usually reduced in proportion to the granulocytes. Platelets are reduced and of small and uniform size. There is a variable reduction in the lymphocyte count between individuals, sometimes the count being normal or even increased so that the total white cell count is normal or near normal, but more commonly the lymphocyte count is reduced. There is sometimes a fall in the CD4:CD8 ratio but this is by no means universal and seems to be non-specifically related to infections or multiple transfusions. Abnormal cells are not seen. The bone marrow aspirate is normally easily obtained, typically with many fragments which appear hypocellular ($>75\%$ fat). The cell trails are hypocellular with a relative increase in lymphocytes and plasma cells and other non-haemopoietic forms. Remaining haemopoietic precursors are normal in appearance. In the early stages of aplastic anaemia, haemophagocytosis may be prominent. In a high proportion of cases the hypocellularity of the marrow is patchy with quite extensive areas of cellular marrow remaining. The bone marrow aspirate may, under these circumstances, be misleadingly cellular. A trephine biopsy (sometimes more than one) is necessary to assess cellularity properly.

The bone marrow trephine shows the fat replacement of marrow with or without the remaining islands of cellularity (Fig. 4.1). Non-haemopoietic cells remain, sometimes giving the impression of a chronic inflammatory infiltrate. Reticulin fibres are scanty, commensurate with the degree of hypocellularity. The most common mistake in the diagnosis of aplastic anaemia is to make the diagnosis on the basis of a bloody tap for an aspirate in the presence of pancytopenia without obtaining adequate trephine specimens.

Special tests may be of interest but little use in the diagnosis and prognosis of aplastic anaemia. Ferrokinetic studies using ^{59}Fe usually show a prolonged iron clearance. Iron utilization is always decreased and the failure of utilization reflects the severity of the aplasia. ^{52}Fe studies confirm the poor iron clearance, most of the iron being taken up by the liver, and the ^{52}Fe scan may demonstrate well the patchy nature of the marrow failure, with islands of active erythropoiesis being seen in an otherwise non-erythropoietic marrow.

Assays of committed haemopoietic precursors show a uniform reduction in aplastic anaemia. Following recovery of peripheral blood counts the CFU-GM most commonly remain low, while BFU-E may show full recovery. Patients who respond to antilymphocyte globulin (ALG) tend to show an early increase in BFU-E, which may be transient, compared with patients who do not respond.

Clinical Presentation

The clinical features derive from the decrease in peripheral blood cells and are non-specific. The patient may be feeling completely well at the time when easy bruising or petechiae appear or may have a more or less prolonged period of feeling tired from anaemia. Sometimes infection is the presenting feature but this seems to be less common in idiosyncratic aplastic anaemia than bleeding manifestations. The spleen, liver and lymph nodes are not enlarged and jaundice is only a feature in those patients with post-hepatitic aplasia who have a prolonged cholestatic phase after the infection.

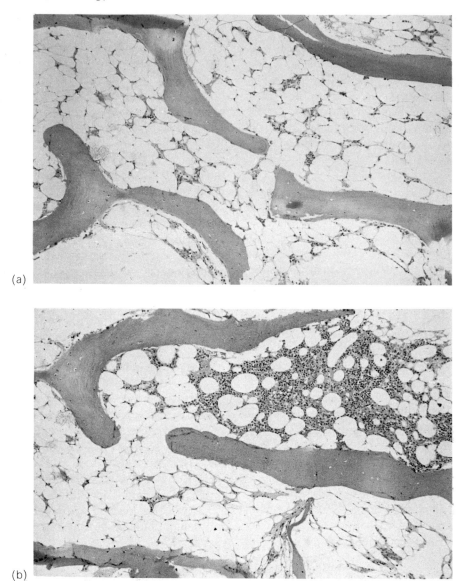

Fig. 4.1. *Aplastic anaemia trephine biopsy. (a) Replacement of normal cellular marrow by fat spaces; normal cellularity occupies only 5% of medullary space. (b) A patch of apparently normal cellularity remaining in the marrow of a patient with severe aplastic anaemia (× 200).*

At presentation it is necessary to take a detailed drug, occupational and symptomatic history to try to establish any aetiological agent so that this may be avoided in the future. Unfortunately, this is not always easy—it is difficult to dissuade someone who may have been exposed to industrial chemicals, for example, to give up their work on the possibility that the chemicals just might be involved in the cause of the disease.

Clinical Course

The clinical course is modified by the transfusion support and antibiotic therapy which the patient receives. There are some events which may interrupt the clinical course apart from the catastrophies associated with the low platelet count and neutropenia. The proliferative capacity of the marrow is greatly reduced but the marrow also appears to be unstable in that abnormal clones of cells, PNH, myelodysplastic or leukaemic, may appear during the disease, sometimes all three in the same individual. Furthermore, the degree of aplasia may vary. Several different patterns may be recognized in patients treated only with support.

1. *Stable aplastic anaemia.* The patient presents with a degree of pancytopenia which remains constant over a long period of time (months or years). In general the greater the degree of pancytopenia the worse the prognosis, which has led to many attempts to categorize that group of patients with the worst prognosis. This has led to the concept of 'severe aplastic anaemia' (SAA), the criteria for which are shown in Table 4.3. Patients with this degree of pancytopenia have about a 1 in 10 chance of surviving for 1 year when treated only with support. Patients with lesser degrees of pancytopenia, particularly those with a relative preservation of granulocytes, have a better prognosis, but clearly this is not a stepwise progression but a continuous spectrum. In either case, patients who do survive after the prolonged period of stable low counts may show a spontaneous improvement and eventually recover.

2. *Progressive or fluctuating aplasia.* A minority of patients may present with minor degrees of pancytopenia or deficiency in particular of one cell line, but over the succeeding months or years the aplasia gradually becomes more profound. Sometimes the cytopenias vary from month to month, often becoming greater following viral infections. This may be seen in its most marked form in patients who present with amegakaryocytic thrombocytopenia which progresses over a period of years to true aplastic anaemia (see below).

3. *Unstable aplasia.* Some patients may show an improvement in peripheral counts which may then be found to be associated with abnormal clones. PNH clones appear in some 10–20% of patients with prolonged aplastic anaemia, though the majority of these are only detected in the laboratory by the Ham's test and are not of clinical significance. In a few patients, frank haemolytic PNH may appear accompanied by a fall in the neutrophil alkaline phosphatase, a rise in reticulocyte, neutrophil and platelet counts and an increase in marrow cellularity. In others, myelodysplastic haemopoiesis appears with hypogranular neutrophils in the peripheral blood and a dysplastic, cellular marrow. Acute leukaemia may later develop or may appear after a period of apparent normal haemopoiesis.

The above syndromes have been separated on clinical grounds; they probably do not represent different pathogenetic disorders.

Treatment of Aplastic Anaemia

The treatment of aplastic anaemia depends on providing total support for the patient whilst awaiting bone marrow recovery and attempts to accelerate that recovery.

Support for the Aplastic Anaemia Patient

This consists of blood product support and the use of antibiotics, both prophylactic and therapeutic.

Table 4.3
Criteria for severe aplastic anaemia

Peripheral blood: two out of three values
  a) Granulocytes $<0.5 \times 10^9/l$
  b) Platelets $<20 \times 10^9/l$
  c) Reticulocytes $<1\%$ (corrected for haematocrit)
Bone marrow trephine
  a) Markedly hypocellular, $<25\%$ normal cellularity
  b) Moderately hypocellular, 25–50% normal cellularity with $<30\%$ remaining cells haemopoietic

Blood product support is mainly with packed red cells and platelet transfusions. Mostly patients are transfused with packed cells as they need them, in the non-bleeding patients about 1 unit per week, given as 3 or 4 units every 3 or 4 weeks. There are advantages in giving white-cell-depleted, filtered blood in that sensitization to platelet transfusions can be delayed by avoiding white cell transfusions and hence the development of HLA-antibodies. Platelet transfusion may be given on the basis of clinical need, but for severe aplastic anaemia patients prophylactic platelet transfusions should be used. Ideally, HLA-matched, white-cell-poor platelets would be used, but this is rarely practicable. Only a proportion of patients will become sensitized to platelet transfusions if random donors are used. Those who are sensitized will have to receive HLA-matched platelets. Family members should be avoided unless bone marrow transplantation has been ruled out as treatment. Platelets (6 units) given twice a week are usually suitable.

Antibiotics may be used prophylactically, particularly in patients with severe neutropenia ($\leq 0.2 \times 10^9/1$). These patients may acquire infection from the gastrointestinal tract (particularly aerobic pathogens) or from the upper respiratory passages. Non-absorbable antibiotics may be used together with antifungal agents to control the former. Strict mouth care with antifungal lozenges and chlorhexidine mouthwash is also of benefit. Patients should be in reverse-barrier isolation whilst in hospital. Fevers should be managed as in every severely neutropenic patient, that is, the prompt administration of broad-spectrum antibiotics, particularly those active against Gram-negative organisms, when fever or signs of infection develop. Treatment should be started after taking appropriate samples for microbiology but before the results are available. The antibiotics should be continued until at least 72 hours of normal temperature has been achieved, but unfortunately, in the severely neutropenic patient, infection is rarely eradicated and all too frequently fevers return after stopping the therapy. The most frequently used antibiotic regimens are an aminoglycoside (e.g. amikacin or netilmicin) with a β lactam penicillin (e.g. piperacillin or azlocillin), or monotherapy with ceftazidime or other suitable third generation cephalosporin.

Restoration of Marrow Activity

As mentioned above, spontaneous remission of aplastic anaemia may occur but this may not take place for several months or even years and the majority of patients with SAA die from the complications of neutropenia or thrombocytopenia before this can occur. Bone marrow transplantation is a therapeutic option open to younger patients who have an HLA-matched sibling donor and is discussed in detail below. Immunosuppressive therapy with antilymphocyte globulin (ALG) or high-dose methyl prednisone (HDMP) has also proved to be effective in increasing the remission rate in aplastic anaemia.

Antilymphocyte Globulin

The use of ALG in the treatment of aplastic anaemia was pioneered by George Mathé and his colleagues in Paris in the 1960s and developed by Bruno Speck in Basel. Using an experimental model of rabbits with benzene-induced aplastic anaemia, Speck showed that anti-rabbit-lymphocyte globulin and mismatched marrow infusion could rescue these animals from the aplasia. Later clinical trials showed that it was unnecessary in humans with acquired aplastic anaemia to give the marrow infusion. The benefit of ALG in promoting marrow recovery in aplastic anaemia was later confirmed in randomized trials conducted in the United States.

Preparations of ALG. ALG is available from a number of commercial companies. The antihuman lymphocyte globulin is raised either in horses or in rabbits. The immunization is obtained by injecting lymphocytes derived from the thymus or from thoracic duct lymphocytes or mixtures of the two. Some preparations are called antilymphocyte globulin (ALG), others are antithymocyte globulin (ATG), but there is no evidence that the specificity or effectiveness of different preparations warrants such distinctions. The partially purified immunoglobulin is absorbed with a variety of other cells— red cells, platelets and tissue cells—to leave a crude preparation of polyclonal ALG. The resulting preparations have the antigenic properties of foreign proteins and also have variable antiplatelet and antineutrophil activity. The final product may be marketed according to biological activity or as milligrams of protein. The producer's instructions should be followed for dosage.

Administration of ALG. ALG is somewhat sclerosing to veins and should be given through an intravenous line into a large vessel, preferably a central line. A test dose of the preparation should be given before starting the full dosage to test for anaphylaxis. It is preferable to give a small dose (10 mg in 100 ml of saline) intravenously over half an hour under monitored conditions rather than to use a skin test. The latter usually produces large reactions from the cytotoxic nature of the material and it is difficult to distinguish this reaction from a true allergic reaction. Providing the patient is not allergic, the full dose may be administered, starting on the same day as the test dose. Because of the antiplatelet activity of some preparations, platelets should be given before and after the infusion, though not during the ALG. The full dose is given over about 16 hours. Reactions are common, perhaps more so with horse antihuman lymphocyte preparations than with rabbit. Fever, rashes, hypotension, hypertension and occasionally the development of a positive direct antiglobulin test have been reported. These effects can usually be ameliorated by slowing the rate of infusion and giving corticosteroids, piriton and pethidine. Although the test carried out should exclude patients with anaphylaxis, massive pulmonary haemorrhage and capillary leak have been seen occasionally during the first day of administration of the full dose. The ALG is given on each of five successive days; there seems to be no benefit from a more prolonged course.

Serum sickness. Serum sickness occurs in about three-quarters of the patients given ALG. Some 7 days after the administration of the ALG, fever, rash and severe joint pains may appear. Proteinuria may be seen but frank renal failure has not yet been reported. The syndrome responds to corticosteroids, requiring high doses for about 7 days. Some centres reasonably give prophylactic corticosteroids when the syndrome is expected. The patients should thus be kept under observation until the risk of serum sickness is over, usually 2–3 weeks from the start of ALG treatment.

Androgens and ALG. Historically androgens, or anabolic steroids, were the first specific form of therapy used in aplastic anaemia. They have a temporary benefit in the management of Fanconi's anaemia (see below) and appeared to be effective in some cases of acquired aplastic anaemia, some patients being androgen dependent. It is not clear whether they are important in obtaining remission in patients treated with ALG. One randomized trial showed no benefit from androgens but the numbers in this trial were rather small and no definite conclusions could be drawn. A European trial is in progress which may well answer this question. The androgens are usually given in high dose (for example 2.5 mg/kg per day of oxymetholone), starting after the period of serum sickness. Side-effects include virilization, prostatic enlargement, salt retention and hepatotoxicity, including the development of peliosis hepatis and/or hepatocellular carcinoma after prolonged usage. If there is no response after 6 months, the androgens should be stopped. If there is a response, androgens should be slowly reduced, first to an alternate day therapy and then increasing the interval between large doses.

Response to ALG. Figure 4.2 shows the survival of patients with aplastic anaemia treated with ALG according to different clinical presentations. Patients who respond to the first course of ALG usually show the first signs of response within 4 months. An increased MCV of the red cells suggests early stressed erythropoiesis and is a good prognostic factor. Patients with severe aplastic anaemia respond less well than other patients, particularly if the neutrophil count is less than 0.2 $\times 10^9/1$ at the time of treatment. There is a suggestion that patients with a long history before ALG is given respond less well than those given the treatment early, but these may constitute a self-selecting group of poor-risk patients. Age does not seem to be a factor in response.

Further treatment. If there is no response to ALG after 4–6 months, a second course may be tried, using rabbit ALG if horse ALG has been used in the first instance and vice versa. Response rates to the second course are marginally less than that seen after the first course. Overall, about 50–60% of patients will respond to ALG. However, the marrow does not usually return entirely to normal and some degree of cytopenia may persist for several years, although the patient may not require transfusion support.

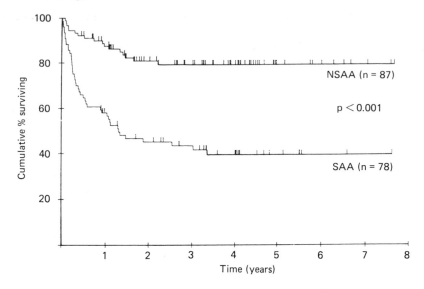

Fig. 4.2. *Survival of patients with aplastic anaemia treated with ALG ± andro-gens according to disease status at time of therapy. (NSAA: non-severe aplastic anaemia; SAA: severe aplastic anaemia.) Results from UK co-operative study, 1987.*

Relapse may occur in 10–15% of responders, either with the reappearance of aplastic anaemia or with the development of PNH.

Alternative Forms of Immunosuppression

High-dose Methylprednisolone

HDMP, 20 mg/kg per day for 3 days, reducing steadily over the next month, has been used as an alternative to ALG. Results from the European Bone Marrow Transplant Group suggest that the response rate is similar to that seen with ALG but toxicity is high and the period of hospitalization longer with HDMP than ALG. It may be a useful form of therapy for patients who relapse after two or more courses of ALG. There seems to be no clear advantage in combining HDMP with ALG.

Cyclosporin

There have been various reports of patients with aplastic anaemia who have responded to cyclo-sporin after failure with ALG. Data are not yet available on randomized trials of cyclosporin ver-sus ALG or in combination with ALG. Again, it may be reasonable to try cyclosporin for patients who fail to respond to ALG.

Monoclonal Anti-T Cell Antibodies

One randomized study from America failed to show any benefit from using monoclonal anti-T cell anti-bodies in place of ALG. The role of this form of treatment is uncertain at present.

Splenectomy

Sporadic reports of improvement following splen-ectomy for aplastic anaemia have appeared over the years and the Basel group has noted this in con-junction with ALG, particularly for patients who have become resistant to platelet transfusions. Clearly, under these circumstances there is a major risk in this operation and so far no statistical benefit has been demonstrated.

Growth Factors

The newly available growth factors, GM-CSF, G-CSF and IL-3, may be of value in the manage-ment of aplastic anaemia but so far there are no clinical data. It is possible that they may produce a small but important rise in neutrophils, but whether they will produce a more sustained improvement in marrow activity will have to await the results of clinical trials.

BONE MARROW TRANSPLANTATION

In this section general principles of bone marrow transplantation are discussed, followed by its results in aplastic anaemia. Results of bone marrow transplantation in other diseases appear in the appropriate chapters.

The idea that normal bone marrow might be used to replace diseased or destroyed marrow in a variety of diseases has been around for many years. Animal experiments had already demonstrated that it was possible to rescue mice from the effects of otherwise lethal irradiation by injecting syngeneic, allogeneic or even zenogeneic haemopoietic cells after the irradiation. These important early observations demonstrated that intravenously administered haemopoietic cells could establish haemopoiesis in the recipient providing the recipient was sufficiently immunosuppressed to accept the graft. The term 'radiation chimera' was coined to describe irradiated animals who accepted donor haemopoietic cells. 'Chimerism' is now used to describe the condition in which there has been complete replacement of the recipient's haemopoietic and immune systems from a donor; 'mixed chimerism' where the replacement is partial. Nearly all attempts at bone marrow transplantation in humans in the early days failed, with the exception of the identical twin transplants. Successful allogeneic transplants only became possible after the identification of the human leucocyte antigen (HLA) system and the improvement in support therapy, antibiotics and blood products, which reduced the problems of engraftment and enabled the patient to be kept alive long enough for the graft to take. The major problems of human bone marrow transplantation, namely rejection, graft-versus-host disease (GvHD) and problems of support, were recognized long before the first successful allogeneic transplants were carried out for severe combined immunodeficiency (SCID) in 1968 by Robert Good and colleagues, and for acute leukaemia and aplastic anaemia by E. Donnall Thomas and co-workers in 1969.

Indications for Allogeneic Bone Marrow Transplantation

The indications for bone marrow transplantation may be considered in two parts—the first relating to the disease, the second to the transplant itself. In the first case, the questions to be asked are whether the disease for which transplantation is proposed can be cured if the patient can be sufficiently treated so that rescue with bone marrow transplantation is essential, and whether alternative successful therapies exist. The second consideration refers to the state of the recipient, age, general health, presence or absence of infections, and the availability of a suitable donor. The diseases for which bone marrow transplantation offers at least as good a chance of cure compared with other treatments are given in Table 4.4. At the present time this only applies to patients who are under 50 years of age who have an HLA-identical donor. In the rare event of a patient having an identical twin donor, the age limit may be higher. The problems of age in relation to allogeneic transplants are related particularly to the increased incidence of graft-versus-host disease in older patients.

Graft Rejection and Graft-versus-Host Disease

Graft rejection is a problem common to all organ transplants and a considerable degree of immunosuppression of the recipient is required to overcome it. The special problems of bone marrow transplantation relate to the mirror image of graft rejection, namely graft-versus-host disease. The immunocompetent cells, which in the recipient can mount a rejection attack, are also present in the bone marrow of the donor and can, if established in a graft, promote a reaction characterized by cytotoxic action against a variety of organs, most prominently the skin, the gastrointestinal tract and the liver. There is clearly a reciprocal relationship between graft-versus-host disease (GvHD) and graft rejection. Measures which reduce the former may promote the latter and vice versa. GvHD is immunosuppressive through cytotoxic action on host lymphocytes. In both rejection and GvHD, T-

Table 4.4

Indications for bone marrow transplantation from HLA-matched sibling donor

Disease groups	Subtypes	Time of transplant
Malignant		
Leukaemias	Chronic granulocytic leukaemia	1st chronic phase 2nd chronic phase after lymphoblastic transformation
	Acute myeloid leukaemia	1st remission Early 1st relapse 2nd remission
	Acute lymphoblastic leukaemia	Poor risk c-ALL 1st remission c-ALL 2nd remission B-ALL 1st remission T-ALL poor risk 1st or 2nd remission
	Myelodysplastic syndrome	During stable phase
Non-malignant		
Marrow failure	Aplastic anaemia	Severe aplastic anaemia < 20 years old Patients less than 50 years old with very severe aplastic anaemia (neutrophils $< 0.2 \times 10^9/l$)
Inherited disorders	β thalassaemia major	Before severe transfusion siderosis Failed chelation therapy
	Fanconi's anaemia	At presentation of pancytopenia Before transfusion dependent
	Storage diseases likely to be cured by haemopoietic graft—including macrophages	Before neurological complications
	Inherited immunodeficiency disorders	
	Osteopetrosis	In infancy in severe cases

helper and cytotoxic T cells are involved in the reaction. It is conventional to discuss these two problems of bone marrow transplantation separately, but it should be appreciated that the two are closely linked.

Prevention of Graft Rejection

Even with genotypic matching of the major histocompatibility complex (MHC), rejection will occur in the immunocompetent recipient unless immunosuppression is given as well. In the management of diseases other than aplastic anaemia, immunosuppression is combined with cytotoxic therapy to eliminate diseased cells, either as antileukaemic therapy or to eradicate the recipient's marrow to make way for the new haemopoiesis. This combination of immunosuppression and cytotoxic therapy is usually referred to as 'conditioning'. A number of agents have become standard for immunosuppression, depending on the disease for which transplantation is carried out.

Cyclophosphamide

Cyclophosphamide was adopted early in bone marrow transplantation as an effective immunosuppressive agent following rat experiments by George Santos and colleagues in the 1960s. Cyclophosphamide at a dose of 50 mg/kg per day intravenously for 4 days has been used alone in immuno-suppression of patients with aplastic anaemia, though the rejection rate with this regimen is un-acceptably high unless additional post-graft immunosuppression is given, especially in multiply transfused patients (see below). Cyclophosphamide is usually used in lower total dose in combination with total body irradiation (TBI) in the condit-ioning of patients with malignant disease, 60 mg/kg per day for 2 days usually being preferred.

Cyclophosphamide is given intravenously, usually in 250–500 ml saline over 0.5–1 hour. Side-effects include nausea and vomiting, usually rela-tively mild, haemorrhagic cystitis, cardiomyopathy, fluid retention and alopecia. The haemorrhagic cystitis may be prevented or greatly modified by giving mesna (2-mercapto-ethane sulphonate) in-travenously to neutralize the effects of metabolites of cyclophosphamide in the urine. The mesna is given at a dose of 40% of the cyclophosphamide (w/w) an hour before the cyclophosphamide and repeated at 3, 6, and 9 hours afterwards, each dose given intravenously over 30 minutes. This regimen is repeated on each day the cyclophosphamide is given. Children require a higher dose of mesna than adults. The cardiotoxicity of cyclophosphamide is not usually a problem at the doses quoted unless there is already cardiac damage. When used in patients who have already received high doses of anthracyclines, careful cardiac monitoring is ad-vised. Late haemorrhagic cystitis (after 20 days) may occur in transplant patients but is probably related to virus infections (particularly adenovirus) rather than to cyclophosphamide

Total Body Irradiation

Total body irradiation (TBI) is an effective immunosuppressive agent. It is used in the condit-ioning of patients with leukaemia both for its immunosuppressive effect and its antileukaemic action. There is a fairly narrow 'window' of TBI dose where ablation of the patient's own marrow and, hopefully, leukaemic cells occurs without un-acceptable toxicity to other organs. The dose rate, fractionation of the total dose and possibly the nature of the ionizing radiation used may all affect the actual position and size of the window. The upper acceptable level is set by toxicity in the lungs,

gastrointestinal tract and central nervous system.

There is still much discussion about the optimum way in which radiation should be delivered. The original Seattle regimen was to give 1000 cGy midline dose from opposing cobalt sources at about 5 cGy per minute. This produces considerable immediate toxicity with vomiting and gastrointesti-nal disturbance. Other groups use a linear acceler-ator and give a lower total dose (750 cGy) at a higher dose rate (up to 26 cGy/min). More recently, fractionation of the whole body irradiation has been used, giving up to 1600 cGy in 200-cGy fractions twice daily. A higher dose rate is usually used. Fractionation undoubtedly makes the im-mediate toxicity more acceptable but there is insuf-ficient evidence to be sure whether it is equally effective as an antileukaemic agent or whether long-term toxicity is reduced.

The major toxic effects of radiation may be divided into immediate and late. The immediate effects include nausea, vomiting, diarrhoea, a rise in the serum amylase, sometimes with abdominal pain suggestive of pancreatitis, salivary gland swelling and skin erythema. Diarrhoea may be delayed in onset for a few days and may be severe. The most serious late effect is radiation pneumonitis which has to be distinguished from other causes of inter-stitial pneumonitis (see below), and lung shielding may be used to reduce the dose to the lungs in non-malignant conditions. Other late effects are endo-crine abnormalities and cataracts. Patients who receive TBI are sterile, thyroid function may be reduced and growth is inhibited in children. There may be some intellectual impairment in children, especially if they have received irradiation for CNS prophylaxis in acute lymphoblastic leukaemia.

There is also debate about the time at which TBI should be administered. Traditionally it has been given after cyclophosphamide in the days immedi-ately preceding the infusion of bone marrow, but it may be that giving it earlier, perhaps a week before the marrow, may improve the immunosuppressive effects.

Total Lymphoid Irradiation

Problems of graft rejection, particularly in patients who receive marrow which has been depleted of T lymphocytes to avoid GvHD, have led to a hunt for improved methods of immunosuppression. Following observations on the immunosuppressive effects of irradiation in Hodgkin's disease, Slavin and colleagues have investigated the use of total lymphoid irradiation (TLI). In this technique the mantle and inverted-Y fields familiar in the treatment of Hodgkin's disease are irradiated, thus avoiding the greater part of lung toxicity. It is too early to assess the advantages of TLI in matched sibling transplants. In aplastic anaemia patients up to 1600 cGy TLI in 200-cGy fractions have been given, together with cyclophosphamide, with a reduction in graft failure rate.

Busulphan

Because of the long-term effects of TBI on growth, development and fertility, there is a reluctance to use it for non-malignant conditions, especially in children. Busulphan, 3.5–4 mg/kg per day on 4 days before giving cyclophosphamide, was introduced by Santos and colleagues from John Hopkins Hospital as an alternative. The combination of busulphan and cyclophosphamide appears to be an effective way of eradicating abnormal marrow to make space for the transplant, particularly in genetic disorders such as thalassaemia and the mucopolysaccharidoses. The toxicity of busulphan in these doses is not well documented. Pulmonary fibrosis may occur but its relationship to the drug and its dose is not clear. Fluid retention and haemorrhagic cystitis may be problems, particularly when cyclophosphamide is given as well.

Other Agents

A variety of immunosuppressive agents have been used to increase the immunosuppression achieved with cyclophosphamide alone. ALG and procarbazine were favoured during the early years of transplantation for aplastic anaemia. It is not clear whether the addition of these agents does reduce graft failure. More recently, interest has returned to the use of specific anti-T cell monoclonal antibodies given in vivo to the recipient. Toxic side-effects possibly related to lysis of the target lymphocytes and complement activation are marked. The approach is very interesting but so far there are insufficient data to assess the effect of specific immunosuppression in the recipient.

Cyclosporin

Cyclosporin is an immunosuppressive agent which is not toxic to the haemopoietic system. It was introduced into the management of patients transplanted for aplastic anaemia as additional immunosuppression to prevent graft rejection. There appeared to be a considerable reduction in graft failure when compared to the use of methotrexate, which was used post-graft to reduce GvHD. In aplastic anaemia cyclosporin is continued for at least 6 months following bone marrow transplantation. It was also hoped that cyclosporin might reduce the incidence of GvHD but its use in that respect seems to be limited by toxicity.

Graft-versus-Host Disease

GvHD is mediated by immunocompetent T cells in the bone marrow transfused which react against recipient cells carrying different surface antigens not detected by HLA and DR matching from the donor.

In the classical GvHD animal model the antigen differences occur in the major histocompatibility antigens. In human bone marrow transplants the major histocompatibility antigens are matched as far as possible so the disease is thought to be a consequence of reaction against minor and so far unidentified histocompatibility antigens. GvHD will only occur in an immunocompromised recipient incapable of rejecting the graft.

GvHD is characterized by fever, skin rash, liver function abnormalities and diarrhoea. In addition there may be profound immunosuppression and reactivation of latent viruses. Other organs may be involved though the pathology is less well defined and GvHD may modify, usually adversely, other complications of transplantation. It is conventional to grade acute GvHD according to the severity of organ damage and the number of systems involved. Death occurs most commonly as a result of infection or occasionally intractable gastrointestinal haemorrhage. In severe acute GvHD there is usually a marked fall in recovering blood counts.

Onset

Acute GvHD may occur at any time up to about 6 weeks following bone marrow transplantation but the majority of cases present between 1 and 3 weeks

Table 4.5

Clinical staging of graft-versus-host disease (Seattle System)

A. Organ involvement

Stage	Skin	Liver	Gut
+	Maculopapular rash <25% body surface	Bilirubin 25–35 μmol/l	Diarrhoea 0.5–1 l/day
+ +	Maculopapular rash >25% body surface	Bilirubin 35–70 μmol/l	Diarrhoea 1–1.5 l/day
+ + +	Generalized erythroderma	Bilirubin 70–150 μmol/l	Diarrhoea 1.5 l/day
+ + + +	Desquamation and bullae	Bilirubin >150 μmol/l	Severe pain Ileus

B. Overall grading

Grade	Degree of organ involvement
1	+ to + + skin rash, no gut involvement, no liver involvement; no decrease in clinical performance
11	+ to + + + Skin rash, + gut and /or liver involvement; mild decrease in clinical performance
111	+ + to + + + skin rash, + + to + + + gut and/or liver involvement; marked decrease in clinical performance
IV	Similar to grade III but with + + to + + + organ involvement and extreme decrease in clinical performance

after the marrow infusion, occasionally even as early as 4 days. Very early GvHD is usually severe. Acute graft-versus-host disease may be graded according to the organs involved and the severity of that involvement. The most commonly used classification is that devised by the Seattle group (Table 4.5). GvHD is more common in older subjects.

Skin Manifestations

A variety of skin conditions may be seen but the most common is a macular erythematous eruption which typically involves the palms and soles as well as the rest of the body. Usually it does not itch but may do so. In severe cases the erythematous lesions coalesce and desquamation and exfoliation occur (Fig. 4.3). Sometimes a syndrome of epidermal necrolysis may be seen. The earliest pathological lesions are single cell necrosis in the basal layer of the epidermis, with 'ballooning' of the damaged cells. Lymphocytes are very scanty in the sections. As the disease progresses the degree of cytolysis increases, eosinophilic bodies are seen and separation of the epidermis occurs.

Hepatic Dysfunction

Typically the patient becomes jaundiced, with marked elevation of the bilirubin, a less marked elevation of the alkaline phosphatase and relatively little disturbance of the hepatic parenchymal enzymes. This typical pattern is often distorted, either by concomitant virus infection, particularly reactivation of cytomegalovirus, or by the effects of drugs. Although the jaundice may be intense, hepatic failure is rarely seen. The hepatic equivalent of basal cell necrosis of the skin is cytolysis of bile duct canaliculi cells.

Gastrointestinal Tract

Diarrhoea is the main consequence of GvHD affecting the gut. It may be a profuse exudative diarrhoea exceeding 10 litres per day in volume. In severe cases abdominal pain is marked. Rectal biopsy shows cytolysis of crypt cells in the early stages, progressing to complete denudation of the gastrointestinal mucosa. Severe, prolonged haemorrhage may develop. Although GvHD of the lower bowel

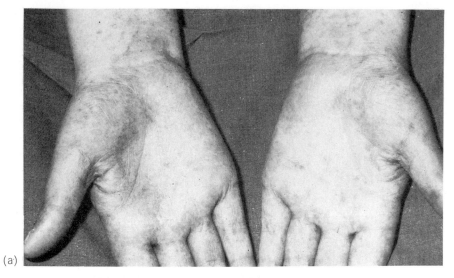

(a)

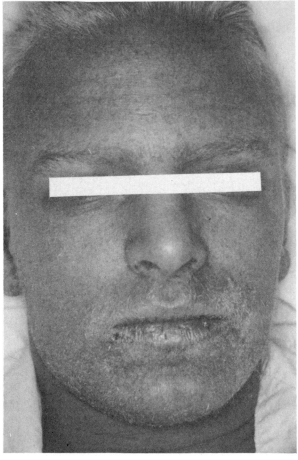

(b)

Fig. 4.3. *Graft-versus-host disease. (a) Typical palmar rash in GvHD grade I. (b) GvHD grade IV: marked exfoliative skin rash in a patient who also had jaundice and severe diarrhoea.*

has been studied most by biopsy, all parts of the gastrointestinal tract below the stomach may be affected.

Lungs

It is not clear what part GvHD plays in the lung pathology seen in bone marrow transplant patients. Both interstitial pneumonitis and obliterative alveolitis may occur in patients with GvHD, but more commonly in patients who have been irradiated than in unirradiated patients. When no viral or other infective pathogen is found it seems probable that GvHD is playing a part in the pathogenesis of the disease.

Prevention of Acute GvHD

Two major approaches have been made to the prevention of acute GvHD.

1. *Post-graft immunosuppression.* Methotrexate and cyclosporin are the two immunosuppressive agents which have been used most extensively, initially as single agents, more recently in combination to prevent or moderate acute GvHD. The incidence of GvHD remains high, 60–80% in most series, but the severity is probably reduced by the use of these drugs. Nevertheless, acute GvHD remains the single greatest transplant-related cause of death for bone marrow transplant patients. Both drugs have disadvantages, methotrexate because of its cytotoxic action, delaying peripheral blood recovery and aggravating mucositis, cyclosporin through its nephrotoxicity and tendency to produce hypertension. When used in combination, cyclosporin is started the day before the bone marrow is infused (day −1), 5 mg/kg per 12 hours by continuous infusion. This dose is continued for 2 days and then reduced to 2.5 mg/kg per 12 hours, the dose being modified in the light of renal or hepatic toxicity. Methotrexate, 10 mg/m², is given on days +1, +3, +9. Cyclosporin is continued by mouth once the gastrointestinal effects of conditioning have settled and is tailed off after 6 months, except for patients transplanted for aplastic anaemia, who continue for 1 year.

2. *T cell depletion of donor marrow.* More recently, attempts have been made to reduce or eliminate acute GvHD by removing the cells responsible for the disease from donor marrow before the marrow is infused into the recipient—so-called ex-vivo T cell depletion. Many techniques have been developed to achieve this end, physical, chemical and immunological; immunological methods are probably the most widely used. Specific monoclonal antibodies directed against T cells are added to the collected marrow and death of the lymphocytes is achieved either through complement lysis (human or rabbit complement as appropriate to the antibody) or by conjugating the antibody to a cell toxin. Most methods will achieve a 2–4 log. kill (that is, leaving 1 in 100 to 1 in 10 000 cells). Acute GvHD is prevented or reduced in intensity by such treatment but at the cost of increased graft failure and, in some studies, increased leukaemic relapse. Certainly in aplastic anaemia, for patients conditioned only with cyclophosphamide, the graft failure rate becomes unacceptable. T cell depletion followed by a successful graft makes for the easiest of allogeneic transplants, but so far the results have not been accompanied by increased long-term survival. Perhaps such improvement will come from using increased immunosuppression in the recipient, particularly through the use of monoclonal antibodies in vivo at the time of and after the bone marrow transplant.

Treatment of Acute GvHD

Significant acute GvHD requires treatment. The skin rash, diarrhoea and liver disorders may all respond to high dose methyl prednisone therapy, starting at 10 mg/kg per day and reducing the dose steadily after 3 days. However, there are difficulties with this treatment, particularly in patients receiving cyclosporin at the same time. Fluid retention, hypertension and seizures occur, particularly, though not exclusively, in children. It is necessary to monitor fluid balance carefully and to reduce or stop cyclosporin if there are problems. Infection may develop, including reactivation of cytomegalovirus or with opportunist infections, and lead to fatal pneumonitis. Diarrhoea may not respond to corticosteroids, though abdominal pain usually settles. In this case massive support with fluids and blood may be required for a prolonged period. Azathioprine and in 1–1 vivo monoclonals may be tried.

Acute GvHD may progress to a chronic form with skin fibrosis and oedema leading to contractures and a scleroderma-like picture. Thalidomide has been used in therapy.

Pneumonitis

Respiratory failure is a devastating complication of bone marrow transplantation. It is most common in patients who have received radiation, who have acute GvHD and in whom cytomegalovirus (CMV) infection or pneumocystis infection can be documented. The development of interstitial pneumonitis most probably does not depend on a single cause but is multifactorial. The use of co-trimoxazole post transplant has reduced the incidence of pneumonitis due to *Pneumocystis carinii* but treatment of established CMV infection is so far disappointing.

Cytomegalovirus Infection

This is perhaps the most devastating infection in the post-transplant patient. The virus, one of the herpesvirus group, is present as a latent virus in a majority of adult patients in most countries. Activation of the virus, or new infection in the previously unexposed recipient, may lead to pneumonitis which is usually fatal. Other manifestations include hepatitis and ulceration in the gastrointestinal tract, including the oesophagus. The virus may be recovered from the urine or found intracellulary in the circulating leucocytes. Diagnosis of CMV pneumonitis may be made from detection of the virus in sputum or bronchial washings. Open lung biopsy is rarely required. There is some evidence that CMV pneumonitis is an immunopathological process, that is, the clinical disease develops as the body mounts an antibody-mediated immune response. Control of infection in normal circumstances is probably achieved through cellular immune responses.

There are four possible combinations of donor and recipient with respect to CMV infection. Where both donor and recipient are negative for CMV antibodies, indicating no previous infection, CMV may be avoided by giving CMV-negative blood products. Other combinations are both donor and recipient positive for CMV antibodies; donor negative, recipient positive; and recipient negative, donor positive. There may be some transferred immunity because in some studies recipients of .transplants from CMV-positive donors, particularly if the recipient is CMV negative, have

fewer problems from CMV pneumonitis than when the donor is CMV negative. Prophylactic acyclovir has been found to reduce the incidence in some studies.

Treatment is unsatisfactory. Trials using hyperimmune globulin injections have failed to show convincing benefits. Drugs are being developed with activity against CMV, especially gancilovir, but so far there has been little clear-cut evidence of cure of established CMV pneumonitis. Drugs such as Phoscarnet and DHPG may be effective in the prevention of pneumonitis from a reactivated CMV infection before pneumonitis is established.

Haemopoietic Recovery after Bone Marrow Transplantation

Marrow recovery is usually indicated by the appearance of neutrophils and reticulocytes in the peripheral blood 10–20 days after marrow infusion and acceptable levels of neutrophils and platelets are usually achieved by 20–30 days. Late bone marrow failure may still occur and falls in the peripheral blood counts often accompany virus infections or acute GvHD. Once the neutrophil count has exceeded $0.5 \times 10^9/1$ and the patient no longer requires platelet transfusion, he or she may leave the protected environment, usually to be discharged from hospital; the patient is still considerably immunosuppressed. Erythropoietic recovery may be greatly delayed in ABO-mismatched transplants and the patients may also suffer temporary autoimmune haemolytic anaemia.

Immune Reconstitution

Immune reconstitution is much slower than haemopoietic recovery, though it may be difficult to demonstrate by in-vitro tests exactly where the defects lie. Patients remain at risk from virus infections for 1 or 2 years post-transplant, and herpes virus infections, both herpes simplex and herpes zoster, are common, the former in the early stages, the latter from 6 weeks after transplant. Both respond to acyclovir, which should be given promptly. Contact with other viruses, measles for example, should be covered by giving appropriate passive immunization. Post transplant, particularly in patients with cGvHD, there is an immune defect similar to that seen in splenectomized patients, with a risk of overwhelming pneumococcal or meningococcal sepsis. For this reason many centres give prophylactic penicillin V for 2 years following bone marrow transplant, or longer if the patient has chronic GvHD.

Response to active immunization is not optimal for at least 2 years after the transplant, but at that time a re-immunization programme should be considered using killed vaccines or toxoids. Transfer of such immunity is best achieved by immunizing both the donor and the recipient pre-transplant.

Bone Marrow Transplantation for Severe Aplastic Anaemia

Allogeneic bone marrow transplantation from HLA-matched sibling donors was first used for patients with severe aplastic anaemia by E. Donall Thomas, Rainer Storb and colleagues in Seattle in 1969. Since then, several hundreds of such transplants have been carried out. The overall survival in recent studies is 60–80%. The clearest indication for such a transplant is the younger patient (less than 20 years old) with severe aplastic anaemia, particularly if the neutrophil count is $<0.2 \times 10^9/1$. For such patients, bone marrow transplantation has a better long-term survival than immunosuppressive treatment. For other patients, immunosuppression offers a similar survival rate and there is a case for offering immunosuppression

first with transplantation reserved for those patients who fail to respond to ALG. Unfortunately the chance of a successful transplant may be reduced in these patients, due to the risk of graft failure in patients who have received multiple platelet and blood transfusions.

Comparisons of survival after immunosuppression and bone marrow transplantation are shown in Figure 4.4.

INHERITED APLASTIC ANAEMIA

A number of inherited disorders are associated with bone marrow failure (Table 4.6). Fanconi anaemia is the most common of these and, together with dyskeratosis congenita, the best characterized. The other disorders are less well characterized and their identity, particularly as separate inherited diseases, is not clear.

Fanconi Anaemia

In 1927, Fanconi in Switzerland described a family in which three brothers developed aplastic anaemia. The brothers also had microcephaly, abnormal skin pigmentation, internal strabismus and genital hypoplasia. Further families and cases were described which led to the recognition of a particular inherited disorder named after Fanconi, though there is heterogeneity of both clinical and genetic features.

Table 4.6
Constitutional aplastic anaemia

Disorder	Inheritance	Associated features
Fanconi anaemia	Autosomal recessive	Skeletal, skin, renal etc.
Dyskeratosis congenita	Sex linked Some families autosomal recessive	Nail, skin atrophy
Xeroderma pigmentosa	Autosomal recessive	Sensitive to u.v. light Late onset pancytopenia
Pancytopenia at birth	?	Abnormal thumbs Responds to corticosteroids
Shwachman's syndrome	Autosomal recessive	Exocrine pancreatic abnormalities Dwarfism Usually neutropenia only

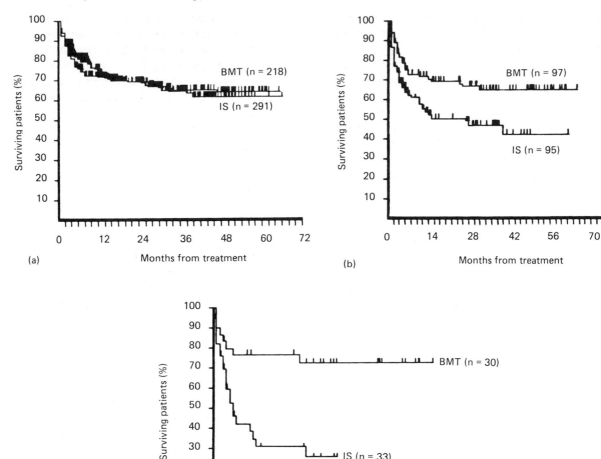

Fig. 4.4. *(a) Comparison of bone marrow transplantation (BMT) with immuno-suppression (IS) in the treatment of aplastic anaemia. (b) Effect of low neutrophil count ($<0.2 \times 10^9/l$) on survival following BMT or IS ($p<0.01$). (c) Survival of patients with aplastic anaemia who have $<0.2 \times 10^9/l$ neutrophils and are infected at time of treatment. (Data from cumulative European Bone Marrow Transplant Group, 1987.)*

Genetics

The disorder appears to be inherited as an autosomal recessive disease with variable penetrance, though there are some features which suggest that the disease may not be inherited in a simple Mendelian fashion. All races are affected.

Consanguineous marriages are more frequent in Fanconi anaemia families, as would be expected with an autosomal recessive inheritance, but males are more commonly affected than females (2:1), shared haplotypes of the HLA system are common between parents, and within a family siblings may be disparate in the expression of haematological abnormalities, some affected members having only the skeletal and skin abnormalities while others have the aplastic anaemia.

The underlying gene defects are not known but cytogenetic analysis reveals an increase in chromatid abnormalities in both stressed and unstressed cultures of a variety of cell lines, including skin fibroblasts and lymphocytes as well as marrow cell cultures. These chromatid abnormalities are non-specific, that is, they occur in normal cell lines but at a much lower frequency than in Fanconi anaemia. Gaps, breaks, reduplications, exchanges, translocations and constrictions may be present in increased numbers, particularly when the cells are exposed to DNA cross-linking agents (Fig. 4.5). The lymphocytes are highly susceptible to transformation by the SV40 virus and are slightly more sensitive to ionizing radiation than normal cells. The most marked effect is seen with the bifunctional alkylating agents,

mitomycin C and diepoxybutane (DEB). Chorionic villus cells show the same sensitivity to the blastogens and may be used for antenatal diagnosis. The increased chromatid abnormalities have been taken to indicate a defect in DNA repair and to underlie the increased incidence of malignant disease in these patients.

Clinical Features

The typical features of Fanconi anaemia are characteristic but are not expressed in all patients (Table 4.7). The children are born with low birth weight at term and do not grow well, mostly being below the 10th centile. Microcephaly, microphthalmia and small mouth and jaw give the classical patient a typical appearance. The skin may show a generalized hyperpigmentation with increased patches of pigment (café-au-lait patches) and other areas of depigmentation. Internal

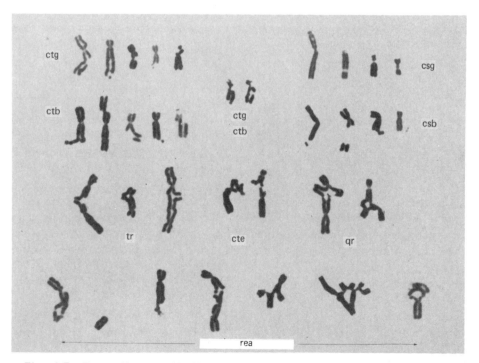

Fig. 4.5. *Fanconi's anaemia. Chromosome aberrations from a peripheral blood mononuclear cell preparation stressed with mitomycin C. (ctg, chromatid gap; ctb, chromatid break; csg, chromosome gap; csb, chromosome break; cte, chromatid exchange; tr, triradial; qr, quadriradial rea, rearrangement.) (Courtesy of Dr M. Orlanda, Guy's Hospital.)*

Table 4.7
Clinical features of Fanconi's anaemia

Common findings	Low birth weight
	Short stature
	Microcephaly
	Microphthalmia
	Microstomia
	Skeletal abnormalities, particularly of thumbs and radii
	Hypoplastic hypothenar eminences
	Generalized increased pigmentation of skin
	Patches of hyperpigmentation
	Patches of depigmentation
	Cryptorchism
	Abnormalities of renal anatomy:
	horseshoe kidneys
	pelvic kidney
	Strabismus
	Hyper-reflexia
Uncommon associations	Mental retardation
	Vascular malformations
	Growth hormone deficiency

strabismus is common. Males may have undescended testes, and horse-shoe kidney or pelvic kidney is common. Mental retardation is uncommon. Skeletal abnormalities affect mainly the hands and forearms. Absent or hypoplastic thumbs and absent radii are the most usual findings.

Vascular abnormalities with hypoplastic veins may be present, a feature to be recognized when trying to insert a central venous catheter at the time of bone marrow transplantation. Cardiac abnormalities, however, are not increased.

At birth the blood count is usually normal and features associated with bone marrow failure do not usually present until the child is 5–10 years old, though in some families bone marrow failure occurs later. Symptoms of anaemia or bruising or nose bleeds are the most commonly seen as initial signs of marrow failure. Sometimes children are investigated for short stature and the haematological abnormalities come to light during this time.

Haematological Features

A low platelet count is the most common presenting haematological finding. A modest fall in platelet count may antedate the development of full marrow failure by several years. Anaemia then gradually becomes apparent, the granulocytes being the last affected cell line. In typical cases the bone marrow becomes hypoplastic between the ages of 5 and 10 years with replacement of haemopoietic tissue by fat cells. Macrophage activity is prominent during the development of marrow failure, with erythrophagocytosis and iron deposition in macrophages.

The marrow failure appears to be at the stem cell level, with reduction in CFU-GM and BFU-E even before pancytopenia occurs. There is no evidence for an immune-mediated inhibition of haemopoiesis nor of failure of growth factors, though haemopoiesis is normally stimulated by the presence of anabolic steroids (see below).

There is a high incidence of acute leukaemic

transformation in the marrow of these children. Acute myeloid leukaemia is the normal development but acute megakaryocytic and erythroleukaemic changes have been described. As many as 10% of patients may develop this complication and the incidence might be even higher if the children did not die from the effects of pancytopenia before this could occur. Some sufferers may present with acute leukaemia without going through an obvious pancytopenic stage. The diagnosis may be suspected from physical examination or from finding the typical chromatid abnormalities in lymphocyte or skin culture.

Clinical Course

As indicated above, the bone marrow failure is usually progressive and patients come to require blood and platelet transfusions. Other malignancies apart from acute myeloid leukaemia are more common in these patients than normal, particularly of the gastrointestinal tract and skin. Rarely, patients may enter remission, usually about the time of puberty, with normalization of blood counts. If left untreated, the majority of patients die from haemorrhage or transformation to acute leukaemia.

Treatment

Apart from transfusion support, treatment consists of anabolic steroids and/or bone marrow transplantation.

Anabolic steroids. Most children show improvement in all haematological indices following treatment with anabolic (androgenic) hormones. The haemoglobin is often normalized but there is also a substantial improvement in the platelet count. The dose of hormone used to achieve remission is large (e.g. 2.5 mg/kg oxymetholone), and treatment is attended by all the unwanted side-effects of androgen treatment, which are particularly distressing in children. In addition to secondary sexual changes in boys and virilization in girls, behavioural changes may be marked, with hyperactivity and aggression developing. Hepatic complications are marked, with cholestatic jaundice, peliosis hepatis and hepatocellular carcinoma (Fig. 4.6) occurring in many patients who receive anabolic steroids over a period of a year or more. Remission is usually androgen dependent and rarely lasts more than 2 years before complications occur, so that treatment with these agents is mainly used to gain time to obtain a bone marrow donor for patients who do not have a normal HLA-identical sibling.

Bone marrow transplantation. The chance of finding an HLA-identical sibling donor for patients with Fanconi anaemia is less than for children with acquired aplastic anaemia. The ratio of affected to unaffected children in families appears to be higher than expected on a simple autosomal recessive inheritance. Clearly the affected siblings cannot be used as donors. The increased incidence of shared haplotypes between parents makes it important to

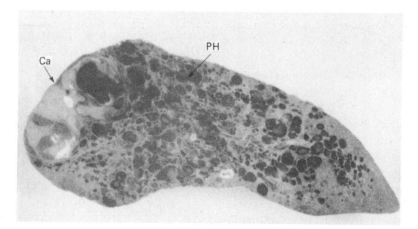

Fig. 4.6. *Fanconi's anaemia Liver showing peliosis hepatis (PH) and hepato-cellular carcinoma (Ca) from a patient treated for 3 years with anabolic steroids.*

examine their HLA-types as potential donors. Donors who are heterozygous for the Fanconi gene seem to be satisfactory as bone marrow donors.

The increased sensitivity of cells from patients with Fanconi anaemia to alkylating agents and radiation has led to a modification of the conditioning regimen for bone marrow transplantation from that used for acquired aplastic anaemia. Low dose cyclophosphamide, 5 mg/kg per day × 4, is combined with relatively low dose total body irradiation, 500 cGy in a single fraction or 200 cGy × 3 in fractionated irradiation. Cyclosporin may be used as post-transplant immunosuppression. T cell depletion leads to a marked increase in graft failure and it is not yet clear how the pre-graft conditioning can be increased to overcome this problem.

When HLA-matched sibling donors have been used, about 80% of the transplants are successful and normal haemopoiesis is restored. Other features such as growth retardation are, of course, not altered and it is important to discuss this with families before commencing a transplant.

Where non-HLA-identical sibling donors have been used results are less successful. Phenotypic matched transplants using parents or unrelated donors probably have an acceptable success rate, possibly as good as the genotypic match allowing for the delay which normally accompanies this type of transplant. Mismatched transplants have a success rate of the order of 20% and the problems associated with T cell depletion mean that graft-versus-host disease is the main cause of death in patients so treated.

Dyskeratosis Congenita

This condition is a sex-linked disorder characterized by nail and skin atrophy and progressive bone marrow failure which usually develops during the third or fourth decade of life but may present earlier. Families in which girls are affected are seen, suggesting a different form of inheritance in some families. Chromosomes are normal and patients do not show the same sensitivity to radiation or alkylating agents as do patients with Fanconi anaemia. Bone marrow transplantation may be used as for patients with acquired aplastic anaemia. There are reports of a late, fatal, vasculitic disease occurring in these patients several years after apparently successful bone marrow transplantation.

Other Congenital Disorders

There are a number of poorly characterized congenital conditions associated with pancytopenia and bone marrow failure. Occasionally newborn infants are seen who have pancytopenia with or without abnormalities of the thumbs who respond to treatment with corticosteroids, rather like a variant of Diamond–Blackfan syndrome (see (p. 107). Shwachmans syndrome may be associated with pancytopenia rather than isolated neutropenia. Patients with progressive pancytopenia in the absence of skeletal or growth abnormalities may be suffering from variants of Fanconi anaemia and chromosome analysis should be made on the lymphocytes of all children presenting with aplastic anaemia to exclude this possibility.

BENZENE-INDUCED APLASTIC ANAEMIA

Chronic exposure to benzene used as a solvent produces a pancytopenia associated with a hyperplastic and dysplastic marrow which may later become leukaemic or, more rarely, be associated with aplastic anaemia. Benzene has been used experimentally to produce aplastic anaemia in rabbits. Benzene itself is now rarely used as a solvent, having been replaced by non-aromatic organic solvents, but it is still encountered in the petroleum industry and benzene derivatives are ubiquitous in occupations such as photographic development. However, the evidence that these compounds produce aplastic anaemia at the low concentrations permitted by industrial safety guidelines is lacking, although there is some evidence that low dose benzene (10 parts per million) may have an effect on erythropoiesis.

MALIGNANT APLASTIC ANAEMIA

Acute Lymphoblastic Leukaemia

This may present as aplastic anaemia, particularly though not exclusively in childhood. The aplasia is not distinguishable from true aplastic anaemia on haematological grounds but there are some clinical observations which raise the possibility that the aplasia is a prodrome of ALL. Fever and documented infection are a more common presentation than in aplastic anaemia. The platelets tend to be relatively better preserved compared to the neutrophils than in acquired aplasia. The spleen is frequently enlarged, though it may be only just palpable or evident only on ultrasound. The aplasia usually lasts 3–6 weeks, when spontaneous or corticosteroid-induced 'remission' occurs. The ALL usually follows after a period of apparently normal haemopoiesis, often 1–3 months after recovery. The phenotype of the ALL does not differ from primary ALL and the prognosis is not affected.

Acute Myeloid Leukaemia

Acute myeloid leukaemia (AML) may present in a similar way to ALL in childhood with a period of aplasia, but this is much less common. Rarely, AML may present with a relatively stable degree of aplasia which may persist for several months before the blood becomes frankly leukaemic. In these patients suspicion may be aroused by finding occasional circulating blasts in the peripheral blood or in a buffy coat preparation, by a low neutrophil alkaline phosphatase (NAP) and by the presence of an excess of myeloblasts in the cells remaining in the bone marrow. It is important to be aware of this possibility in the differential diagnosis of aplastic anaemia because these patients are probably best treated by early bone marrow transplantation where an HLA-identical sibling donor is available, using TBI and some additional chemotherapy. Patients without a donor may be supported with blood transfusion until they become frankly leukaemic. Attempts to produce remission are often, but not always, unsuccessful because the aplastic marrow remains aplastic.

Hypoplastic Myelodysplastic Syndrome (MDS)

Some patients with MDS may present with a hypoplastic marrow. The remaining haemopoietic cells usually show the changes of MDS with hypogranular neutrophils, micromegakaryocytes and marked dyserythropoietic changes. Where bone marrow transplantation is appropriate, TBI as well as cyclophosphamide 60 mg/kg per day × 2 should be used.

SINGLE LINEAGE BONE MARROW FAILURE

Pure Red Cell Aplasia

Failure of erythropoiesis may be an inherited or an acquired disorder. The acquired disorder may be primary or secondary and may be transient or chronic. Whatever the cause, red cell aplasia is characterized by anaemia and reticulocytopenia with reduction of red cell precursors in the marrow. The marrow usually shows a complete absence of red cell precursors but some forms of either the inherited or acquired disease may be associated with the absence of the later forms of erythropoietic precursors—a picture of maturation arrest.

Congenital Pure Red Cell Aplasia— Diamond–Blackfan Syndrome

Children with this disorder are born with anaemia and reticulocytopenia. The inheritance is not clearly established, most probably it is a recessive condition with variable penetrance. Associated abnormalities may be present, particularly triphalangeal thumbs.

Haematology

There is anaemia and reticulocytopenia. The bone marrow aspirate most commonly shows an absence of erythrocyte precursors, though some infants show a 'maturation arrest'. Culture of peripheral blood or bone marrow mononuclear cells shows a variable pattern. Some cases produce normal numbers of BFU-E whereas in others BFU-E are absent. There is some suggestion that patients with BFU-E respond better to corticosteroid treatment.

Clinical Features and Treatment

The clinical features, apart from any skeletal abnormalities, are those of anaemia. The majority of Diamond–Blackfan patients will respond to treatment with corticosteroids, though there is a substantial minority who require long-term transfusion support.

Once the diagnosis is established, infants should receive corticosteroid therapy, prednisolone 20 mg daily, to achieve remission. Response is normally prompt, with reticulocytes appearing within 7–10 days. Once the haemoglobin level has risen the steroids should be reduced steadily. Prolonged high dose steroids lead to complications of severe growth retardation, diabetes and infection, the normal consequences of corticosteroid treatment. These problems can be overcome in some part by using intermittent therapy. Alternate-day corticosteroids permit better growth but, if possible, steroids should be given on a weekly basis with 1 or 2 weeks between courses.

For patients who do not respond to corticosteroid therapy or for whom the side-effects are unacceptable, a prolonged transfusion regimen or bone marrow transplantation is the main alternative. Cyclosporin has been reported to produce remission in a few patients. Recurrent transfusions need to be supplemented by iron chelation therapy from an early age (as with patients with thalassaemia) to avoid iron overload.

A few patients show progressive enlargement of the spleen with a prolonged transfusion course and splenectomy may be indicated if features of hypersplenism develop or if the transfusion requirements increase. Occasionally remission may follow splenectomy.

The pathogenesis of the condition is unknown. The response to prednisone or cyclosporin suggests the possibility of an immune basis but this has never been fully demonstrated.

Acquired Pure Red Cell Aplasia

Failure of erythropoiesis may occur as a primary acquired event or may be associated with other disorders (Table 4.8). The condition presents as anaemia with reticulocytopenia and bone marrow lacking erythrocyte precursors.

Primary Acquired Pure Red Cell Aplasia

The majority of patients with this rare condition are aged between 20 and 50. They have symptoms of a slowly progressive anaemia. There are no additional physical findings. The Coombs' test may be weakly positive but it is not normally possible to demonstrate a humoral inhibitor to erythropoiesis in the peripheral blood or cellular inhibition in the marrow. About half the patients respond to treatment with corticosteroids and some to cyclosporin. The remainder are transfusion dependent and require iron chelation therapy.

Secondary Acquired Pure Red Cell Aplasia

Thymoma.   Between a third and half of the patients with acquired pure red cell aplasia have a thymoma. The majority show spindle cell

Table 4.8
Pure red cell aplasia

Type	Syndromes	Examples
Inherited	Diamond–Blackfan syndrome	
Acquired	Primary, idiopathic	
	Autoimmune	Acquired hypogammaglobulinaemia
		Systemic lupus erythematosus
		Associated with other immune cytopenias
	Thymoma	
	Lymphocyte disorders	T.cell lymphocytosis (large granular lymphocytes)
		Chronic lymphocytic leukaemia
		Lymphoma
	Drug induced	Immune
		Cytotoxic

morphology but some have a lymphoma. The tumour may most commonly be diagnosed on plain x-ray but tomography or CT scanning may be required. There may be associated abnormalities of other systems linked to the thymoma, for example myasthenia gravis.

The response to thymectomy is unpredictable. About half the patients respond to surgery but some relapse later. Some patients develop pure red cell aplasia only after removal of the thymoma and some show no response. Corticosteroids together with azathioprin may be tried in non-responders but frequently are ineffective. Other forms of immunosuppression including ALG, cyclosporin and vincristine have been tried with occasional success. It is worth trying these agents in succession in resistant cases.

Neutropenia Associated with Marrow Failure

There are a number of disorders in which neutropenia appears to be caused by failure of production of granulocytes rather than their peripheral destruction, but it should be emphasized that immune neutropenia, often drug induced, is much more common than production failure. The bone-marrow-derived neutropenias may be congenital or acquired.

Congenital Neutropenias

These are mostly poorly characterized and collectively are rare. Three main groups may be distinguished—reticular dysgenesis, Kostmann's syndrome and congenital benign neutropenias of childhood.

Reticular Dysgenesis

This is an extremely rare disorder with total failure of all white cells, both lymphocytes and granulocytes, associated with aplasia. The infants die shortly after birth of overwhelming sepsis.

Kostmann's Syndrome

Severe neutropenia is usually identified in the first month or so after birth as a result of recurrent infections, mainly of the throat, ears or skin though urinary tract or gastrointestinal infections are not uncommon. The peripheral blood shows a marked or complete neutropenia though eosinophils, basophils and monocytes are well preserved and often increased. Lymphocytes are normal. The bone marrow is cellular with a marked decrease in neutrophil precursors. There is some discussion about granulocyte-colony-forming cells, but in at least some cases these seem to be present. The children often survive with the help of repeated antibiotic therapy, and bone marrow transplantation has been carried out successfully. Spontaneous remission in the teens has been reported but in most cases the disease is fatal with a high incidence of acute leukaemia. The inheritance is probably autosomal recessive.

Congenital Benign Neutropenia of Childhood

This name is given to cover what are probably several different disorders characterized by neutropenia, active marrow with absence of granulocytes and their later precursors, and preservation of macrocyte function. Eosinophils are not increased. As the name implies, most children do well with the help of antibiotics. Various subgroups of the syndrome have been reported, including some families with dominant inheritance. The spleen may enlarge as the child gets older but, at least in my experience, patients do very poorly after splenectomy, with a high incidence of over-whelming sepsis. In some families the neutropenia is accompanied by immunoglobulin deficiency and treatment of the latter often reduces the rate of infections considerably.

Acquired Neutropenia

Some drugs produce neutropenia apparently by a direct toxic effect on the bone marrow or possibly through immune processes affecting the committed precursor cells. Virus infections may be followed by prolonged neutropenia, lasting many years or even life long. Rubella seems to be particularly liable to cause this syndrome.

Drug-induced Neutropenia

Carbimazole probably produces neutropenia more commonly through a toxic action on granulocyte precursors than by a peripheral antibody-mediated mechanism. Once the neutropenia develops it may take up to 6 weeks to recover following withdrawal of the drug. Metiamide, the first of the H-2 antagonists, also produced an unacceptably high incidence of neutropenia. Its successors, cimetidine and ranitidine, appear to be free of this complication, possibly because, unlike metiamide, they are not concentrated in the marrow.

Acquired Neutropenia of Unknown Cause

Prolonged neutropenia may arise spontaneously or following a viral infection, particularly rubella. There are several clinical syndromes. Patients who have a reduction in monocytes as well as neutrophils tend to suffer many infections, whereas those that have a monocytosis have a relatively benign disorder. In some cases the neutrophil count 'cycles', with a fixed periodicity, normally between 21 and 28 days. The monocytes often fluctuate in the opposite direction. The bone marrow is usually cellular with a marked reduction in granulocyte precursors, though there may be 'maturation arrest' at the metamyelocyte or promyelocyte stage. The appearance of the marrow may vary from time to time in the same individual, as may the number of granulocyte colonies obtained in vitro. In a few cases chronic prolonged neutropenia may slowly progress to a full marrow failure. Treatment is mainly symptomatic with management of infection by antibiotics.

Amegakaryocytic Thrombocytopenias

Thrombocytopenia with absent megakaryocytes may be congenital or acquired.

Congenital Amegakaryocytic Thrombocytopenia

Two main groups of infants may be identified though it is not clear whether they are totally separate disorders. In the first group the amegakaryocytic thrombocytopenia is associated with total absence of the radius (TAR), whereas in other children it is an isolated phenomenon.

Death from haemorrhage is most likely to occur at birth or in the first year of life but if the infant can be supported with platelet concentrates during the first year, the outlook may improve. Bone marrow

transplantation from an HLA identical sibling has been carried out successfully.

Acquired Amegakaryocytic Thrombocytopenia

This may develop at any age and result in a prolonged thrombocytopenia. The condition may remain stable for many years or may progress to total aplasia, a myelodysplastic syndrome or an acute myeloid leukaemia may develop. The marrow in the early stages is normal or hypercellular with absent megakaryocytes. Treatment is supportive, though isolated case reports have suggested an improvement with antilymphocyte globulin.

Cytopenias Associated with Chronic T Cell Lymphocytosis

A variety of single cell cytopenias have been reported in association with a proliferation of morphologically mature T lymphocytes, usually showing the features of large granular lymphocytes (LGL). Neutropenia is the most common cytopenia, thrombocytopenia next and pure red cell aplasia next. Multiple cytopenias have been described. The lymphocytes usually have the phenotype, E^+, $CD1^-$, $CD3^+$, $CD8^+$, $CD4^-$ and may or may not express HLA-DR. The lymphocyte population expansion is clonal and probably represents a malignant disease, but the lymphocyte population and the accompanying cytopenia may remain stable for many years (see also Chapter 15). A more generalized immune disorder is indicated in some of these patients who develop arthropathy with positive rheumatoid factor. Splenectomy may be indicated in patients with large spleens. Chemotherapy has been used but the most efficacious regimens have not been determined.

DYSERYTHROPOIESIS

Dyserythropoiesis is caused by defects in erythropoiesis which lead to the production of abnormal erythroid cells—some of these cells are destroyed within the marrow during maturation, whilst those which reach maturity and enter the circulation may show morphological abnormalities, and are liable to have a shortened lifespan. Conditions which may be referred to as dyserythropoiesis include a wide range of diseases which primarily affect either the nucleus or the cytoplasm. Examples where the nucleus is affected are vitamin B_{12} and folate deficiencies (see Chapter 3). In these cases there is a defect in DNA production due to enzymatic abnormalities in the pathways of pyrimidine and purine synthesis.

Disorders which primarily involve cytoplasm include disturbances in haemoglobin production which may be due to impaired availability of any component of the haemoglobin molecule. The most common cause is iron deficiency. When there is an adequate amount of iron available but it is not utilized, sideroblastic anaemia may occur: there is failure of mitochondrial synthesis of protophorphyrin with accumulation of iron within the mitochondria seen as ring sideroblasts (see Chapter 2). Impairment in globin synthesis results in thalassaemic syndromes (see Chapter 7). It is apparent that dyserythropoiesis is a very common phenomenon and is associated primarily or secondarily with a large number of different diseases which seem to have little in common with each other to justify their inclusion in a single category. The term is, however, a useful one as it suggests an important aspect of the pathogenesis of the anaemias, and indicates the fact that there is an interrelationship of the various aspects of the erythropoietic mechanism, whereby a defect at any stage will lead to a similar end-result.

Morphological Features

These include binuclearity and multinuclearity, asynchrony between nuclear and cytoplasmic maturation and premature nuclear extrusion; nuclear budding, fragmentation and degeneration (karyorrhexis); and various abnormalities of mitosis. There is also persistence of intercellular connection by cytoplasm and abnormalities of the cytoplasm itself, such as vacuolation, basophilic stippling and the presence of an excessive amount of siderotic granules. The extent to which these abnormalities are apparent in a bone marrow varies considerably between cases, but all the features can be seen readily in certain conditions, e.g. megaloblastic anaemias, and AML, FABM6 or myelodysplasia.

By electron microscopy other structural abnormalities are revealed (Fig. 4.7). Anomalies of nuclear division include incomplete separation of nuclei, which ranges from slight indentations, to deep clefts in the nuclear substance, to chromatin bridges between two nuclei, or the nuclei might be completely divided but the cells remain joined by cytoplasmic junctions, with a persistent spindle bridge containing microtubules.

In the cytoplasm, siderotic material is prominent, both free-lying and in mitochondria, whilst the mitochondria themselves are swollen with disintegrating internal structure, and loss of normal configuration. Microtubules similar in size to those of the spindle bridge are found within the cytoplasm and there is persistence of endoplasmic reticulum and stacks of annulated lamellae occur adjacent to the nucleus. The nuclear membrane itself is abnormal and loses its integrity, so that one sees mitochondria and cytoplasmic vesicles in the nuclear area and, conversely, oozing of nuclear material into the cytoplasm. The nuclear pores are widened and contain disintegrating structures. The picture of dyserythropoiesis is completed by the ribosomal anomalies. Some cells have few or no ribosomes, in others ribosomes may not have characteristic distribution in the cytoplasm, but may instead be found in arrays attached to the nuclear membrane.

Other Indications of Dyserythropoiesis

Ferrokinetic studies show an accelerated clearance of plasma iron with a decreased erythrocyte incorporation in the order of 25–50%, and there is an accumulation and retention of the iron in the bone marrow (Fig. 4.8). A useful parameter of ineffective erythropoiesis is the serum bilirubin. An unconjugated hyperbilirubinaemia is observed in many dyserythropoietic conditions and this is evidence of increased haemoglobin catabolism. High carbon monoxide production in the absence of peripheral blood haemolysis is a pointer to ineffective erythropoiesis. Intramedullary destruction of cytoplasm results in the liberation of various enzymes, notably lactic dehydrogenase and aldolase, and destruction of nuclear material leads to an increased level of uric acid.

Congenital Dyserythropoietic Anaemia

In addition to the non-specific phenomenon of dyserythropoiesis described above, there is a group of disorders of variable severity with recessive inheritance, known as congenital dyserythropoietic anaemias. They are characterized by chronic anaemia with a relatively low reticulocyte count, jaundice and haemosiderosis. Peripheral blood films show anisocytosis, poikilocytosis and irregularly crenated and contracted cells. The marrow shows one of three patterns (Figs. 4.9–4.11).

Type I. Megaloblastic changes, macrocytosis, internuclear chromatin bridges, but binuclearity not prominent; pro-erythroblasts and basophilic erythroblasts especially affected.

Type II. Binuclearity, especially of late erythroblasts, multinuclearity, pluripolar mitoses, karyorrhexis.

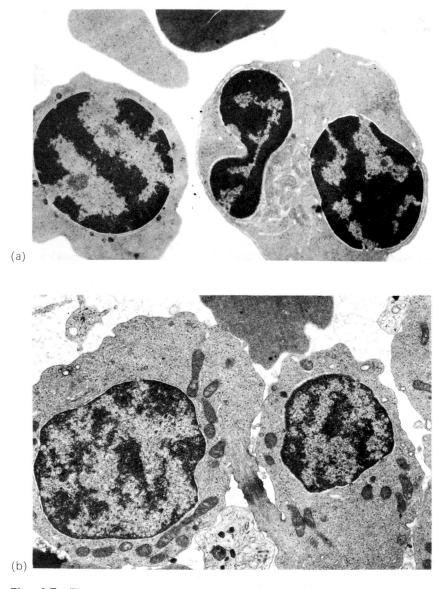

(a)

(b)

Fig. 4.7. *Electron microscope appearances of erythroblasts showing features of dyserythropoiesis.*

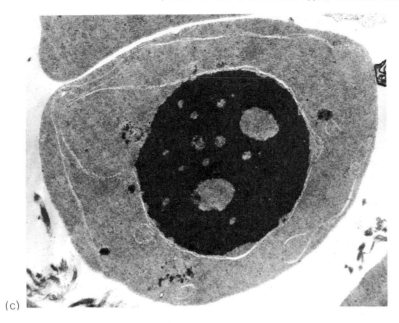

(c)

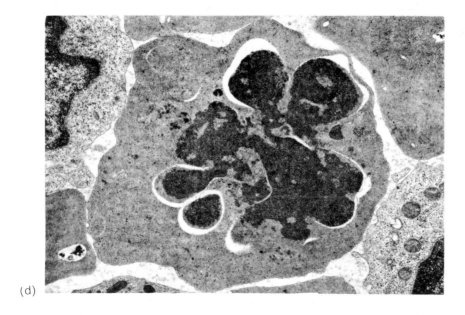

(d)

Fig. 4.7c d

Type III. Multinuclearity with up to 12 nuclei, gigantoblasts, macrocytosis.

There is an overlap between types I and II and there are variants of each type.

CDA Type II

Type II will be described first as it is the most common type of CDA. It is transmitted as an

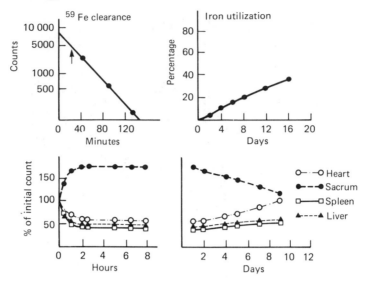

Fig. 4.8. *Ferrokinetic study in dyserythropoiesis following intravenous injection of ^{59}Fe. Plasma clearance was rapid ($T_{1/2} = 23$ min) and iron utilization was reduced. Surface counting showed concentration of the iron in bone marrow (sacrum).*

autosomal recessive disease; the geographical distribution of the recorded cases suggests a particularly high frequency in North-West Europe, in Italy and in North Africa. The clinical manifestations include a variable degree of jaundice, hepatomegaly and splenomegaly, cirrhosis and diabetes, even in patients who have neither been transfused nor treated with iron; a few patients have been mentally retarded. The serum iron and transferrin saturation are increased.

CDA II has an eponym, HEMPAS—hereditary erythroblast multinuclearity with positive acidified serum—because of the unique feature that the red cells are haemolysed by some acidified normal sera but, unlike PNH where lysis in the acidified serum test is due to marked sensitivity to complement, in HEMPAS there is a specific antigen on the erythrocytes and only sera which contain an IgM anti-HEMPAS antibody in sufficient amount (about 30% of normal people) will induce lysis of HEMPAS cells. HEMPAS is readily distinguished from PNH because lysis does not occur when the patient's own serum is used (Table 4.9, p.118) and also because lysis occurs with only about one-third of normal sera. Another point of difference is that lysis may be enhanced if the cell–serum mixture is

chilled before it is incubated at 37°C. Furthermore, sucrose lysis is negative.

In common with other types of dyserythropoiesis, there is enhanced I and i antigen activity, demonstrated in vitro by increased agglutination and by a positive cold-antibody (anti-I) lysis test (Table 4.9).

CDA II shows the ultrastructural abnormal features described above. In addition, there is a characteristic peripheral arrangement of endoplasmic reticulum giving the appearance of a 'double membrane' (Fig. 4.12a).

There is a defect in the glycoprotein of the cell membrane with decreased glycosylation of bands 3 and 4.5 and reduced sialic acid. The fundamental defect has not yet been elucidated.

CDA Type I

CDA I has been identified far less frequently than CDA II. It has an autosomal recessive inheritance; no method is available to identify heterozygous subjects. Haematologically it differs from type II by its bone marrow morphological appearance, and electron microscopy shows a high proportion of cells with 'Swiss cheese' nuclear abnormality (Fig.

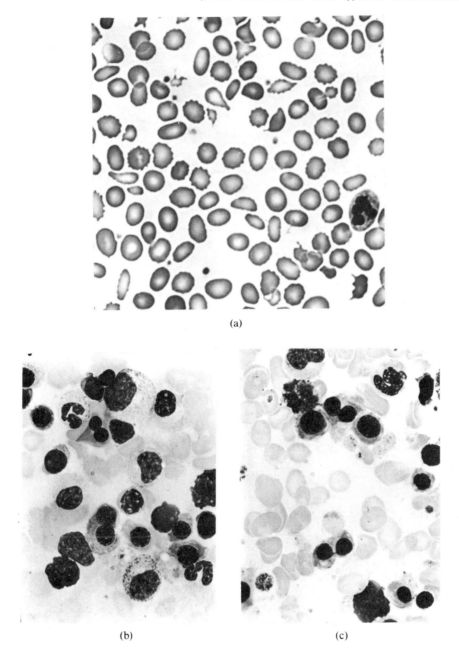

Fig. 4.9. *Morphology of blood and bone marrow in congenital dyserythropoietic anaemia type I.*

4.12b). Serological reactions are negative, especially in the acidified serum lysis test. It has been suggested that the primary defect is in the nucleoprotein or the nuclear membrane, with various secondary effects, including failure of protein synthesis and altered globin chain synthesis.

CDA Type III

Type III is the rarest form. It is notable for the multinuclearity and gigantoblasts in the bone marrow. Indeed, the erythroblasts are especially remarkable for being present with up to 12 nuclei in a

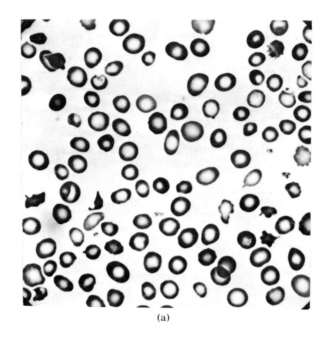

(a)

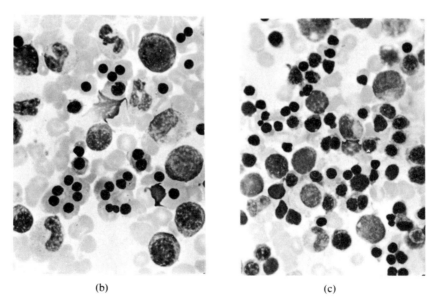

(b)   (c)

Fig. 4.10. *Morphology of blood and bone marrow in congenital dyserythro-poietic anaemia type II (HEMPAS).*

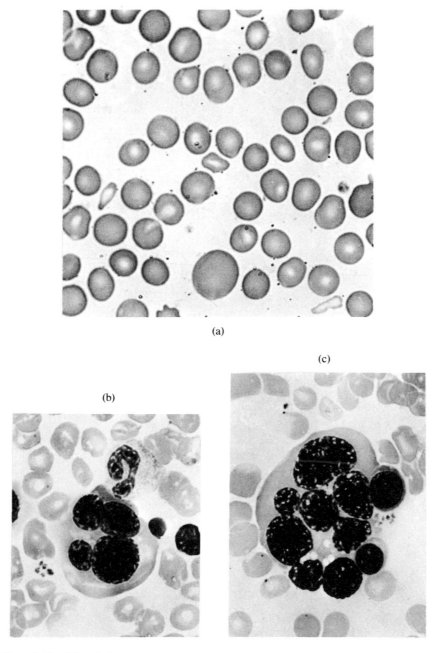

Fig. 4.11. *Morphology of blood and bone marrow in congenital dyserythropoietic anaemia type III.*

Table 4.9

Comparison of in-vitro lysis tests in different diseases

| | Acidified-serum test | | Anti-I | | Anti-i | | Sucrose lysis test |
	Donor serum	Patient serum	Lysis	Agglutination	Lysis	Agglutination	
Normal adult	−	−	−	±	−	−	−
PNH	+++	++	++++	+	±	±	+++
Congenital dyserythropoietic anaemia							
Type I	−	−	±	±	−	−	−
Type II	+ (with selected sera)	−	++	++	++	++	−
Type III	−	−	++	++	++	++	−
Secondary dyserythropoiesis	−	−	++	+++	+	+++	−

The results shown indicate common types of reaction, but degree of positivity varies in individual cases.

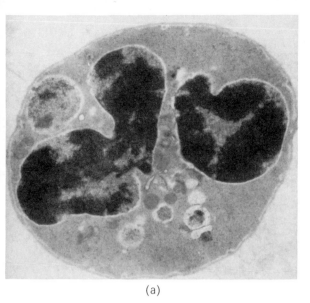
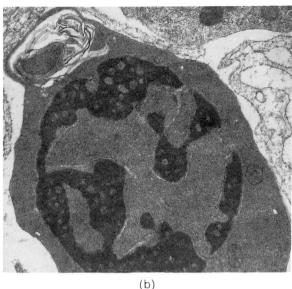

(a)   (b)

Fig. 4.12. *Electron microscope appearances of erythroblasts in congenital dys-erythropoietic anaemia (a) type II and (b) type I.*

cell (see Fig. 4.11). Morphologically the condition is more likely to be confused with erythroleukaemia than with other types of CDA, but the clinical picture is of a mild anaemia with good prognosis, and there is no granulocytopenia or thrombocytopenia.

As with other types of CDA, there is ineffective erythropoiesis. In the few cases studied, the red cells have been strongly haemolysed by both anti-I and anti-i sera but the acidified-serum lysis test has been negative.

SELECTED BIBLIOGRAPHY

Aplastic Anaemia

Camitta B. M., Thomas E. D., Nathan D. G. *et al.* (1976). Severe aplastic anemia: a prospective study of the effect of early marrow transplantation on acute mortality. *Blood*, **48**, 63–70.

Gordon-Smith E. C. (1987). Treatment of severe aplastic anemia by bone marrow transplantation. *Hematological Oncology*, **5**, 255–263.

Marsh J. C. W., Hows J. M., Bryett K. A. *et al.* (1987). Survival after antilymphocyte globulin therapy for aplastic anemia depends on disease severity. *Blood*, **70**, 1046–1052.

Speck B., Gluckman E., Haak H. L., van Rood J. J. (1977). Treatment of aplastic anaemia by antilymphocyte globulin with or without allogeneic bone marrow infusion. *Lancet*, **ii**, 1145–1148.

Storb R., Prentice R. L., Thomas E. D. (1977). Marrow transplantation for treatment of aplastic anemia. An analysis of factors associated with graft rejection. *New England Journal of Medicine*, **296**, 61–66.

Williams D. M., Lynch R. E., Cartwright G. E. (1973). Drug-induced aplastic anemia. *Seminars in Hematology*, **10**, 195–223.

Bone Marrow Transplantation (General)

Blume K. G., Petz L. D. (Eds.) (1983). *Clinical bone marrow transplantation*. New York, Edinburgh, London: Churchill Livingstone.

Moller G. (Ed.) (1985). *Graft versus host reaction. Immunological Reviews*, No. 88. Copenhagen: Munksgaard.

Fanconi's Anaemia

Auerbach A. D., Adler B., Chaganti R. S. K. (1981). Prenatal and postnatal diagnosis and detection of Fanconi anemia by a cytogenetic method. *Pediatrics*, **67**, 128.

Fanconi G. (1967). Familial constitutional panmyelocytopathy, Fanconi's anemia. I. Clinical aspects. *Seminars in Hematology*, **4**, 233.

T Cell Lymphocytosis

Newland A. C., Catovsky D., Linch D. *et al.* (1984). Chronic T cell lymphocytosis: a review of 21 cases. *British Journal of Haematology*, **58**, 433–446.

Reynolds C. W., Foon K. A. (1984). T gamma lymphoproliferative disease and related disorders in human and experimental animals. A review of the clinical, cellular and functional characteristics. *Blood*, **64**, 1146.

Dyserythropoiesis

Fukuda M. N., Papayannopoulou T., Gordon-Smith E. C., Rochart H., Testa U. (1984). Defect in glycosylation of erythrocyte membrane proteins in congenital dyserythropoietic anaemia type II (HEMPAS).

British Journal of Haematology, **56**, 55–68.

Lewis S. M., Verwilghen R. L. (1973). Dyserythropoiesis and dyserythropoietic anemias. *Progress in Hematology*, **8**, 99–129.

Lewis S. M., Verwilghen R. L. (Eds.) (1977). *Dyserythropoiesis.* London: Academic Press.

Porter R., Fitzsimons D. W. (Eds.) (1976). *Congenital disorders of erythropoiesis.* Ciba Foundation Symposium 37 (new series). Amsterdam: Elsevier/Excerpta Medica/North Holland.

Wickramasinghe S. N., Pippard M. J. (1986). Studies of erythroblast function in congenital dyserythropoietic anaemia, type I: evidence of impaired DNA, RNA, and protein synthesis and unbalanced globin chain synthesis in untrastructurally abnormal cells. *Journal of Clinical Pathology*, **39**, 881–890.

Chapter 5

THE HAEMOGLOBINOPATHIES

J. S. WAINSCOAT

The study of haemoglobin has been of major importance in biology and medicine. Haemoglobin and myoglobin were the first proteins to have their three-dimensional structures determined, and they have played a key role in understanding the relationships between protein structure and function.

Sickle cell anaemia became the prototype molecular disease with the demonstration in 1949 by Pauling that HbS could be electrophoretically separated from HbA. The subsequent discovery by Ingram in 1957 that HbS was caused by a single amino acid substitution was of historic significance to the development of studies of molecular pathology of disease.

Over the last ten years there has been an explosion in knowledge of the human genome at the DNA level. The globin genes were amongst the first genes to be cloned and sequenced, and the molecular basis of many of the thalassaemia disorders has been determined. Prenatal diagnosis of the severe thalassaemia disorders by DNA analysis is now feasible. Unfortunately there have been no major therapeutic advances in recent years for thalassaemia or sickle cell anaemia. This serves to highlight the major challenge ahead, which is the correction of these serious haemoglobin disorders by gene therapy.

HAEMOGLOBIN

Structure and Function

The haemoglobin molecule has four globin subunits, each covalently linked at a specific site to a haem group, consisting of an iron atom surrounded by a porphyrin ring. The transport of oxygen by haemoglobin is dependent on the ability of ferrous iron to combine reversibly with molecular oxygen instead of being irreversibly oxidized.

The haemoglobin molecule undergoes structural changes ('breathes') during oxygen uptake and release (Fig. 5.1). Upon deoxygenation the β chains rotate apart by about 0.7 nm. This conformational change is responsible for many of the functional properties of haemoglobin. Deoxyhaemoglobin is in the taut (T) configuration, stabilized by the presence of salt bonds. The addition of a ligand such as oxygen results in the salt bonds being broken, and the full liganded haemoglobin is in the relaxed (R) configuration.

Haemoglobin binds oxygen in the lungs and delivers it to the tissues, and although oxygen can dissolve directly in the plasma, this is insufficient to sustain life. Myoglobin in voluntary muscle stores oxygen and releases it when needed for metabolic oxidation. It is structurally related to haemoglobin but has a single protein chain with a linked haem group (Fig. 5.2). The essential features of this oxygen-transport system are summarized below.

1. Haemoglobin has a high affinity for oxygen in the lungs, and a low affinity for oxygen in the tissues.

2. Myoglobin has a higher affinity for oxygen than haemoglobin at low oxygen concentrations.

3. Haemoglobin transports carbon dioxide back to the lungs where it is expelled.

4. Haemoglobin releases its oxygen preferentially to exercising muscle rather than to resting muscle.

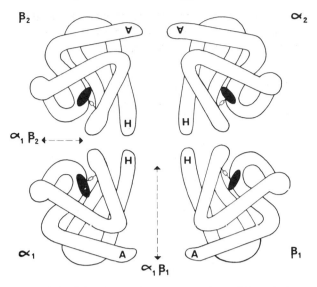

Fig 5.1. *Diagrammatic representation of the relationship between the α and β chains in the haemoglobin tetramer. The α1 β1 (α2 β2) contact is the stabilizing contact; the α1 β2 (α2 β1) is the contact across which the β chains slide during oxygenation and deoxygenation.*

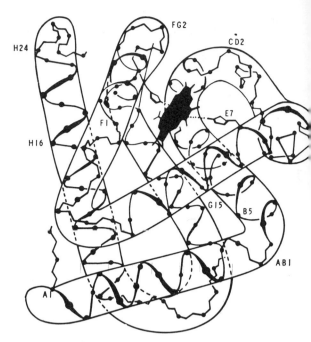

Fig. 5.2. *Diagrammatic representation of the tertiary configuration of the myoglobin of sperm whale showing: helical segments A–H; interhelical segments A, B etc., and position of haem group (black) in haem pocket. (Adapted from Dickerson, 1964.)*

The oxygen saturation curve of myoglobin is hyperbolic, which is to be expected from the one-to-one association of myoglobin and oxygen (Fig. 5.3). The oxygen saturation curve of haemoglobin is a sigmoid shape as a result of the effect of oxygen binding on the interaction between its subunits. The binding of oxygen to the haem groups is dependent on the oxygenation state of the other three haem groups. The first oxygen binds weakly to haem whereas the binding of the three successive molecules is increasingly strong. Effectively this results in most haemoglobin molecules carrying no oxygen (deoxyhaemoglobin) or four oxygens (oxyhaemoglobin). This process can also be considered in terms of the two haemoglobin conformations, deoxy (T) and oxy (R). During the oxygenation of the haemoglobin molecule there is a sudden change from the T to the R configuration, at which point the oxygen affinity of the partially liganded molecule suddenly increases.

Deoxyhaemoglobin has a higher affinity for protons than does oxyhaemoglobin and, therefore, under acidic conditions the equilibrium between deoxy- and oxyhaemoglobin shifts in favour of

deoxyhaemoglobin. This phenomenon is known as the Bohr effect.

$$HbO_2 + H^+ \rightleftharpoons HbH^+ + O_2$$

The Bohr effect serves a physiologically useful purpose since oxygen dissociates from haemoglobin when muscle acidity indicates it is needed. Three other naturally occurring substances—carbon dioxide, chloride ions and 2,3-diphosphoglycerate (2,3-DPG)—bind to deoxyhaemoglobin better than to oxyhaemoglobin, thus favouring release of oxygen from oxyhaemoglobin. Carbon dioxide has two effects on haemoglobin function. First, it results in the formation of carbonic acid:

$$CO_2 + H_2O \rightleftharpoons HCO_3^- + H^+$$

This leads to a reduced oxygen affinity due to a pH fall (the Bohr effect). Carbon dioxide can also bind to free amino groups on haemoglobin to form carbamino complexes:

$$RNH_2 + CO_2 \rightleftharpoons RNHCOO^- + H^+$$

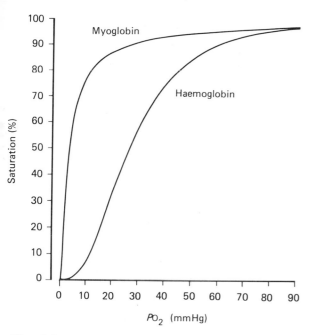

Fig. 5.3. *The oxygen dissociation curves of haemoglobin and myoglobin.*

Deoxyhaemoglobin forms carbamino complexes more readily than oxyhaemoglobin and hence oxygen affinity is reduced.

Protons and carbon dioxide act quickly to alter oxygen dissociation. However, a longer term control of oxygen release results from the interaction of haemoglobin with 2,3-DPG. The binding of 2,3-DPG to haemoglobin may be represented by the following equation:

$$Hb\,DPG + 4O_2 \rightleftharpoons Hb(O_2)_4 + DPG$$

The preferential binding of 2,3-DPG to deoxyhaemoglobin explains its effect in reducing oxygen affinity. Individuals living at high altitudes have higher levels of 2,3-DPG in their red cells than those at lower altitudes. In the fetus, the transfer of oxygen across the placenta is helped by the increased oxygen affinity of HbF in comparison to HbA. This difference is accounted for by the fact that 2,3-DPG binds less well to the γ chains of HbF than to the β chains of HbA.

Genetic Control of Human Haemoglobin Synthesis

All human haemoglobins have a similar tetrameric structure consisting of two α-like globin chains and two β-like chains; each globin chain is associated with one haem molecule. The haemoglobins found at various stages of development are:

embryonic

(to 8 weeks) $\zeta_2\varepsilon_2$ Hb Gower I

            $\zeta_2\gamma_2$ Hb Portland

            $\alpha_2\varepsilon_2$ Hb Gower II

fetal	$\alpha_2\gamma_2$ HbF	85%
	$\alpha_2\beta_2$ HbA	5–10%
adult	$\alpha_2\beta_2$ HbA	97%
	$\alpha_2\delta_2$ HbA$_2$	2.5%
	$\alpha_2\gamma_2$ HbF	0.5%

The α-like globin chains are ζ and α; the β-like globin chains are ε, γ, δ and β. The ζ is the first α-like chain to be expressed, followed by α. The β-like pathway has two switches, firstly ε to γ and, later, γ to β.

Fetal haemoglobin (HbF) is the major haemoglobin from the eighth week of gestation until term. HbF is a mixture of two molecules which differ by one amino acid residue in their γ chains; residue 136 is either glycine or alanine. The γ chains which contain glycine or alanine at position 136 are called Gγ and Aγ chains respectively, and are coded for by different genes. In adults HbA is the predominant haemoglobin, although there is a minor component, HbA$_2$, which has α chains combined with δ chains.

The globin chains are coded for by structural genes in the α- and β-globin gene clusters. Interestingly, in both gene clusters the genes are arranged in the same order (5′ to 3′) as they are expressed sequentially during development.

The α-globin gene cluster is located on the short arm of chromosome 16, the gene order is 5′ ζ2-$\psi\xi$1-$\psi\alpha$2-$\psi\alpha$1-α2-α1 3′ (Fig. 5.4). The two functional α-globin genes (α2 and α1) are separated from an embryonic α-like gene (ζ2) by three non-functional pseudogenes ($\psi\zeta$1, $\psi\alpha$2 and $\psi\alpha$1), the normal α-genotype is written $\alpha\alpha/\alpha\alpha$. The β-globin gene cluster is located on the short arm of chromosome 11, the gene order is 5′ε-Gγ-Aγ-$\psi\beta$-δ-β3′ (Fig. 5.5). The pseudogenes $\psi\zeta$1, $\psi\alpha$2, $\psi\alpha$1, ζ and $\psi\beta$ are structurally closely related to functional globin genes but contain mutations which prevent their expression.

Scattered along both gene clusters every hundred bases or so are single base changes, many of which

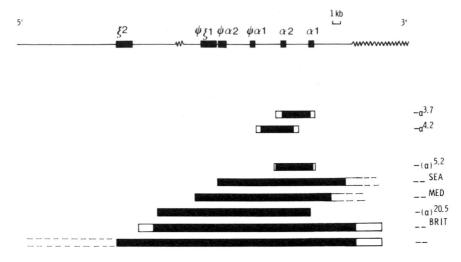

Fig. 5.4. *The α-globin gene cluster showing the various deletions responsible for α thalassaemia. The* $-\alpha^{3.7}$ *and the* $-\alpha^{4.2}$ *deletions give rise to* α^+ *thalassaemias, the other deletions to* α^o *thalassaemia. (SEA, South East Asia; MED, Mediterranean; BRIT, Britain.)*

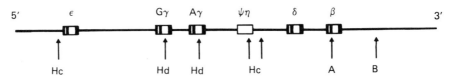

Fig. 5.5. *The β-globin gene cluster showing the position of various common restriction endonuclease polymorphic sites. (Hc, Hinc II; Hd, Hind III; A, Ava II; B, Bam H1.)*

give rise to sites which are either recognized by restriction enzymes or which remove previously existing ones. The standard nomenclature designates the presence of a restriction site by a plus (+) symbol and its absence by a minus (−) symbol. The restriction fragment length polymorphisms (RFLPs) generated by these sites are inherited in Mendelian fashion and can be used as linkage markers to identify chromosomes which carry thalassaemia or other mutations. The combination of the various RFLPs along one chromosome is referred to as a haplotype.

All globin genes have three exons (coding regions) and two intervening sequences, or introns (non-coding regions; Fig. 5.6). The initial RNA is transcribed from both the introns and exons. Sub-

sequently this transcript is processed by capping (the addition of methylated guanine) of the 5′ end, splicing out of the sequences transcribed from the introns, and polyadenylation of the 3′ end (the addition of about 200 adenine residues).Thus the RNA now enters the cytoplasm as messenger RNA (mRNA) and the process of translation can begin producing globin chains.

Although the introns and the 5′ and 3′ flanking sequences do not code for protein they are of functional importance. For example, the comparison of many genes has shown that sequences at exon–intron boundaries are important for accurate and efficient splicing. 5′ to each globin gene is the promoter which consists of those sequences which are necessary for the accurate and efficient initiation

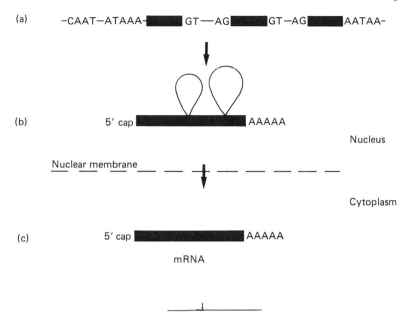

Fig. 5.6. *Prototype globin gene showing the three exons as solid blocks. (a) The CAAT and TATA boxes 5' to the gene and the invariant dinucleotides at the start and end of the introns (GT/AG). (b) The nuclear processing of the transcribed RNA, which occurs before export to the cytoplasm of mature mRNA (c).*

of transcription. Comparison of sequences 5' to functional genes of different species has revealed conserved sequences in this region. The first such sequence is AT rich and is sometimes known as the TATA box. The sequence begins at position −28 to −31 base pairs (by convention, nucleotides 5' to the gene are numbered as minus the number from the first transcribed nucleotide). The second conserved sequence is a pentanucleotide segment CCAAT, otherwise known as the CAAT box, found at around position −70. Finally, the 3' flanking regions of globin genes all have the sequence AATAAA, which gives rise to the sequence AAUAAA in the RNA transcript and is believed to be a recognition site for cutting the primary transcript about 20 nucleotides downstream from this signal, and for the addition of the Poly A 'tail'. Mutations have now been described in all these critical sequences giving rise to types of thalassaemia.

Increased HbF in Adult Life

Many inherited disorders of the β-globin gene cluster give rise to increased levels of HbF (see below). However, acquired disorders may occasionally be associated with raised levels of HbF. These disorders are usually associated with acute erythroid expansion such as recovery after marrow transplantation, chemotherapy-induced marrow aplasia, or transient erythroblastopenia in childhood. The levels of HbF very rarely exceed 10%.

STRUCTURAL HAEMOGLOBIN VARIANTS (Table 5.1)

The haemoglobin variants (other than sickle cell haemoglobin) may be classified into the following categories: haemoglobins with increased oxygen affinity, haemoglobins with decreased oxygen affinity, unstable haemoglobins and M haemoglobins.

SICKLE CELL DISEASE

Haemoglobin SS Disease

Geographic Distribution

The β^S gene occurs widely throughout Africa, parts of Asia, the Arabian peninsula and parts of

Table 5.1

Types of structural haemoglobin variants

HbS: the sickle syndromes

Unstable haemoglobins

Abnormal oxygen affinity haemoglobins
  High affinity
  Low affinity

  M haemoglobins

Structural variants with thalassaemia phenotype
(a) α thalassaemia:
    Chain termination mutants (Hb–Constant Spring)
    extreme instability (Hb–Quong Sze)
(b) β thalassaemia:
    Hb–Lepore ($\delta\beta$ fusion)
    Abnormal mRNA processing (HbE)

Southern Europe. In Africa there are two areas with very high frequencies of β^S, one including Nigeria and Ghana and the other Gabon and Zaire. In these areas approximately one-third of all births are AS heterozygotes. The other areas with high frequencies of the β^S gene are the eastern part of Saudi Arabia and parts of East Central India. Recent genetic studies suggest that the β^S mutation may have arisen independently in Africa and Asia and that subsequent selection pressure by malaria has resulted in the observed high frequencies.

Pathophysiology

Sickle cell disease is caused by a single base mutation of adenine to thymine which results in a substitution of valine for glutamic acid at the sixth codon of the β-globin chain.

Early experiments showed that concentrated cell-free solutions of sickle haemoglobin gel when deoxygenated. A model for the aggregation of deoxyhaemoglobin S molecules has been put forward which incorporates the sequential steps of nucleation, growth and subsequent alignment of the molecules into microfibrils. It is now believed that the formation of more or less parallel microfibrils causes red cell membrane damage resulting in the classic sickle red cell deformity. These deformed and rigid cells may cause obstruction to blood flow in the microcirculation.

The outcome of physical studies of this process has been the recognition of the importance of the concentration of sickle haemoglobin within red cells. It has been proposed that the rate of gelation of HbS varies as to the 15th power of its concentration. Such studies have suggested that it may be clinically useful to delay the sickling process long enough after deoxygenation to allow the red cells to pass through the capillaries into the larger veins. It has been estimated that a 10% reduction in deoxyhaemoglobin S concentration could increase this delay time by greater than tenfold. Hence therapeutic agents which delay but do not abolish the sickling process are potentially valuable.

Diagnosis

This is usually not difficult. SS disease patients have recurrent painful crises, marked anaemia, fixed sickle cells on the blood film (Fig. 5.7), and greater than 80% HbS. The differential diagnosis of SS disease is set out in Table 5.2. Individuals with the compound heterozygosity S/D have to be distinguished since HbD comigrates with HbS on haemoglobin electrophoresis at pH 8.9. It is necessary to repeat the electrophoresis at low pH (e.g. pH 6.2 on agar) to separate the two variants. In addition, two forms of sickle cell–β thalassaemia have to

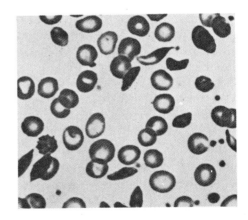

Fig. 5.7. *Peripheral blood appearances of a patient homozygous for HbS (sickle cell anaemia). Many irreversibly sickled cells and occasional target cells are present.*

Table 5.2
The differential diagnosis of homozygous sickle cell (SS) disease (adapted from Bunn and Forget, 1985)

Diagnosis	Clinical severity	PCV	Red cell morphology	Electrophoresis
SS	Marked	0.18–0.30	Target cells 2–30% ISCs	80–95% S 2–20% F 2–4% A_2
$S\beta^0$ thalassaemia	Moderate	0.20–0.35	Hypochromic, target cells, microcytic, rare ISCs	80–95% S 0% A 1–15% F 3–6% A_2
$S\beta^+$ thalassaemia	Mild	0.25–0.40	Microcytic, target cells, rare ISCs	55–75% S 10–30% A 1–13% F 3–6% A_2
SD	Moderate	0.20–0.30	Target cells, frequent ISCs	~ 50% S ~ 50% D

be recognized. In the Mediterranean region, β thalassaemia is common, whereas the incidence of sickle cell trait is low and therefore S/β thalassaemia is the most common type of sickling disorder observed. The S/β^+ thalassaemia genotype gives rise to the production of 20–30% HbA and is usually associated with a milder disease. The differential diagnosis between SS and S/β^0 thalassaemia is more difficult since the elevation of HbA_2 may not be accurately measured. Microcytic red cells observed in S/β^0 thalassaemia may also be found in SS disease when associated with α thalassaemia (particularly $-\alpha/-\alpha$). Hence family studies may be required for confirmation.

Clinical Aspects

The clinical features of SS disease are those of a chronic haemolytic anaemia complicated by intercurrent infections and sickle cell crises. However, it should be emphasized that patients with SS disease have a very variable and unpredictable clinical course. Some patients die of overwhelming infection in infancy, whereas others may have a relatively normal lifespan. Studies are in progress to determine the genetic and environmental factors which

interact to give rise to this clinical spectrum. The impact of environmental conditions on the disease is shown most dramatically by the almost total absence of SS disease in adult rural Africans due to a very high childhood mortality rate.

The possible influence of genetic factors is shown by the relatively mild clinical course of SS disease patients from parts of the Arabian peninsula, Iran and India. These patients have raised levels of HbF, although the mode of inheritance is still not clear.

Patients usually present in infancy with anaemia and jaundice. However, they may occasionally present with the so-called hand and foot syndrome. This is a painful dactylitis with swelling of the fingers or feet which may cause selective growth defects of one or more digits. During early infancy splenomegaly can be noted, although in most cases this gradually resolves due to repeated infarction of the spleen (autosplenectomy).

Anaemia

The anaemia is caused by marked reduction in red cell lifespan due to an increased rate of red cell destruction. Hence, if red cell production ceases—albeit temporarily—a dramatic fall in haemoglobin results. Aplastic crises in sickle cell anaemia are usually associated with infection, particularly due to parvovirus infection, and therefore more than one sibling may be affected. The anaemia may also be exacerbated by folic acid deficiency; this should be prevented by supplements.

Growth and Development

Sickle cell disease children in the United States have significantly delayed growth and maturation compared with black controls; SS and S/β^0 thalassaemia patients show a greater growth delay than SC and S/β^+ thalassaemia patients. By the end of adolescence the sickle cell disease children have almost caught up with controls in height but not in weight. Boys and girls both have delays in sexual maturation, although most do achieve full sexual maturation.

Infection

In young children with SS disease, pneumococcal septicaemia and meningitis are major causes of death. Septicaemia has a fulminant course with a mortality rate of around 50%. Pneumococcal prophylaxis should begin at 6 months with penicillin therapy. Unfortunately, pneumococcal vaccine cannot be relied upon as the sole prophylactic measure in these children since the vaccine may not be effective against all pneumococcal serotypes. Osteomyelitis is also more common in sickle cell anaemia. Staphylococci are the most common bacteria responsible for this complication, but SS and S/βthal patients also have a peculiar susceptibility to Salmonella osteomyelitis.

SS patients are often troubled by chronic skin ulcers around the ankle which are often slow to heal and may become recurrent. If simple measures are not effective, blood transfusions to keep the HbS level below 50% are usually helpful in healing the ulcers.

Sickle Cell Crisis

A sickle cell crisis in young children is often associated with a bacterial or viral infection, although in older children and adults this association is often absent. The factors which precipitate the majority of painful crises remain unknown, although factors such as environmental cold, dehydration, physical or emotional stress may be held responsible. Some patients have frequent severely painful crises whereas others have only rare painful crises.

Chest Syndrome

The 'chest syndrome' is a common complication of SS disease. The patients experience a sudden onset of pleural pain with fever. There is great difficulty in distinguishing pulmonary infection, infarction due to local sickling or pulmonary embolism, hence the use of the term 'chest syndrome'.

Splenic Sequestration

Acute splenic sequestration is one of the major causes of death of children with SS disease under the age of 2 years. The pathophysiological basis for this condition remains puzzling, but essentially the circulating red cells are trapped in the spleen causing circulatory collapse. Therapy is symptomatic but recurrent attacks may be prevented by splenectomy.

Organ Damage

Many organs may suffer damage in sickle cell disease. Infarcts of bone are common, with, e.g. avascular necrosis of the femoral head. In children a dactylitis is common, leading to unequal growth of digits (the 'hand-foot' syndrome). Cholelithiasis is very common, as would be expected in a chronic haemolytic anaemia. Hepatic damage may result from transfusion-related hepatitis or from hepatic infarcts. Renal failure is uncommon, but mild renal impairment is common in SS disease patients in the fourth or fifth decade. Proliferative sickle retinopathy is a complication of vaso-occlusion in the peripheral retina. Priapism occurs occasionally in both prepubertal and post-pubertal patients. Iron overload is not a problem unless frequent blood transfusions are given.

Central Nervous System

The most important CNS complication of SS disease is stroke. The majority of strokes occur in children in whom they are caused by cerebral infarcts. Although most patients survive their first stroke, it is important to realize that there is a high recurrence rate of second strokes in these patients. Many clinics now maintain children after stroke on a hypertransfusion regime which is effective in preventing a further stroke.

Treatment

There has been major progress in the understanding of the molecular pathology of sickle cell disease over the last two decades. Unfortunately this has not resulted in any advance in treatment of the disease. Therefore, at the present time the important aspect of treatment is really supportive care.

General Measures

The identification of newborns with SS is very valuable since it enables the parents to receive appropriate advice on the care of their child. In particular, the parents should be alerted to the need for early detection of infections and their prompt treatment. General hygiene measures should be encouraged to avoid infected leg ulcers. Patients should be warned to avoid hypoxia resulting from high altitudes, air travel or anaesthesia. In hot weather they should be encouraged to maintain an adequate fluid intake, and also warned against sudden exposure to the cold.

Infection

Prophylactic penicillin, e.g. 250 mg orally twice daily, may reduce the frequency of infections and crises, and is often prescribed for children with recurrent crises. Antibiotics should also be given to patients at the first signs of infection, especially to children. Pneumococcal vaccine has an important role but does not protect against all serotypes of pneumococcus. It is hoped that effective vaccines may be developed for Haemophilus and Meningococcus. Antimalarial prophylaxis should be given if indicated.

Anaemia and Transfusion Therapy

Generally patients tolerate their anaemia well, and blood transfusion is only indicated in special circumstances. If blood transfusions are given to prevent sickling, it is important to make certain that over 50% of the circulating red cells are of donor origin. The risks of blood transfusion are well known and include hepatitis, iron overload and red cell sensitization. Exchange transfusion may be indicated at times of increased risk such as pregnancy and surgery.

Painful Crisis

The management of the painful crisis consists of treatment of any associated infection, rehydration and adequate pain relief. SS patients cannot produce concentrated urine and are, therefore, prone to dehydration. In practice fluids should be given intravenously. The adequate relief of pain is extremely important and often pethidine or morphine is required as initial therapy. In the United Kingdom the risk of addiction is low, although in the United States patients have become dependent on narcotics. It should be stressed that such worries should not result in patients receiving inadequate pain relief. It has been shown that alkali therapy is not effective in the treatment of acute painful crises. Oxygen is often given, although there is no evidence it is beneficial unless there is significant hypoxia. Exceptionally, if a patient has a very bad patch of frequent crises, it may be considered justifiable to prevent further crises by a transfusion programme.

Surgery

Major surgery has an increased risk for SS patients. For major planned surgery it is advisable to lower the HbS level to around 20% either by an exchange transfusion or, alternatively, by repeated transfusions without withdrawal of blood. During surgery, special care should be taken with hydration, acid–base balance and oxygenation.

Antisickling Drugs

The history of the use of antisickling drugs in sickle cell disease should encourage caution about claims for therapeutic benefits of such agents and at the present time there is no antisickling drug of clinical value.

Knowledge of the sickling process has given some insight into the properties required of an antisickling drug. The drug should increase the oxygen affinity of haemoglobin, thus favouring the oxyconformation, or it should interfere with the intermolecular contacts involved in deoxyhaemoglobin polymerization. One compound, cyanate, was initially investigated with enthusiasm for its use in treating sickle cell anaemia. Patients treated with the drug were found to have higher haemoglobin levels with increased oxygen affinity. Unfortunately the drug was found to cause a peripheral neuropathy and its use was abandoned.

Another experimental approach which is currently being investigated is the use of 5-azacytidine to stimulate γ chain production. It was noted that the rise in HbF levels seen in baboons made acutely anaemic could be amplified by the administration of 5-azacytidine. Since active genes are demethylated, it was argued that the mechanism of this rise in HbF is related to demethylation of the γ genes. However, hydroxyurea, which is not a demethylating agent, also increases γ chain production in anaemic monkeys. It remains possible that 5-azacytidine acts by killing late red cell precursors leaving earlier precursors which have higher γ-globin gene expression to undergo terminal differentiation. To date, the increases in HbF levels observed in SS patients given 5-azacytidine have been modest. A most important consideration for clinical use is that 5-azacytidine may be carcinogenic.

Contraception and Pregnancy

Barrier methods of contraception are generally recommended for SS disease patients in view of the associated risks of thromboembolism. If these methods are unacceptable, intrauterine devices or medroxyprogesterone acetate may be considered as alternatives.

Pregnancy in SS disease women carries a higher rate of abortions and stillbirths than normal pregnancy and is associated with an increased maternal morbidity. Recently there has been a reduction in morbidity during pregnancy and this has been attributed to the policy in pregnancy of partial exchange transfusion or hypertransfusion. So far there has been no published controlled trial of exchange transfusion in pregnancy, and it remains possible that recent improvements in morbidity result from better general antenatal care.

Interaction of α Thalassaemia and SS Disease

In the US black population and many West African populations, about 30% of individuals are α thalas-

saemia 2 heterozygotes ($-\alpha/\alpha\alpha$), and about 2% are homozygotes ($-\alpha/-\alpha$). Therefore, both these types of α thalassaemia will be seen in SS disease patients, and the application of gene mapping has enabled them to be identified and characterized. It has been found that the coinheritance of α thalassaemia (particularly the $-\alpha/-\alpha$ genotype) has marked effects on the red cell indices but little effect on the vaso-occlusive complications of SS disease. There is evidence that in some populations the coinheritance of α thalassaemia may be associated with a slightly longer survival in SS disease patients.

Sickle Cell Trait

Diagnosis

Sickle cell trait (AS) individuals have normal blood counts, although some may have a small number of target cells on the blood film. The diagnosis is made by a positive test for sickling (metabisulphite slide test or a solubility test) and by haemoglobin electrophoresis. The characteristic pattern is 60% HbA and 40% HbS. The proportion of HbS decreases slightly with the coinheritance of α thalassaemia.

Clinical Features

Individuals with sickle cell trait (AS) have normal growth, development, and normal exercise tolerance. The benign nature of AS is demonstrated by the fact that its frequency is the same in US black professional football players as in the general US black population. Nevertheless, a number of clinical abnormalities have been reported to occur at a somewhat higher frequency in AS heterozygotes; these include splenic infarction at high altitude, haematuria, and bacteruria and pyelonephritis in pregnancy. General anaesthesia should not entail any special risks and even the application of a tourniquet to an injured extremity is usually well tolerated despite the theoretical risk of sickling.

Haemoglobin SC Disease

Since HbC is the second most common Hb variant in individuals of African ancestry (see below), the compound heterozygotes HbSC are found in US

Blacks. Higher frequencies have been noted in the parts of West Africa where it may be more common in adults than HbSS due to the high childhood mortality of the latter.

Clinically, HbSC is generally a mild sickling disorder with a typical Hb level of around 110 g/l. The patients have normal growth and development patterns. Although the complications of SC disease are generally less severe than those of SS disease, there are some exceptions, for example proliferative retinopathy is more common in SC disease. Other complications which are not reduced are aseptic necrosis of the femoral head, bone marrow embolism, and haematuria from renal medullary infarction.

It has been assumed that the sickling tendency in SC disease is due to copolymerization of S with C. However, there is no evidence for this hypothesis and it seems more likely to relate to a higher haemoglobin S content in red cells of individuals with HbSC disease than is found in the red cells of those with sickle cell trait (HbAS).

Haemoglobin C

This abnormal haemoglobin is caused by a substitution of lysine for glutamic acid at the sixth position of the β-globin chain. Haemoglobin C has a relatively restricted geographic distribution in West Africa, predominantly in Ghana and Upper Volta where up to a quarter of the population are AC heterozygotes (HbC trait). The frequency in US Blacks is much lower at around 2%, as would be expected since slaves were transported to the New World from a wider region of Africa. Haemoglobin C trait individuals are symptomless. The blood film shows target cells but not in such profusion as in homozygous CC individuals. The haemoglobin electrophoresis pattern shows 40% HbC and 60% HbA. Patients homozygous for HbC have a mild haemolytic anaemia. They often have splenomegaly and, as in other chronic haemolytic disorders, cholelithiasis and 'aplastic crises' may occur. The blood film is very striking in that most of the red cells are target cells. Haemoglobin electrophoresis shows HbC greater than 90%, with slightly increased HbF; HbA is absent and HbA_2 is undetectable since it comigrates with HbC.

The D Haemoglobins

The original HbD was a haemoglobin variant which co-migrated with HbS but did not sickle (HbD–Punjab or HbD–Los Angeles). Subsequently, other variants have been described with the same electrophoretic mobilities; these are all known as HbD qualified by the relevant place name of their discovery. Although none sickle by themselves, they may sickle in combination with HbS; the compound heterozygotes having a mild sickling disorder. Individuals who are compound heterozygotes for HbD/β thalassaemia have a mild anaemia in contrast to those with HbE/thalassaemia (see below) and HbS/β thalassaemia.

Haemoglobin E

Haemoglobin E is the second most common haemoglobin variant. It is found in South East Asia, with high gene frequencies in Thailand and Burma.

The β^E mutation, in addition to causing a structural haemoglobin variant, can be regarded as a β^+ thalassaemia defect since it gives rise to abnormal mRNA processing (see p. 137). AE heterozygotes have microcytic red cells with a MCV of around 70 fl. The coinheritance of α thalassaemia (very common in this population) will reduce the MCV further. Haemoglobin electrophoresis shows 30% HbE, the remainder being HbA. On routine electrophoresis, HbE co-migrates with HbC on cellulose acetate or starch gel at pH 8.6. However, C and E can be separated at pH 6.2 on citrate agar. The important interaction is HbE/β thalassaemia which is very common in parts of South East Asia. This results in a thalassaemia disorder which has a variable clinical severity but which is often as severe as homozygous β thalassaemia.

Haemoglobins with Increased Oxygen Affinity

Patients with high oxygen affinity haemoglobins usually present with an unexplained isolated erythrocytosis with a normal white count and platelet count (Hb–Chesapeake, an α-chain variant, was the first characterized example). Although the demonstration of an abnormal band on haemoglobin electrophoresis can provide strong evidence in favour of this diagnosis, a normal electrophoretic pattern does not exclude it since some variants migrate normally on either cellulose acetate or starch gels at pH 8.6. Around twenty variants have been described which give rise to this syndrome. Most of them have amino acid substitutions at critical sites: either at the $\alpha_1\beta_2$ interface or at the C-terminal end of the β chain. The vast majority of patients do not require treatment, although occasional patients have been reported to benefit from venesection.

Haemoglobins with Decreased Oxygen Affinity

A small number of haemoglobin variants with decreased oxygen affinity (such as Hb–Kansas) have been reported. The affected individuals with some of these variants have had mild anaemia which presumably is related to oxygen being more readily available to the tissues in contrast to the polycythaemia found in the high oxygen affinity variants.

Unstable Haemoglobins

The unstable haemoglobins are those variants whose instability is sufficient to cause clinically recognizable haemolysis. They are inherited as autosomal dominants. Interestingly, a proportion of unstable haemoglobins have presented as spontaneous mutants. Their most characteristic feature is their heat instability. If a dilute haemoglobin solution is heated at 50 °C for 15 minutes, most of the haemoglobin appears as a precipitate. A similar phenomenon can be induced by isopropanol. Only about half of the unstable haemoglobin variants can be detected by haemoglobin electrophoresis.

These disorders generally present as a congenital Heinz body haemolytic anaemia (CHBA), Heinz bodies resulting from denaturation of unstable haemoglobins. The Heinz bodies attach to the inner surface of the red cell membrane and decrease the pliability and filterability of the red cell. The membrane-bound Heinz bodies are removed by the spleen, explaining why the number of Heinz bodies increases markedly after splenectomy. At the molecular level there are several causes of instability, including the disruption of the α helix by the insertion of proline, substitution of an amino acid side chain which is too small or too large, introduc-

tion of a charged group inside the molecule and, finally, deletion of residues.

The clinical picture of patients with CHBA is very diverse. Some patients, for example those with Hb–Zurich, have very little haemolysis unless they are exposed to an oxidant stress such as treatment with a sulpha drug. Haemolysis may also be exacerbated in these patients by viral or bacterial infection. Occasionally the patient may present in an aplastic crisis due either to folate deficiency or infection. As expected for a chronic haemolytic state, there is an increased frequency of gallstones.

Most patients do not need any specific treatment other than general supportive care such as folic acid supplementation, avoidance of oxidant drugs and prompt treatment of infections. Since the spleen sequesters CHBA red cells, it would be anticipated that splenectomy would be beneficial in severe cases of CHBA, although this has not always been the case. One approach to this problem is to be guided by the past experience of the results of splenectomy on individuals with the same variant.

M Haemoglobins

In 1948, Horlein and Weber described a four-generation family in which congenital cyanosis was transmitted as an autosomal dominant trait. The haemolysates were found to have absorption spectra similar to methaemoglobin. Horlein and Weber showed that the abnormality was in the globin and not the haem part of haemoglobin, making this family the first reported example of an abnormal globin causing a familial haemoglobinopathy.

The M haemoglobins favour the methaemoglobin or oxidized iron state (Fe^{3+}) and usually present as cases of familial cyanosis with an autosomal dominant inheritance. Those presenting at birth probably have an α chain variant, whereas the β chain variants present at around 6 months when β chain synthesis has replaced γ chain synthesis. The diagnosis is made from absorption spectra of the haemolysate and by haemoglobin electrophoresis; the differential diagnosis is congenital methaemoglobinaemia (diaphorase I deficiency) which has a recessive inheritance pattern. Usually the α chain M haemoglobins constitute around 25% and the β chain M haemoglobins around 40–50% of the total haemoglobin.

The Hb concentration and red cell indices are usually normal. However, some individuals with Hb–Hyde Park or Hb–Saskatoon have a mild compensated haemolytic state since these two haemoglobins are also slightly unstable.

There is no specific treatment for individuals with M haemoglobins, rather it is important to prevent them suffering unnecessary investigations or receiving inappropriate treatment.

THALASSAEMIAS

The thalassaemias are genetic disorders of haemoglobin synthesis characterized by a reduction in the synthesis of particular globin chains. They constitute one of the most common single gene disorders occurring in a broad geographical region stretching from the Mediterranean through the Middle East and India to South East Asia. They also occur sporadically in most populations.

Classification of the Thalassaemias

The thalassaemias are classified according to the particular globin chain which is produced at a reduced rate, the commonest types being α, β and $\delta\beta$ thalassaemia. There is also the group of disorders known as hereditary persistence of fetal haemoglobin (HPFH) in which there is persistent excessive γ-globin chain synthesis in adult life.

In many populations in which thalassaemia is common, there is also a high prevalence of structural haemoglobin variants. These may interact with thalassaemia determinants giving rise to a wide clinical spectrum of thalassaemia syndromes. Such cases require careful and sometimes sophisticated laboratory analysis for their correct elucidation. Nevertheless, it should be emphasized that a complete family study by standard haematological techniques is often very informative.

The α Thalassaemias

Alpha-globin is one of the two chains in both fetal ($\alpha_2\gamma_2$) and adult ($\alpha_2\beta_2$) haemoglobin and, therefore, α thalassaemia results in defective fetal and adult haemoglobin production. In the fetus, excess γ chains form γ_4 tetramers (Hb–Barts), whereas in adults the excess β chains form β_4 (HbH). However, the degree of chain imbalance in most cases heterozygous for α thalassaemia is not sufficient to result in easily detectable levels of Hb–Barts or HbH (Table 5.3).

Two systems of classification for α thalassaemia have been used. The first denotes the severe heterozygotes as α thalassaemia 1, and the mild heterozygotes as α thalassaemia 2. Gene-mapping studies have shown that the α thalassaemia 1 phenotype may result from the loss of the two normal α-globin genes from one chromosome ($--/\alpha\alpha$) or one from each chromosome ($-\alpha/-\alpha$), whereas the α thalassaemia 2 phenotype may result from a single α-globin gene deletion ($-\alpha/\alpha\alpha$). The more recent classification uses the term α^0 to indicate a total absence of α-globin production from one chromosome, and the term α^+ to indicate a reduced but not absent production of α-globin from the affected

Table 5.3
The α thalassaemia syndromes

Type of thalassaemia	Heterozygote	Homozygote	Molecular defect
α-thalassaemia-1	Thalassaemia minor 5–10% Hb–Barts at birth	Hb–Barts hydrops 80% Hb–Barts	Deletion of both α-globin genes
α-thalassaemia-2	Thalassaemia minor or silent 1–2% Hb–Barts at birth	Thalassaemia minor 5–10% Hb–Barts at birth	Deletion of one α-globin gene
Hb–Constant Spring	Silent 0.5–1% Hb–Constant Spring 1–2% Hb–Barts at birth	Thalassaemia minor 5–6% Hb–Constant Spring	α chain termination mutation

chromosome. In these two different nomenclatures it may be helpful to note that α thalassaemia 1 and α^0 thalassaemia are phenotypically equivalent, as are α thalassaemia 2 and α^+ thalassaemia.

The two important clinical forms of α thalassaemia are the Hb–Barts hydrops fetalis syndrome $(--/--)$ and HbH disease $(-\alpha/--)$. Figure 5.8 shows the inheritance of HbH disease.

Hb–Barts Hydrops Syndrome

This syndrome is observed most frequently in South East Asia and in parts of the Mediterranean. The affected infants are either stillborn between 28 and 40 weeks gestation or survive only for a few hours if born alive. They show the characteristic appearance of hydrops fetalis and have haemoglobin levels in the region of 50–80 g/l. The haemoglobin is made up of 80% Hb–Barts and about 20% Hb–Portland and there is a complete absence of HbF and HbA. The parents of these infants are obligatory carriers of α^0 thalassaemia. The syndrome may be diagnosed prenatally if suspected (see below).

HbH Disease

HbH disease is found most commonly in South East Asia and to a lesser extent in the Middle East and in some of the Mediterranean island populations.

The clinical picture of HbH disease is very variable. However, the usual features are an anaemia (70–100 g/l), splenomegaly and often hepatomegaly. Nearly all the patients have normal physical development, although a proportion have thalassaemic facies. Extramedullary haematopoiesis of the sort observed in homozygous β-thalassaemia does not occur. The commonest complication is the development of severe splenomegaly with hypersplenism. Splenectomy in such cases usually results in levels of haemoglobin 20–30 g/l higher than preoperatively. The patients are not generally transfusion dependent and do not develop iron overload.

The peripheral blood film shows hypochromia, microcytosis, poikilocytosis, polychromasia and target cells. Incubation of their red cells with brilliant cresyl blue reveals the presence of inclusion bodies which are precipitates of HbH. Haemoglobin electrophoresis shows a pattern of HbA, H, A_2 and Barts. The level of HbH ranges from 5% to more than 40% of the total haemoglobin. HbH and Barts are best detected by electrophoresis at pH 6.0 to 7.0 since they are unique in migrating anodally in acid pH conditions. As expected, studies of globin chain synthesis on peripheral blood reticulocytes show a marked globin chain synthesis

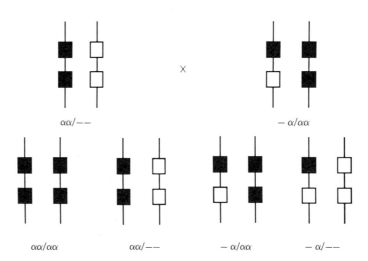

Fig. 5.8. *Inheritance of HbH $(-\alpha/--)$ disease. Normal α-globin genes are shown by closed boxes, and deleted or otherwise inactivated α-globin genes by open boxes.*

imbalance with α/β synthesis ratios ranging between 0.2 and 0.4 (normal ratio 1.0).

Acquired HbH Disease

There is also an acquired form of HbH occasionally observed in association with the preleukaemia syndromes. In this condition the red cells show a dimorphic picture with normal and hypochromic populations. The latter population of cells generates HbH inclusions on incubation with brilliant cresyl blue.

HbH Disease and Mental Retardation

In this rare syndrome the individual suffers from HbH disease and mental retardation. Family studies show that one parent has α^+ thalassaemia whereas the other parent is normal. Hence it is probable that the affected individuals have inherited the α^+ chromosome from one parent and have a de novo α^0 thalassaemia mutation on the other chromosome 16, resulting in HbH disease. However, the de novo mutation not only inactivates the α-globin genes but must also affect another, as yet unidentified, gene which is important for normal mental development.

α Thalassaemia Carrier States

It is difficult to identify α thalassaemia carrier states by standard haematological studies. Individuals possessing only two of the normal four α-globin genes $(--/\alpha\alpha$ or $-\alpha/-\alpha)$ usually have low red cell indices, an elevated red cell count and, on incubation with brilliant cresyl blue, occasional cells containing HbH inclusions may be seen. At birth the MCV and MCH are reduced and raised levels of Hb–Barts (3–10%) are detected in umbilical cord blood.

Those individuals with a single α-globin gene deletion $(-\alpha/\alpha\alpha)$ are more difficult to detect since, although the mean red cell indices of a large group of individuals with the $-\alpha/\alpha\alpha$ genotype are lower than the mean of a group of normals $(\alpha\alpha/\alpha\alpha)$, there is considerable overlap of values between the two groups. Globin chain synthesis studies characteris-

tically show α/β-globin chain production ratios of 0.7 in the α^0 thalassaemia group $(--/\alpha\alpha)$. These ratios are only slightly reduced in the α^+ thalassaemia group with a single α-globin gene deletion $(-\alpha/\alpha\alpha)$ and hence cannot be relied on to make the diagnosis.

A common problem is the individual with a hypochromic microcytic anaemia which is not due to iron deficiency and in whom the level of HbA_2 is normal. Once other causes of iron-refractory hypochromic anaemia such as sideroblastic anaemia have been excluded, α thalassaemia is the probable diagnosis particularly if the RBC count is high $(> 5.5 \times 10^{12}/l)$. Rarely, in some patients (particularly those of Greek origin), the HbA_2 level is normal in heterozygous β thalassaemia. A more definitive diagnosis may be made by globin chain synthesis studies and by gene mapping.

Molecular Basis of the α Thalassaemia Defects

Deletion Type

The majority of cases of α thalassaemia are caused by gene deletions; these remove one or both α-globin genes leading to α^+ and α^0 thalassaemia respectively (see Fig. 5.5). The single α-globin gene deletions are thought to arise by unequal crossing-over events. The 3.7 kilobase (kb) deletion involves recombination between both α genes leaving a single α-globin gene. This particular mutation is very common in many populations, occurring at frequencies of up to 60% in some Asian Indian and Saudi Arabian populations. The single α-globin deletion $(-\alpha/)$ is the only form of α thalassaemia commonly found in Blacks, the absence of α^0 thalassaemia defects $(--/)$ explaining the rarity of HbH disease $(-\alpha/--)$ in this population. The 4.2-kb deletion removes the complete $\alpha2$ globin gene. Individuals with chromosomes representing the reciprocal crossovers have triplicated α-globin gene arrangements $(\alpha\alpha\alpha/)$ and have been found at low frequencies in many populations.

The α^0 deletions range in size from those which remove part of the $\alpha1$ gene and the whole of the $\alpha2$ gene to those removing the entire α gene cluster. Interestingly, one specific deletion has been found to be responsible for many of the rare cases of α thalassaemia which occur in the British.

Non-deletion Type

Non-deletion α thalassaemia defects are defined by the absence of major deletions on gene mapping. One such α^+ thalassaemia results from the loss of five bases following the G of the invariant GT within the donor (5′) splice site in the first intron of the $\alpha2$ gene. A Hpa1 restriction enzyme site is removed and hence this is a type of α thalassaemia which can be identified directly by restriction enzyme analysis.

Hb–Quong Sze is a rare variant which results from a change of codon 125 from CTG (leucine) to CCG (proline). This amino acid change causes the globin molecule to be unstable, resulting in an α thalassaemia phenotype. Another group of α^+ thalassaemias results from single base mutations in the α^2-globin gene termination codon. An amino acid is coded for at the normal stop codon position and an α-globin chain variant is produced with 31 additional amino acid residues at the C terminal end. Hb–Constant Spring, a common variant in parts of South East Asia, is the best known example of this class of mutations and is produced in very low quantities, thus explaining the resulting α^+ thalassaemia phenotype.

The β Thalassaemias

The β thalassaemias are characterized by reduced (β^+) or absent (β^0) synthesis of β-globin. Unlike the α thalassaemias, the majority of β-thalassaemias are caused by point mutations rather than by gene deletions. Over 40 mutations are now known to cause β thalassaemia, the majority of these having been defined within the last 3 years. The rapid elucidation of the molecular basis for many of the β thalassaemia mutations has been helped by the development of an efficient strategy for cloning different thalassaemic genes. This development arises from the discovery that, within a given population, different mutations tend to be associated with different restriction enzyme haplotypes. The picture which has emerged is that each major population group, for example the Mediterranean, Asian Indian or Chinese groups, has its own spectrum of β thalassaemia mutations.

Gene Deletion

The first example of a gene deletion causing β thalassaemia was reported in patients of Indian origin. This deletion removes 600 base pairs from the 3′ end of the β-globin gene and is easily identified by restriction enzyme analysis, thus enabling the direct detection of the mutation in carriers which may facilitate prenatal diagnosis.

Transcriptional Mutants

The promoter sequences including the CAAT and the TATA boxes are important for transcription (see Fig. 5.6). Several β thalassaemia mutations have been described which result from single base substitutions within these sequences. These generally lead to a modest reduction of β chain production and hence result in a mild β^+ thalassaemia.

RNA Processing Mutants

The majority of β thalassaemia mutations can be classified under this heading. The initial RNA product results from the transcription of both the introns and the exons. This RNA has to be processed before it is exported to the cytoplasm as functional mRNA. A β^0 thalassaemia results if the normal splicing is abolished. For example, those mutations which alter the two invariant nucleotides at the start or end of the introns (5′-GT/AG-3′) result in a total absence of normal splicing and an absence of β-globin production.

Other mutations have been described which cause β-thalassaemia by creating alternative splicing sites. One of these is a G to A substitution at position 110 of intron 1 (the common Cypriot β^+ thalassaemia mutation). The mutation creates an AG sequence at this position which behaves as an alternative 3′ splice site. Studies of the expression of this mutant gene have shown that the first intron is incorrectly spliced in about 90% of the mRNA because of the new 3′ splice site created by the point mutation (Fig. 5.9). The remaining 10% of the mRNA is correctly spliced and translated to synthesize normal β-globin.

Mutations in the coding sequences may also result in abnormal RNA processing. The substitution of G to A in codon 26 gives rise to the common

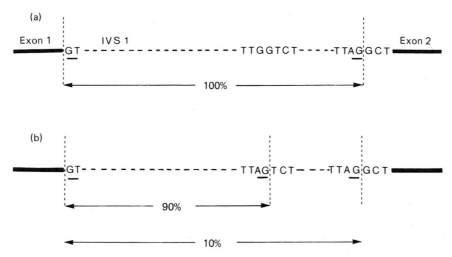

Fig. 5.9. *The splicing pattern (a) in normal chromosomes, and (b) in β^+ IVS 1–110 thalassaemia in which only 10% normal splicing occurs.*

structural variant HbE, which is associated with a mild β thalassaemia phenotype. The reason seems to be that this substitution causes the sequence around it to be recognized as an alternative splice site.

Non-functional RNA

Some β thalassaemia mutations give rise to non-functional RNA and hence to β^0 thalassaemia. These may be caused by either nonsense or frameshift mutations. Nonsense mutations are single nucleotide substitutions in codons which create an in-phase termination codon such that translation of the mRNA stops at the altered codon. For example, in the β^0 thalassaemia (β^0 39) which is common in Sardinia, the substitution of C by T in codon 39 introduces the termination codon UAG in β-globin mRNA. Several other β thalassaemias are now known to result from nonsense mutations.

The mRNA sequence is deciphered in triplets of bases (codons) which code for individual amino acids. Frameshift mutations (deletions or insertions of one, two or more than three nucleotides) put this reading frame out of phase, and result in the sequence at some point reading as a premature termination codon which stops translation at this point. For example, one β^0 thalassaemia gene described in an Asian Indian patient has a deletion of a single nucleotide (C) in the third position of codon 41. This causes an altered reading frame of the mRNA with an in-phase termination codon (UGA) in a position corresponding to codons 60–61, hence no functional β-globin is produced.

Heterozygous β Thalassaemia

Typically, individuals heterozygous for β^0 or β^+ thalassaemia are asymptomatic with slightly reduced haemoglobin levels and low red cell indices (typically for a man, Hb 110–130 g/l, MCH 18–22 pg). The red cell count is usually $> 5.5 \times 10^{12}$/l. Occasionally, β thalassaemia heterozygotes do have red cell indices close to the lower end of the normal range due to the coinheritance of α thalassaemia which reduces the globin chain imbalance. The single most important diagnostic feature of an individual with heterozygous β thalassaemia is a raised level of HbA$_2$ (4.0–7.0%). Many β thalassaemia heterozygotes have minor elevations of HbF (1–3%), probably resulting from some degree of cell selection.

Homozygous β Thalassaemia

In homozygous β thalassaemia there is either a total absence or a marked reduction of β-globin chains, leading to excessive α-globin chains which precipitate out in the red cell precursors causing extensive

Table 5.4

The haematological characteristics of the homozygous and heterozygous states of different β thalassaemias

Thalassaemia type	Homozygote	Heterozygote
β^0 39	Thalassaemia major HbF 98%, HbA$_2$ 2%	Thalassaemia minor HbA$_2$ 3.5–7.0%
β^+ IVS1–110 (Cypriot)	Thalassaemia major HbF 70–90%	Thalassaemia minor HbA$_2$ 3.5–7.0%
β^+ IVS1–6 (Portuguese)	Thalassaemia intermedia HbF 15–30%	Thalassaemia minor HbA$_2$ 3.5–7.0%

The $\beta^0$39 and β^+ IVS1–110 are given as typical examples of β^0 and β^+ thalassaemia respectively. The β^+ IVS1–6 is given as an example of a mild β^+ thalassaemia.

intramedullary destruction of red cell precursors with consequent marked expansion of the bone marrow. In addition there is some increased destruction of peripheral blood red cells. The anaemia is thus predominantly dyserythropoietic, with a haemolytic element. Red cells containing increased levels of HbF survive selectively, and this largely explains the high level of HbF found in the peripheral blood (Table 5.4).

Homozygous β^0 or β^+ thalassaemia usually presents as a severe anaemia in the first or second year of life, necessitating regular blood transfusions for survival. This condition is generally referred to as thalassaemia major. A later presentation suggests that the child may run a somewhat milder clinical course (thalassaemia intermedia).

Haematology

The blood film of untransfused homozygous β thalassaemia is grossly abnormal (Fig. 5.10). The red cells show very marked anisocytosis and poikilocytosis. Although most of the cells are very hypochromic, curiously some cells appear to have normal haemoglobinization. Nucleated red cells are always very numerous.

It is important to carry out haemoglobin electrophoresis before the child's first blood transfusion to determine accurately the type of haemoglobin synthesized. In homozygous β^0 thalassaemia, haemoglobin electrophoresis shows a complete absence of HbA, small amounts of HbA$_2$, with the

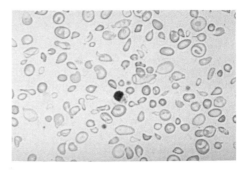

Fig. 5.10. *Peripheral blood appearances of a 7-year-old patient suffering from thalassaemia major. Pale, thin target cells and normoblasts are present; post-splenectomy (× 700)*

remainder (around 98%) consisting of HbF. The equivalent haemoglobin pattern of homozygous β^+ thalassaemia is more variable, with HbF levels around 60%, although a wide range can be found. Patients with relatively low percentages of HbF usually have inherited mild types of β^+ thalassaemia such as the 'Portuguese' β thalassaemia (see Table 5.4).

Clinical Findings

The clinical features of homozygous β thalassaemia are very dependent on the treatment the affected child receives. The neglected child with its protuberant abdomen, poor musculoskeletal development and spindly legs looks very much like a child with malignant disease. The typical thalassaemic facies with skull bossing, hypertrophy of the maxilla and prominent malar eminences are well known. There are marked radiological changes of the skull (the 'hair on end' appearance), long bones and hands. The child is likely to experience serious complications including recurrent infections, spontaneous fractures, hypersplenism, leg ulcers and later a variety of syndromes relating to tumour masses resulting from extramedullary haemato-poiesis.

Treatment with regular blood transfusions dramatically atlers this clinical picture: the child generally remains well and grows normally until the age of 10 or 11. After this age complications relating to iron overload begin to appear, including hepatic, cardiac and endocrine disturbances. The first change noted is often a failure or reduction in the pubertal growth spurt often associated with failure of sexual maturation. Diabetes mellitus, hypo-thyroidism and hypoparathyroidism are also fre-quent. Before regular chelation was introduced, deaths in the second and third decades occurred almost invariably as the result of iron overload, involving the myocardium in particular. It is still too early to know the prognosis of children treated from an early age by iron chelation with regular subcutaneous desferrioxamine (see p. 53). Never-theless, there are grounds for optimism that the children who comply with the treatment will have a much improved prognosis.

Thalassaemia Intermedia

Thalassaemia intermedia describes the clinical syn-drome in which patients are symptomatic and thus more severely affected than β thalassaemia hetero-zygotes but have a clinically milder disorder than typical transfusion-dependent thalassaemia major. Interactions of thalassaemia with structural haemo-globin variants can give rise to this picture. Ho-wever, the most important category is that of the clinically mild forms of homozygous β thalas-saemia, that is, individuals with an anaemia, a haemoglobin pattern consistent with homozygous β thalassaemia, and whose parents both have eleva-ted levels of HbA$_2$.

The genetic factors involved in the production of clinically mild homozygous β thalassaemia are

Table 5.5
Thalassaemia intermedia

Homozygous β thalassaemia
   Homozygous mild β^+ thalassaemia
   Coinheritance of α thalassaemia
   Enhanced propensity for γ chain production

Heterozygous β thalassaemia
   Coinheritance of additional α-globin genes
   ($\alpha\alpha\alpha/\alpha\alpha$, or $\alpha\alpha\alpha/\alpha\alpha\alpha$)

$\delta\beta$ thalassaemia and HPFH
   Homozygous $\delta\beta$ thalassaemia
   Heterozygous $\delta\beta$ thalassaemia/β thalassaemia
   Homozygous Hb–Lepore (some cases only)

listed in Table 5.5. The importance of the deleter-ious effects of excess α-globin chains on the patho-physiology of β thalassaemia has already been emphasized. The coinheritance of α thalassaemia has been found to ameliorate the clinical picture of homozygous β thalassaemia. The resulting clinical outcome depends on whether one or two α-globin genes are deleted, and whether the patient has β^0 or β^+ thalassaemia. The deletion of a single α-globin gene ($-\alpha/\alpha\alpha$) in a patient homozygous for β^0 thalassaemia makes little clinical difference, where-as the deletion of two α genes ($-\alpha/-\alpha$, or $--/\alpha\alpha$) in a patient homozygous for β^+ thalas-saemia usually gives rise to the clinical picture of thalassaemia intermedia.

It has long been considered that some patients must be homozygous for mild forms of β^+ thalas-saemia, that is, those mutations in which β-globin chain production is not so severely reduced. A well characterized example is the Portuguese β^+ thalas-saemia mutation which results from a T to C mutation at position 6 in the first intron of the β-globin gene. This mutation affects a splice consen-sus sequence but still allows a significant degree of normal splicing and hence β-globin chain produc-tion to occur. Patients homozygous for this β thalassaemia are found scattered throughout the Mediterranean region. They are generally mildly affected, some being diagnosed for the first time in early adulthood. Their chief haematological charac-teristic is a HbF level of around 20%, which is low for a homozygous β^+ thalassaemia patient.

Many cases of clinically mild forms of β^+ thalassaemia have been observed in black populations. One common mutation is an A to G change in the promoter region at position -29. Homozygotes for this mutation are mildly anaemic although not transfusion dependent. Finally, some patients with mild disease have inherited an enhanced propensity for HbF production. This is clearly seen in those homozygous β^0 thalassaemia patients with haemoglobin levels around 100 g/l consisting of over 95% HbF. Some of these cases have one parent with an elevated level of HbF and it is probable that an HPFH determinant has been inherited. However, in many cases the parents do not have elevated levels of HbF and it is now believed that these cases have inherited an HPFH-like determinant which is only expressed under conditions of erythropoietic stress such as thalassaemia.

Management of the Thalassaemias

Transfusion

In the early days, blood transfusion was given simply to sustain life. Since the mid 1960s 'hypertransfusion' has become the accepted practice, which means the Hb level is kept above 100 g/l at all times. It rapidly became apparent that children regularly transfused to maintain good Hb levels had fewer intercurrent illnesses. To achieve the most benefit from the hypertransfusion programme it must be started early in life. More recently, supertransfusion (keeping the PCV above 0.35) has been advocated to be a further improvement on hypertransfusion. Interestingly, the blood requirements of this approach seem to be no more than with hypertransfusion, possibly because the more complete suppression of the bone marrow reduces blood to the marrow and reticuloendothelial system. As with any transfusion programme, there is a risk of transfusion-related infections including hepatitis, cytomegalovirus and AIDS. It is hoped that the introduction of screening tests in blood donors for anti-HIV antibodies will virtually eliminate the last-mentioned risk. Occasionally isoimmunization to minor blood group antigens causes difficulties in cross-matching blood. It is, therefore, valuable to genotype all new cases before transfusion is given. Febrile reactions due to sensitization to white blood cells are common but may be reduced by using blood depleted of white cells

(washed or frozen and washed or preferably filtered. p. 284).

Splenectomy

Children maintained on a transfusion programme from an early age may not develop splenomegaly. However, splenomegaly often does occur and worsens the anaemia by causing haemodilution. For this reason it is important to keep good records to detect any increase in transfusion requirement. In addition, splenomegaly may also occasionally cause problems due to pressure effects or to splenic infarcts. The decision as to whether to perform splenectomy is not always straightforward. In practice, isotopic studies are not very helpful and the decision must be taken on clinical grounds, particularly an increasing transfusion requirement.

Splenectomy is usually avoided before the age of 5 years on account of the high risk of septicaemia. Pneumococcal vaccine is given before splenectomy, and afterwards it is advisable to maintain children on penicillin for at least 5 years. Splenectomy should also be carefully considered for children with possible thalassaemia intermedia. A milder clinical outcome of homozygous β thalassaemia may be suspected if the child's first blood transfusion is given over the age of 2 years. Such children may occasionally become transfusion independent following splenectomy, running Hb levels of 60–90 g/l.

Iron Chelation

Desferrioxamine was introduced in the 1960s and has remained the iron-chelating agent of choice. Initially it was given intramuscularly and the results were disappointing. In the mid 1970s it was shown to be much more effective when given as a slow continuous infusion. Subsequently the practical form of administration was found to be by means of a battery-operated pump as a continuous subcutaneous infusion through a butterfly needle. The usual dose in older children is 2 g (20–40 mg/kg) over 12 hours, but ideally the dose is best worked out from dose–response experiments. The early results of this therapy given to young children are encouraging. However, the effect on lifespan will not be known for some years to come. (The principles of iron chelation are further discussed in Chapter 2.)

Hormone Replacement

In general, hormone replacement is not effective in the treatment of sexual underdevelopment, presumably because there is target organ unresponsiveness caused by either siderotic or hypoxic damage. Occasionally hormones may be helpful in treating the delayed puberty of patients with thalassaemia intermedia.

Bone Marrow Transplantation

Bone marrow transplantation from an HLA-identical sibling has now been used in several centres to effect a cure for homozygous β thalassaemia. There is no doubt that haematopoiesis is restored to normal in successful transplants. Nevertheless, there is a significant morbidity and mortality of around 20% associated with this procedure. The dilemma is that, with modern iron chelation and good general management, patients can be given at least 20 years of reasonable life. In addition there is always the hope that a more definitive therapy may be developed during this time. The decision to go ahead with transplantation must be based on a realistic awareness of all the facts and full discussion with the patient's family.

Gene Therapy

There is no immediate prospect of gene therapy in thalassaemia since there are still a number of significant steps to be achieved. It is unlikely that thalassaemia will be one of the first disorders corrected by gene therapy since tissue-specific and regulated globin gene expression is necessary. Immuno-deficiency states such as adenosine deaminase deficiency are better candidates since these are disorders caused by a lack of a single chain polypeptide that undergoes no intracellular processing, and also in these cases tissue-specific regulation of gene expression may not be so important. Nevertheless, the rate of progress in understanding regulatory sequences and factors is very rapid and it is realistic to hope for gene therapy for diseases such as thalassaemia before the end of this century.

THE δβ THALASSAEMIAS AND HEREDITARY PERSISTENCE OF FETAL HAEMOGLOBIN

Hereditary persistence of fetal haemoglobin (HPFH) and δβ thalassaemia are genetic disorders characterized by reduction of both δ- and β-globin chain production and increased levels of HbF. HPFH heterozygotes have normal red cell indices, balanced α/non α-globin synthesis ratios and approximately 25% HbF, whereas δβ thalassaemia heterozygotes have microcytic red cells, globin chain imbalance and 10–15% HbF. However, there is overlap between these two conditions, and molecular studies have shown that both are commonly due to gene deletions within the β-globin gene complex.

Deletion Disorders

The δβ thalassaemias are found in most racial groups, although in all populations these are rare as compared to the β thalassaemias. They result from deletions of the δ- and β-globin genes (Fig. 5.11).

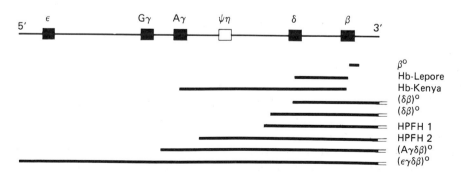

Fig. 5.11. *The deletions responsible for the Indian form of deletion β⁰ thalassaemia, Hb–Lepore, Hb–Kenya and some of the many deletions described causing δβ thalassaemia and HPFH.*

There is considerable variation in the size of the deletions, and also in the position of their 5' and 3' ends. The present classification of these disorders is based on which genes are deleted. Thus, if a deletion extends 5' removing the Aγ gene, the notation is $(A\gamma\delta\beta)^0$, whereas if both γ genes are intact the notation is $(\delta\beta)^0$.

The important clinical features of $\delta\beta$ thalassaemia is that it is milder than β thalassaemia since there is some compensation for the lack of β-chain production by enhanced γ-chain production. Individuals homozygous for this condition have the clinical phenotype of thalassaemia intermedia, with haemoglobin levels in the 80–110 g/l range consisting of 100% HbF.

Some HPFH syndromes result from gene deletions which seem to be similar to those causing $\delta\beta$ thalassaemia, although it remains unclear why some large gene deletions produce $\delta\beta$ thalassaemia and some HPFH. The two different forms of deletion HPFH in Blacks have the same phenotype. Heterozygotes have normal haematological findings, with 15–30% HbF evenly distributed among their red cells. The homozygotes have 100% HbF, with red cell changes similar to those of heterozygous β thalassaemia.

Non-deletion Disorders

γ-Globin Gene Upstream Mutations

There are also examples of HPFH which are not associated with any form of gene deletion. These conditions have variable levels of HbF. Several of them have now been shown to have mutations within the promoter region of the particular γ gene which has increased expression (Gγ or Aγ).

The best known examples are the Greek and the $G\gamma\beta^+$ HPFH. The Greek form is characterized by the production of 10–20% HbF in heterozygotes, of which 90% is Aγ. Molecular cloning and sequencing has demonstrated a substitution of A for G at position −117 of Aγ gene, which is only two nucleotides upstream (5') from the conserved CAAT box. The $G\gamma\beta^+$ form found in American Blacks has also been shown to have a mutation in the promoter region, in this case at position—202 of the Gγ gene.

High HbF Determinants Unlinked to the β-Globin Gene Cluster

Family studies of some cases of HPFH have shown that there is a high HbF determinant which segregates independently from the β-globin gene cluster. The nature of this genetic determinant is at present unknown.

γδβ Thalassaemia

The γδβ thalassaemias are caused by gene deletions of γ, δ and β genes. Only heterozygotes for this type of thalassaemia have been observed. They are characterized by neonatal haemolysis and haematological changes of β thalassaemia, with a normal haemoglobin A_2 level in adults.

PRENATAL DIAGNOSIS OF THE HAEMOGLOBINOPATHIES

The haemoglobinopathies (including thalassaemia) are the commonest single gene disorders and constitute a huge public health problem in many parts of the world. Many countries are now involved in programmes for the prenatal diagnosis of these disorders, particularly for sickle cell anaemia and β-thalassaemia.

Fetal Blood Sampling

The majority of prenatal diagnoses have been made using fetal blood sampling, although diagnosis by fetal DNA analysis is now becoming more widely applied. Prenatal blood sampling is performed late in the second trimester and in vitro globin chain synthesis is measured to determine directly the products of the mutant gene loci. This technique is relatively safe and reliable. The major disadvantage is the long period of uncertainty for the mother and, if indicated, an often difficult therapeutic abortion at 20 weeks gestation or later. Nevertheless, this approach has led to a major decline in the incidence of new cases of β thalassaemia in several populations.

DNA Analysis

Fetal DNA can be obtained either from amniotic fluid cells (midtrimester) or by chorion villus sampling (CVS), either by the transcervical approach (9–11 weeks of pregnancy) or by the trans-abdominal approach (up to 15 weeks of pregnancy). Chorion villus sampling has the advantage of a relatively early termination if indicated, although the fetal loss rate is currently of the order of 4% which is higher than the risk from amniocentesis.

Most prenatal diagnosis laboratories are switching from fetal blood sampling to DNA analysis, either by oligonucleotide probes in countries where the majority of cases of β thalassaemia are caused by a single mutation (such as the β39 nonsense mutation in Sardinia), or by a combination of oligonucleotide analysis, direct detection by gene mapping and linkage analysis of DNA polymorphisms (see below).

Haemoglobin Disorders Detectable By Gene Mapping

Many of the α thalassaemias result from gene deletions which are readily detectable by gene mapping, as discussed previously. However, there are only two large deletions causing β thalassaemias out of the known 40 or so described mutants. The remainder are single base changes or deletions or insertions of one, two or four bases. Some of these base changes do, however, alter a recognition site for a particular restriction enzyme. Thus digestion of DNA will yield different sized restriction fragments in the abnormal as compared to normal DNA. The major haemoglobinopathy which is amenable to this approach is the β^S mutation. A particular enzyme, Mst II, identifies the A to T change that characterizes this mutation. Unfortunately many of the β thalassaemia mutations cannot be diagnosed in this way. Perhaps the β39 nonsense mutation is the commonest directly detectable β thalassaemia mutation (by restriction enzyme analysis with Mae 1).

RFLP Linkage Analysis

Restriction fragment length polymorphisms (RFLPs) are caused by single base changes which are found as normal variants scattered along the globin gene clusters. In the β-globin gene cluster there are many possible patterns (haplotypes) of RFLPs of which a relatively small number are common. RFLPs, can be used for prenatal diagnosis by first establishing in a family study the linkage of the normal and abnormal β-globin genes to particular haplotypes. Subsequently fetal DNA can be studied, the haplotypes analysed and the linkage of the haplotypes determined from the family study. This approach has two general limitations. Firstly, linkage may only be established if the couple already has an affected or normal child, or alternatively if grandparents can be studied. Secondly, if the parents are homozygous for a particular haplotype, it is impossible to determine linkage.

Rarely, this approach may give an erroneous result due to either non-paternity or to a cross-over event between the polymorphic markers studied and the β-globin gene.

Oligonucleotide Probes

Conventional gene probes are several hundred bases long and too large to detect a single base difference in a mutant gene. However, short probes consisting of 17–19 nucleotides can be synthesized which are capable of detecting single base changes. In practice, two oligonucleotide probes are synthesized, one directed against the normal sequence and one against the abnormal sequence. Normal DNA only hybridizes to the normal probe, and DNA homozygous for a particular mutant will only hybridize to its complementary probe. DNA heterozygous for a mutant will hybridize to both the normal and the mutant probe. Oligonucleotide probes can be synthesized for the common mutations that exist in a particular population providing a feasible method of prenatal diagnosis.

Gene Amplification

In 1985 Saiki published a new method for the enzymatic amplification of DNA sequences. This method has already had a major impact in many areas of molecular biology and is likely to become very important worldwide in the prenatal diagnosis

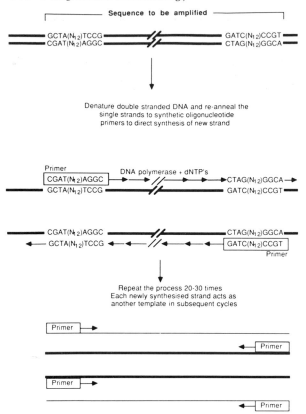

Fig. 5.12. *Schematic representation of the polymerase chain reaction. The primers flank the sequence of interest and are complementary to opposite DNA strands. The repeated cycles of amplification result in an increase of target DNA sequence of more than 200 000 fold.*

ated. Target DNA sequences of up to 2.5 kilobase pairs can be amplified.

In prenatal diagnosis the relevant gene, for example, the β-globin gene in the diagnosis of the β-thalassaemias, is first amplified and subsequently a variety of techniques may be used in the characterization of the amplified sequence. The most simple is the restriction enzyme digestion of the amplified DNA and gel electrophoresis for mutations such as β^s which alter particular restriction enzyme recognition sites. More commonly, oligonucleotide probes (see above) will be used for the detection of specific mutations. It seems likely that such probes can be labelled with non-radioactive markers which may allow this technology to be practised more widely in those countries where the haemoglobinopathies are most prevalent.

A further extension of this technique is the direct genomic sequencing of the amplified DNA which obviates the need for constructing haplotypes for prenatal diagnosis of β-thalassaemia, and also offers a useful method for the discovery of rare mutations. However, the major advantage of the PCR technique is that it is now feasible to screen large numbers of samples for particular mutations.

of genetic disorders since it allows the sequence analysis of very small clinical samples.

The polymerase chain reaction (PCR) technique is illustrated in Figure 5.12. It depends on the use of a pair of DNA primers which flank the particular region of interest and hybridize to opposite strands. The DNA is amplified progressively as the cycle of heat denaturation, annealing of the primers to their complementary sequences, and extension of the annealed primers with DNA polymerase is repeated. There is an exponential accumulation of the amplified sequence at approximately 2^n, where n is the number of cycles. Recently the results have been significantly improved with the use of the heat-resistant Taq polymerase. The use of Taq polymerase has also enabled the technique to be autom-

SELECTED BIBLIOGRAPHY

Bunn H. F., Forget B. G. (1985). *Haemoglobin: Molecular, genetic and clinical aspects.* Philadelphia: W. B. Saunders.

Collins F. S., Weissman S. M. (1984). The molecular genetics of human haemoglobin. *Progress in Nucleic Acid Research and Molecular Biology*, **31**, 315–462.

Dickerson R. E. (1964). In *The proteins*, 2nd edn. (Ed. H. Neurath.) New York: Academic Press.

Dickerson R. E., Geis I. (1983). *Haemoglobin.* New York: Benjamin/Cummings.

Higgs D. R., Weatherall D. J. (1983) Alpha thalassaemia. In *Current topics in hematology*, pp. 37–97. (Eds. S. Poinelli and S. Yachnin.) New York: Alan R. Liss.

Hill A. V. S., Wainscoat J. S. (1986). The evolution of the α and β-globin gene clusters in human populations. *Human Genetics*, **74**, 16–23.

Livingstone F. B. (1985) *Frequencies of hemoglobin variants.* Oxford: Oxford University Press.

Thein S. L., Weatherall D. J. (1987). Approach to the diagnosis of β-thalassaemia by DNA analysis. *Acta Haematologica*, **78**, 159–167.

Wainscoat J. S. (1987). The origin of mutant β-globin genes in human populations. *Acta Haematologica*, **78**, 154–158.

Wainscoat J. S., Thein S. L., Weatherall D. J. (1987). Thalassaemia intermedia. *Blood Reviews*, **1**, 273–279.

Weatherall D. J. (Ed.) (1983). *The thalassaemias: Methods in haematology*. Edinburgh: Churchill Livingstone.

Weatherall D. J., Clegg J. B. (1981). *The thalassaemia syndromes*, 3rd edn. Oxford: Blackwell Scientific, Publications.

Weatherall D. J., Old J. M., Thein S. L., Wainscoat J. S., Clegg J. B. (1985). Prenatal diagnosis of the common haemoglobin disorders. *Journal of Medical Genetics*, **22**, 422–430.

Chapter 6

INHERITED HAEMOLYTIC ANAEMIAS

L. LUZZATTO

This chapter deals with genetically determined disorders of the red cell (other than haemoglobin disorders) which cause its premature destruction. Whereas the primary genetic changes underlying these disorders are mostly heterogeneous, many of the manifestations are quite similar since they result mainly from the increased rate of red cell destruction and from the consequent hyperactivity of the erythroid component of the bone marrow. Therefore the description of individual conditions will be prefaced with a brief consideration of red cell metabolism and the pathophysiology of haemolysis.

DEFINITIONS

Haemolysis means that the destruction of red cells is accelerated above its normal rate. Any condition in which this takes place can be defined therefore as a **haemolytic disorder**. Because of the considerable reserve capacity of the bone marrow (up to six times if fully effective), partly due to increased cellularity of existing haemopoietic marrow and partly to expansion of haemopoietic marrow down the long bones, increased red cell destruction is often completely matched by increased production, resulting in **compensated haemolysis**. When the rate of haemolysis exceeds the maximum erythropoietic capacity of the bone marrow, or when the latter is impaired, e.g. when the disease process affects marrow red cell production or if there is iron or folate deficiency, this results in **haemolytic anaemia**. Since in any haemolytic disorder, with or without anaemia, the consequences of haemolysis are always present, and since haemolytic disorder and

haemolytic anaemia may coincide, even in the same patient at different times, the two terms are often used, somewhat loosely, as though they were interchangeable. However, the distinction between haemolytic disorder and haemolytic anaemia is obviously of great clinical significance and must always be borne in mind.

CLASSIFICATION

Because of the unique structural and functional specialization of the mature red cell, the impact on it of exogenous or endogenous changes is relatively monotonous: the cell will be destroyed prematurely. According to the site of the primary change, haemolytic disorders have been traditionally classified as being due either to **intracorpuscular** or to **extracorpuscular** causes. According to the nature of the primary change, haemolytic disorders have also been classified as **genetic** or **acquired**. These two classifications correlate almost completely with each other in that extracopuscular causes are usually acquired whereas intracorpuscular causes are usually inherited. One notable exception is paroxysmal nocturnal haemoglobinuria, a disease in which an intracorpuscular defect is acquired as a result of a somatic mutation (see Chapter 7).

Although in every cell all molecules and organelles are naturally interdependent, it is convenient to consider the red cell as a receptacle for a large amount of haemoglobin contained in a plasma membrane, the stability of which is maintained by an appropriate metabolic machinery. Unfavourable genetic changes in any of these components may cause haemolysis. Accordingly, haemolytic disorders can be classified into three major groups:

1. abnormal haemoglobin (see Chapter 5),
2. abnormal membrane (including the cytoskeleton),
3. abnormal metabolism (enzymopathies).

This chapter will deal with groups (2) and (3).

RED CELL PHYSIOLOGY AND HAEMOLYSIS

A normal red cell lifespan requires maintenance of its normal biconcave disc shape. This in turn requires structural integrity of the membrane and of the cytoskeleton and sufficient energy supply for active transport of sodium and potassium (the cation pump). Thus we can expect that genetic changes affecting either the structure of the membrane–cytoskeleton complex or any of the enzymes involved in the supply of chemical energy may result in haemolysis. Whilst the range of possible underlying genetic changes is very wide, two general points must be kept in mind in analysing their consequences.

1. By comparison with other somatic cells, the mature erythrocyte has a much more limited biochemical machinery. In the course of its differentiation and in parallel to perfecting its oxygen-carrying role it has given up its nucleus and with it the capacity to make RNA; it has given up ribosomes and thus the capacity to make protein; it has given up mitochondria and with them the most efficient mechanism for ATP production, namely cytochrome-mediated oxidative phosphorylation. As a result, red cell survival must rely entirely on preformed proteins and on ATP produced by glycolysis (Table 6.1).

2. Since normally red cells have a finite lifespan, their ageing is a physiological process. Although we do not have a complete understanding of what normally causes their demise after about 120 days in the circulation, haemolysis can be regarded as an acceleration of the ageing process.

RED CELL METABOLISM

Glycolysis

As a result of the trimming of its biochemical armamentarium (see above), the metabolism of the mature erythrocyte can be visualized more easily than that of most other cells in the body. Basically, the red cell feeds on plasma glucose and excretes lactate and pyruvate; specific molecules are present in the red cell membrane for the transport of these molecules. By contrast, the intermediate metabolites are all negatively charged phosphorylated sugars to which the membrane is impermeable. The entire process of conversion of glucose to pyruvate gives a net yield of two molecules of ATP per molecule of glucose (Fig. 6.1). The supply of plasma glucose to the red cells can be regarded generally as inexhaustible and the rate-limiting steps for glucose

Table 6.1

Some characteristics of erythroid cells at various stages of maturation

	Normoblast	Reticulocyte	Mature erythrocyte
DNA synthesis and cell division	+	0	0
RNA synthesis	+	0	0
RNA and ribosomes present	+	+	0
Protein synthesis	+	+	0
Mitochondria and cytochromes present	+	+	0
Krebs' tricarboxylic acid cycle	+	+	0
Embden–Meyerhof pathway	+	+	+
Pentose–phosphate pathway	+	+	+

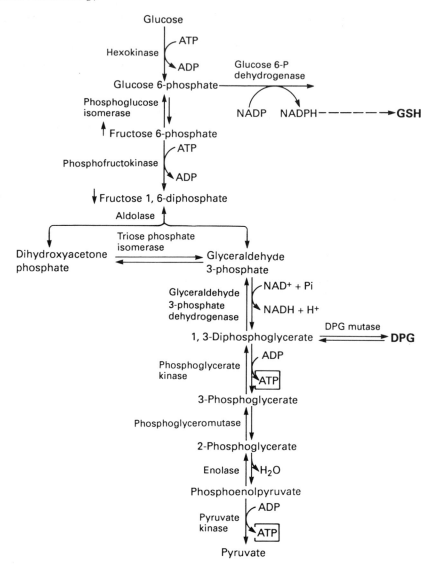

Fig. 6.1. *The glucose metabolism of red blood cells. Glucose and pyruvate are transported across the red cell membrane. Pyruvate is in equilibrium with lactate. Deficiency of almost any of these enzymes can lead to haemolytic anaemia (see Table 6.12). ADP, adenosine diphosphate; ATP, adenosine triphosphate; Pi, inorganic phosphate; NAD$^+$ and NADH, oxidized and reduced forms of nicotinamide adenine nucleotide; GSH, reduced glutathione; DPG, 2,3-diphosphoglycerate.*

metabolism in them are the two phosphokinase enzymes, hexokinase (HK) and phosphofructokinase (PFK). Much of the ATP produced by glycolysis is used up by the energy-requiring active transport of cations—the cation pump, the main structural component of which is the membrane-bound sodium- and potassium-dependent ATPase. This enzyme tightly couples the hydrolysis of one molecule of ATP to the outward transport of 3Na$^+$ and the inward transport of 2K$^+$.

Redox Reactions

Whereas maintenance of the normal shape of the red cell requires a normal operation of the ion pump, maintenance of haemoglobin in a functional state requires reductive potential. Some of this is provided by glycolysis in the form of reduced nicotinamide adenine dinucleotide (NADH). Indeed, the finding that genetically determined deficiency of NADH diaphorase causes methaemoglobinaemia (Chapter 5) is good evidence that this enzyme is normally responsible for regeneration to haemoglobin of the small amount of methaemoglobin which is produced all the time in red cells. However, in the course of methaemoglobin formation, highly reactive and highly toxic oxygen radicals are also formed, such as OH' and O_2^-. These in turn produce hydrogen peroxide, which is itself toxic and must be quickly detoxified by conversion to water by the glutathione-dependent enzyme glutathione peroxidase (GSHPX) (Fig. 6.2). Hydrogen peroxide is formed also in other reactions (including the metabolism of a variety of drugs) and therefore GSH must be constantly regenerated by glutathione reductase (GSSGR), a reduced nicotinamide adenine dinucleotide phosphate (NADPH) linked flavoenzyme. NADPH in turn is produced by the two consecutive reactions catalysed by glucose 6-phospate dehydrogenase and 6-phosphogluconate dehydrogenase (G6PD), (6PGD). Because in other cells G6PD and 6PGD divert a portion of the metabolic flow of G6PD from glycolysis to the production of pentose required for nucleic acid synthesis, this pathway is referred to as the pentose phosphate shunt. The physiologically important role of G6PD and 6PGD in these cells is the supply of NADPH, and not the supply of pentose.

Nucleoside Metabolism

Glucose is the main metabolic fuel of the erythrocyte, but it is not the only one. Purine nucleosides can enter red cells and, through the action of nucleoside phosphorylase, pentose phosphate is produced and becomes able to enter the glycolytic pathway (Fig. 6.3). The best evidence for the physiological role of these compounds has accrued from

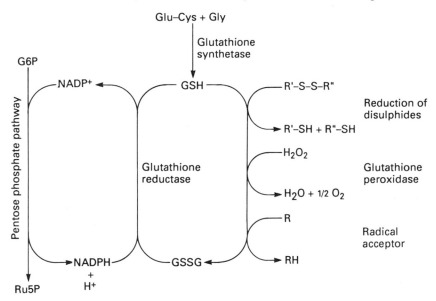

Fig. 6.2. *Glutathione—a tripeptide of glutamic acid (Glu), cysteine (Cys) and glycine (Gly)—is responsible for reduction of a variety of disulphides, for hydrogen peroxide detoxification (see also Fig. 6.13) and for formation of mixed disulphides (these three roles are shown on the right). All these processes convert reduced glutathione (GSH) to oxidized glutathione (GSSG) which needs NADPH to be reduced back to GSH. The red cell membrane is not permeable to GSH but when GSSG accumulates some of it 'leaks' out and is lost to the red cell.*

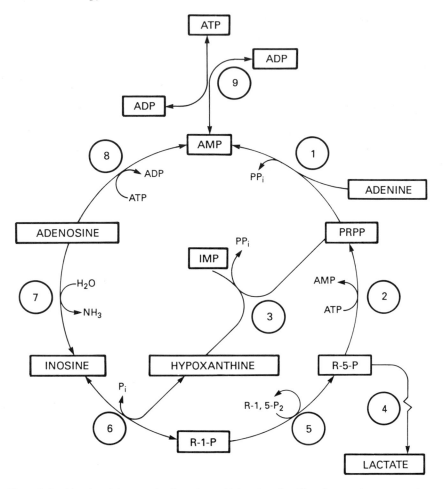

Fig. 6.3. *Nucleoside metabolism in red blood cells. Numbers refer to reactions catalyzed by (1) adenine phosphoribosyl transferase, (2) ribosephosphate pyrophosphokinase, (3) hypoxanthine–guanine phosphoribosyl transferase, (4) enzymes of the terminal pentose phosphate and Embden–Meyerhof pathways, (5) phosphoribomutase, (6) purine nucleoside phosphorylase, (7) adenosine deaminase, (8) adenosine kinase, (9) adenylate kinase. This diagram shows how the red cell can produce ATP from adenine outside glycolysis, thus explaining the beneficial effect of adenine addition on blood storage. (Reproduced from Paglia and Valentine (1981), with permission.) (PRPP, phosphoribosyl pyrophosphate; R-5-P, ribose-5-phosphate; R-1-P, ribose-1-phosphate; R-1,5-P$_2$, ribose-1,5-diphosphate; PP$_i$, pyrophosphate; P$_i$, inorganic phosphate; IMP, inosine monophosphate.)*

work on red cell storage, leading to the use of adenine in blood preservation. Since adenine is effective in preventing the deterioration of red cells during storage, even in the presence of excess glucose, it must mean that the fuel value of these two compounds is additive, presumably because adenine bypasses the hexokinase bottleneck. Adenosine is also important because it is in a balance with ADP and ATP via adenosine kinase and adenylate kinase (Fig. 6.3). Nucleotides and nucleosides also arise endogenously as a result of the degradation of RNA which takes place gradually during erythroid cell maturation and only becomes complete when the reticulocyte becomes an erythrocyte.

Metabolic Regulation

Some compounds play a key controlling role in the metabolic machinery of the red cell and it is useful to identify them because their levels may be altered in pathological conditions.

Diphosphoglycerate

Diphosphoglycerate (DPG) is the major regulator of the haemoglobin–oxygen dissociation curve. Increase in DPG is associated with a shift to the right in that curve (see Chapter 5), entailing an increased rate of oxygen delivery to the tissues. This phenomenon has emerged as a major general mechanism of adaptation to anaemia. By contrast, a decrease in DPG is associated with a shift to the left of the oxygen dissociation curve—an increased oxygen affinity. The steady state level of DPG depends on a balance between reactions which produce and reactions which remove DPG (Fig. 6.4). These reactions are closely intertwined with glycolysis and therefore they constitute an interface between glycolysis itself and haemoglobin.

Adenosine Triphosphate

ATP in the red cell is the prime product of glycolysis and at the same time it also regulates this pathway, mainly through its interaction with PFK, of which it is both a substrate and an inhibitor. This means that when the ATP level is high its production by glycolysis will slow down—a good example of feedback inhibition. By contrast, when the ATP level falls, PFK inhibition is relieved and the rate of glycolysis increases, thus readjusting the ATP level upwards. The control of PFK by ATP conforms to a common pattern whereby a metabolic pathway, in this case glycolysis, is regulated at the level of one of its early steps. It is noteworthy, however, that the reaction involved is PFK rather than hexokinase (HK). In this way control is exerted distally rather than proximally to G6P, and therefore NADPH production, when needed, can proceed without being limited by the rate of glycolysis (see Fig. 6.1).

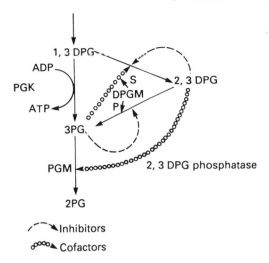

Fig. 6.4. *The metabolism of 2,3 diphosphoglycerate (DPG) in red blood cells. The level of DPG is seen to depend on the balance between its synthesis from 1,3-DPG and its hydrolysis to 3-PG. The two enzyme activities catalyzing these two reactions are referred to as DPG synthase and DPG phosphatase respectively, but, interestingly, the same enzyme protein is endowed with both activities. The official name for this enzyme is now bisphosphoglycerate synthase–phosphatase, but in this diagram we have retained the better known designation diphosphoglycerate mutase (DPGM), with the (S) and (P) indicating the synthase and phosphatase roles respectively. The vertical sequence of reactions is just a section of glycolysis (see Fig. 6.1). The triangular pathway on the right can be seen as a shunt from glycolysis and is sometimes referred to as the Rapoport–Luebeing shunt (or cycle, because it can be read as a circle, going, for instance, from 3-PG back to 3-PG). Note that for each molecule of 1,3-DPG shunted away from the 'regular' glycolytic pathway there is one molecule of DPG synthesized, but at the expense of failing to produce one ATP molecule. The curved arrows indicate that 3-PG is a cofactor of DPGM(S) and 2,3-DPG is a cofactor of PGM (they can be regarded as coenzymes because each one is regenerated in the course of the respective reaction). Finally, it should be mentioned that, to complicate matters, PGM has a weak DPGM(S) activity and a significant DPGM(P) activity. In normal red cells DPGM is much more abundant than PGM and therefore the role of the latter in DPG metabolism is probably negligible. This role, however, may become significant in DPGM-deficient red cells (see Table 6.12). PGK, phosphoglycerate kinase; PGM, (51 phosphoglycerate mutase).*

The NADP/NADPH System

The NADP/NADPH system is crucial for the provision of reducing potential. In the steady state most of the coenzyme is in the NADPH form. This compound is a potent inhibitor of G6PD and this is another example of feedback control, since G6PD produces NADPH. When NADPH is oxidized, for instance to regenerate GSH, G6PD inhibition is relieved and more NADPH is formed. Thus, regulation again takes place at the level of the first of the two NADPH-supplying reactions.

THE MEMBRANE, THE CYTOSKELETON AND THE SHAPE OF THE ERYTHROCYTE

The general organization of the red cell membrane is broadly similar to that found in other cells as it consists of a lipid bilayer in which a number of **integral membrane proteins** are embedded. However, an important and specific feature of the red cell is that its membrane is extensively and tightly connected with the complex network of fibrous proteins within the cytoplasm which form the cytoskeleton. This feature is related in turn to two essential structural-functional characteristics of the red cell, namely, the biconcave disc shape and its high deformability. The membrane alone would make a quasi-spherical cell; the anchorage to the cytoskeleton produces the discoid shape while at the same time providing the degree of elasticity required to maintain deformability.

A description of the membrane structure is given in Chapter 8. Here, suffice it to say that the membrane consists of approximately 50% protein and 50% lipid. All the red cell lipid is in the membrane and it consists of about one-half phos-

Table 6.2

Proteins of the red cell membrane and cytoskeleton

Name	Electrophoretic band*	Molecular weight (kd)	Number of molecules per red cell ($\times 10^5$)	Location/ function	Chromosomal assignment	Gene cloned
Spectrin α	1	240	2	CS; form hetero-dimers, tetramers	1q22–1q25	Yes
β	2	220	2			Yes
Actin	5	42	5	CS; forms protofila-ments of 10–13 monomers	7pter–q22	Yes
'Band'	4.1	78	2	Crosslinks spectrin heterodimers	1p32–1pter	Yes
Ankyrin	2.1	210	1	Links spectrin to band 3		
'Band'	3	95	10	IMP; anion transport; links to ankyrin		
Glycophorin A PASI, 2		29	4	IMP; sialoglyco-protein	4q28–q31	Yes

IMP, integral membrane protein; CS, cytoskeleton; *, as currently numbered on SDS-gels.

pholipid and one-half cholesterol. The membrane cholesterol is to some extent exchangeable with plasma cholesterol. The surface area of the red cell is about $140\ \mu m^2$: a sphere of the same volume ($\simeq 90$ fl) would have a surface area of about $95\ \mu m^2$. The 'excess' membrane area ($\simeq 45\ \mu m^2$) is related to the discoid shape and confers on the red cell the required deformability. The major cytoskeletal protein is spectrin (Table 6.2). The role of the cytoskeleton in determining red cell shape is proven by the fact that red cell ghosts stripped of the membrane by the use of detergents (e.g. Triton) retain their discoid shape. The role of spectrin within the cytoskeleton is proven by the fact that mice homozygous for a spectrin-deficiency mutation have spherical red cells. This evidence is paralleled in humans by the finding that structural mutations in spectrin or in other proteins that anchor spectrin to the membrane or spectrin molecules to each other are also associated with abnormal red cell shapes (see Tables 6.2 and 6.5).

Red Cell Ageing and Haemolysis

A characteristic feature of extravascular haemolysis is acceleration of normal red cell breakdown—rather than a process otherwise unknown to the body. Indeed, it is probable that in many haemolytic disorders premature destruction of abnormal red cells results from the fact that they age faster than normal.

The precise structural/functional change in normal red cells which is recognized by macrophages as the signal for their removal is not yet known. Death normally occurs in the whole of the reticuloendothelial system, with the bone marrow macrophages as quantitatively the next important site. However, we do have abundant information on what changes take place as red cells age (Table 6.3). From the physical point of view, normal red cells become gradually denser; this is associated with loss of water, increased MCHC, tendency to sphering and increased osmotic fragility. With respect to electrolytes, loss of K^+ and increase in intracellular Na^+ suggest a deterioration in membrane function which may be due directly to gradual loss in activity of the ion pump. From the biochemical point of view, a most characteristic phenomenon is the exponential decrease in activity of many intracellular enzymes (Fig. 6.5). It is clear that all these changes are interrelated and it is difficult to discern whether a particular alteration is causal, but it is obvious that changes in metabolites are secondary to changes in enzyme activities. Indeed, it seems reasonable to surmise that each protein in the red cell decays according to a time course which is determined within that particular environment by its own intrinsic stability, which in turn will depend on the structure of the protein. Thus, ageing of a red cell can be visualized as resulting from the ageing of its proteins until one or more of these falls below a

Table 6.3
Examples of changes occurring in ageing red cells

	Increased in old cells	*Decreased in old cells*
Haemoglobin	Glycosylated Hb	Diphosphoglycerate, p_{50}
Membrane	Osmotic fragility Na^+ Binding of IgG	Sialic acid K^+ Lipid and protein
Enzymes		Hexokinase Glucose-6-phosphate dehydrogenase Pyruvate kinase Others
General	Cell density Sphericity	Deformability Disc-like shape

These changes presumably result from decreased efficiency of the cation pump in the membrane.

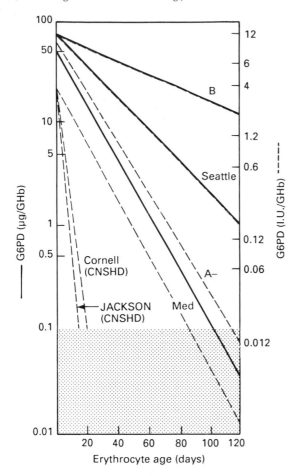

Fig. 6.5. *The activity of G6PD, as of many other red cell enzymes, is age dependent. The top line refers to normal G6PD (B). The other lines refer to genetic variants of G6PD associated with enzyme deficiency. The top of the dotted area represents the threshold below which red cells become non-viable. For the Mediterranean variant the full line and the broken line represent a fall in immunochemical reactivity and in enzyme activity respectively. (Reproduced from Luzzatto and Testa (1978), with permission.)*

threshold level incompatible with red cell viability. It is possible that the proteins which are crucial are those that determine the structure and function of the membrane and that intracellular enzymes do not normally control red cell survival. However, when an enzyme is reduced in amount, or in stability, this enzyme may limit red cell survival.

This pathophysiological situation is critical in haemolysis associated with enzymopathies.

General Pathophysiology of Haemoloytic Disorders

Accelerated extravascular destruction of red cells will cause: (a) an excess of their breakdown products, and (b) a bone marrow response. It is convenient therefore to consider under these two headings how we can find evidence of haemolysis. Intravascular haemolysis which occurs only in acquired haemolytic anaemias is considered later.

Increased Red Cell Destruction

Increased red cell destruction causes release of larger than normal amounts of haem. When the spleen is an important site of red cell destruction (as in hereditary spherocytosis), it may enlarge and become palpable. The iron released from haem enters the plasma pool and contributes to increased transferrin saturation (Fig. 6.6). The protoporphyrin is catabolized to bile pigments, causing hyperbilirubinaemia, clinically manifest as jaundice. Bilirubin enters the plasma where it binds to albumin and is transported to the liver. Unconjugated bilirubin (being poorly water soluble) is tightly bound to protein, whereas conjugated bilirubin is soluble. It then separates from albumin and enters the parenchymal cell where it is conjugated as a diglucuronide. Bilirubin is secreted in the bile and 'pigment' gallstones are common in chronic haemolytic disorders. The conjugated bilirubin enters the intestine where it is converted to urobilinogen by intestinal bacteria. Urobilinogen (stercobilinogen) is excreted in the faeces; it is reabsorbed and partly excreted in the urine and partly in bile. Normal adults excrete from 50 mg to 300 mg each day.

Laboratory Findings

The blood film does not show any unique set of changes in congenitally determined haemolytic anaemias. However, by looking at red cell morphology, it is possible in general to infer that haemolysis is going on, especially when it is brisk. It is common to see very marked anisocytosis, bizarre poikilocytes, contracted red cells, red cell fragments and marked polychromasia. The difficulty these

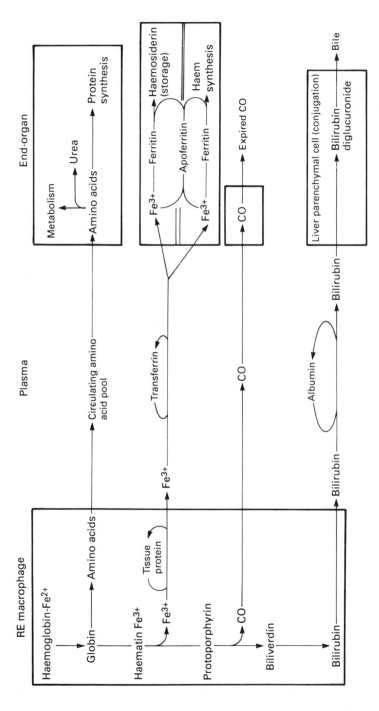

Fig. 6.6. *The catabolism of haemoglobin. When time-expired red cells are removed from the circulation by macrophages the main component which needs processing is haemoglobin. Most of its building blocks are recycled: thus, amino acids released by proteolytic enzymes enter the plasma; haem iron also enters the plasma bound to transferrin (if haemolysis is excessive, it will accumulate as ferritin and haemosiderin). The only major component which goes to waste is the porphyrin moiety of haem which is degraded to bilirubin and excreted in the bile. Carbon monoxide (released upon opening of the porphyrin ring) is excreted through the lungs; and urobilinogen (a further catabolite of bilirubin) is excreted in urine and faeces: either can be used to quantitate the rate of haemolysis.*

cells have in negotiating the microvasculature, together with anoxia due to anaemia, may account for the ankle ulcers which occur in some cases (e.g. severe hereditary spherocytosis). More specific morphological changes will be mentioned in the respective sections. Bilirubin levels in the plasma usually lie between 30 μmol/l and 50 μmol/l in haemolytic anaemia. Higher levels suggest a sudden increase in haemolysis, some form of liver damage, or an unsuspected bilirubin transport defect such as Gilbert's disease. The bilirubin is unconjugated (indirect van den Bergh reaction) and bound to albumin. In this form bilirubin is unable to pass through the glomerular membrane and therefore does not appear in the urine.

Increased Urobilinogen Excretion

The excess bilirubin excreted in the liver results in increased urobilinogen in the urine and stools. Urobilinogen gives a red colour with Ehrlich's reagent, which provides a useful qualitative test. Quantitative estimation of urobilinogen or stercobilinogen in faeces, however, is not useful in the routine diagnosis of haemolytic anaemia because of the wide normal range and technical difficulties in collection and estimation.

Reduced Haptoglobins

The normal plasma haemoglobin level is less than 4 mg/dl, though the normal range varies according to the care with which samples are withdrawn from patients. Plasma haemoglobin is normally bound by the plasma haptoglobins. Haptoglobin has an exquisite affinity for haemoglobin, of which it can bind about 125 mg haemoglobin/dl plasma. The complex so formed is rapidly cleared from the blood by the reticuloendothelial system so that the total plasma haptoglobin falls in the presence of haemolysis. The liver has limited ability to synthesize haptoglobin, and low or absent haptoglobins are therefore found in many chronic haemolytic states. Return to normal levels takes about a week after haemolysis has subsided.

Shortened red Cell Survival

Various methods are available for measuring the lifespan of red cells, of which radioactive chromium (^{51}Cr) tagging is the most widely used (see also Chapter 1). The isotope binds to the β chain of haemoglobin. The lifespan may be expressed in terms of the time taken for half the ^{51}Cr to disappear from the circulation (normal range 25–32 days) or the appropriate mathematical calculations may be made to express the mean cell life (MCL). This cannot be regarded as a routine method because it entails some radiation to the patient and because it requires serial blood sampling over a period of days or weeks, making the procedure lengthy, expensive, and not always easy or desirable, especially in children. Therefore ^{51}Cr red cell survival studies are not indicated if diagnosis of a haemolytic anaemia is established. It must also be realized that this procedure alone does not usually help to clarify the cause for haemolysis (except when coupled with cross-transfusion studies which can show whether haemolysis is due to an intracorpuscular or an extracorpuscular cause). A ^{51}Cr red cell survival study does, however, remain the 'gold standard' when the existence of haemolysis is in doubt or when it seems useful to quantitate it. When combined with scanning, it may also be useful in determining the dominant site of red cell destruction.

Changes in Iron Metabolism

In extravascular haemolysis, iron accumulates in the reticuloendothelial system; the serum iron and ferritin may be increased. In some cases, excess iron is absorbed, especially if there is ineffective erythropoiesis or if the patient is a carrier of a haemochromatosis gene.

Increased Red Cell Production

Reticulocytosis

In the face of a normal or decreased number of circulating red cells, there is increased erythropoietic activity, giving a reticulocytosis. The reticulocyte develops in the bone marrow following the extrusion of the nucleus from the normoblastic precursor cell. Its release from the bone marrow is a complex process and under normal circumstances only reticulocytes which have been present for some 24–48 hours in the marrow are deformable enough to leave the marrow. However, under the stimulus of anaemia, the structure of the marrow may be modified so that earlier reticulocytes, or even normoblasts, may leave the marrow and appear in the peripheral blood. Once the reticulocyte leaves the marrow it exists for about 2 days in the peripheral blood. The characteristics of the reticulocyte are derived from the remaining RNA and intracellular organelles which persist for a while after extrusion from the marrow (see Table 6.1). The persistent RNA stains slightly bluish with Romanovsky stains, giving rise to polychromasia, and precipitates and stains purple with methyl violet or other vital dyes, producing a reticular pattern. In normal blood, reticulocytes constitute 0.2–2% (in absolute numbers, $10–80 \times 10^9/l$). A reticulocyte count of more than $100 \times 10^9/l$ is evidence of increased erythropoietic activity. The degree of reticulocytosis gives a crude indication of the extent of this increase, although the correlation between reticulocytosis and haemolysis is not linear, partly because during episodes of haemolysis reticulocytes may be prematurely released from the bone marrow and may take longer than normal to mature to erythrocytes. The 'shift' reticulocytes appear larger than normal reticulocytes, and inclusions such as Howell–Jolly bodies or basophilic stippling are common. In infants and when haemolysis is severe,

erythroblasts may also appear in the peripheral blood, sometimes in large numbers.

Bone Marrow

Bone marrow aspiration in haemolytic disorders usually shows increased cellularity with marked erythroid hyperplasia without disturbance of the other cell lineages. The myeloid:erythroid ratio is often reversed. In general, bone marrow aspiration is not necessary for the diagnosis of haemolytic anaemia. It may be indicated, however, in order to rule out associated or complicating pathology or in the evaluation of special intercurrent events, for instance when an aplastic crisis or severe folate deficiency is suspected.

Increased erythropoietic activity entails physical expansion of marrow spaces in bones, especially if the anaemia is chronic and congenital. This is shown by an increase in active marrow along the shafts of long bones such as the femur and the humerus and in severe cases also in metacarpal bones and phalanges of the fingers (Fig. 6.7) and in tarsal and metatarsal bones. In addition to the extension of marrow down the long bones, there may be widening of the marrow cavity of the central skeleton, particularly the skull and ribs. In extreme cases this produces frontal bossing and the 'hair on

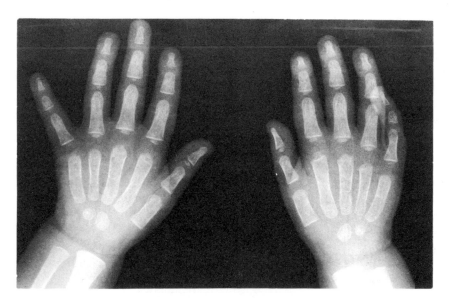

Fig. 6.7. *Bone marrow expansion in the bones of the hands of a child with severe anaemia due to pyruvate kinase deficiency.*

end' appearance of the skull x-ray. These changes, however, are never as severe as they are in thalassaemia major, when the effects of peripheral haemolysis are compounded by those of ineffective erythropoiesis. Increased bone marrow activity can also be revealed by studies with radioactive iron (see Chapter 1). Extramedullary haemopoiesis occurs in thalassaemia major and some acquired haemolytic anaemias but is unusual in the hereditary disorders of red cell membrane or metabolism.

Platelets and Granulocytes

In chronic haemolysis, platelets are often in the high normal range, but are not usually above normal unless the spleen has been removed. The granulocyte count may also be raised and, in severe haemolytic states, metamyelocytes may be seen in the blood.

INTRAVASCULAR HAEMOLYSIS

In most haemolytic anaemias the extra destruction of red cells is effected by macrophages of the RE system, and its site is therefore extravascular. In some conditions, however, the nature of the red cell abnormality or of the exogenous agent damaging the red cells (Table 6.4) is such that they are lysed within the bloodstream (intravascular haemolysis). This entails release of haemoglobin in the plasma (haemoglobinaemia) which is followed, once the renal threshold for haemoglobin is surpassed, by haemoglobinuria. This sign can be quite dramatic, and it is described by the patient as the urine resembling port wine or Coca cola, or simply as 'passing blood'. It is, of course, important to differentiate haemoglobinuria from haematuria: this can be done by microscopic examination of a centrifuged urine sediment, which will show red cells or red cell ghosts with haematuria but not with haemoglobinuria. The haemoglobin is partially degraded by the renal tubular cells, and the urine sediment, stained for iron, will subsequently reveal haemosiderin and this persists for up to 6 weeks after a single episode. The recognition of haemoglobinuria and haemosiderinuria is important, because by indicating intravascular haemolysis, they drastically restrict the differential diagnosis of haemolytic anaemia (Table 6.4). In chronic intravascular haemolysis, iron deficiency may occur. In the blood, free haem may be bound to specific proteins (haemopexins) or to albumin. In either case, oxidation occurs, producing methaem

Table 6.4

Haemolytic anaemias associated with intravascular haemolysis

Condition	Comments	Diagnostic test
Mismatched blood transfusion	Usually ABO incompatibility	Repeat crossmatch
G6PD deficiency	After exogenous trigger (*e.g.* fava beans)	Assay for enzyme
PNH	Intermittent course	Ham test
PCH	Usually after viral infection	Donath–Landsteiner antibody
Autoimmune haemolytic anaemia	Unusually severe	Direct Coombs' test
Septicaemia	*Clostridium welchii,* typically after septic abortion	Blood culture
Blackwater fever	Rare complication of *Plasmodium falciparum* malaria	Examine blood film for malaria

G6PD, glucose 6-phosphate dehydrogenase, PNH, paroxysmal-nocturnal haemoglobinuria; PCH, paroxysmal cold haemoglobinuria.

(haemin) or methaemalbumin, which have characteristic absorption spectra and may cause a brownish appearance of plasma. The Schumm's test amplifies the spectral effects of methaemalbumin but is too sensitive for routine use in the investigation of intravascular haemolysis.

SOME GENERAL NOTES

'Aplastic Crisis'

This phrase refers to the common clinical observation that patients with any kind of congenital haemolytic anaemia may experience a sudden and catastrophic fall in haemoglobin level concomitant with infection. The peripheral blood shows a reticulocytopenia and the bone marrow an absence of late red cell precursors (aplastic crisis is rather a misnomer since it is only the red cell precursors which are affected). The 'switch-off' in red cell production lasts 24–72 hours. If such an event occurs in a patient with a normal red cell lifespan, the effect is unnoticed; but in patients with haemolytic anaemia, in whom the red cell lifespan may be 20 days or less, the effects are serious and potentially fatal. Following the demonstration that aplastic crises in sickle cell anaemia can be attributed to a parvovirus, similar evidence has been obtained also in PK deficiency and in other chronic haemolytic anaemias. The mechanism of parvovirus-induced erythroblastopenia is not yet known and the possibility cannot be excluded that other infectious agents may also cause aplastic crises. It is important to distinguish these crises from reduced marrow output due to folate deficiency which is likely to occur in severe chronic haemolytic anaemias due to increased breakdown of folate coenzymes and therefore increased demands for the vitamin.

Dangers of Splenectomy

Splenectomy in patients with haematological disorders is more hazardous than when it is carried out, for instance, because of traumatic rupture of the spleen. The immediate dangers of abdominal surgery—infection and deep vein thrombosis—are compounded by the location of the spleen under the left side of the diaphragm. Thus, splenectomy often causes collapse of the lower lobe of the left lung and a rise in platelets, often to over $1000 \times 10^9/l$. In patients with PK deficiency and in those with other chronic haemolytic anaemias in whom the anaemia is not fully corrected by the operation, the platelet count may remain very high for several years, if not for life. The major danger, however, is of overwhelming post-splenectomy infection (OPSI). Catastrophic infection with encapsulated organisms—*Streptococcus pneumoniae* or *Neisseria meningitis*—can cause death within a few hours. It is possible that the spleen is responsible for the early production of IgM antibody directed against thymus-independent antigens of these organisms. Fortunately these organisms are highly sensitive to penicillin. It is good practice to vaccinate all patients with antipneumococcal vaccine before splenectomy and to give them penicillin V daily by mouth after splenectomy. The penicillin administration is continued for at least one year after splenectomy in all patients, when the risk of OPSI is greatest. For children, who have an increased risk of OPSI compared with adults, penicillin continues until they leave school. Finally, *Plasmodium falciparum* malaria is extremely life threatening in splenectomized subjects. Therefore, in malaria-endemic areas one ought to be even more cautious than elsewhere in recommending splenectomy. Once this is done, rigorous antimalarial prophylaxis must be kept up for life.

GENETIC ABNORMALITIES OF THE RED CELL MEMBRANE

Hereditary Spherocytosis

Definition

This condition—a congenital disorder characterized by spherocytic red cells with a short lifespan—has been the first form of haemolytic anaemia to be identified as genetically determined. Classically it is defined by the triad of spherocytosis, increased osmotic fragility and dominant inheritance. In addition, the beneficial response to splenectomy is so uniform that it has been regarded almost as a diagnostic criterion. However, it must be borne in mind that the degree of spherocytosis is variable, changes in osmotic fragility are not always unambiguous, sporadic cases occur, and other haemolytic anaemias respond to splenectomy. Therefore the diagnosis of hereditary spherocytosis (HS) is not always easy.

Clinical Manifestations

The majority of patients with HS present in childhood or as teenagers. However, rarely, the diagnosis is made when investigating a neonate with persistent jaundice or, at the opposite end of the spectrum, it has been made as late as at the age of 60 in a previously asymptomatic person. This wide variation in the age of presentation indicates in itself the characteristically wide spectrum of severity of HS. Within this spectrum the most consistent findings are, in order of frequency, jaundice, an enlarged spleen, and anaemia. In about one-third of patients the haemolysis is well compensated and the haemoglobin may be within the normal range; perhaps because of this, a classical phrase to describe patients with HS is that they may be 'more yellow than sick'. Cholelithiasis, although regarded in conventional terms as a complication, is found so commonly in HS that it can be regarded as part of the clinical picture: indeed, it is not unusual for HS to be diagnosed while investigating a patient who has gallstones at an unusually young age. As in other congenital haemolytic anaemias, it is useful from the clinical point of view to distinguish the *steady state* from intercurrent *episodic changes*. Each patient tends to have a certain level of haemoglobin and of bilirubin and it is useful to establish these steady-state values for each individual so that reference can be made to them. The common complications of HS are: (a) leg ulcers which are attributed to inadequate perfusion of the skin as a result of decreased red cell deformability. (b) gallstones which are the rule rather than the exception but which are often asymptomatic; and (c) aplastic crises (see p. 159).

Role of the Spleen

The best evidence that the spleen adversely affects the HS red cells is the therapeutic efficacy of splenectomy. After splenectomy one sees not only a decrease in the rate of haemolysis (and therefore an amelioration of the anaemia, if present), but also a decrease in the number of circulating spherocytes. Yet splenectomy certainly cannot have cured the abnormal red cell. The most likely explanation is that the spleen, apart from being a major site of red cell destruction, also adversely affects the viability of HS red cells in a special way. Most probably this is due to a combination of two phenomena. First, because HS red cells have decreased deformability, they are retained in the splenic pulp for an unduly long time; second, the red cells find in the splenic pulp especially unfavourable environmental conditions, particularly an acid pH and a low glucose concentration. These conditions (mimicked in vitro in the autohaemolysis test without added glucose) will cause failure of the cation pump (which was already working overtime because of the abnormal membrane), with consequent loss of water and loss of the red cell discoid shape. This closes a vicious circle, whereby transit through the spleen will produce spherocytes and the decreased deformability of spherocytes prolongs the transit time from the splenic pulp to the splenic vein. Thus splenectomy removes the major site of haemolysis. It is especially beneficial in HS because the unique anatomy of the spleen is liable to cause damage to HS red cells more than to most other genetically abnormal red cells.

Laboratory Tests

The first and foremost approach to the diagnosis of HS is the examination of the peripheral *blood film*, showing significant numbers of spherocytes (Fig. 6.8). A spherocyte is identified as an orthochromic–hyperchromic red cell with absence of central pallor and a reduced diameter (cells without central pallor but with increased diameter and a polychromatic tinge are reticulocytes). For the correct appreciation of spherocytes it is essential to look at the thin portion of the film where cells are just touching, not at the extreme tail end (or at the thick part) of the film, where central pallor is often not seen in a majority of cells even with normal blood. In the best portion of almost every film a few spherocytes can be found. Therefore, it is suggested that a proportion of greater than 1–2% is to be regarded as 'significant' spherocytosis. Spherocytes are not only abnormal in shape; they also have is a shift to the right of the entire curve or, more frequently, of only part of the curve (Fig. 6.9), indicating the presence of at least a fraction of cells which are abnormally prone to osmotic haemolysis. This is not seen in every case, however, and one way to make the test more sensitive is to pre-incubate the blood at 37°C for 24 hours. This produces a shift in the curve which is usually more pronounced in HS than in a control sample. A tail of cells more resistant than normal correlates with the increased reticulocytosis.

The osmotic fragility test has several drawbacks: (a) it is a laborious test and must be carried out on fresh defibrinated blood; (b) it is not specific for HS: increased fragility is also found, for instance, in AIHA; and (c) it is insufficiently sensitive: it is estimated that between 10% and 25% of patients with genetically proven HS have normal osmotic fragility, even after pre-incubation.

Gottfried and Robertson (1974) introduced a procedure to overcome the first difficulty in which red cells are lysed by the addition of glycerol, and a

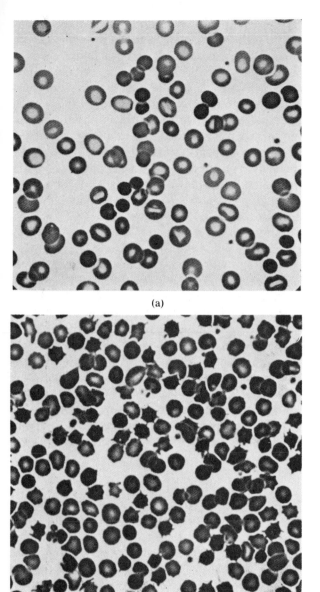

Fig. 6.8. *Blood film in hereditary spherocytosis: (a) before splenectomy; (b) after splenectomy.*

decreased water content and this explains why HS is one of the few conditions in which the MCHC is increased (sometimes to 37 g/dl), or at least is in the upper part of the narrow normal range (33–35 g/dl). A good way to quantitate spherocytosis is by means of the *osmotic fragility* test, which must be carried out by a rigorous technique and must always include a control run in parallel. The typical finding

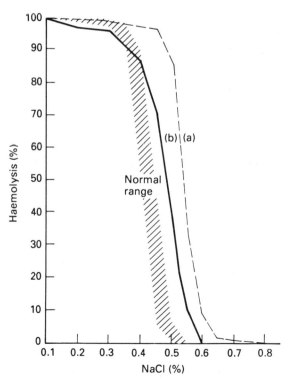

Fig. 6.9. *Osmotic fragility of fresh red cells from a patient with hereditary spherocytosis: (a) before splenectomy; (b) 4 years after splenectomy.*

subsequent modification of this method has become known as the acidified glycerol lysis time (AGLT: Zanella *et al.*, 1980). Unlike the classical osmotic fragility test, which measures the extent of haemolysis when red cells are equilibrated with a certain salt concentration, this test measures the rate of haemolysis (usually expressed as the time required for 50% lysis: normal values > 1800 seconds). It is simple and fast and can be carried out on blood stored for up to 48 hours in acid citrate dextrose (ACD). In the hands of some investigators it has been claimed to detect 100% of patients with HS. This 'high yield', with clear demarcation between normal subjects and HS patients, requires a rigorous control of experimental conditions, especially the pH of the lysis solution. However, the AGLT is still not specific because it is positive in patients with autoimmune haemolytic anaemia (AIHA), in some patients with chronic renal failure or with leukaemia and, surprisingly, in normal pregnant women. Recently, Acharya *et al.* (1987), have shown that some anomalies can be eliminated by standardizing the temperature at 28°C. It would be very desirable for the AGLT to be more widely used, with these precautions, in order to establish its value further.

Autohaemolysis

Various modifications of this test have been used, all based on the original work of Selwyn and Dacie (1954) in the investigation of congenital haemolytic anaemias. The principle of the test is simply to measure the extent of haemolysis that takes place when whole defibrinated blood is incubated under sterile conditions for 48 hours. Under these conditions red cell metabolism depends on the glucose present in the serum, and in normal blood less than 2% of red cells will haemolyse in 48 hours—less than 0.5% if extra glucose is added (see Table 6.5). In HS the rate of glucose consumption is much increased and therefore autohaemolysis is abnormally high without added glucose but it is restored to normal or near-normal when glucose is added (partial or complete correction). In haemolytic anaemias caused by deficiency of a glycolytic enzyme, autohaemolysis is also abnormal but extra glucose does not help much, since it cannot be utilized due to a metabolic block (little or no correction).

Although the autohaemolysis test is crude and non-specific, it remains a very useful screening test in the diagnosis of haemolytic anaemia, for several reasons. First, if the test is entirely normal, an intrinsic red cell abnormality is very unlikely. Second, a great strength of the test lies in the fact that the glucose addition serves as an internal control. Correction of excessive autohaemolysis by glucose means that glucose metabolism in itself is normal and points therefore to increased glucose requirement, most probably ascribable to a membrane defect. Poor correction by glucose means that glycolysis itself is abnormal (Table 6.5).

Diagnosis

When all the criteria listed under the definition are met, the diagnosis of HS is straightforward, and this is true in at least 50% of cases. The importance of finding evidence of HS in a first-degree relative,

Table 6.5

The autohaemolysis test

Condition	Lysis in a typical case (%)	
	No addition	+ 27 mmol glucose
Normal	1.7	0.15
Hereditary spherocytosis	10.1	1.3
Pyruvate kinase deficiency	5.5	6.1
G6PD deficiency with CNSHA*	2.9	1.8

*In the much more common forms of G6PD deficiency without chronic non-spherocytic haemolytic anaemia (CNSHA) the autohaemolysis test is normal.

even if asymptomatic, cannot be overemphasized. In the remaining cases, two main sorts of diagnostic problems arise.

1. If spherocytosis is prominent, the main differential diagnosis is acquired haemolytic anaemia. If the direct antiglobulin test is positive, the diagnosis is AIHA. If the direct antiglobulin test is negative and family data are negative or unobtainable, an acute presentation will favour in general an acquired disorder, and a search for an underlying cause is necessary. For instance, the coexistence with spherocytes of red cell fragments and poikilocytes may suggest a microangiopathic process. An acute febrile illness might suggest a rare infectious cause for haemolysis (e.g. *Clostridium. welchii* septicaemia). On the other hand, the finding in the patient's past record of a previously unnoticed reticulocytosis or borderline high MCHC and the persistence of spherocytosis after the acute illness is over will favour a diagnosis of HS.

2. When spherocytosis is not prominent but there is evidence of a chronic, probably congenital, haemolytic disorder, the differential diagnosis is between HS and any other intrinsic red cell abnormality. Paroxysmal nocturnal haemoglobinuria (PNH) can be excluded by the Ham test. Enzymopathies are uniformly recessive and therefore a negative family history and even negative family studies do not help to differentiate between HS due to a new mutation and an enzymopathy. It is in these circumstances that the laboratory tests discussed above may be very helpful. In enzymopathies, unlike in HS, the osmotic fragility is usually normal or decreased; and autohaemolysis is almost invariably not only abnormal but also not fully corrected by glucose addition.

Management

Hereditary spherocytosis cannot be cured. As in many other genetic disorders, however, the aim we can set ourselves is to minimize the consequences of the genetic abnormality. In this respect, because of the special role exerted by the spleen in the pathophysiology of HS, the mainstay of management is splenectomy. In view of the wide spectrum of severity of HS, it is debatable whether this surgical procedure ought to be adopted in mild cases.

However, most haematologists agree that, once the diagnosis of HS is firmly established, splenectomy is indicated in order to prevent complications, particularly cholelithiasis and aplastic crises. What is more debatable is the timing of splenectomy. In children one tries to avoid splenectomy before the age of five, except when haemolytic anaemia is very severe (it rarely is in HS). When the diagnosis is first made in an adult there is usually no good reason to postpone splenectomy. Possible exceptions would be the few patients found to have HS when they are in their fifth decade or beyond (usually because HS has been diagnosed in a younger member of the family) and who have lived happily with HS until then. In these cases the decision must rest with judgement of the individual case.

With pre-splenectomy, at any age, it is usual to give pneumococcal vaccination, and post-splenectomy to give regular penicillin prophylaxis (e.g. 250 mg oral penicillin b.d.) for at least 2 years to prevent pneumococcal infections (see later). Treatment of folate deficiency, aplastic crises or gallstones is similar to that for other haemolytic states.

Pathogenesis

The study of the pathogenesis of HS serves as a good example of how the trail from phenotype to genotype must be explored step by step to elucidate the basic genetic disorder.

Step I: From the clinical phenotype to its cellular basis. The combination of spherocytosis and an enlarged spleen was compatible, in principle, either with an abnormal spleen damaging normal red cells (extracorpuscular defect) or with abnormal red cells being destroyed in the spleen and thus causing its enlargement (intracorpuscular defect). The controversy persisted for nearly half a century until Dacie and Mollison (1943) demonstrated normal survival of red cells in HS patients and decreased survival of HS red cells in normal subjects. Thus, the defect is *intracorpuscular*.

Step II: Defining the nature of the intracorpuscular defect. Numerous studies of red cell enzymes in HS have found either normal or high levels (the latter presumably due to a younger than normal red cell population) and they have consistently failed to reveal any enzyme deficiency. By contrast, studies of ion composition and transport have demonstrated a decreased intracellular potassium concentration and an increased sodium efflux. Analyses of membrane lipids have shown an essentially normal composition but an abnormally high rate of loss of phospholipid and cholesterol upon incubation of HS red cells in vitro under a variety of conditions. In addition, the abnormal shape of the HS red cell is retained after cell ghosts are treated with non-ionic detergents such as Triton. All of these data suggest strongly that the defect is in the membrane–cytoskeleton complex.

Step III: Identifying the primary lesion. The most consistent abnormality emerging from detailed studies of the red cell membrane in HS has been a quantitative reduction in spectrin. Thus, one might be tempted to think that HS is caused by decreased spectrin synthesis. However, one cannot lightly assume that this is necessarily the case because spectrin loss might be in turn secondary to some other lesion. At the moment, the pertinent data can be summarized as follows. (1) The degree of spectrin deficiency varies between 20% and 40%—it is up to 70% in the rare recessive type of HS (see below). (2) Spectrin deficiency is quite specific in the sense that normal levels have been found in a variety of haemolytic disorders (other than HS), including acquired autoimmune haemolytic anaemia in which red cell morphology and osmotic fragility changes are similar to those of HS, (3) There may be a crude correlation between the degree of spectrin deficiency and the clinical severity of HS. (4) In some individual cases there has been evidence of qualitative changes in the tail end of either α- or β-spectrin and this is associated with impaired binding to the band 4.1 protein. (5) Genetic analysis in some families has shown that HS does not co-segregate with a DNA polymorphism in the α-spectrin gene, indicating that the mutation responsible for HS is probably not at that genetic locus.

Genetic Heterogeneity

The above data, together with the well-recognized variability in the clinical severity of HS, suggest that HS must arise, in deficient families, from more than one primary lesion. This inference has been reinforced by the relatively recent discovery that some cases conforming to the classical phenotype of HS exhibit recessive rather than dominant inheritance (Agre *et al.*, 1982). Because dominant inheritance has been regarded as part of the definition of HS, one would tend to assume that these cases must constitute a very small proportion of all patients with HS. However, for about 20% of HS patients, both parents are normal and it has been generally assumed that these cases are due to new mutations. It is possible instead that some of them may have the recessive form of HS. Because the latter tends to be severe, this explanation ought to be considered especially with severe HS from asymptomatic parents. Very recently it has been shown that these asymptomatic parents do have a slight decrease in red cell spectrin. Heterogeneity of a Mendelian genetic disorder may signify either that the underlying mutation is not always at the same locus or that there are multiple allelic mutations at the same locus. It would not be surprising if in HS both occurred. In cases with qualitative changes in spectrin the mutation must reside within the coding region of the respective α- or β-spectrin structural gene. In cases with spectrin deficiency but no qualitative changes the mutation might be in a noncoding region of one of the spectrin structural genes (it could still be β-spectrin in the families in which HS does not segregate with α-spectrin), or it might be in a different gene altogether. In cases with recessive inheritance the mutation is likely to be in a different gene than in those with dominant inheritance. Thus, step III is not yet completed in HS. However, a possible pathogenetic sequence can be visualized (Fig. 6.10).

Hereditary Elliptocytosis

This disorder is defined in a way similar to HS by the characteristic shape of the red cells (Fig. 6.11). The clinical manifestations and pathophysiology are similar to those of HS. The diagnosis is often easier because the finding of a large proportion of elliptocytes in the blood film is virtually pathognomonic. Elliptocytes are seen in iron deficiency but the differentiation is usually easy because in this condition they are fewer in numbers, associated with other sorts of poikilocytes and the picture is microcytic hypochromic. In some cases of hereditary elliptocytosis (HE), however, especially in

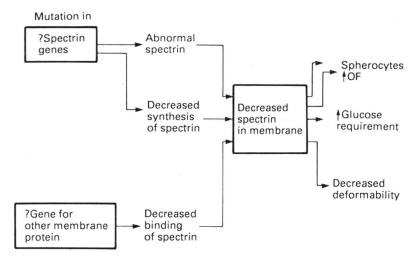

Fig. 6.10. *Pathogenesis of hereditary spherocytosis. A partly hypothetical diagram, amining to illustrate how each of the different primary lesions (left) can, through different mechanisms (centre), lead to one common outcome—decreased amount of spectrin associated with the red cell membrane (spectrin is, more exactly, a filamentous cytoskeletal protein lining the cytoplasmic face of the membrane). The deficiency of spectrin is in turn responsible for the various characteristic morphologic, physical and metabolic abnormalities of HS red cells (right).*

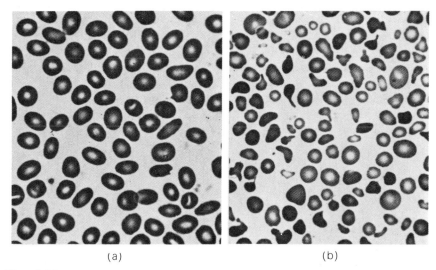

(a)　　　　　　　　　　　　(b)

Fig. 6.11. *(a) Hereditary elliptocytosis trait: the majority of the cells are oval in shape. (b) Homozygous hereditary elliptocytosis: this is the blood film from a son of the patient in (a).*

infants (neonatal pyropoikilocytosis), the morphology is remarkably similar to that of iron deficiency, and definitive diagnosis, as in many genetic disorders, must be backed up by family studies. As in HS, autohaemolysis in HE is increased and

corrected by glucose, but the osmotic fragility curve is not helpful for diagnosis.

The variable clinical and morphological expression of HE has led to a classification of various subtypes of this condition (see Table 6.6). Recognition of different forms is of practical importance because HE with little or no haemolysis does not require treatment, whereas the more severe forms usually associated with clinical splenomegaly benefit from splenectomy—usually in a rather dramatic way, just as in HS. The identification of the primary molecular lesion has been more successful in HE than in HS and it has clarified the relationship between the expression of the defect in heterozygotes and in homozygotes (Table 6.6). A substantial proportion of cases are due to structural changes in α-spectrin. This includes the non-haemolytic form, designated in the older literature as benign ovalocytosis. The mapping of the α-spectrin gene to the long arm of chromosome 1 (see Table 6.2) explains the well-established genetic linkage of this form of HE to the rhesus blood groups.

Homozygous elliptocytosis presents as a severe haemolytic anaemia with splenomegaly and bizarre red cell morphology, including microspherocytes, small dense cells of other shapes, elliptocytes and poikilocytes (pyropoikilocytes).

Other Congenital Membrane Abnormalities

A variety of familial haemolytic anaemias have been reported which, on grounds of direct or indirect evidence, can be attributed to a genetically abnormal red cell membrane. In a proportion of these families the most conspicuous morphological feature has been the presence of large numbers of **stomatocytes** and therefore the term hereditary stomatocytosis has been used. In several cases marked changes in red cell sodium and potassium have been demonstrated. When sodium gain causes high MCV and low MCHC the red cells appear swollen and this has been referred to as **hydrocytosis**. When potassium loss causes low MCV and high MCHC the red cells appear shrunken and this has been referred to as **xerocytosis**. A satisfactory classification of these disorders will clearly require an identification of the underlying primary genetic lesion. The multitude of names is rather confusing, but it appears likely that most of these disorders are closely related to HS and HE (see for instance

Table 6.6
Different forms of elliptocytosis

Sub type of hereditary elliptocytosis (HE)	Genetic status	Degree of haemolysis	Example of known molecular lesion	Remarks
Common				
Non-haemolytic	Heterozygote	Absent	Structurally abnormal α-spectrin	One parent has similar picture
Mild	Heterozygote	Minimal	Glycoprotein C deficiency	One parent has similar picture
Intermediate	Heterozygote	Moderate		One parent has similar picture
Severe	Heterozygote	Severe		One parent has HE; sometimes both
Pyropoikilocytosis	Homozygote	Severe	Structurally abnormal α-spectrin	Usually both parents asymptomatic, or one has HE
Spherocytic	Heterozygote	Mild		
	Homozygote	Severe	Absence of protein 4.1	Deletion revealed at DNA level (Conboy *et al.*, 1986)
Stomatocytic	Not well defined	Absent or mild		Common in Melanesians ?Protects against malaria

stomatocytic HE in Table 6.6). This is supported by the fact that in these conditions anaemia, if present, responds to splenectomy, although not always completely. One looks forward to the day when the classification of red cell membrane abnormalities will consist of a list of defined changes in individual proteins.

A usually mild haemolytic anaemia is associated with the rare, but serologically uniquely characterized abnormality which goes under the name of **Rh-null disease**, in which all rhesus antigens are missing (see Chapter 9). This condition proves that the membrane protein(s) carrying the rhesus antigenic determinants is (or are) essential for the function of the red cell membrane.

All disorders mentioned thus far in this section are known or presumed to be caused by primary changes in one of the proteins of the membrane or of the cytoskeleton, with lipid abnormalities, if any, being secondary. On the other hand, in rare cases primary lipid abnormalities can affect markedly red cell morphology and red cell viability. Abetalipoproteinaemia causes strikingly spiculated red cells referred to as **acanthocytes.** In this condition autohaemolysis in vitro is abnormal (correctable by glucose) but there is little evidence for haemolytic anaemia in vivo. By contrast, in genetically determined deficiency of lecithin-cholesterol acetyl transferase (LCAT deficiency), there are large numbers of target cells and haemolytic anaemia, presumably due to excess cholesterol in the red cell membrane.

RED CELL ENZYMOPATHIES

Glucose-6-Phosphate Dehydrogenase Deficiency

Electrophoretic variants of G6PD with normal activity have long been known as a good example of genetic polymorphism of human enzymes. For historical reasons the most common normal type is called G6PD B. An electrophoretically fast-moving, non-deficient variant common in Africa is referred to as G6PD A; it has no known clinical significance, and it should not be confused with the G6PD deficient variant A − (see below).

Whereas HS can be only defined as a clinico-haematological entity which may result from mutations at various genetic loci, only some of which are as yet elucidated, G6PD deficiency is defined directly and unambiguously by its very name. G6PD is a dimeric enzyme of a single polypeptide chain of about 59 kd, encoded in an X-linked locus mapped to the telomeric region of the X-chromosome, very near the factor VIII gene (band Xq 28). The gene has recently been cloned and sequenced and thus the complete amino acid sequence has now become known (Persico *et al.*, 1986).

Genetics and Epidemiology

Biochemical evidence had already indicated that G6PD deficiency results from a variety of mutant alleles of its structural gene. Recently this has been confirmed by cloning the G6PD gene from G6PD-deficient subjects and identifying point mutations causing such amino acid replacements. These mutations may cause decreased catalytic activity or decreased stability of the enzyme, or both. G6PD deficiency is common in many human populations, particularly, of subtropical and tropical regions (see Fig. 6.12), with the exception of autochthonous Americans. In addition, as a result of recent migrations, G6PD has become widespread in many other areas, including Great Britain, North America and South America. The prevalence of G6PD deficiency varies widely, from being very rare in the indigenous populations of Northern Europe, to frequencies of about 20% in parts of Southern Europe, Africa and Asia, and up to 40% in certain areas of the Middle East. Because the G6PD gene is X-linked, the frequency of G6PD deficiency is quite different in males and in females (Table 6.7). It is commonly stated that deficiency in women is more rare; this is true for homozygotes but not for heterozygotes who also can have clinical manifestations. Indeed, it must be remembered that because of the phenomenon of X-chromosome inactivation, heterozygotes have two populations of red cells, normal and G6PD deficient. The proportions of the two cell populations are quite variable and obviously susceptibility to haemolysis will be greater when the size of the deficient population is larger.

Clinical Features and Management

The manifestations of G6PD deficiency may be acute or chronic. The large majority of subjects with G6PD deficiency are asymptomatic until an acute

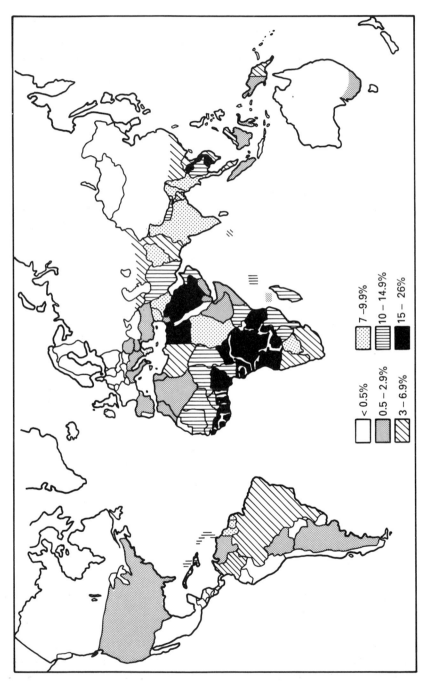

Fig. 6.12. *Geographic distribution of G6PD deficiency (reproduced with permission of the World Health Organization. Geneva.)*

Table 6.7

Frequency of G6PD deficiency in the two sexes in various populations

Examples	Overall frequency of G6PD-deficient gene, Gd⁻	G6PD-deficient people (%)		
		Males (hemizygotes)	Females Heterozygotes	Homozygotes
I	0.0001	0.1	0.02	$\simeq 0$
II	0.01	1.0	2.0	0.01
III	0.2	20	32	4.0

The three examples represent idealized populations, which might correspond rather closely, for instance, to England (I), Northern Italy (II) and Nigeria (III). The frequencies in males and females are in Hardy–Weinberg equilibrium.

episode takes place. Very few subjects have a chronic haemolytic anaemia which varies from mild to severe. This considerable clinical heterogeneity results directly from a vast genetic heterogeneity (see below). Indeed, all of the G6PD-deficiency variants that occur with high frequency in various populations are as a rule asymptomatic and they are clinically important only because of the risk of acute haemolytic anaemia (HA). By contrast, chronic haemolytic anaemia is the expression of other genetic variants, which are quite rare in any population.

Acute Haemolytic Anaemia

The fact that G6PD deficiency is usually asymptomatic must mean that a level of G6PD enzyme activity of 20% of normal (or even less, i.e. as low as 3%) is sufficient for normal red cell function and survival under ordinary circumstances. It is only when some exogenous factor imposes an extra stress on the red cells that the rate of supply of NADPH becomes inadequate and haemolysis takes place. Thus acute HA associated with G6PD deficiency is a typical example of interaction between an intracorpuscular and an extracorpuscular factor, neither of which would by itself cause haemolysis.

Three types of trigger have been identified, namely fava beans, infection and drugs (Table 6.8). Whatever the agent, the haemolytic attack has a number of common features which make it fairly easy to recognize, provided one is alert to the possibility (Table 6.9). The severity of haemolysis can vary from causing mild anaemia and jaundice requiring only a few days of bed rest, to severe, life-threatening anaemia requiring urgent blood transfusion. In general, but not always, haemolysis is less severe with the African variant A⁻ (when sometimes it subsides even when the trigger is still present) than it is with the variants more prevalent in the Mediterranean, the Middle East and South-East Asia.

Massive haemoglobinuria is seen most frequently in children with favism, but some degree of haemoglobinuria is always present in an attack, and it is especially useful in the differential diagnosis. Renal failure associated with haemoglobinuria is very rare in children, but it is not infrequent in adults, perhaps in those who have some previously unrecognized renal damage. Its management does not differ from that of acute renal failure from other causes, and occasionally haemodialysis may be required. Withdrawal of a potentially offending drug is obviously indicated, because while in some cases haemolysis has been found to be self-limiting, this is not necessarily true for all drugs or for all variants. Treatment of an underlying infection which may have triggered haemolysis is also obviously mandatory.

An unsolved riddle is why fava bean ingestion is not always followed by a haemolytic attack in G6PD-deficient individuals. Recent evidence suggests that the offending agent may be the glucoside divicine, or its aglycone isouramil. The amount of divicine varies widely in different cultivars of *Vicia faba*, and with the way the fava beans are consumed. Favism has been reported with fresh beans, dried beans, canned beans and frozen beans;

Table 6.8

Drugs to be avoided in G6PD deficiency *

Antimalarials	*Analgesics*
Primaquine (can be given at reduced dos-	Acetylsalicylic acid (aspirin)—moderate
age, 15 mg/daily or 45 mg twice weekly	doses can be used
under surveillance)	Acetophenetidin (phenacetin), safe altern-
Pamaquine	ative—paracetamol
Sulphonamides and sulphones	*Antihelminthics*
Sulphanilamide	β naphthol
Sulphapyridine	Stibophan
Sulphadimidine	Niridazole
Sulphacetamide (Albucid)	
Salicylazosulphapyridine	*Miscellaneous*
(Salazopyrin)	Vitamin K analogues (1 mg of menaph-
†Dapsone	thone can be given to babies)
†Sulphoxone	†Naphthalene (mothballs)
Glucosulphone sodium (Promin)	Probenecid
Septrin	Dimercaprol (BAL)
	Methylene blue
Other antibacterial compounds	Toluidine blue
Nitrofurans	
Nitrofurantoin	
Furazolidone	
Nitrofurazone	
Nalidixic acid	

* This list is compiled on the basis of data available for patients with the 'A–' variant of G6PD deficiency. It can be generally assumed to be applicable to patients from Africa and of African descent. For patients with the Mediterranean type of G6PD deficiency, or with an unknown variant, or with CNSHA, the following should also be added: acetanilide, chloramphenicol, chloroquine (may be used under surveillance when required for prophylaxis or treatment of malaria), mepacrine, p-amino salicylic acid and thiazosulphone. Many other drugs may produce haemolysis in particular individuals.

† These drugs may cause haemolysis in normal individuals if taken in large doses.

however, it is commonest when the beans are eaten fresh and raw. It has also been suggested that the oxidative damage may depend on how much iso-uramil is released by glycosidases present in the bean itself or in the intestinal tract of the consumer.

Neonatal Jaundice

It has been well documented in Greece, Sardinia, Nigeria, Thailand, Singapore and elsewhere that G6PD-deficient babies are more prone to neonatal jaundice (NNJ) than G6PD-normal babies. The association between G6PD deficiency and NNJ is sufficiently strong (Table 6.10) to make the former the most common cause of the latter in these and probably in other parts of the world. However, the nature of the causal link is not entirely clear, because at least one-half of G6PD-deficient babies do not develop NNJ. We must postulate that an additional genetic, developmental or acquired factor interacts with G6PD deficiency to bring about NNJ. Sometimes a drug given to the mother nearing delivery or to the newborn baby may be the culprit: in such cases the situation is similar to that of acute haemolytic anaemia (as just described), with the added risk contingent to any hyperbili-rubinaemia in the neonatal period; but in most cases an offending agent cannot be pinpointed. The hy-perbilirubinaemia tends to develop late, when com-pared to NNJ caused by Rh isoimmunization, and it is frequently far in excess of what can be ac-counted for by haemolysis, suggesting that the

Table 6.9
Characteristic features of haemolytic attack in G6PD deficiency

Phase	Clinical	Laboratory
Acute	Abrupt onset	
	Malaise, prostration	
	Pallor	Anaemia; Heinz bodies; reticulocytosis; G6PD deficient
	(Abdominal pain)	
	Fever	Leucocytosis
	(Hypotension)	
	Dark urine	Haemoglobinuria; haptoglobin absent
		Haemoglobinaemia
		Methaemalbuminaemia
	Jaundice	Hyperbilirubinaemia
	(Renal failure)	↑Urea ↑Creatinine
Recovery	Gradual but rapid	Reticulocytes peak day 5–8
	Urine clears in few days	G6PD increases but rarely to normal range
	Jaundice clears in 1–2 weeks	

Table 6.10
Association between G6PD deficiency and jaundice in male newborns

Groups of newborns	n	G6PD deficiency
		%
Normal	500	22.5
Mild jaundice (bilirubin 150–200)	38	45
Severe jaundice (bilirubin > 230)	70	60
Admitted with kernicterus	20	78

Data collected in Ibadan, Nigeria.
Bilirubin values in μmol/l.

handling of unconjugated bilirubin by the liver may be subnormal, perhaps as a result of low G6PD in the hepatocyte. The treatment of G6PD-associated NNJ does not differ from that of NNJ from other causes, namely, phototherapy in most cases and exchange transfusion in severe cases (see Luzzatto and Meloni, 1986). With good management, full recovery without sequelae is the rule.

Chronic Haemolytic Anaemia

Rare individuals have a G6PD mutation producing an enzyme variant which is so severely abnormal qualitatively, or so severely deficient quantitatively, that they suffer from life-long anaemia. Morphologically, the anaemia is normocytic and normochromic, with reticulocytosis and no excess of spherocytes. Hence it is usually referred to as chronic non-spherocytic haemolytic anaemia (CNSHA) and its features in the steady state are not significantly different from those of CNSHA caused by other enzyme abnormalities, such as pyruvate kinase deficiency. However, not surprisingly, it carries the risk of acute hyperhaemolytic exacerbations triggered by the same agents that can cause acute HA in G6PD deficiency (see Table 6.8). Diagnosis requires only a G6PD assay. Most patients are well adjusted to their anaemia and usually require no treatment except folic acid supplements. The bone marrow shows erythroid hyperplasia without evidence of ineffective erythropoiesis and therefore there is no indication for a chronic blood transfusion regimen. However, blood transfusion may be required in episodes of acute 'aplastic' or hyperhaemolytic crisis. Although in general there is no evidence for selective red cell destruction in the spleen, splenectomy has been beneficial in some patients.

Laboratory Diagnosis

Several tests can be used to identify G6PD deficiency in red blood cells. Some of them are very simple and especially suitable for handling large numbers of samples, as in population studies, and they are appropriately referred to as screening tests. The most widely used have been brilliant cresyl blue decolorization test, the methaemoglobin reduction test and an ultraviolet spot test. Although each one of these can be made semiquantitative, they can be fully relied upon only to tell us whether a blood sample is deficient or not, and from the diagnostic point of view nothing else is necessary. Thus, hemizygous deficient males and homozygous deficient females will be identified, the threshold being a G6PD activity of about 20% of normal. If a screening test indicates deficiency or is doubtful, the ideal follow-up test for definitive diagnosis is quantitation of G6PD activity by a spectrophotometric assay.

There are two clinical situations in which quantitation is especially important. First, during a haemolytic attack the oldest red cells (with least G6PD activity) are destroyed selectively and therefore the surviving red cells have a relatively higher (but still deficient) G6PD activity. This increases further as a reticulocyte response sets in over the following days (recovery phase). During this time a screening test might yield a false-normal result and, rarely, even a quantitative test might do so. In such cases the best counsel is to repeat the test a few weeks later. Alternatively, the oldest remaining cells can be isolated by differential centrifugation and they can be shown to have low G6PD activity. The same approach can be used if the situation is further complicated by the patient having been transfused (although a pre-transfusion sample should have been saved!). Secondly, the diagnosis of heterozygous females can be especially difficult: indeed, in extreme cases it can only be done by family studies. However, from the practical point of view it must be borne in mind that the probability of clinically significant haemolysis in a heterozygote roughly correlates with the proportion of G6PD-deficient

red cells in her blood. Therefore, if a normal level of G6PD activity is found in a heterozygote, she is unlikely to be at risk of G6PD-related haemolysis. On the other hand, the diagnostic problems mentioned above with respect to the haemolytic and recovery phases will be compounded in the case of a heterozygote.

Pathophysiology

G6PD-deficient red cells are more susceptible than normal red cells to oxidative damage. The reason for this is that NADPH, produced by G6PD, is required for regeneration of glutathione (GSH) which, in turn, detoxifies hydrogen peroxidase via GSH peroxidase (Fig. 6.13). Oxidative damage can be caused by bacteria producing hydrogen peroxide or by a variety of chemicals (see Table 6.8) or by divicine present in fava beans, thus explaining how these exogenous agents can trigger a haemolytic attack.

Biochemical analysis has shown that G6PD deficiency is vastly heterogeneous, with over 200 different variants having been identified. The variants underlying CNSHA are different from those which are associated only with acute HA and are otherwise asymptomatic. Patients with CNSHA usually have a 'sporadic' variant, i.e. the underlying mutation is probably different in each unrelated patient. Of the variants underlying acute HA, many are common in a particular population, i.e. they are polymorphic, but different variants are found in different parts of the world (see Table 6.11).

The difference between these two groups of variants must lie in the fact that the latter provide the red cell with enough residual G6PD activity to be compatible with nearly normal red cell survival except when an oxidative agent adds insult to injury. By contrast, in patients with CNSHA the residual G6PD activity is inadequate even under basal condition. In determining whether a G6PD variant will cause CNSHA or will only be exposed to the risk of acute HA, at least two main features seem to be important: the level of residual activity of the enzyme and its kinetic properties (quantity and quality). Variants associated with CNSHA have, as a group, lower residual enzyme activity than variants which are usually asymptomatic. By contrast, the latter often have increased substrate affinities,

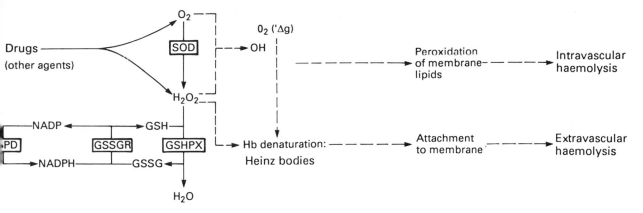

Fig. 6.13. *Mechanism of haemolysis in G6PD deficiency*

Table 6.11
G6PD deficiency in some human populations

Country	Approximate frequency range of G6PD deficiency in males (%)	Most common G6PD variants present
Greece	4–35	Mediterranean, Athens-like, Orchomenos, Union-Markham
Southern Italy	2–22	Mediterranean, Sassari, Cagliari, Seattle-like
Nigeria	18–25	A⁻
Thailand	3–14	Mahidol, Canton, Union, Hong-Kong
Papua New Guinea	1–29	Markham; many others

meaning that they can operate at practically normal rates at physiologically low substrate concentrations. Of the two substrate-binding constants, K_m^{NADP} and K_m^{G6P}, the latter seems to be more critical.

The exact mode whereby oxidative damage eventually leads to haemolysis is not yet completely elucidated. On the one hand, haemoglobin denaturation (manifested in the formation of Heinz bodies) affects the physical properties of red cells which are then destroyed or fragmented in the reticuloendothelial system. On the other hand, lipid peroxidation may sufficiently disturb the structure of the membrane to cause red cell destruction directly. It is tempting to ascribe to the first and to the second mechanism respectively the extravascular haemolysis and the intravascular haemolysis which are both seen in G6PD deficiency, even though this correlation may not be perfect in vivo.

What is clear is that intravascular haemolysis dominates the clinical picture in acute HA whilst extravascular haemolysis predominates in CNSHA.

Pyruvate Kinase Deficiency

Pyruvate kinase (PK) deficiency has emerged as the most common red cell enzymopathy after G6PD deficiency. It is, however, a rare disease with an estimated prevalence of less than 1 in 10 000 and, unlike G6PD deficiency, it does not have a widely different prevalence in different parts of the world. The inheritance of PK deficiency is autosomal recessive and, because of the rarity of PK deficiency, many patients probably inherit from their parents two different mutant allelic genes—in which case they ought to be referred to as genetic compounds rather than as homozygotes. On the other hand, if a patient is the offspring of a consanguineous marriage, the two parental genes are likely to be identical by descent and the patient is a true homozygote (Fig. 6.14).

Clinical Features

There is considerable variation in the presentation, severity and response to treatment of different patients with PK deficiency. Most patients are found to be jaundiced or anaemic in infancy or childhood. Occasionally the disorder is so mild that it is not diagnosed until adult life. Siblings with PK deficiency tend to have a similar age of onset and a similar clinical course (Fig. 6.15). Most patients show moderate to severe anaemia with haemoglobin levels between 4 g/dl and 10 g/dl. Because of the lowered oxygen affinity of the blood (resulting from high diphosphoglycerate), symptoms from anaemia may be less than would be expected: one patient with a haemoglobin of approximately 8–9 g/dl regularly enjoyed cross-country running. As with most haemolytic anaemias, anaemia is often exacerbated during infections. Aplastic crises have been described in PK deficiency.

The bilirubin level in the serum is related to the rate of haemolysis and to liver function; clinical jaundice is usual and may increase during infections. Jaundice in the neonatal period is not uncommon and exchange transfusions may be required. Gallstones are a common result of the hyperbilirubinaemia, with all the attendant potential complications of biliary colic and cholecystitis.

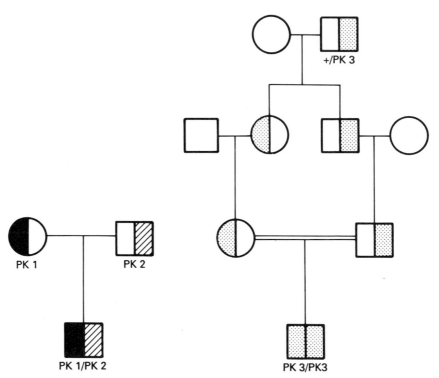

Fig. 6.14. *Inheritance of pyruvate kinase (PK) deficiency. In the pedigree at the left, two unrelated parents, heterozygous for PK deficiency, produce a PK-deficient offspring who is heterozygous for two different abnormal alleles (PK1/PK2). In the pedigree at the right, two first cousin parents, both having inherited the same PK-deficient allele (PK3) from the same grandfather, produce an offspring who is a true homozygote for PK deficiency. There is no evidence that either genetic status is clinically more severe than the other. The pedigree at the right, however, highlights the fact that this enzymopathy, like any other recessive condition, will be much more common in communities with a high rate of inbreeding.*

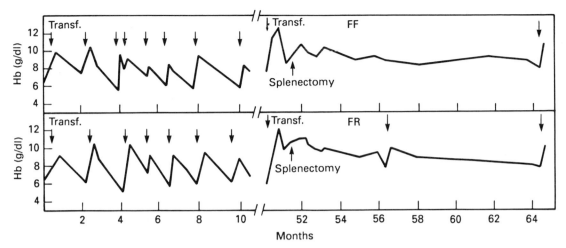

Fig. 6.15. *Long-term haematological follow-up of two sisters with pyruvate kinase (PK) deficiency. FF (top) was diagnosed at the age of 7 and FR (bottom) at the age of 5. It is seen that both patients had severe anaemia and were transfusion dependent. After splenectomy their haemoglobin levels stabilized in the range of 8–9 g/dl and they required blood transfusion only occasionally in concomitance with intercurrent viral infection, such as influenza.*

The spleen is usually enlarged but the increase in size is only slight to moderate; even in severe cases the spleen is rarely enlarged beyond the umbilicus. Marked enlargement of the spleen or a firm spleen together with enlargement of the liver suggests haemosiderosis.

Although there may be a widening of the marrow cavities, skeletal changes are not prominent, except for frontal bossing. As with all congenital anaemias, growth is impaired if there is severe, continuing anaemia but otherwise children develop normally.

Women with PK deficiency seem to tolerate pregnancy well and there is no increase in perinatal mortality or miscarriage. However, there is often a fall in haemoglobin during pregnancy greater than is seen in normal women and occasionally transfusions may be necessary. Folate deficiency may also develop during pregnancy.

Diagnosis

The blood film pre-splenectomy shows a fairly uniform macrocytosis. Bizarre 'prickle' cells may be present but are much more frequent post-splen-

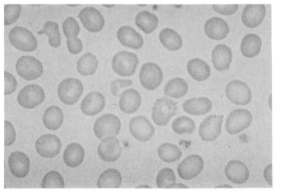 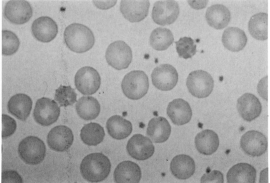

Fig. 6.16. *Blood film in pyruvate kinase (PK) deficiency before (left) and after (right) splenectomy.*

Table 6.12

Genetic and biochemical features of enzymes, deficiency of which can cause haemolytic anaemia

Group	Enzyme	Known number of genetic loci	Number of subunits in active enzyme	Predominant enzyme form in RBC	Chromosome localization	Gene cloned	Severity of haemolytic disorder	Other systemic manifestations	Relative frequency (PK = 100)
Glycolytic enzymes	Hexokinase (HK)	3	4	HK-1	10		++	No	3
	Glucose phosphate isomerase (GPI)	1	2	Common	19cen–q13		+ to ++++	Sometimes	20
	Phosphofructokinase (PFK)	3	4	M,L	Icenq 32; 21q 22		++	Yes	10
	Aldolase (ALD)	3	4	A	?		+	Yes	2
	Triose phosphate isomerase (TPI)	1	2	Common	12p13	Yes	+++	Yes	9
	2,3-Diphosphoglycerate mutase (DPGM)					Yes		No	4
	Phosphoglycerate kinase (PGK)	1	1	Common	X913	Yes	+ to ++++	Yes	4
	Pyruvate kinase (PK)	3	4	L	15q22–qter		+ to ++++	No	100

Table 6.12 (*Continued*)

Group	Enzyme	Known number of genetic loci	Number of subunits in active enzyme	Predominant enzyme form in RBC	Chromosome localization	Gene cloned	Severity of haemolytic disorder	Other systemic manifestations	Relative frequency (PK =100)
Glutathione metabolism	Glucose 6-phosphate dehydrogenase (G6PD)	1	2–4	Common	Xq 28	Yes	+ to + + + +	No	
	Glutathione synthetase (GSHS)				?		+	Sometimes	
	Glutamylcysteine synthetase (GCS)				?		+	Sometimes	
	Glutathione reductase (GSSGR)				8p21.1	Yes	(+)	No	
	Glutathione peroxidase (GSHPX)				3p13–q12		+	No	
Nucleotide metabolism	Adenylate kinase (AK)	3		AK-1	9q34		+	No	
	Adenosine deaminase (ADA)	1		Common	209q13.2–qter	Yes	+	No	
	Pyrimidine 5'-nucleotidase (P5'N)			Unique			+ +	No	

ectomy (Fig. 6.16). The reticulocyte count is usually moderately raised, but post-splenectomy it is markedly raised, sometimes to 50% or more.

In PK deficiency, as in other glycolytic enzyme abnormalities, the autohaemolysis test is abnormal, with poor correction by glucose (see Table 6.5). Definitive diagnosis requires a quantitative spectro-photometric PK assay and the results are not always straightforward. Affected homozygotes usually have values of 5–20% of the normal mean, but there are two main problems. (a) From the technical point of view, it must be noted that white cells have 10–100 times more PK activity than red cells. It is essential therefore to remove white cells completely before lysing the red cells. (b) From the biological point of view, an abnormal PK may have activity within the normal range when assayed in excess of substrates (as it usually is). Therefore it is appropriate to carry out tests at different substrate concentrations, as recommended by Beutler (1977). Finally, PK is an enzyme dependent on red cell age: PK deficiency may be difficult to pick up in the face of reticulocytosis. Family studies will usually clarify this problem because heterozygous parents have no haemolysis and may, paradoxically, have lower PK than the patient.

Treatment

As with all patients with severe chronic haemolysis, folic acid (5 mg daily) should be given regularly. Unless superimposed iron deficiency is present, iron administration should be avoided since some degree of haemosiderosis is usual.

Repeated or occasional blood transfusions may be necessary, especially during exceptional stress, for example infection and pregnancy. Since, however, there is no evidence of ineffective erythro-poiesis, attempts to keep the haemoglobin near normal values should not be made. In the neonatal period exchange transfusions may be needed, as in severe neonatal jaundice from any other source.

Splenectomy often leads to some improvement of the clinical condition of patients with PK deficiency (see Fig 6.14). Therefore, this procedure is advisable for all those who require frequent transfusions. Patients who develop complications of hyperbili-rubinaemia should also be considered for splen-ectomy, although the effect upon the bilirubin level is not nearly so marked as it is in HS. Patients who do not require repeated transfusions despite con-tinuing anaemia probably do not require splen-ectomy.

Deficiencies of other Glycolytic Enzymes

Apart from PK deficiency, all other enzymopathies involving glycolytic enzymes are very rare.

More often than not, the biochemical diagnosis is made in a specialized laboratory on a sample received from far away. Because the samples tested are highly selected through secondary and tertiary referral, it is impossible to give a meaningful esti-mate of absolute prevalence rates, which are prob-

Table 6.13
Mechanisms of enzymopathies

	Decreased catalytic activity	Abnormal kinetics	Instability	Reduced synthesis
Glucose 6-phosphate dehydrogenase (G6PD)	+	+	+	
Pyruvate kinase (PK)		+		
Glucose phosphate isomerase (GPI)	+	+	+	+
Haemoglobin analogy	HbM	Abnormal Hbs with high or low O_2 affinity	Unstable Hbs	Thalassaemias

ably of the order of around one in a million. In order to obtain at least a rough idea of the relative frequencies of these enzymopathies, a survey was carried out by correspondence*. From this survey it emerged that deficiencies of glucose phosphate isomerase (GPI), PFK and triose phosphate isomerase (TPI) are probably somewhat more common than the others (Table 6.12). The clinical haematological manifestation in all of these enzyme deficiencies is that of a life-long haemolytic anaemia of variable severity. An important consideration is that enzyme deficiency is often expressed not only in erythrocytes but in other somatic cells as well. To what extent this takes place depends, amongst other things, on the existence of several isoenzymes which are differentially expressed in different tissues. For instance, the hexokinase of red cells (HK-1) is encoded in a different gene from that expressed in other cells and therefore HK-1 deficiency only affects red cells. By contrast, the same phosphoglycerate kinase (PGK) locus is expressed in all cells and therefore PGK deficiency causes not only haemolytic anaemia but also serious neurological manifestations. The same is true for patients with TPI deficiency, who usually succumb in infancy to severe CNS disease (see Table 6.11). At least one case of aldolase deficiency was associated with glycogen storage because the same aldolase isoenzyme is expressed in red cells and hepatocytes. Space does not permit the discussion of details of these rare enzymopathies; some features of clinical findings, pathogenesis and secondary metabolic changes in red cells are summarized in Tables 6.12–6.14. The two different genetic situations of true homozygosity and of combined heterozygosity, outlined for PK deficiency, also apply to these enzymopathies. An exception is PGK deficiency which, because the respective gene is X-linked, has been seen only in hemizygous males. The blood film in glycolytic enzyme deficiencies is invariably abnormal but the abnormalities are not usually specific* (Fig. 6.17). Similarly, the autohaemolysis

*I am very grateful to the following investigators who have offered an opinion on this matter: H. Arnold (Freiburg, Germany); E. Beutler (La Jolla, USA); P. Boiron (Paris, France); S. Miwa (Tokyo, Japan); J. Rosa (Paris, France); Staal (Utrecht, Holland); W. Valentine (Los Angeles, USA); J. L. Vives-Corrons (Barcelona, Spain); A. Zanella (Milano, Italy).

Table 6.14

Mechanism of haemolysis in some erythrocyte enzymopathies

Deficient enzyme	Changes in metabolites				Likely cause of haemolysis	Associated pathophysiological changes
	ATP	DPG	GSH	Other		
Hexokinase (HK)	↓			G6P	Inadequate energy supply	Hb–O_2 affinity ↑
Glucose phosphate isomerase (GPI)		↓		G6P	?Inhibition of HK	
Phosphofructokinase (PFK)		↑↓		FDP	?	Hb–O_2 affinity ↑
Pyruvate kinase (PK)	↓	↑		PEP	Inadequate ATP production	Inhibition of HK, PFK
Glucose 6-phosphate dehydrogenase (G6PD)			↓	NADPH/NADP ↓	H_2O_2 toxicity	Glutathione reductase (GSSGR) ↑
Glutathione synthetase (GSHS)			↓↑		H_2O_2 toxicity	
Pyrimidine 5'-nucleotidase (P5'N)			↑	Nucleotides	?Inhibition of HK	PRPPK ↓

G6P, glucose 6-phosphate; FDP, fructose disphosphate; PEP, phosphoenol pyruvate; NADPH, reduced NADP; NADP, nicotinamide adenine dinucleotide phosphate.

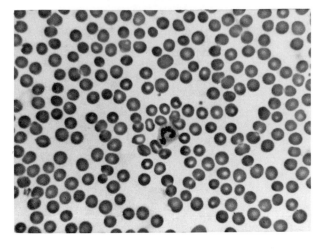

(a)

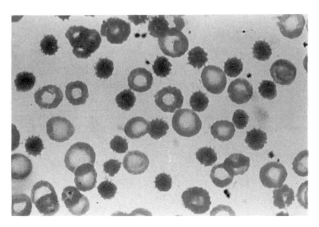

(b)

Fig. 6.17. *Blood films in two enzymopathies: (a) glucose phosphate isomerase (GPI) deficiency (by courtesy of Dr H. Arnold); (b) triose phosphate isomerase (TPI) deficiency (by courtesy of Dr J-L Vives Corrons).*

test is usually abnormal with little correction by glucose; but a specific diagnosis must rely on specific enzyme assays.

With respect to management, those patients who survive childhood are usually relatively well adjusted to their anaemia. Therefore there is little rationale for a hypertransfusion regimen, and blood

transfusion treatment is best reserved for intercurrent episodes of exacerbation of anaemia. The role of splenectomy is controversial, but in practice this is the only therapeutic option available and some patients have benefitted from it.

Pathogenesis

Although each enzymopathy is different, there are a limited number of mechanisms whereby an inherited change can cause enzyme deficiency (see Table 6.13). Thus far, only a few instances have been elucidated at the molecular level, but as more normal genes are cloned it will become easier to identify mutations in patients. This is turn will clarify where the critical regions are in the structure of each enzyme, just as has been the case for haemoglobin.

Although it is not surprising that if a glycolytic enzyme is deficient the red cell will be destroyed prematurely, the precise sequence of events leading to haemolysis is not always clear. In general, and in view of the features of red cell metabolism outlined in the first section of this chapter, we can expect that either failure of energy generation (ATP) or the failure of reductive potential (NADPH) will cause failure of the red cell. At the same time, changes in other metabolites can influence the pathophysiological state of enzyme-deficient red cells (see Table 6.13).

Pyrimidine 5′ Nucleotidase Deficiency

This enzymopathy was discovered by Valentine *et al.* (1974) whilst investigating patients with congenital haemolytic anaemia of previously unknown aetiology. Indeed, the enzyme (P5N) itself was discovered through the study of these patients. Experience in several specialized centres suggests that P5N deficiency, though rare, may be more common than all glycolytic enzyme deficiencies except PK. In contrast to other enzymopathies, red cell morphology is relatively characteristic in that it exhibits prominent basophilic stippling; indeed, this finding strongly suggests the diagnosis once thalassaemia has been excluded. The basophilic stippling is attributed to inhibition of breakdown of ribonucleoproteins present in reticulocytes as a consequence of the impaired dephosphorylation of pyrimidine nucleotides which normally are hydrolysed by P5N.

Patients with P5N deficiency usually have moderate anaemia (e.g. HB 10 g/dl), reticulocytosis, hyperbilirubinaemia and splenomegaly. Splenectomy has been of limited benefit. The mechanism of haemolysis in vivo is not clear. In vitro autohaemolysis is increased with little or no correction by glucose. Final diagnosis requires P5N assay or the demonstration of a markedly increased pool of pyrimidine nucleotides in a red cell lysate.

It is noteworthy that the best known acquired haemolytic anaemia associated with basophilic stippling, namely lead poisoning, turns out to be associated with acquired P5N deficiency because lead is a potent inhibitor of this enzyme. Thus, lead poisoning can be regarded as a phenocopy of P5N deficiency.

A Systematic Approach to Diagnosis

In many cases the exact diagnosis of a congenital haemolytic anaemia can be made quite promptly by conventional haematology and common sense. For instance, in a Southern European or African boy reporting sudden haemoglobinuria following sulphonamide administration, G6PD deficiency can be obviously suspected and quickly diagnosed by the appropriate specific assay with all 'screening' tests being conveniently bypassed. By contrast, in a middle-aged Scandinavian woman with low-grade haemolysis of uncertain duration and a moderately enlarged spleen, it would be wise to rule out immune haemolytic anaemia and congenital spherocytosis before embarking on an extensive (and expensive!) battery of enzyme assays. At any rate, a general systematic approach is recommended (see

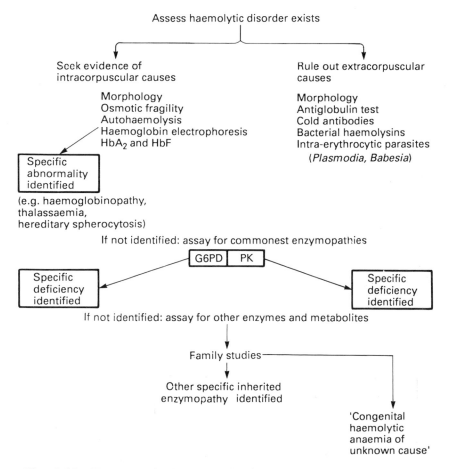

Fig. 6.18. *Flow sheet in the diagnosis of congenital haemolytic anaemia.*

diagrammatic summary in Fig. 6.18). In spite of all tests available, a small number of congenital haemolytic anaemias still defy explanation, even in the most highly specialized centres. Whilst this consideration is sobering, it is also stimulating because it suggests that something that we do not yet know still remains to be learnt about the physiology and pathophysiology of the red cell.

SELECTED BIBLIOGRAPHY

Several of the detailed reviews on the main topics of this chapter which are listed here supply extensive lists of references. In addition, only recent primary papers are listed here.

Acharya J., Ferguson I. L. C., Cassidy A. G., Grimes A. J. (1987). An improved acidified glycerol lysis test (AGLT) used to detect spherocytes in pregnancy. *British Journal of Haematology*, **65**, 343–345.

Agre P., Asimos A., Casella J. F., McMillan C. (1986). Inheritance pattern and clinical response to splenectomy as a reflection of erythrocyte spectrin deficiency in hereditary spherocytosis. *New England Journal of Medicine*, **315**, 1579–1583.

Agre P., Orringer, E. P., Bennett V. (1982). Deficient red-cell spectrin in severe recessively inherited spherocytosis. *New England Journal of Medicine*, **306**, 1155–1161.

Beutler, E., Blume K., Kaplan J. C., Lohr G., Ramot B., Valentine W. N. (1987). ICSH: recommended methods for red cell enzyme analysis. *British Journal of Haematology*, **35**, 331–340.

Conboy J., Mohandes N., Tchernia G., Kan Y. W. (1986). Molecular basis of hereditary elliptocytosis due to protein 4.1 deficiency. *New England Journal of Medicine*, **315**, 189–224.

Dacie J. V. (1985). *The haemolytic anaemias*, 3rd edn., Vol. 1. Edinburgh: Churchill Livingstone.

Dacie J. V., Mollison P. L. (1943). Survival of normal erythrocytes after transfusion to patients with familial haemolytic anaemia (acholuric jaundice). *Lancet*, **i**, 550–552.

Gottfried E. L., Robertson N. A. (1974). Glycerol lysis time as a screening test for erythrocyte disorders. *Journal of Laboratory and Clinical Medicine*, **83**, 323–333.

High S., Tanner M. J. A. (1987). Human erythrocyte membrane sialoglycoprotein β. The cDNA sequence suggests the absence of a cleaved N-terminal signal sequence. *Biochemical Journal*, **243**, 277–280.

Luzzatto L., Meloni T. (1985). Hemolytic anaemia due to glucose 6-phosphate dehydrogenase deficiency. In *Current therapy in hematology–oncology* 1985–86. (Eds. M. C. Brain and P. C. Carbone). Toronto: C. V. Mosby.

Luzzatto L., Testa U. (1978). Human erythrocyte glucose 6-phosphate dehydrogenase: structure and function in normal and mutant subjects. *Current Topics in Haematology*, **1**, 1–70.

Paglia D. E., Valentine W. N. (1981). Haemolytic anaemia associated with disorders of the purine and pyrimidine salvage pathways. *Clinics in Haematology*, **10**, (1), 81–98.

Palck J. (1987). Hereditary elliptocytosis, spherocytosis and related disorders: consequences of a deficiency or a mutation of membrane skeletal proteins. *Blood Reviews*, **1**, 147–168.

Persico M., Battistuzzi G., Mareni C.; Nobile C., D'Urso M., Toniolo D., Luzzatto L. (1982). Genetic variants of human glucose 6-phosphate dehydrogenase (G6PD): studies of turnover and G6PD-specific mRNA. In *Advances in red cell biology*, pp. 309–318 (Eds. D. J. Weatherall, G. Giorelli and S. Gorino). New York: Raven Press.

Persico M. G., Toniolo D., Nobile C., D'Urso M., Luzzatto L. (1981). cDNA sequences of human glucose 6-phosphate dehydrogenase cloned in pBR322. *Nature*, **294**, 778–780.

Persico M. G., Viglietto G., Martini G., Toniolo D., Paonessa G., Moscatelli C., Dono R., Vulliamy T., Luzzatto L., D'Urso M. (1986). Isolation of human glucose 6-phosphate dehydrogenase (G6PD) cDNA clones; primary structure of the protein and unusual 5′ non-coding region. *Nucleic Acids Research*, **14**, 2511–2522.

Selwyn J. G., Dacie J. V. (1954). Autohemolysis and other changes resulting from the incubation in vitro of red cells from patients with congenital hemolytic anemia. *Blood*, **9**, 414–438.

Valentine W. N., Fink K., Paglia D. E., Harris S. R., Adams W. S. (1974). Hereditary hemolytic anaemia with human erythrocyte pyrimidine 5′-nucleotidase deficiency. *Journal of Clinical Investigation*, **54**, 866–879.

Zanella A., Izzo C., Rebulla P., Zanuso F., Perroni L., Sirchia G. (1980). Acidified glycerol lysis test: a screening test for spherocytosis. *British Journal of Haematology*, **45**, 481–486.

Chapter 7

ACQUIRED HAEMOLYTIC ANAEMIAS

E. C. GORDON-SMITH AND J. HOWS

The acquired haemolytic anaemias are usually divided into two main categories according to the mechanism by which haemolysis is produced. In the immune haemolytic anaemias antibodies are the main agents in the premature destruction of red cells. The non-immune acquired haemolytic anaemias include a wide variety of agents and mechanisms which shorten the red cell survival.

IMMUNE HAEMOLYTIC ANAEMIA

Immune haemolysis is an important cause of acquired haemolytic anaemia. Antibodies produced in vivo against red cell antigens may be alloantibodies or autoantibodies. A simple classification of immune haemolytic anaemia is given in Table 7.1. Red cell autoantibodies may be formed in association with pathological processes which alter the normal immune response, including autoimmune disease, infections, lymphoproliferative disorders, and drug reactions. Alloimmune haemolytic anaemia may follow incompatible blood transfusions, presenting as an immediate or delayed haemolytic transfusion reaction. Another important cause of alloimmune haemolysis is the transplacental transfer of maternal alloantibody to the fetus, presenting as haemolytic disease of the newborn. These alloimmune haemolytic anaemias are described in Chapter 10.

The increased use of allogeneic transplantation for renal, hepatic, cardiac and bone marrow disease has led to recognition of alloimmune haemolytic anaemia due to the production of donor-derived red cell antibodies in the recipient by sensitized donor lymphocytes transferred in the allograft.

Table 7.1

Classification of immune haemolytic anaemias

A. Autoimmune haemolytic anaemias
1. *Warm antibody type*
(i) Idiopathic
(ii) Associated with:
   autoimmune disease
   lymphoproliferative disorders
   other malignancies
   drugs
   infections

2. *Cold antibody type*
(a) Cold agglutinin syndromes
(i) Idiopathic (cold haemagglutinin disease)
(ii) Associated with:
   infections
   lymphoproliferative disorders
(b) Paroxysmal cold haemoglobinuria

B. Alloimmune haemolytic anaemias
1. Haemolytic transfusion reactions
2. Haemolytic disease of the newborn
3. Allograft associated

C. Drug-induced immune haemolytic anaemia
1. Drug absorption mechanism
2. Membrane modification mechanism
3. Immune complex mechanism

Finally, drug-specific antibodies may lead to immune haemolysis, either through absorption of the drug on to the red cell membrane or due to the adherence of drug-specific immune complexes to the red cell membrane and the activation of complement.

AUTOIMMUNE HAEMOLYTIC ANAEMIA

Pathogenesis of Immune Red Cell Destruction

The severity of the anaemia due to immune red cell destruction depends on three main factors.

1. Structural and functional characteristics of the antibody.

2. The efficiency of the in-vivo effector mechanisms for the destruction of red cells sensitized by antibody and complement.

3. The capacity of the bone marrow to compensate for increased red cell destruction.

Antibody Characteristics

Important antibody characteristics which influence the site and intensity of red cell destruction in autoimmune haemolytic anaemia (AIHA) can be evaluated in the immunohaematology laboratory.

Immunoglobulin Class.

Red cell autoantibodies are detected on the red cell surface in AIHA by the direct antiglobulin test (DAT). Monospecific antihuman globulin reagents for IgG, IgM, IgA, C_3c and C_3d are routinely available. In addition, reagents specific for the different IgG subclasses exist but are difficult to standardize.

Warm-type AIHA. IgG antibodies predominate and the most frequent reaction patterns detected by the DAT are:
   (a) IgG,
   (b) IgG and complement,
   (c) complement only.

Cold-type AIHA. In cold agglutinin syndrome IgM red cell autoantibodies predominate. Although the cold-reacting IgM elutes off the patient's red cells in vitro, complement remains bound and will be detected as C_3d in the DAT. In paroxysmal cold haemoglobinuria (PCH) the cold antibody detected is IgG (Donath Landsteiner antibody). As with the cold agglutinin syndrome, in PCH complement is activated and is detectable by the DAT.

Thermal Range

The clinical picture seen in AIHA depends on the thermal range of the red cell autoantibodies.

Warm-type AIHA. Serum antibody is detectable by the indirect antiglobulin test (IAT) at 37°C in 50–60% of cases of warm AIHA and in $> 90\%$ of cases when the red cell membrane of the reagent red cells is modified with proteolytic enzymes (e.g. papain). A subtype of warm AIHA has been defined where although antibody activity in the serum and red cell eluate is maximal at 37°C, there is a significant cold agglutinin component. Both the warm and cold antibodies detected in this variant tend to be lytic in vitro. This variant, sometimes known as 'mixed'-type AIHA, usually occurs in patients with systemic lupus erythematosus or lymphoproliferative disorders and should not be confused with cold agglutinin syndrome. It is often associated with severe haemolysis and a chronic relapsing course.

Cold-type AIHA. Cold agglutinin syndrome is characterized by cold agglutinins in the patient's serum which may agglutinate normal cells to a titre of > 1024 at 4°C. Not all patients with a raised cold agglutinin titre have AIHA. The diagnosis should only be considered if there are clinical signs of haemolysis and the DAT is positive. Cold agglutinins are usually complement-fixing IgM antibodies which are lytic in vitro and may cause intravascular lysis in vivo. Changes in the in-vitro lysin titre and thermal range reflect clinical changes better than the thermal range and titre of the cold agglutinins. In PCH the Donath Landsteiner antibody reacts in vitro below 20°C. When the temperature is raised to 37°C in the presence of complement, lysis occurs. This biphasic activity is diagnostic of PCH and may be demonstrated in the Donath Landsteiner test.

Complement Activation (see also Chapter 8)

Red cell autoantibodies activate complement through the classical pathway. Antibody binding to two adjacent antigenic sites on the red cell membrane is required before C_1 is activated. A single pentameric IgM molecule can bind two antigenic sites and activate complement, whereas two monomeric IgG molecules forming a 'doublet' are required. In general, IgM molecules are more likely to activate complement in vivo and in vitro than IgG. IgG_1, IgG_2 and IgG_3 can activate complement; IgG_3 is the most efficient, followed by IgG_1, IgG_4 and IgA molecules do not activate complement.

In AIHA the complement activation process usually stops at the C_3 stage. C_3b becomes bound to the red cell membrane where further enzymic cleavage of the C_3b molecule occurs, leading to the formation of inactive C_3d. Recent work from Lachman's group indicates that in patients with idiopathic cold agglutinin syndrome the final breakdown product on circulating red cells is antigenically distinct from C_3d and is designated C_3d,g.

Specificity of Red Cell Autoantibodies

Warm-type AIHA. In most cases antibody detected in the patient's serum or red cell eluate is panreactive when tested against a routine panel of group O red cells, the antibody reacts with basic membrane compounds present on virtually all red cells. Specificity within a particular blood group antigen system is sometimes found, most often the rhesus system, e.g. autoanti-e, Occasionally, specificity may be demonstrated using rare red cells lacking high frequency red cell membrane antigens (e.g. Rh^{null}, En^{a-}, WrG^-, U^- cells).

Cold-type AIHA. In cold agglutinin syndrome anti-I specificity is usually seen; occasionally anti-i specificity is detected and in rare cases anti-Pr specificity is found. In PCH the Donath Landsteiner antibody has anti-P specificity, which can only be checked if rare pp cells are available.

Effector Mechanisms for Immune Red Cell Destruction in vivo

Two main effector mechanisms exists in vivo: these are cell-mediated immune red cell destruction and complement-mediated intravascular haemolysis. Cell-mediated red cell destruction predominantly causes the symptoms and signs of extravascular haemolysis.

Cell-mediated Immune Red Cell Destruction

Human macrophages and monocytes have cell surface receptors for Fc portion of IgG and for antigenic determinants present on activated C_3 molecules. Cellular immune red cell destruction is mediated through these receptors. Other cell types, including neutrophils and lymphocytes, have Fc and C_3 receptors. However, macrophages are the most important cells involved in immune red cell destruction in vivo. Macrophages are found in the reticuloendothelial system within the spleen, liver and bone marrow.

Fc Receptor Mechanism

Human macrophages have receptors for the Fc portion of IgG_1 and IgG_3 molecules but not for IgG_2, IgG_4, IgM or IgA. Therefore only IgG-coated cells are destroyed by the Fc receptor mechanism. Clinically this is most important in warm AIHA, where in 70–75% of cases the autoantibodies are predominantly IgG. Phagocytosis is the most important process activated by the Fc receptor; however, in vitro a process called antibody-dependent cell-mediated cytotoxicity (ADCC) can be demonstrated and is Fc receptor dependent. The contribution of ADCC to immune red cell destruction in vivo is uncertain.

The Role of the Spleen

The splenic vasculature is adapted to make the spleen an efficient filter for such particles as effete red cells, bacteria and immune complexes.

As blood passes through the central arteries towards the red pulp, the branches of the central artery have a plasma-skimming effect which raises the haematocrit of the blood within the central artery. Red cells delivered to the splenic cords of the red pulp come into close contact with the splenic macrophages. The low plasma concentration and lack of free plasma IgG molecules allow the red-cell-bound IgG to interact preferentially with the macrophage Fc receptors, leading to phagocytosis. In some cases partial phagocytosis takes place and spherocytes are formed.

Spherocytic red cells lack deformability and may be phagocytosed during their passage across the walls of the splenic sinuses into the sinus lumen. Alternatively the damaged red cells may escape into the sinus lumen and pass into the systemic circulation. Damaged cells can be identified on the peripheral blood smear as 'spherocytes', although they tend to be less regular in shape than the spherocytes seen in hereditary spherocytosis.

The Role of the Liver

The Kupffer cells are macrophages present in the liver sinusoids. These cells bear Fc receptors similar to those of the splenic macrophages. However, the blood flow through the liver sinusoids is rapid compared with that of the spleen and there is no plasma-skimming effect. These conditions are not optimal for Fc-receptor-mediated immune red cell destruction. Hence IgG-coated red cells are preferentially destroyed in the spleen, unless the cells are also heavily coated with C_3 (see below).

C_3 Receptor Mechanisms

Two types of C_3 receptor have been identified on human macrophages—CR_1 and CR_3. CR_1 is specific for an antigenic site in the C_3c region of C_3b which is not exposed on native C_3. The breakdown product of C_3b ($_iC_3b$) is also a major ligand for the macrophage CR_1 receptor and is the only ligand for the CR_3 receptor. Immune adherence of C_3-coated red cells to macrophages occurs mainly through the CR_1 receptor, whereas the CR_3 receptor triggers phagocytosis. In cold AIHA characterized by IgM cold agglutinins, antibody binds to red cells in the peripheral circulation where the temperature may be as low as 10–$20°C$. Complement activation occurs and leads to irreversible binding of C_3 to the red cell membrane. Interactions between red-cell-bound C_3 derivatives and macrophages are the main mechanism for immune red cell destruction in cold AIHA characterized by IgM cold agglutinins but also occurs in warm AIHA due to complement-fixing IgG and IgM antibodies.

The Role of the Spleen

Native C_3 present in plasma is not a ligand for macrophage CR_1 and CR_3 receptors. Therefore the high haematocrit present in the red cell pulp does not lead to enhanced destruction of C_3-coated red cells in the spleen.

The Role of the Liver

The largest concentration of C_3 receptor-bearing macrophages is present in the liver sinusoids so the liver is the major site of trapping and phagocytosis of C_3-coated red cells. However, if massive splenomegaly is present, the spleen becomes an important site of destruction.

Complement-mediated Intravascular Haemolysis

Intravascular complement-mediated haemolysis is a minor mechanism for red cells destruction in most patients with AIHA, and occurs by activation of the classical pathway. The details of complement activation and the final membrane attack sequence are described in Chapter 8.

Intravascular Haemolysis in Warm-type AIHA

This is unusual but may be due to IgG or IgM autoantibodies. In some cases lysis of enzyme-treated pooled O cells can be demonstrated; in-vitro lysis of normal pooled O cells is rare.

Intravascular Haemolysis in Cold Agglutinin Syndrome

Attacks of intravascular haemolysis may be precipitated if the patient is exposed to the cold. Often lytic as well as agglutinating antibody with a high thermal range can be demonstrated in vitro.

Intravascular Haemolysis in PCH

In PCH the autoantibodies are IgG but despite this activate complement very efficiently both in vivo and in vitro. The initial presentation of PCH is often with an episode of brisk intravascular haemolysis. Cell-mediated immune red cell destruction plays a minor part in this disorder.

Other Factors Influencing Immune Red Cell Destruction in vivo

Bone Marrow Function

The ability of the marrow to increase erythropoietic activity in AIHA may be impaired. Firstly, autoantibodies against reticulocytes and erythroblasts as well as mature red cells may be produced; secondly, a relative lack of folic acid may lead to ineffective megaloblastic erythropoiesis; thirdly, the marrow may be infiltrated by lymphoproliferative disease.

Reticuloendothelial Function

The severity of cellular immune red cell destruction depends overall on macrophage function. In systemic lupus erythematosus (SLE), macrophage function may be reduced by the clearance of immune complexes, a process known as reticulo-endothelial blockade. In patients with methyldopa-induced AIHA, the drug has been shown to reduce reticuloendothelial clearance of IgG-sensitized red cells, a finding which explains why many patients with a strongly positive DAT due to methyldopa do not have a haemolytic anaemia.

Hypocomplementaemia

Partial protection from complement-mediated lysis may occur in patients with chronic cold agglutinin syndrome where continuous complement activation leads to relative complement deficiency. In SLE, hypocomplementaemia is common and may also be partially due to complement activation. In addition there is a strong association between SLE and the occurrence of null alleles for the C_2 and C_4 genes which causes a genetically determined complement deficiency.

Clinical Features

Warm-type AIHA

Presentation is variable but most patients complain of weakness and lethargy. Occasionally the onset of the illness is sudden with rapidly developing anaemia and, in older patients, heart failure. Mild jaundice is usually noted. Total bilirubin levels of > 90 μmol/l suggest co-existing liver dysfunction due to biliary tract obstruction from pigment gallstones. Excess urobilinogen is found in the urine. Haemoglobinuria and haemosiderinuria are uncommon as intravascular haemolysis is infrequent. Splenomegaly is often but not invariably noted clinically. The peripheral blood film is characterized by spherocytosis, polychromasia (Fig. 7.1), circulating nucleated red cells and, in some cases, red cell agglutination. The DAT test is positive except in very rare cases where it appears that the amount of antibody on the red cell surface is insufficient to be detected by the conventional DAT test.

Evans' Syndrome

A small subgroup of patients with warm AIHA develop thrombocytopenia with platelet autoantibodies during their illness. This is known as Evans'

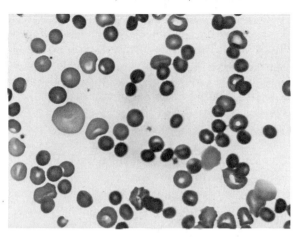

Fig. 7.1. *Autoimmune haemolytic anaemia—warm type. Intense microspherocytosis with large reticulocytes (× 1200).*

syndrome. The thrombocytopenia does not always occur during the haemolytic phase of the disease and should be managed in the same way as other patients with autoimmune thrombocytopenia (see Chapter 22). Episodes of immune neutropenia and pancytopenia have also been documented in patients with AIHA.

Idiopathic Warm AIHA

In approximately 30% of patients with warm-type AIHA no associated disease is found. A careful drug history should be taken, Hodgkin's disease, non-Hodgkin's lymphoma (NHL), chronic lymphocytic leukaemia (CLL) and autoimmune disease should be excluded clinically and by appropriate laboratory investigations.

Treatment

Corticosteroids. Initial treatment is with oral corticosteroids, e.g. prednisolone 1–2 mg/kg per day, and with folic acid supplements. The initial dose of prednisolone should be reduced after 10–14 days according to response and reducing doses continued for approximately 3 months.

Transfusion in warm AIHA. All patients, but especially the elderly, with initial haemoglobin of < 8 g/dl should be carefully monitored and urgent blood transfusion considered if the haemoglobin continues to fall or incipient heart failure develops. If the specificity of the autoantibody is known, donor blood lacking the relevant antibody should be given. Otherwise, the least incompatible blood should be used, but donor red cells are likely to have a shortened survival, similar to that of the patient's own red cells.

Splenectomy is considered if response to the initial 3–month trial of corticosteroids is unsatisfactory. Patients with predominantly IgG-coated red cells respond best to splenectomy. Post-splenectomy, about 50% of patients achieve a complete remission and in the remainder haemolysis becomes easier to manage with immunosuppressive drugs. Prophylactic penicillin V 250 mg b.d. should be given to prevent overwhelming post-splenectomy infection with pneumococci or meningococci. Penicillin prophylaxis should be continued until immunosuppressive treatment is stopped or for a minimum of 2 years. In children penicillin is continued up to the age of 18. Additional protection should be given by administering polyvalent pneumococcal vaccine after discontinuing immunosuppressive therapy.

Azathioprine 1–1.5 mg/kg per day orally may be used in patients who respond poorly to corticosteroids and when splenectomy is contraindicated. In patients who continue to haemolyse post-splenectomy, azathioprine may have a steroid-sparing effect. Azathioprine should be given for at least 3 months as response is usually not seen for 4–6 weeks.

Cyclophosphamide. Low-dose cyclophosphamide 1–1.5 mg/kg per day may be used in place of azathiaprine, although the side-effects include the risk of haemorrhagic cystitis and of myelodysplasia and/or acute myeloid leukaemia following long-term administration.

Cyclosporin. Oral cyclosporin may be tried in resistant cases. A few therapeutic successes have been recently reported. An oral dose of 3 mg/kg twice daily is given. Close monitoring of renal function and trough plasma cyclosporin levels is necessary: trough cyclosporin levels of 80–150 ng/ml are satisfactory. Response may not be seen for 2–3 months.

Thymectomy. This has been carried out in a few infants who developed AIHA in the first year or two of life. Some, but not all, have benefitted.

Systemic Lupus Erythematosus

IgG and C_3 immune complexes may become absorbed on to the red cell surface and are detected by the DAT and often haemolysis occurs. Initial treatment of AIHA in SLE is the same as for idiopathic warm AIHA. However, the spleen is important for clearing circulating immune complexes in SLE and there is some evidence that splenectomy may worsen the haemolysis and other manifestations of the disease.

Warm AIHA and Other Autoimmune Diseases

The most frequent disease associations reported are with rheumatoid arthritis and ulcerative colitis.

Warm AIHA in the Lymphomas and CLL

The commonest associations are with B cell CLL, low-grade B cell non-Hodgkin's lymphoma and Hodgkin's disease. The autoantibodies formed are polyclonal and usually IgG. It is most likely that the formation of red cell autoantibodies in this group is secondary to immune dysregulation rather than antibody production by the malignant clone. Initial treatment is with corticosteroids and appropriate cytotoxic therapy for the lymphoproliferative disease.

Warm AIHA Due to Drugs

Warm AIHA has most frequently been associated with methyldopa although mefenamic acid, L-dopa and procainamide are reported. Approximately 20% of all patients receiving methyldopa develop a positive DAT but only 1–2% of patients develop haemolytic anaemia. The DAT always detects IgG alone on the red cell surface and the autoantibodies often show rhesus specificity (e.g. anti-e or -c). It is not certain whether drug-induced alteration of red cell antigens or modulation of the immune response by the drug is responsible for methyldopa-induced AIHA. In haemolytic cases the drug should be stopped and folic acid supplements given. The haemolysis generally stops within 1–2 weeks of withdrawing the drug, although the DAT may remain positive for several months.

Other Malignancies

Warm AIHA has been reported with various common carcinomas. However, it is not certain whether this represents a true disease association. Dacie reports a definite association between ovarian carcinoma and warm-type AIHA.

Warm AIHA and Viral Infections

Occasionally warm AIHA is reported after viral illnesses in children, but rarely in adults. Haemolysis is usually brisk but self-limiting. It is possible either the virus alters the antigenicity of the red cell membrane which stimulates 'auto' antibody formation or that the antiviral antibodies cross-react with antigens on the red cell surface. A third possibility is that immune complexes form between the virus and specific antibodies and that the complexes are secondarily absorbed on to the red cell membrane leading to immune red cell destruction.

Cold-type AIHA—Cold Agglutinin Syndromes

The clinical features seen in the cold agglutinin syndrome vary with the pathogenesis of the disorder. Serological tests are useful in investigating the cause and in clinical management. The serological characteristics of the antibodies found in the cold agglutinin syndromes are shown in Table 7.2.

Table 7.2

Serological characteristics of cold agglutinins in the cold agglutinin syndromes

	Anti-I	Anti-i
Idiopathic (CHAD)†	M	
Secondary to lymphoproliferative disorders	M	M
Secondary to infection:		
Mycoplasma pneumoniae	P	
infectious mononucleosis	P	P

M, monoclonal; P+, polyclonal.
†Rarely, a monoclonal anti-P antibody may be present.

Idiopathic Cold Haemagglutinin Disease

Cold haemagglutinin disease (CHAD) is primarily seen in the elderly and runs a chronic and usually benign course. Purplish skin discolouration (acrocyanosis), maximal over the extremities, may be present in cold weather. Acrocyanosis is due to stasis in the peripheral circulation secondary to red cell agglutination. On warming, the skin colour returns to normal or temporary erythema may be seen. This sequence distinguishes acrocyanosis from Raynaud's syndrome. Mild jaundice and splenomegaly may be observed. The cold agglutinins are monoclonal IgM kappa but serum electrophoresis may not reveal a monoclonal band due to the low concentration of antibody in the serum. CHAD may be thought of as a premalignant B cell monoclonal proliferation which only presents clinically because of the specificity of the monoclonal antibody for red cell surface antigens.

In the laboratory, spontaneous agglutination of the blood is frequently observed both macroscopically and on the peripheral blood film. Automated blood cell counters detect red cell agglutinates and may compute erroneously high MCV values. The DAT shows C_3d only on the red cell surface, indicating in-vivo complement activation. The IgM cold agglutinins are not detected by the DAT because they elute from the red cell surface in vitro.

Treatment

General. All patients should avoid cold exposure, and electrically heated gloves and socks are available for use in the winter. Folic acid supplements should be given to those patients with active haemolysis. When possible, patients should spend the winter in a warm climate!

Corticosteroids. These are usually ineffective in CHAD and carry a high complication rate in the elderly.

Alkylating Agents: Oral chlorambucil may be given to decrease antibody production in patients with active haemolysis. Intermittent regimens, e.g. chlorambucil 10 mg daily for 14 days every 4 weeks, or continuous regimens of chlorambucil 2–4 mg daily are effective. Long-term treatment should be avoided because of the risk of myelodysplasia and acute myeloid leukaemia.

Splenectomy. In CHAD, C_3-coated red cells are mainly destroyed in the liver or by intravascular haemolysis if the cold antibodies have a high thermal range. These factors suggest that splenectomy is unlikely to be helpful in the control of haemolysis in CHAD unless massive splenomegaly is present. Plasma exchange immediately before splenectomy has been used to lower the cold antibody titre in order to reduce the risk of exacerbating haemolysis during surgery.

Cold Agglutinin Syndrome and Lymphoproliferative Disorders

Occasionally the cold agglutinin syndrome is seen in patients with B-cell lymphomas or CLL. In these cases the cold antibody is monoclonal and the product of the neoplastic clone. The serological specificity of the cold antibody is either anti-I or anti-i. Treatment for haemolysis is along the same lines as for CHAD. However, additional chemotherapy or irradiation may be necessary for the treatment of the lymphoproliferative disorder.

Cold Agglutinin Syndromes and Infections

These can occur in patients of all ages, including children. Haemolysis occurs 2–3 weeks following the acute infection. The cold antibodies are IgM and are polyclonal or oligoclonal with both kappa and lambda light chains present. IgG cold antibodies have rarely been documented. Both anti-I and anti-i specificity is seen on serological testing (see Table 7.2). The most frequent infections responsible for cold agglutinin syndrome are pneumonia due to *Mycoplasma pneumoniae* and infectious mononucleosis. The cold antibody is stimulated by the infective agent and cross-reacts with determinants on the red cell membrane. Less frequently, cases have been documented following listeria or toxoplasmosis. In most cases the haemolysis is mild and self-limiting. Recovery occurs as the titre and thermal range of the cold antibodies diminish. All patients should avoid cold exposure and, in rare cases of severe haemolysis, treatment in a specially heated room is necessary. Transfusion is occasionally indicated and blood should be given through a blood warmer. As the condition is self-limiting, immunosuppressive treatment is rarely required.

Paroxysmal Cold Haemoglobinuria

Paroxysmal cold haemoglobinuria (PCH) is rare and makes up 5–10% of the cold autoimmune haemolytic anaemias. The syndrome usually occurs in children following acute viral infections, although the original cases were described in congenital and tertiary syphilis by Donath, Landsteiner and Ehrlich. A history of cold exposure is not always obtained and presentation is with sudden intravascular haemolysis characterized by haemoglobinuria, abdominal pain, pallor and prostration.

The cold antibody is a polyclonal IgG antibody (the Donath Landsteiner antibody); it is biphasic, reacting with red cells at below 20°C in the peripheral circulation and causing lysis by complement activation as the red cells are returned to the central circulation. The antibody has specificity for the P antigen and in vitro will not lyse rare pp cells.

Treatment

Patients should be nursed in a specially heated room. Haemolysis is self-limiting but transfusion is often necessary. As rare pp cells are seldom available for transfusion, ABO and Rhesus compatible P-positive blood is usually given.

DRUG-INDUCED IMMUNE HAEMOLYTIC ANAEMIA

Drug-induced immune haemolytic anaemias are rare, apart from relatively common autoimmune haemolysis caused by methyldopa. The antibodies formed are drug specific and are not specific for red cell membrane components, in contrast to the true autoantibodies induced by methyldopa. The diagnosis of drug-induced haemolytic anaemia should be made in three stages:

1. diagnosis of a DAT-positive haemolytic anaemia,
2. careful drug history,
3. serological demonstration of drug-specific antibody which interacts with red cells.

Pathogenesis

Drug Absorption Mechanism (Hapten Mechanism)

Penicillin is the prototype drug although cephalosporins and tetracyclines have also been implicated. Drugs in this group readily form hapten–carrier complexes with plasma proteins which enhance drug-specific antibody production. It has been estimated that 90% of individuals receiving penicillin produce clinically insignificant IgM antipenicillin antibodies. When high-dose intravenous penicillin is administered the drug is absorbed on to the red cell surface where it becomes non-specifically attached to red cell surface proteins. A minority of patients on high-dose intravenous penicillin therapy (>1 mega unit daily) develop high titre IgG antipenicillin antibodies which attach to the drug bound to the red cell surface and cause predominantly extravascular haemolysis. The clinical picture is variable and occasionally severe intravascular haemolysis occurs.

Membrane Modification Mechanism

Cephalosporin, in addition to the drug absorption mechanism, can cause a positive DAT by modifying red cell membrane components. As a result a variety of plasma proteins, including immunoglobulin and complement, may attach through a non-immune mechanism to the red cell membrane. This may result in the finding of a positive DAT but rarely causes immune haemolytic anaemia.

Immune Complex Mechanism (Innocent Bystander Mechanism)

Several drugs have been reported to cause immune haemolytic anaemia by this mechanism. Most frequently reported are rifampicin, phenacetin, quinine, quinidine, nomifensine, hydrochlorthiazide and chlorpropramide. Hapten–carrier complexes are formed between these drugs and plasma proteins, leading to the production of drug-specific antibodies. Once drug antibodies are present, reintroduction of the drug causes immune complexes to form which are absorbed on to the red cell membrane and complement activated.

Classically haemolysis occurs on the second or subsequent exposure to the drug and may develop within minutes or hours of drug ingestion. Severe intravascular haemolysis may occur with fever, rigors or nausea and, in extreme cases, acute renal failure.

Serological Diagnosis of Drug-Induced Immune Haemolytic Anaemia

1. *Drug absorption and membrane modification mechanisms.* The DAT is usually positive with IgG_1, or IgG and C_3 on the red cell surface. The red cell eluate and serum do not react against normal or enzyme-modified red cells. Warm-reacting drug-specific antibody in the eluate and serum is only detected after preincubation of the test red cells with the appropriate drug.

2. *Immune complex mechanism.* The DAT is usually positive but may be negative if performed immediately after a brisk 'episode' of haemolysis. The red cell eluate is not reactive, even in the presence of the drug. The drug-specific antibody is best detected by preincubating patients' serum with drug in solution to allow immune complexes to form. The preincubated serum is then tested against normal and enzyme-modified groups of cells in the presence of fresh complement. In some cases, e.g. nomifensine, the antibodies may be specific for metabolities rather than the parent drug. Drug metabolite antibodies may be detected by preincubating drug metabolite obtained from the serum or urine of a volunteer who has taken the drug with the patient's serum. A simplified summary of the serological investigation of a patient with suspected drug-induced immune haemolysis is shown in Table 7.3.

THE NON-IMMUNE ACQUIRED HAEMOLYTIC ANAEMIAS

Haemolysis and haemolytic anaemia are the consequences of a wide variety of acquired ills and so do not lend themselves readily to a precise classification. Classification is useful if it helps clinically to arrive at a correct diagnosis and hence management, or if it helps with understanding pathogenesis and, at a more removed stage, treatment. With the acquired haemolytic anaemias it is more helpful to

Table 7.3
Serological investigation of drug-dependent antibodies

Immune complex mechanism
*Pre-incubation reaction mixture**

PS	AB	S	Drug	N or ET	Result	Interpretation
+	+	−	+	+	+	Drug antibody present
					−	No drug antibody
+	+	+	−	+	+	Allo or auto red cell antibody present
−	+	−	+	+	−	Negative control

Drug absorption and membrane modification mechanisms
Pre-incubation reaction mixture

N	S	Drug	PE or PS	Result	Interpretation
+	−	+	+	+	Drug antibody present
				−	No drug antibody
+	+	−	+	+	Auto or allo red cell antibody present
+	−	+	−	−	Negative control

N = normal red blood cells; ET = enzyme-treated red blood cells; PS = patient serum; PE = patient eluate; AB = fresh antibody serum; S = saline; drug = drug or drug metabolite solution.
* Patient eluate not reactive even after pre-incubation with drug (see text).

have a classification based on causes rather than mechanisms, with the different pathways forming a subclassification. The main groups of agents causing haemolysis are: infections, vascular disorders (mechanical disorders), chemical and physical agents, and disorders affecting the red cell membrane. This classification is shown in Table 7.4.

Infections Causing Haemolytic Anaemia

A wide variety of infections may produce haemolytic anaemia, either through direct invasion of the red cells and alteration of their properties leading to intravascular or extravascular haemolysis, or indirectly through changes in the circulation. Such relationships between infection and the red cell may be a primitive protective mechanism against infections or for the clearance of immune complexes, but in modern medicine the consequences of the infection predominate.

Malaria

Falciparum malaria is one of the most common causes of anaemia in the world. Many factors lead to the anaemia and include marrow suppression, hypersplenism and red cell sequestration as well as haemolysis. Haemolysis has two main components, extravascular destruction of parasitized cells in the reticuloendothelial system, particularly the spleen, and intravascular lysis when the sporozoites break out of the red cells.

Blackwater Fever

The syndrome of acute intravascular haemolysis often accompanied by acute renal failure is an uncommon but devastating complication of falciparum malaria. The condition was first described in whites who were treated with quinine and the importance of the association was stressed. More recently it has been recorded in blacks in areas

Table 7.4
Non-immune acquired haemolytic anaemia

Cause	Examples	Mechanisms
Infections	Malaria Babesiosis Bartonella	Intracellular organisms
	Meningococcal sepsis Pneumococcal sepsis Gram-negative sepsis	Microangiopathic haemolysis
	Haemorrhagic fevers	
	Clostridium perfringens	Enzymatic toxins
Chemical and physical agents	Drugs Industrial/domestic substances Burns Drowning	Oxidative haemolysis Membrane damage Osmotic lysis
Mechanical lysis	Diffuse intravascular coagulation Vasculitis	Microangiopathic haemolytic anaemia
	Cardiac prostheses	'Foreign surface' haemolysis
Acquired membrane disorder	Liver disease	Lipid abnormalities
	Paroxysmal nocturnal haemoglobinuria	Somatic mutation

which had previously been free from malaria and it seems probable that it is related to the degree of parasitaemia and lack of immunity. Immune lysis due to quinine and the presence of G6PD deficiency have to be excluded when faced with a patient presenting with malaria and intravascular haemolysis. The onset is acute, with marked haemoglobinaemia, a rapid fall in haemoglobin, haemoglobinuria and swift progression to oliguric renal failure. Fever, abdominal pain and renal pain are usual. The kidneys show changes of acute tubular necrosis; hypotension consequent on hypovolaemia is common and pulmonary and cerebral complications may ensue. In half the cases parasitaemia is marked but in other cases parasites may be scanty, perhaps because with the acute haemolysis the parasite count drops. The red cell count may fall below $1 \times 10^{12}/l$ within 24 hours. Intravascular coagulation does not seem to be an important mechanism in this haemolysis.

Immediate treatment is directed to correction of fluid and electrolyte loss, counteracting the ana-emia and eradication of the parasite. Renal dialysis is often required and may have to be continued for a month or more. Subsequent attacks of falciparum malaria in affected patients are likely to produce further episodes of blackwater fever so scrupulous prophylaxis is essential for patients who have recovered from one episode.

Babesiosis

Infection with the intraerythrocytic protozoan *Babesia* is rare and mostly confined to patients who have been splenectomized, at least in the European variety. *Babesia* are tick-borne organisms, the tick in Europe being *Ixodes vicinus* associated with cattle, in America *Ixodes dammini* associated with rodents and deer.

In splenectomized patients the disease has an acute onset and is usually fatal. There is a 1–3-day period of malaise, sometimes with vomiting and diarrhoea, followed by high fever, rigors, jaundice, acute intravascular haemolysis, haemoglobinaemia, haemoglobinuria, renal failure and death. In non-splenectomized patients in North America the disease tends to be self-limiting, though intravascular haemolysis may occur.

The diagnosis is made from the peripheral blood where the parasites, looking very similar to *P. falciparum*, are seen in the red cells. The history of possible exposure to the vector or zoonotic host and the absence of travel to malarial areas by a splenectomized subject may indicate the diagnosis. Pentamidine and chloroquine have been recommended as treatment, but their effectiveness is unknown. Exchange transfusion and renal support offer the main chance of recovery.

Toxoplasmosis

Infection with *Toxoplasma gondii* acquired in utero may produce haemolysis and a syndrome similar to haemolytic disease of the newborn. In adults toxoplasma rarely causes haemolysis except perhaps in severely immunosuppressed patients.

Oroya Fever (Bartonella bacilliformis)

Infection with *Bartonella bacilliformis* is found only in the Western Andes of Peru and neighbouring countries. The organism is intracellular, and Gram negative, rod shaped in the acute attack, coccoid during recovery. In non-immune people there may be intense haemolysis, partly intravascular, partly through erythrophagocytosis. The diagnosis is made on the peripheral blood. The organism is killed promptly by chloramphenicol, tetracyclines, penicillin or aminoglycosides.

Clostridium perfringens

Clostridium perfringens (previously called *welchii*) septicaemia may cause intense intravascular haemolysis with prominent microspherocytosis and evidence of intravascular haemolysis. The spherocytosis may be the result of membrane loss caused by the lipases and proteinases which the organism produces.

Bacterial Infections

Certain bacterial infections may cause diffuse intravascular haemolysis (DIC) and a secondary micro-angiopathic haemolytic anaemia. Mengingococcal and pneumococcal infections are particularly liable to produce this result but other Gram-negative septicaemias have the same effects.

Psittacosis and Yersinia enterocolitica infections have also been described as causing microangiopathic haemolytic anaemia. Usually the intravascular haemolysis is mild and its effects trivial in relation to the other effects of the sepsis.

Viral Infections

Viruses which produce the syndrome of haemorrhagic fever may cause haemolytic anaemia. Dengue, yellow fever as well as the West African haemorrhagic fevers may each cause intravascular haemolysis.

Haemophagocytic Syndromes

A wide variety of infectious agents have been described in patients who have pancytopenia, jaundice, haemolysis and proliferation of histiocytes in the bone marrow, spleen and liver. The condition is difficult to separate from malignant proliferation of histiocytes. Viruses are often suspected but firmer diagnoses have been made in patients infected with Mycobacteria, Pneumocystis or Gram-negative organisms. The majority of such patients are immunosuppressed.

Mechanical Haemolytic Anaemias

The relationship between the cellular elements of the blood, coagulation system, the fibrinolytic system and the endothelial lining of the blood vessels is clearly intimate and complex. The integrity of the red blood cell is readily destroyed by contact with abnormal endothelial surfaces, though not all abnormalities of the vessels cause haemolysis. The common mechanism, if there is one, seems to be contact between the erythrocyte and the abnormal surface, with some degree of adherence. Direct mechanical breakdown caused by shear stress probably is not important. There are two major situations in which intravascular haemolysis occurs characterized by the presence of fragments of red cells in the peripheral blood. These are 'cardiac haemolysis' and microangiopathic haemolytic anaemia (MAHA).

Cardiac Haemolytic Anaemia

This syndrome was so called because it nearly always followed cardiac surgery in which prosthetic valves, patches or vessels were inserted. More recent cardiac surgical techniques, using new materials, homografts or xenografts, have made the condition much less common than it used to be. The condition is recognized by intravascular haemolysis and fragmentation of red cells (with a normal platelet count) after appropriate surgery. The two factors which appear to be required are artificial material in the bloodstream and turbulent blood flow to bring the red cells in contact with the material. There are certain situations where the haemolysis may be of considerable clinical importance.

1. *Periprosthetic or perivalvular leaks.* If, after insertion or repair of the mitral valve, a leak occurs around the prosthesis or through a suture track around the valve, there may be intense intravascular haemolysis unaccompanied by any haemodynamic effects. The lesion may be so trivial that few signs indicate its presence, but there is no cure except re-operation. A particular difficulty is that in this case fragmentation of red cells in the blood film may be minimal, though spherocytes may be seen. However once immune haemolytic anaemia is excluded, the diagnosis can scarcely be anything else in a patient who has had mitral valve surgery.

2. *'Ambulatory haemolysis'.* A patient who has undergone valve replacement may show only slight evidence of haemolysis whilst recovering from the operation yet develop significant anaemia after discharge. It seems likely that in these cases the increased cardiac output, associated with increased physical activity after discharge, causes increased turbulent blood flow and increased lysis. Should iron deficiency develop and compound the anaemia, the condition may be aggravated. Iron replacement and advice about the level of activity may prevent or delay the need for further surgery.

3. *Valve failure.* Some of the valves used in the early days of prosthetic valves were liable to changes in shape (ball variance) after a period of use. Significant haemolytic anaemia may then develop and require a replacement operation.

Microangiopathic Haemolytic Anaemia

The phrase is used to describe intravascular haemolysis with fragmentation of red cells caused by destruction of the red cells in an abnormal microcirculation. Proof of microscopic abnormality in the blood vessels is often lacking in patients who do not have a *post mortem*, and MAHA should be considered a clinical syndrome. The three major pathological lesions which may give rise to MAHA are diffuse intravascular coagulation, platelet aggregation and vasculitis. The vessel abnormalities may be generalized or localized to particular organs. Some of the more well documented causes of MAHA are shown in Table 7.5. It is helpful only to describe in detail a few well-defined clinical syndromes associated with MAHA.

MAHA and Malignant Disease

Fragmentation of red cells with chronic intravascular haemolysis may occur in malignant disease with or without evidence of acute intravascular haemolysis. The lysis of the cells may occur either within the abnormal blood vessel of the primary tumour or as a result of metastatic tumour emboli. If there is invasion of the tumour into large blood vessels, MAHA may be marked (as in haemangiopericytoma), but fragmentation may also occur with relatively small and undetected primary cancers. A blood film which shows evidence of MAHA together with leucoerythroblastic changes is virtually diagnostic of malignant disease with secondary deposits in the bone marrow.

In acute leukaemia, particularly, but not exclusively, promyelocytic leukaemia (M3), there may be intense intravascular coagulation which may be accompanied by MAHA. The coagulation abnormality dominates the clinical picture and the syndrome is detailed in Chapter 14.

MAHA and Infection

Infections, particularly septicaemias, may provoke intravascular coagulation and MAHA. Some examples have been given in the previous sections. In meningococcal and pneumococcal infections the

Table 7.5
Causes of microangiopathic haemolytic anaemia

Disease	Microangiopathy
Haemolytic uraemic syndrome of childhood	Endothelial-cell swelling, microthrombi in renal vessels
Haemolytic uraemic syndrome with bacterial infection (especially *Esch. coli* (0157)	Endotoxaemia, microthrombi in renal arteries
Thrombotic thrombocytopenic purpura	Platelet plugs, microaneurysms, arteriolitis
Renal cortical necrosis Acute glomerular nephritis	Necrotizing arteritis
Pre-eclampsia	Fibrinoid necrosis
Vasculitis Polyarteritis nodosa Wegener's granulomatosis Systemic lupus	Arteritis
Homograft rejection	Microthrombi in transplanted organ
Meningococcal sepsis	Endotoxaemia, diffuse intravascular coagulation
Carcinomatosis	Abnormal tumour vessels, intravascular coagulation—local or diffuse
Primary pulmonary hypertension	Abnormal vasculature
Cavernous haemangioma ((Kasabach–Merritt Syndrome)	Local vascular changes and thrombosis

coagulation and bleeding problems are more important than the haemolysis. A combination of malignant disease with Gram-negative sepsis may produce marked haemolysis. Some infections may produce a chronic state of partially compensated intravascular haemolysis and marked red cell fragmentation.

The Haemolytic Uraemic Syndrome
(see also pages 605, 667)

The haemolytic uraemic syndrome (HUS) is an acquired disorder, mainly affecting infants and children, whose main features are intravascular haemolysis, renal failure and thrombocytopenia. The syndrome was first described in Europe, in 1955, by Gasser and colleagues who found that the kidneys of such patients who died showed renal cortical necrosis. Brain and others emphasized the

fragmentation of red cells and the presence of microangiopathic haemolytic anaemia and suggested that diffuse intravascular coagulation played a major role. It now seems probable that localized, rather than diffuse, microangiopathy, mainly in the glomerular capillaries, is the major cause of the syndrome and that the microangiopathy is produced primarily by an abnormal interaction between platelets and the vascular endothelium.

Incidence

The syndrome is most common in infants and young children, the majority of reported cases being less than 4 years old. The complete syndrome is rare after puberty, the closely related syndrome of thrombotic thrombocytopenic purpura (TTP) being more common in teenagers and young adults (see below). Cases may be sporadic or occur in clusters in time and space suggesting an epidemic.

Aetiology

The cause of HUS is not fully understood, but both host and environmental factors appear to play a part. The abnormal platelet–endothelial response may, in some patients, be related to abnormalities of prostacyclin (PGI_2) production which normally limits platelet adherence to the vascular endothelium, though the evidence for this as a universal defect in the syndrome is not conclusive. The occurrence of the syndrome in different members of families suggests constitutional and genetic factors are important. In epidemic outbreaks various infective agents have been implicated, including viruses, rickettsiae and bacterial infections. The syndrome has followed immunization but in the majority of patients no specific agent has been identified. HUS may occur in epidemic form following infection with *Escherichia coli* 0157 (endotoxin producing).

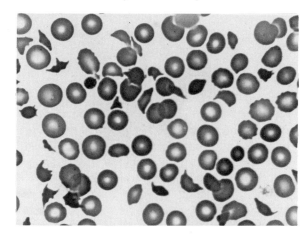

Fig. 7.2. *Microangiopathic haemolytic anaemia. Peripheral blood from a patient with haemolytic uraemic syndrome. Fragmented, contracted and distorted red cells with reduced platelets (× 1200).*

Clinical Features

The syndrome may arise de novo or follow a systemic illness with fever and diarrhoea. The latter is the more common presentation, with fever, bloody diarrhoea and vomiting lasting a day to 2 weeks preceding the onset of jaundice, haemoglobinuria, proteinuria, hypertension and uraemia. Anaemia and thrombocytopenia develop and purpura or petechial haemorrhages are common. In a proportion of cases oliguria follows. Central nervous system involvement is variable, many cases showing no CNS signs, but convulsions or coma may develop, particularly in children with fever and marked hypertension. The presentation is usually of a subacute illness rather than acute prostration.

Laboratory Findings

The typical blood film shows fragmentation of red cells with thrombocytopenia (Fig. 7.2). Polychromasia may be marked. The platelet count is often severely reduced, with most patients having counts fewer than $50 \times 10^9/l$. The bone marrow is cellular and appropriate responses to the haemolysis and thrombocytopenia develop. The urea and creatinine levels are raised, and hyperbilirubinaemia consistent with the haemolysis is seen. Coagulation abnormalities are variable and may be subtle but some abnormality is nearly always present. Prothrombin time (PT), partial thromboplastin time with kaolin (PTTK) and the thrombin time (TT) should be measured, though they are not always prolonged. There is usually some increase in fibrin degradation products but not always above the level expected in acute renal failure. In some cases there is more florid evidence of DIC. The fibrinogen turnover is usually increased but fibrinogen levels may be normal. The urine shows the presence of free haemoglobin but red cells and casts are usually present as well.

Management

The mainstay of treatment is support, with additional efforts to halt the syndrome and allow recovery before irreversible renal failure ensues.

Dialysis, either peritoneal or haemodialysis, should be instituted early in the presence of obvious renal failure and may be continued for 2 or 3 weeks, with eventual recovery of renal function. Control of hypertension is most important. Red cell transfusions are usually required but platelet transfusions are rarely needed, and there is still debate as to whether platelet transfusions are likely to make the condition worse. If there is evident dangerous bleeding with severe thrombocytopenia and laboratory changes of DIC, replacement therapy will have to be given and may be an indication for heparin therapy to halt the thrombotic process. In the presence of DIC, antithrombin III levels may be reduced and heparin relatively weak as an anticoagulant. Nevertheless, heparin should be used in moderate doses (equivalent to 20 000 units in 24 hours for an adult) rather than achieving full anticoagulant control. As soon as the DIC process stops, the antithrombin III level will rise rapidly.

Other forms of therapy which have been tried are corticosteroids and agents which inhibit platelet adherence, including aspirin, dipyridamole and prostacyclin analogues. Results have been disappointing and no definite conclusions may be drawn about their effectiveness.

Plasma exchange is effective in many cases of TTP and should be tried in cases of HUS which do not rapidly reverse, but data on its therapeutic benefit are not available.

Prognosis

The acute mortality of the syndrome varies from about 5% to 30%, more recent reports showing the lower figure as support measures improve. About one-third of patients recover completely, with normal renal function and blood pressure, one-third have persistent hypertension and may later develop chronic renal failure, and one-third have persistent oliguric renal failure. The prognosis is closely related to the degree of renal failure at the time of presentation. In a few cases recurrent episodes of HUS occur, sometimes going on to a TTP-like illness as the child gets older. This is more common where there is a family history or where there is evidence of an immune systemic abnormality. The relapsing cases usually respond to plasma exchange or infusion of fresh frozen plasma.

Thrombotic Thrombocytopenic Purpura
(see also page 667)

Thrombotic thrombocytopenic purpura (TTP) is a clinical syndrome characterized by the pentad of fever, anaemia, thrombocytopenia, neurological disorders and renal abnormalities. The pathological changes which produce the syndrome are of platelet aggregation in small blood vessels. The disease is of unknown aetiology so other conditions which produce similar clinical features have to be excluded, particularly infections and malignant diseases associated with DIC and systemic lupus erythematosus.

Clinical Features

The condition is rare but devastating, with a mortality of over 50% in conservatively managed cases. In most instances the syndrome is sporadic but familial cases have been described. Both sexes are affected equally and there may be a peak incidence in adolescents and young adults. In females it may develop during pregnancy, when it must be differentiated from pre-eclampsia.

The onset is usually sudden, with the development of fever and neurological disturbance. The more common neurological features include convulsions, coma, transient or permanent paralysis and bizarre psychiatric disorders including hallucinations. Purpura often develops early, sometimes preceding neurological signs, more commonly appearing subsequently. Anaemia is variable but sometimes there is evidence of marked haemolysis with a rapid fall in haemoglobin, haemoglobinuria and jaundice. Renal failure is not common at presentation and evidence of renal damage, though virtually always present, is subtle and determined by laboratory investigations. In some cases episodes of haemolysis and thrombocytopenia are always accompanied by hypertension, in other cases the blood pressure remains normal or variable.

Typically the syndrome runs a fluctuating route. Severe neurological signs may suddenly disappear and a confused or even comatose patient become lucid and apparently normal, only to relapse with the same or different neurological features within hours or days. Occasionally there is a history of neuropsychiatric disorders occurring over a period of months or years which may indicate previous subacute episodes. Some patients have a history suggestive of HUS during childhood.

Laboratory Findings

The main haematological features are of microangiopathic haemolytic anaemia with thrombocytopenia. The blood film shows fragmented and contracted red cells with polychromasia and thrombocytopenia. The degree of anaemia varies considerably from case to case, with many cases showing only an elevation of plasma haemoglobin as a sign of intravascular haemolysis. A neutrophil leucocytosis is common but not inevitable. The bone marrow shows an increased cellularity with normal morphology.

Coagulation abnormalities are slight in most cases and normal PT, PTTK and TT are usual. Occasionally there are more substantial changes compatible with some DIC. Marked changes should raise the possibility of other diagnoses, bacterial sepsis, malignant disease or coagulation disorders associated with pregnancy.

Proteinuria is an almost universal feature of the disorder, though it may be intermittent. Uraemia and a raised creatinine tend to develop late in the syndrome and oliguria is uncommon.

Pathology

Pathological changes in small blood vessels and changes in various organs are most commonly described from post-mortem material. Proof of microangiopathy may be difficult to obtain in life and various procedures have been recommended, including gingival biopsy and careful examination of blood vessels in marrow trephines.

The cardinal lesions are microthrombi present throughout the capillary bed and small vessel bed of affected organs. The thrombi are mainly composed of platelet plugs with a variable amount of hyaline degeneration and fibrin deposition (Fig. 7.3). There may be some aneurysmal dilatation of small vessels associated with thrombi. In some cases changes suggestive of SLE may be seen with perivascular 'onion skin' appearance in the spleen and thickening of the glomerular basement membrane with a 'wire loop' appearance. In such cases the syndrome obviously merges into SLE itself.

Pathogenesis

The cause of the syndrome is unknown but there is considerable current interest in the relationship between platelets and the vascular endothelium in these patients. In some cases a deficiency of a serum factor which promotes prostacyclin production by vascular endothelium has been detected. This concept is supported by the recovery of some patients

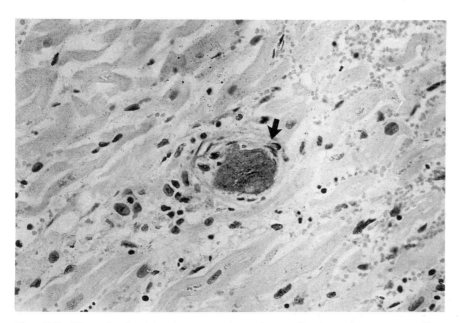

Fig. 7.3. *Thrombotic thrombocytopenic purpura. Sections from myocardium showing platelet plug in capillary stained with monoclonal antibody to type IIb glycoprotein, demonstrated by indirect immunofluorescence × 100. (Courtesy of Dr Margaret Burke.)*

following infusion of fresh frozen plasma (see below), but the precise nature of the serum factor is not defined. In other cases immune complexes have been detected in the circulation but immunoglobulin and complement are not detected in the thrombotic plugs.

Treatment

TTP is an unpredictable disease and patients should be managed in places where full intensive care facilities are available. Support, including ventilation and haemodialysis where required, should be maximal. Recovery may occur even in patients who have been comatose for days or weeks and who have developed renal failure, though it must be admitted that this is uncommon. The main urgent measure in the current treatment of TTP is plasma exchange with replacement using fresh frozen plasma (FFP) as well as plasma protein fraction and platelets. Plasmapheresis should be carried out daily with 5-litre exchanges until a response is achieved. If the patient responds rapidly to plasma exchange, maintenance with infusions of FFP without exchange may be possible. Response is indicated by clearing of neurological signs, a rise in platelet count, cessation of haemolysis and normalization of blood pressure. The response to FFP may be swift (within 12 hours) but repeated infusi-

ons of FFP may be needed to sustain remission, sometimes for months (Fig. 7.4). Patients with a history of previous attacks of TTP or HUS or those with a family history of similar disorders are more likely to respond to FFP alone than are patients who present for the first time with an acute attack.

The recommendation that patients should be treated first with plasma exchange rather than simply trying FFP and reserving plasma exchange for those who fail to respond may be challenged. The reasoning is that the syndrome may be rapidly and unpredictably fatal and that some patients respond only to exchange and may die whilst waiting for a response to FFP. However, there is bound to be a delay in setting up the plasma exchange and it would seem prudent to give FFP or blood before starting the first exchange. Cryoprecipitate and plasma protein fraction are not able to maintain remission in patients who require FFP.

A substantial proportion of patients do not respond to either FFP or plasma exchange. The rarity of the condition and the tendency to publish successful cases mean that it is impossible to quantify this proportion, but it is probably between 25% and 50% of cases. Corticosteroids and heparin have each been used in the past. Heparin is dangerous in the thrombocytopenic patient and probably ineffective in true TTP. Corticosteroids are also of doubtful benefit. Antiplatelet drugs, which ought

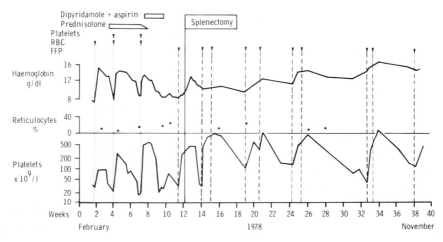

Fig. 7.4. *Thrombotic thrombocytopenic purpura. Response to various therapeutic efforts. Platelets and haemoglobin respond to fresh frozen plasma (FFP) and blood transfusions of red cells (RBC) or platelets. Response is predictable and repeatable. The patient eventually recovered fully.*

theoretically to be of benefit, have mainly been disappointing. Infusions of prostacyclin analogues or drugs which promote prostacyclin synthesis may be of benefit, mainly in patients who respond to FFP.

Splenectomy has been used with variable outcome in TTP. A few patients respond dramatically with a sustained and apparently permanent remission but others show no response. Sudden death due to cardiac microthrombi is one of the end-states of the disorder which may occur at any time and may even occur during surgery. In desperate and unresponsive cases splenectomy may even be considered.

Thrombotic thrombocytopenic purpura may be triggered by a variety of stimuli, of which infection and pregnancy have already been mentioned. It is therefore essential to search diligently for such a trigger and remove it. There is a strong case for considering the early use of broad-spectrum antibiotics, particularly in patients with high and persistent fever. Patients may also relapse during therapy if they acquire an infection. Pulmonary and urinary tract infections are not uncommon. It may not be necessary to terminate pregnancy in patients who respond well to plasma exchange or FFP infusion, but in patients who do not respond promptly termination is normally achieved, either spontaneously or therapeutically. Termination does not always halt the disease.

March Haemoglobinuria

Haemoglobinuria following running has been documented for about 100 years. Davidson demonstrated that its origin was mechanical, with destruction of red cells occurring in the feet, and that it could be cured by running with soft shoes or on soft ground. The disorder may arise in joggers and is benign except that it may lead to extensive invasive investigations unless recognized. The blood film does not show any red cell fragmentation or consistent abnormality. Occasionally haemoglobinuria after running is accompanied by nausea, abdominal cramps and aching legs and for enthusiastic athletes with this condition there may be mild splenomegaly and jaundice.

CHEMICAL AND PHYSICAL AGENTS

Oxidative Haemolysis

Oxidative substances may cause haemolysis in people with normal red cell metabolism and normal HbA if the oxidative stimulus is large enough. The major causes of oxidative haemolysis in normal subjects are shown in Table 7.6. The features of oxidative haemolysis are dependent on the main sites of oxidative attack, whether on the membrane of the red cell, the globin chains or the haem group.

Chronic Intravascular Haemolysis with Heinz Bodies

Dapsone and salazopyrine (salicylazosulphapyridine) will cause oxidative, intravascular haemolysis in normal subjects if taken in high enough dosage. Red cells show the 'bite' abnormality of the chemically damaged cell (Fig. 7.5). Heinz bodies may be absent or scanty in patients with an intact spleen. Dapsone is used in the treatment of leprosy, where G6PD-deficient subjects may receive the drug, and in the treatment of dermatitis herpetiformis, in which functional hyposplenism occurs. Heinz bodies appear in the latter case, acute intravascular haemolysis in the former.

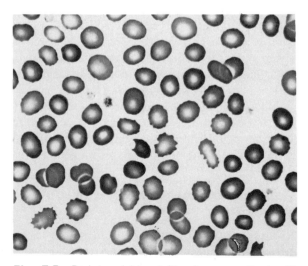

Fig. 7.5. *Peripheral blood film from a patient with phenacetin-induced haemolysis, showing anisocytosis and occasional chemically damaged cell ('bite' abnormality).*

Table 7.6
Substances causing oxidative haemolysis and/or methaemoglobinuria in normal people

Substance	Use	Remarks
Dapsone	Leprosy; dermatitis herpetiformis	Chronic Hb haemolysis: slow acetylators more susceptible
Maloprim	Antimalarial	Methaemoglobinaemia in NADH Met-Hb-depleted subjects
Salazopyrine	Ulcerative colitis	Chronic Hb haemolysis
Phenazopyridine	Analgesic in urinary tract infections	Methaemoglobinaemia
Menadiol	Water-soluble vitamin K analogue	Haemolysis and kernicterus in infants
Nitrites	Fertilizer; present in well-water and some vegetable juices	Methaemoglobinaemia in infants
Nitrates	Amylnitrate, butyrl nitrite: abused as recreational	Methaemoglobinaemia
Chlorate	Sodium chlorate: a weed killer	Acute i.v. haemolysis; renal failure 30 g fatal
Arsine	Gas produced in smelting and other industrial processes	Acute i.v. haemolysis; renal failure

Haemosiderinuria may be detected in patients taking these drugs and there may be polychromasia and macrocytosis. Haemolysis is usually well compensated and there is no need to stop the treatment because of the haemolysis unless the anaemia is severe. A dose reduction may sometimes be needed.

Methaemoglobinaemia is uncommon unless the patient is partially deficient in NADH methaemoglobin reductase. The gene for this abnormality may not be very uncommon and it may account for some people becoming cyanosed after taking dapsone-containing antimalarial preparations.

Methaemoglobinaemia With or Without Haemolysis

Nitrites in water or vegetable juices may cause methaemoglobinaemia in infants who have a physiological impairment of the reducing systems. Well-water which comes from land with an excess of nitrites and which is used to reconstitute artificial feeds has produced cyanosis in infants. Cases have also been described following enthusiastic feeding of juice from carrots grown on organically fertilized land and of spinach juice—spinach has a high concentration of nitrogen-fixing bacteria on its leaves.

Nitrate drugs also produce methaemoglobinaemia and have proved fatal when taken in high enough dosage for 'recreational' purposes.

Water-soluble analogues of vitamin K (menadiol-sodium-diphosphate) cause haemolysis with or without methaemoglobinaemia in infants and in utero if given to the mother during the third trimester. Fat-soluble vitamin K preparations must be used if required in these situations.

Methaemoglobinaemia due to oxidative drugs may be treated with intravenous methylene blue in doses of 1–2 mg/kg. Ascorbic acid by mouth may also be used. These measures are ineffective in G6PD-deficient patients and when very strong oxidant substances are implicated. In these circumstances methylene blue should be avoided because it acts as an oxidant and makes the condition worse.

Acute Intravascular Haemolysis, Methaemoglobin-aemia and Renal Failure

These occur following exposure to strong oxidizing substances which are found mainly in industrial or horticultural pursuits. Sodium chlorate is a popular weed killer; Arsine is a gas which is produced in various industrial settings. Acute intravascular haemolysis with haemoglobinuria develops. The serum becomes brown, often very dark so that blood cells cannot be seen in anticoagulated preparations, due to the presence of methaemalbumin, methaemoglobin and free haemoglobin. Oliguric renal failure usually develops over about 24 hours. The blood film shows microspherocytosis and bizarre forms.

Plasma exchange and renal dialysis are the mainstays of treatment, methylene blue being ineffective. Poisoning with arsine is usually reversible with these measures. Chlorate poisoning is more difficult, 30 g being a generally fatal dose. It is mostly ingested deliberately in suicide attempts.

Acquired Disorders of the Red Cell Membrane

The mature red cell does not have the capacity for repair of its membrane. The lipids of the membrane are in equilibrium with the lipids of the plasma and changes in ratio of free cholesterol to phospholipids in plasma may affect the red cell shape and in some instances lead to haemolysis. This is most commonly seen in liver disease, but other inherited lipid disorders may affect the red cell secondarily.

Liver Disease

Some degree of shortening of the red cell survival occurs in most cases of acute hepatitis, cirrhosis and Gilbert's disease, but anaemia is not present and there is only a slight rise in reticulocytes which may not be detectable. Biliary obstruction is associated with the appearance of target cells and fulminant hepatitis with acanthocytosis, both consequent on changes in the plasma lipid composition.

Zieve's syndrome is an uncommon disorder, seen mainly in alcoholics, comprised of intravascular haemolysis and acute abdominal pain. The patients usually have cirrhosis and jaundice. The cause is unknown but is probably related to lipid changes in the blood. Spherocytes are seen in the peripheral blood.

Wilson's disease may present as acute intravascular haemolysis. This is probably not a membrane disorder but consequent on the high levels of copper ions in the blood. The haemolysis may antedate the development of hepatic or neurological features but Keyser–Fleischer rings are usually present. The blood film may show spherocytosis. The diagnosis is made once the condition is suspected. Apart from caeruloplasmin deficiency, the patients have a specific aminoaciduria.

Hereditary Acanthocytosis (a- β-lipoproteinaemia)

This rare inherited deficiency of low-density lipoproteins is characterized by retinitis pigmentosa, steatorrhoea, ataxia and mental retardation. The haemolysis which occurs is of minor importance to such patients but the blood film may indicate the diagnosis, the red cells showing marked acanthocytosis.

Vitamin E Deficiency

Deficiency of vitamin E may occur in infants fed a diet rich in polyunsaturated fatty acids. There is haemolysis with contracted cells and a thrombocytosis. Oedema may be present. Vitamin E is an antioxidant and oxidative damage to the red cell membrane is thought to be the cause of the haemolysis.

Paroxysmal Nocturnal Haemoglobinuria

Paroxysmal nocturnal haemoglobinuria (PNH) is a rare but fascinating disorder which is probably derived from a somatic mutation arising in a marrow which is already damaged so that the PNH stem cells have a selective growth advantage. Its clinical features of haemoglobinuria occurring the morning after sleep brought it to the attention of physicians from an early time and it has many eponyms, of which Machiafava–Michaelis syndrome is perhaps the best known. It also has the distinction of being the first disease whose clonal nature was demonstrated by the use of G6PD enzyme analysis by Luzzatto and colleagues in Nigeria in 1970.

Clinical Features

Two main types of PNH may be distinguished on clinical grounds—'classical haemolytic' PNH, in which the haemolysis is the main feature, and 'laboratory' PNH, where the clone of PNH cells is identified by laboratory tests but where the haemolytic effect is trivial in relation to the general marrow disorder. Syndromes in between occur.

Haemolytic PNH is very rare in infants and young children, is most common in adolescents and young adults up to the age of 40, and the incidence declines thereafter. It is much more common in the Far East than in Western countries. Males and females are affected equally.

Typically the condition presents as haemoglobinuria which is noticed in the first micturition after sleep, the urine clearing during the day (Fig. 7.6), but there are many other presentations so that the diagnosis may be missed for months or years. Abdominal pain, often severe, intermittent and unrelated to meals, is one such presentation which may lead to extensive gastrointestinal investigations and even psychiatric referral if the diagnosis is missed. Thrombotic complications are common (see below) and may be the presenting feature. The condition may arise on the background of aplastic anaemia, and clinical features associated with that disease may predominate. Rarely, the patient presents features of iron deficiency due to chronic intravascular haemolysis. The presentation is occasionally of acute haemolysis occurring during an infection. PNH may arise during the course of another blood disorders, most commonly aplastic anaemia, sometimes after a period of apparent remission. There are no specific physical findings other than those of haemolytic anaemia or secondary to thrombosis. Splenomegaly occurs in some patients.

Laboratory Findings

These depend to some extent on the background of marrow disorder on which the PNH develops but there are some common features and the condition is defined by the sensitivity of the PNH cells to complement lysis.

The peripheral blood shows anaemia, polychromasia, neutropenia and thrombocytopenia. The last two are variable in degree but in the majority of cases are reduced below the limit of normal. Thrombocytopenia is sometimes marked, even when there is a thrombotic presentation. The red cell morphology is often abnormal, though no specific changes are seen. Tear-drop poikilocytes may be present without any suggestion of extramedullary haemopoiesis. The reticulocyte count, though normally elevated, is less than would be expected for the degree of anaemia. The neutrophil alkaline phosphatase score is decreased. Haemo-

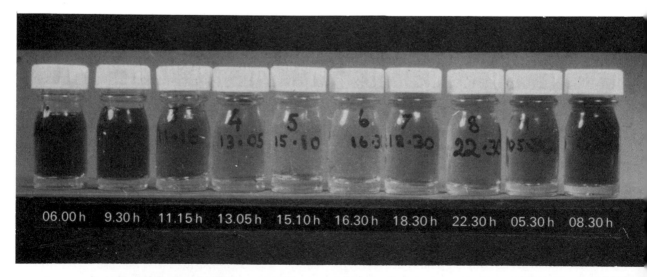

Fig. 7.6. *Paroxysmal nocturnal haemoglobinuria. Serial urine samples starting at 06.00 h, showing clearing of haemoglobinuria during the day and return at night*

globin may be present in the urine, though it may be intermittent. Haemosiderinuria is present.

Acidified-Serum Lysis Test (Ham–Dacie Test)

Acidification of normal serum activates the alternate pathway of complement. The characteristic feature of PNH red cells is their sensitivity to lysis by complement. PNH red cells incubated with serum acidified to pH 6.4 will lyse both with normal and autologous serum. Heating the serum to 56°C before incubation inactivates the complement and lysis does not occur, even with acidification. Only a proportion of the red cells lyse and the amount of lysis is not always a good indication of the severity of the disease, the result also depending on the amount of complement present in a particular serum. A positive acidified-serum lysis test is also found in congenital dyserythropoietic anaemia (CDA type 11, HEMPAS) but the test is negative in autologous serum in this condition (see p. 114).

Other Tests of Complement Sensitivity

The sucrose lysis test and the thrombin lysis test are each positive in PNH because the tests activate the classical pathway of complement. The sucrose lysis test may be positive in other disorders, such as aplastic anaemia and myelofibrosis, and is less specific than the Ham–Dacie test. It is a useful screening test. Lysis by cold antibody (anti-I) is also increased in PNH because the cells present a high concentration of I antigen on their surface.

The bone marrow in PNH presents many different abnormalities depending on associated disorders (see below). Most commonly in haemolytic anaemia the marrow is cellular, but less so than would be expected from the degree of pancytopenia observed. There are no other diagnostic features.

Pathogenesis

PNH is a clonal disorder which appears to be a somatic mutation. It is a stem cell disorder, as shown by abnormalities of granulocytes and platelets, though these are less easy to demonstrate than those of the red cells. The basic defect is not known but the clinical features derive from the membrane

abnormalities produced. The membrane of the red cells shows several features, including diminished acetylcholinesterase concentration and increased I and i antigen expression, which are probably not important in the pathogenesis of the haemolysis. It has been shown that there is also a decrease in an important enzyme, decay-accelerating factor (DAF), which inactivates C3a bound to the red cell. The absence of this protein may explain the sensitivity of the cells to complement lysis but is unlikely to be the consequence of the somatic mutation itself. More recently, an anchoring phosphatidylinositol which is common to several surface proteins including DAF and acetylcholinesterase, has been shown to be deficient in PNH (Selvaraj *et al.*, 1988).

It has been repeatedly mentioned that PNH usually develops on the background of damaged marrow. Some of the associations are described below, but even where haemolysis predominates with an active marrow, culture of committed precursor cells shows a decrease in CFU-C and BFU-E which are not complement sensitive. As described below, PNH may be cured by infusion of normal syngeneic stem cells without any cytotoxic therapy, suggesting that the PNH has a growth advantage when other stem cells are damaged in some way.

Associated Bone Marrow Disorders

PNH is most commonly associated with evidence of hypoplasia of the bone marrow. The PNH may precede, accompany or follow the development of aplastic anaemia. A PNH population may appear transiently and not produce any haematological effects. Haemolytic PNH may occur after recovery from aplastic anaemia. It has also been described in patients with inherited aplastic anaemia. The next most common association has been with myelosclerosis. Malignant conditions, Ph-negative CGL and erythroleukaemia have also been the background in which PNH develops. PNH itself may terminate with the development of acute leukaemia.

Course of PNH

PNH may evolve in many different ways. The condition may remain stable for decades, with a regular transfusion requirement. Iron overload is uncommon because of the urinary iron loss. The PNH clone may disappear after several years. Acute leukaemia may develop. Aplastic anaemia may ensue.

Thrombotic complications are the most devastating of the effects of PNH. There is a particular tendency for thrombosis to occur in the splanchnic vessels or the hepatic veins but cerebral or femoral thromboses are recorded. The abdominal pain of PNH is thought to be caused by thrombosis, and infarction of the bowel has been recorded. Thrombosis of the hepatic veins causes the Budd–Chiari syndrome, a justly feared complication of PNH.

Infections may occur secondary to granulocyte functional abnormalities.

Treatment

Treatment is unsatisfactory. This is a chronic disorder for which support measures, both haematological and psychological, are more important than any definitive treatment. Blood transfusion is the major factor. Red cells should be given after removal of white cells to reduce transfusion reactions. White cell depletion may be obtained by washing the red cells or by using commercial filters which remove white cells. Iron deficiency may develop but iron supplements should be used with caution. The increase in haemopoiesis produced by iron may increase the production of PNH cells and increase intravascular lysis. This does not matter by itself but there may be an increased risk of thrombosis.

Thrombosis has to be treated by anticoagulation despite the presence of thrombocytopenia. The Budd–Chiari syndrome is the most devastating thrombotic complication. It may arise piecemeal with preceding veno-occlusive disease of the liver. This may be identified by increasing size of the liver and confirmed by ultrasound of the liver. High-dose heparin may halt the process. Tissue plasminogen activator has been used successfully to reverse the Budd–Chiari syndrome in the early stages.

Anticoagulants should be continued for life once the thrombosis is under control: even if the PNH clone disappears, the veins will have been damaged by the thrombosis.

High-dose corticosteroids probably stabilize the red cell membrane against complement lysis but the dose required is unacceptable for long-term treatment and the efficacy of these drugs in preventing thrombosis is unclear. Heparin has an anticomplementary action but is not suitable for long-term management and the effect is weak.

Bone marrow transplantation will cure PNH provided the patient does not die as a result of treatment. A few cases of syngeneic, identical twin transplants have been described. Remarkably, the recipients have recovered even though no cytotoxic chemotherapy has been given.

In such a disease, with a median survival of 10 years and with the possibility of spontaneous remission, the effectiveness of any treatment is difficult to assess. A clear marker would be the prompt disappearance of the PNH clone, but so far no treatment, other than bone marrow transplantation, has achieved this. Careful, sympathetic management is all that is available for most patients.

SELECTED BIBLIOGRAPHY

Dacie J. V. (1967). *The haemolytic anaemias III. Secondary symptomatic haemolytic anaemias.* London: J. & A. Churchill.

Dacie J. V. (1967). *The haemolytic anaemias IV. Drug induced haemolytic anaemias etc.* London: J. & A. Churchill.

Gordon-Smith E. C. (1980). Drug induced oxidative haemolysis. *Clinics in Haematology*, **9:3**, 557–586.

Karmali M. A., Petric M., Lim C. *et al.* (1985). The association between idiopathic haemolytic uremic syndrome and infection by verotoxin-producing *Escherichia coli. Journal of Infectious Diseases*, **151**, 775–782.

Kwan H. C. (1987). Thrombotic microangiography I and II. *Seminars in Hematology*, **2** and **3**.

Oni S. B., Osumkoya B. O., Luzzatto L. (1970). Paroxysmal nocturnal haemoglobinuria: evidence for monoclonal origin of abnormal red cells. *Blood*, **36**, 145–152.

Pagbura M. K., Schreiber R. D., Muller-Ebahard H. J. (1983). Deficiency of an erythrocyte membrane protein with complement regulatory activity in paroxysmal nocturnal haemoglobinuria. *Proceedings of the National Academy of Science USA*, **80**, 5430–5434.

Perrin L. H., Mackey L. J., Miescher P. A. (1982). The haematology of malaria in man. *Seminars in Hematology*, **19**, 70–82.

Petz L. D. (1980). Drug induced immune haemolytic anaemia. *Clinics in Haematology*, **9:3**, 455–482.

Petz L. D., Garraty G. D. (1980). *Acquired immune haemolytic anaemias*. New York, Edinburgh, London: Churchill Livingstone.

Rosse W. F., Parker C. J. (1985). Paroxysmal nocturnal haemoglobinuria. *Clinics in Haematology*, **14**, 105–125.

Selvaraj P., Rosse W. F., Silber R., Springer T. A. (1988). The major Fc receptor in blood has a phosphatidyl-inositol anchor and is deficient in paroxysmal nocturnal haemoglobinuria. *Nature*; **333**: 565–7.

Chapter 8

BLOOD GROUP SEROLOGY

MARCELA CONTRERAS AND ANATOLE LUBENKO

It is sometimes thought that a worker in blood transfusion is merely a provider of 'safe' blood if and when the clinician requests it. Indeed, in many ways this is true, and a great deal of effort and thought goes into the Blood Transfusion Service. However, the subject of blood groups and problems of blood transfusion are extremely interesting in their own right and their solutions have much to offer to haematology in general. Blood group serology should, in a broad sense, include the study of antigenic molecules present on the various cellular and soluble components of whole blood together with that of the antibodies and lectins that recognize them and their interactions. However, blood group serology is in practice restricted to red cell antigens and their interactions with specific antibodies. In this narrower sense, the complexities of HLA, granulocyte, platelet and plasma protein determinants are not considered as falling within the blood group serologist's realm, even though all of them are genetically polymorphic and play a role in blood transfusion.

The narrower definition of blood group serology encompasses: (i) the determination of the phenotype of red cells using antibodies and reagents of known specificity; (ii) the search for and identification of antibodies using red cells of known phenotype; and (iii) compatibility testing of patients' sera against cell samples from donor units of the same ABO and RhD groups. Currently, approximately two million units of blood are transfused to patients each year in the UK alone.

The data gathered by blood group serologists hold a wider interest than those of workers in blood transfusion alone. For example, blood group serology can help the haematologist to establish the origin of immune haemolytic states as drug induced, alloimmune or frankly autoimmune. For the paediatrician, serological data can help to distinguish congenital from immunologically induced haemolytic syndromes of the newborn. In forensic science, blood group serology can prove a valuable tool in problems of identity and parentage.

Since most blood group systems are inherited as autosomal dominant Mendelian characters, blood group serology has proven to be an extremely useful tool for linkage studies and chromosome mapping. The wide tissue distribution of some red cell antigens has led to the study of their involvement in neoplastic, microbial and parasitic diseases. Further, studies of the membrane defects of some hereditary antigenic deficiencies have helped our understanding of the basic structure of the erythrocyte membrane.

The aim of this chapter will be to provide an introduction to blood group serology and to include such parts of immunology and biochemistry as can contribute to our understanding of blood group antigens, antibodies and antigen–antibody reactions.

THE RED CELL MEMBRANE AND CHEMISTRY OF BLOOD GROUP ANTIGENS

An overview of the chemistry of the red cell membrane is essential in order to understand the physical and chemical bases of blood group serology.

The red cell membrane is composed of about 40% w/w lipids and up to 10% carbohydrates, the remainder being proteins. The exact arrangement of its components is controversial, but most people follow the ideas of Singer and Nicolson (1972). A diagram based on their work is shown in Fig. 8.1.

The lipids of the red cell membrane can be subdivided into 60% w/w phospholipids, 30% w/w neutral lipids (mainly cholesterol) and 10% w/w glycolipids. The phospho- and glycolipids play a role in the structure of the membrane and are thought to be important in the maintenance of red cell shape. These lipids have a molecular arrangement reminiscent of a tuning fork, with the hydrophobic fatty acids forming the 'prongs' and the polar group the 'handle'. They are arranged in a bilayer with the 'prongs' pointing inwards and the hydrophilic 'handle' pointing outwards in contact with the aqueous solutions of the plasma or cytoplasmic surface of the membrane (Fig. 8.1). Cholesterol is inserted in between the other lipids. This arrangement allows the interior of the membrane to be in a semifluid state and the whole membrane to be very flexible. The lipid bilayer does not allow the passive transfer of ions.

The carbohydrates are attached to the lipids and proteins and occur only on the external surface of the membrane. They are composed of monosaccharides, the majority being hexoses.

About 20–40% of the proteins of the membrane are released relatively easily (e.g. by changing the ionic strength of the medium) and are therefore not very firmly attached (peripheral proteins). The remaining 60–80% are released only after drastic treatment with detergents or bile salts; these integral proteins penetrate the lipid bilayer. After red cell membranes have been treated with the detergent sodium dodecyl sulphate, the proteins can be separated electrophoretically on polyacrylamide gels according to their molecular size. If the gel is stained for protein, up to eight bands are seen, as shown in Fig. 8.2. Bands 1 and 2 are proteins that are easily released by a low ionic strength medium. They are monomers and dimers of the contractile protein spectrin, which form a network of tetramers on the inner surface of the membrane contributing to the maintenance of the red cell shape. Band 5 (actin) links the spectrin tetramers together. Band 3, the anion channel, is a dimer linked to the cytoskeleton through ankyrin (band 2.1). Band 6 and band 4.1 are also associated with band 3 on the inner side of the membrane.

If the polyacrylamide gel is stained for carbohydrate (PAS stain), four or five bands are seen (Fig. 8.2). These bands contain two major glycoproteins. The first, α sialoglycoprotein (αSGP), or glycophorin A, is found as a dimer and monomer in PAS 1 and 2 bands respectively. The second, δ SGP, or glycophorin B, is found in the PAS 3 band. The PAS 4 band contains dimers of α and δ SGPs. An

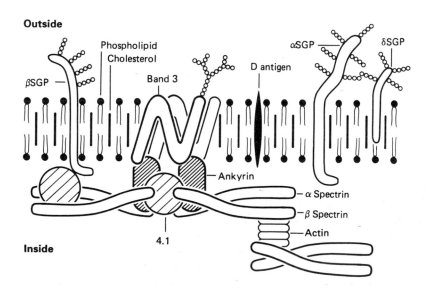

Fig. 8.1. *Diagram of a cross-section of the red cell membrane.*

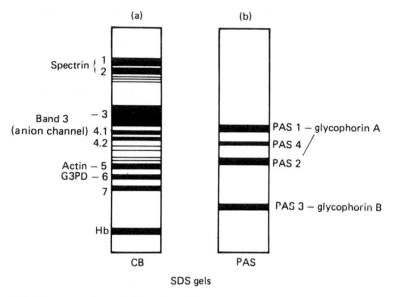

Fig. 8.2. *The proteins of the red cell membrane after separation by electrophoresis in sodium dodecyl sulphate (SDS) gels: (a) stained for protein (Coomassie blue, CB), (b) stained for carbohydrate (periodic acid-Schiff's reagent, PAS).*

additional band, PAS 2, consists of β SGP, or glycophorin C. The α SGP has been extensively studied and its amino acid sequence determined. The other SGPs have been partially sequenced. The outer portion of the SGPs contains all the carbohydrate of these molecules (60% w/w) and extends far beyond the lipid bilayer, allowing charged groups or receptors to extend some distance into the plasma. The α and β SGPs extend through the whole of the lipid bilayer. On the other hand, δ SGP only partly penetrates the bilayer (see Fig. 8.1).

Blood group antigens have been found in both the protein and the carbohydrate component of membrane glycoproteins and in glycolipids. The RhD and Fy^a antigens have been ascribed to minor membrane proteins with molecular weights in the 29 000–40 000 range in monomeric form, whereas the MN and Ss antigens are found on the larger, major membrane proteins α and δ SGP respectively. Antigens of the P, P$_1$ and P^k series, together with ABH, Le and Ii antigens, are found in the carbohydrate portion of glycolipids. ABH antigens have also been found on the polysaccharide cluster attached to band 3. Apart from the antigens on integral membrane components, some can be adsorbed passively from plasma, e.g. Lewis, Chido, Rogers. Others, like the M and N antigens, arise from interactions between the carbohydrate hapten and its protein carrier.

The role of interaction of lipid with protein is unclear; full expression of RhD has been shown to require the presence of phospholipid.

The precise structure of only a handful of blood group antigens is known with any certainty; these are mainly carbohydrate antigens. Further structural details of selected known antigens are given in Chapter 9.

ANTIGENS

Originally, an antigen was defined as that part of a molecule or particle that is bound by a specific antibody. More recently, it has become customary to define an antigen as a substance that can stimulate an immune response (immunogenicity). Immune responses can be either positive or negative. Positive responses lead to the production of antibodies (humoral immunity) and/or proliferation of immunocompetent cells (cellular immunity) that can bind and eliminate their stimulatory antigen. In negative responses, the cells that mediate humoral and cellular immune responses are rendered non-responsive. This state is described as acquired immunological tolerance and is important in preventing autoimmune disease, as well as in establishing the 'take' or acceptance of transplanted syngeneic and allogeneic tissues.

The hallmark of the adaptive immune response is its specificity: specific immunocompetent cells and/or antibodies are produced that can distinguish molecules that differ only by two or three atoms, e.g. TNP versus DNP. As described later, even the difference between the blood group A and B antigens is minimal. However, sometimes antibodies can react with antigens similar to, but not identical with, the stimulatory antigen (cross-reactivity). As far as is known, specific immune responses to human red cells are mediated by antibodies only; *specific* cell-mediated immunity to red cell allo- or autoantigens has not been described.

The parts of an antigen that bind to antibodies or cellular receptors are called antigenic epitopes or determinants, and the parts of the antibody that bind them are called paratopes. Most antigens that occur naturally are of large molecular weight and each antigenic molecule may have several different or several identical epitopes. As antibodies are specific for the individual epitopes and not for the antigen as a whole, antisera will usually be a collection of antibodies specific for different regions of the antigen in question arising from different clones of immunocompetent cells (polyclonal antibodies); such antibodies can sometimes be distinguished serologically by anti-idiotype reagents (see below).

The Significance of Blood Group Antigens

Antigens exist only insofar as antibodies can be made that define them. The function of the membrane structures bearing antigenic determinants is by and large unknown; only the band 3 membrane glycoprotein, which bears a dendritic polysaccharide with ABH antigenic activity, has a known physiological role. This protein, with most of its mass in the lipid bilayer, mediates the passive transport of polar molecules (Cl^-, HCO_3^-) across the non-polar bilayer, thus providing an anion channel.

The differences between the epitopes of various red cell antigens are very small—just one or two sugars or one or two amino acids. The meaning of these differences is unknown and there is little evidence to suggest that one antigen confers any significant advantage over another. Indeed, an abundant major membrane molecule can be completely absent and yet the red cell still functions quite normally. One of the major transmembrane proteins, α SGP or glycophorin A, of which there are approximately 500 000 copies per red cell, is absent in rare individuals with missing M and N antigens such as M^k or in En^a-negative subjects. This absence profoundly affects the charge of the red cell but does not affect its lifespan or function at all. The δ SGP, or glycophorin B, may be absent in people with missing S and s antigens, again without any apparent effect on the red cell lifespan. Major carbohydrate antigens are absent in the Bombay and Tj(a−) or pp subjects who lack all ABH and P antigens respectively; their red cells are normal.

In contrast, absence of a less abundant minor membrane protein can have profound effects on the structure and function of the red cell. Rh_{null} individuals, who have a total absence of Rh antigens, all show chronic haemolysis which is usually mild and may be compensated for by increased red cell production. The red cells are more 'leaky' than normal and have a shortened lifespan. The blood film usually shows some spherocytic and stomatocytic red cells. In the Kell system, the very rare persons of the McLeod phenotype, who lack the Kx antigen, have very depressed Kell antigens and a mild chronic haemolytic process with some acanthocytes in the blood film.

On the other hand, the absence of antigens can be beneficial, as in the Fy(a−b−) phenotype. It has been shown that the Duffy antigens (Fy^a and/or Fy^b) are used as receptors by the *Plasmodium vivax* to penetrate red cells. Fy(a−b−) subjects predominate amongst Negroes, who are therefore resistant to *P. vivax* malaria. This parasite will no longer penetrate Fy(a+) or Fy(b+) red cells that have been coated with anti-Fy^a, anti-Fy^b or treated with proteases which destroy Fy antigens.

ANTIBODIES

Antibodies are immunoglobulins (Ig) produced by the B lymphocytes of the adaptive immune system in response to an antigen for which they exhibit specific binding.

Depending on the origin of the antigenic stimulus, antibodies can be termed: (i) alloantibodies when produced by an individual against epitopes present in another individual, (ii) autoantibodies when reactive with determinants present on the individual's own antigens, (iii) heteroantibodies when produced against antigenic determinants present on the cells of another species. The first two are the antibodies encountered routinely in the blood bank; heteroantibodies can be used as antiglobulin sera or typing reagents when raised in animals against human antigens.

There are five classes of immunoglobulin: IgM, IgG, IgA, IgD and IgE. Antibodies with specificity for blood group antigens are found only in the IgG, IgM and IgA classes. IgA antibodies play a minor role in blood group serology as they only appear as alloantibodies together with IgM and/or IgG. Some of the biochemical and biophysical differences between IgG, IgM and IgA are listed in Table 8.1.

Biochemistry of Immunoglobulins

Figure 8.3 shows a diagram of the basic immunoglobulin molecule. This is made up of four polypeptide chains arranged as two L (or light) chains and two identical H (or heavy) chains. The light and heavy chains are usually held together by S–S bonds. IgG and serum IgA molecules are mainly monomers of this basic immunoglobulin structure; secretory IgA is mainly dimeric. IgM molecules are pentamers, with the basic immunoglobulin molecules held together by S–S bonds and a J (joining) chain (Fig. 8.4).

There are two distinct types of light chain, kappa (κ) and lambda (λ). These are common to all immunoglobulin classes. Either of these chains may combine with any heavy chain, but in any one immunoglobulin both light chains are of the same type and are identical: hybrid molecules do not occur. Kappa chains occur in about 65% and lambda chains in about 35% of the normal immunoglobulins in each class. On the other hand, each class has an immunologically distinct heavy chain: γ for IgG, μ for IgM, α for IgA, δ for IgD and ε for IgE (Fig. 8.4). The heavy chain also determines the immunoglobulin subclass. There are four subclasses of human IgG (IgG1, IgG2, IgG3 and IgG4

Table 8.1
Biological and physical properties of the major serum immunoglobulins

	IgG	IgM	IgA
Molecular forms	or $\gamma_2\kappa_2$ / $\gamma_2\lambda_2$	or $[\mu_2\kappa_2]_5.J$ / $[\mu_2\lambda_2]_5.J$	or $\alpha_2\kappa_2{}^\dagger$ / $\alpha_2\lambda_2$
Molecular weight (daltons)	150 000	900 000	160 000†
Sedimentation coefficient	7S	19S	7S†
Plasma concentration (mg/ml)			
Adult	7.3–23.7	0.47–1.47	0.61–3.3
Newborn	Slightly higher	~0.1	Undetectable
Percentage intravascular	44	80	40
Fractional catabolic rate (%/day)	7	18	33
$T_{\frac{1}{2}}$ (days)	23	5	6
Effect of reducing agents	0*	↓↓↓	0
Serological behaviour	Non-agglutinating	Agglutinating	Usually non-agglutinating

*0.01 mol/l dithiothreitol (DTT) or 0.1 mol/l 2-mercaptoethanol (2-ME) may convert IgG into agglutinins.
† 10% of serum IgA is found as 9S–10S dimers, in $[\alpha_2\kappa_2]_2.J$ or $[\alpha_2\lambda_2]_2.J$ forms, with mol. wt = 330 000.

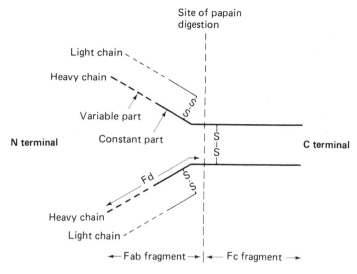

Fig. 8.3. *Structure of the basic immunoglobulin molecules.*

with γ1, γ2, γ3 and γ4 heavy chains), and two IgA subclasses (IgA1 and IgA2, with α1 and α2 chains).

Analyses of various light chains from different sources show that while the amino acid sequence differs in one half of the chain (variable region), in the other half the sequence remains remarkably constant (constant region) between light chains of the appropriate kappa or lambda groups. Similarly, in the corresponding heavy chain there is a variable region and a constant region when different chains are analysed.

Papain can split the basic Ig molecule into three fragments at a site near the S–S bonds holding the heavy chains together (see Fig. 8.3). One fragment contains the carboxyl terminal ends of the heavy chains and is called the Fc fragment. The other two are called Fab fragments; each consists of the N terminal end of the heavy chain (Fd portion) and the whole of the light chain and contains the antigen binding site of the molecule.

Repetition of amino acid sequences within the heavy chain constant regions indicates that there are either three (for IgG and IgA) or four (for IgM, IgD, IgE) constant region domains for H chains. These are designated C_H1, C_H2, C_H3 etc. In contrast, there is only one constant region domain for light chains and only one variable region domain for heavy and light chains. The segment between the C_H1 and C_H2 domains is called the hinge region.

This area imparts flexibility to the immunoglobulin molecule so that antigen binding sites can span varying distances.

The vast majority of the differences between antibodies of differing specificities occur in three or four short amino acid sequences in the L and H chain variable regions respectively. These hypervariable sequences contact the antigen on binding and provide the basis of antibody specificity.

The remaining sequences within the variable region are known as the framework determinants. These are believed to provide the general skeleton of the antigen-recognizing region, within which variations in and between hypervariable sequences generate specificity for the different antigens bound by different antibodies.

Amino acid sequences within framework and hypervariable segments can sometimes be recognized by specific antisera, usually from another species, raised by deliberate immunization with a particular antibody. The sequences recognized are referred to as idiotopes, and the sera that define them are called anti-idiotypes. The idiotype of the particular immunoglobulin molecule represents the sum of all the idiotopes of all its framework and hypervariable sequences.

The binding of anti-idiotype sera which recognize idiotopes within hypervariable sequences of the immunizing immunoglobulin can be inhibited by

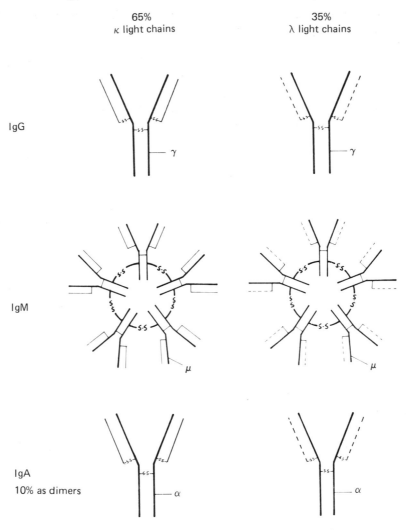

65%
κ light chains

35%
λ light chains

IgG

γ

γ

IgM

μ

μ

IgA
10% as dimers

α

α

Fig. 8.4. *Structure of IgG, IgM and IgA molecules.*

the specific hapten recognized by that immunizing antibody. This is because contact between the hapten and the hypervariable sequences blocks the access of the anti-idiotype serum. In contrast, binding of anti-idiotypes to framework determinants of the immunizing antibody is usually not blocked by the binding of the hapten recognized by that antibody.

The great diversity in the repertoire of antibodies that can be generated by the immune system is a direct reflection of the immune system's ability to generate variations within the three hypervariable sequences. This ability is partly genetic in origin and arises from the random selection and joining of several separate genetic elements (minigenes) from a large array of variable region DNA sequences. These minigenes produce a single intact variable region gene coding for the final variable region amino acid sequence.

The minigenes are comprised of: (1) a large number of V region sequences, with approximately 150 κ chain, 125 λ chain and 500 or so heavy chain variable region genes. Each of these genes is arranged in exons, the random joining of which provides the variations that generate the first hypervariable sequence; (2) in heavy chains only, approximately 10 to 20 D ('diversity') genes; and (3) in both heavy and light chains, five or six J ('joining') genes.

The random joining of V–J genes in light chains and V–D–J genes in heavy chains during ontogeny of the immune response generates the second and third hypervariable sequence, and provides an additional somatic contribution for increasing the repertoire of the immune system. Following V–J/V–D–J joining, which is achieved by splicing together of certain DNA sequences and deletion of others during B cell maturation, further increase in antibody diversity can be achieved by mutation in the spliced V gene DNA of mature B cells during their proliferation in an ongoing immune response. Further details of this DNA rearrangement in the immune response are given in Chapter 12.

Biological and Physical Properties of Immuno-globulins

Immunoglobulins are essentially multifunctional. Not only do they bind antigen, but they also perform various other functions depending on antibody class. Most of these additional functions reside on the Fc fragment and are listed in Table 8.2. The most important include: (a) complement fixation ($IgM > IgG3 > IgG1 > IgG2$) (IgA does not bind complement in the classical pathway); (b) binding to Fc receptors of reticuloendothelial cells, in particular monocytes and macrophages ($IgG3 \gg IgG1$); (c) transplacental passage: there appears to be preferential active transport of IgG1 relative to other IgG subclasses.

Some functions can be ascribed to particular domains, e.g. C_H2 or C_H2/C_H3 for complement (Clq) binding and control of catabolic rate; C_H3 for binding to the Fc receptors of macrophages and monocytes; $C_H2 + C_H3$ for binding to staphylococcal protein A (IgG3 does not bind) and to the Fc receptors on placental syncytium trophoblast and lymphocytes.

For blood group specific antibodies, these class-dependent biological functions contribute to their clinical significance. In the majority of cases, antigen–antibody binding does not cause red cell destruction per se; immune-mediated red cell destruction is usually a consequence of these secondary effector functions.

Since only IgG passes the placental barrier, only IgG blood group antibodies can cause haemolytic disease of the newborn. However, only IgG1 and IgG3 will mediate significant immune red cell de-

Table 8.2
Effector functions of the different immunoglobulin isotypes*

	IgG1	IgG2	IgG3	IgG4	IgA1	IgA2	SeIgA	IgM	IgE
Complement fixation: Classical pathway	+ +	+	+ + +	−	−	−	−	+ + + +	−
Complement fixation: Alternative pathway	−	−	−	−	+[†]	+ +	−	−	−[†]
Placental transfer	+	+	+	+	−	−	−	−	−
Lymphocyte/macrophage FcR binding	+	−	+	−	−	−	−	−	?[§]
Mast cell binding	−	−	−	(?)	−	−	−	−	+ + +
Binding to *Staph. aureus* protein A	+	+	−	+	−	−	−	−	−

* No biological function has been ascribed to IgD, but it may be intimately involved in maturation of B cells into competent effector cells and/or memory cells.

[†] Aggregated molecules can activate the alternative pathway.

[§] Human IgE has been reported to bind to macrophages.

Se IgA = secretory IgA.

struction. The IgG level in cord blood will be much the same as the level in the mother (IgG1 slightly higher). The passively transferred maternal IgG gradually disappears from the infant after birth and is almost gone by 3 months of age. The serum of newborn infants contains a small amount of IgM of fetal origin but almost no IgA; the production of IgA and IgG starts at about 1–2 months of age.

There are many ways of separating IgG and IgM molecules using sophisticated physical methods, e.g. gel filtration, affinity chromatography, etc. However, in routine serology, IgG is easily distinguishable from IgM by treating sera with mild reducing agents such as 2-mercaptoethanol (2-ME) or dithiothreitol (DTT) at low concentrations. These agents split the S–S bonds which link the IgM subunits, thereby rendering them non-agglutinating. IgA is either slightly affected or not affected by such reducing agents.

BLOOD GROUP ANTIBODIES

There are several terms that have been used in the past and are still sometimes used to describe different types of blood group antibodies. These are naturally occurring and immune antibodies, cold and warm antibodies, and complete (or saline) and incomplete antibodies. They will be described now and an attempt made to correlate these terms with the class of immunoglobulin involved.

Naturally Occurring and Immune Antibodies

Antibodies are called naturally occurring when they are produced without any obvious stimulus such as pregnancy, transfusion or injection of blood. However, these antibodies are not present at birth and, in the case of anti-A and anti-B, start to appear in the serum of children with the appropriate ABO groups at about 3–6 months of age. Moreover, ABO antibodies are probably all produced in response to antigens of bacteria, viruses and other substances which are inhaled or ingested; many gram-negative organisms have antigens which are structurally similar to the A and B antigens. In spite of this probable antigenic stimulus, the term 'naturally occurring' is retained because these antibodies are 'non-red cell induced.' Immune blood group antibodies are only produced after pregnancy or following transfusion or injection of blood or blood group substances.

Cold and Warm Antibodies

Cold antibodies give higher agglutination titres at low temperatures (0–4°C) and many of them will not agglutinate the appropriate cells at all at 37°C. Most naturally occurring antibodies are cold reacting. Some, such as naturally occurring anti-A and anti-B, have a wide thermal range and will still react at 37°C, but the titre will be much higher at 0–4°C. Cold antibodies which fail to react above 30°C are of no clinical significance and can be ignored for blood transfusion purposes.

The thermal optimum of warm antibodies is often said to be 37°C and this implies that higher titres are obtained at this temperature. However, some warm antibodies will also agglutinate the appropriate cells at 4°C, but the antigen–antibody reaction will take much longer to reach equilibrium at this lower temperature. Most immune antibodies are warm reacting. Any red cell antibody reacting above 30°C should be considered potentially destructive in vivo.

Complete and Incomplete Antibodies

Complete antibodies agglutinate red cells when they are suspended in saline. They are often called saline antibodies in laboratory parlance. Conversely, incomplete antibodies will not agglutinate the appropriate saline-suspended red cells. However, lack of visual agglutination does not mean that the antibodies have not bound to their antigen, and it can be shown that they have reacted by using antiglobulin reagents (see below). Most naturally occurring antibodies are cold reacting, complete and of the IgM class. On the other hand, immune antibodies are always warm reacting; most are incomplete IgG antibodies, but some may be complete and IgM. Exceptionally, IgG complete antibodies can be found.

Monoclonal Antibodies

Animal sera have, in general, been a poor source of blood grouping reagents. Deliberate immunization of laboratory animals to produce blood group specific heteroantibodies has had limited success since only a few polyclonal specificities have been made in rabbits, goats and chickens. The most useful reagents have been anti-A, -B, -M, -N, -s, -P_1, -Le^a, -Le^b and -LW.

The advent of monoclonal antibody technologies has partly offset this deficiency in polyclonal antibodies. By fusing the spleen cells of immunized mice or rats with drug-sensitive myeloma cells and selecting for drug-resistant hybrids, it has been possible to establish permanently growing cell lines in tissue culture that secrete antibodies of desired specificities. Several murine hybrids secreting human blood group specific monoclonal antibodies have now been established, many of which were raised using immunogens other than intact red cells, e.g. anti-A, -B, -Le^a, -Le^b, -M and -N.

Unfortunately, attempts to produce human monoclonals by the cell fusion approach have been of limited success due to the lack of suitable human myelomas. Nevertheless, human monoclonal antibodies specific for RhD and the ABO blood group antigens have been obtained by the alternative approach of transforming isolated peripheral blood lymphocytes from immunized individuals with the Epstein–Barr virus (EBV). Monoclonal antibodies of murine and human origin are rapidly replacing polyclonal blood grouping reagents in everyday ABO and RhD grouping.

Lectins

Lectins are sugar-binding proteins extractable from plants and lower vertebrate animals which are useful tools for routine and experimental blood group serology. They combine with simple sugars (e.g. fucose, galactose, N-acetyl-galactosamine) present on the glycolipids and glycoproteins of cell membranes and body fluids. Extracts from several thousand plant species have been investigated for red cell binding properties, but only a small minority can agglutinate human erythrocytes. Most of such lectins do so irrespective of target cell phenotype; hence only a handful are used with any regularity in blood group serology. The three most commonly used blood group specific lectins are extracts from *Dolichos biflorus* (the Hyacinth bean), *Vicia graminea* (Horse Gram) and *Ulex europaeus*

(Common Gorse), which have anti-A_1, anti-N and anti-H specificities respectively. Several other lectins have proven valuable in investigating red cell polyagglutinability. In addition to blood grouping, lectins are also used for determining ABH secretor status, separating mixtures of red cells, and for partially purifying and identifying blood group active membrane glycoproteins.

Lectins are not immunoglobulins, and are not produced as a result of a specific immune response. They do not possess the uniform molecular structure of immunoglobulins. Some exist as simple monomers (e.g. *Ulex*), while others are polymers (e.g. *Dolichos*).

The lectins used in blood grouping are highly specific. For example, *Ulex* and *Dolichos* recognize L-fucose and N-acetyl galactosamine respectively. This specificity does not depend solely upon the presence of the particular sugar, but is also influenced by its orientation and conformation, nature of the carrier molecule, and the number and distribution of reactive molecules on the red cell membrane. There are only seven sugars on the red cell membrane in various combinations with each other and their lipid and protein carriers; the similarities in these combinations lead to cross-reactivity of many lectins.

COMPLEMENT

Complement consists of a series of proteins, mainly enzymes, present in fresh plasma as inactive precursors which react sequentially with each other to form products that are important in the immune destruction of cells, bacteria etc. In complement activation, there are two stages of relevance. The first stage, in which the early components of complement participate, is the generation of the active form of the third component, C3b, which leads to the coating, or opsonization, of the cell with a large amount of protein. There are two pathways in which active C3b may be generated: the classical and alternative pathways. The second stage is the lytic stage. In this, activation of the proteins of the membrane attack complex (MAC), components C5 through to C9, leads to the destruction of red cells in the circulation.

In general terms, the complement sequence is somewhat like the clotting sequence. Activation of one component or group of components leads to the generation of enzyme activity for the next. However, in order to lead to haemolysis, the activated components in the plasma must bind to the red cell membrane (except C1 which binds only to a specific binding site on the antibody) and they do this with varying degrees of efficiency. Moreover, some activated components, for example C1, C4 and C3, have specific inactivators in the plasma as well as (for C3b and C4b) in the red cell membrane itself, and even though these components bind to the red cell membrane their active life may be very short (half-life ($T_{1/2}$) of 2–25 minutes). As a consequence the whole sequence may not be completed and there may be no haemolysis; in these cases, however, early components can be detected on the red cell surface with suitable antiglobulin sera.

Complement components in the classical pathway are called C1, C2, C3 etc. in their native form. Apart from C4, which is activated before C2 and C3, the components are activated sequentially according to their numerical order. Complement components in the alternative pathway include Factor B, Factor D and properdin. When the native forms of these products become activated they are written as $\overline{C1}$, $\overline{C2}$, Factor $\overline{D}$ or, in the case of C4, C3, C5 and Factor B, as $\overline{C4b}$, $\overline{C3b}$, $\overline{C5b}$ and Factor $\overline{Bb}$. In the activation of these last classical components, small molecular weight fragments C4a, C3a, C5a are released which have important chemotactic and anaphylactic activity. C3a and C5a lead to most of the initial symptoms in severe haemolytic transfusion reactions.

The Opsonization Phase of the Complement Sequence

The Classical Pathway (Fig. 8.5)

Several substances can activate the classical pathway: antigen–antibody complexes, enzymes (trypsin, plasmin, lysosomal enzymes), endotoxins, low ionic strength media, etc. Only one molecule of IgM on a cell membrane is necessary to activate the

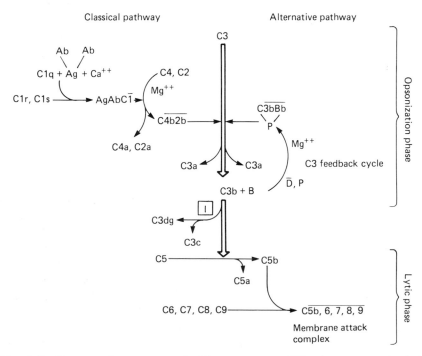

Fig. 8.5. *The complement cascade. The component C3b plays a central role in the classical and alternative pathways.*

complement system, and at least two of the five IgM subunits must attach to the cell membrane for activation to occur. On the other hand, at least two IgG molecules must combine with antigens very close together on the cell membrane to bring about complement activation.

The first component of complement is a complex of three protein molecules, Clq, Clr and Cls. After complement-fixing antibodies have bound to their red cell antigens (EA is often used to denote the resulting erythrocyte–antibody complex), Cl-binding sites are exposed on the Fc fragments. If two such sites are sufficiently close together (approximately 25–40 nm), the Cl complex is fixed through its Clq subunits. Clq is a complex molecule with six immunoglobulin-binding sites. Binding of Clq activates Clr, which in turn cleaves the third molecule, Cls, yielding the active enzyme form of the Cl complex which is held together by calcium. In the presence of EDTA or other chelating agents, the complex falls apart and the whole process of complement fixation will not occur.

Cls can now activate sequentially C4 and C2 in the presence of magnesium, generating a second enzyme, C4b2b, called C3 convertase.

The cell-bound C4b2b can optimally activate several thousand C3 molecules. Since C3 is present in large amounts (100–150 mg/100 ml) in the serum, the fixation of C3 can considerably increase the globulin coating of the red cells. While C3b is still intact, opsonized red cells will adhere to monocytes and macrophages through their C3b receptors and may then be phagocytosed. C3b coating of IgG-sensitized cells neutralizes the inhibitory effect of free plasma IgG on macrophage immune-adherence and amplifies erythrophagocytosis 100-fold. Thus C3b-coated, IgG-sensitized cells are destroyed mainly in the liver (see Chapter 10). However, the active phase of C3 is transient because it is rapidly degraded by an enzyme (C3b inactivator, C3bINA or Factor I) and its accelerator (βIH or Factor H) so that only C3dg remains on the red cell surface. C3dg is an end-product of the complement sequence and, by occupying the C3 sites, can prevent the further binding of C3b and therefore the haemolysis of the red cell. C3dg, unlike C3b, is not capable of adhering to macrophages and monocytes so that cells coated with C3dg may return to the circulation and will be resistant to further lysis. This explains the existence of a population of C3dg-coated cells refractory to lysis in cold haem-agglutinin disease (CHAD).

C4b2b3b-coated cells can trigger the fixation of C5, C6, C7, C8 and C9 onto normal red cells in close proximity and bring about their lysis.

The Alternative Pathway (Fig. 8.5)

The alternative mechanism does not necessarily involve antibody and represents non-specific 'innate' immunity. The proteins of the alternative pathway form a feedback loop for the conversion of C3 to C3b; the latter is both a product and reactant of this loop (Fig. 8.5).

The alternative pathway can be activated by aggregated IgA, zymosan, bacterial cells or lipopolysaccharides. Initiation of the alternative pathway is a two-step process: (i) binding of C3b to an activator, and (ii) interaction of bound C3b with neighbouring surface structures. Initially, spontaneously generated fluid phase C3b interacts with Factor B to form a complex. Factor B is activated through cleavage by the protease Factor D, releasing a fragment (Ba) into the plasma and yielding a transient alternative C3 convertase C3bBb. The latter can be stabilized by properdin. Although properdin is no longer implicated in initiating the alternative pathway, it is essential for preventing the dissociation of C3bBb by Factor H.

The alternative C3 convertase splits serum C3 into C3a and C3b which attaches to the cell surface and can then combine with more Factor B and D, thereby restarting the feedback loop. The amount of C3b deposited by the alternative pathway is low due to the small amount of convertase generated and to the inefficient deposition of C3b from plasma. This contrasts with the vast numbers of C3b molecules generated by the classical pathway. Either source of C3b is indistinguishable; both act on C5 to start the lytic phase.

The classical and alternative pathways cannot be separated from each other in vivo; the alternative pathway amplifies the classical pathway because when C3b is generated, Factors B and D may be activated and complexed with it to generate further C3b.

The Lytic Phase of the Complement Sequence
(Fig. 8.5)

The lytic phase starts with the activation of C5 by C3b, yielding membrane-bound C5b and fluid phase C5a. This step is followed by non-enzymatic interaction of C5b with C6, C7, C8 and C9. These molecules adhere to each other to form the membrane attack complex and insert themselves into the lipid bilayer of the red cell membrane. C8 catalysed by C9 produces lesions in the membrane that can be seen with an electron microscope. These lesions appear as protein-lined cylinders in the red cell membrane and are about 10 nm in diameter. They form pores through which ions and water can enter. The osmotic pressure exerted by haemoglobin draws water into the cell until it swells and bursts.

Optimum Temperature and pH for Complement Lysis

Many of the active complement components are enzymes and as such are very sensitive to changes in pH and temperature. The optimum pH for haemolysis to occur is 6.8 and the optimum temperature is 32–37°C. At temperatures below 15°C the red cell cannot be haemolysed by complement and it is assumed that the last stages of complement fixation do not occur. However, the early stages of complement fixation can occur at 15°C and the components can be detected on the red cell surface with anti-complement sera.

The Ability of the Antibody to Bind Complement

Why some antibody molecules bind complement easily and others do not is not fully understood, but several factors seem to be important. (i) The immunoglobulin class and subclass of the antibody are relevant, as discussed later. (ii) At least two Clq-binding sites, properly aligned and close together are necessary for complement fixation. One molecule of IgM antibody carries several Clq-binding sites whereas one molecule of IgG antibody carries only one, and will therefore need another molecule of IgG alongside it (IgG doublet) in order to fix Clq. Therefore, for IgG antibodies to cause lysis by complement, there must be many more of them

available. Hence, it has been shown that only one molecule of IgM anti-sheep red cell antibody is needed to lyse a sheep red cell, but at least 700–1000 molecules of IgG antibodies are needed to ensure that the two IgG molecules are aligned so that the whole process of the complement sequence can start. (iii) If the antigen site density is low or moderate, it may be difficult for two IgG molecules to be properly aligned, however much antibody is available. This may partly explain the poor performance of IgG antibody molecules in complement fixation compared with IgM. (iv) Flexibility at the hinge region is important; the wider the angle at the Y junction, the greater the ability of the IgG antibody to fix complement. (v) A single antibody molecule must be bound to more than one antigen site before complement fixation can occur. This provides another explanation for the poor performance of IgG in complement fixation.

In red cell destruction caused by complement-fixing lytic antibodies, the number of red cells which can be rapidly destroyed is limited only by the amount of antibody and complement available. In ABO-incompatible transfusions there may be no surviving A or B red cells in the circulation within 1 hour of transfusion. However, if antibodies are only weakly or partially able to fix complement (most anti-Jk^a, anti-Kell, anti-Fy^a), red cell destruction will be predominantly extravascular and will proceed more slowly. Anti-Le^a will destroy only a proportion of transfused Le(a+) red cells intravascularly; the remaining cells will have normal survival (see Chapter 9). This explains the two component red cell survival curves seen when labelled Le(a+) cells are injected into subjects with anti-Le^a.

CLINICAL SIGNIFICANCE OF RED CELL ANTIBODIES

The clinical significance of different red cell antibodies depends partly on their destructive capacity and partly on their frequency. For example, anti-Tj^a (anti-PP$_1$P^k) is a very potent haemolysin, but due to its great rarity it is of minimal importance in blood transfusion practice. Alternatively, ABO and RhD antibodies are by far the most significant due to their high frequency and destructive activity.

Several factors influence immune red cell destruction in vivo. These include the following.

a) Plasma concentration and avidity of the antibody.

b) Thermal amplitude of the antibody.

c) Immunoglobulin class and subclass. The complement-fixing ability of most warm-reacting IgM antibodies makes them clinically significant. Of the IgG subclasses, IgG3 has the most practical importance because of its ability to fix complement and its avidity for the Fc receptors of mononuclear phagocytic cells, the effector cells of in vivo extravascular immune red cell destruction.

d) Antibody specificity. Several warm-reacting antibodies are incapable of causing in vivo red cell destruction, e.g. anti-Ch, anti-Rg, anti-Cs^a and most examples of anti-Xg^a and anti-Yt^a.

e) Antigen density on the red cell membrane. The likelihood and degree of sensitization of a red cell with antibody and complement increase with the number of antigen sites on the membrane.

f) Volume of incompatible red cells transfused. A small volume of incompatible red cells will be destroyed more rapidly than a large volume from the same donor. Larger volumes of cells exhaust the circulating antibody available and saturate the reticuloendothelial system (RES). This difference is important in interpreting ^{51}Cr survival tests which employ small volumes of red cells and which therefore might overestimate the destruction of larger volumes.

g) Presence of antigen in donor plasma. Antigens such as Lewis, Chido and Rogers are primarily in plasma and secondarily adsorbed onto red cells. The free antigen in plasma, especially when whole blood is transfused, will react with the antibody and inhibit its binding to red cells. Hence, cross-match-compatible blood unscreened for Lewis is transfused to patients with Lewis antibodies. Furthermore, when Lewis-positive blood is transfused to patients with antibodies, the cells lose their Lewis antigens and become Le(a−b−). For this reason, Lewis antibodies are unable to cause delayed haemolytic transfusion reactions.

h) Activity of RES macrophages. The ability of RES macrophages to remove sensitized red cells varies between individuals. Splenectomy and drugs such as corticosteroids will decrease the clearance of sensitized cells.

i) Sensitivity of red cells to complement. Patients with paroxysmal nocturnal haemoglobinuria (PNH) have red cells which are highly sensitive to lysis by complement activation.

j) Extent of complement activation. Some antibodies are regularly complement binding and others rarely or not at all. Of the complement-binding antibodies, a few (e.g. anti-A, anti-B, anti-Tj^a) will activate the complement cascade through to C9, but for most (e.g. anti-Fy^a, -Jk^a, -Kell) the cascade is interrupted at the C3 stage. Red cells coated with IgG and C3b will be destroyed extravascularly in the liver. As a rule, Rh antibodies do not fix complement.

BLOOD GROUP ANTIGEN–ANTIBODY REACTIONS

In blood group serology the interaction between the antigen sites on the cells and the corresponding antibody is normally detected by observing agglutination of the cells concerned. Agglutination is the result of the cross-linking of individual red cells by antibody molecules and can be thought of as occurring in two stages. The first stage is the fundamental reaction; that is, the combination of the antibody molecules with their specific antigen sites. The second stage is the actual linkage of the individual antibody-coated red cells.

First Stage of Agglutination: Combination of Antibody with Antigen

The combination of antigen with antibody cannot be observed directly, but arises from the fit of the antigen into a structurally complementary site within the antibody molecule. The resulting complex is then stabilized by various short-range forces between the chemical groups of the antigen-binding site in the antibody and the antigen itself. These weak short-range forces include ionic attraction (e.g. between COO^- and NH_3^+), hydrogen bonding (e.g. between –OH, –NH$_2$ and –CO), van der Waals forces and hydrophobic interactions. Individually, these forces are weak; however, when in close apposition, the simultaneous formation of a large number of bonds stabilizes antigen binding. The greater the interface between antigen and antibody, the stronger are the binding forces generated and the greater the affinity of the antibody for its specific antigen.

The association of antigen (Ag) with antibody (Ab) is reversible and obeys the law of mass action, so that, at equilibrium:

$$(Ag) + (Ab) \underset{k_2}{\overset{k_1}{\rightleftharpoons}} (AgAb)$$

where k_1 and k_2 are rate constants of association and dissociation respectively. Hence, at equilibrium:

$$K = \frac{k_1}{k_2} = \frac{(AgAb)}{(Ag)(Ab)}$$

where K is the equilibrium constant for the reaction and reflects the strength of association between antigen and antibody. The greater the value of K, the greater the amount of antigen–antibody complex formed.

Factors Affecting the First Stage of Agglutination

Factors that affect the equilibrium constant include pH, ionic strength and temperature.

pH

Most antibodies are not affected by changes in pH within the range 5.5–8.5. However, this is not true for all antibodies, and in order to make one day's work comparable with the next, routine serology should be carried out with saline buffered to pH 7.0–7.4. Below pH 4 and above pH 9, antigen–antibody complexes are largely dissociated and the antibody can be recovered in the supernatant. This is the basis of some elution techniques.

Ionic Strength of the Medium

In saline of normal ionic strength, the ionized groups of both antigen and antibody are partially neutralized by oppositely charged ions in the medium. By lowering the ionic strength while maintaining tonicity, the ions become exposed and theoretically there should be an increase in attraction. Decreasing the ionic strength increases the rate of association (k_1) of antigen with antibody but has little effect on their rate of dissociation (k_2). For example, a 1000-fold increase in k_1 with a threefold

fall in k_2 has been observed for anti-D by reducing the ionic strength to 0.03 mol/l. Low ionic strength solutions (LISS) containing 0.03 mol/l NaCl in a solution of sodium glycinate are used routinely in many blood banks to increase the speed and sensitivity of pretransfusion tests. Regrettably, LISS can lead to failure in detection of some clinically important antibodies, e.g. some anti-K.

Low ionic strength solutions are also used to coat red cells with complement components via the alternative pathway, e.g. a few drops of fresh whole blood can be taken into 1–2 ml of 10% sucrose, incubated for 10 minutes at 37°C and washed, to provide control cells coated with C3 and C4 for the antiglobulin test. For this reason, the use of LISS under uncontrolled conditions can lead to unwanted positive direct and indirect antiglobulin tests.

The Temperature of the Reaction

The effect of temperature on antigen–antibody reactions includes: (i) an alteration in the equilibrium constant of the antibody, and (ii) an alteration of the rate of encounter. With warm antibodies, the equilibrium constant is not changed by changes in temperature, but decreasing the temperature from 37°C to 4°C slows the rate of reaction twentyfold. With cold antibodies, on the other hand, there is an increase in the equilibrium constant with decreasing temperature, and even though the rate is reduced, stronger reactions and higher titres are found at lower temperatures.

Factors that Affect the Second, or 'Visual', Stage of Agglutination

These include the degree of contact of the antibody-coated red cells with each other, the span of the antibody molecules, the electrical charge of the red cells, the location and density of the antigen sites on the red cells, and the capacity of the antibody to bind complement after reacting with the antigen.

Degree of Contact of Antibody-Coated Cells

It is obvious that the antibody molecules cannot form bridges between individual cells until the cells are close together. This contact can be achieved by allowing the cells to settle by gravity, and full settling does not occur in a saline–serum medium until 1 or 2 hours have elapsed. Settling can always be speeded by centrifugation. However, as red cell drifts mimicking agglutination may be formed, it is best to centrifuge at quite low speeds for not more than 1 minute.

In colloidal medium (e.g. albumin), settling of the red cells occurs after 3–6 hours of incubation of serum and cells. However, if albumin is added to the mixture after centrifugation, incubation times can be reduced to 1 hour; this is the basis of albumin addition techniques.

The Electrical Charge of the Red Cells

Red cells suspended in 9 g/1 NaCl are negatively charged, and because of this charge and the repulsive force that it generates, there is always a gap between individual red cells. The minimum distance of approach of unsensitized cells is approximately 18 nm between their actual membranes. This is considerably greater than the maximum distance between the two valencies of an IgG molecule (12 nm). IgM antibody molecules, with a greater distance (approximately 30 nm) between the antigen-combining sites, are able to bridge this gap and thus cause agglutination of appropriate cells in saline. Conversely, untreated IgG anti-D in saline cannot cross-link two D-positive cells even though some of these antibodies are attached by one arm to the D antigen. Cells coated in this way approach each other to within 6 nm between the Fc ends of the coating IgG. Agglutination of IgG-coated cells can then be brought about by various agents that bring them closer together or by molecules that cross-link coating IgG.

The treatment of cells with proteases (trypsin, papain, bromelin, ficin) or neuraminidase removes negatively charged neuraminic acid from the red cell membrane. Proteases, but not neuraminidase, also remove membrane glycoproteins, thus enabling enzyme-treated cells to come sufficiently close together to allow agglutination by IgG antibodies.

The explanation for agglutination of appropriate red cells by incomplete antibody in albumin media is not well understood. It used to be thought that such media also lowered the effective negative charge of the red cells, or that they increased the dielectric constant of the medium. It is now thought that albumin increases the interfacial tension of red cells thus allowing them to aggregate more easily.

Until recently, it was thought that red cells were kept apart by their zeta potential and that the second stage of agglutination was achieved by factors which affect this potential. The negative charge of the cell surface attracts a cloud of tightly bound counterions and a second layer of more diffuse counterions. The difference in electrostatic potential between the inner and outer limits of this diffuse layer of counterions is the zeta potential. Several authors have produced good evidence to dispute this theory, and it is now not necessary to invoke the zeta potential theory to explain agglutination.

The Span of the Antibody Molecule

As discussed above, the distance between the antigen-binding sites of a single antibody molecule is a critical factor in the second stage of agglutination. The span of an IgG molecule can be increased by mild reduction and alkylation, which opens up the hinge region by cleaving S–S bonds. Therefore IgG antibodies treated in this way can be used as direct saline agglutinins and in effect are available as 'saline' reagents from commercial companies.

The Location and Density of Antigen Sites

The fourth factor that affects the second stage of agglutination is the number of antigen sites on a single red cell and therefore the number of possible sites for antibody combination. IgG anti-A, anti-B, anti-M and anti-N may agglutinate the appropriate red cells in saline; this may be due to the comparatively high number of the corresponding antigen sites (see Chapter 9). For those antigens that protrude from the cell surface (e.g. ABO, MN, Ii), agglutination by the corresponding antibodies will occur more readily than for antigens embedded in the membrane (e.g. Rh).

The number of antigen sites is, for some blood group systems, a reflection of the genotype; *MM* cells will carry twice the number of M antigens as *MN* cells and will be more readily agglutinated by the appropriate antibody (dosage effect). In other systems, e.g. ABO, dosage is not apparent.

The Capacity of the Antibody to Bind Complement

The last factor that affects the second stage of agglutination is the ability of antibody to bind complement after reacting with its antigen. Here it should be remembered that if an antibody binds complement, there may be no agglutination. The simplest explanation for this absence of agglutination is that the added presence of complement molecules, close to the antibody, prevents the antibody molecules from linking up individual cells. This lack of agglutination can be very important. For instance, in grouping or compatibility tests, anti-A and anti-B in patient's fresh serum may cause partial lysis of the red cells and no agglutination of the unlysed cells. If this lysis is not noticed, the test may be read as negative and grossly incompatible blood might be regarded as compatible.

The Use of Enzyme-Treated Red Cells

Several proteases (papain from papaya, trypsin from calf spleen, bromelin from pineapple, ficin from figs) are used under strictly standardized conditions to treat red cells and potentiate agglutination. Since there are no important qualitative differences between these enzymes, the one chosen for routine use is largely a matter of personal preference.

Whether or not enzyme treatment of the red cells enhances agglutination by an antibody depends on the nature of the appropriate antigen. Agglutination by Rh, Lewis, P_1, Kidd, and Ii antibodies is enhanced regardless of whether the antibodies are IgM or IgG. Most examples of anti-Kell are not enhanced with enzyme-treated cells. Some antibodies may no longer agglutinate enzyme-treated cells that carried the relevant antigens before enzyme treatment. These protein antigens, destroyed by proteases, include M, N, S, Fy^a, Ch^a, Rg^a, Pr and Tn (see Chapter 9).

DETECTION OF RED CELL ANTIGEN–ANTIBODY REACTIONS

Manual Methods

There are various ways of detecting antigen–antibody reactions in vitro. The most widely used methods include the following.

Direct Agglutination

Most IgM antibodies will directly agglutinate the appropriate red cells suspended in saline. This method is used routinely for ABO grouping.

Indirect Agglutination

Apart from ABO, antibodies against most blood group antigens are IgG and will not bring about direct agglutination of red cells. However, such antibodies can be detected with the aid of agents that enhance agglutination, e.g. proteases, albumin and other colloids, and aggregating agents such as polybrene. When proteases are used, more reproducible and reliable tests are achieved if the cells are enzyme-treated before incubation with the relevant serum. Although the antiglobulin technique is also an indirect agglutination technique, its importance in blood group serology warrants a separate section.

The Antiglobulin Test or Coombs' test

The antiglobulin test (AGT) is used to detect incomplete antibodies that do not cause direct agglutination of red cells carrying the corresponding antigen when suspended in saline. The technique can be used to test directly, with an antiglobulin reagent, for the presence of immunoglobulins or complement components that have been bound to the red cells in vivo—the direct antiglobulin test (DAGT). Secondly, the test can be used to detect incomplete antibodies in the patient's serum by adding the appropriate test red cells and then, after incubation and thorough washing, testing them for the presence of immunoglobulins or complement components bound to their surface in vitro by adding an antiglobulin reagent. This is the indirect antiglobulin test (IAGT). It is essential for both the DAGT and IAGT that the red cells are washed three to four times with a large volume of saline before adding the antiglobulin reagent, as any free IgG or complement will neutralize the anti-IgG or anti-complement reagent and lead to false negative reactions.

Antiglobulin serum was originally made by injecting animals, usually rabbits, sheep or goats, with human serum. The animal's immune system is able to differentiate very well between the large collection of foreign proteins that make up human serum, and under optimum conditions an animal can make distinct antibodies against a wide variety of serum proteins. Of particular relevance to the antiglobulin test are antibodies against IgG and complement, which should always be present in so-called broad spectrum antiglobulin serum. The anti-IgG component is essential for pretransfusion antibody screening and cross-matching since the vast majority of clinically significant antibodies are IgG. The anti-complement component is needed for the detection of occasional examples of weak complement-binding antibodies (e.g. some anti-Jk[a]) and for the detection of in vivo complement coating of red cells, i.e. in the direct antiglobulin test. Currently, antiglobulin reagents are made in animals by injecting purified or partially purified plasma proteins, and the minimum basic composition of a broad spectrum reagent is a blend of anti-IgG, anti-C3 and anti-C4. Antibodies against IgA and IgM are not necessarily always present in a broad spectrum reagent. Pure anti-IgA and anti-IgM serum can be made by injecting the appropriate purified immunoglobulin and removing any antibody against light chains by absorption.

Most IgM blood group antibodies are complete antibodies and can be detected more readily by direct agglutination. On those occasions when it is desirable to detect subagglutinating amounts of IgM active at 37°C, the lack of anti-IgM in broad spectrum reagents can be offset by the ability of the IgM antibody to fix complement in the presence of fresh serum. Moreover, since only a few molecules of IgM are needed to start the complement sequence and can then lead to the binding of many hundreds of molecules of C3, the agglutination of complement-coated cells by anti-complement sera may be a very sensitive method of detecting IgM antibodies. Of course, complement-fixing IgG antibodies will also be detected with anti-complement sera, but in most cases they can effectively be detected by anti-IgG. However, there are exceptional examples of complement-fixing IgG red cell alloantibodies (e.g. anti-Jk[a]) which are not detectable with anti-IgG, and anti-complement is essential for their identification.

The advent of monoclonal antibody technology has led to the production of excellent antiglobulin reagents, particularly anti-C3d. Although the current standard antiglobulin sera against the four IgG subclasses are polyclonal, monoclonal antibodies are now available and look promising.

Broad spectrum antiglobulin reagents composed of anti-IgG and anti-C3/C4 are perfectly suitable for pretransfusion testing, including the cross-match. However, for those rare cases of autoimmune haemolytic anaemia where IgA or IgM autoantibodies are the only immunoglobulins coating the red cells, it is necessary either to include anti-IgA and anti-IgM in the broad spectrum reagent, or to test separately with these monospecific antisera when the direct antiglobulin test is negative with a conventional broad spectrum reagent.

Standardization of Anti-human Globulin Serum

All currently available antiglobulin reagents, monospecific or broad spectrum, are standardized by the producer and issued prediluted for immediate use.

Antiglobulin reagents standardized for use in haemagglutination tests should not agglutinate red cells after incubation with compatible serum, regardless of their ABO type, i.e. they should be free of unwanted antibodies, especially anti-species. The antiglobulin reagent should not agglutinate washed red cells taken from units of blood intended for transfusion nearing the end of their shelf-life (i.e. 5 weeks in CPD-A or in SAG-M). The final dilution of the anti-IgG component should be sufficient to allow the optimal detection of weak examples of incomplete non-complement-fixing IgG alloantibodies (e.g. anti-D, anti-c) coated onto heterozygous (single antigen dose, e.g. Dd or Cc) target cells. The anticomplement component (namely anti-C3d) should be optimized so that all complement-binding alloantibodies are detected, but not so strong that stored cells, with traces of bound C3d and C4d, react non-specifically. Hence the anti-C3c activity should exceed the activity of anti-C3d as well as the activity of any (non-essential) anti-C4d that might be present.

The exhaustive standardization of raw reagents produced from animals immunized with whole human serum that used to be undertaken is now only of academic interest, especially since modern reagents are either raised by immunizing with purified proteins or are of monoclonal origin. However, when new batches of antiglobulin reagents are acquired by a laboratory, they should be subjected to a minimum standardization with several IgG antibodies of different specificities and several complement-binding antibodies to ensure that all are detectable. Each laboratory should have a battery of sera stored for the purpose of testing new batches of anti-human globulin serum (AHGS). Modern reagents should not have the problem of prozoning, i.e. lack of agglutination of IgG-coated cells due to a marked excess of anti-IgG; a saturating amount of anti-IgG would bind to and completely cover all the coating IgG molecules on the red cells, so that too few IgG sites would be available for cross-linking of red cells by anti-IgG; hence agglutination of IgG-coated cells would not occur. In practice, antiglobulin sera are a blend of several optimally diluted batches of monospecific reagents.

In addition, laboratories should confirm that on each day of use, the AHGS is reacting according to the manufacturer's specifications with control red cells coated weakly with IgG, and the container should be inspected visually for abnormal appearance and cloudiness. The control IgG-coated cells are the same cells that are used routinely in the laboratory to check the validity of negative antiglobulin tests, i.e. the weakly coated cells are added to each tube giving a negative result followed by repeat centrifugation and reading, to confirm that the AHGS in the tube has not been neutralized by residual unbound IgG not removed during washing.

Inhibition of Agglutination

Expected agglutination reactions with known antigens and antibodies can be neutralized by soluble antigens of the appropriate specificity. For example, the saliva of group A secretors inhibits the agglutination of group A cells by anti-A. Hydatid cyst fluid with P_1P^k activity can be used to confirm the specificity of anti-P_1 sera.

Haemolysis

Red cell lysis indicates a positive antigen–antibody reaction mediated by complement-fixing antibodies. A pink or red-coloured supernatant after settling or centrifugation of red cell–antibody mixtures is an indication of red cell lysis.

Absorption and Elution Tests

Specific antibodies can be removed from serum by absorption with red cells carrying the corresponding antigen. Bound antibodies can be subsequently recovered from the washed, sensitized red cells (elution) using organic solvents (e.g. ether, chloroform, xylene), heat treatment, freeze–thaw, low pH, etc.

Specialized Methods

These include radiolabelling and enzyme-linked immunosorbent assays (ELISA) used for the estimation of the number of antigen sites on red cells and when more sensitive antiglobulin techniques are required.

The essence of both approaches is the use of a labelled antiglobulin: for radiometric assays, ^{125}I is usually used to 'tag' the antiglobulin molecules, whereas, in the case of ELISA, enzymes are attached covalently (i.e. conjugated) to the antiglobulin (Fig. 8.6).

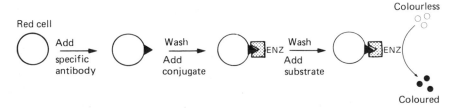

Fig. 8.6. *The ELISA for cell-bound antibodies. The antibody being detected is represented by the solid triangle, and the conjugate by the stippled 'peg' with its covalently attached enzyme (ENZ); substrate is represented by the closed and open circles, for coloured and colourless derivatives respectively.*

The execution of these assays requires antibody-coated cells or particles to be incubated with the labelled antiglobulin reagent. After incubation, excess unbound antiglobulin is washed away, and bound, labelled antiglobulin then measured. For radiometric assays, this is achieved by simply counting radioactivity in a Gamma counter; for ELISA tests, the bound enzyme conjugate is detected through the enzyme's ability to modify its particular substrate. Usually, the modified substrate will change its colour (Fig. 8.6) upon modification, and the colour intensity of the modified substrate can then be accurately assessed using a spectrophotometer.

Automated Techniques

Fully automated blood grouping and antibody screening are carried out in transfusion centres where large numbers of donor samples are tested daily. Machines based on two alternative techniques are available: (i) continuous flow machines, with the disadvantage of carry-over from one sample to another, e.g. Technicon Autogrouper 16C; and (ii) machines based on discrete analysis, where each reaction takes place in individual cuvettes, e.g. Groupamatic models.

Both types of machines are designed to detect agglutination reactions produced on mixing red cells with plasma or reagents. For blood grouping, antisera of known specificity (usually anti-A, -B, -A,B and anti-C + D, -D and -D + E) are used. For antibody screening, plasma from the test samples is mixed with at least one group O cell, usually a Kell positive, R_1R_2 (i.e. *CDe/cDE*) cell, to detect Rh antibodies, as well as one group A_1, A_2 and B rr (i.e. all three *cde/cde* or Rh negative) cell for the detection of ABO agglutinins in the reverse ABO grouping. All four screening cells are enzyme-treated to facilitate sensitive and rapid detection of Rh and ABO antibodies.

In continuous flow machines, each of the above typing sera and screening cells is run in a separate channel consisting of glass coils and plastic tubes, with the test samples being added sequentially to the channels and separated from each other by air bubbles. The length of the coils and the flow rate dictate the length of the incubation time of cells with serum. As the sample mixtures are decanted at the end of the channel, agglutinated red cells are detected photometrically with a laser beam.

In the discrete analysis system of the Groupamatic models, test samples are mixed with typing sera and screening cells in individual plastic cuvettes housed in a disc-shaped holder. This approach minimizes the 'carry-over' between test samples inherent in the Autogrouper approach. After incubation and agitation of the cuvette holder, agglutinates in the bottom of the cuvette can be distinguished from dispersed unagglutinated cells by comparing the transmission of laser light at peripheral and central regions of the cuvette.

The single channel AutoAnalyzer (Technicon), which operates on continuous flow principles, is used for quantitation of anti-D or anti-c, especially in antenatal serology, and for antibody detection. There are several different methods to quantitate the anti-Rh(D) concentration in samples from antenatal patients and immunized volunteers, as well as in plasma pools used for the manufacture of anti-D immunoglobulin. Manual titration, the commonest method, is simple but only provides rough semiquantitative estimates of the concentration of anti-D. Radioisotope methods give more accurate estimates and do not require standards, but their sensitivity is poor and they are too laborious for routine use. On the other hand, quantitative haemagglutination methods using single-channel AutoAnalyzers and appropriate anti-D standards are sensitive (0.02 i.u. anti-D/ml), relatively simple, objective, rapid, of acceptable reproducibility and amenable to routine use and standardization. Reactants are introduced into the system at preselected rates and flow continuously. The mixtures of serial dilutions of serum, Rh(D)-positive cells and other reagents are divided into small segments by air bubbles which reduce the carry-over between samples. The red cells are aggregated non-specifically by a variety of substances (e.g. methylcellulose), enabling anti-D molecules (IgG, IgM, or IgA) to bind to specific D sites on adjacent cells, causing specific immunologic agglutination which is further enhanced if these cells are enzyme treated. The reaction mixtures are then pumped through a series of coils at set temperatures to allow the desired incubation of the segments. A suitable diluent such as citrate is added to break up the non-specific aggregates, leaving the true antibody-mediated agglutinates unaffected. The agglutinates are then sedimented and removed while the remaining un-agglutinated red cells are haemolysed by a detergent. The optical density (OD) of the haemolysate is measured and recorded; the change in OD is proportional to the amount of Hb, and thus inversely proportional to the number of agglutinated cells removed. This means that anti-D sera will cause a reduction in OD, the extent of which will reflect the antibody concentration.

Microtitre Plate Methods

Semi-automated blood grouping and antibody screening can be performed using microtitre plates in those laboratories that are not large enough for cost-effective automation (i.e. less than 80 000–100 000 samples/year). Microplates can also be used for extended phenotyping of red cells, antibody identification, large-scale screening for rare red cells and antibodies, etc. A single microplate is equivalent to 96 short test tubes, and the same basic principles of agglutination apply. The advantages of these techniques include enhanced sensitivity, speed of performance, reduced reagent requirements, simplicity, and reduced requirements for laboratory space and expensive equipment. Plate readers are available that can be linked to computers for easy and accurate record keeping. Fully automated microplate systems are being developed.

Blood Grouping

In order to avoid potential fatalities due to errors in ABO grouping, it is essential that ABO-typing reagents have suitable potency and are standardized appropriately. According to the British Pharmacopaeia, ABO grouping reagents must have a potency at least one-quarter of the appropriate relevant WHO International Standard. In practical terms, this means that anti-A and anti-B reagents should have a minimum titre of 1 in 8 against selected A_2B (i.e. weak A antigen) and A_1B (i.e. weak B) cells respectively; even when diluted 1:8, they should still be capable of giving macroscopic agglutination of 2% red cell suspensions after a 1.5–2-hour incubation. Furthermore, they must be sufficiently avid so as to agglutinate an equal

volume of a 5–10% v/v suspension of the above selected cells within 30 seconds when undiluted reagents and test cells are mixed on a tile. Similarly, anti-A,B should have a titre of at least 1 in 32 against A_2 cells in tube tests; in tile avidity tests, A_x cells must be agglutinated within 2 minutes of mixing. Similarly, anti-D reagents should have adequate potency in order to detect all RhD-positive cells.

Blood-grouping reagents should be free of unwanted antibodies and should have been exhaustively tested with an extensive panel of cells, to exclude common and rare specificities (anti-Bg, anti-Vw, anti-Wr^a etc.), before they are issued for routine use.

Strict adherence to the manufacturers' instructions for each reagent is essential. Standard operational procedures should include: writing out the worksheet prior to testing, labelling all tubes, microplates, slides etc., recording results immediately after reading, repeating discrepancies, using adequate controls.

ABO grouping has an in-built control in the reverse grouping (serum check, see Chapter 9). However, controls for RhD typing must always be used in order to prevent an Rh-negative patient being mistyped as RhD positive. At least two potent anti-D reagents should be used in Rh typing.

Antibody Screening and Identification

Patients' sera should be screened against 2–3 unpooled group O cells from selected individuals known to carry the following antigens between them: D, C, E, c, e, M, N, S, s, P_1, Le^a, Le^b, K, k, Fy^a, Fy^b, Jk^a, Jk^b. Ideally, one cell should be R_1R_1 (*CDe/CDe*) and the other R_2R_2 (*cDE/cDE*); if possible, homozygous expression of Fy^a and Jk^a should be present on one of the cells.

The techniques employed for antibody screening need only include the indirect antiglobulin test (IAT) and the use of enzyme-pretreated cells. Saline tests are not essential. All incubations should be performed at 37°C; antibodies reacting at lower temperatures are of no clinical importance.

It is recommended that an autologous control is used, either as a DAGT or by incubating patient's serum with patient's cells, in the methods used for antibody screening. All tests should follow a standard procedure so that any member of staff can take over and complete a colleague's work if necessary. Blood bankers should not forget that the main aim of blood group serology is to provide hazard-free transfusions.

SELECTED BIBLIOGRAPHY

General

Mollison P. L., Engelfriet C. P., Contreras M. (1987). *Blood transfusion in clinical medicine*, 8th edn. Oxford: Blackwell Scientific Publications.

Immunology

Golub E. S. (1987). *Immunology: a synthesis*. Sunderland, Massachusetts: Sinauer Associates.

Roitt I., Brostoff J., Male D. (1985). *Immunology*. London, New York: Gower Medical.

Roitt I. (1988). *Essential immunology*, 6th edn. Oxford: Blackwell Scientific Publications.

Red Cell Membrane

Anstee D. J., Mawby W. J., Tanner M. J. (1982). Structural variations in human erythrocyte sialoglycoproteins. In *Membranes and transport, a critical review*, pp. 427–433. (Ed. A. Martonossi). New York: Plenum Press.

Marchesi V. T. (1979). Functional proteins of the human red cell membrane. *Seminars in Hematology*, **16**, 3–20.

Schrier S. L. (1985). Red cell membrane biology—introduction. *Clinics in Haematology*, **14**, 1–12.

Singer S., Nicolson G. (1972). The fluid mosaic model of the structure of cell membranes. *Science*, **175**, 720–731.

Complement

Lachmann P. J., Hughes-Jones N. C. (1984). Initiation of complement activation. In *Complement*, pp.147–184 (Ed. H. J. Müller-Eberhard and P. A. Miescher). New York: Springer-Verlag.

Ross G. D. (Ed.) (1986). *Immunobiology of the complement system. An introduction for research and clinical medicine*. London: Academic Press.

Antigen–Antibody Reactions

AABB (1982). *Seminar on antigen–antibody reactions revisited* (Ed. C. A. Bell). Arlington, Virginia: American Association of Blood Banks.

Oss C. J. Van, Absolom D. R. (1984). Haemagglutination and the closest distance of approach of normal, neuraminidase- and papain-treated erythrocytes. *Vox Sanguinis*, **47**, 250–256.

Lectins

Bird G. W. G. (1981). Lectins and polyagglutination. In *Clinical practice of blood transfusion*, pp. 131–147 (Eds. L. D. Petz and S. N. Swisher). New York: Churchill Livingstone.

Chapter 9

ANTIGENS IN HUMAN BLOOD

MARCELA CONTRERAS AND ANATOLE LUBENKO

In this chapter our discussion will centre on red cell antigens and their antibodies, and these will be described under the various blood group systems. However, there are many other antigenic structures in human blood which can stimulate the production of antibodies in recipients of blood transfusions: leucocyte antibodies are an important source of febrile transfusion reactions in patients who have had multiple transfusions; lymphocytotoxic HLA antibodies and, rarely, platelet antibodies may be a cause of failure of the platelet count to rise after platelet transfusions. Thus a short description of leucocyte and platelet antigens will be included. Antibodies against plasma protein antigens may lead to urticarial or anaphylactic transfusion reactions and these will be considered briefly.

There are at least 300 red cell antigens that can be recognized with specific antisera. Many blood group antigens are assigned to blood group systems. Antigens that are the product of alleles at a single locus or at closely linked loci constitute a blood group system. The 16 most important blood group systems are listed in Table 9.1. Each of these systems is inherited quite independently from all the other systems.

THE INHERITANCE OF BLOOD GROUPS

In normal people, the nucleus of all somatic cells contains 46 chromosomes arranged in 23 pairs (22 pairs of autosomes and 1 pair of sex chromosomes). Inherited characteristics such as blood group antigens are controlled by genes which are carried on these chromosomes. Each chromosome of a pair (homologous chromosomes) contains genes which affect the same characters, and these are arranged in a similar order on both chromosomes. In the germ cells, a process of reduction division (meiosis) reduces the chromosomes to 23, so that in the ova and in the spermatozoa there is only one representative chromosome from each pair. This is the haploid state. Fusion of the ovum and the spermatozoon leads to pairing of their chromosomes so that each inherited characteristic in the offspring is controlled by at least two genes, one from the mother and one from the father.

The two genes that control one character can be the same or different. Alternative genes occupying the same locus or site on homologous chromosomes are known as alleles or allelomorphic genes. If the two genes for a character are identical, the person is said to be *homozygous* (e.g. *DD*) for that character. If the two genes are different, the person is said to be *heterozygous* (e.g. *Dd*). In some blood group systems, the red cells of subjects who are homozygous for a given gene (e.g. *MM*) carry more antigen than the cells of those subjects who are heterozygous (e.g. *MN*); this difference in antigen sites can often be detected serologically and is referred to as dosage. The actual genetic make-up of the individual for a specific character is known as the genotype. If the effects of the genes can be observed directly, the resulting observation is known as the phenotype. It is conventional to distinguish genotypes from phenotypes by italicizing *genes* and *genotypes* (e.g. A_1, *CDe*, Fy^a) but not antigens or phenotypes (i.e. A_1, CDe, and Fy^a). With few exceptions, blood group antigens can, after the age of about 2 years, be determined easily and objectively. These antigens remain virtually

Table 9.1

Red cell antigens in humans (adapted from Race and Sanger, 1975)

System	Most important antigens	Approximate number of antigens
ABO	A_1, A_2, B, H*	More than 10
MNSs	M, N, S, s, U	>26
Rhesus	D, C, E, c, e, G	45
Lutheran	Lu^a, Lu^b	17
Kell	K, k, Kp^a, Kp^b, Js^a, Js^b	22
Lewis	Le^a, Le^b	3 or 5
Duffy	Fy^a, Fy^b	5
Kidd	Jk^a, Jk^b	3
Diego	Di^a, Di^b	2
Cartwright	Yt^a, Yt^b	2
Auberger	Au^a, Au^b	1
Dombrock	Do^a, Do^b	2
Colton	Co^a, Co^b	3
Sid	Sd^a	1
Scianna	Sc1, Sc2	2
Xg	Xg^a	1
Indian[†]	In^a, In^b	2
Very frequent or public antigens	Vel, Ge, Lan, JMH	28
Very infrequent or private antigens	Bp^a, Rd, Sw^a, Wr^a	More than 40
Other antigens	P, P_1, P^k	
	I, i	
	Bg (HLA on red cells)	
	Chido, Rg (C4 markers)	
	Kn^a, Cs^a, Yk^a, McC^a	

*H is genetically independent from the system.
[†]Its status as a blood group system is not officially recognized.

Chromosome Mapping and Linkage

Characteristics found to be associated through several generations are considered to be governed by genes within measurable distance of each other on the same chromosome (linkage). The nearer the loci, the closer the linkage. Linked loci at some distance from each other may be separated by crossing-over, which occurs at the first meiotic division. Loci on the same chromosome, regardless of measurable linkage, are syntenic, e.g. *Rh* and *Fy* are syntenic but unlinked on chromosome 1, whereas *Rh* and *Sc* are syntenic and closely linked on chromosome 1. Alleles at loci on different chromosomes or alleles far apart on the same chromosome segregate independently. The terms *cis* and *trans* help to describe the positional relationship of the genes to each other: genes occupying loci on the same chromosome are positioned *cis* to one another, while genes on opposite chromosomes of a pair are positioned *trans* to each other.

During the last 10 years, most blood group systems have been assigned to chromosomes, and the particular location within the chromosome is known for many. The following assignments have been established: *Fy*, *Rh*, *Sc* and *Rd* to chromosome 1; *Jk* and *Co* to chromosome 2; *MNSs* to chromosome 4; *HLA*, *Ch* and *Rg* to chromosome 6; *ABO* to chromosome 9; *Le*, *Lu*, *Se*, *H* and *LW* to chromosome 19 and *Xg* to the X chromosome.

Phenotypes and Genotypes

Blood group antigens are stable characteristics controlled by genes inherited in a simple Mendelian manner. Serological techniques do not test for the presence or absence of a gene itself, but for the gene product. A gene is *expressed* when its product can be observed. Genes expressed only in the homozygous state are recessive. Genes expressed in the heterozygous state in the presence or absence of expression of their allele are dominant. Codominance is the state in which two different alleles are equally expressed; most blood group genes are codominant (e.g. *A* and *B*). Silent genes, or amorphs, are those with no observable expression (e.g. *O*).

Sometimes a particular genotype can be recognized directly from the phenotype, e.g. an MN individual must have the genotype *MN*. Similarly, a group AB individual must have the genotype *AB*. Figure 9.1 depicts the chromosomes carrying the *M* and *N* genes. Either *M* or *N* can occupy each locus. Because there are antisera for both the M and N antigens, the phenotype may be M + N −, M + N + or M − N +. These can be translated into genotypes directly (*MM*, *MN* or *NN*, respectively). In some phenotypes it is not possible to distinguish between two different genotypes; for example, in a group A individual, the distinction cannot be made between the two possible different genotypes *AO* and *AA*. However, the correct genotype can sometimes be determined by suitable family studies, and one such family is shown in Fig. 9.2, where the mother must be *AO* as her first child is group O.

Similarly, in the Rh system, the allele of the gene controlling the D antigen is called *d*. However, *d* is either an amorph or just the absence of D. When *D* is absent from both chromosomes, a subject is said to be *dd*. As with the ABO blood group system, the heterozygote *Dd* can be determined by suitable family studies. On the other hand, it is not difficult to type for the other antigens determined by closely linked Rh genes such as *C* and *c*; *E* and *e*. Then, from the phenotypes, the probable *DD* or *Dd* geno-

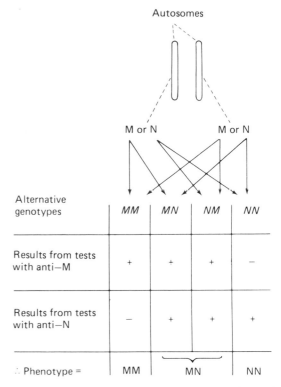

Fig. 9.1. *Diagram showing how two alternative genes at each locus of the chromosome pair can give rise to three possible genotypes. The phenotype is the same as the genotype because the products of each gene can be determined.*

type can be deduced from tables of the frequency of these combinations. To be meaningful, these tables must have been compiled from studies of families within the population under study. For example, if the phenotype of a man is CcDee, his likely genotype will be *CDe/cde*, as this genetic combination is the most frequent one in the English population and hence more frequent than the other possible genotype *cDe/Cde* (see Table 9.10).

Gene Expression, Interactions and Genetic Pathways

Some blood group antigens, if proteins, are the direct products of their genes, e.g. Rh, Kell. Others, especially carbohydrates, e.g. ABO, Lewis, P, result from the action of enzymes (transferases) on the appropriate substrate or precursor substance. These substrates are usually the products of genes

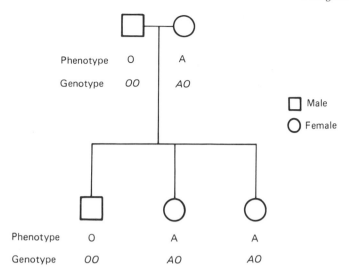

Fig. 9.2. *A family study from which the ABO genotypes of all the family members can be determined.*

located at unlinked loci—e.g. H, the product of the *H* gene (chromosome 19), is the substrate that can be converted to A or B antigens by the action of *A* or *B* transferases (chromosome 9).

If genes coding for the precursor substances are absent, then the final blood group antigen will not be expressed even if the appropriate genes coding for the final product are present, e.g. in the absence of the *H* gene, *A* or *B* cannot be expressed since no substrate is available for the relevant transferases (see Fig. 9.4 for biochemical pathway).

X-linked Inheritance

So far, only one red cell antigen, Xgᵃ, is known which shows X-linked inheritance. The phenotypes are Xg(a+) and Xg(a−). The incidence of Xg(a+), 70% in males and 90% in females, gave the first indication that the gene controlling the Xgᵃ antigen was on the X chromosome. Since normal males have X and Y sex chromosomes and normal females have two X chromosomes, it follows that the inheritance of an X-linked character obeys certain rules. An Xg(a+) man must be hemizygous for *Xgᵃ* since he has only one X. He will pass *Xgᵃ* only to his daughters, who receive his X chromosome, and not to his sons, who receive his Y chromosome. An Xg(a+) woman may be heterozygous or homozygous for *Xgᵃ*. If she is heterozygous, and her

consort is Xg(a−), half the children will by Xg(a+) and half will be Xg(a−).

The inheritance of Factor VIII is also sex linked. In Factor VIII deficiency, a haemophiliac father will pass the abnormal gene on the X chromosome to all his daughters, making them carriers of the disease. However, his sons will not be haemophiliacs provided their mother is not a carrier.

Blood Group Antigens in Problems of Parentage and Identity

Blood groups are almost, but not quite, as individual as fingerprints. Some antigens are not fully developed at birth, and some antigens are peculiar to newborn infants. There are also well-defined differences in the incidence of blood group antigens between people of different races.

In problems of parentage, the determination of blood group antigens can either exclude a putative father or can give an estimate of the likelihood of paternity. Usually it is the paternity that is in dispute and the main principles which govern exclusion from paternity are as follows: firstly, the man is excluded if both he and the mother lack an antigen which is present in the child; and, secondly, the man is excluded if antigens which he must pass on to his offspring are not present in the child.

Paternity tests should always be left to experts who are constantly engaged in this work; they are definitely not the province of the general haematologist. With the large number of genetic markers presently available, including HLA, the likelihood of excluding a wrongly accused male from paternity of a given child is of the order of 98%. With DNA fingerprinting this likelihood reaches 99.9%.

THE ABO SYSTEM

The importance of a blood group system in blood transfusion lies in the frequency of its antibodies and in the possibility that such antibodies will destroy incompatible red cells in vivo. The ABO system was the first to be recognized, and remains the most important. The reason for this is that almost all persons over the age of about 6 months have anti-A and/or anti-B in their serum if they lack the corresponding antigen on their red cells. Thus, if we consider the incidence of ABO blood groups in the UK (Table 9.2), transfusions given without regard to ABO groups would result in incompatibility about once in every three times.

The Antigens of the ABO System

Table 9.2 is compiled from the data of Dobson and Ikin (1946) and ourselves. As shown, the majority of human bloods can be grouped into six main ABO

Table 9.2
Incidence of the ABO groups in the UK

Blood group	Incidence (%) United Kingdom (n = 190, 177)*	Blood group	Incidence (%) Southern England (n = 52 636)†
O	46.68	O	44.94
A	41.72	A$_1$	30.82
		A$_2$	10.27
B	8.56	B	10.14
AB	3.04	A$_1$B	2.64
		A$_2$B	1.19

*Airmen.
†North London blood donors.

phenotypes, although several other rare, weak variants can be distinguished serologically. The incidence of ABO groups varies very markedly in different parts of the world and in different races. Even in a country as small as the United Kingdom there is some variation between north and south, and cities in some areas with a large immigrant population will reflect racial differences. In such areas, the blood groups of the patient population do not necessarily reflect those of the predominantly Caucasian blood donors.

The Subgroups of A

The distinction between the A$_1$ and A$_2$ subgroups is made by using anti-A$_1$, which will agglutinate A$_1$ but not A$_2$ red cells. Anti-A$_1$ can be obtained in several ways. It can be made by absorbing anti-A (from group B people) with A$_2$ red cells; secondly, and more commonly, it can be made from a saline extract of the seeds of the hyacinth bean, *Dolichos biflorus*. Finally, it is found in the serum of some A$_2$ and A$_2$B persons (Table 9.3). Anti-A$_1$ is not used routinely in most laboratories since it is not necessary to distinguish group A$_1$ from group A$_2$ bloods for most recipients.

There is no specific antibody for A$_2$ red cells; if anti-A is absorbed with A$_1$ cells, all the antibody is removed. Group B serum can therefore be thought of as containing two antibodies, anti-A, which agglutinates both A$_1$ and A$_2$ red cells, and anti-A$_1$, which agglutinates only A$_1$ red cells. The anti-A component of group O serum also has both antibodies (Table 9.3).

The presence of the A$_2$ gene cannot be determined by routine serology in the presence of A$_1$, but of people who are genotypically *AO* or *AB*, approximately three possess the A$_1$ gene for every one who possesses A$_2$ (see Table 9.2).

The difference between the A$_1$ and A$_2$ subgroups is partly quantitative: the red cells of A$_1$ and A$_1$B subjects have more A antigen sites than those of A$_2$ and A$_2$B subjects, respectively. There is some evidence that there may be qualitative differences between A$_1$ and A$_2$ cells also: (i) Hakomori and other workers have obtained more polymorphic types of blood group A determinants from A$_1$ red cells than from A$_2$ red cells, and (ii) A$_2$ and A$_2$B people sometimes have anti-A$_1$ in their serum. However,

Table 9.3
ABO grouping

Agglutination of test cells with known				Agglutination by test serum of known			ABO group or phenotype of test sample	Possible genotype
Anti-A	Anti-A₁	Anti-B	Anti-A,B*	A cells	B cells	O cells		
O	O	O	O	+	+	O	O	OO
+	+	O	+	−	+	O†	A₁	A₁A₁, A₁O or A₁A₂
+	O	O	+	−/+§	+	O	A₂	A₂A₂, A₂O
O	O	+	+	+	O	O†	B	BB, BO
+	+	+	+	O	O	O†	A₁B	A₁B
+	O	+	+	−/+§	O	O	A₂B	A₂B

*Anti-A,B (group O serum) is not used routinely in some laboratories
†Occasionally some group A₁ and A₁B individuals may have weak ant -H in their plasma.
§The serum from a proportion of A₂ (1–8%) and A₂B (22–35%) individuals will agglutinate A₁ red cells.

these qualitative differences must be very subtle for there is also evidence that A_2 red cells can absorb out *all* the anti-A from group B serum if the absorption is continued at 0–4°C for a sufficient length of time.

For practical purposes, A_2 can be regarded as a weaker form of A_1. Table 9.4, taken from the work of Economidou *et al.* (1967), shows quantitative differences in the number of A antigen sites on A_1 and A_2 red cells. The same table shows that when both the A and B antigens are present together, there are fewer sites for each than when either is present alone. The practical importance of this lies in the fact that the A antigen of an A_2B person may give an extremely weak reaction with anti-A which is sometimes missed in routine grouping tests. Moreover, if the same person's serum contains anti-A_1 and is tested in the reverse grouping only with A_1 and not A_2 red cells, the person will be grouped as B. This is the commonest technical error in ABO grouping tests, and, apart from using potent anti-A reagents in routine blood grouping, *the serum of all so-called group B bloods should be tested with both A_1 and A_2 red cells.*

The H Antigen

Table 9.3 shows O cells as having no antigens in the ABO system. However, they do possess the H antigen, the precursor upon which the products of the *ABO* genes act. The *H* gene segregates independently from *ABO*. The H antigen is present to some extent on all red cells regardless of the ABO group (except 'Bombay' red cells), but the amount of H antigen varies with the ABO group as follows: $O > A_2 > A_2B > B > A_1 > A_1B$.

'Bombay' Phenotypes

The *H* gene is absent in the Bombay phenotype; such individuals are *hh*. Their red cells are not agglutinated by anti-A or anti-B, but are not group O since they are not agglutinated by anti-H either. The serum of Bombay subjects contains anti-H, anti-A and/or anti-B. In the heterozygous state *Hh*, the *H* gene is dominant and therefore the parents and offspring of Bombay individuals have H and red cells of normal ABO phenotype.

The first 'Bombay' individual was discovered in Bombay in 1952 and a second proposita with an

Table 9.4

Number of A and B antigen sites on red cells of various A and B groups (data from Economidou *et al.* 1967)

Blood group of red cell	Approximate numbers of A antigen sites
A₁ adult	1 000 000
A₁ cord	300 000
A₁B adult	500 000
A₁B cord	220 000
A₂ adult	250 000
A₂ cord	140 000
A₂B adult	120 000

Blood group of red cell	Approximate number of B antigen sites
B adult	700 000
A₂B adult	400 000

extensive pedigree was published by Levine and co-workers in 1955, part of which is shown in Fig. 9.3. Three siblings apparently lacked the A, B and H antigens. However, from their mother and father they could have inherited either *BO* or *OO* genes. The first child of the Bombay proposita gives a clue

to the possible explanation. She is group AB and her father is group A. Her mother must have inherited the *BO* genes, which she was somehow unable to express, but could pass on to her children. It was postulated, therefore, that this affected sibling and presumably her two sisters lacked a gene which controlled a precursor of the A and B antigens and thus her normal *B* gene could not be expressed.

Development of the A, B and H Antigens

The A and B antigens can be detected on the red cells of very young fetuses but their reactions are weaker than those of adult red cells. Table 9.4 shows that the number of A and B antigen sites is less on cord red cells than on adult red cells. Similarly, the H antigen is less well developed at birth than in adult life. After birth, the agglutinability of red cells with anti-A, anti-B and anti-H increases until about 3 years of age, and thereafter, in health, remains stable throughout life.

The Distribution of the A and B Antigens

A and B antigens are not confined to red cells. There is evidence that they are present on white cells,

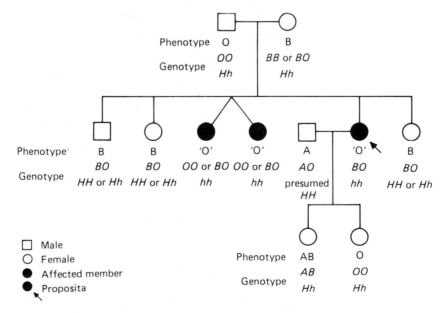

Fig. 9.3. *The pedigree of a family with the 'Bombay' blood group (after P. Levine et al., 1955).*

platelets, epidermal and other tissue cells. They are also present in an alcohol-soluble form in plasma of people of suitable ABO groups whether they are secretors or non-secretors, and in the saliva and secretions of ABH secretors (see below).

Rare ABO Variants

Rare ABO variants are usually disclosed because an expected ABO antibody is missing. Thus, a sample typed as group O that has anti-B but no anti-A will usually prove to be a weak A variant. The presence of weak A or B antigens can be demonstrated either by using potent antisera or by absorption and elution.

Rare ABO variants can arise in three ways.

1. *Rare genetic variants of ABO.*

A_3. This type of blood is recognized by the characteristic mixed field appearance of agglutination with anti-A and most anti-A,B sera; the mixed field consists of small agglutinates in a sea of unagglutinated cells. The cells are not agglutinated by anti-A_1. A similar pattern of agglutination may be seen with blood group chimeras, other mixtures of blood and some phenotypic changes that occur in leukaemia. It has been estimated that A_3 is found about once in every 1000 Danish group A bloods.

A_x. A_x cells are agglutinated weakly or not at all by anti-A but are agglutinated quite strongly by most anti-A,B sera. A_x subjects usually have anti-A_1 but not anti-A in their serum. Saliva from A_x secretors contains H but no A.

There are various other subgroups of A (e.g. A_4, A_5, A_z, A_{el} etc.) but they are all extremely rare in Britain and will not be discussed further.

Similar subgroups of the B antigen have been recognized. The red cells of such subjects are agglutinated weakly or not at all by anti-B and anti-A,B; these are all rare and not as well defined as the A subgroups.

2. *Variants due to the action of other genes.* All these variants are extremely rare. The best known examples are the 'Bombay' bloods. Various independently segregating modifier genes, recessive or dominant, have also been described.

3. *Variants due to the action of the environment.*

Leukaemia. An apparent weakening of the A antigen in persons known to be of the A_1 group and who were suffering from various forms of leukaemia (usually acute myeloid) has been described. The A antigen has been shown to revert to almost normal in some patients in remission. Similar weakenings of B, H, I and D antigens have also been described.

The acquired B antigen. B-like antigens may occasionally be acquired by group A persons suffering from bowel infections. Most of the patients described in the literature had carcinoma or strictures of the large bowel. Red cells with an acquired B antigen are agglutinated by some anti-B but not others; they are not agglutinated by the patient's own anti-B. The antigen arises through the action of bacterial deacetylases which convert the A antigen into galactosamine, which is structurally very similar to the B antigen (galactose, see later).

ANTIBODIES OF THE ABO SYSTEM

Anti-A and Anti-B

Sera taken from people over the age of about 6 months which do not contain the expected A and B antibodies (see Table 9.3) are very rare and they should be thoroughly investigated. The person may have blood of a rare subgroup of A or may be a blood-group chimera, or may have a congenital absence of IgM.

It is likely that the ABO antibodies arise in response to A- and B-like antigens present on bacterial, viral or animal molecules which enter the body in various ways. Titres of ABO antibodies vary considerably depending on the techniques used. Generally, the majority of normal adult sera have saline anti-A titres in the range 32–2048 and anti-B titres in the range 8–512.

Immune anti-A and anti-B can be produced by persons of the appropriate ABO groups after immunization with suitable red cell, or blood group substances. Immune anti-A and anti-B can also arise following the use of various vaccines and inoculations for the prophylaxis of infections. Here, the A-like antigens come from the hog pepsin digest used in their preparation.

Naturally occurring anti-A and anti-B are cold antibodies in that they react better at lower temperatures than at 37°C. There is always some IgM component to the antibody and, in group A and B persons, the antibodies are almost entirely IgM. However, the antibodies from group O persons even before immunization usually have some IgG anti-A,B. After appropriate immunization the thermal characteristics of the antibodies change, but group A and B persons continue to produce antibodies that are mainly of the IgM class, although some IgG is usually made. Most group O persons, however, readily produce IgG as well as IgM anti-A,B. This correlates with the well-known fact that mothers of children with ABO haemolytic disease of the newborn are usually group O. Some IgA anti-A or anti-B is produced following immunization with A or B substances. Table 9.5 shows some of the differences in the serological properties of immune and naturally occurring anti-A and anti-B. The table also gives an indication of ways of detecting IgG anti-A or anti-B in the presence of IgM anti-A or anti-B; this has relevance to ABO haemolytic disease of the newborn, as discussed in Chapter 10.

Dangerous Universal Donors

Good practice in pretransfusion testing requires compatibility testing which consists of incubating the patient's serum with the donor's red cells. Group O red cells will not be agglutinated by the anti-A and anti-B in the serum of group B and A patients. Therefore, group O red cells can be given to A, B or AB recipients and were formerly inappropriately called 'universal donor' red cells.

However, group O donors have anti-A and anti-B in their plasma which will react with the recipient's A or B cells. Normally, if group A, B or AB recipients are transfused with a relatively small number of group O units, and if these contain naturally occurring antibodies only, these antibodies will be diluted out and neutralized by the plasma of adult recipients. However, if the transfused units contain immune antibodies, this neutralization and dilution effect may be insufficient and may lead to a marked destruction of the A or B red cells of the recipient, causing a severe haemolytic transfusion reaction. For this reason the practice of transfusing group O blood to non-O recipients should be strongly discouraged. Moreover, in the UK there is usually a shortage of group O blood, and not infrequently a surplus of group A blood. In the vast majority of cases, including emergencies, there is enough time to do a rapid ABO group on the patient's cells, which will allow the transfusion of group-specific blood. This matter is discussed again in Chapter 10.

Anti-A$_1$

Anti-A$_1$, reactive at room temperature (18–22°C), can be found in the serum of 1–8% group A$_2$ and 22–35% group A$_2$B persons. Most of these antibodies are more of a nuisance in compatibility tests than of clinical importance, for they will not often agglutinate A$_1$ red cells at temperatures of 30°C and above and so are unlikely to result in increased in

Table 9.5
Some properties of immune and naturally occurring anti-A and anti-B

	Naturally occurring	Immune	
	IgM	IgM	IgG
Complement binding (at 37°C)	+ +/+ + +	+ + +	+ +
Agglutination of appropriate cells	+ + +	+ + +	+ + +
Cross the placenta	0	0	+ + +
Enhanced by anti-IgG	0	0	+ + +
Inhibited by A or B substance (e.g. saliva)	+ + +	+ + +	0*
2-ME† or DTT‡ sensitive	+ + +	+ + +	0

*IgG ABO antibodies are inhibited only by large amounts of specific substances.
†Mercaptoethanol.
‡Dithiothreitol.

vivo red cell destruction. Anti-A_1, reactive at 30 °C but not at 37 °C, may lead to some in-vivo destruction of A_1 red cells, but these antibodies are uncommon. Very rarely, anti-A_1 that will still agglutinate A_1 red cells at 37 °C may lead to massive destruction of A_1 red cells in vivo. The appropriate group A_2 or A_2B blood should be crossmatched in these rare instances.

Anti-H

Several forms of anti-H exist.

1. *Clinically significant 'true' anti-H* occurs in the serum of persons with 'Bombay' blood and is very rare. When it does occur it is very important from the point of view of selecting blood for transfusion; since the antibody is active at 37 °C, only 'Bombay' blood can be transfused.

2. *Normal incomplete cold 'antibody'* is present in all normal sera. This is not an immunoglobulin and, as it does not react at temperatures over 12 °C, it is of no importance in selecting blood for transfusion. It binds complement to red cells in vitro at low temperatures and can be detected with anticomplement serum.

3. *Anti-H and anti-HI*, commonly found in the serum of group A_1, B and A_1B persons, give similar patterns of agglutination with adult and cord red cells. Anti-H is inhibited by secretor saliva, and anti-HI is not. Although these antibodies agglutinate O red cells at 20 °C, they do not usually agglutinate them at temperatues above 30 °C. Very occasionally, anti-H/anti-HI are found which will cause rapid destruction of at least some of the transfused O red cells. However, these antibodies will not usually interfere with the survival of transfused cells if A_1, B or A_1B donor units are chosen for A_1, B or A_1B recipients whose serum contains clinically significant anti-H or anti-HI.

ABH SECRETOR STATUS

The majority of the British population are secretors of the appropriate A, B and H substances and have these antigens in all their body fluids. The saliva is normally tested in order to determine secretor status; group A, B or AB individuals who are secretors have the corresponding ABH antigens in their saliva. Approximately 20% of people are non-secretors and lack these antigens in their body fluids regardless of the ABO group on their red cells.

The term secretor applies to the H antigen together with the appropriate A and B antigen, which are present in a water-soluble form in secretions. The gene responsible for secretion, *Se*, can be regarded as an operator gene which causes the H antigen, and as a consequence the appropriate A and B antigens, to be expressed in all body fluids. *Se* is active in homozygotes and heterozygotes and thus non-secretors must be homozygous for the allele, *se*.

BIOCHEMISTRY AND BIOSYNTHESIS OF ABH, LEWIS AND P ANTIGENS

The structure and biosynthetic pathways of ABH, Lewis (Le), and P antigens are intimately related, and the understanding of the genetics and serology of Le and P can be made much easier by first discussing the underlying biochemistry.

ABH Antigens

The structure of the soluble A, B and H antigens is known in some detail because it is easy to obtain them in large quantities from saliva and other body fluids (e.g. ovarian cyst fluid) in a state of relative purity. These soluble antigens have the same basic common structure; the same 15 amino acids make up the protein backbone and the same four sugars form side-chains off this backbone. Thus, the soluble A, B and H antigens are glycoproteins and the differences in the terminal sugars determine the specificity of these three antigens:

a) L-fucose for H,
b) L-fucose + N-acetyl-D-galactosamine for A, and
c) L-fucose + D-galactose for B.

The cellular A, B and H antigens are on glycoproteins and glycolipids. The latter form part of the paragloboside series. Their structure at its simplest (the carbohydrate chains may be more complicated and may branch) is shown in Table 9.6. It can be seen that these structures have the same terminal

Table 9.6

Glycolipids of the red cell membrane with A, B, H, P_1, P and P^k specificity

Structure	Antigen specificity	Chemical name
Paragloboside series		
βGal(1–4)βGlcNAc(1–3)βGal(1–4)Glc-CER	—	Paragloboside
βGal(1–4)βGlcNAc(1–3)βGal(1–4)Glc-CER 2 | 1 α-L-Fuc	H	
αGalNAc(1–3)βGal(1–4)βGlcNAc(1–3)βGal(1–4)Glc-CER 2 | 1 α-L-Fuc	A	
αGal(1–3)βGal(1–4)βGlcNAc(1–3)βGal(1–4)Glc-CER 2 | 1 α-L-Fuc	B	
αGal(1–4)βGal(1–4)βGlcNAc(1–3)βGal(1–4)Glc-CER	P_1	
Globoside series		
βGal(1–4)Glc-CER	—	Lactosylceramide
αGal(1–4)βGal(1–4)Glc-CER	P^k	Trihexoxylceramide
βGal NAc(1–3)αGal(1–4)βGal(1–4)Glc-CER	P	Globoside

Abbreviations: Gal, galactose; GlcNAc, N-acetylglucosamine; Glc, glucose; CER, ceramide; Fuc, fucose, GalNAc, N-acetylgalactosamine.

immunodominant sugars as the carbohydrate chains of the soluble A, B and H glycoproteins. From the biochemistry of the A, B and H antigens, it can be seen that A and B are the same as H but with an additional different sugar molecule each. Hence, the ABO determinants are oligosaccharides synthesized on glycoproteins and glycolipids by specific transferases which are the products of the *ABO* genes. The *O* allele is an amorph not producing an active transferase. Compared with A or B, group O cells have more H, which is the acceptor substrate for *A* and *B* transferases. As illustrated in Fig. 9.4, two types of carbohydrate chain endings serve as acceptors for the *H* fucosyl transferase. Type 1 chains have β-galactose (β-Gal) joined through $1 \rightarrow 3$ linkage to N-acetylglucosamine (GlcNAc). Type 2 chains have a $1 \rightarrow 4$ linkage between these two sugars. *A* and *B* transferases attach α-N-acetylgalactosamine (α-GalNAc) and α-galactose (α-Gal), respectively, by a $1 \rightarrow 3$ linkage to the terminal β-galactosyl residue of Type 1H and Type 2H, thus masking H specificity.

ABH-active carbohydrates can be highly branched structures carrying H, A and/or B specificities on the same molecule. Secretory glycoproteins possess both Type 1 and Type 2 chains, whilst red cells synthesize Type 2 chains only. Plasma glycolipids, passively adsorbed onto the red cells, are assumed to have only Type 1 chains. Lewis antigens are also carried on Type 1 chains.

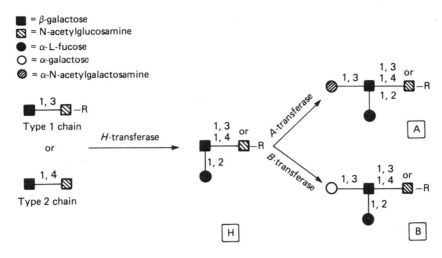

Fig. 9.4. *Biosynthetic pathway of the ABH antigens. (R = rest of molecule.)*

Biochemistry of the Lewis Antigens

The Lewis antigens in saliva and plasma are glycoproteins and glycolipids respectively and are made up of the same basic ingredients as the A, B and H antigens. The terminal fucose molecules that give specificity to H, Le^a and Le^b antigens are shown in Fig. 9.5.

The Le^a antigen arises from the addition of an α-L-fucose in a $1 \rightarrow 4$ linkage to the subterminal N-acetylglucosamine of Type 1 chains by the *Le* transferase. This enzyme cannot use Type 2 chains as acceptors since C4 of N-acetylglucosamine is blocked in such chains. If the *H* transferase (in the presence of *Se*) has already added its fucose to Type 1 chains, the presence of the *Le* transferase leads to the formation of Le^b. Therefore, Le^b is a hybrid antigen of Le^a and H, requiring the presence of *Se*, *H* and *Le* genes (Fig. 9.5). Hence all Le(b+) individuals are secretors. Once Le^a is formed, it cannot serve as acceptor for the *H* transferase. A and B transferases cannot add their corresponding sugars to Le^b structures. Although *ABH* transferases cannot act on chains carrying Lewis specificity, *Le* transferases can use chains with ABH specificities to produce complex antigens such as ALe^b etc.

Biochemistry of the P Groups

The red cells of almost all people have globoside, which forms about 75% of the glycolipid of the membrane and carries the P antigen. In Britain, 79% of these people will also have the P$_1$ antigen, a structure in the paragloboside series of glycolipids. The 21% of people who lack the P$_1$ antigen but have globoside (P) are called P$_2$. Two other very rare phenotypes occur: the first, P^k, lacks globoside and has in its place large amounts of trihexosylceramide; the second, p[Tj(a−)], lacks both globoside and trihexosylceramide. P^k red cells can have the P$_1$ antigen but p red cells cannot (Table 9.6).

Biosynthetic Pathways of ABH, Lewis and P Antigens

As stated above, ABH, Lewis and P specificities are carried on glycosphingolipids, and ABH and Lewis are also carried on glycoproteins. The specificities on glycosphingolipids arise from lactosylceramide (Fig. 9.6). Although the relevant transferases for the P groups have not been isolated, at least two pathways must be involved. The first leads to the synthesis of P$_1$ and the second to P^k and P. It is clear from Fig. 9.6 that P^k and P$_1$ arise from the action of α-galactosyl transferases on different substrates. In contrast, P is produced by the action of a β-GalNAc transferase which uses P^k (CTH) as a substrate. It should also be obvious that *ABH* and *Le* transferases compete for the same precursor substances as the transferases of the P groups (see left arm of Fig. 9.6).

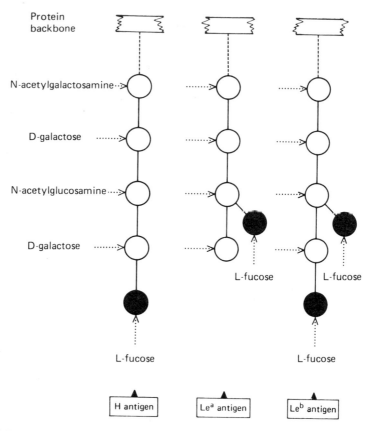

Fig. 9.5. *Diagram of the terminal sugars that give specificity to the soluble H, Le^a and Le^b antigens. Note that the Le and H gene products are both L-fucosyl transferases.*

THE LEWIS SYSTEM

Lewis was the seventh blood group system to be discovered. However, it is discussed here after ABO because the soluble A, B, H, and Lewis antigens are all chemically and biosynthetically related and because the expression of the Lewis antigens on the red cells depends on the presence or absence of the soluble H antigen.

The Antigens of the Lewis System

The Lewis system differs from all other blood group systems. It is primarily a system of soluble antigens, present in secretions (saliva etc.) and plasma; the Lewis antigens on red cells are adsorbed passively from the plasma, and the constant presence of plasma is needed to maintain Lewis on the red cells, which in adults will be Le(a+b−), Le(a−b+) or Le(a−b−).

The *Le* gene codes for the expression of Lewis and has a silent allele *le*. As discussed above, although *Le* and *Se* are inherited independently, Lewis phenotypes are affected by the ABH secretor status, and the expression of the Le^b antigen requires the presence of both *Le* and *Se* genes (see p. 241 and Table 9.7). An individual who inherits the gene *Le* will be Le(a+b−) if he is a non-secretor (*sese*). An individual who inherits *Le* will be Le(a−b+) if he is a secretor (*SeSe* or *Sese*). An individual who is *lele* will be Le(a−b−) regardless of secretor status. In Whites, the frequencies are approximately 20% Le(a+b−), 75% Le (a−b+) and 5% Le(a−b−).

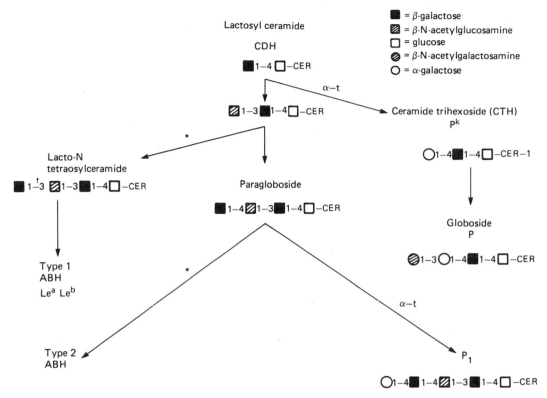

Fig. 9.6. *Biochemical pathways for the formation of ABH, Lewis, P_1, P^k and P on Type 1 and 2 chains in glycolipids. CER, ceramide; α–t, α–galactosyl-transferase; for abbreviations see text and Table 9.14. *For details of these pathways see Fig. 9.4. †Type 1 chain (1–3 linkage). ‡Type 2 chain (1–4 linkage).*

If saliva and serum or plasma are examined for the presence of Lewis and ABH antigens, one of four results will be found as illustrated in Table 9.7, which shows the relationship between ABH secretion and the presence or absence of Lewis antigens.

The Relationship between the Lewis Antigens on the Red Cells and Secretor Status

The secretor status of an individual is determined by his or her ability to secrete ABH antigens in saliva and other body fluids. From Table 9.7, it can be seen that all persons whose red cells group as Le(a−b+) have the H antigen in their saliva and are therefore ABH secretors. However, although the vast majority of people who are secretors have red cells which group as Le(a−b+), a minority of ABH secretors will group as Le(a−b−) if they are

lele. Similarly, all persons whose red cells group as Le(a+b−) are non-secretors but not all non-secretors have red cells which group as Le(a+b−): the red cells of those non-secretors whose genotype is *lele,* group as Le(a−b−).

Adsorption of the Lewis Substances onto Red Cells

Sneath and Sneath (1955) suggested that the Lewis antigens on the red cells were simply adsorbed from the plasma. They showed that Le(a+b−) and Le (a−b+) red cells after incubation in vitro in Le(a−b+) and Le(a+b−) plasma respectively, reacted as Le(a+b+). Moreover, Le(a+b−) and Le(a−b+) red cells incubated in Le(a−b−) plasma lost their Lewis antigens into the plasma. Similarly, in transfusion practice, if Le(a+b−) or Le(a−b+) blood is transfused to an Le(a−b−) person, the transfused

Table 9.7

The Lewis system and secretion of ABH

Genotype		Saliva Le^a	Le^b	ABH	Serum Le^a	Le^b
SeSe or *Sese*	*LeLe* or *Lele*	+	+ +	+ +	(+)	+ +
SeSe or *Sese*	*le/le*	−	−	+ +	−	−
sese	*Lele* or *Lele*	+ + +	−	−	+ +	−
sese	*lele*	−	−	−	−	−

red cells will gradually lose the Le^a or Le^b antigens and will group as Le(a−b−) within a week of transfusion.

Development of Lewis Antigens on the Red Cells

At birth, the Lewis antigens are poorly developed and cord blood specimens usually group as Le(a−b−). Thereafter, there is a gradual development of Lewis antigens starting with Le^a and followed by Le^b. Tests on young children may be confusing because many may group as Le(a+b+) and it seems that all children possessing the *Le* gene at some time express the Le^a antigen on their cells even though most will eventually group as Le(a−b+). The definitive adult Lewis phenotype may not be reached until the age of 4–5 years.

The Antibodies of the Lewis System

Anti-Le^a occurs fairly frequently, although only 5% of the British population lack the *Le* gene and can therefore make this antibody. From one careful study in Denmark, it was calculated that 1% of the population (or 20% of the people potentially able to make anti-Le^a) did, in fact, make the antibody. In Negroes the incidence of *lele* is very much higher. In

Nigeria, where about 30–40% of the population group as Le(a−b−), Lewis antibodies active at 22 °C or above are found in about 10% of random sera.

Anti-Le^b commonly accompanies anti-Le^a. Pure anti-Le^b is rather uncommon; it is made by people who are non-secretors of the H antigen and whose red cells group as Le(a−b−). Very rarely, it can be made by people whose red cells group as Le(a+b−). Anti-Le^b occurs in two forms: as the more common anti-Le^{bH}, which is inhibited by secretor saliva (i.e. saliva that contains the H antigen) and only agglutinates specifically A_2 Le(b+) and O Le(b+) red cells; and as anti-Le^{bL}, which is inhibited only by saliva that contains the Le^b antigen and agglutinates all Le(b+) cells regardless of their ABO groups. Anti-Le^{bL} is the antibody that should be used as a typing reagent.

Serological Characteristics of Lewis Antibodies

Lewis antibodies are almost always predominantly IgM, even after deliberate stimulation with Lewis substances. These antibodies usually agglutinate the appropriate cells at 20 °C. The agglutination is rather fragile and it may be necessary to add EDTA to the serum (to prevent complement binding) or to centrifuge the cell–serum mixture to enhance agglutination. The agglutination has a characteristic appearance: the red cell clumps are often joined by strings of single red cells, like beads in a necklace.

All Lewis antibodies bind complement and will sometimes lyse the appropriate cells directly. More often, they will lyse these cells only after treatment with enzymes. Usually, the antibody does not agglutinate red cells of appropriate Lewis groups in a saline medium at 37°C, but can be detected at this temperature by the indirect antiglobulin test using anti-complement. Apart from being haemolytic, Lewis antibodies can be lymphocytotoxic and can contribute to renal graft rejection.

Clinical Significance of Lewis Antibodies

Lewis antibodies are the commonest single cause of positive results in pretransfusion antibody screening tests. They occur without obvious stimulation by transfusion or pregnancies, and so can be found the first time a serum is tested. Most of these antibodies, even though they give positive results by the indirect antiglobulin test, would cause little or no destruction of crossmatch-incompatible blood if transfused. However, occasionally anti-Le^a (but not anti-Le^b) can cause severe transfusion reactions with haemoglobinaemia and haemoglobinuria. The strength of Lewis antibodies is clinically important: Lewis antigens in the plasma of 'incompatible' blood will completely neutralize antibody of low titre.

In routine practice, a patient possessing anti-Le^a which gives positive results at 37°C with units of blood of the same ABO group should be given Le(a−) blood. However, anti-Le^b very seldom reacts at 37°C with ABO-identical blood. It is therefore recommended that ABO-compatible blood untyped for Le^b be crossmatched for patients with anti-Le^b. On those extremely rare occasions when anti-Le^a is accompanied by anti-Le^b which also gives positive results at 37°C, it may be very difficult to obtain the necessary Le(a−b−) blood in sufficient quantities. In those cases, in the absence of Le(a−b−) blood, whole blood should be given, or the plasma from the respective donations should be given beforehand in order to neutralize the antibodies and enable potentially incompatible blood to be transfused. Alternatively, plasma from ABH secretors can be given before the blood transfusion. By the time the antibodies reappear, the transfused blood will have lost the original Lewis antigens and will have developed the same Lewis group as the recipient, i.e. Le(a−b−).

Lewis antibodies do not cause haemolytic disease of the newborn: firstly, because they are almost always IgM and, secondly, newborn infants group as Le(a−b−).

P BLOOD GROUPS

The P groups were discovered by Landsteiner and Levine in 1927 using suitably absorbed sera of rabbits injected with human red cells. About 75% of subjects tested were positive for the character, now called P_1, which is inherited as a Mendelian dominant. P_1 frequency varies in different populations, and P_1 negatives are called P_2. The system has been expanded to include five phenotypes (see Table 9.8).

Table 9.8
The P groups (after Race and Sanger, 1975)

Phenotype	Antigens on red cells	Antibodies in serum	Approximate European frequency (%)
P_1	P_1, P (P^k)*	None	79
P_2	P (P^k)*	Often anti-P_1	21
P_1^k	P_1, P^k	Anti-P	⎫
P_2^k	P^k	Anti-P	⎬ Very rare
p [Tj(a−)]	None	Anti-PP$_1$P^k	⎭

*P^k has been detected on P_1 and P_2 cells.

The P_1 antigen is weakly expressed at birth and its strength varies considerably in adults. For this reason, identification of anti-P_1 can be difficult as panel cells will have varying expression of this antigen.

The biochemistry of P_1, P and P^k has shown that they are not the products of alleles at a single locus (Fig. 9.6). Antigens of the P system have been detected on other cells: P_1 and P on fibroblasts and lymphocytes and P^k on fibroblasts.

In all P^k, all p and a proportion of P_2 subjects, the appropriate antibodies seem to be present whenever the antigen is absent (see Table 9.8). Anti-P_1 is a common naturally occurring antibody, but, unlike anti-A and anti-B, it rarely causes transfusion reactions since it is usually a cold IgM antibody, not often reacting at temperatures above 30°C. Potent anti-P_1 can be found in patients with fascioliasis or with hydatid disease, and, like anti-P^k, can be inhibited by hydatid cyst fluid (a useful tool for confirmation of such antibodies). Anti-P and anti-PP_1P^k, which occur in the sera of the rare people who are P^k and p respectively, are usually strong IgM plus IgG antibodies and are often lytic at 37°C. These antibodies cause severe haemolytic reactions if blood of the appropriate P group is not transfused. The IgG component of anti-PP_1P^k is IgG3 and has been associated with early abortion in p women. Anti-PP_1P^k has caused haemolytic disease of the newborn (HDN).

The Donath–Landsteiner antibody is found in patients suffering from paroxysmal cold haemoglobinuria. It usually has anti-P specificity and reacts with all cells except the rare P^k and p. Unlike the other antibodies in the P groups, it is always IgG and is, of course, an autoantibody (see also Chapter 7).

THE Ii ANTIGENS

The Ii groups are difficult to understand since the antigen I cannot be regarded as being controlled by a gene allelic to that controlling i: when a person is said to be of the i group, the red cells will still be agglutinated to some extent by anti-I. It might be more helpful to think of I and i as both occurring on all cells, with sometimes the I antigen and other times the i antigen more available for agglutination with the appropriate antisera.

The red cells from almost all adults are agglutinated strongly and to a high titre by most I antibodies and only relatively weakly by most i antibodies; such red cells are called 'adult I'. The red cells from cord blood samples give the opposite results with these two antisera and are called 'cord i'. As the child matures, the agglutinability of its red cells with anti-I increases and with anti-i decreases, so that at about 18 months of age they give the expected reactions of adult cells. Very rarely, some adults will be found whose red cells react extremely weakly with anti-I and strongly with anti-i; such cells are called 'adult i'. This phenotype is inherited.

In many haematological disorders with a high proportion of reticulocytes and young red cells (thalassaemia, megaloblastic anaemia, sideroblastic anaemia, hereditary spherocytosis, paroxysmal nocturnal haemoglobinuria, some aplastic and dyshaemopoietic anaemias, etc.), the agglutinability of the patient's red cells by anti-i is increased without a reciprocal decrease in the agglutinability by anti-I.

Anti-I and anti-i recognize various structures that constitute the inner portions of the ABH-active carbohydrate chains. These antibodies react optimally when the ABH determinants are removed. In view of the chemical structure of Ii, some anti-I and anti-i cross-react with ABH and P antigens (anti-AI, anti-BI, anti-HI, anti-P_1I).

The Ii antigens are present on neutrophils and lymphocytes and are also widely distributed on the cells of other animals.

Anti-I

Anti-I, as a cold autoagglutinin with a titre of 16–32 at 4°C and an upper limit of activity at about 15°C, occurs in almost all normal adults and 60% of cord blood samples. Most adult i have alloanti-I in their serum and in these people the thermal range may extend up to about 30°C.

An increase in the thermal range of autoanti-I, so that there is agglutination of the patient's own and other adult ABO-compatible red cells at 20°C, is not uncommon and occurs in a variety of disorders and after blood transfusions. In these patients the direct antiglobulin test is negative and the antibodies do not react at 30°C or above. A transient increase in strength, titre and thermal range of anti-I regularly occurs after infections with *Mycoplasma pneumoniae* and perhaps other organisms causing atypical pneumonia, and occasionally leads to the development of acute haemolysis; such patients have a positive direct antiglobulin test.

Patients suffering from chronic cold haemagglutinin disease also give a positive direct antiglobulin test. The autoantibody nearly always has anti-I specificity (see also Chapter 7) and is monoclonal, whereas other examples of anti-I are usually polyclonal. All anti-I are IgM and complement binding. Their reactions are enhanced by using enzymes or albumin techniques.

Anti-i

Anti-i is found transitorily in the serum of many patients suffering from infectious mononucleosis. Very occasionally, the titre and thermal range of this antibody may be sufficient to lead to the development of acute haemolysis, particularly if the patient's red cells are for any reason more agglutinable than normal with anti-i. These patients have a positive direct antiglobulin test. Autoanti-i is only found in pathological conditions and may occasionally be the antibody specificity in chronic cold haemagglutinin disease. Patients with this type of antibody often have an underlying reticulosis. Anti-i has the same properties as anti-I.

Changes of ABH, Lewis and I in Malignancy

Gastrointestinal adenocarcinoma can lead to loss of A and B antigens through loss of the corresponding transferases; this is sometimes accompanied by increase in H, Le^b, I and i. Aberrant expression of A in group O or B patients is likely to be due to the A-like, cross-reactive Forssman antigen. In haematological malignancy, changes in ABH expression are caused by depression or loss of *H* transferases in haemopoietic tissue.

THE Rh SYSTEM

The Rh (from Rhesus) blood group system was the fourth system to be discovered, yet it is the second most important in blood transfusion. This is not because Rh antibodies, as in ABO, are present when the Rh antigen is absent, but because RhD antibodies are formed readily when RhD-positive blood is transfused to an Rh-negative person. Moreover, since these immune antibodies are normally IgG, they are able to cross the placental barrier and lead to haemolytic disease of the newborn (HDN).

In 1939, Levine and Stetson reported that an antibody was present in the serum of a patient after a severe reaction to transfusion of her husband's blood. This antibody agglutinated the red cells of 85% of ABO-compatible donors. In 1940, Landsteiner and Wiener reported that by injecting guinea-pigs and rabbits with Rhesus monkey red cells, they had made an antibody that not only agglutinated Rhesus monkey red cells but also the red cells of 85% of people of European origin. These two antibodies were originally thought to be the same, and the human antibody was therefore called Rhesus. Many years later, it was realized that the human antibody (now called anti-Rh$_0$ or anti-D) did not identify the same antigen as the rabbit and guinea-pig rhesus antibody. It was by then too late to change the name of the whole system, so Levine suggested that the antigen defined by the original Rhesus antibody be called LW in honour of Landsteiner and Wiener, and the antibody anti-LW.

The Antigens of the Rh System

RhD, due to its high immunogenicity, is by far the most important Rh antigen. This is due to the ability of anti-D to cause severe HDN and haemolytic transfusion reactions.

The Rh System in Terms of Rh Positive and Rh Negative

For most clinical purposes, individuals can be classified as those who are Rh positive (have the D antigen) and those who are Rh negative (lack the D antigen).

The Expansion to Include Cc and Ee

In 1941, it was realized that the Rh groups could not be explained by only one antigen and its alternative.

By the end of 1943, four antisera were available, and Fisher, studying tables of their reactions, noticed that two of them appeared to give antithetical results. He proposed that the antigens recognized by these two antisera, and therefore the genes controlling them, were allelic and he called them C and c. He gave further letters, D (the original Rh antigen) and E, to the antigens recognized by the other two antisera and postulated that each had an alternative which he called d and e respectively. Thus, the Rh antigens were envisioned as being controlled by three closely linked genes on each homologous chromosome, and it was predicted that the Rh gene complex of one chromosome could be made up in eight different combinations or haplotypes, i.e. *cDe, cde, CDE, CdE, cDE, cdE, CDe* or *Cde*. Rh has now been assigned to chromosome 1, and the order of the genes is thought to be *DCE* because of the relative frequency of the eight different haplotypes, and because of the existence of antigens such as G, which links C with D, and compound antigens such as Ce, ce, etc., which link C with E.

Fisher's postulated anti-e was discovered in 1945. However, anti-d was never found, and d is thought of as the absence of D rather than an antigen capable of stimulating antibodies. All eight Rh haplotypes have now been found and other Rh antigens have also been discovered, e.g. C^w determined by an allele of *C* and *c*.

In contrast to Fisher, Wiener postulated that the Rh antigens are determined by allelic genes at a single locus rather than three genes, however closely linked, e.g. R^1 rather than *CDe*. In practice, most workers in England use the CDE nomenclature for writing and the Wiener shorthand nomenclature for speaking (Table 9.9). In the shorthand nomenclature, R stands for the presence of D and r for its absence.

The approximate incidence of the Rh gene complexes in this country, taken from Race and Sanger (1975), is shown in Table 9.9. It will be seen that the first three complexes form 94% of the total and so combinations of these three will give the commonest genotypes. These are shown in Table 9.10. Genotype frequencies vary considerably in different parts of the world. For instance, *rr* varies from about 35% in the Basques to 0% in Japanese and Chinese.

Table 9.9

The incidence of the Rh gene complexes in the British population

Nomenclature		Approximate incidence
CDE	Wiener	(%)
CDe	R^1	41
cde	r	39
cDE	R^2	14
cDe	R^0	3
C^wDe	R^{1w}	1
cdE	r''	1
Cde	r'	1
CDE	R^Z	Very rare
CdE	r^y	

Table 9.10

Commonest Rhesus genotypes in the British population

Nomenclature CDE	Wiener	Approximate incidence (%)
CDe/cde	R^1r	31
CDe/CDe	R^1R^1	16
cde/cde	rr	15
CDe/cDE	R^1R^2	13
cDE/cde	R^2r	13
cDE/cDE	R^2R^2	3

Determination of the Probable Rh Genotype

It was mentioned on page 232 that if a person's Rh phenotype was known, the probable genotype could be discerned and its likelihood calculated from tables of genotype frequencies within the same population. In people of European origin, the phenotype is usually determined initially with anti-D, anti-C, anti-E and anti-c. If there is no agglutination with anti-E, the phenotype is assumed to be ee. If there is agglutination with anti-E, anti-e is used to distinguish between EE and Ee. The phenotype determinations and the genotypes that they most commonly represent are shown in Table 9.11. The incidence of these genotypes in unselected persons and fathers of children with Rh haemolytic disease

Table 9.11

Determining the Rh genotype in the British population

Reactions with					Rh phenotype	Common alternative genotypes	Rh genotype incidence (%) in	
Anti-C	Anti-c	Anti-D	Anti-E	Anti-e			Unselected persons	Father of infants with Rh HDN
+	+	+	−		CcDee	*CDe/cde* *CDe/cDe*	94 6	79 21
+	−	+	−		CCDee	*CDe/CDe* *CDe/Cde*	96 4	99 1
−	+	+	+	+	ccDEe	*cDE/cde* *cDE/cDe*	94 6	79 21
−	+	+	+	−	ccDEE	*cDE/cDE* *cDE/cdE*	86 14	96 4
+	+	+	+	+	CcDEe	*CDe/cDE* { *CDE/cde* *cDE/Cde* *CDe/cdE* *CDE/cDe*	90 10	97 3

of the newborn is also shown. When these determinations are done, it is very important that the ethnic origin of the person is known; figures for one population will not apply to people of other populations.

Variations in Antigen Strength and Site Density with Phenotype

In most blood group systems, the red cells of a person who is homozygous at the loci controlling a red cell antigen will react more strongly with the appropriate antisera than the red cells of a person who is heterozygous at the same loci. Thus the red cells of persons who are homozygous for the gene controlling the C antigen, i.e. genotypically *C/C*, give stronger reactions with anti-C than the red cells of persons who are heterozygous for the same gene, i.e. genotypically *C/c*. Similarly, this dosage effect occurs with the c, E and e antigens, but is only partly true for D. Table 9.12, taken from the work of Rochna and Hughes-Jones (1965), shows the number of D antigen sites on red cells of different phenotypes as estimated by using ^{125}I-labelled anti-IgG to quantitate bound IgG anti-D. The number of antigen sites for E, c and e has also been estimated, and there are more c than D sites per red cell.

Other Rh Antigens and Phenotypes

The C^w Antigen

This is a rare antigen occurring in about 2% of Whites. The specific antibody, anti-C^w, either occurs together with anti-C or, more rarely, alone. Like most Rh antibodies, anti-C^w can cause haemolytic transfusion reactions and haemolytic disease of the newborn.

The G Antigen

This occurs in all people who have C and almost all who have D. Very rarely, persons can be found with the D antigen but lacking G and, equally rarely, the converse may occur (r^G). Anti-G usually occurs with anti-D (see page 253) and it is essential that anti-D typing reagents do not contain anti-G, which may lead to mistyping of Cde/cde (r′r) women of child-bearing age as D positive.

D^u

This is a weak form of D and therefore cells that type as D^u should, to all intents and purposes, be regarded as D positive. D^u cells have fewer D sites per red cell than normal D-positive cells. There are different grades of D^u and high-grade D^u can occasionally stimulate the production of anti-D when whole units of blood are transfused to D-negative subjects. In Britain, D^u is commonly accompanied by the C or E antigen, and the gene complex cD^{u}e (R_o^u) is rare. In some populations, for instance Nigerians, 8% of those typed as Rh negative are, in fact, D^u. It is therefore essential that modern typing reagents detect most of the weak forms of D in routine grouping.

Numerous laboratories spend a great deal of time and effort on elaborate tests to detect D^u and few have questioned the rational basis of these tests. The consequences of mistyping a low-grade D^u as D negative are minimal: (i) if the blood is from a donor and it is transfused to a negative recipient, no anti-D is formed due to the poor immunogenicity of low-grade D^u; (ii) if D^u blood is given to a recipient with preformed anti-D, slight haemolysis is a possibility; (iii) if the recipient's red cells are misclassified as D negative, Rh-negative blood will be wasted with no harm to the recipient; (iv) misclassification in pregnant women will lead to unnecessary but harmless use of anti-Rh(D) immunoglobulin; (v) if a newborn is mistyped, the mother will not be given the required anti-D prophylaxis although sensitization is unlikely and there are only anecdotal cases of

Table 9.12
Variation in number of antigen sites with different Rh phenotypes (data from Rochna and Hughes-Jones, 1965)

Rh phenotype	Most probable genotype	Number of D antigen sites
CcDee	CDe/cde	9 900–14 600
ccDee	cDe/cde	12 000–20 000
ccDEe	cDE/cde	14 000–16 000
CCDee	CDe/CDe	14 500–19 300
CcDEe	CDe/cDE	23 000–31 000
ccDEE	cDE/cDE	15 800–33 300

maternal sensitization due to pregnancy with D^u children.

Points in favour of abolishing D^u tests or D typing by the indirect antiglobulin technique altogether are: (i) they may lead to the dangerous misclassification of a D-negative recipient as D positive; (ii) the D^u test does *not* detect all examples of D^u; up to 15% of D^u samples (very low grade) may be missed by IAGT.

Elevated D

Certain Rh phenotypes can give strong agglutination reactions with incomplete anti-D when cells are suspended in saline, e.g. $-D-/-D-$ cells and Rh-positive En(a−) cells.

D Variants

It is generally assumed that the D antigen is a mosaic of several epitopes, and that the majority of Rh-positive individuals have normal D antigens with all epitopes present. Very occasionally, persons who have an apparently normal or a weak D antigen (D^u) will make anti-D after stimulation with foreign D-positive red cells. This anti-D does not agglutinate their own red cells and these people can be regarded as having a part or an epitope of the normal D antigen missing completely. Such phenotypes are called D variants or D categories. In D^u variants, the remaining epitopes of the D mosaic are often weakly expressed, and since most anti-D reagents contain antibodies against all parts of the D antigen, such variants will be difficult to distinguish from persons with a normal D^u antigen (i.e. with all epitopes of D but in smaller quantities). Occasionally, the red cells of D variants and D^u variants will give negative results by the indirect antiglobulin test with otherwise potent and specific incomplete anti-D sera. On the other hand, normal D^u cells will be agglutinated by all incomplete anti-D by IAGT. The classification of D variants can only be made by reference laboratories.

Table 9.13

Nomenclature of the Rh antigens

Numerical	CDE	Wiener	Numerical	CDE	Wiener
Rh 1	D	Rh_0	Rh 23	Wiel, D^W	
2	C	rh′	24	E^T	
3	E	rh″	25	LW	
4	c	hr′	26	'Deal', c-like	
5	e	hr″	27	cE	
6	f, ce	hr	28	—	hr^H
7	Ce	rh_i	29	'Total Rh'	
8	C^W	rh^{W1}	30	Go^a	
9	C^X	rh^X	31	—	hr^B
10	V, ce^s	hr^V	32	$\bar{R}^N$	
11	E^W	rh^{w2}	33	R_0^{Har}	
12	G	rh^G	34	Bas	
13	} D variants {	Rh^A	35	$\bar{R}^N$-like (1114)	
14		Rh^B	36	Be^a	
15		Rh^C	37	Evans	
16		Rh^D	38	Duclos	
17	—	Hr_0	39	C-like autoantibody	
18	—	Hr	40	Tar	
19	—	hr^s	41	Ce-like	
20	VS, e^s		42	Ce^s, hr^H-like	
21	C^G		43	Crawford	
22	CE		44	Nou	
			45	Riv	

Variants of the e Antigen

These are common in Negroes, amongst whom the whole Rh system shows many rare alleles when compared with Europeans.

Compound Antigens

There are many other Rh antigens, particularly those that are the products of two theoretically separable genes, for example *ce* (*f*), *Ce*, etc., and antibodies against these compound antigens are known. Table 9.13 gives some idea of the complexity of the Rh system and shows the latest nomenclature in which the various antigens are just given as numbers to facilitate computerization (Rosenfield *et al.*, 1962), as well as the CDE and Wiener notation.

The LW Antigen

LW is the antigen that was detected by the original animal anti-Rhesus monkey serum of Landsteiner and Wiener. It is associated with the D antigen, at least in adults, because the original anti-Rhesus serum (now called anti-LW) would, after suitable absorption and elution, distinguish between D-positive and D-negative adults. However, it is not the same as D because the animal anti-Rhesus serum will not distinguish D-positive from D-negative cord blood. Moreover, persons who type as D positive may become transiently LW negative and, when transfused or pregnant, may make anti-LW. However, only people whose red cells group as Rh_{null} lack LW antigens completely (see below). LW is polymorphic and the *LW* genes (the common *LW^a* and rare *LW^b*) are inherited independently of *Rh*.

Rh_{null} Cells

Rh_{null} cells lack all CDE and LW antigens. Rh_{null} cells may give false negative results with anti-S, anti-s and anti-U by IAGT. Rh_{null} subjects suffer from a chronic compensated haemolytic stomatocytic anaemia of varying degrees of severity. Their red cells may show increased agglutinability with anti-i and have increased osmotic fragility. Rh_{null} cells have been shown to lack two membrane proteins: the

Rh(D) polypeptide, a transmembrane protein attached to the cytoskeleton, and another polypeptide found in all normal red cells irrespective of RhD status.

There are two ways in which the Rh_{null} phenotype can be inherited. In the first, the amorph type

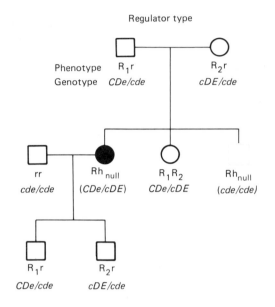

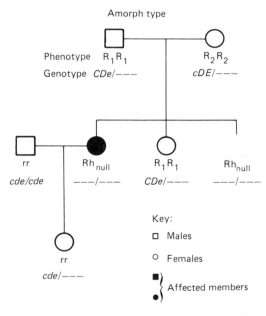

Fig. 9.7. *Family trees showing the modes of inheritance for the two types of Rh_{null}. In the regulator type Rh_{null}, the genes are present, as shown in brackets, but not expressed.*

(the rarer of the two), both parents possess only half the expected number and quantity of Rh antigens and therefore have an amorphic gene complex $(- - -)$ at one locus controlling the CDE antigens. The Rh_{null} phenotype results when the offspring are homozygous for these amorphic genes $(- - -/- - -)$ and, provided the spouse of an Rh_{null} person has normal Rh antigens, their offspring will again have half the number of functional Rh genes (Fig. 9.7). In the second, the regulator type, both parents have two normal Rh haplotypes (although they may or may not be weaker than normal) and are thought to be heterozygous for an abnormal 'regulator' gene; this recessive gene is not part of the locus controlling the CDE antigens. The Rh_{null} phenotype results when the children are homozygous for this abnormal regulator, but because this gene in the heterozygous state does not cause any abnormality of expression of the *CDE* genes, the children of Rh_{null} people of the regulator type will have normal Rh antigens (see Fig. 9.7). The parents of both types of Rh_{null} individuals are usually consanguineous.

Partially deleted Rh phenotypes have been described that lack some of the genes of the Rh haplotype, e.g. $-D-/-D-$; $C^w D-/C^w D-$ etc. These are very rare and have enhanced D.

Development and Distribution of the Rh Antigens

The Rh antigens are well developed at birth. They have not been found on cells other than red cells.

ANTIBODIES OF THE Rh SYSTEM

Naturally Occurring Antibodies

Anti-E is often naturally occurring, and about half the E antibodies found may occur without a history of pregnancy or transfusion. Occasionally, naturally occurring anti-D and anti-C^w are found in patients and blood donors. Such antibodies react optimally with enzyme-treated cells or in the Technicon AutoAnalyzer.

Immune Antibodies

The whole clinical importance of the Rh system lies in the readiness with which anti-D arises after stimulation by pregnancy or transfusion. *Due to prophylaxis of Rh immunization with anti-Rh immunoglobulin, the incidence of anti-D has significantly decreased but it still remains the commonest atypical antibody of clinical relevance detected in a routine blood transfusion laboratory.* D is considerably more immunogenic than the other Rh antigens, which have the following order of immunogenicity: $c > E > e > C$.

About 20–30% of anti-D sera also contain anti-C. Usually this anti-C is not a separable antibody, and it is probably anti-G. About 1–2% of anti-D sera also contain anti-E. Anti-C (and anti-G) in the absence of anti-D is very uncommon.

The incidence of other Rh antibodies is much lower, but together they are commoner than the antibodies against K (Kell) which is the most immunogenic antigen after D. In routine screening, pure anti-E is the commonest, followed by anti-c, although anti-c is a commoner cause of HDN. This is probably because about half the anti-E are weak, naturally occurring antibodies. Anti-e, like anti-C, is very rare. The vast majority of Rh antibodies are IgG and do not fix complement. IgM anti-D is very rare but very useful as a rapid typing reagent. Anti-D may be occasionally partly IgA. Recently, monoclonal human IgG and IgM anti-D have been produced by culture of EBV-transformed lymphocytes from immunized donors.

Experimental Immunization of Rh-Negative Volunteers

The realization that D-negative women unsensitized to the D antigen, who had just had a D-positive child, could be protected from forming anti-D by the passive injection of IgG anti-D soon after delivery has been a powerful stimulus for experimental work on D-negative volunteers. About 90% of D-negative people will make anti-D after the transfusion of a large volume of Rh(D)-positive cells, and 70% will respond to repeated small volumes. Responders to D can usually be revealed from survival curves after a single injection of ^{51}Cr-labelled D-positive cells. Serological methods are relatively insensitive to detect very low levels of anti-D.

ABO-incompatible D-positive red cells are less likely to stimulate the production of anti-D than

ABO-compatible D-positive red cells when injected into a D-negative recipient. Two explanations have been offered for this protection. First, it might be due to competition for the antigens so that the red cells are taken up by anti-A or anti-B-forming cells and are thus unavailable for anti-D-forming cells. Secondly, it might be that anti-A and anti-B bring about intravascular lysis with sequestration of the red cell stroma predominantly in the liver which is an unfavourable site for antibody formation. Neither of these explanations is very satisfactory, and the reason for the protection afforded by ABO-incompatible red cells remains uncertain. This protection is the basis of the lower incidence of maternal Rh sensitization when mother and infant are ABO incompatible.

It has been shown that 20 μg (100 i.u.) of anti-D immunoglobulin given intramuscularly will give complete protection from immunization by 1 ml of concentrated D-positive red cells. This figure is the basis for the standard dose of 100 μg (500 i.u.) anti-D Ig given post-partum in the UK, as it will cover the vast majority of transplacental haemorrhages (TPH). A dose of 3.2–4.0 mg of anti-D will protect a D-negative recipient against the consequences of the inadvertent transfusion of a unit of D-positive blood (200 ml of red cells).

The mechanism of protection by anti-D immunoglobulin is not really known. Two explanations have been suggested. The first is that the passively administered antibody leads to phagocytosis of antibody-coated red cells and their rapid destruction in the spleen before they can combine with receptors on immunologically competent cells. The second is a central mechanism by which the Fc fragment of the antibody combined to antigen might give a suppressive or inactivating signal to the immunocompetent cells. It has been calculated that the amount of passive antibody needed to protect the recipient from antibody formation is much less than that needed to cover all the D antigen sites on the injected Rh-positive cells.

Source of Anti-D for Immunoprophylaxis

Anti-D is usually obtained from volunteer men and from women who are unable to bear children, preferably already immunized by transfusion or pregnancy. Those with low levels of anti-D are deliberately restimulated with D-positive red cells from carefully selected accredited donors matched for all red cell antigens other than Rh. Plasma from these donors is harvested by apheresis and sent to a fractionation plant.

Immunization by Pregnancy

Nevanlinna has shown that even after five or more pregnancies the incidence of antibody formation in D-negative women is only about 10%. This figure is much less than that following injection of D-positive blood, and there are three explanations for this discrepancy. First, not all D-negative women have D-positive children. It can be calculated that in Britain about 10% of matings will result in a mother who is D negative carrying a D-positive fetus, and that only 47% of D-negative women pregnant for the second time will be carrying a second D-positive child. Second, not all pregnancies are ABO compatible, and, as stated earlier, ABO incompatibility protects against Rh antibody formation. Prior to Rh immunoprophylaxis, the first ABO-compatible, D-incompatible infant resulted in the primary immunization of about 17% of Rh-negative women. In about half these women, the antibodies appeared within 6 months of delivery, and in the other half the antibodies became detectable by the end of the second pregnancy if the child was D positive. Finally, no fetal cells or too few fetal cells may get into the mother's circulation to stimulate antibody formation.

Fetal red cells can be detected in a sample of maternal blood by the acid elution method of Kleihauer, which depends on the fact that fetal haemoglobin is more resistant to elution in an acid medium than adult haemoglobin. Thus fetal haemoglobin is retained in the cell, which stains darkly with the counterstain, while adult haemoglobin elutes and the mother's red cells appear colourless. About 80% of fetal red cells can be recognized by this technique. Fetal red cells can frequently be detected in the mother's circulation, particularly during the last trimester of pregnancy and after delivery. In about 85% of blood samples taken soon after delivery, the proportion of fetal cells to adult cells is less than 1 in 20 000 (equivalent to a TPH of less than 0.5 ml). In only two to three samples per 1000 deliveries will the incidence of

TPH be of the order of 10 ml of whole blood (5 ml of red cells), or more. Such women will not be protected by the standard anti-D dose of 100 μg, and they should be carefully assessed so that additional anti-Rh Ig can be given if necessary. All laboratories should standardize the conditions of the acid elution method in order to estimate more accurately the absolute amount of fetal red cells present in the maternal circulation.

Immunization by Abortion, Miscarriage and Obstetric Intervention

Abortion and miscarriage may lead to immunization of D-negative women, and obviously the incidence is greater if the abortion occurs in the second trimester than in the first. Amniocentesis, chorionic villus sampling and other obstetric manoeuvres can also lead to immunization of Rh-negative women carrying a Rh-positive fetus.

Details on the prevention of Rh sensitization are discussed in Chapter 10.

THE MNSs SYSTEM

This was the second blood group system to be discovered by Landsteiner and his colleagues in 1927. Due to its polymorphism, it is a useful blood group system in forensic medicine and paternity testing, but remains relatively unimportant in blood transfusion.

The Antigens of the MNSs System

M and *N* are inherited as codominant Mendelian traits giving rise to three common genotypes, *MM*, *MN* and *NN*. The *Ss* locus also consists of two codominant alleles closely linked to *MN*. In Northern Europeans, haplotype frequencies are $MS = 0.25$; $Ms = 0.28$; $NS = 0.08$ and $Ns = 0.39$ (Race and Sanger, 1975). There are several rare variants of M and N and also many rare antigens are linked genetically to M and N. There are also silent alleles; the rare En(a$-$) cells lack MN, and M^kM^k lack both MN and Ss antigens. About 2% of West African and 1.5% of American Negroes are S$-$s$-$ and most of these are U$-$ (almost all Caucasians are U$+$).

The MN antigens are carried on the α sialoglycoprotein (αSGP) or glycophorin A (see Fig. 8.1, Chapter 8), a transmembrane polypeptide with 16 sialic acid-rich oligosaccharides. M and N differ in amino acids at positions 1 and 5 of the external amino terminus of αSGP. There are $0.5-2 \times 10^6$ molecules of αSGP per cell, but their total absence in En(a$-$) people does not affect red cell function or survival. The negative charge of the red cells is mainly due to the ionized COOH groups of sialic acid (neuraminic acid), which is mostly carried on the oligosaccharides of αSGP and can be removed with neuraminidase. Hence En(a$-$) cells have reduced negative charge and behave as if they have been enzyme treated.

The δSGP, or glycophorin B (see Fig. 8.1), carries the S and s determinants, which differ from each other in the amino acid at position 29. The amino-acid sequence at the amino terminal of δ is identical to that of the N-specific αSGP and accounts for the reactivity of MM cells, provided they are S$+$ and/or s$+$ (i.e. provided they have δSGP) with anti-N. This specificity has been termed 'N'.

Pasvol *et al.* (1982) demonstrated that α and δSGP are required for erythrocyte invasion by *Plasmodium falciparum*. They suggested that specific binding between the parasite and an oligosaccharide cluster is needed for attachment. Two receptors (sialic acid-dependent and independent) seem to be required for *P. falciparum* invasion.

The Antibodies of the MNSs System

Anti-M is an uncommon antibody which reacts with about 80% of random ABO-compatible samples. It is usually a naturally occurring antibody, more common in infants than adults, but can be immune and has been described as the cause of haemolytic disease of the newborn.

Anti-N is also rare and reacts with about 70% of random samples. It is nearly always a cold IgM antibody. At low temperatures, anti-N reacts with and can be completely absorbed by all MM cells except the rare M$+$N$-$S$-$s$-$; this is because δSGP has the same N terminal amino acids as αSGP in N$+$ red cells. Since S$-$s$-$ red cells lack δSGP, they will not carry 'N'. Useful anti-N lectin can be prepared from the seeds of *Vicia graminea*.

Both anti-M and anti-N react more strongly

when the appropriate antigen is present in double dose, i.e. MM or NN, than when the red cells are MN.

Another N-like antibody (anti-Nf) has been described in certain patients undergoing renal dialysis. Anti-Nf can occur in persons of any MN group; it is a cold antibody, and although it may cause confusion in cross-matching tests, it is usually of little clinical importance. It has been reported, however, to cause hyperacute renal graft rejection. The Nf antigen arises from the effects of minute amounts of formaldehyde (used to sterilize the dialyser coil) on the patient's red cells. These changed cells stimulate anti-Nf which can cross-react with normal red cells.

Anti-S, the rarer anti-s and even rarer anti-U are usually immune, IgG. They can cause HDN and have been implicated in haemolytic transfusion reactions. Anti-U only occurs in some Negroes who are S−s−; it reacts with all cells that have the S or s antigens and with 16% of cells that are S−s−. Finding compatible blood for a patient with anti-U may prove difficult as less than 1% of Negroes and practically no Whites are U negative.

The Use of Enzyme-Treated Cells to Detect MNSs Antibodies

Human anti-M and anti-N will not agglutinate the appropriate red cells after they have been treated with proteolytic enzymes. Anti-S reacts variably and anti-s may be enhanced when the appropriate cells have been treated with certain proteases.

THE LUTHERAN BLOOD GROUP SYSTEM

The incidence of the Lutheran antigens, called Lu^a and Lu^b, in the English population is as follows:

Lu(a+b−)	0.1%
Lu(a+b+)	7.5%
Lu(a−b+)	92.4%

Anti-Lu^a is an uncommon antibody, and the Lu^a antigen is usually absent from antibody screening cells. Anti-Lu^a has the tendency to appear only transiently and, even though it is an immune antibody, it is usually IgM. The clinical significance of this antibody is doubtful. The agglutination of Lu(a+) red cells by anti-Lu^a has a characteristic appearance similar to that of A_3 red cells with anti-A, i.e. small clumps of agglutinates in a sea of unagglutinated cells.

Anti-Lu^b is also very rare, occasionally partly IgA, and has caused delayed haemolytic transfusion reactions. It is unclear whether anti-Lu^b can cause HDN.

THE KELL BLOOD GROUP SYSTEM

The antigens of the Kell blood group system include K (Kell) and k (Cellano), Kp^a (Penny) and Kp^b (Rautenberger), and Js^a and Js^b (the Sutter antigens). The Kell genes are a set of three closely linked genes like the Rh genes. The Kell antigens are on glycoproteins; they are inactivated by ZZAP (mixture of DTT and papain) and by AET.

The incidence of the K and k antigens in English people is as follows:

K+k−	0.2%
K+k+	8.7%
K−k+	91.1%

The K antigen does not occur with any frequency in Negroes. Js^a is extremely rare in Caucasians, but the Js^a antigen is present in about 20% of Negroes. Very rarely, all the antigens of the Kell system may be missing and such people are said to have the blood group K_o.

Kx is thought to be an 'underlying' Kell antigen whereas K, k, Kp^a, Kp^b, Js^a, and Js^b are final determinant antigens. The cells from a healthy blood donor McLeod (since found to have a compensated acanthocytic haemolytic anaemia) were found to react extremely weakly with antisera against these final determinant antigens. Occasionally, boys with sex-linked chronic granulomatous disease (CGD) are found to have a similar phenotype to that of McLeod, and a similar abnormality in the peripheral blood film. These patients, when transfused with normal blood, can make an antibody which reacts with all cells including K_o but not with their own red cells. This antibody is called anti-KL. A separate specificity, anti-Kx may be prepared by elution after anti-KL is absorbed onto K_o cells. The red cells of the McLeod phenotype and from some patients with sex-linked CGD will not react with anti-Kx.

It was previously postulated that neutrophils of all patients with sex-linked CGD lacked the Kx antigen, which is supposedly present on the neutrophils of all normal subjects (including McLeod) without CGD. However, this belief has been recently disproved by the finding of Branch et al. (1985) that granulocytes from all individuals lack Kx. The same authors have questioned the hypothesis that Kx is a precursor of the Kell antigens, since DTT treatment enhances the expression of Kx on normal red cells without affecting the expression of the 'final' Kell antigens. It must be said that most boys with CGD have normal Kell antigens and a normal blood film, but the small proportion that do not are important because of the antibodies that they may produce after transfusion.

Anti-Kell is an important antibody in Britain; it is nearly always immune and often IgG and complement binding. It has been the cause of haemolytic transfusion reactions and HDN. The Kell antigen stimulates the formation of anti-Kell in about 10% of Kell-negative people who are given one unit of Kell positive blood. This makes K the next most immunogenic antigen after the D antigen. About 0.1% of all cases of HDN are caused by anti-Kell; most of the mothers will have had previous blood transfusions. Anti-Kell is best detected by the indirect antiglobulin test; this antibody does not always give agglutination of the appropriate enzyme-treated red cells, or of cells suspended in LISS.

Anti-k is a very rare antibody which reacts with 99.8% of random blood samples. It is always immune and has been incriminated in some cases of mild haemolytic disease of the newborn.

Anti-Js^a, anti-Js^b, anti-Kp^a and anti-Kp^b are all rare immune antibodies that are best detected by the indirect antiglobulin technique.

THE DUFFY BLOOD GROUP SYSTEM

Duffy consists of two antigens, Fy^a and Fy^b, controlled by allelomorphic genes on chromosome 1. The incidence in Britain is as follows:

Fy(a+b−)	20%
Fy(a+b+)	46%
Fy(a−b+)	34%

About 70% of Negroes are negative with both anti-Fy^a and anti-Fy^b and are homozygous for the

silent allele *Fy*. Interestingly, the Fy(a−b−) red cell phenotype confers resistance to penetration by *Plasmodium vivax*. In West Africa, where other forms of malaria are common, *P. vivax* does not occur and it is tempting to speculate that the high incidence of Fy(a−b−) persons arose by natural selection when the parasite was previously prevalent.

Anti-Fy^a is not infrequent and is found in previously transfused patients who have usually already made other antibodies. It is an IgG antibody, often complement fixing, and can cause haemolytic transfusion reactions but seldom HDN. It is best detected by IAGT and normally will not agglutinate the appropriate red cells if they have been treated with proteases. Anti-Fy^b is very rare and is always immune.

THE KIDD BLOOD GROUP SYSTEM

Kidd has two alleles, *Jk^a* and *Jk^b*, with the very rare silent allele *Jk*. The incidence in the English population is as follows:

Jk(a+b−)	25%
Jk(a+b+)	50%
Jk(a−b+)	25%

Anti-Jk^a is uncommon and anti-Jk^b is very rare, but they may both cause severe transfusion reactions and haemolytic disease of the newborn. Kidd antibodies have often been implicated in delayed haemolytic transfusion reactions; they are IgG and predominantly complement fixing but may be difficult to detect. The antiglobulin test is the best method of detection, and reactions will be enhanced if the appropriate cells have been protease-treated or if fresh serum is added as a source of complement. Kidd antibodies tend to disappear rapidly after stimulation and patients who have made them should always be given an antibody card.

THE Di, Yt, Xg, Do, Sd AND Co BLOOD GROUP SYSTEMS

Diego (Di)

Two antigens, Di^a and Di^b, have been described. The corresponding antibodies are immune and extremely rare. Di^a is of very low incidence in Whites but is not uncommon in Mongoloids.

Cartwright (Yt)

The incidence of Yt^a and Yt^b in Europe is as follows:

Yt(a + b −)	91.9%
Yt(a + b +)	7.9%
Yt(a − b +)	0.2%

Anti-Yt^a and anti-Yt^b are immune, extremely rare, and most are of no clinical significance.

Xg

The importance of this blood group system, which is controlled by genes carried on the X chromosome, has already been mentioned (see p. 233). Only one antigen is known, Xg^a. Anti-Xg^a is a very rare immune antibody, best detected by IAGT, and not known to affect red cell survival.

Dombrock (Do)

Two antigens, Do^a and Do^b, have been described. Approximately 64% of North Europeans are Do(a +). The antibodies are extremely rare, immune and are best detected by IAGT.

Sid (Sd)

Only one antigen, Sd^a, is known. Over 90% of people have the antigen but only about 10% react strongly with anti-Sd^a. The antigen is also present in saliva and other body fluids; the best method of Sd^a typing is by inhibiting the agglutination of known strong Sd(a +) red cells by anti-Sd^a with saliva from the people to be typed. Only about 4% of people fail to secrete the antigen and about half of these Sd(a −) subjects have some detectable anti-Sd^a in their serum. The antibody is IgM, naturally occurring, and is of clinical importance only when 'strong' Sd(a +) cells are transfused.

Cad was originally described as a polyagglutinable cell, but was later shown to be a very strong form of Sd^a. The structure of the Cad antigen is very similar to the A antigen; hence Cad + cells will be agglutinated by *Dolichos biflorus* extracts, regardless of their ABO group.

Colton (Co)

Two antigens, Co^a and Co^b, have been described and their incidence in Britain is as follows:

Co(a + b −)	90.5%
Co(a + b +)	9.0%
Co(a − b +)	0.5%

Colton antibodies are immune and extremely rare.

ANTIGENS WITH A HIGH AND LOW INCIDENCE

There are many other antigens either with a very high incidence (public antigens), for example Vel and Lan, or with a very low incidence (private antigens), e.g. Wr^a, that have not yet been assigned to blood group systems.

By definition, a low frequency antigen is one that occurs in less than 1 in 400 individuals of a given population. They are usually found as unexpected reactions in compatibility testing or by deliberate screening. Some of them have been implicated in HDN.

Antibodies to low frequency antigens are usually naturally occurring, and sometimes occur with appreciable frequency. These antibodies may sometimes cause problems when present in blood grouping reagents; if present in anti-D reagents, an Rh-negative woman carrying the relevant low frequency antigen will be mistyped as Rhesus positive.

For those rare individuals lacking a high incidence antigen who have formed the corresponding antibody, provision of compatible blood can be a problem and it may be necessary to approach the National or International Panels of Rare Donors for compatible blood.

Wright (Wr^a)

The incidence of Wr^a is only about 0.1%. However, naturally occurring anti-Wr^a is present in approximately 1% of blood donors. For some unknown reason, anti-Wr^a is often found in the serum of patients who have made other antibodies or who are suffering from autoimmune haemolytic anaemia. Many are often detected as incompatibilities in the crossmatch.

The Bg or the Bennett–Donna–Goodspeed antigens reflect the presence of HLA antigens on red cells. The clinical significance of anti-Bg is disputed.

POLYAGGLUTINABLE RED CELLS

Erythrocyte polyagglutination is the agglutination of red cells irrespective of blood group by most sera from normal adults, optimally at room temperature. Autologous polyagglutinable red cells are not agglutinated by the patient's own serum. The abnormality is a property of the red cells, not of the sera, in contrast to panagglutination which is the agglutination of most red cells by one particular serum.

There are two classes of polyagglutinable red cells: acquired and inherited. The acquired forms can be subdivided into: (i) microbial, due to either the passive coating of red cells with bacteria or their products, or to the action of microbial enzymes on the red cell surface (T, Tk, acquired B); and (ii) non-microbial, which is thought to be due to somatic mutation (Tn polyagglutination). There are two types of inherited polyagglutination: Cad and HEMPAS.

Polyagglutination used to occur predominantly in vitro as a result of enzymes from bacteria contaminating the blood. However, these days most types occur in vivo. Lectins are required for the diagnosis of different types of polyagglutination (see Table 9.15).

T Activation

T activation occurs transiently in some patients with an obvious microbial infection, e.g. *Vibrio cholerae, Clostridium perfringens, Diplococcus pneumoniae,* various streptococci and the influenza virus. These microbes produce neuraminidase which removes negatively charged N-acetylneuraminic acid (NANA or sialic acid) from the oligosaccharides of membrane SGPs (Table 9.14) to expose the hidden T antigen (galactose linked to N-acetylgalactosamine), with an accompanying loss of the negative surface charge. For T polyagglutination to occur, microbial neuraminidase must be present in amounts large enough to neutralize the enzyme inhibitors normally present in plasma; the

Table 9.14
Biochemistry of T, Tk and Tn antigens

```
Serine/threonine——GalNAc                     Tn
                     |
                   NeuNAc

Serine/threonine——GalNAc——Gal                T

Serine/threonine——GalNAc——Gal                Normal
                     |        |
                   NeuNAc   NeuNAc            (Oligosaccharide
                                              chain of SGP)

A, B or H chains
        endo-β-galactosidase
                 ↓
R-GlcNAc-Gal-GlcNAc-Gal-GalNAc* A
                        |
                      Fuc                      Tk
```

*If GalNAc is replaced by Gal, group B specificity is obtained.
Abbreviations: Gal, galactose; GalNAc, N-acetylgalactosamine; NeuNAc, N-acetylneuraminic acid (NANA); GlcNAc, N-acetylglucosamine; Fuc, fucose.

same is true for other forms of enzymic polyagglutination.

Most adult sera contain naturally occurring cold-reacting IgM, complement-fixing anti-T, and the majority of cases of T activation are detected by the discrepancy in results of cell and serum ABO grouping. Thus T activation is unlikely to be detected in group AB subjects and is most easily detected in group O individuals. The correct ABO group can be obtained from tests at 37°C.

T polyagglutination may be associated with: (i) haemolytic anaemia; (ii) haemolytic transfusion reactions (especially in children) due to anti-T in transfused plasma; (iii) haemolytic uraemic syndrome.

The identification of T-activated cells can be made using a lectin from the peanut, *Arachis hypogaea* (Table 9.15).

Tk Activation

Tk activation, like T activation, is also transient and associated with infection. Endo-β-galactosidases produced by *Bacteroides fragilis*, various *Clostridia*, *Candida albicans*, etc., remove β-galactose from ABH polysaccharide chains exposing N-acetylglucosamine (see Table 9.14), with the consequent depression of ABH antigens, without affecting the amount of sialic acid of the red cell. Tk cells are specifically agglutinated by BS II lectin, an extract from *Bandeiraea simplicifolia* (Table 9.15). These cells are also agglutinable by peanut lectin.

Tn Activation

Tn activation, unlike T and Tk, is a persistent abnormality not associated with infection and is caused by an abnormal clone of stem cells arising by somatic mutation. It is often associated with other haematological abnormalities such as chronic haemolytic anaemia, leucopenia or thrombocytopenia, but it may be present in normal subjects. Patients may lose the abnormality spontaneously. Somatic mutation would lead to a deficiency of the galactosyl and the sialyl transferases that elongate the oligosaccharide chains on αSGP, so that many of the chains end at N-acetylgalactosamine, the immunodominant sugar of Tn (see Table 9.14). This loss results in a depression of M and N antigens and a loss of sialic acid and of negative charge similar to that found in T activation. Only some of the red cells are agglutinated by the anti-Tn present in all normal adult sera, giving the mixed field appearance. The platelets also show two populations: Tn + and Tn −. *Salvia sclarea* lectin agglutinates Tn-activated cells specifically, and the exposed N-acetylgalactosamine molecules can be detected with *Dolichos biflorus* lectin in people who are not group

Table 9.15

Some differences between T, Tk, Tn and Cad red cells

	Red cells			
	T	*Tk*	*Tn*	*Cad*
MN antigens	↓	Normal	↓	Normal
ABH antigens	Normal	↓	Normal	Normal
Glycine soja lectin	+	−	+	+
Arachis hypogaea lectin	+ +	+	−	−
Bandeiraea S. II lectin	−	+	−	−
Salvia sclarea lectin	−	−	+	−
Dolichos biflorus lectin (other than Group A)	−	−	+	+
Polybrene* solution	−	+	+^{MF}	+

*Polybrene is a positively charged polymer which agglutinates cells with a negative charge and fails to aggregate NANA-deficient cells.
MF = mixed field.

A. The serological differences between the various types of polyagglutination is shown in Table 9.15.

Acquired B

Acquired B is a rare transient condition that, strictly speaking, is not a form of polyagglutination. The condition occurs in patients with carcinoma of the colon, some infections, and in healthy people. It is probably caused by microbial deacetylases, as described on p. 237. Cells with acquired B react optimally with the anti-B of group A_2 people.

Blood Transfusion and Polyagglutination

Polyagglutination may cause problems not only in blood grouping but also in the consequences of transfusion. According to Bird, transfusions of whole blood or plasma are contraindicated, especially in children, because of the potential danger arising from antibodies to polyagglutinable red cells in donor plasma. Bird recommends the transfusion of washed red cells and that all patients who group as AB, particularly very young babies, be carefully studied to exclude polyagglutination.

WHITE CELL AND PLATELET ANTIBODIES

The HLA System

The HLA antigens constitute the major histocompatibility complex (MHC) or system, which is controlled by a small region on chromosome 6. HLA antigens (human leucocyte antigens or histocompatibility locus A) are also called tissue or transplantation antigens. They play an important role in the outcome of tissue grafts and can facilitate acute graft rejection. The ABO system also has a major influence on the survival of transplanted tissue, but the expression of ABO and HLA varies widely in different tissues, e.g. vascular endothelium is rich in such markers whereas hepatocytes are devoid of them. Hence ABO is also regarded as a major histocompatibility system. However, there are several additional loci (including those of blood groups) distributed throughout the genome which can lead to chronic rejection. These are the minor histocompatibility loci.

The major histocompatibility complex codes for three types of proteins.

Class 1 antigens are the products of the *HLA-A, B* and *C* loci, which consist of a large MHC-encoded transmembrane glycoprotein non-covalently linked to a small peptide, β_2-microglobulin, encoded by a locus outside the MHC (Fig. 9.8). Class 1 antigens are present on all nucleated cells (except spermatozoa and placental trophoblast) and platelets. Class 1 antigens are the major targets of rejection following organ transplantation. Some class 1 antigens are present on red cells, with varying degrees of expression.

Class 2 antigens consist of two different (α and β), non-covalently linked transmembrane glycoproteins (Fig. 9.8). They are the products of the HLA-D region and its closely associated loci (DR, DP and DQ), and are restricted to B lymphocytes, activated T cells, macrophages, monocytes, dendritic cells and early haemopoietic cells.

Class 3 antigens are those complement components (C4, C2, Bf) coded by the MHC. Chido (Ch) and Rodgers (Rg) are serological determinants of C4 and, although they can be detected on normal red cells, they are best defined by inhibition of agglutination of C4-coated cells.

The order of the MHC genes on chromosome 6 is *HLA-A, HLA-C, HLA-B, Bf, C2, C4, HLA-D* (Fig. 9.9). These loci are closely linked, with a recombination rate of approximately 1%. The *HLA-A, HLA-B, HLA-C* and *HLA-D* loci are the most polymorphic loci in humans, as can be seen in Table 9.16. Clearly defined antigens are designated by a number following the letter that identifies their locus, e.g. HLA-A1 and HLA-B5. The use of the prefix 'w' implies workshop status or conditional characterization of an antigen. The numbering of the HLA-A and HLA-B antigens does not follow a logical sequence because, originally, clearly defined individual antigens were not identified as being the products of two separate loci.

Since the HLA loci are closely linked, the HLA genes on a chromosome are inherited as a single entity, referred to as a haplotype. The number of possible haplotypes in humans is very large and consequently the number of possible genotypes is unimaginable. Every individual will have a maternal and a paternal haplotype, each of which can be transmitted to their offspring en bloc. In a

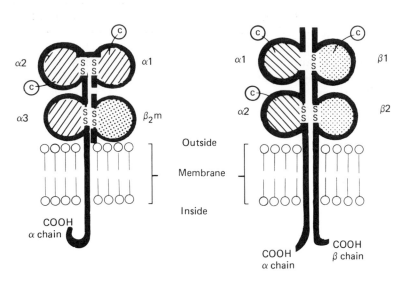

Fig. 9.8. *Structure of HLA class 1 and 2 molecules. Small circles denote carbohydrate moieties; individual domains of α and β chains are designated α1, α2 or β1, β2 etc.*

Table 9.16
Complete listing of recognized HLA specificities

HLA-A	HLA-B	HLA-C	HLA-D	HLA-DR	HLA-DQ*	HLA-DP†
A1	B5	Cw1	Dw1	DR1	DQw1	DPw1
A2	B7	Cw2	Dw2	DR2	DQw2	DPw2
A3	B8	Cw3	Dw3	DR3	DQw3	DPw3
A9	B12	Cw4	Dw4	DR4		DPw4
A10	B13	Cw5	Dw5	DR5		DPw5
A11	B14	Cw6	Dw6	DRw6		DPw6
Aw19	B15	Cw7	Dw7	DR7		
A23(9)	B16	Cw8	Dw8	DRw8		
A24(9)	B17		Dw9	DRw9		
A25(10)	B18		Dw10	DRw10		
A26(10)	B21		Dw11(w7)	DRw11(5)		
A28	Bw22		Dw12	DRw12(5)		
A29(w19)	B27		Dw13	DRw13(w6)		
A30(w19)	B35		Dw14	DRw14(w6)		
A31(w19)	B37		Dw15			
A32(w19)	B38(16)		Dw16	DRw52		
Aw33(w19)	B39(16)		Dw17(w7)	DRw53		
Aw34(10)	B40		Dw18(w6)			
Aw36	Bw41		Dw19(w6)			
Aw43	Bw42					
Aw66(10)	B44(12)					
Aw68(28)	B45(12)					

Table 9.16 (*Continued*)

HLA-A	HLA-B	HLA-C	HLA-D	HLA-DR	HLA-DQ*	HLA-DP†
Aw69(28)	Bw46					
	Bw47					
	Bw48					
	B49(21)					
	Bw50(21)					
	B51(5)					
	Bw52(5)					
	Bw53					
	Bw54(w22)					
	Bw55(w22)					
	Bw56(w22)					
	Bw57(17)					
	Bw58(17)					
	Bw59					
	Bw60(40)					
	Bw61(40)					
	Bw62(15)					
	Bw64(14)					
	Bw65(14)					
	Bw67					
	Bw70					
	Bw71(w70)					
	Bw72(w70)					
	Bw73					
	Bw4					
	Bw6					

*DQ was formerly DC or MB.

†DP was formerly SB.

Numbers in parentheses indicate earlier designations or broad specificities before the antigens were split, e.g. A9 has now been split into antigens A23 and A24. HLA-Bw4 and HLA-Bw6 are very broad or public specificities which include many splits. These shared antigenic determinants contribute to extensive cross-reactivity.

free-breeding population, the frequency with which two alleles occur together is given by the product of the individual gene frequencies. However, in the HLA system, certain haplotypes occur much more often in a given population than would be expected on the basis of the product of the individual gene frequencies. For example, the frequency of the haplotype *HLA-A1-B8-DR3* in Caucasians is significantly higher than expected. Such deviation from expectation is called linkage disequilibrium.

The HLA-D region has now been divided into three subregions, each encoding a different family of genes: *DR*, *DQ* (previously known variously as *DC*, *DS*, *MB* and even *LB-E*) and *DP* (previously called *SB*). Products of the *DR* and *DQ* genes are recognized serologically; those of *DP* by a test similar to the MLC which involves T-cell proliferation of primed lymphocytes as a response to test cells.

The application of recombinant DNA technology to the expanded HLA-D region has revealed that DR molecules arise from the product of a single invariant α gene linked to three polymorphic β genes which code for the serologically defined DR specificities. The products of two of the different β genes are associated with particular HLA-DR specificities; the third β gene is considered to be a

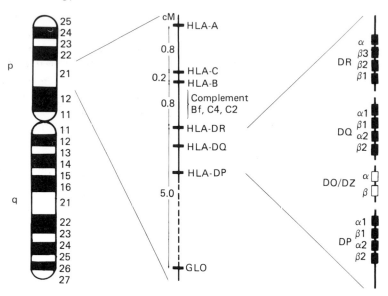

Fig. 9.9. *Chromosome 6 and maps of the HLA and HLA-D loci.*

pseudogene. In contrast to DR, DQ molecules arise from two α genes (DQα1 and DQα2) linked to two β genes (DQβ1 and DQβ2). Although both DQ α and β genes are polymorphic, the three known serologically defined DQ specificities appear to arise from the β genes. As expected of closely linked genes, there is strong linkage disequilibrium between *DQ* and *DR* genes with, in Caucasian populations, *DQw1* being associated with *DR1*, *DR2* and *DRw6*, while *DQw2* is associated with *DR3* and most *DR7*. Similarly, there is disequilibrium between the specificities coded for by DRβ1 and DRβ2. Like DQ, the DP region codes for two α and two β genes. However, only one pair of αβ genes codes for the six known DP antigens (DPw1–6); the other pair of genes seems not to be expressed.

Although the main interest in HLA is in its role as a histocompatibility system, the scope of HLA has expanded to include numerous other applications: (i) immune recognition and immune responsiveness, (ii) association with certain diseases (e.g. HLA-B27 and ankylosing spondylitis), (iii) outcome of platelet and granulocyte transfusions, and (iv) problems of parentage and identity.

Methods for the Detection of HLA Antigens

The HLA-A, -B, -C and -DR antigens can induce the formation of antibodies by transfusion, preg-

nancy or transplantation. Hence all class 1 and some of the class 2 antigens can be detected by serological techniques using appropriate target cells (lymphocytes) and HLA typing reagents, usually derived from sera of multiparous women, although more recently some monoclonal reagents have become available.

HLA-A, -B and -C antigens are determined using the two-stage lymphocytotoxicity test. Briefly, lymphocytes are separated from whole blood by density gradient centrifugation, then antiserum of known specificity is incubated with the isolated lymphocytes. In the second stage, complement is added. Cells carrying the relevant antigen(s) will bind antibody and complement, which will damage the cell membrane; the dead cells can be visualized by adding a suitable vital dye, such as trypan blue or eosin, which is not taken up by living cells. The test has been miniaturized in order to conserve antisera and lymphocytes as, in view of the extreme polymorphism of HLA, a large number of reaction mixtures are needed for HLA typing.

Although class 1 antigens are clearly distinguishable from each other, some appear to be closely related serologically: cross-reactivity. Particularly strong cross-reactivity exists between HLA-A2 and -A28, and between HLA-A1, -A3 and -A11. In cases of cross-reactivity it is therefore essential to use several typing sera for each antigen.

The antigens of the HLA-D region can be determined by the following methods. (i) Serological techniques similar to the lymphocytotoxicity test, but on separated B lymphocytes and using sera absorbed with platelets, which do not carry class 2 antigens. These techniques detect the HLA-D related (DR) and DQ antigens. (ii) Serological techniques, on unseparated lymphocytes, employing two-colour fluorescence to detect DR antigens on B cells. B cells carry immunoglobulin on their surface and will stain bright green with fluorescein-labelled AHG serum; when the cytotoxicity test is then performed on such stained cells, killed B cells will also fluoresce red with ethidium bromide. (iii) Cellular techniques: with the exception of HLA-DR and DQ, class 2 antigens can only be detected by their participation in cell-to-cell interaction. The test generally used is called the mixed lymphocyte reaction (MLR) or mixed lymphocyte culture (MLC). When lymphocytes from two unrelated individuals are incubated together in culture, the different cell surface antigens stimulate the lymphocytes to enlarge, proliferate and transform into blast cells, and produce DNA. This lymphocyte stimulation can be measured within 5–7 days of culture by the incorporation of ^{3}H-thymidine into the dividing cells and monocytes. The T cells proliferate in response to antigens carried on B cells. If the cells of one of the individuals are prevented from dividing, by treatment with mitomycin or x-irradiation, while still capable of stimulating the untreated cells of the other individual, unidirectional stimulation will occur (**one-way MLC**). Typing for HLA-D antigens is accomplished by using a panel of inactivated stimulator cells that are homozygous for *HLA-D* (homozygous typing cells); failure to react means that the test cells carry the same HLA-D antigens as the homozygous typing cells. Since the MLC takes several days to perform, it can be used for selecting bone marrow transplant donors or living related kidney donors, but it is not practical for the selection of cadaveric grafts.

An alternative cellular technique is primed lymphocyte typing (PLT), which was derived from the MLC as a faster typing method. If the cells in the MLC are left in culture for approximately 2 weeks, the stimulator cells die and the responder cells cease to proliferate. However, the responder cells have been primed, and hence they will undergo faster (i.e.

24 h) proliferation than in the original MLR when re-exposed to the same HLA-D associated antigen that was present on the original stimulator cells. PLT is the method used to define DP (originally SB) antigens and it will not give the same pattern of reactions as MLC, i.e. it will not define HLA-D antigens, but rather HLA-D-associated antigens.

The above serological and cellular techniques have revealed an extensive polymorphism that exists in class 1 and class 2 molecules, and which arises because of variation *within* the protein-coding portions (exons) of class 1 and class 2 genes. The application of recombinant DNA technology has revealed further heterogeneity in the HLA locus which arises from variations in the DNA *outside* the protein-coding portions of HLA (at least, class 2) genes, i.e. variation in the intervening nucleotide sequences (introns) between the structural genes. The latter variability is identified on the basis of differences in the size of DNA fragments that hybridize with radiolabelled complementary DNA (cDNA) probes, specific for the HLA locus, after digestion of native DNA with nucleotidases known as restriction enzymes. This size difference (i.e. polymorphism) between these enzyme-derived fragments (restriction fragments) reflects the difference in the length of nucleotide sequences of the various fragments and is known as an RFLP (restriction fragment length polymorphism). Restriction fragments arise because of the presence of particular nucleotide sequences repeated along a single stretch of DNA that can be recognized and cleaved by a specific nucleotidase; if few cleavage sites are present, longer DNA fragments are produced. Hence hybridization with a cDNA probe specific for a particular gene will reveal an RFLP only if restriction sites on either side of the gene recognized are absent in some individuals whilst being present in others. Interestingly, RFLPs detected with the enzyme Pstl in *HLA-DQ* genes have been found to correlate quite strongly with DQ markers defined by serological means or by T-cell proliferation.

Neutrophil-specific Antigens

Neutrophils carry not only class 1 MHC antigens but also neutrophil-specific antigens, as shown in Table 9.17. These antigens are clinically important in: (i) alloimmune neonatal neutropenia (NA1,

Table 9.17
Neutrophil-specific antigens

Locus	Antigens	Phenotype frequency (%)	Genotype frequency
NA	NA1	61.2	0.32
	NA2	89.6	0.68
NB	NB1	90.8	0.72
	NB2	67.9	0.17
NC	NC1	94.5	0.80
ND	ND1	98.5	0.88
NE	NE1	22.9	0.12
9	9a*	62.6	0.39
HGA-3	HGA-3a, 3b, 3c, 3d, 3e		
GA, GB, GC			
GR	Gr1, Gr2		

*According to Lalezari, 9a and NB2 are the same.

NA2, NB1, NC1); (ii) febrile transfusion reactions (NA1, NA2, NB1, NB2 and other unidentified granulocyte-specific antigens); (iii) pulmonary reactions caused by the passive transfer of granulocyte antibodies in donor plasma (NA2); (iv) autoimmune neutropenia (ND1 and NE1 have only been defined by autoantibodies).

The techniques used to detect neutrophil-specific antigens and antibodies include EDTA-dependent leucoagglutination, indirect immunofluorescence, cytotoxicity, opsonization, chemiluminescence, radioactive antiglobulin test and the use of *Staph*. protein A.

Platelet-specific Antigens

Platelets carry ABO, HLA class 1 and platelet-specific antigens (see Table 9.18). The class 1 antigens are important in the refractoriness to random donor platelet transfusions, although occasionally platelet-specific antigens may be involved. Platelet-specific antigens have been responsible for alloimmune neonatal thrombocytopenia, post-transfusion purpura (almost exclusively Pl^{A1}) and occasionally for febrile transfusion reactions.

Typing for platelet-specific antigens is difficult since most antisera are contaminated with HLA antibodies. The techniques used for platelet serology include agglutination, platelet suspension immunofluorescence (PSIFT), radioactive

Table 9.18
Platelet-specific antigens

System	Alleles	Phenotype frequency (%)	Genotype frequency
Pl^A	Pl^{A1} (Zwᵃ)	97.6	0.855
	Pl^{A2} (Zwᵇ)	26.8	0.155
Ko	Ko^a	14.3	0.074
	Ko^b	99.4	0.923
Pl^E	Pl^{E1}	>99.9	0.968
	Pl^{E2}	5.0	0.025
Bak (=Lek)	Bak^a	90.8	0.696
DUZO	$DUZO^a$	18.0	0.094
Pen		>99.9	
Yuk	Yuk^a	1.7	0.008
	Yuk^b	>99.9	0.992

*Most of the frequencies apply to the Dutch population.

anti-globulin test (PRAT), ELISA, ^{51}Cr-release, complement fixation test (CFT), etc.

PLASMA PROTEIN ANTIGENS AND ANTIBODIES

Many of the components of human plasma may be antigenic when whole blood or plasma is transfused. Problems associated with such antibodies are one of the less well investigated areas in blood transfusion. Urticarial reactions following the transfusion of blood or plasma components are not infrequent, although the culprit protein is only rarely disclosed. Antibodies to Factor VIII are not known to cause transfusion reactions although they will cause refractoriness to the transfusion of Factor VIII. Antibodies to IgA can lead to serious reactions (see Chapter 10). Antibodies to IgG determinants may cause problems in blood grouping, but their role in transfusion reactions is debatable.

Gm Antigens

Gm antigens are the polymorphic antigens on the heavy chains of IgG (γ chains), present mainly on the Fc region with a few on the Fd piece. There are a large number of different Gm antigens and they are inherited in groups, like the Rh antigens CDE. Within one group, antigens that appear to be controlled by allelomorphic genes in one population are inherited together as a haplotype in another population. IgG myeloma proteins have shown that different antigens are associated with different IgG subclasses, e.g. four different determinants have been described for IgG1, thirteen for IgG3 and none for IgG4.

Routine typing for Gm antigens is carried out using test serum to inhibit the agglutination of Rh-positive red cells coated with selected IgG Rh antibodies of known Gm status by Gm-specific antibodies.

Gm Antibodies

Gm antibodies are found:

(i) in the sera of patients with rheumatoid arthritis: these antibodies, known as 'Raggs' (rheumatoid agglutinators), are usually of high titre, but are often non-specific or multispecific and are commonly autoantibodies;

(ii) in the sera of patients who have received transfusions, injections of immunoglobulin or have been pregnant: these antibodies, known as 'SNaggs' (serum normal agglutinators), are usually of lower titre than Raggs but are often monospecific; these can be used as typing reagents;

(iii) in children between the ages of 6 months and 5 years who are genetically incompatible with their mothers' IgG, and in some normal adults.

SELECTED BIBLIOGRAPHY

General

Mollison P. L., Engelfriet C. P., Contreras M. (1987). *Blood transfusion in clinical medicine*, 8th edn. Oxford: Blackwell Scientific Publications.

Red Cell Antigens

Branch D. R., Gaidulis L., Lazar G. S. (1985). Human granulocytes lack red cell Kx antigen. *British Journal of Haematology*, **59**, 505–512.

Contreras M., Lubenko A. (1984). Red cell blood group systems. In *Immunohaematology* (Eds. C. P. Engelfriet, J. J. van Loghem and A. E. G. Kr. von dem Borne). Amsterdam: Elsevier.

Dobson A., Ikin E. W. (1946). The ABO blood groups in the United Kingdom: frequencies based on a very large sample. *Journal of Pathology and Bacteriology*, **58**, 221–227.

Economidou J., Hughes-Jones N. C., Gardner B. (1967). Quantitative measurements concerning A and B antigen sites. *Vox Sanguinis*, **12**, 321–328.

Levine P., Robinson E., Celano M., Briggs O., Falkinburg L. (1955). Gene interaction resulting in suppression of blood group substance B. *Blood*, **10**, 1100.

Pasvol G., Jungery M., Weatherall D. J., Parsons S. F., Anstee D. J., Tanner M. J. A. (1982) Glycophorin as a possible receptor for *Plasmodium falciparum*. *Lancet*, **ii**, 947–950.

Race R. R., Sanger R. (1975). *Blood groups in Man*, 6th edn. Oxford: Blackwell Scientific Publications.

Rochna E., Hughes-Jones N. C. (1965). The use of purified ^{125}I-labelled anti-γ globulin in the determination of the number of D antigen sites on red cells of different phenotypes. *Vox Sanguinis*, **10**, 675.

Rosenfield R. E., Allen F. H. Jr, Swisher S. N., Kochwa S. (1962). A review of Rh serology and presentation of a new terminology. *Transfusion*, **2**, 287–312.

Sneath J. S., Sneath P. H. A. (1955). Transformation of the Lewis groups of human red cells. *Nature* (Lond.) **176**, 172.

HLA

Bodmer W. F. (1984). The HLA system, 1984. In *Histocompatibility testing* (Eds. E. D. Albert, M. P. Baur and W. R. Mayr). Heidelberg: Springer-Verlag.

Crumpton M. J. (Ed.) (1987). HLA in medicine. *British Medical Bulletin*, **43**, 1–245.

Dausset J., Cohen D. (1984). HLA at the gene level. In *Histocompatibility testing* (Eds. E. D. Albert, M. P. Baur and W. R. Mayr). Heidelberg: Springer-Verlag.

Govaerts A., Dausset J. (1984). The major histocompatibility complex of man (HLA system). In *Immunohaematology* (Eds. C. P. Engelfriet, J. J. van Loghem and A. E. G. Kr. von dem Borne). Amsterdam: Elsevier.

Hayry P., Koskimies S. (Eds.) (1987). Proceedings of the 11th International Congress of the Transplantation Society. *Transplantation Proceedings* **19**, (Book 1), 639–902.

White Cell and Platelet Antigens

Aster R. H. (1984). Platelet antigen systems. In *Immunohaematology* (Eds. C. P. Engelfriet, J. J. van Loghem and A. E. G. Kr. von dem Borne). Amsterdam: Elsevier.

Lalezari P. (1984). Granulocyte antigen systems. In *Immunohaematology* (Eds. C. P. Engelfriet, J. J. van Loghem and A. E. G. Kr. von dem Borne). Amsterdam: Elsevier.

Protein Antigens

Giblett E. (1969). *Genetic markers in human blood*. Oxford: Blackwell Scientific Publications.

Van Loghem E. (1984). Genetic markers of immunoglobulins. In *Immunohaematology* (Eds. C. P. Engelfriet, J. J. van Loghem and A. E. G. Kr. von dem Borne). Amsterdam: Elsevier.

Polyagglutinability

Bird G. W. G. (1981). Lectins and polyagglutination. In *Clinical practice of blood transfusion* (Eds. L. D. Petz and S. N. Swisher). New York: Churchill Livingstone.

Chapter 10

CLINICAL BLOOD TRANSFUSION

MARCELA CONTRERAS AND PATRICIA HEWITT

In this chapter, some of the special problems involved in transfusing patients are considered. Aspects of blood donation and collection are discussed first, and subsequent sections deal with preparation, storage and use of blood components. Pretransfusion testing of the recipient's blood is covered next, followed by complications of blood transfusion. The chapter ends with a description of haemolytic disease of the newborn (HDN).

THE BLOOD DONOR

'Blood donation shall in all circumstances be voluntary . . . financial profit must never be a motive for the donor or for those collecting the donation.'

These statements sum up the attitude of the World Health Organization and the International Society of Blood Transfusion towards the principle of blood donation.

In general, blood donation should be by healthy adults between the ages of 18 and 65. These age limits may vary slightly worldwide, but the lower is set to take account of the high iron requirements of adolescence. The upper limit is necessary because over that age there is an increase in medical conditions which might make blood donation more hazardous, or in the probability of coincidental accidents which may be attributed to the act of giving blood. Pregnant and lactating women are not accepted as donors, again because of high iron requirements.

Measures to Protect the Donor

Volume of Blood Taken

Modern blood collection packs are designed to hold 450 ml $\pm$ 45 ml of blood, mixed with 63 ml of anticoagulant. The ratio of anticoagulant to blood must be maintained at the optimal level (1:7), and donations of less than 405 ml or more than 495 ml of blood should not be issued for clinical use. Healthy donors can generally withstand the loss of 450 ml of blood without any ill-effect, but those who weigh less than 105–110 1b (47.5–50 kg) are more likely to faint, as this amount represents a greater proportion of the total blood volume. Thus 'underweight', otherwise healthy, donors should not give full blood donations but may donate 250 ml of blood into specially designed 'paedipacks', containing the appropriate volume of anticoagulant.

Haemoglobin Estimation

A donation of 450 ml of blood contains approximately 200 mg of iron, which is lost to the body. All donors are tested before donation to exclude anaemia. A convenient method, widely used, depends upon the specific gravity of a drop of blood (taken by means of a finger prick). An estimate of the Hb value can be made depending upon whether the drop of blood sinks in a copper sulphate solution of known specific gravity. A solution of specific gravity 1.055 approximates to a Hb level of 135 g/l (the standard for male donors); the equivalent for females is 1.053 (Hb of 125 g/l). This method tends to underestimate the Hb value and may lead to unnecessary rejection of donors. On the other hand, the specific gravity of whole blood does not solely depend upon the Hb content of red cells, and a pathological rise in plasma protein level or total white cell count (e.g. myeloma, chronic myeloid leukaemia) may lead to an anaemic donor passing the Hb test. Some transfusion centres use an additional method of Hb determination for donors who fail the $CuSO_4$ test; a relatively inexpensive portable haemoglobinometer can reduce the number of unnecessary rejections by up to 30%.

Donation Intervals

In general, donors are not bled more often than twice a year (unless the red cells are replaced) so that iron stores are not reduced. Studies have shown depletion of iron stores in those who give three or four donations per year, but that iron deficiency anaemia is uncommon except in female donors of child-bearing age. For this reason, donation intervals of 6 months are standard in the United Kingdom, but some donors are able to donate more frequently without any significant iron depletion. When it is standard practice to take donations at intervals shorter than 6 months, it is recommended that iron supplements are given.

Hazards of Blood Donation

The most common hazards of blood donation are fainting and venous spasm. Fainting is reported in between 2% and 5% of all donors but is especially common in young people and in those donating for the first time, particularly if nervous or apprehensive. A sympathetic approach by transfusion centre staff, enforcement of an adequate rest period, and constant vigilance to detect warning signs of an impending vasovagal attack can help avert this problem. Once a faint occurs, standard treatment of rest in a horizontal position and elevation of the legs is usually sufficient. Delayed faints occurring after a donor has left the clinic are potentially hazardous and a contraindication to further donations. Infection of the venepuncture site should be avoided by meticulous attention to skin cleansing and aseptic techniques. All blood collection packs are manufactured as integral sets, each needle is sterile and used only once. No pack should be re-used (even on the same donor) if the initial venepuncture attempt fails. Bruising of the arm may occur, particularly where a donation has been difficult; firm pressure over the site and explanation to the donor are usually sufficient. In the very rare event of arterial puncture, elevation of the limb and firm pressure over the site should be combined with prolonged rest if a whole donation has been taken,

as the rate of blood donation under such circumstances is usually very rapid.

Measures to Protect the Recipient

A number of diseases have the potential to be transmitted by transfusion of blood or its components. Donor selection criteria and subsequent testing of all donations are designed to prevent such transmission.

Hepatitis

Hepatitis A is rarely transmitted by transfusion. Any donor who has been in contact with a case or who develops hepatitis A is deferred for 6 months.

Hepatitis B was formerly a frequent sequel to blood transfusion and the most common cause of death post-transfusion. Currently, all blood donations are tested for the presence of hepatitis B surface antigen (HBsAg) by very sensitive third-generation techniques able to detect at least 1 ng of HBsAg per ml of serum (e.g. RIA, ELISA). These techniques take a few hours to perform; for emergencies there are other rapid, slightly less sensitive techniques such as reverse passive haemagglutination (RPHA).

When serum from an individual with hepatitis B virus (HBV) is ultracentrifuged and examined with the electron microscope, three main types of particle are seen. The large (about 42 nm diameter) Dane particles are the actual virus. A central nucleocapsid core has its own antigenic specificity, HBc. The core contains double-stranded DNA and DNA polymerase, and is surrounded by a lipoprotein coat carrying the surface antigen (HBs). The other two types of particles are 20-nm rods and spheres and represent overproduction of surface antigen material. The HBe antigen is in soluble form and is present in the incubation period, during acute infection, and during the first years of the carrier phase. HBe is a marker of infectivity.

Individuals with a history of jaundice may be accepted as donors one year after the illness. Effective screening for HBsAg is available and donors with a past history of jaundice are no more likely than the general population to have markers of past hepatitis B infection. In addition, clinical jaundice may be due to causes other than hepatitis B, therefore there is no sense in rejecting all people who give a history of clinical jaundice. The majority of donors who are positive for HBsAg have no such history, and prior to 1984 predominantly belonged to two groups: (1) young male homosexuals, and (2) donors from areas endemic for hepatitis B infection (the Mediterranean, Africa, Near East and Far East). The former group has been virtually eliminated from donor panels by aggressive publicity and donor education (see below—HIV infection). The incidence of HBsAg in first-time blood donors in London was approximately 1 in 500 (1 in 1000 in other parts of the UK) before rigorous publicity aimed at excluding donors in groups at risk for HIV infection. It is now much lower. The rate in established donors (i.e. new infections) has also decreased from the previous pre-existing very low figure of 1 in 40 000.

Although the transmission of HBV by blood and blood components has been virtually eliminated, it is not possible to exclude all donors capable of transmitting the hepatitis B virus, as the sensitivity of presently available techniques may allow as many as 10^8 HBsAg particles per millilitre to remain undetected. HBsAg-positive subjects are permanently barred from donation, but should be followed up, as they have an increased risk of developing chronic liver disease and hepatoma.

Non-A, non-B (NANB) hepatitis is a common sequel to blood transfusion in the United States. Although apparently much less common in Britain, there is undoubtedly under-reporting of cases. At least two viruses with different incubation periods (short and long) seem to be involved. Some recipients develop clinical hepatitis, but many others manifest only abnormal liver function tests (mainly elevation of ALT) and hence may go undetected. As there is at present no serological marker of NANB hepatitis, this is a diagnosis of exclusion, and other causes of post-transfusion hepatitis, such as cyto-megalovirus (CMV) and Epstein–Barr virus (EBV) infection should be eliminated.

Syphilis

It is mandatory that each donation is tested by a serological test for syphilis. Any donation from an individual giving a positive result is discarded. Although *Treponema pallidum* does not survive well at 4°C, and blood is likely to be non-infective after 4 days refrigeration, storage does not affect the positive serology. The organism is more likely to be transmitted in platelet concentrates, due to their storage conditions and short shelf-life. Subjects with positive tests are permanently debarred from donation, even after effective therapy. Passive transmission of the antibody to a recipient is unacceptable.

Malaria

Malarial parasites remain viable in blood stored at 4°C, and are easily transmitted by blood transfusion. In some endemic areas all recipients are treated with antimalarial drugs. In non-endemic areas there is a real risk of failure to recognize post-transfusion malaria, due to the rarity of the infection. This fact, combined with increasing travel to tropical areas, necessitates the careful vetting of blood donors by direct questioning and, in some centres, by tests for malarial antibodies. Donors who have lived in endemic areas or have had an attack of malaria can be accepted; their fresh plasma is used, but the red cells will not be used. Visitors who have recently travelled to a tropical area are asked to wait 3–6 months after the visit before donating blood.

Cytomegalovirus (CMV)

Post-transfusion cytomegalovirus infection is not uncommon. Most cases are subclinical, but the syndrome of post-transfusion glandular fever-like illness is well recognized, especially after the transfusion of large amounts of fresh blood (e.g. during cardiac surgery). The infection is characterized by fever, splenomegaly, and atypical lymphoid cells in the peripheral blood with a negative Paul–Bunnell test. The usually benign course of cytomegalovirus infection in recipients has meant that, until recently, there has been no necessity to screen donors for evidence of past infection. However, immunosuppressed individuals are at great risk from potentially fatal pneumonitis or disseminated cytomegalovirus infection. Seronegative blood and cellular components should be provided for these recipients. The groups at particular risk are: premature babies weighing < 1500 g, bone marrow transplant recipients, pregnant women (the fetus is at risk). In such cases, if the patient (and the tissue donor) or the mother (in the case of babies) lacks evidence of past CMV infection, then anti-CMV seronegative blood and blood components should be provided. This may produce logistic problems, especially with platelet supplies, as the incidence of antibodies to CMV in the UK adult population is 50–60%. Although only a small number of antibody-positive donors may be capable of transmitting the infection, there is no test for infectivity. Thus the white cells from all seropositive donors should be considered as potentially infectious. Plasma from donors who have high titre anti-CMV can be used for the preparation of CMV immunoglobulin.

HIV (HTLV-III/LAV) Infection

The causative agent of acquired immune deficiency syndrome (AIDS) has been known variously as HTLV-III (human T cell lymphotropic virus type III), ARV (AIDS-associated retrovirus) and LAV (lymphadenopathy-associated virus). It has now been agreed by members of the International Committee on the Taxonomy of Viruses that the virus should be renamed 'human immunodeficiency virus' (HIV), and thus this term will be used throughout. The classical descriptions and the vast majority of the literature on AIDS refer to HIV-1; recently, a second retrovirus capable of causing AIDS and named HIV-2 has been described, mainly in West Africa.

It is now accepted that HIV can be transmitted both in cellular and plasma components. Of the recipients of blood or blood products, those who have the highest probability of infection have been transfused with unheated, non-pasteurized pooled plasma products. Thus HIV infection has become an important sequel to transfusion of Factor VIII concentrates to haemophiliacs. In a pattern not unlike that of hepatitis B and NANB, frequently transfused haemophiliacs have become infected by transfusion of concentrates prepared from pools of plasma contaminated by HIV. A proportion of these recipients have developed AIDS and died; others have various manifestations of HIV infection

(lymphadenopathy, immune thrombocytopenia, haemolytic anaemia, neuropathy) and the remainder are asymptomatic. In contrast to the hepatitis B and NANB viruses, HIV is heat labile, especially when in solution, and prolonged heat treatment of Factor VIII concentrates appears to be an effective means of protecting haemophiliacs from infection —although too late for the majority who were receiving regular Factor VIII therapy in the late 1970s and early 1980s.

Albumin solutions are pasteurized, and carry no risk of HIV transmission. Similarly, intramuscular immunoglobulin preparations are rendered safe from HIV infectivity by the manufacturing process.

Blood and all fresh blood components (platelets, white cells, single donor plasma, fresh frozen plasma and cryoprecipitate) are capable of transmitting HIV. When this risk became apparent in 1982/83, blood transfusion services throughout the Western world began issuing information for donors, including the advice that certain groups of individuals were recognized to be 'at risk' of HIV infection, and should therefore cease blood donation. These include male homosexuals and bisexuals, intravenous drug abusers and prostitutes. The sexual partners of these individuals and of haemophiliacs treated with blood products should also be excluded. In addition, large areas of sub-Saharan Africa have a high incidence of HIV seropositivity and AIDS in the general population, and natives from these areas and their partners should also be considered 'high risk'. Donor education and encouragement of those in high-risk groups to self-exclude themselves from blood donation are highly cost-effective in the prevention of transmission of HIV infection by blood transfusion.

In most HIV-infected subjects, antibody develops within 1–2 months and it coexists with the virus thereafter. Hence, HIV seropositivity is an indicator of infectivity. During 1985, tests became available which allowed screening of blood donations for the presence of antibody to HIV. The tests which lend themselves most readily to the rapid mass screening required in blood transfusion are all based on an enzyme-linked immunosorbent assay (ELISA), using either a competitive or an antiglobulin technique, and examples of each are currently being used in British blood transfusion centres. Particle agglutination tests look promising. As many of the commercially available kits have some false positive reactions, due mainly to cross-reactivity, confirmatory tests using alternative methodology should be employed before a positive result is reported.

Routine screening of all blood donations came into practice in the UK in October 1985. Combined with the well-established donor education and self-deferral scheme, this screening has reduced the already small risk of the transfusion of a contaminated donation even further. At the time of writing, the number of cases of AIDS due to transfusion of blood or fresh blood components from British donors is three. These were all transmitted before anti-HIV screening came into practice. There are more cases of seroconversion to anti-HIV positivity in recipients of blood or blood components and the number of transfusion-related cases of AIDS is likely to increase (because of the possible long incubation period between infection with HIV and symptoms of illness) before the benefit of routine screening of blood donations is seen. In addition, more examples of asymptomatic 'carriers' are likely to be identified through follow-up of previous recipients of blood from donors now identified as seropositive by screening. The incidence of HIV antibodies in British blood donors is less than 1 in 50 000, and there is no doubt that aggressive donor education has contributed to this very low rate by excluding high-risk groups.

Other Diseases

There are no other protozoal or microbiological diseases which can be screened for and which cause problems in the context of blood transfusion in Britain, although diseases such as Chagas' can cause significant problems for the blood transfusion services in other countries.

Other Unsuitable Donors

As donors should be fit, healthy individuals, no donations should be accepted from those who have ever suffered from cancer, diabetes, heart or kidney disease. Those with severe allergic disorders should not give blood because recipients may develop temporary hypersensitivity reactions due to passively transfused antibodies.

Minor Red Cell Abnormalities

Donors with minor red cell abnormalities such as thalassaemia trait, sickle cell trait and hereditary spherocytosis, are perfectly acceptable providing that the Hb screening test excludes anaemia. Red cells containing HbS have a limited survival under conditions of reduced oxygen tension and should not be transfused to newborn infants and patients with hypoxia or sickle cell disease. Blood from donors with G6PD deficiency survives normally unless the recipient is given oxidant drugs.

Laboratory Tests on Blood Donors

Laboratory tests are performed on pilot tubes taken at the time of donation, to avoid entering the sterile blood pack.

All blood donors are tested at each donation for syphilis, HBsAg and anti-HIV. ABO and Rhesus (D) grouping is determined routinely on each occasion. Where large numbers of donor samples are tested daily, blood grouping is automated. In England and Wales, blood that is Rh(D) negative is further tested with anti-C and anti-E, and only blood which is C, D and E negative (i.e. Rh phenotype cde/cde) is labelled Rh negative. There are strong arguments for abandoning this practice (as has already been done in some transfusion centres) as C and E are weakly immunogenic in the absence of D, and these antigens are not taken into account when selecting blood for Rh(D)-positive individuals who are C or E negative. It is thus inconsistent to take account of C and E antigens for Rh(D)-negative recipients.

All donations should also be tested for the presence of potent atypical red cell alloantibodies, against at least two group O red cells selected to represent all the most common blood group antigens. The incidence of clinically significant red cell alloantibodies in blood donors is very low (0.3%) compared with the incidence in potential recipients (1.5–2%). Donations with potent alloantibodies should not be issued to hospitals. Group O blood for emergency or 'flying squad' use which may be given to ungrouped recipients should in addition be tested for high titre anti-AB; if present, the blood should be labelled 'for group O recipients only'.

Autotransfusion

Anxiety over transfusion-transmitted infection in general and HIV infection in particular has roused public interest in the subject of autotransfusion. There are three different options for autologous transfusion.

1. *Predeposit*, where blood is taken from the potential recipient in the weeks immediately prior to the planned transfusion (which almost always occurs in relation to surgery) and stored in the liquid state until needed.

2. *Haemodilution*, where blood is taken immediately prior to surgery once the patient has been anaesthetized and reinfused at the end of the operation.

3. *Salvage*, where lost blood is collected and reinfused, often with the use of a mechanical 'cell-saver', during heavy blood loss.

The first alternative (predeposit) is usually implied when the term autotransfusion is used. In theory this is the ideal option for a patient who requires blood transfusion—the infectious complications of transfusion should be totally abolished, as should the immunological problems arising from exposure to foreign antigens. There are, however, a number of factors which reduce the likelihood of autotransfusion being suitable for more than a small proportion of recipients. Firstly, the individual must be fit to donate blood. It is often said that anyone who is considered well enough to undergo an anaesthetic is also fit enough to give blood. However, only a proportion of recipients receive transfusion during surgery, and autotransfusion cannot be an option for those who require transfusion because of chronic anaemia, malignancy, leukaemia, severe blood loss, trauma and many other conditions. Thus autotransfusion is restricted to those adult patients who are likely to need modest (2–4 units) blood replacement during elective surgery and who are sufficiently fit to donate preoperatively. Orthopaedic and gynaecological surgery are two situations most likely to fulfil these requirements. Unfortunately, such surgery cannot always be planned for a definite date some weeks in advance—last-minute cancellations do occur all too often and in those cases the blood could be wasted. Liquid stored blood has a limited shelf-life and it may be logistically very difficult to organize the provision of sufficient blood to coincide with the day of surgery. In an ideal world, every patient having elective surgery would be given in advance a definite date for the operation which would allow the necessary arrangements for the autologous blood to be made. The logistics of provision of autologous blood require that this is a hospital-based procedure (at least in the UK), and already hard-pressed medical and laboratory staff will have extra work and expense in running such a service.

Larger amounts of autologous blood can only be provided if the blood is stored in a frozen state between donation and transfusion. This is an extremely expensive and labour-intensive exercise and there are few who would consider that this approach can be justified in view of the many other financial pressures on the National Health Service.

In summary, although autotransfusion is the best form of transfusion, it is likely to prove an expensive option that will benefit only a small proportion of recipients of blood.

The practice of storing autologous blood in the frozen state for the 'eventuality of transfusion requirements' in the future is totally contrary to the principles of a National Blood Transfusion Service and should only be justified for those exceptional individuals with rare groups for whom it is impossible to find compatible blood at short notice (e.g. OR_h or Bombay, pp, etc.).

Directed Donations

Donations which are sought by one individual for transfusion to him/herself from named selected donors (usually friends or relatives) are termed directed donations. In the United States, and to the lesser degree the UK, demands or requests for directed donations have been made in the wake of the AIDS publicity. Such requests are often made by individuals for whom autotransfusion is not possible. Experience in the United States has shown that most requests come from individuals who have never donated blood themselves and neither have their selected donors. There is no evidence to suggest that such donors will be 'safer' than those recruited through the transfusion service. Indeed, the fact that the donor has been 'chosen' by someone to whom he/she is known makes it very difficult for that person to refuse, even if in a 'high-risk' group for HIV infection.

Directed donations completely contravene the ethics of blood transfusion: that blood donation should be anonymous and for altruistic causes. As such, directed donations should be actively discouraged.

THE STORAGE OF BLOOD

When blood is stored in a liquid state there is a progressive loss of viability of the red cells, and of red cell ATP, and depletion of 2,3-diphosphoglycerate (2,3-DPG). Modern anticoagulants used for collection of blood have been developed to attempt to reduce these changes to a minimum.

Anticoagulants and Solutions for Red Cell Preservation

Heparin

This is a very safe anticoagulant, and does not affect the pH of blood, but is only useful for blood that is to be used immediately. On storage, heparin is gradually broken down and the blood clots. In doses of 2250 i.u. per 500 ml of blood, heparin is preferred in some hospitals as the anticoagulant for blood for neonatal cardiac surgery, to avoid the problems of citrate toxicity in small babies. The use of heparinized blood for exchange and intrauterine transfusion has been largely replaced by CPD-A blood, less than 72 hours old.

Acid Citrate Dextrose Solution

Acid citrate dextrose (ACD) solution was introduced as the standard preservative solution for blood during the Second World War. Citrate provides anticoagulation, dextrose provides energy for the synthesis of phosphate compounds (DPG and ATP), and acid reduces the lysis of red cells and subsequent leakage of K^+. The pH of the solution is approximately 5.0, and after admixture the pH of the blood is 6.9–7.0. As ACD is hypotonic, the cells swell and have increased osmotic fragility. The shelf-life for ACD blood was 21 days; it has now been replaced by citrate phosphate dextrose (CPD) and is only used in automated plasmapheresis of donors.

Citrate Phosphate Dextrose Solution

The constituents of citrate phosphate dextrose (CPD) are shown in Table 10.1. CPD contains relatively less citric acid than ACD, is isotonic, and has a pH of 5.6 (pH after mixing with blood is 7.1). The pH of blood stored in CPD falls less than in ACD; thus 2,3-DPG is better maintained (falling to 25–35% of the original level after 3 weeks' storage). Post-transfusion survival of red cells stored in CPD solution is slightly better than that of ACD-stored cells, and the shelf-life can be extended to 28 days.

Citrate Phosphate Dextrose Adenine (CPD-A) Solution

The addition of 'rejuvenating' agents or purine nucleosides (adenosine, inosine) to standard anticoagulant solutions has been shown to improve the viability of red cells significantly. Adenosine is effective in restoring the ATP content of stored red cells; inosine restores the 2,3-DPG content. Adenosine is potentially toxic, although rapidly deaminated to inosine in the circulation. Inosine catabolism can raise serum uric acid levels. Hence, neither compound is used in routine practice, but adenine has been found to have a beneficial effect similar to that of adenosine, without its side-effects. CPD-A solution has a final concentration of 0.25 mmol/l adenine and a slightly higher dextrose content than standard CPD. Red cell viability is well maintained for up to 5 weeks (see Table 10.1).

Optimal Additive Solutions (OAS)

Optimal additive solutions (OAS) have been developed to improve the viability of plasma-depleted red cells on storage, by maintaining both ATP and 2,3-DPG levels. Saline adenine glucose mannitol (SAG-M and ADSOL) medium has been shown to provide good red cell storage conditions and is increasingly being introduced in Britain. A multiple blood collection pack is used. The blood donation is taken into the main pack which contains standard CPD anticoagulant. Plasma or platelet-rich plasma

Table 10.1.

Anticoagulant solutions for red cell preservation

	CPD	CPD-A1
Citric acid (monohydrate)	3.27 g	3.27 g
Trisodium citrate (dihydrate)	26.3 g	26.3 g
$NaH_2PO4.H_2O$	2.22 g	2.22 g
Dextrose	25.5 g	31.9 g
Adenine	—	0.275 g
Water to	1000 ml	1000 ml
pH of solution	5.6–5.8	5.95
Volume per 450 ml of blood	63 ml	63 ml
Shelf-life of red cells	21–28 days	35 days
2,3-DPG level at 1 week	Normal	Normal

CPD, citrate phosphate dextrose solution; CPD-A1, citrate phosphate dextrose adenine solution.

is transferred into an empty satellite pack; the latter is further separated into plasma and platelets; 100 ml of SAG-M medium, contained in another satellite pack, is added to the packed red cells (i.e. in a closed system). The resulting red cells have flow characteristics equivalent to plasma-reduced blood, and a storage life of 35 days. Using this method, maximal amounts of plasma can be removed from blood donations for the manufacture of Factor VIII and albumin, thus helping to meet the self-sufficiency targets for plasma products. At the same time, both platelets and an improved red cell product can be obtained.

Storage Changes of Blood

Loss of red cell viability is the most important practical consideration. Progressive loss of viability varies according to the anticoagulant used, and the time limit for storage of blood is set taking this into consideration. After transfusion of stored red cells, a proportion is removed from the circulation within the first 24 hours. The remainder appear to survive normally. With increased length of storage, a greater proportion of red cells is removed within the first 24 hours. The destruction at 24 hours of more than 30% of the total number of cells transfused is considered unacceptable.

Depletion of ATP is progressive during storage of red cells, leading to changes in red cell shape (discs to spheres), loss of membrane lipid, and increased rigidity. These changes can be partially reversed by incubation with purine nucleosides, and reduced by addition of adenine at the time of collection. ATP seems to be an important determinant of red cell viability, though not the only one.

Reduction in 2,3-DPG during storage is less severe in CPD blood than ACD blood, and DPG levels are normal in CPD and CPD-A1 blood at 1 week. Reduced red cell DPG levels increase the oxygen affinity of Hb, and the oxygen dissociation curve is shifted to the left. Thus, less oxygen is given up to the tissues, until the red cell 2,3-DPG level is restored to normal approximately 24 hours after transfusion. The clinical significance of the low DPG level of stored red cells is only likely to be an important consideration in recipients with severe anaemia or coronary artery insufficiency. Even in massive transfusion of stored blood, depletion of red cell DPG can probably be well tolerated if cardiac function is satisfactory.

Electrolyte changes are the result of equilibration of sodium and potassium levels across the cell membrane once active transport has been halted by the cooling of blood to 4°C. There is rapid restoration of levels after transfusion.

The pH of blood decreases rapidly with storage, but most recipients can cope with the acid load during transfusion without ill-effect.

Frozen Red Cells

Red cells can be stored for a prolonged period without damage if glycerol is added before freezing. Thawed red cells must be washed free of glycerol before transfusion. This method of storage is expensive and time consuming but is invaluable as a means of storing rare blood (banks for frozen rare cells have been established for this purpose). In addition, freezing, thawing and washing is an efficient way of removing plasma, platelets, and leucocytes from red cells (see p. 285).

BLOOD COMPONENTS (Fig. 10.1)

Platelet Concentrates

Platelets do not survive well in stored blood. For all practical purposes, there are no viable platelets remaining in blood stored for 48 hours at 4°C. Blood donations should be kept at room temperature after collection and platelets separated as soon as possible. Each single-donor platelet concentrate should contain a minimum of 5.5×10^{10} platelets resuspended in 50 ml of plasma. Although function is maintained when platelet concentrates are stored at 4°C, post-transfusion survival is poor, and any haemostatic effect is short-lived. Storage at 20–22°C is therefore preferred. Platelets prepared in conventional blood packs have a shelf-life of 72 hours which can be extended to 5–7 days with new plastics used in 'extended storage' platelet packs. These allow the diffusion of oxygen into the pack, which, in combination with constant gentle agitation and the suspension in 50 ml of plasma, reduces the rate of fall of pH.

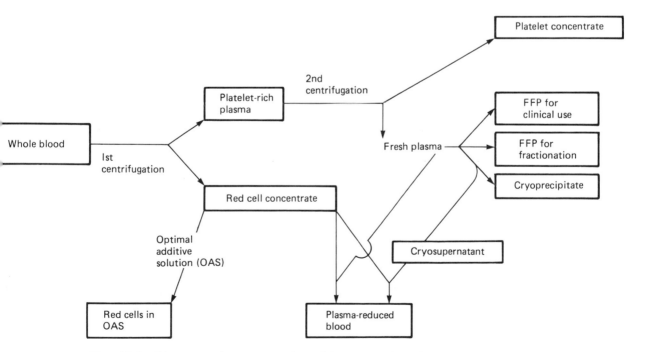

Fig. 10.1. *Diagrammatic representation of the preparation of components from whole blood. Items in boxes represent final components. (FFP = fresh frozen plasma.)*

A larger number of platelets, equivalent to 5–6 single-unit concentrates, may be obtained from one donor by an apheresis procedure lasting approximately 2 hours. These concentrates are invaluable for the treatment of refractory thrombocytopenic patients requiring HLA-matched platelets. However, they are expensive to produce and extremely demanding on both staff and donors. A large HLA-typed donor panel is needed in order to provide HLA-compatible platelets.

Frozen platelets can be preserved in dimethyl sulphoxide (DMSO) or glycerol. The platelet recovery is lower than with fresh preparations but the post-transfusion survival is normal.

Granulocyte Concentrates

Granulocytes are extremely labile; they must be separated from whole blood immediately after collection and transfused within hours of preparation. Granulocytes prepared from routine blood donations (buffy coats) are heavily contaminated with red cells, and the number of concentrates required to produce a therapeutic dose (at least 1×10^{10} granulocytes) for an adult make this technique impractical as a routine procedure. Preparation of granulocyte concentrates by apheresis is the only satisfactory means of achieving a therapeutic dose for an adult neutropenic patient. Sedimenting agents (gelatin, HES) and/or steroids must be added to the blood or given to the donor in order to obtain an adequate yield, unless the donor has chronic myeloid leukaemia.

Fresh Frozen Plasma

This plasma has been separated from red cells within 6 hours of blood collection, and immediately frozen. A longer delay leads to reduction of the labile Factors V and VIII. The fresh frozen plasma (FFP) contains all coagulation factors, and should be stored at $-30\,^{\circ}\mathrm{C}$ or below for up to 12 months. When needed, the plasma is thawed rapidly at $37\,^{\circ}\mathrm{C}$ and should then be transfused without delay.

Single Donor Plasma/Cryoprecipitate Poor Plasma (Cryosupernatant)

The former term refers to plasma separated from whole blood at any time after 18 hours of donation. The latter term is used for the remaining plasma after the removal of cryoprecipitate. Both these components lack the labile coagulation factors but may be used interchangeably with FFP in most instances. They should be stored, refrigerated, for 5 days, or frozen at $-30\,^{\circ}\mathrm{C}$ or below for up to 12 months.

Cryoprecipitate

Cryoprecipitate is prepared from blood within 6 hours of collection. Plasma is separated, frozen, and allowed to thaw (classically, at $4\,^{\circ}\mathrm{C}$, overnight). The Factor VIII and fibrinogen are left as a precipitate which is then refrozen with approximately 15 ml of plasma, and stored at $-30\,^{\circ}\mathrm{C}$ or below for up to 12 months. Each unit should contain a minimum of 80 i.u. of factor VIIIC. In addition, there is approximately 150 mg or more of fibrinogen, together with fibronectin, von Willebrand's factor and some Factor XIII in each concentrate. When needed, cryoprecipitate is thawed at $37\,^{\circ}\mathrm{C}$; several single donations are pooled, and administered to the patient without delay.

THE RECIPIENT

Laboratory Tests

Group and Screen

The ABO and Rh(D) group of all potential recipients should be determined before transfusion. No other blood groups are routinely tested or matched for when selecting blood for transfusion. The need for blood is rarely so urgent that there is insufficient time to determine the ABO and RhD group before transfusion. Rapid testing need only take 5–10 minutes.

The patient's serum should also be tested for the presence of atypical red cell antibodies, using at least two individual (not pooled) group O red cells selected to represent, between them, all the common red cell antigens. At least two sensitive techniques should be used: an indirect antiglobulin test (IAGT) and an enzyme method and/or a polybrene technique. If a positive result is obtained, further investigation using a red cell panel to identify the antibody is required.

If red cell grouping and antibody screening are performed routinely when the patient is seen in the out-patient department (in the case of planned surgery), or as soon as surgery is contemplated, then the last-minute problems caused by incompatibilities first detected on a crossmatch procedure can largely be avoided. The advantages to both potential recipients and laboratory staff are obvious, especially when there is a previous history of pregnancy or transfusions. Only a small proportion (1–1.5%) of potential recipients will have clinically significant red cell alloantibodies other than anti-D. However, routine pretransfusion antibody screening will allow blood bank staff to identify those samples which need detailed investigation well in advance of the planned transfusion.

Blood for transfusion is selected to be of the same ABO and RhD groups as the recipient. If a clinically significant red cell alloantibody/ies is present in the recipient, units of blood lacking the relevant antigen/s are selected.

Compatibility Testing (Crossmatch)

The donor red cells are routinely tested against the recipient serum in order to detect any potential incompatibilities. The crossmatch will provide a means of checking the ABO compatibility of donor and recipient. If an antibody screen has been performed, then the crossmatch should be as simple as possible and two techniques will suffice (saline immediate spin and IAGT) in order to cover clerical or technical errors. The antiglobulin test can be performed in a medium of saline, albumin or low ionic strength solution (LISS). The last-mentioned decreases the incubation time and increases the sensitivity for some antibodies. It is pointless to carry out tests at room temperature, as clinically insignificant cold antibodies will be detected, especially when LISS or albumin is used. The detection of such antibodies often causes much confusion and inconvenience to the recipient (cancellation of planned surgery). Any clinically significant antibody will react at 37°C, and the techniques chosen should take this into account.

The adoption of a group and screen policy can reduce the number of compatibility tests performed if used in combination with a blood-ordering policy. Each hospital blood bank should have its own list based on a retrospective comparison of units of blood crossmatched and used for each elective surgical procedure. All patients expected to undergo surgery have blood samples taken for grouping and antibody screening. If no atypical alloantibodies are detected, routine compatibility testing is reserved for those cases where the need for blood is fairly certain. Operations where blood requirement is unusual (such as hysterectomy and cholecystectomy) are not covered by crossmatched blood. If blood is unexpectedly needed, an abbreviated crossmatch (using an immediate spin technique to ensure ABO compatibility) may safely be employed with minimal risk to the recipient. When atypical antibodies have been detected, antigen-negative blood should be crossmatched prior to surgery even if the surgical procedure is unlikely to require blood.

Antenatal Testing

All women should have blood samples taken at booking and at 28 weeks gestation for blood grouping and antibody screening (see p. 278). Much of the emergency compatibility testing for possible caesarean sections and exchange transfusions can be avoided by antibody screening near term.

Repeated Transfusions

For patients requiring repeated transfusions with an interval of more than 48 hours, fresh blood samples should always be tested. A clinically significant antibody may be stimulated in an anamnestic response by the recent transfusion, and will not be detected unless fresh samples are tested. Severe haemolytic transfusion reactions due to failure to observe this simple rule still occur, and many could be avoided. A direct antiglobulin test should also be performed on the red cells of the fresh sample to detect any alloantibodies attached to donor red cells and not free in the serum.

Massive Transfusion

When the total blood volume has been replaced within a short period (24 hours or less), compatibility testing becomes academic. In such cases the most likely problem is interdonor incompatibility, but all donor sera should have been screened at the transfusion centre for the presence of potent atypical antibodies. When a pretransfusion antibody screen on the recipient has failed to detect the presence of atypical antibodies and a number of units of blood have been crossmatched without problem, then compatibility testing may be omitted, apart from the immediate spin check on ABO compatibility (for possible labelling errors). If a pretransfusion screen reveals the presence of an atypical antibody, the blood selected should be negative for the relevant antigen. Once transfusion has commenced, the antibody may be 'diluted out' and compatibility testing may no longer be reliable, unless the original serum sample is used for all testing.

Transfusion in Autoimmune Haemolytic Anaemia

Ideally, patients with autoimmune haemolytic anaemia (AIHA) should not be transfused since it is difficult, and often impossible, to provide compatible blood and the allogeneic stimulus of blood transfusion often enhances autoantibody formation. In most cases the benefits expected of a transfusion will be short-lived since donor cells will usually be affected as much as the patient's own red cells by the autoantibodies. The adverse effects of any additional haemoglobinuria and haemoglobinaemia secondary to the haemolysis of donor cells must be considered by the clinician when deciding to transfuse. However, if transfusion is imperative for patients with a history of past transfusions or pregnancies, special serological techniques should be used to exclude the presence of alloantibodies which may be masked by autoantibodies.

Patients with cold-type AIHA seldom require blood transfusion, and when they do it is not difficult to find compatible units of blood provided all tests are done at 37 °C. On the other hand, in patients with warm-type AIHA, it is sometimes difficult to type the cells and all units crossmatched are frequently incompatible by standard serological techniques. If the patient's cells are heavily coated with Ig and/or complement, it will be necessary to elute by heat or ZZAP (DTT plus a proteolytic enzyme) before typing the cells with saline-reacting reagents.

In the absence of a recent transfusion within the last 3 months, several methods are available for the detection of alloantibodies in patients with a past history of transfusions or pregnancies. (1) Titration of the serum against a fully typed red cell panel: differences in reactivity of the serum against different panel cells suggest the presence of an alloantibody. (2) Autoabsorption of the patient's serum using the patient's own cells after the antibody coating them in vivo has been eluted by heat or chemical reagents. Once the autoantibody has been absorbed, any underlying alloantibody can be detected with the aid of a red cell panel. Crossmatching should be performed with the autoabsorbed serum. (3) Differential or selective alloabsorption using three cells of known Rh phenotype (R_1R_1, R_2R_2 and rr) and negative between them for the most immunogenic red cell antigens. The absorbed sera are then tested against a panel to detect any possible residual alloantibody and they are also used for crossmatching.

The autoabsorbed serum can then be tested for the presence of underlying alloantibodies and used for crossmatching. If the autoantibody appears to have specificity for a particular red cell antigen (for example, one of the Rh antigens), then antigen-negative blood should be selected for crossmatching. On occasions, the autoantibody may not be totally removed by repeated autoabsorptions and it may be necessary to transfuse blood which cannot be shown to be totally compatible in vitro; in such cases the donor red cells should at least be as compatible as the recipient's own.

COMPLICATIONS OF BLOOD TRANSFUSION

The frequency of the complications of blood transfusion will vary inversely with the care exercised in the preparation for, and the supervision of, the transfusion.

Although the majority of side-effects are mild, the overall incidence of complications is estimated at 2–5%. Fatalities (although difficult to quantify accurately) are not unknown and are mainly due to failure to identify the donor or recipient correctly. It follows that transfusions of blood and blood components should only be prescribed when there is a definite clinical indication.

Table 10.2
The complications of blood transfusion

Immunological
Sensitization to red cell antigens
Haemolytic transfusion reactions
    Immediate
    Delayed
Reactions due to white cell and platelet antibodies
    Febrile transfusion reactions
    Post-transfusion purpura
Reactions due to plasma protein antibodies
    Urticaria
    Anaphylaxis

Non-immunological
Transmission of disease
Reactions due to bacterial pyrogens and bacteria
Circulatory overload
Thrombophlebitis
Air embolism
Transfusion haemosiderosis
Complications of massive transfusion

The complications of blood transfusion can be conveniently divided into immunological and non-immunological (Table 10.2).

Immunological Complications

Sensitization to Red Cell Antigens

As only the ABO and RhD antigens are routinely matched in blood transfusion, there is always a possibility of sensitization to other red cell antigens (more likely in multitransfused patients). The consequences may be negligible, but could lead to haemolytic disease of the newborn, difficulty with compatibility testing, and haemolytic transfusion reactions.

Haemolytic Transfusion Reactions

These are the result of premature destruction of red cells—almost always donor red cells destroyed as a consequence of the reaction with immune antibodies in the recipient. Such reactions may occur immediately after the transfusion, or may be delayed for anything up to 2–3 weeks.

Immediate Haemolytic Transfusion Reactions

Destruction of recipient red cells should be avoidable. In practice, the only likely instances are when group O donor blood with high titre anti-A and/or anti-B is transfused to a recipient of group A, B, or AB. Group O blood should not be used routinely for non-O recipients for this reason; furthermore, this practice leads to unnecessary shortages of group O blood. If unavoidable, the group O blood must first be screened for the presence of high-titre anti-A, B and if present that blood should never be used for non-O recipients. In general, ABO-compatible cryoprecipitate, fresh frozen plasma, and platelet transfusions should also be selected for all recipients, but especially for children because of their smaller blood volume.

Destruction of donor red cells is brought about by antibodies in the recipient. This is the most dangerous type of transfusion reaction; it may be fatal, but in all cases it should be avoidable. Very rarely is there a laboratory error where antibodies in the recipient's plasma are not detected (or there is insufficient time to complete an antibody screen or compatibility test). These reactions are usually due to clerical or administrative errors—failure to confirm the identity of the patient when taking samples, mislabelling of the sample of blood, or failure to perform proper checks before transfusing the blood. The serious consequences of such failures emphasize the need for meticulous checks at all stages, and set procedures for checking should always be followed.

Haemolytic antibodies are generally IgM or IgG complement-binding. The binding of such antibodies to antigen on the red cell activates the full complement cascade (see Chapter 8), and lysis of the red cell occurs in the circulation (intravascular haemolysis).

Macrophages in the RE system have receptors for the Fc fragment of IgG1 and IgG3; the binding of IgG-coated cells to these receptors is inhibited by free IgG in plasma. There are no receptors for IgM on macrophages. Red cells sensitized by IgG1 and/or IgG3 antibodies which do not activate the full complement cascade are removed extravascularly (phagocytosis or cytotoxicity) by mononuclear phagocytic cells, predominantly in the red pulp of the spleen where the plasma is largely excluded. On the other hand, cells coated with IgG or IgM antibodies which activate complement up to C3 only, adhere to the C3b receptor on macrophages. The presence of C3b on red cells greatly enhances the extravascular destruction of IgG-coated cells. The binding to C3b receptors is not inhibited by native C3 in plasma, and consequently cells coated with IgG and C3b are destroyed predominantly in the liver, where there are abundant macrophages and a generous blood flow. Some of the C3b-coated cells are destroyed by phagocytosis or cytotoxicity, but a proportion re-enter the circulation coated with C3dg and are resistant to further lysis (Fig. 10.2).

The features of an immediate haemolytic trans-fusion reaction will vary according to a number of factors: whether the red cells are destroyed within the circulation or in the RE system, the strength,

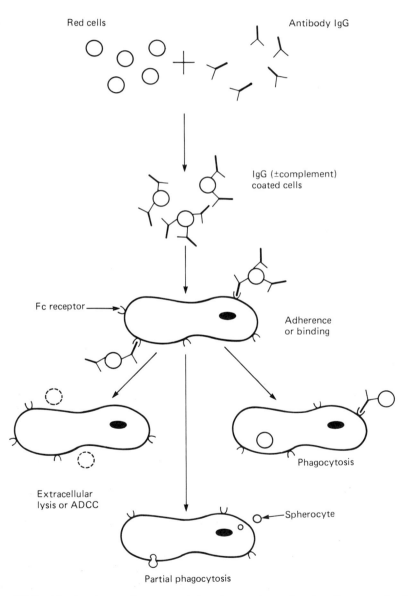

Fig. 10.2. *Mechanisms of extravascular destruction of red cells coated with IgG1 or IgG3 (±C3b)*

class and subclass of antibody, the nature of the antigen, the number of incompatible red cells transfused, and the clinical state of the patient. When antibodies are present in the circulation in low titres and a large volume of incompatible blood is given, all circulating antibody will bind to the incompatible red cells, coating them weakly without destroying them. There will then be no antibody detectable in the serum for a number of days until secondary antibody production is stimulated by the immune challenge. On the other hand, in the presence of an overloaded or poorly functioning RE system, large volumes of sensitized incompatible red cells can be present in the circulation with minimal or no premature removal.

Intravascular red cell destruction is the most dangerous type of haemolytic transfusion reaction; it is associated with activation of the full complement cascade and is practically always due to ABO-incompatible blood transfusions (haemolytic anti-A and/or anti-B present in donor or recipient). The mortality rate in such ABO-incompatible cases is up to 10%. The symptoms in the recipient are usually dramatic and severe, and most are due to anaphylatoxins C3a and C5a liberated during complement activation (see Chapter 8). These molecules cause smooth muscle contraction, platelet aggregation and release of vasoactive amines and hydrolases from mast cells and granulocytes respectively. Typically, within less than 1 hour of the start of the transfusion, the patient complains of heat in the vein, throbbing in the head, flushing of the face, chest tightness, nausea and lumbar pain. These symptoms are usually accompanied by tachycardia and hypotension. In severe cases there is profound hypotension and collapse. Rigors and pyrexia usually follow. These initial symptoms may of course be modified or abolished in anaesthetized or heavily sedated patients. Intravascular destruction of red cells brings about liberation of thromboplastin-like substances which activate the coagulation cascade and lead to disseminated intravascular coagulation (DIC). The bleeding diathesis and increased destruction of red cells (which may eventually involve the recipient's cells) further exacerbate the problem.

Intravascular destruction of red cells liberates haemoglobin into the circulation. Once haptoglobins are saturated, haemoglobin will also appear in the urine. If haemoglobinuria is very severe, haemosiderinuria may be seen. Renal complications consist of acute renal failure with oliguria and anuria, possibly the result of hypotension and/or the action of activated complement. It is no longer accepted that renal failure is directly due to haemoglobinuria.

The above symptoms, with some attenuations, may also be seen occasionally after the transfusion of lysed red cells (overheated, or subject to extreme cold due to poor storage conditions), haemolysis of cells due to mechanical problems during administration, and injection of 5% dextrose with the transfused red cells. Severe fulminant toxic symptoms leading to death can be seen after the transfusion of infected blood. Haemoglobinaemia and haemoglobinuria may also follow transfusion of blood to a patient with active autoimmune haemolysis, due to an increase in the number of red cells in the circulation, which will be subject to the immune process.

Not all ABO-incompatible transfusions lead to severe haemolytic reactions; if the anti-A or anti-B is weak, mild symptoms with no haemoglobinuria are seen.

Immediate extravascular destruction of red cells may be accompanied by hyperbilirubinaemia, occasionally mild haemoglobinaemia (in severe cases), fever, and failure to achieve the expected rise in Hb level. The signs and symptoms are less severe and dramatic than in intravascular haemolysis and usually appear more than 1 hour after the start of transfusion. However, there may be no signs or symptoms of extravascular haemolysis. Renal failure is very rare, even when the antibody binds the earlier components of the complement cascade, but is non-lytic. The mortality is extremely low, but in an already sick patient the added complication of a transfusion reaction may contribute to death.

The diagnosis and management of immediate haemolytic transfusion reactions consist of termination of the transfusion immediately the patient develops signs or symptoms of a haemolytic transfusion reaction. The circulating blood volume should be restored and the blood pressure and urinary flow maintained. Blood samples must be taken for investigation of haemoglobinaemia, bilirubinaemia, full blood count with platelet count, haptoglobins, coagulation studies and serological investigations. The last mentioned should include a direct antiglobulin test, repeat antibody screen and repeat compatibility testing against red cells of all the units transfused (all packs of transfused units should be returned to the blood bank). Pretransfusion samples should be tested in parallel. A sample should be sent for bacteriological testing and all urine passed during the first 24 hours measured and examined for haemoglobin. Subsequent management depends upon awareness of the possible complications, and prompt therapy if these occur. If the patient develops only a rise in temperature unaccompanied by other symptoms, red cell incompatibility is unlikely and the transfusion should be slowed but need not be stopped.

Immediate haemolytic transfusion reactions can always be prevented. They are more often the result of clerical and administrative errors (failure to check labels, to identify the patient correctly, etc.) than of mistakes in laboratory techniques. If such a mistake does occur, the clerical, administrative and technical procedures in blood transfusion must be carefully reviewed.

Delayed Haemolytic Transfusion Reactions

Such reactions are not predictable. In the majority of cases, an individual has been previously sensitized to one (or more) red cell antigen(s) by transfusion or pregnancy. No antibody is detectable in routine pretransfusion testing, but the transfusion of blood containing the antigens to which the recipient has previously been sensitized provokes a brisk anamnestic response characteristic of the secondary immune response. Within days, the antibody level has risen and the transfused cells are removed from the circulation. The peak of the reaction usually occurs within 7–10 days of the transfusion — at a time when the recipient may already have left hospital.

The clinical features of this type of reaction are the triad of fever, hyperbilirubinaemia, and anaemia. The fall in Hb level will of course depend upon the number of transfused red cells carrying the relevant antigen.

The possibility of delayed haemolytic reactions underlines the importance of always taking fresh serum samples for antibody screening and compatibility testing if a transfusion has been given more than 48 hours previously. Awareness of this complication may avoid unnecessary investigations to exclude infection when fever develops after a transfusion.

Reactions Due to White Cell and Platelet Antibodies

Febrile Transfusion Reactions

Febrile reactions, due most frequently to sensitization to granulocyte-specific antigens and more rarely to platelet antigens, are the most common type of immunological reaction to blood transfusion. Antibodies may be directed against HLA antigens or white cell and platelet-specific antigens; they are stimulated by previous transfusions or pregnancies. Characteristically, the onset of the reaction is delayed until 30–90 minutes after the start of the transfusion (depending upon the strength of antibody and the speed of transfusion). A rise in temperature may be the sole symptom, but occasionally the recipient complains of chills or headache and even rigors. There is no associated hypotension, lumbar pain or chest discomfort. These reactions are more usually troublesome than dangerous, except in very sick patients.

The management of a simple, mild febrile transfusion reaction is to slow the rate of transfusion and treat the patient with aspirin (unless the drug is contraindicated). Antihistamines are of no benefit. Although it is usually not necessary to discontinue the transfusion, more blood is probably wasted by premature termination of a transfusion because of a simple febrile reaction than for any other reason.

When a patient requiring repeated transfusions has a history of simple febrile reactions, the simplest measures should be taken first — a slow rate of transfusion and antipyretics. If symptoms recur with repeated transfusions, tests for HLA antibodies (lymphocytotoxicity) and for granulocyte antibodies (leucoagglutinins, immunofluorescence, ELISA, etc.) should be performed. If these are negative, platelet antibodies should be sought. Patients with troublesome symptoms in whom white cell antibodies have been demonstrated should be given white cell-depleted blood. The simplest and cheapest method is centrifugation with removal of the buffy coat layer. This will remove 80–90% of the white cells and will be sufficient for many patients with low-titre antibodies. If symptoms persist, more sophisticated techniques such as filtration of blood through a specific nylon or cotton-wool leucocyte-depletion filter must be applied. If all else fails, frozen-thawed red cells, containing less than 2% of the original white cells, should be administered.

There is no place for prophylactic administration of white-cell-depleted blood, except in cases where prevention of sensitization to HLA/leucocyte/platelet antigens is essential (i.e. possible future consideration for bone marrow transplantation, especially in patients with aplastic anaemia).

Reactions due to passive transfer of leucoagglutinins in donor plasma consist of pulmonary infiltrates of white cells accompanied by chills, fever, cough and dyspnoea. The donors involved are normally multiparous women who should be removed from the donor panel.

Post-transfusion Purpura

Post-transfusion purpura is a rare complication of blood transfusion. Characteristically, there is a sudden onset, 7–10 days after transfusion, of severe thrombocytopenia. The patient always has a history of previous blood transfusions or pregnancies (thus it is far more common in women). The most usual cause is the presence in the recipient of an antibody (anti-Pl^{A1}) against the platelet-specific antigen Pl^{A1}. The patient's platelets type as Pl(A1 negative). It appears that the antigen–antibody reaction between recipient's antibody and donor platelets causes both transfused and autologous platelets to be prematurely destroyed, either by the formation of immune complexes ('innocent bystander' mechanism), or by cross-reaction of the causative antibody with the patient's own platelets. The disease is self-limited, but in severe cases or if bleeding occurs, prompt plasma exchange is the therapy of choice. There have been recent reports of response to high-dose intravenous immunoglobulin.

Reactions Due to Plasma Protein Antibodies

Urticarial and Anaphylactic Reactions

Mild urticarial reactions unaccompanied by other symptoms are not uncommon during blood trans-fusion. Severe anaphylactic reactions accompanied by dyspnoea, wheezing, collapse and shock are rare and potentially fatal. The majority of severe reactions are associated with the presence of anti-IgA in an IgA-deficient recipient. These antibodies react with IgA in the transfused plasma, and complement is activated with the consequent liberation of anaphylatoxins. Milder reactions may be associated with anti-IgA of limited specificity, reaginic antibodies (in donor or recipient) or, rarely, with Gm antibodies. Mild reactions may be treated effectively with antihistamines, and do not always recur. There is no necessity to avoid transfusion of standard 'bank blood' unless symptoms are recurrent and severe. However, if an anaphylactic reaction occurs, the recipient should be examined for the presence of plasma protein antibodies. If anti-IgA is detected, blood and components from IgA-deficient donors should be used. Very rarely, washed cells may be indicated for patients with serious urticarial or severe hypersensitivity reactions due to non-IgA antibodies.

Non-Immunological Complications

Transmission of Infectious Agents

This has been covered earlier in this chapter. The morbidity and mortality caused by the transmission of agents such as hepatitis viruses, HIV, malaria and CMV are at present the major serious complications of blood transfusion.

Reactions Due to Bacterial Pyrogens and Bacteria

The presence of bacteria in transfused blood may lead to either febrile reactions in the recipient (due to pyrogens) or to the far more serious manifestations of transfusion of infected blood.

Bacterial pyrogens are very rarely the cause of reactions with present-day methods of manufacture and sterilization of fluids and disposable equipment. Infection of stored blood is also extremely rare, but leads to a very high mortality rate in recipients. Skin contaminants are not infrequently present in freshly donated blood but these organisms (predominantly staphylococci) do not survive storage at 4°C. However, a number of Gram-negative psychrophilic, endotoxin-producing contaminants found readily in dirt, soil, and faeces (pseudomonads, coliforms) may very rarely enter a unit and grow readily under the storage conditions of blood (and even more rapidly at room temperature). Transfusion of heavily contaminated blood will usually lead to sudden, dramatic symptoms with collapse, high fever, shock, and haemorrhagic phenomena (due to disseminated intravascular coagulation). These symptoms resemble, and are worse than, those of ABO incompatibility. Prompt recognition of the cause and administration of broad-spectrum intravenous antibiotics are vital. The diagnosis should be confirmed by direct microscopic examination of the blood, and blood cultures at 4°C, 20°C and 37°C.

Prevention of this potentially disastrous complication of blood transfusion rests on stringent observation of procedures for aseptic techniques in blood donation (and in the manufacture of anticoagulant solutions and packs). Packs should never be opened for sampling, and the unit should be transfused within 24 hours if any open method of preparation has been used (for example washed red cells, frozen-thawed blood). Blood should always be kept in accurately controlled refrigerators (with alarms) maintained strictly at 2–6°C, and a unit of blood should never be removed and taken to the ward until it is required. The practice of obtaining multiple units of blood for the same patient, and leaving unused units at room temperature (or in uncontrolled ward refrigerators) until needed, must not be tolerated. All units should be inspected for haemolysis and clots before transfusion.

Circulatory Overload

All patients except those who are actively bleeding or fluid depleted will experience a temporary rise in blood volume and venous pressure after the transfusion of blood and/or plasma. In young people with normal cardiovascular function, this will not cause any embarrassment providing the total volume given and the transfusion rate are not excessive. In contrast, pregnant women, patients with severe anaemia, and the elderly with compromised cardiovascular function will not tolerate the increase in plasma volume, and acute pulmonary oedema may develop. In order to reduce this likelihood, concentrated red cells should be given slowly (over 4–6 hours). Patients with severe chronic anaemia and cardiac failure may require partial exchange transfusion. In less severe cases, diuretics (oral or intravenous frusemide) should be given at the start of the transfusion and only one or two units of concentrated red cells should be transfused in any 24-hour period. The patient should be observed carefully for early signs of cardiac failure (raised jugular venous pressure, basal crepitations in the lungs) and symptoms of pulmonary oedema (dry cough and breathlessness). For this reason alone, transfusions should be given during the daytime, when staff are able to monitor the patient closely. Overnight transfusions should be avoided wherever possible for the patient's benefit, let alone that of the staff. If circulatory overload occurs, the transfusion should be discontinued, the patient propped upright and intravenous diuretics given. Emergency venesection for fluid overload should not be necessary if all precautions have been taken.

Thrombophlebitis

Thrombophlebitis is a complication of indwelling venous cannulae, and not specifically related to blood transfusion. Patients who require long-term blood transfusion should have cannulae removed at the earliest opportunity. It is far better to perform a fresh venepuncture each day than to lose a precious peripheral vein from thrombophlebitis.

Air Embolism

This is now practically unknown as blood and blood components are administered in plastic bags.

Transfusion Haemosiderosis

Haemosiderosis is a very real complication of repeated blood transfusions, and is being seen more commonly as long-term blood transfusion therapy improves the survival of patients suffering from previously lethal disorders. It is most commonly seen in thalassaemic individuals who now commence transfusions in early childhood. Each unit of blood has approximately 200 mg of iron, while the daily excretion rate is about 1 mg and the body has no way of excreting the excess. Unless a patient is actively bleeding, and therefore losing iron, iron accumulation is inevitable. It has now become routine to give thalassaemic patients the chelating agent desferrioxamine. This does not completely overcome the iron load administered with blood, but has substantially delayed the onset of problems due to haemosiderosis (see Chapter 2).

Transfusion of neocytes or young red cells looked promising as a means of decreasing the frequency of transfusions and of reducing the iron load. However, this practice is expensive and time consuming and the results have not been as favourable as expected.

Complications of Massive Transfusion

Massive transfusion is usually defined as the replacement of the total blood volume within a 24-hour period. Although a number of different problems may result from changes which occur in stored blood, it should not be forgotten that any patient who needs a massive blood transfusion is by definition already seriously ill. Too much attention may be paid to the theoretical problems caused by metabolic changes in stored blood, and not enough regard of the underlying clinical condition.

Although the transfusion problems encountered in cardiac surgery were in the past similar to those of massive transfusion, the volume of blood transfused to most patients is now insufficient to merit the routine administration of fresh blood or FFP. Where postoperative bleeding occurs, it is usually due to platelet dysfunction and/or reduced numbers. Platelet transfusions are then indicated.

Replacement of the total blood volume will inevitably lead to dilution of platelets. Blood effectively has no functional platelets after 48 hours storage, and once 8–10 units of blood have been given to an adult, thrombocytopenia will usually be seen. This will vary from patient to patient, and bleeding due to a slightly low platelet count will not always occur, so that routine administration of platelets after a set number of units of blood is wasteful practice. Regular monitoring of the platelet count in these situations is far more helpful, and platelet administration may then be judged on the clinical condition and the platelet count.

Although coagulation factors will also be diluted as stored blood is administered, blood that has been stored for less than 14 days has haemostatically adequate levels of all coagulation factors. Factors V and VIII are the most labile, but in conditions of 'stress', Factor VIII is released from endothelial cells so that administration of Factor VIII is not usually necessary in these circumstances. If blood stored for longer than 14 days is given, or if plasma-reduced blood has been used, then replacement of coagulation factors with fresh frozen plasma may become necessary. Treatment should be monitored by coagulation studies, and arbitrary administration of FFP should be discouraged. Disseminated intravascular coagulation (DIC) associated with massive transfusion is most usually due to the underlying condition and prolonged shock, and not due to transfused blood per se. Metabolic changes in stored blood include low pH, hypocalcaemia, and hyperkalaemia. The reduced oxygen-carrying capacity of stored blood becomes significant only after 21 days storage (for CPD-A1 blood), and is due to low 2,3-DPG levels (see p. 276). Although excess citrate in transfused blood could theoretically cause toxicity, metabolism in the liver is usually rapid. In practice, the only situations in which citrate toxicity is a real problem are with extremely rapid transfusion (one unit every 5 minutes) or in infants having exchange transfusion with blood stored in citrate for longer than 72 hours. Hypocalcaemia and hyperkalaemia are usually transient and rapidly corrected once the transfused blood is circulating. Acidosis is not usually significant; citrate metabolism leads to an alkalosis. However, if a patient is severely shocked and undertransfused, acidosis may be a clinical problem. All these changes due to stored blood are exacerbated by hypothermia. Cardiac irregularities, in particular ventricular fibrillation, may result from transfusion of large quantities of cold blood. Thus a blood warmer and keeping the patient warm may be the most important measures to prevent the complications of massive transfusion. Unfortunately this inevitably reduces the speed at which blood can be transfused, which may be a serious disadvantage when rapid transfusion is needed.

The most important consideration in massive blood transfusion is to replace blood loss quickly and adequately. Too little blood too late has far more serious consequences than has massive blood transfusion.

HAEMOLYTIC DISEASE OF THE NEWBORN

Haemolytic disease of the newborn (HDN) is a condition in which the lifespan of the infant's red cells is shortened due to maternal alloantibodies against paternal antigens on the child's erythrocytes. Maternal IgG can pass across the placenta into the fetal circulation, thus IgG red cell alloantibodies can gain access to the fetus. If the fetal red cells contain the corresponding antigen, binding of antibody to red cells will occur. When the antibody is of clinical significance (e.g. anti-Rh, anti-Kell, anti-Jk^a), the coated cells will be prematurely removed by the reticuloendothelial system. The effects on the fetus/newborn may vary, according to the characteristics of the maternal alloantibody.

The IgG antibodies giving rise to HDN most commonly belong to the Rh or ABO blood group systems. The importance of Rh HDN is explained by the great immunogenicity of the D antigen. However, antibodies against antigens in almost all the blood group systems (e.g. Kell, Duffy, Kidd etc.) and against the so-called public and private antigens have been culprits in cases of HDN. On the other hand, Lewis and P_1 antibodies are usually IgM and do not lead to HDN as IgM cannot cross the placenta. Furthermore, the Lewis antigens are not fully developed at birth.

All women who have had previous pregnancies or blood transfusions have had the opportunity to be immunized against foreign red cell antigens, but alloantibodies may be found in those with no such history, either because the antibodies are naturally occurring, or because a spontaneous abortion early in a previous pregnancy has been unrecognized as such. All maternal blood samples must be tested for the presence of atypical red cell antibodies early in pregnancy (usually at the booking visit) and again at 28–32 weeks gestation. Where clinically significant red cell alloantibodies are detected, the strength of the antibody and the rate of rise (if any) of the titre during pregnancy must be carefully monitored by regular blood sampling — monthly during the first two trimesters, and then fortnightly until term.

Haemolytic disease due to anti-D tends to be more severe than that due to any other alloantibody. The next important in terms of frequency and severity is that due to anti-c. Anti-A and anti-B in group O mothers are common causes of HDN (1 to 150 births), but the disease is usually mild, death in utero is unknown, and exchange transfusion after birth is rarely required.

Clinical Features

In its least severe form, HDN causes a mild haemolytic anaemia in the newborn. The infant's red cells, coated with maternal IgG alloantibody, are removed prematurely from the circulation, causing hyperbilirubinaemia (maximal on the second to third days of life) and mild anaemia during the second week of life. More severely affected infants show severe hyperbilirubinaemia in the neonatal period, a condition which was called icterus gravis neonatorum. Unless the jaundice is treated promptly, bilirubin impregnates the basal ganglia and neurological damage occurs — a condition known as kernicterus. This condition may be fatal, or lead to serious neurological deficit with deafness, mental retardation, choreoathetosis and spasticity. In severely affected infants, profound anaemia develops in utero, and intrauterine death may occur at any time from the 18th week of gestation, depending upon the antibody strength. Affected fetuses are pale and oedematous with marked ascites. The placenta is bulky, swollen, and friable. This condition is known as hydrops fetalis, and had a high mortality rate until intrauterine blood transfusion and improved intensive care facilities for very premature babies were introduced.

The blood film of a fetus affected by HDN shows polychromasia and increased numbers of nucleated red cells. In most cases (except a few due to ABO antibodies) the direct antiglobulin (Coombs') test on the infant's cells is positive due to IgG coating.

Rh Haemolytic Disease of the Newborn

Until the early 1970s (when Rh immunoprophylaxis was introduced), 0.5–0.75% of all births gave rise to babies affected by Rh HDN. Anti-D accounted for over 90% of all cases. Although HDN due to anti-D has been reduced significantly, it remains important. The disease due to anti-D is more severe than that due to any other alloantibody (e.g. anti-c, anti-K, anti-E). Of all infants affected by Rh HDN,

10–20% died in utero or in the early neonatal period before effective therapy was possible. Over 50% of affected infants need treatment during the neonatal period. Hence, early detection of maternal alloantibodies and regular assessment of changes of antibody titre are prerequisites for a successful outcome.

Antenatal Assessment of Maternal Blood

Rarely, anti-D may develop in a first pregnancy in a woman who has had no previous transfusions. It is not common for the antibody to reach high levels, and it is not usually detectable before 28 weeks. Conversely, in women who have had previous pregnancies or transfusions, anti-D may be detectable early in pregnancy, and regular monitoring of the level is necessary in order to plan the type and timing of intervention best. At present, the most objective means of quantitating anti-D levels routinely is with the AutoAnalyzer and not by manual titration. The ABO, Rh groups and antibody screen should be performed in all pregnant women at booking. In Rh-negative women and Rh-positive women with no history of transfusion or a prior pregnancy, the testing should be repeated once more at about 28 weeks. Rh-negative women in second or subsequent pregnancies, and all women who have had previous transfusions, should be screened more often—at approximately 28 weeks and 34 weeks.

All Rh-negative women should have their sera retested at term to confirm the Rh group and the absence of immunization to the D antigen. Unsensitized women should be given prophylactic anti-Rh(D) immunoglobulin if the infant is Rh(D) positive.

The strength of any anti-D present in the maternal serum correlates approximately with the clinical severity of the HDN, But this is also affected by factors such as IgG subclass, rate of rise of antibody and past history. As a rough guide, levels below 1.0 i.u./ml (0.2 μg/ml) require no action; whereas a level of 10 i.u./ml (2.0 μg/ml) usually reflects a seriously affected infant, as does a level above 5 i.u./ml (1.0 μg/ml) and rising rapidly. These latter two situations and any history of previously affected infants would be taken as an indication for amniocentesis.

Amniocentesis and Amniotic Fluid Analysis

The severity of the haemolytic process on the fetus may be assessed by ultrasound and by measurement of the bile pigments in the amniotic fluid. Normal amniotic fluid is clear or straw coloured, but becomes bright yellow when the infant is suffering from haemolysis. The quantity of bile pigment is estimated by spectrophotometry. The optical density of normal amniotic fluid over the range of wavelengths 400–600 nm forms a smooth curve when plotted on semi-logarithmic graph paper. The amniotic fluid from an infant suffering from HDN shows a greatly increased optical density with a peak at about 450 nm (Fig. 10.3). The increase in density at this wavelength over the normal optical density is the measurement of severity. In 1961, Liley produced a chart relating the optical density at 450 nm to the length of gestation. This chart is

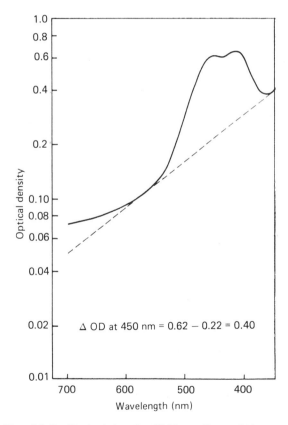

Fig. 10.3. *Optical density (OD) readings of the amniotic fluid from a Rh-immunized woman at the 26th week of pregnancy, plotted on semi-log graph paper.*

divided into three zones. The lowest zone indicates either an RhD-negative or unaffected RhD-positive infant, the midzone a mild/moderately affected infant, and the highest a severely affected infant. Serial measurements are a useful guide to the progress of the disease (Fig. 10.4).

Amniocentesis carries a small risk of immunizing a previously unsensitized RhD-negative woman carrying an RhD-positive fetus, due to leakage of fetal blood into the maternal circulation. Similarly, pre-existing antibody levels may be 'boosted' by a new stimulus to fetal RhD-positive red cells. More rarely, immunization to, or boosting of, other clinically significant red cell alloantibodies may occur. Furthermore, although the risks are small in experienced hands, there are possible adverse effects on the fetus (e.g. puncture of fetal vessels).

Antenatal Maternal Plasma Exchange

Women with high levels of anti-D may be treated, with varying degrees of success, during pregnancy with plasma exchange with the object of decreasing their anti-D levels. Unfortunately, no controlled trials of this form of therapy have been performed.

Intrauterine Transfusion

This method of treatment involves injection of antigen-negative donor red cells into the infant in utero, either into the peritoneal cavity, or directly into the fetal umbilical vessels. Direct intravascular transfusion may be achieved via fetoscopy as early as 18 weeks, and is carried out in very few specialized centres. Intraperitoneal transfusions are usually not technically possible until 24 weeks of gestation. If ascites is already present, absorption of the red cells into the fetal circulation is slow.

The donor blood for intrauterine transfusion is usually group O Rh(D) negative. The blood should be white cell free (to avoid the risk of graft versus host disease), of the desired haematocrit and less than 72 hours old.

Premature Delivery

Modern neonatal intensive care units have dramatically increased survival rates of very premature infants (born at 28–30 weeks gestation). With this increasing success, planned premature delivery is usual for severely affected and moderately affected infants likely to need exchange transfusion.

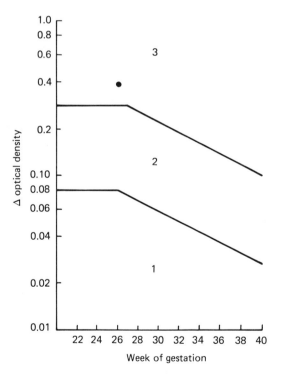

Fig. 10.4. *Graph, according to Liley (1961), adapted for earlier stages of pregnancy, on which the optical density increment can be plotted according to gestational age. There are three areas. An increment falling into area 1 indicates a Rh-negative or unaffected Rh-positive child; an increment falling into area 2 indicates haemolytic disease of intermediate severity; and an increment falling into area 3 indicates a severely affected infant and impending fetal death. The solid dot marks the optical density increment from Fig. 10.3.*

Assessment of Severity in the Newborn

Cord blood samples should be taken at delivery. The direct antiglobulin test (DAGT) will be positive, but is not a useful indication of severity or need for therapy. The best simple criterion of severity is the cord Hb level, and this is much more useful than a sample taken a few hours after birth, when rapid haemodynamic changes are occurring. The normal range of cord Hb is 136–196 g/l; most affected infants with levels in this range do not require exchange transfusion and more than 50% of affected babies have a level in the normal range. The probability of survival diminishes with the fall in cord Hb; where the Hb is below 120 g/l, exchange transfusion will be necessary. It may also be indicated for a rising bilirubin level after birth — dependent upon the rate of rise and the immaturity of the infant. If no exchange transfusion is necessary, phototherapy may be given to reduce the rise in bilirubin levels. Later, 'top-up' transfusions of red cells may be required at 2–3 weeks of age.

The infant's ABO and RhD group should be determined on the cord blood sample. If intrauterine transfusions have been given, the ABO and Rh groups may be those of the donor, and the DAGT may be negative.

Exchange Transfusion

Exchange transfusion is effective therapy for the pathophysiological process underlying HDN, removing both sensitized infant's red cells and plasma with maternal antibody directed against these cells. It also treats the results — anaemia and hyperbilirubinaemia. An exchange transfusion of one total blood volume will replace approximately 75% of the infant's red cells. It is usual to replace relatively large volumes of blood (e.g. 200 ml/kg) in small aliquots via an umbilical vein catheter. The donor blood should be ABO compatible with mother and fetus, and lack the antigen against which the maternal antibody is directed. A compatibility test should be performed against maternal serum. For most infants, CPD-A1 blood less than 72 hours old is adequate.

ABO Haemolytic Disease of the Newborn

In 20% of births a mother is ABO incompatible with her fetus. In A and B subjects the anti-B and anti-A are predominantly IgM, so that problems are usually restricted to group O mothers possessing IgG anti-A,B. In 15% of all pregnancies in Caucasians, a group O mother is carrying a group A or B fetus, but the incidence of ABO HDN requiring treatment is extremely low, and exchange transfusion is rarely necessary (roughly 1 in 3000 infants).

The low incidence of infants requiring treatment for ABO HDN is in contrast with the situation in Rh HDN. Furthermore, ABO HDN is found as frequently in the first pregnancy as in later pregnancies and, conversely, may not affect later pregnancies after a first child has been affected. However, severely affected infants are likely to be followed by severely affected children in subsequent pregnancies. Thus ABO HDN differs significantly from Rh HDN, where a first pregnancy is usually unaffected (unless there has been prior immunization by abortion or transfusion), and where subsequent Rhesus-incompatible infants are affected to an equal degree or more severely. The majority of newborns affected with Rh HDN require some form of therapy. The lack of severity of ABO HDN can be accounted for by the widespread occurrence of A and B antigens, not only on red cells but in plasma and on other cells. Maternal IgG ABO antibodies will be partially neutralized by these extra-erythrocytic antigens. Furthermore, the A and B antigens are not fully developed in the infant. Thus, only small amounts of the maternal antibody are bound to infant red cells, and clinical sequelae are usually mild.

Serological Findings

a) The mother is usually blood group O, and IgG anti-A and anti-B can be demonstrated directly after inactivating or inhibiting the IgM component with a reducing agent (2ME or DTT). Where infants are affected and require therapy, the maternal IgG anti-A or anti-B is almost always present in a titre greater than 64.

b) The infant will be group A or B and the DAGT may be positive, only weakly positive or negative. If a drop of whole blood from the cord is rocked gently on a tile, spontaneous agglutination will be seen in most cases, especially if the cells are suspended in ABO-compatible plasma. Eluates from the red cells will give positive results with suitable adult cells by the IAGT. Examination of the infant's blood film may show spontaneous agglutination of the red cells, spherocytosis (not seen in Rh HDN), reticulocytosis, polychromasia, and increased numbers of nucleated red cells.

Treatment

Severe anaemia is uncommon. Occasionally, hyper-bilirubinaemia may be serious enough to threaten kernicterus, and in this situation exchange trans-fusion is necessary, using group O donor blood with low titre anti-A,B or, ideally, group O red cells suspended in group AB plasma from ABH secretors.

Haemolytic Disease of the Newborn Due to Other Antibodies

The antibodies encountered most commonly are anti-c and anti-K (both usually due to previous maternal blood transfusions). The disease is usually less severe than that caused by anti-D, but assessment and treatment of the infant are along the same lines. If exchange transfusion is required, blood that lacks the appropriate antigen should be given.

Prevention of Haemolytic Disease of the Newborn

The major success in the reduction in the incidence of HDN in the last 15 years is the result of the decrease in cases due to anti-D. Other antibodies now account for a greater relative proportion of total cases. The reduction has been achieved by the routine administration of 500 i.u. (100 μg) anti-RhD immunoglobulin within 72 hours of delivery to all RhD-negative mothers of RhD-positive infants. Extra doses of 125 i.u. (25 μg) per additional millilitre of red cells may be required for the small number of women (<1%) who experience a trans-placental bleed greater than that covered by the standard dose (4 ml of packed cells). It is critical that a Kleihauer acid-elution test for detection and quantitation of fetal red cells is performed on a maternal blood sample taken after delivery. Failure of protection may be due to insufficient dose, failure to administer the dose (e.g. early discharge), or rare cases where primary immunization has already occurred during the pregnancy. Anti-Rh(D) immunoglobulin is also indicated after abortion or miscarriage (a dose of 250 i.u. is sufficient for gestations up to 20 weeks) and all procedures which might lead to a transplacental bleed (amniocentesis, external version, threatened miscarriage, chorionic villus sampling). Despite prophylaxis, new cases of

sensitization to the D antigen still occur. Some may be due to an early unrecognized abortion, some to clerical and administrative errors (incorrect grouping of mother or child, or errors in the recording of groups), and most are now due to immunization during pregnancy. Approximately 0.8% of Rh-negative women carrying an Rh-positive fetus experience primary Rh immunization during pregnancy. In order to reduce the number of cases further, anti-RhD immunoglobulin should be given during pregnancy (usually 500 i.u. at 28 and 34 weeks) to all RhD-negative women without any live children. This antenatal prophylaxis would significantly reduce a small incidence of new cases of anti-D in women to a smaller level, but, on the current figures, will not totally eliminate the problem.

SELECTED BIBLIOGRAPHY

Barbara J. A. J. (1983). *Microbiology in blood transfusion.* Bristol: John Wright.

Bayer W. L. (Ed.) (1984). Blood transfusion and blood banking. In *Clinics in haematology*, Vol. 13. London: W. B. Saunders.

Bowell P. J., Wainscoat J. S., Peto T. E. A., Gunson H. H. (1982). Maternal anti-D concentrations and outcome in rhesus haemolytic disease of the newborn. *British Medical Journal*, **285**, 327–329.

Bowman J. M. (1985). Controversies in Rh prophylaxis. Who needs Rh immune globulin and when should it be given? *American Journal of Obstetrics & Gynecology*, **151**, 289–294.

Clarke C. A., Mollison P. L., Whitfield G. A. (1985). Deaths from rhesus haemolytic disease in England and Wales in 1982 and 1983. *British Medical Journal*, **291**, 17–19.

Contreras M., Barbara J. A. J. (1985). Acquired immuno-deficiency syndrome and blood transfusion. *Journal of Hospital Infection*, **6**, Suppl. C, 27–34.

Engelfriet C. P., von dem Borne A. E. G. Kr., van der Meulen F. W., Fleer A., Roos D., Ouwehand W. H. (1981). Immune destruction of red cells. In *Seminar on immune-mediated cell destruction*, pp. 93–130 (Ed. C. A. Bell). Chicago: American Association of Blood Banks.

Heaton A., Miripol J., Aster R., Hartman P., Dehart D., Rzad L., Grapka D., Davisson W., Buchholz D. H. (1984). Use of Adsol(R) preservation solution for prolonged storage of low viscosity AS-1 red blood cells. *British Journal of Haematology*, **57**, 467–478.

Högman C. F., Åkerblom O., Hedlund K., Rosen I., Wiklund L. (1983). Red cell suspensions in SAGM medium. *Vox Sanguinis*, **45**, 217–223.

Liley A. W. (1961). Liquor amnii analysis in management of pregnancy complicated by rhesus sensitization. *American Journal of Obstetrics and Gynecology*, **82**, 1359.

Mollison P. L., Engelfriet C. P., Contreras M. (1987). *Blood transfusion in clinical medicine*, 8th edn. Oxford: Blackwell Scientific Publications.

Mollison P. L. (1985) Antibody-mediated destruction of foreign red cells. In *Antibodies: Protective, destructive and regulatory role*, pp. 65–74 (Eds. F. Milgrom, C. J. Abeyounis and B. Albini). Basel: Karger.

Moore B. P. L., Beal R. W. (Eds.) (1984). *Socio-economic aspects of blood transfusion Vox Sanguinis* Supplement. Basel: Krager.

Nicolaides K. H., Rodeck C. H., Mibashan R. S. (1985). Obstetric management and diagnosis of haematological disease in the fetus. In *Haematological disorders in pregnancy*, pp. 775–805. (Ed. E. A. Letsky). *Clinics in Haematology*, **14**. London: W. B. Saunders.

Petz L., Swisher S. N. (1981). *Clinical practice of blood transfusion*. New York: Churchill Livingstone.

Robinson A. E. (1984). Principles and practice of plasma exchange in the management of Rh haemolytic disease of the newborn. *Plasma Therapy*, **5**, 7–14.

Tovey L. A. D., Townley A., Stevenson B. J., Taverner J. (1983). The Yorkshire antenatal anti-D immunoglobulin trial in primigravidae. *Lancet*, **2**, 244–246.

WHO (1984). *Resolutions, recommendations and decisions on blood transfusion*. Geneva: League of Red Cross and Red Crescent Societies.

Chapter 11

GRANULOCYTES, MONOCYTES, AND THEIR BENIGN DISORDERS

J. M. GOLDMAN

The application of new techniques has added considerably to our knowledge of leucocyte structure and function in the last 20 years. For example, the neutrophil granulocyte has been studied extensively by electron microscopy, and its kinetics and mechanisms of phagocytosis and bacterial killing have received much attention. The eosinophil has been studied in detail and much is now known of its surface properties and granular constituents. The lymphocytes, so recently described as 'phlegmatic spectators watching the turbulent activities of the phagocytes', are now known to comprise a highly heterogeneous population of cells with a variety of specific surface receptors and differing responsiveness to antigens and other mitogenic agents.

In parallel with studies of the mature leucocytes, the techniques of experimental haematology, involving particularly in-vitro cell culture and transplantation studies in animal systems, have contributed greatly to our understanding of the regulation and function of haemopoietic stem cells and the pathways along which they differentiate.

STEM CELLS AND MYELOPOIESIS

Stem Cells (Fig. 11.1)

A continuously proliferating population of cells requires the existence of a stem cell. The concept of the bone marrow stem cell has become rather confused, in part because the same term is used by workers with very different approaches to the problem. The stem cell as a *kinetic entity* may be defined as a self-renewing precursor cell that can at times differentiate to form the next cell in the series. In theory, stem cells may divide either symmetrically or asymmetrically to form one differentiating cell and one further stem cell. Which of these mechanisms operates in the bone marrow of humans is unknown. The myeloid stem cell as a *morphological entity* remains a subject of dispute. There is evidence that it may resemble a small lymphocyte both residing in the marrow and circulating at times in the peripheral blood, but equally it may appear as a larger cell with a more 'active' nucleus and more abundant cytoplasm. The stem cell as a colony-forming unit (CFU) is a useful functional definition derived from experimental work with mice. If a mouse is 'lethally' irradiated and then transfused with bone marrow or peripheral blood leucocytes from a syngeneic animal, the mouse survives and discrete colonies of haemopoietic cells of donor origin appear in the spleen after about 7 days. Each colony may contain maturing cells of granulocyte, erythroid or megakaryocyte lineage, yet all appear to be the progeny of a single stem cell. The cell (CFU-s) that forms these mouse spleen colonies may therefore be regarded as a pluripotential stem cell. In humans, the observation that the acquired Ph[1] chromosomal abnormality that characterizes chronic granulocytic leukaemia is identifiable in erythroid and megakaryocyte precursors and in some lymphoid cells as well as in cells of granulocyte lineage is circumstantial evidence that a pluripotential stem cell is present in the marrow in humans, but no direct proof comparable to the mouse spleen colony assay is available.

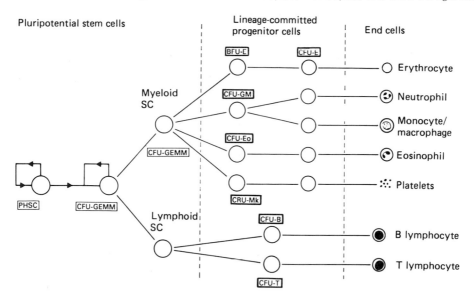

Fig. 11.1. *Schematic representation of the developmental pathway for haemo-poietic cells in humans. The arrows indicate the presumed potential for self-renewal. Note that the term CFU is essentially synonymous with the possibly more accurate CFC (colony-forming cell). The cell marked PHSC is approximately equivalent to the spleen colony-forming cell (CFUs) assayable in the lethally irradiated mouse (or rat) model system.*

(PHSC, pluripotential haemopoietic stem cell; SC, stem cell; CFU–GEMM, colony-forming unit, granulocytic-erythroid-macrophagic-megakaryocytic (also known as CFU–mix); BFU–E, burst-forming unit, erythroid; CFU–E, colony-forming unit, erythroid; CFU–GM, colony-forming unit, granulocyte–macrophage; CFU–Eo, colony-forming unit, eosinophilic; CFU–Mk, colony-forming unit, megakaryocytic; CFU–B, colony-forming unit, B lineage; CFU–T, colony-forming unit, T lineage.)

Though the pluripotential stem cell of human bone marrow cannot be cultured in vitro, a number of systems have been developed that permit proliferation in vitro for limited periods of precursor cells already committed to differentiation. In semi-solid media, such as agar or methyl cellulose, a human bone marrow cell can be detected that is capable of giving rise to colonies containing small numbers of granulocytic, monocytic, erythroid and megakaryocytic progeny. The cell forming these colonies has been named CFU–GEMM or CFU–mix. It is not clearly equivalent to a stem cell because its capacity for self-renewal is negligible. A series of more mature myeloid progenitor cells can be assayed in human bone marrow or peripheral

blood. These include a progenitor cell committed to leucocyte differentiation (CFU–GM, previously CFUc), which proliferates and forms colonies of mature granulocytes and macrophages after incubation for 7–14 days under the influence of appropriate regulatory molecules, designated collectively colony-stimulating factors (CSF) or colony-stimulating activity (CSA). The addition of erythropoietin to the culture system leads to proliferation of a relatively primitive erythroid-committed progenitor cell, designated an erythroid burst-forming unit (BFU–E), which in turn produces small groups, or 'bursts', of more mature erythroid colony-forming units (CFU–E). Progenitor cells capable of giving rise to colonies containing eosinophils

(CFU–Eo) or megakaryocytes (CFU–Mk) can also be recognized in the marrow or blood with appropriate culture conditions.

Haemopoietic Growth Factors (Haemopoietins) (Fig. 11.2)

As a result of the development of the semisolid culture systems for clonal growth of haemopoietic cell colonies referred to above, a number of specific regulatory glycoproteins have been recognized which are essential for progenitor cell survival and proliferation. Though the nomenclature is still somewhat confusing, four factors have been defined that regulate the proliferation of murine colonies and four comparable factors in human culture systems (Table 11.1)

These glycoproteins are produced by specific cells. G–CSF, M–CSF and GM–CSF are produced principally by stromal cells and cells of the monocyte/macrophage series. The major source of inter-

leukin-3 is activated T lymphocytes. The mechanism of action of the granulocyte–macrophage colony-stimulating factors is not yet precisely defined, but each factor has a specific receptor on the surface of the corresponding progenitor cell target. Individual progenitor cells may exhibit receptors for more than one haemopoietin simultaneously. Presumably, binding of the appropriate ligand by one receptor influences cell commitment and leads to reduced expression (down-modulation) of other receptors. In-vitro studies show that they also maintain progenitor cell viability and can promote activation of mature granulocytes and monocytes.

The physiological function of the granulocyte–macrophage regulatory molecules is likewise not yet fully defined. They are probably produced principally within the marrow cavity from stromal cells in response to stimulation by interleukin-1 (IL-1) and tumour necrosis factor (TNF), produced by macrophages and T lymphocytes which act locally to modulate granulopoiesis and monocytopoiesis.

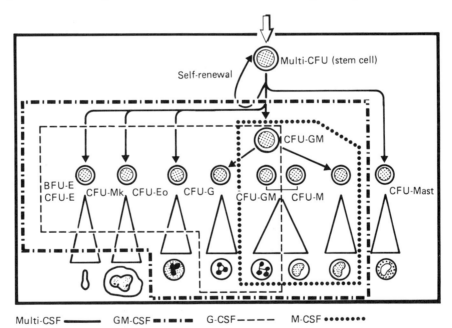

Fig. 11.2. *Biological specificity for the different haemopoietins. The cell responsive to each of the different haemopoietins is included within the respective boundaries. (Modified, with permission, from a scheme proposed by D. Metcalf.) CFU–G, granulocyte-committed colony forming unit; CFU–M, macrophage-committed colony forming unit; GM–CSF, granulocyte–macrophage colony stimulating factor; G-CSF, granulocyte colony stimulating factor; M-CSF, macrophage colony stimulating factor. (For other abbreviations, see Fig. 11.1.)*

Table 11.1

The known myeloid regulatory growth factors (haemopoietins)

Species	Name (synonym)	M_r	Chromosomal localization of gene	cDNA cloned
Murine				
	GM–CSF (CSF–α)	23	11	Yes
	G–CSF (CSF–β)	25	—	Not yet
	M–CSF (CSF–1)	40–70	—	Not yet
	Multi–CSF (burst-promoting activity, interleukin-3)	23–30	11	Yes
Human				
	GM–CSF	22	5q 23–32	Yes
	G–CSF	20	17q 21	Yes
	M–CSF	70	5q 33–1	Yes
	Interleukin-3 (Multi-CSF)	18	5q 23–q31	Yes

M_r, relative molecular mass.

In animals and humans treated with cytotoxic drugs, injection of recombinant factors regularly expedites the recovery of blood granulocyte numbers. The obvious question arises as to whether the pathogenesis of the myeloid leukaemias may be explained in part by autocrine production of one or other growth factor or by altered responsiveness of a progenitor cell to a growth factor. However, most myeloid leukaemia cells require apparently physiological levels of appropriate regulatory molecules for proliferation in vitro, and the recombinant factors will have to be used with great caution in the management of leukaemia or after bone marrow transplantation in humans if the recovery of normal haemopoiesis is to be expedited without also stimulating leukaemic cell proliferation.

Bone Marrow Stroma

The fact that normal haemopoiesis proceeds only in intramedullary sites implies the existence of a specific haemopoietic microenvironment. Thus the bone marrow consists of haemopoietic cells closely packed between stromal cells and blood vessels. The stromal cells constitute an ill-defined entity that includes endothelial cells, fibroblasts, fat cells and macrophages. The stromal cells collectively support haemopoiesis but the precise contribution of the different components cannot readily be assessed. Study of bone marrow stroma was, however, greatly facilitated by the introduction in 1977 by Dexter and colleagues in Manchester of a culture system that supports the proliferation in vitro of murine and, to a lesser extent, of human haemopoietic cells for weeks or months (Dexter, 1979). In this system a primary inoculum of marrow cells is used to establish a stromal layer that adheres to the surface of a plastic tissue culture flask. When the adherent layer is fully established, a second inoculum of marrow cells is added to the stromal layer; the latter proliferates and produces differentiated progeny that are released into the supernatant culture medium. Thus CFU–GEMM, CFU–G, BFU–E and CFU–GM are produced for long periods without the need for exogenously provided growth factors, which are presumably produced by the adherent layer. The culture conditions can be modified by addition of growth factors or drugs or by other methods designed to stimulate or inhibit the regulatory role of the stromal cells.

The marrow fibroblast looks superficially like its counterpart derived from other sites. It adheres to plastic and glass surfaces and produces collagen types I and III. Marrow fibroblasts can be cultured in vitro as discrete colonies derived from fibroblast colony-forming cells (CFU–F). They release M–CSF, GM–CSF and G–CSF in response to stimulation by IL-1 and TNF. Fat cells can be propagated in vitro and are also adherent to glass and plastic surfaces. They are particularly numerous in cultures to which hydrocortisone has been added. Their biological function is unknown, but the unsaturated fatty acids they contain may act as non-specific stimulators of haemopoiesis. The macrophages that form part of the marrow stroma resemble macrophages derived from other tissues. They may produce fibronectin, acid phosphatase and non-specific esterases. They have surface receptors for Fc and C3. The endothelial cells also adhere to glass and plastic surfaces but are much more 'rounded' than marrow fibroblasts. They produce type IV collagen and express factor-VIII-related antigen. Endothelial cells derived from human umbilical cord produce colony-stimulating activity, but marrow endothelial cells may or may not behave in the same way.

Very little is known of the origins of the marrow stromal cells. Earlier evidence suggested that they were all derived, together with haemopoietic cells, from a common stem cell; more recent studies suggest that haemopoiesis and stromal cell proliferation are discrete. The fibroblast may give rise to the fat cell, as well as the endothelial cell. The macrophage is presumably derived directly from the stromal stem cell. These speculative relationships are set out in Fig. 11.3.

Neutrophil Kinetics (Fig. 11.4)

Myeloblasts, promyelocytes and myelocytes all undergo mitotic division but the metamyelocyte is an end-stage cell that matures further but no longer divides. The total mass of marrow granulocytes can therefore be divided into an early mitotic pool in which cell division, growth and maturation take place, ending at the myelocyte, a subsequent maturation pool that ends with the mature neutrophil, and a storage pool of mature neutrophils residing in the marrow. These pools all overlap to some extent. The use of isotopic labels, in particular diisopropyl phosphofluoridate (DF^{32}P), has contributed greatly to our knowledge

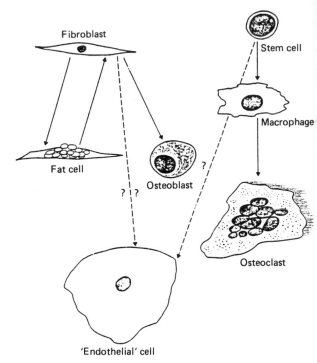

Fig. 11.3. *Proposed relationships between 'non-haemopoietic' cells in the marrow. (Adapted from Barrett and Gordon (1985), with permission.)*

of granulocyte kinetics. Measurements with this label suggest that the average time required for a myelocyte to complete a generative cycle in a human is 1 day. Thereafter the time taken to traverse the post-mitotic maturation and storage pools in the marrow and enter the blood is about 10 days. It has been calculated that the storage pool contains 9×10^9 cells/kg body weight and this represents a reserve of band and segmented neutrophils 13 times the number in the blood (7×10^8/kg).

In normal circumstances, neutrophils are released into the blood at the rate of 16×10^8 cells/kg per day. Various factors control the rate of their release and there may be a negative-feedback control, possibly mediated humorally by mature neutrophils. A delay in such feedback could account for the oscillation in neutrophil numbers over 2 or 3 weeks observed in healthy persons, and an unexplained accentuation of this oscillation could be the cause of cyclical neutropenia.

The total blood granulocyte pool (TBGP) has two components: a circulating granulocyte pool

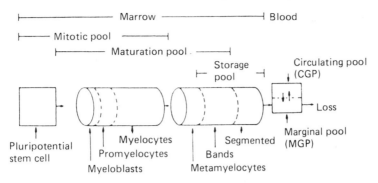

Fig. 11.4. *A model of neutrophil granulocyte kinetics in normal human subjects. (CGP, circulating granulocyte pool; MGP, marginated granulocyte pool.) (Reproduced from Boggs (1967), with permission.)*

(CGP) and a marginated granulocyte pool (MGP). The latter consists of cells that 'marginate' along and adhere to the walls of capillaries and small venules while the axial stream of a large vessel contains cells in the CGP. Granulocytes are lost from the TBGP when they pass into the tissues. They die there in presumed subclinical infection or migrate out of the tissues in body secretions (saliva, urine, gut). There is a small loss from cell senescence and consequent destruction in the reticuloendothelial system. In contrast to the lifespan in the marrow of the maturing and mature granulocyte, estimated to be about 11 days, the time spent in the circulation (blood transit time) is extremely short, with a $T_{1/2}$ of 6–8 hours.

Although there is some diurnal variation in granulocyte counts, leucocyte numbers are maintained within remarkably narrow limits during health. Leucocytes are subdivided into five cell types on the basis of nuclear shape and the presence and type of cytoplasmic granules, namely neutrophil, eosinophil and basophil granulocytes, monocytes and lymphocytes.

GRANULOCYTES

Morphology and Maturation (Fig. 11.5)

The myeloblast is the earliest identifiable precursor of the mature granulocyte. It is usually found in small numbers in the bone marrow but is absent from the peripheral blood in health. In preparations stained by a Romanowsky method, the cell is of variable size (10–18 μm) and has a large round or oval nucleus with one to five pale-blue nucleoli; the remaining nucleoplasm is evenly dispersed without definite aggregation of chromatin or forms a fine meshwork. The cytoplasm is scanty and basophilic and can be seen to contain in the more mature myeloblast a few rather angular azurophilic (reddish-purple) or primary granules. These average 350 nm in size and show acid phosphatase and myeloperoxidase activity. The primary granules become more frequent as the cell matures. Occasionally in acute leukaemia, some of the primary granules coalesce to form one or more rod-like cytoplasmic inclusions known as Auer bodies. These bodies are thin and needle-like, measuring 200–1000 nm in length; they stain in the same way as the primary granule, and electron microscopy (Fig. 11.5) often reveals features of a crystal with a periodic structure. They are regarded as diagnostic of leukaemic myeloblasts (or possibly also of monoblasts). As the cytoplasm of the maturing cell becomes more abundant, a new type of granule, designated secondary or specific, makes its appearance; these granules at first stain darkly and lie over the nucleus (14–20 μm) as well as in the cytoplasm. As long as it retains nucleoli, this cell with secondary granules is regarded as a promyelocyte.

The myelocyte is a somewhat smaller cell (12–18 μm) but the cytoplasm remains more prominent than in the myeloblast. The nucleus is still round or is slightly indented, but nucleoli are now absent; the nuclear chromatin has become more coarse and specific granules may still overlie it. The cytoplasm of the cell has lost some of its basophilia and becomes pink and contains increas-

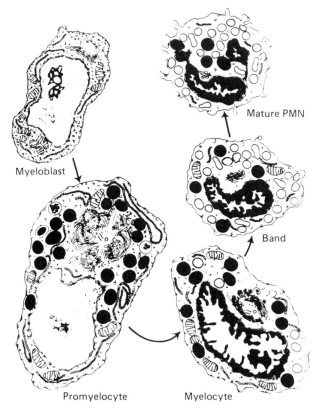

Myeloblast

Mature PMN

Band

Promyelocyte

Myelocyte

Fig. 11.5. *Diagrammatic representation of the different stages in the maturation of neutrophil granulocytes (PMN). Note the absence of granules in the myeloblast, the prominent Golgi area in the promyelocyte with densely staining primary granules and the appearance of secondary granules at the myelocyte stage. Note also that the staining characteristics of the granules in this diagram are different from those represented in Figs 11.10 and 11.11. (Reproduced from Bainton and Farquhar (1966), with permission.)*

mature polymorphonuclear granulocyte is a smaller cell (10–14 μm), with nuclear material divided into three or four segments which are joined by thin strands of chromatin. It was at one time proposed that the number of nuclear segments correlated with the age of the cell, but this is probably not the case. Both types of granule are present in the cytoplasm of the mature neutrophil.

A characteristic nuclear appendage may be identified in 2–3% (range 1–17%) of neutrophils obtained from normal women. This so-called drumstick appendage is a round or oval mass of dense chromatin (about 1.5 μm in diameter) lying separate from the main nuclear material but attached to a nuclear lobe by a slender chromatin thread. It is the neutrophil analogue of the Barr body identifiable adjacent to the nuclear membrane in normal female somatic cells. It should not be confused with the occasional presence of fragmented nuclear material separated from the main lobes by much thicker bands of chromatin; these have no sex specificity.

Cells of the granulocytic series have been studied extensively by electron microscopy. They are illustrated in Figs 11.6, 11.7, 11.10 and 11.11; the contrasting appearances of monocytes and lymphocytes are shown in Figs 11.8 and 11.9 respectively. The myeloblast contains prominent nucleoli, small mitochondria and indistinct Golgi apparatus; the last-mentioned becomes more prominent as the cell matures. The primary granules typically appear round and are dense after staining with uranyl acetate. The specific granules are more variable in size and shape and often appear elongated like rice grains; after staining they are less dense to electrons. Although both types of granule appear to be formed in the Golgi complex, the primary granules apparently emerge from the concave or proximal face of the complex, whereas the secondary granules make their appearance somewhat later from the convex or distal face. Little is known of the functional differences of the two types of granules. The mature polymorph shows many granules as membrane-bound structures of varying size and electron density; they are evenly distributed in the cytoplasm but seldom appear less than about 100 nm from the cell surface. Mitochondria are now scarce and generally small and elongated when present. Ribosomes and rough endoplasmic reticulum are seen even more rarely.

ing numbers of specific granules. The latter average 500 nm in size and can be identified as neutrophilic, eosinophilic or basophilic. Unlike the primary granule, the specific or secondary granule lacks myeloperoxidase but is apparently rich in alkaline phosphatase (Table 11.2).

The development of nuclear indentation marks the transition from myelocyte to metamyelocyte, and the specific granules in the cytoplasm become more numerous. The nucleus then becomes kidney shaped and as it elongates further and bends, the cell comes to be known as a 'band' form. The fully

Table 11.2

Properties of neutrophil leucocyte granules

	Primary	*Secondary*
Shape	Round	Elongated
Size (nm)	350	300–600
Appearance		
Light microscopy (Romanowsky)	Reddish-purple (azurophilic)	Grey-blue (neutrophilic)
Electron microscopy (uranyl acetate)	Dense	Less dense
Contents	Myeloperoxidase	Alkaline phosphatase
	Acid phosphatase	Lysozyme
	β-galactosidase	Aminopeptidase
	β-glucuronidase	Lactoferrin
	Chymotrypsin-like cationic proteins	
	Elastase	
	Collagenase	

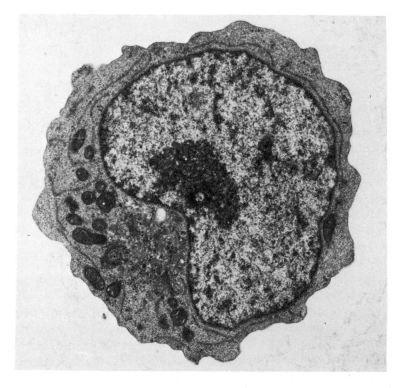

Fig. 11.6. *Electron micrograph of a myeloblast showing finely dispersed nuclear chromatin and a large nucleolus. Small granules are visible in the region of the Golgi apparatus.*

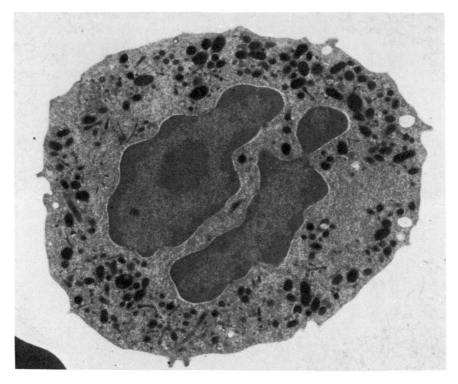

Fig. 11.7. *Electron micrograph of a mature neutrophil with segmented nucleus and abundant cytoplasmic granules, heterogeneous in size and density.*

Biochemistry

Leucocytes have many metabolic pathways in common with other mammalian cells. They synthesize protein and break it down and they can produce lactic acid, lipids, nucleotides and nucleic acids. Granulocytes appear to depend very heavily for the supply of energy on glycolysis; the mature neutrophil has relatively few mitochondria and the citric acid cycle (Krebs' cycle) is less important than in other cells. Phagocytosis results in an increased rate of glycolysis and appears to be equally efficient under aerobic and anaerobic conditions. The killing of certain ingested micro-organisms does, however, depend on availability of molecular oxygen, although this oxygen requirement may be for oxygenase systems rather than for respiration. Thus, under aerobic conditions neutrophils deficient in myeloperoxidase behave like normal neutrophils under anaerobic conditions and are defective in killing certain species of bacteria and fungi.

The granulocyte is an important source of one of the vitamin B_{12}-binding proteins, transcobalamin I (and III). Serum levels of B_{12} and the B_{12}-binding capacity are greatly raised in conditions in which there is proliferation of granulocyte precursors, of which chronic granulocytic leukaemia is the prime example (see Chapter 3).

Neutrophil Cytochemistry

The granules that can be seen by light and electron microscopy are all probably lysosomes which, although present in other cells, are particularly well developed in cells of the granulocytic series. Lysosomes are small bag-like organelles containing enzymes that are synthesized in ribosomes of the cell endoplasmic reticulum; the enzymes are then packaged in the Golgi area and surrounded by a single lipoprotein membrane. These enzymes (hydrolases) are capable of degrading organic material

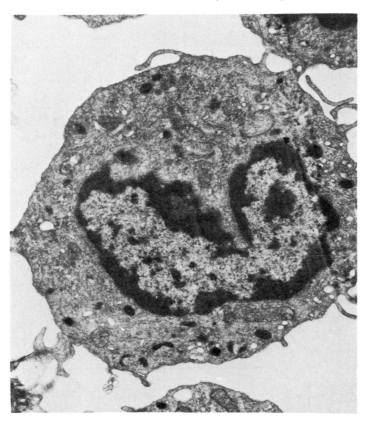

Fig. 11.8. *Electron micrograph of a monocyte showing idented nucleus, cytoplasmic granules and numerous small vacuoles.*

including proteins, fats, carbohydrates and nucleic acids, and the cell cytoplasm is normally protected from their hydrolytic action by the lipoprotein membrane. After bacteria or other particles have been phagocytosed, the contents of the organelles are discharged into the phagocytic vesicle (phagosome) and may digest and destroy its contents. The term secondary lysosome is sometimes used to describe the phagosome that contains enzymes after fusion with the primary lysosome; it should not be confused with the secondary or specific granule.

Granulocyte lysosomes have been studied most extensively in the rabbit, but many of the findings have been shown to apply to humans also. The primary granules are rich in myeloperoxidase and contain acid phosphatase, β-galactosidase and esterase as well as chymotrypsin-like cationic proteins, elastase and collagenase. The secondary granules lack myeloperoxidase but are relatively rich in lysozyme and aminopeptidase. They also contain lactoferrin, an iron-binding protein which has some bacteriostatic potential and may be involved in the physiological control of granulopoiesis.

A number of lysosomal enzymes are of particular interest. Lysozyme (muramidase) was first demonstrated in 1922 by Alexander Fleming by virtue of its remarkable capacity to lyse the cell walls of certain bacteria, notably *Micrococcus lysodeikticus.* This enzyme, a cationic protein with a molecular weight of 14 000–15 000 daltons is widely distributed through the animal and bacterial world. In humans it appears to originate from the specific granules of the granulocyte (as well as from the granules of monocytes and tissue macrophages) and is released from these cells to appear in small amounts in the serum, tears, urine, and other body secretions. Serum and urine levels may be unusually

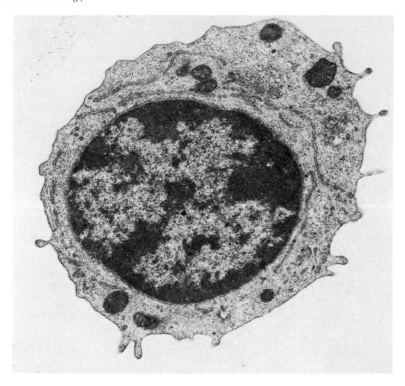

Fig. 11.9. *Electron micrograph of a 'mature' lymphocyte with clumped nuclear chromatin and several mitochondria.*

high in acute myelomonocytic and monocytic leukaemias; in some of these patients the lysozymuria may be associated with renal tubular damage, loss of potassium in the urine and systemic hypokalaemia.

Mature neutrophils show considerable alkaline phosphatase activity in their cytoplasm and this neutrophil alkaline phosphatase (NAP) is thought to be associated with secondary granules, though recent studies suggest that it may be more closely linked with a membrane-related organelle distinct from both primary and secondary granules. NAP can be quantitated by biochemical or histochemical methods and very low levels are usually characteristic of Ph¹-positive chronic granulocytic leukaemia (see Chapter 16). Low levels are also less regularly a feature of leucocytes from patients with acute myeloid leukaemia and paroxysmal nocturnal haemoglobinuria. Levels of NAP are usually somewhat raised in aplastic anaemia and in leucocytosis of pyogenic origin; they may be extremely high in leukaemoid reactions as well as in polycythaemia vera and myelofibrosis.

The myeloperoxidase present in the mature neutrophil seems to play an important role in the killing of certain micro-organisms. A rare hereditary deficiency of neutrophil myeloperoxidase has been reported in which there is impaired killing of *Candida albicans* and the patients suffer from susceptibility to systemic infection with this organism.

Neutrophil Function

Phase contrast studies of fresh preparations of leucocytes reveal that myeloblasts are capable of slow snail-like motion in some situations and the myelocyte exhibits the same low-grade locomotion. Polymorphonuclear cells, however, are highly motile and at body temperature move in an amoeboid fashion, generally in the same direction for some length of time. The cell first projects an ectoplasmic pseudopodium and the granule-

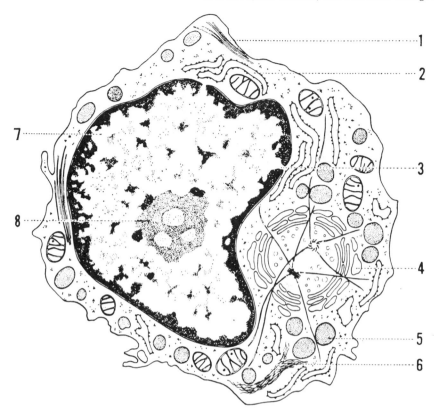

Fig. 11.10. *Diagram of the electron microscopic appearance of a normal mye-loblast. 1, Microtubules; 2, rough endoplasmic reticulum; 3, nuclear pore; 4, Golgi body vacuole; 5, azurophilic granules; 6, microfibrils; 7, nucleus; 8, nucleolus.*

containing endoplasm then flows into it. The intracellular basis for this motility is not well understood. Ultrastructurally the hyaline ectoplasm of the neutrophil contains fine filaments (microfibrils) which have been identified as actin polymers. Moreover, materials with the structural and enzymic characteristics of myosin have been identified in the neutrophil cytoplasm, so the molecular mechanism underlying neutrophil motility may resemble that of muscle contraction. Another cytoplasmic structure that may be concerned in motility is the microtubule. Unlike solid actin filaments, microtubules are hollow fibres with a larger diameter, 24 nm, and are composed of a different protein, tubulin. The tubulin may have the capacity to contract. Microtubules are primarily localized in the neutrophil endoplasm and appear to insert into the region of the actin filaments at the cell periphery.

Neutrophil migration in vivo is directed, at least in part, by a variety of chemical substances designated collectively chemotaxins. One class of chemotaxins is formed directly by such bacteria as *Escherichia coli* or staphylococci. However, the principal mechanism by which chemotaxins are generated involves the activation of serum complement. Antibody reacting with the surface of a microbe sequentially activates steps in the complement system with the generation of C3a and C5a, low molecular weight fragments with chemotactic activity. In addition, a complex of complement proteins acting later in the haemolytic sequence, C567, also acts as a chemotaxin. The activation of Hageman factor, occurring during the clotting process, produces two active chemotactic products, kallikrein and plasminogen activator. Lymphokines also have the ability to attract neutrophils.

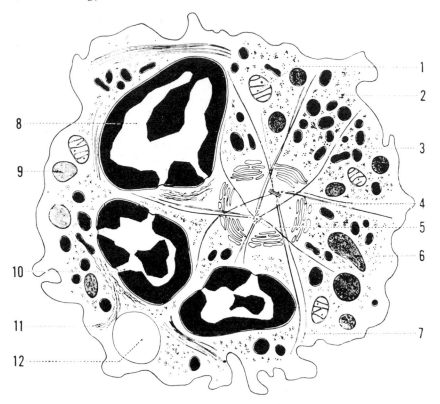

Fig. 11.11. *Diagram of the electron microscopic appearance of a mature neutro-phil granulocyte. 1, Mitochondria; 2, glycogen; 3, dense granules; 4, Golgi body; 5, centriole; 6, less dense granules; 7, microtubules; 8, nuclear lobe; 9, granule; 10, nuclear pore; 11, microfibrils; 12, contractile vacuole.*

(Figs 11.10 and 11.11 are reproduced by courtesy of Marcel Bessis, and originally appeared in Proceedings of the International Conference of Leukaemia-Lymphoma *(1968), Lea & Febiger.)*

Finally, neutrophils that have ingested particulate matter themselves release a factor with the capacity to attract other neutrophils in the absence of serum.

The only proven useful function of the neutrophil is to phagocytose and kill micro-organisms. When a small particulate object, such as a bacterium, comes into contact with the surface of the phagocytosing cell, it appears to sink into the cytoplasm and be engulfed with the help of the amoeboid action of the cell's pseudopodia. Opsonins may aid the ingestion at this stage and phagocytosis does not occur in the absence of complement and certain divalent cations (Ca^{++}, Mg^{++}). After ingestion of the particle, there is a sharp increase in oxygen consumption and release of hydrogen peroxide. Within the cell the particle is surrounded by a membrane, probably formed from the cell's cytoplasmic membrane, and within a very short time (less than 1 minute at $37°C$) the contents of various lysozomal organelles are discharged into this phagocytic vesicle, or phago-some. Organic materials are thus digested and most bacteria are killed; nevertheless, certain bacteria including *Mycobacterium tuberculosis* can, on oc-casion, survive phagocytosis and be discharged alive from the cell. 'Degranulation' accompanies phagocytosis and the cytoplasm may appear com-pletely devoid of granules after a number of particles have been ingested.

The precise mechanism by which a neutrophil kills an ingested micro-organism is not well under-stood. A variety of killing, or 'cidal', mechanisms are known but their relative importance in relation to the killing of individual microbes is difficult to define. Indeed, it is likely that microbial killing reflects 'collaboration' of different mechanisms and the neutrophil probably has a degree of functional redundancy—it can kill a microbe in a number of different ways. The identified mechanisms can be divided into those that depend on oxygen and those that do not (Table 11.3).

Oxygen-dependent Mechanisms

Phagocytosis by neutrophils is accompanied by a burst of oxygen consumption. Glucose is utilized at this stage by one of two main pathways, the Embden–Meyerhof pathway, which reduces NAD to NADH, and the hexose monophosphate shunt, which regenerates NADPH from NADH. The final step in microbial killing by oxygen-dependent mechanisms is thought to involve the generation of oxygen radicals which may be directly lethal to the micro-organism. Radicals are molecules which contain a single unpaired electron; they are unstable and thus seek to gain or lose an electron to restore stability. Either NADH or NADPH could act as a source of reducing equivalents for an oxidase system probably localized in the membrane of the phagocytic vacuole. Alternatively, the transfer of electrons could involve an electron-transfer chain, which includes a recently described cytochrome located in the plasma membrane. Either way, molecular oxygen is reduced sequentially by the addition of electrons, first to form the superoxide radical,

Table 11.3
Microbicidal mechanisms in the polymorph neutrophil

Oxygen dependent
Myeloperoxidase–H_2O_2-halide
H_2O_2
Superoxide anion
Hydroxyl radical
Singlet oxygen

Oxygen independent
Acid
Lysozyme
Lactoferrin
Cationic proteins

---

then hydrogen peroxide (H_2O_2) and finally hydroxyl radicals.

There are, however, sources of H_2O_2 other than those involving glucose metabolism. Certain bacterial species such as pneumococci, streptococci or lactobacilli, which lack catalases, can provide H_2O_2. This bacterial source of H_2O_2 may make a significant contribution to the bactericidal capacity of the neutrophil, especially when endogenous production of H_2O_2 is defective, as in patients with chronic granulomatous disease (see later). It has been suggested that hydrogen peroxide forms the substrate for myeloperoxidase, which is present in the primary granules and can oxidize a halide such as iodide or chloride to iodine or a chloramine, and that these agents then damage the microbial wall. It is notable, however, that most individuals lacking neutrophil myeloperoxidase have no increased risk of infection, so other mechanisms of microbial killing must be equally important.

A further oxygen radical that may be important in the microbicidal mechanism of the cell is singlet oxygen, a highly reactive species with the same molecular formula (O_2) as atmospheric or 'triplet' oxygen but differing from it in the distribution of its electrons and therefore its magnetic properties. In this electronically 'excited' state, singlet oxygen emits light (chemiluminescence) until it reverts to its triplet ground state. Singlet oxygen is found in the phagocytosing cell and may be formed by the myeloperoxidase system or independently of it; it seems to have potent microbicidal activity.

Whatever the relative importance of the different oxygen radicals, the precise mechanism of bacterial killing is still speculative. It may involve the incorporation of iodine or Cl^- into the bacterial cell wall, which would then alter its permeability and result in cell death.

Oxygen-independent Mechanisms

Exposure of intact neutrophils to an oxygen-free environment does not abolish 'cidal' activity, suggesting the existence also of oxygen-independent killing mechanisms. The interior of the phagocytic vacuole has a pH that may be 3.0 or lower, and some bacteria are probably killed as a direct result of exposure to this acid environment. Alternatively, lysozyme is active in the absence of oxygen but the number of pathogenic bacteria that it can kill is very restricted. Its prime function is probably the digestion of bacteria already killed by other means. Lactoferrin has bacteriostatic rather than bactericidal activity and may play a role in retarding the growth of ingested micro-organisms. The neutrophil contains a number of proteins that are heat stable, acid resistant and strongly cationic; the most cationic of these have been shown to have esterase activity and so resemble pancreatic chymotrypsin. All these cationic proteins, but particularly those with chymotrypsin-like activity, are potently microbicidal in the absence of oxygen: Gram-positive bacteria seem to be more sensitive to their action than Gram-negative ones.

A small proportion of the neutrophils that circulate in the blood of a normal person have the capacity in vitro to reduce the soluble colourless dye nitroblue tetrazolium (NBT) to an insoluble blue-black precipitate. In patients with systemic bacterial infection, the numbers and proportion of neutrophils capable of performing this reduction are usually increased, often greatly. The reduction is thought to depend on the activity of NADH oxidase which may be more readily available in the neutrophil stimulated by bacteria or bacterial products than in the 'resting' neutrophil. In direct contrast, a congenital defect in this enzyme system is thought to explain the complete absence of neutrophils capable of reducing NBT in vitro in patients with chronic granulomatous disease.

Leucocyte Antigens

Various methods are now available for defining antigenic determinants on leucocytes and detecting antileucocyte antibodies in the serum. Methods based on leucocyte agglutination make use primarily of granulocytes, whereas for the more sensitive cytotoxicity tests lymphocytes are the usual target cell. Leucocytes appear to carry the antigens of the ABH system but the status of the Rh factor on leucocytes remains unclear. Granulocytes and lymphocytes both carry the antigens of the HLA system and a number of relatively less important histocompatibility antigens have been described; very little is known, however, about the differences in amount of antigen on granulocytes and lymphocytes respectively (see also Chapter 9). Because they carry the HLA and other tissue antigens and are also readily accessible, leucocytes form an excellent target for histocompatibility tests before organ transplantation. Neutrophils and lymphocytes also have a surface glycoprotein leucocyte-function antigen (LFA-1) responsible for cell adhesion.

In addition to antigens shared with other tissues, neutrophils have a number of specific antigens best demonstrated by agglutination in the presence of EDTA. So far six such neutrophil-specific loci have been identified (Table 11.4 and Chapter 9).

Leucocyte isoantibodies of clinical significance arise in two situations. After multiple blood transfusions, agglutinating isoantibodies may be detec-

Table 11.4
Human neutrophil antigens

	Antigens	Techniques for identification
Shared with other tissues	ABH I, i U; Jk^a, Jk^b, Kx 5^{a,b} HLA-A, B	Absorption and elution Cold agglutination Absorption Agglutination Cytotoxicity
Shared with lymphocytes	LFA-1	Cell adhesion
Neutrophil specific	NA1, NA2 NB1 NC1	EDTA-agglutination

ted in the serum and these may provoke pyrexial and allergic reactions on the administration of further leucocyte-rich blood. Alternatively, pregnancy, associated presumably with fetomaternal transfer of blood, may be associated with the production of leucocyte-agglutinating maternal antibody; such antibody may then cross the placenta and on occasion gives rise to neonatal leucopenia. Rarely, leucocyte autoantibodies are found in leucopenic subjects who have never been transfused. Finally, autoantibodies directed against leucocyte nuclear material are occasionally identified; these may have specificity for DNA, nucleoprotein or other nuclear constituents. They are usually seen against a background of generalized autoimmune disturbance, as in systemic lupus erythematosus.

Eosinophils

Eosinophil granulocytes are formed exclusively in the bone marrow and their development from myeloblasts parallels that of the neutrophil granulocyte. Studies with experimental animals suggest that appropriate stimuli acting on T lymphocytes lead to release of a lymphokine, provisionally designated Eo–CSF or eosinophilopoietin, that stimulates eosinophil production in vitro and in vivo.

Eosinophilic differentiation is first observed at the myelocyte stage when the characteristic specific granules make their appearance. The mature eosinophil typically has a two-lobed nucleus but occasionally a small third lobe is interposed between two larger ones. Numerous granules appear to pack the cytoplasm and these are relatively large (600 nm), of uniform size and stain bright yellowish-red by Romanowsky methods. The cytoplasmic membrane is particularly prone to rupture during the production of blood films and granules may then be found some distance from the bare nucleus. When examined by electron microscopy, two kinds of granule are recognizable: the eosinophil myelocyte contains many large spherical granules that appear dense and homogeneous; the granules that predominate in the eosinophil polymorph are equally dense but are smaller and irregular in outline and are packed with haphazardly arranged

crystalloids. If large numbers of eosinophils disintegrate in secretions or exudates, the crystalloids remain intact and coalesce into larger particles known as Charcot–Leyden crystals.

As with the neutrophil, the cytochemistry of the eosinophil granulocyte has been studied more extensively in animals (especially horse and rabbit) than in humans. Both the homogeneous and the crystalline eosinophil granules contain phospholipid and a zinc-rich basic protein. This protein also contains a high proportion of arginine and is responsible for the strong affinity of the granules for acid dyes. Both types of granule contain myeloperoxidase and probably also ribonuclease, nucleotidase, β-glucuronidase and cathepsin. Acid phosphatase and a sulphated acid muco-substance, however, seem to be restricted to the homogeneous granules. Neither type of granule contains lysozyme.

The bone marrow is the only important reserve of eosinophils in the body and mature eosinophils remain there for 3 or 4 days. They then leave the marrow in favour of the bloodstream, but fewer than 1% of the body's eosinophils are to be found in the circulation and the blood transit time is 3–8 hours. In health, eosinophils are found in skin, lungs and gastrointestinal tract. Ultimately they leave these tissues by way of lymphatic channels and are destroyed in the reticuloendothelial system. Their total lifespan after exit from the marrow is 8–12 days.

The precise function of the eosinophil is understood less well than that of the neutrophil. Their preferential location at epithelial surfaces implies a role in the defence of the host against attack by foreign materials, but their activities seem in no way immunologically specific. Eosinophil release from the marrow and migration are under humoral control, and histamine may be the physiological stimulus. Like neutrophils, eosinophils are active, motile and capable of phagocytosis; they can be attracted chemotactically by a number of substances, all of which are proteins, complex polysaccharides or a complex of these.

They will respond to the injection of such a substance (e.g. a helminthic extract) by margination, diapedesis and migration to the site of injection; repeated injection produces a progressive increase in tissue and blood eosinophilia. They may also migrate in response to foreign antigen and then may phagocytose antigen–antibody complexes. Chemical- and antigen-induced eosinophil migration (eosinotaxis) can be blocked by the administration of ACTH or adrenal cortical hormones, which also eventually deplete the marrow of their eosinophil reserves.

They differ from neutrophils in that they may be the critical effector cell in antibody-mediated attack on metazoan parasites. Experimentally, degranulating eosinophils can be seen surrounding the parasite and the cationic protein of the granules may be directly toxic to it.

Basophils

Basophil granulocytes are very numerous in the blood of some amphibia but relatively few are present in the blood of humans. The nucleus of the mature basophil resembles that of a neutrophil but the cell cytoplasm is filled with large, coarse metachromatic granules that appear black or purplish-black with Romanowsky stains. They usually completely fill the cytoplasm and overlie the nucleus. These granules appear to be water soluble and in poor preparations the cell may show only vacuoles in place of its granules. Like neutrophils and eosinophils, basophils are extremely motile and their appearance in the blood is merely a stage in their transit from the marrow to the tissues.

Larger cells bearing a certain resemblance to and often confused with basophil granulocytes are found in the bone marrow and most other tissues; their numbers are increased in these sites in certain pathological conditions, including Waldenström's macroglobulinaemia and lymphomas. These *mast* cells differ from basophils in that they possess packed granules of more uniform size; these crowd the cytoplasm but do not usually overlie the nucleus. The latter is often small, quite round and eccentrically placed.

The granules of the basophil contain histamine, kallikrein, myeloperoxidase, esterases and proteases and three sulphated mucopolysaccharides, chondroitin sulphate, dermatin sulphate and heparin sulphate. The basophil surface membrane expresses receptors for IgG, C' and IgE. Binding of IgE causes the cell to degranulate and release histamine and other contents involved in the mediation of immediate-type hypersensitivity reactions. Their heparin content and the presence of large numbers of basophils in the healing phase of inflammation suggest that they may have a role in the prevention of coagulation of blood or lymph in obstructed tissues. The granules also contain hyaluronic acid and produce and release serotonin. The fact that mast cell granules are not water soluble and the finding of distinct differences on electron microscopy suggest that basophil and mast cell granules are of differing chemical composition.

MONOCYTES

The monocyte seen in a Romanowsky-stained preparation of peripheral blood is a large cell (14–20 μm) with an often somewhat peripherally placed nucleus. The nuclear shape is very variable: it may be round, oval or notched or it may be folded or convoluted with overlapping lobes. It has a very delicate lace-like distribution of chromatin. There are no nucleoli. The cytoplasm is usually abundant and appears greyish or muddy blue; it contains variable numbers of very fine pink or lilac granules which are rather smaller than the typical granules of the polymorphonuclear neutrophil. Electron microscopic studies (see Fig. 11.8) suggest that the unstimulated monocyte is a resting cell with dispersed ribosomes and inactive Golgi area; the cytoplasmic membrane is distinguished by the presence of a large number of finger-like projections at the surface; these may be the electron microscopic counterpart of the membrane 'ruffling' seen by light microscopy. Monocytes move with a characteristic motion; the cell contour is often irregular and wavy and the surface seems to be in constant oscillating motion as the cell slides forward.

Kinetics

The majority of monocytes are formed in the bone marrow. The marrow monoblast is indistinguishable on morphological grounds from a myeloblast but gives rise to a large cell with indented nucleus which is termed a promonocyte. Labelling studies indicate that the newly formed monocyte leaves the marrow very soon after maturation and, like the neutrophil granulocyte, passes by way of the peripheral blood to the tissues. In mice the blood transit time for monocytes is of the order of 32 hours. On reaching the tissues, the monocyte becomes actively phagocytic and is then called a macrophage. The total number of tissue macrophages greatly exceeds the number of circulating monocytes, perhaps by a factor of 400. Macrophages are especially prominent in the lymph nodes and spleen, in the liver as Kupffer cells and in the pulmonary alveoli. The exact lifespan of the tissue macrophages is not established but its total duration appears to be measured in months rather than in days.

Role in Inflammation

Mononuclear phagocytic cells accumulate at the site of the lesion in both acute and chronic inflammatory conditions. When experimental lesions are produced by the introduction of sterile irritants such as paraffin oil or fibrinogen, the number of macrophages at the site increases rapidly over the first 3 days, and these are derived from the peripheral blood. Similarly, the mononuclear phagocytes that appear in the cutaneous delayed hypersensitivity reaction are derived from circulating monocytes and these in turn originated from bone marrow. The exact function of the macrophage in this reaction remains unclear, but antigen can be identified within the cells in close association with lysosomal organelles; the cell may act both to process antigen to a form acceptable to lymphocytes and to catabolize antigen excess. After a few days, migration of monocytes into the lesion from the blood begins to decline and macrophages already present start to divide; this may then continue for 3 months or longer. Thus it is clear that the macrophage present early in inflammatory lesions is derived from the blood monocyte, but later on it can in some circumstances proliferate locally.

The monocyte can produce IL-1 and TNF in response to endotoxin and so stimulate production of GM–CSF, G–CSF and M–CSF. It is also capable of synthesizing CSFs as well as MIF (macrophage immobilizing factor).

GRANULOCYTE VARIATIONS

A number of conditions in which granulocyte morphology or numbers differ from normal have been recognized in persons with and without clinical problems (Table 11.5); moreover, granulocytes that are morphologically and numerically normal may still exhibit a certain functional defect. Although most of these variations are rare, they have in some instances provided insight into normal leucocyte metabolism and kinetics. Some of these variations will be considered.

Table 11.5
Variations in granulocyte morphology and function

Eponym	Date of description	Inheritance	Features
Pelger–Huët	1928, 1931	Dominant	Bilobed neutrophil nuclei
Hereditary neutrophil hypersegmentation	1939	Dominant	Neutrophil nuclei with 4 or more lobes
May–Hegglin	1909, 1945	Dominant	Döhle bodies in neutrophils, thrombocytopenia and giant platelets
Alder–Reilly	1939, 1941	Recessive	Prominent purple granules in granulocytes, lymphocytes and monocytes
Chediak–Higashi	1943, 1952	Recessive	Giant leucocyte granules, thrombocytopenia
Chronic granulomatous disease	1950	Recessive	Defective neutrophil killing of certain engulfed bacteria

Pelger–Huët Anomaly (Fig. 11.12A)

Pelger, in 1928, described an anomaly whereby neutrophil leucocytes appear to have no more than two lobes. Huët later showed that it was inherited by simple autosomal dominant transmission. The condition is rare and affects 1 in 1000–10 000 people. Typically, bilobed neutrophils are found in the blood in normal numbers and a shift to the left (as may occur in infection) leads to the appearance of many unsegmented cells with round nuclei. Although the anomaly is of interest in studies of inheritance and in tracing the survival of transfused leucocytes, the morphologically abnormal cells show no impairment of function and persons with the anomaly are clinically normal.

Odd bilobed neutrophils that can sometimes be distinguished from the inherited Pelger–Huët cells are found in a variety of conditions including leukaemia, infectious mononucleosis, malaria and in the presence of bone metastases; certain drugs, particularly colchicine, can also induce this so-called pseudo-Pelger change (Fig. 11.12A).

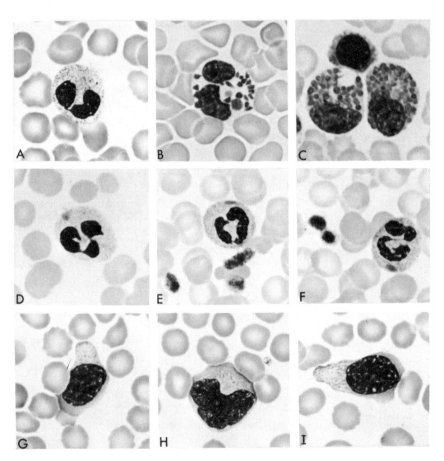

Fig. 11.12. *A. Mature neutrophil from a patient with acute leukaemia showing toxic granulation and pseudo-Pelger changes. B. Neutrophil from a patient with Chediak–Higashi syndrome. C. Two eosinophils and an erythroblast from the marrow of a patient with Chediak–Higashi syndrome. D, E and F. Neutrophils from a patient with May–Hegglin anomaly. Note the cytoplasmic Döhle bodies, seen here as darkly staining inclusions near the plasma membrane, and the giant platelets. G, H and I. Atypical lymphocytes from a patient with infectious mononucleosis.*

Hereditary Hypersegmentation of Neutrophils

This is a rare anomaly in which the majority of neutrophils have four or more lobes. It is inherited by a simple dominant transmission and neutrophil function appears intact. Its main importance is that it should not be confused with the much more common neutrophil hypersegmentation seen in association with deficiency of vitamin B_{12} or folate.

May–Hegglin Anomaly (Fig. 11.12D, E, F)

This uncommon condition, first described by May in 1909 and redescribed by Hegglin in 1945, is characterized by the presence of inclusion bodies in the neutrophil cytoplasm and thrombocytopenia. The inclusion bodies, termed Döhle bodies, are discrete round or rod-shaped cytoplasmic bodies usually 1 μm or 2 μm in length; they stain blue or grey with Romanowsky stains, in contrast to the pinkish cytoplasm of the mature granulocyte. There may be an associated leucopenia or, more regularly, thrombocytopenia; giant platelets are also present. Haemorrhagic manifestations have been described, but in general persons with the anomaly have no clinical problems. One family with May–Hegglin anomaly and a high incidence of leukaemia has been described. The inheritance is autosomal dominant.

Döhle bodies stain an intense red with pyronin, and electron microscopy shows that they contain electron-dense fibrils 5 nm in diameter; the features suggest that they represent RNA and are islands of cytoplasm persisting from an earlier stage in cell development. They may be seen as an acquired phenomenon in scarlet fever, other infections, after severe burns and in normal pregnancy.

Alder–Reilly Anomaly

Alder and Reilly independently described, in 1939 and 1941, an anomaly of neutrophils in which the granules are unduly prominent. The granules take on a deep purple colour with Romanowsky stains and are present in all types of granulocytes as well as in lymphocytes, monocytes and probably cells of other tissues such as osteoblasts. The granules contain a mucopolysaccharide and are therefore thought to represent an abnormality of polysac-

charide storage. The abnormality is often seen in association with gargoylism (Hurler syndrome) and occasionally in amaurotic family idiocy (Tay–Sachs disease).

Myeloperoxidase Deficiency

About one person in 2000 has neutrophils (but not eosinophils) that lack myeloperoxidase. The majority of these individuals have no increased incidence of bacterial infection. Occasional patients with myeloperoxidase have recurrent bacterial infections due to failure of neutrophils to kill bacteria and fungi.

Chediak–Higashi Syndrome (Fig. 11.12B and C)

This curious anomaly gives rise to giant neutrophil granules in children who have poor resistance to infection and a tendency to albinism. It was first described by Higashi in 1943 but its importance was re-emphasized by Chediak in 1952. The giant granules present in the neutrophils are peroxidase positive and represent the coalescence of large numbers of primary granules; the large granules appear in the neutrophils, but single large granules are present also in lymphocytes and monocytes. The secondary granules in the neutrophil are morphologically normal. Bone marrow cells, liver parenchymal cells, adrenal cortical cells and anterior pituitary cells also have very conspicuous granules. In pigment cells the melanin is aggregated into large masses instead of lying diffusely throughout the cytoplasm. The anomaly is inherited as an autosomal recessive.

Those lysosomal enzymes that have been measured appear to be normal and the neutrophil ingests and destroys bacteria normally. Suspicion has therefore focused on the function of the lysosomal membrane, which may be defective. Whatever the defect, children with the anomaly develop leucopenia and thrombocytopenia and show undue susceptibility to infection. They also show partial albinism, with blond hair, pale skin and photophobia. They usually die of infection or haemorrhage in childhood; in those who survive there appears to be an increased prevalence of lymphoma.

Functional Abnormalities

Chronic Granulomatous Disease

Chronic (fatal) granulomatous disease is a congenital disease first recognized in 1950 and characterized by increased susceptibility to infection with certain bacteria. Children afflicted with this disorder suffer from chronic suppurative and granulomatous lesions involving the skin, lymph nodes, pulmonary parenchyma and viscera. They develop hepatosplenomegaly and most eventually die of their disease. No abnormality of immune function has been demonstrated and the children have neutrophils that are normal in number and morphology; the neutrophils appear to be able to phagocytose bacteria normally but they are unable to destroy engulfed micro-organisms of quite low virulence (e.g. staphylococci, many Gram-negative organisms, *Candida albicans*, *Aspergillus fumigatus*). The defect is in the unusual cytochrome b (b_{-245}) which is missing from the cells. This is a heterodimer of α and β chains, both of which are absent. There appears to be defective oxidation within the phagocytic vesicle of reduced nicotinamide adenine dinucleotide; neutrophils of chronic granulomatous disease fail to reduce the yellow dye nitroblue tetrazolium (NBT) to a blue-black formazan in vitro and this forms the basis of a sensitive test for the disease.

The disease is usually inherited on a sex-linked recessive basis. The condition has now been recognized in girls and in these cases, cytochrome b_{-245} is present but functionally inactive.

Shwachman's Syndrome

A syndrome comprising exocrine pancreatic insufficiency with neutropenia, metaphyseal chondrodysplasia, growth retardation and increased susceptibility to infection was described by Shwachman in 1964. Patients and some of their parents have impaired neutrophil mobility and this, with the neutropenia, is presumably the cause of the infections. The conditions appears to be inherited on an autosomal recessive basis.

Lazy Leucocyte Syndrome

The term lazy leucocyte syndrome has been used to describe rare patients with frequent bacterial infections attributed to neutropenia and impaired neutrophil mobility in the absence of other somatic features. The condition is poorly characterized.

Job's Syndrome

This condition was originally described as recurrent subcutaneous staphylococcal abscesses in red-haired girls in association with defects in neutrophil mobility. Patients may suffer also from recurrent infections of the nasal sinuses and lungs and eczematoid rashes. Since the original report, eosinophilia with raised levels of IgE was noted in other patients and the condition was described in boys.

Leucocyte Adhesion Deficiency (see p. 348)

LEUCOCYTOSIS

The term leucocytosis describes an increase in the number of circulating leucocytes, usually above 10 or $11 \times 10^9/l$. Such increases often consist predominantly of one leucocyte type with modest increases in members of other series. The commonest cause of a leucocytosis is an increase in the absolute numbers of neutrophils.

Neutrophilia

Neutrophils do not normally number more than $7.5 \times 10^9/l$ in the peripheral blood. Increases that may be moderate ($15-25 \times 10^9/l$) or occasionally marked (up to $40 \times 10^9/l$) are not unusual in acute infections, especially when caused by pyogenic bacteria. Such infections may be localized in the form of abscesses, or generalized, as in septicaemia. Neutrophil leucocytosis is seen where there is inflammation produced by toxins or infectious agents, neoplasms or burns. It may also be seen following haemorrhage. The peripheral blood shows an increase mainly in mature neutrophils, although there may be some 'bands' and occasional metamyelocytes. Toxic granulations are often present. The presence of a neutrophil leucocytosis in the absence of an identifiable cause may suggest chronic granulocytic leukaemia or, less commonly, myelofibrosis with myeloid metaplasia. Other features, including the presence of immature granulocytes in the peripheral blood, the low NAP and the presence of Ph[1] chromosome, may then be helpful in diagnosis (see Chapter 16).

Leucocytosis is notable for its absence in certain diseases and may then be of diagnostic importance. It is not a usual feature of uncomplicated typhoid fever, tuberculosis or of certain viral infections including measles, mumps and varicella.

Eosinophil Leucocytosis

Eosinophilia is the term applied to an increase in the total number of eosinophils above $440 \times 10^6/l$ in the peripheral blood. The increase is usually moderate but in some cases, especially bronchial asthma, parasitic infections and occasionally in Hodgkin's disease, very great numbers $(20-40 \times 10^9/l)$ of eosinophils are seen. Parasitic infections, particularly when there is invasion of the tissues or bloodstream, are a common cause of mild or moderate eosinophilia in endemic areas. Where parasites are uncommon, eosinophilia is more likely to be due to an allergic condition or to the ingestion of one of a wide variety of drugs. Malignant tumours, especially in the presence of metastatic deposits, may cause moderate or marked eosinophilia and perhaps 5% of patients with Hodgkin's disease have a raised eosinophil count.

Hypereosinophilic Syndrome

The descriptive term hypereosinophilic syndrome (HES) is used for a small number of patients with peripheral blood eosinophilia and other clinical features for which no primary cause has been identified. The patients may have weight loss, fever, rashes, splenomegaly, peripheral neuropathy, oedema, pulmonary abnormalities and a variety of cardiac disturbances, in any combination. The eosinophil count can be very high, up to $100 \times 10^9/l$. In some cases the eosinophils are all morphologically normal; in others, their nuclei may show an increase in segmentation or other abnormalities and their cytoplasm is partially degranulated with prominent vacuolation. The bone marrow shows increased numbers of eosinophils and their precursors but no other specific change. Cytogenetic abnormalities in the myeloid series are not seen. The cardiac damage (Loeffler's endocarditis) may be

associated with eosinophilia of any cause but is seen particularly in HES. It is thought to be due to the direct toxic action of the eosinophil granules on the endomyocardium. Histologically, eosinophils, plasma cells and lymphocytes may be seen infiltrating the myocardium. In the acute phase, arteritis, pericarditis and mural thrombus formation may occur. After months or years there may be subendocardial fibrosis with involvement of the chordae tendineae and valvular incompetence.

Hypereosinophilic syndrome is a chronic disease and patients who do not develop major cardiac complications may survive for many years without undue problems. Treatment, when indicated, is aimed mainly at reducing the eosinophil count, for which purpose corticosteroids, hydroxyurea or vincristine are useful.

The cause of HES is not known. It may be due to a primary abnormality in the eosinophil series or to aberrant production of an eosinophil-stimulating factor. Its relationship to eosinophilic leukaemia is not clear. The latter diagnosis is more appropriate when patients have immature eosinophils present in the blood, cytogenetic abnormalities in the myeloid series or increased numbers of circulating CFU–GM, none of which characterizes HES. Moreover, the occurrence of haematological progression to a blastic phase is consistent with eosinophilic leukaemia but not with HES.

Other causes of eosinophilia are shown in Table 11.6.

Basophil Leucocytosis

Basophil leucocytes normally number up to $0.1 \times 10^9/l$ in the peripheral blood. Young women usually have a slightly higher absolute number than other adults. A basophil leucocytosis is not normally an isolated finding, but is often present in myxoedema and, less frequently, in chickenpox, smallpox and chronic ulcerative colitis. Absolute numbers of basophils are very frequently raised as part of the peripheral blood leucocytosis seen in the myeloproliferative diseases, especially polycythaemia vera and chronic granulocytic leukaemia; an additional rise in the relative numbers of basophils may herald a transformation to the 'blastic' phase of the latter disease.

Table 11.6

Causes of eosinophilia

Allergic reactions: asthma, urticaria, angioneurotic oedema
Parasitic infestation: intestinal parasites (*Ascaris, Taenia,* etc.), tissue
    parasites (trichinosis, filariasis, etc.), visceral larva migrans
Skin diseases: eczema, pemphigus, dermatitis herpetiformis, psoriasis
Drugs (the list is endless)
Loeffler's syndrome
Tropical eosinophilia (possibly microfilarial)
Neoplastic diseases, especially with tumour necrosis; Hodgkin's disease
Following irradiation or splenectomy
Miscellaneous conditions: polyarteritis nodosa, sarcoidosis, scarlet fever,
    chorea, erythema multiforme, eosinophilic granuloma
Hypereosinophilic syndrome
Eosinophilic leukaemia

Lymphocytosis

The term lymphocytosis is applied to an increase above normal in the number of circulating lymphocytes. It is very important to distinguish the raised percentage with normal total numbers of lymphocytes seen when the neutrophil count is low (relative lymphocytosis) from a true lymphocytosis (absolute lymphocytosis) when total numbers exceed $3.5 \times 10^9/l$. Greatly raised numbers of morphologically normal lymphocytes ($25–100 \times 10^9/l$) are seen in infectious lymphocytosis, a rare disease that mainly afflicts children; it usually occurs in small epidemics and may be due to an enterovirus. An absolute lymphocytosis may also be seen in infectious mononucleosis and certain other viral infections, when the presence of 'atypical' forms may be helpful in diagnosis. Infants with pertussis may exhibit extreme degrees of lymphocytosis (up to 150 $\times 10^9/l$). High lymphocyte counts are seen in a variety of chronic infections, especially where chronic granulomas occur. Finally, the most important cause of a high lymphocyte count in adults is chronic lymphocytic leukaemia (Table 11.7).

Monocytosis

A monocytosis is present when the peripheral monocyte numbers rise above $0.8 \times 10^9/l$. Monocytes form an important component of the cellular reaction to the presence of mycobacteria in the tissues, and monocytes are therefore increased in the peripheral blood in tuberculosis. Monocytosis is also seen in subacute bacterial endocarditis and some of the cells in the capillary circulation in this disease may have prominent vacuoles while others may show phagocytosis of erythrocytes or leucocytes. Monocytosis is a not uncommon feature of Hodgkin's disease and is seen also in patients with carcinoma. Increased numbers of monocytes are a diagnostic feature of acute monocytic and acute myelomonocytic leukaemias (see Chapter 14). Other causes are included in Table 11.8.

Table 11.7

Causes of lymphocytosis

Acute infections: infectious mononucleosis, acute infectious lympho-
    cytosis, mumps, rubella, pertussis
Chronic infections: tuberculosis, syphilis, brucellosis, infectious hepatitis
Thyrotoxicosis (usually only relative)
Chronic lymphocytic leukaemia

Table 11.8
Causes of monocytosis

Chronic bacterial infections: tuberculosis, bacterial endocarditis, brucellosis
Other infections: malaria, kala-azar, trypanosomiasis, typhus, Rocky
  Mountain spotted fever
Hodgkin's disease
Monocytic and myelomonocytic leukaemia

Leukaemoid Reactions

Extremely high leucocyte counts are sometimes seen in non-leukaemic conditions including acute infections, intoxications and malignancy. The peripheral leucocyte count may exceed $50 \times 10^9/l$ in these cases and there may be an outpouring of immature forms highly suggestive of leukaemia; such reactions are designated leukaemoid and may be lymphocytic or granulocytic according to the variety of leukaemia simulated. The latter is more common, and the peripheral blood in these cases may show numbers of blast cells, myelocytes and metamyelocytes in addition to numerous mature polymorphs. The neutrophil polymorphs often have an increased number of intensely staining primary granules, usually referred to as toxic granulations. Their cytoplasm is characteristically extremely rich in alkaline phosphatase. Döhle bodies may be seen. Nucleated red cells may appear in the peripheral blood. The platelets are usually normal or increased in number.

The toxic granulations and high NAP are important in establishing the differential diagnosis from leukaemia, which may in other respects be extremely difficult. The term hyperleucocytosis is probably preferable to leukaemoid reaction to describe those cases with extremely high white cell counts without immature forms in the peripheral blood. However, the causes of the two reactions are identical (Table 11.9).

Leucoerythroblastic Reactions

The term leucoerythroblastic anaemia (myelophthisic anaemia) is used to describe a form of anaemia in which nucleated red cells and granulocyte precursors appear in the peripheral blood. There is often irregularity in the size and shape of the red cells. Nucleated red cells are present often in large numbers and these are disproportionately frequent in relation to the number of reticulocytes. The white cell count is normal or moderately raised and the complete spectrum of immature granulocytes, including the occasional blast cell, may be represented in the peripheral blood. The platelet count is normal or reduced.

Leucoerythroblastic anaemia is seen particularly when the marrow is invaded by malignant disease. It is also seen in myelosclerosis and in about 10% of patients with multiple myeloma. Rarer causes are shown in Table 11.10.

Table 11.9
Causes of leukaemoid reactions

Severe infections, especially in children:
  pneumonia, septicaemia, meningococcal meningitis, tuberculosis
  infectious mononucleosis, infectious lymphocytosis, pertussis
Intoxications: eclampsia, severe burns, mercury poisoning
Neoplasia, especially with bone marrow metastases
Severe haemorrhage or haemolysis

Table 11.10
Causes of leucoerythroblastic anaemia

Metastatic carcinoma in the marrow (e.g. from breast, lung, prostate, thyroid)
Myelosclerosis (with myeloid metaplasia); osteopetrosis
Multiple myeloma
Hodgkin's disease
Miscellaneous conditions:
 Miliary tuberculosis
 Thrombotic thrombocytopenic purpura
 Megaloblastic anaemia severe haemolytic anaemia

LEUCOPENIA

Leucopenia is defined as a reduction in the number of leucocytes below $4.0 \times 10^9/l$ in the peripheral blood in Caucasians; in Blacks and the Middle East the lower limit of normal is $3.0 \times 10^9/l$. In these it is due to increased margination. In practice, the major contribution to a leucopenia usually comprises a reduction of neutrophils in the blood. Leucopenia is seen in a number of distinct conditions, most of which are listed in Table 11.11 and will not be separately discussed. The majority of them are covered in detail in other chapters.

A number of agents, including toxic chemicals (such as benzene), ionizing radiation and the cytotoxic drugs used mainly in the treatment of malignant disease, cause predictable depression of the bone marrow. In the case of radiation therapy or cytotoxic chemotherapy, the depression of neutrophils (and platelets) in the peripheral blood may be a limiting factor in their use. Many other drugs are capable of depressing granulopoiesis by a direct effect on the marrow. In some cases the effect appears to be dose related, while in others the depression is only seen in sensitive persons. Usually the neutropenia is reversible on withdrawal of the drug. The principal causes of drug-induced depression of granulocyte production (other than those drugs used in the chemotherapy of cancer and leukaemia) are listed in Table 11.12.

Drug-induced agranulocytosis and the idiopathic neutropenias however merit special attention.

Agranulocytosis

Agranulocytosis is a term now reserved for a reasonably well-defined syndrome characterized by severe infection with marked peripheral neutropenia and believed to be of drug-induced origin. Werner Schultz drew attention in 1922 to an illness seen mainly in middle-aged women and characterized by severe prostration, fever, necrotic lesions in the mouth and throat and near or complete absence of.granulocytes from the peripheral blood. Overwhelming sepsis and death usually ensued. He regarded it as a clinical entity, the cause of which was unknown; in retrospect, many of his cases were probably due to ingestion of the analgesic drug amidopyrine.

Schultz suggested the name agranulocytosis for this symptom complex of fever and sepsis associated with pronounced neutropenia. It is now believed that the mechanism of neutropenia is immunological and parallels quinine-induced thrombocytopenia; in this instance, circulating neutrophils rather than platelets are coated with a drug–antibody complex and are then preferentially removed by the reticuloendothelial system. The bone marrow is active in these cases; there may be granulocytic hyperplasia involving the early cells but the more mature forms (myelocytes, metamyelocytes, bands, polymorphs) are missing. This is not due to a 'maturation arrest' but is in fact a depletion phenomenon, since the maturing cells have emerged prematurely from the marrow or have been destroyed in situ.

Table 11.11
Causes of leucopenia

Infections
    Viral—including infectious hepatitis, influenza, rubella and others
    Bacterial—typhoid fever, brucellosis, miliary tuberculosis
    Rickettsial and protozoal infections (on occasion)

Drugs
    Selective neutropenia
    Agranulocytosis
    Aplastic anaemia

Megaloblastic anaemia

Hypersplenism

Leucoerythroblastic anaemia
    Metastatic carcinoma
    Multiple myeloma, etc

Acute leukaemia

Myelodysplasia

Aplastic anaemia

Cyclical neutropenia

Chronic idiopathic neutropenias

Paroxysmal nocturnal haemoglobinuria

Ionizing radiation and cytotoxic drugs
    Radiotherapy
    Alkylating agents, antimetabolites, etc.

Miscellaneous conditions
    Myxoedema, anaphylactoid shock, hypopituitarism, systemic lupus erythematosus

The syndrome is much less common since the recognition of the role of drugs in its causation. However, occasional cases are still seen and in some no offending drug can be identified. If the infection can be controlled with appropriate bactericidal antibiotics, the neutrophil destruction usually ceases spontaneously and the prognosis for the disease today is good.

Cyclical Neutropenia

Cyclical (or periodic) neutropenia is a rare disorder characterized by episodes of neutropenia occurring at more or less regular intervals. The most commonly reported period of oscillation is 20–21 days, but intervals as short as 14 and as long as 35 days are recorded. There is a cyclical reduction in the granulocyte proliferative pool in the bone marrow followed by the onset of neutropenia; the leucopenia is sometimes less obvious and there may be a compensatory increase in circulating monocytes. The abnormality appears to be in the pluripotent stem cell, as similar fluctuations are seen in the erythroid and megakaryocytic cell lines.

Clinical manifestations usually appear before the age of 10 and may recur regularly thereafter; they include fever, buccal ulceration and skin infections. The severity of the infectious complications is very broadly related to the degree of neutropenia, and other periodic complaints may coexist—arthralgia, abdominal pain, sialorrhoea and mouth ulcer-

Table 11.12

Drugs that may be associated with neutropenia

Analgesics	Amidopyrine, phenylbutazone, oxyphenbutazone
Antimicrobials	Tetracycline, streptomycin, novobiocin, methicillin, chloramphenicol
Anticonvulsants	Diphenylhydantoin
Antihistamines	Chlorpheniramine, promethazine, mepyramine, etc.
Antithyroids	Thiouracil, propylthiouracil, carbimazole
Antidiabetic agents	Carbutamide, tolbutamide, chlorpropamide
Tranquillizers	Promazine, chloropromazine, prochlorperazine, trifluoperazine, meprobamate
Miscellaneous	Allopurinol, barbiturates, chlorothiazides, cimetidine, ethacrynic acid, isoniazid, metronidazole, para-aminosalicylic acid, penicillamine, phenindione

ations. Family studies suggest that the disease may be transmitted as an autosomal dominant. Splenectomy is of little therapeutic benefit but testosterone may be of help.

Immune Neutropenia

Occasionally patients are seen with moderate or severe persistent neutropenia that cannot be attributed to alloantibodies following previous blood transfusion. This may occur in isolation, or in association with other autoimmune or connective tissue disorders. It is occasionally associated with drug therapy (e.g. penicillin). Antibodies against neutrophil-specific antigens (N series) occur in isoimmune neonatal neutropenia, and immune complexes and antibodies against neutrophils and CFU–GM have been detected in autoimmune neutropenias. In general, patients' symptoms are variable and usually mild. They include malaise, pharyngitis, cellulitis and mucosal ulceration. Sooner or later such patients are usually treated with corticosteroids, or high dose intravenous immunoglobulin, with varying success. Splenectomy also may raise the leucocyte count, but loss of the spleen renders the patients more susceptible to bacterial, especially pneumococcal, infection and the decision to operate requires very careful deliberation.

Felty's Syndrome

In 1924, Felty described a syndrome in five adults with rheumatoid arthritis characterized by splenomegaly and neutropenia. Less than 1% of patients with rheumatoid arthritis are affected, but such patients usually have a severe arthritis with frequent extra-articular features, such as nodules and lymphadenopathy. The bone marrow shows increased production of granulocytes and the leucopenia results from destruction or pooling of mature granulocytes in the spleen, since removal of the spleen usually restores the blood leucocyte count to normal. The mechanism underlying the splenomegaly is uncertain. Unfortunately, leucopenic patients with Felty's syndrome, for whom infection is a major problem, may continue to have frequent infections even after the leucocyte neutrophil count has been restored to normal following splenectomy. It seems therefore that loss of the spleen has replaced the neutropenia in rendering the patient susceptible to infection.

A leucocyte-specific antinuclear factor has been described in Felty's syndrome but its titre does not correlate with the leucocyte count and similar antibodies have been detected in patients with rheumatoid arthritis and normal neutrophil counts.

Familial Benign Chronic Neutropenia

This is a benign condition characterized by borderline low neutrophil counts. Patients may suffer from severe periodontal disease and furuncles but other major clinical problems are rare. The prognosis is therefore good. The condition is inherited as a non-sex-linked dominant.

Infantile Genetic Agranulocytosis

This a severe disease described by Kostmann (1956). Infants are born with nearly complete absence of neutrophils from the blood and the marrow shows reduced or absent granulopoiesis. Mortality in the first year of life is considerable. The inheritance appears to be autosomal recessive.

Chronic Idiopathic Neutropenia

Severe reduction in peripheral blood neutrophil numbers (below 1.0×10^9/l) is occasionally seen in otherwise normal adults in whom no predisposing cause can be determined. The marrow is normal and there is no evidence of hypersplenism or auto-immune disease. Such patients do not suffer from frequent infections and the condition is therefore benign.

GRANULOCYTE TRANSFUSIONS

Since 1965, it has increasingly become clear that the transfusion of granulocytes collected from normal donors or from patients with chronic granulocytic leukaemia (CGL) can in the short term be life saving for patients with severe neutropenia complicated by bacterial infection. A consideration of normal neutrophil kinetics and the problems of obtaining adequate numbers of donor granulocytes explains the delay in developing granulocyte transfusions for clinical use as compared with red cell transfusions. If the normal daily production of neutrophils is 16×10^8/kg body weight, or 10×10^{10} for a 60 kg adult, one can calculate that the appropriate replacement number to simulate in a neutropenic individual a 'normal' response to bacterial infection might be 5×10^{11} granulocytes daily or more. As the average normal subject may be expected to have in his circulation only about $1-2 \times 10^{10}$ granulocytes, it is apparent that methods for collecting additional granulocytes normally resident in the donor's marrow storage pool are necessary. Such logic led to the development of extracorporeal circuits incorporating centrifugal blood cell separators. Even with these methods, the number of cells that may conveniently be collected from normal donors is only a fraction of the number that should ideally be transfused.

Techniques for Granulocyte Collection

The original continuous flow blood cell separator, first put to clinical use in 1965, was developed by collaboration between workers at the National Cancer Institute in Washington DC and engineers at the IBM Corporation. The equipment is now marketed by the Cobe Company. To operate the IBM–Cobe cell separator, blood is withdrawn continuously from a vein in the donor's arm and passed to the cylindrical separation bowl, or rotor, sunk into the working surface of the machine. The bowl rotates on a vertical axis and blood after entry is allowed to flow upwards from the base of the bowl towards the horizontal transparent plastic lid. During this process the blood is separated into components on the basis of density—heavy red cells concentrate in an outer ring visible through the lid of the separator, plasma occupies a central position, and leucocytes are concentrated as a buffy coat at the interface between 'inner' plasma and 'outer' packed red cells. From these sites red cells, plasma and buffy coat can each be selectively removed through ports in the plastic lid and the plasma and packed red cells can be recombined and led back to a vein in the donor's other arm. The concentrated leucocytes can be collected into ACD or CPD. The typical collection procedure lasts 2–3 hours but can be prolonged if necessary. Heparin is the usual anticoagulant to prevent clotting in the separator bowl. The Fenwal Company has designed and marketed a machine for collecting granulocytes and platelets—the Fenwal 3000—also based on the centrifugal principle. In this equipment the need for a rotating seal between the rotor and its holder has been eliminated and the components are collected directly into plastic bags.

An alternative machine for collecting granulocytes, also based on the centrifugal principle, was derived by modification of a blood cell separator bowl originally designed for platelet collection. In this system, marketed by the Haemonetics Corporation, the separator bowl is allowed to fill with venous blood but the different components are removed seriatim, first plasma, then platelets, then leucocytes and finally packed red cells. Because the bowl must alternately be filled and emptied, the process is designated intermittent or discontinuous flow centrifugation. Both the continuous flow and the intermittent flow methods yield only low numbers of granulocytes from normal donors unless additional measures are taken (Table 11.13). If a red-cell sedimenting agent is added to the extra-

Table 11.13

Typical leucocyte harvests using different collection methods

System	Donors	Red cell sedimenting agent	Number of cells harvested per procedure ($\times 10^{10}$)	
			Leucocytes	Granulocytes
NCI–IBM	Normal	No	1.0 (0.5–1.5)	0.6 (0.2–1)
	Normal	Yes	2.0 (0.5–5)	1.0 (0.5–2)
	CGL	Yes	—	20 (14–100)
Haemonetics	Normal	No	0.8	0.3
	Normal	Yes	1.6 (1.5–1.7)	1.0 (0.7–1.3)

Results compiled from various sources and standardized to a 3 hour collection procedure. Numbers in brackets are ranges.

corporeal circuit of the separator, the granulocyte yield may be increased by a factor of two or more. For this purpose, hydroxyethyl starch, high molecular weight dextran and modified fluid gelatin (Plasmagel) have all proved very effective. A complementary method of increasing the yield of granulocytes involves the use of a corticosteroid such as dexamethasone or hydrocortisone to 'stimulate' a neutrophil leucocytosis in the donor. The ethics of giving such agents to normal persons can be questioned, but in practice no adverse effects of giving single doses of steroids in this manner have been reported.

Use of Donors with Chronic Granulocytic Leukaemia

The number of granulocytes that can be obtained by leucapheresis of patients with newly diagnosed or high-count chronic granulocytic leukaemia (CGL) may exceed by a factor of 20 or more the numbers obtainable from normal donors. In-vitro tests suggest that the function of CGL cells is only minimally impaired, if at all, so the use of such cells is attractive. In practice, enough cells can be transfused to a leucopenic patient to raise his peripheral count by 5 or even 10×10^9/l and this increase may be sustained for some days. Frequently, enough cells can be obtained from one CGL donor to supply granulocytes for two or more patients in need.

In severely neutropenic patients, especially those with aplastic anaemia, the transfusion of CGL leucocytes including granulocyte precursors may engraft the recipient's bone marrow with Ph-positive cells of donor origin. A substantial blood leucocytosis may result. This by itself would be beneficial for the patient, but it may be associated with graft-versus-host disease and the latter may be lethal. To prevent myeloid engraftment and graft-versus-host disease, it is therefore mandatory to irradiate the CGL donor cells in vitro: 20 Gy (2000 rad) is adequate to prevent lymphoid cell proliferation. The principal objections to the routine use of CGL patients as donors are their relative rarity and the desirability of treating them with easily administered cytotoxic agents, which would preclude their continued use as granulocyte donors.

Indications for and Results of Granulocyte Transfusions

It is extremely difficult to assess the result of a course of granulocyte transfusions in an individual patient. In many febrile patients with acute leukaemia or aplastic anaemia, resolution of fever and clinical improvement seem to coincide with the institution of granulocyte transfusion therapy, but in each case the observed improvement could in reality have been due to other factors, e.g. impending bone marrow recovery, change of antibiotics, increasing endogenous antibody levels. However, a number of randomized clinical trials have been carried out in which some patients received granulocyte transfusions and others did not. Though each of these studies can be criticized for specific errors of design, all lend weight to the impression that transfusing granulocytes to appropriate patients can in some cases lead to control of infection.

It is generally agreed that transfusing granulocytes to patients with neutrophil counts greater than $0.5 \times 10^9/l$ is not useful, perhaps because the small number of donor cells available adds little to those already circulating. Moreover, the value of transfusing granulocytes to patients with viral or fungal infection has not been established. With these provisos, the clinician should consider obtaining and transfusing donor granulocytes to any patients with severe neutropenia who develop serious infections which do not respond to antibiotics. Ideally, granulocyte transfusions once started should be continued for 5 days; in practice it is reasonable to interrupt this expensive procedure when the patient again becomes afebrile, but granulocyte transfusions should be continued for at least five consecutive days before one can conclude that a particular patient's fever is not responsive to such transfusions. In these circumstances it might be desirable to increase the frequency of transfusions to twice or even thrice daily, but available facilities usually preclude this.

Adverse Transfusion Reactions

Ideally, granulocyte donors should be HLA- and ABO-compatible with the prospective recipient. HLA-A and HLA-B antigens are expressed on neutrophils and the blood granulocyte increment at 1 hour after transfusion of donor granulocytes is higher when HLA-compatible than when HLA-incompatible granulocytes are transfused. ABH antigens are probably only weakly expressed on neutrophils and there is no evidence that ABO incompatibility interferes either with in-vivo survival or with clinical efficacy of transfused cells. However, the likelihood that centrifuge-collected granulocytes will be contaminated with appreciable numbers of red cells makes ABO compatibility

between donor and recipient very desirable. To achieve HLA-compatibility when the donor cells are of CGL origin is, of course, almost impossible. In practice, the much greater number of CGL cells that may be transfused probably offsets any impairment of in-vivo function that could be mediated by anti-HLA antibodies in the recipient.

The transfusion of donor granulocytes may be followed by a clinical picture in the recipient resembling a red-cell-related transfusion reaction. The patient may develop fever, rigor, headache, abdominal pain, sweating, dyspnoea and hypotension. Such reaction may be due to serum antibody to donor leucocytes.

In addition to the risk of producing graft-versus-host disease, applicable particularly to CGL cell transfusions but described also following transfusion of normal cells, transfusion of granulocytes can theoretically transmit syphilis, malaria, hepatitis, cytomegalovirus (CMV) and HIV infection. Appropriate screening of potential donors should minimize such risks. CMV is a particular risk in marrow transplant patients.

SELECTED BIBLIOGRAPHY

Bainton D. F., Farquhar M. G. (1966). Origin of granules in polymorphonuclear leukocytes: two types derived from opposite faces of the Golgi complex in developing granulocytes. *Journal of Cell Biology*, **28**, 277.

Barrett A. J., Gordon M. Y. (1985). *Bone marrow disorders: the biological basis of clinical problems*. Oxford: Blackwell Scientific Publications.

Boggs D. R. (1967). The kinetics of neutrophil leukocytes in health and disease. *Seminars in Hematology*, **4**, 359.

Clark S. C., Kamen R. (1987). The human hematopoietic colony-stimulating factors. *Science*, **236**, 1229–1237.

Cline M. J. (Ed.) (1981). *Leukocyte function*. London: Churchill Livingstone.

Dexter T. M. (1979). Cell interaction in vitro. *Clinics in Haematology*, **8**, 453–468.

Golde D. W. (Ed.) (1984). *Haematopoiesis*. London: Churchill Livingstone.

Goldman J. M. (1982). Production and kinetics of the phagocytic leucocytes and their disorders. In *Blood and its disorders*, pp. 601–627 (Eds. R. M. Hardisty and D. J. Weatherall). Oxford: Blackwell Scientific Publications.

Kostmann R. (1956). Infantile genetic agranulocytosis (agranulocytosis infantilis hereditaria). A new recessive lethal disease in man. *Acta Pediatrica Scandinavica*, **45**, (Suppl. 105), 1.

Minchinton R. M., Waters A. H. (1984). The occurrence and significance of neutrophil antibodies. *British Journal of Haematology*, **56**, 521–528.

Nathan D. G., Sieff C. A. (1988). The biologic activities and uses of recombinant granulocyte–macrophage colony stimulating factors. In *Progress in hematology* 15, pp. 1–18. (Ed. E. B. Brown) New York: Grune & Stratton.

Sieff C. A. (1987). Hemopoietic growth factors. *Journal of Clinical Investigation*, **79**, 1549.

Soothill J. F., Segal A. W. (1982). Phagocyte function and its defects. In *Blood and its disorders*, pp. 629–646 (Eds. R. M. Hardisty and D. J. Weatherall). Oxford: Blackwell Scientific Publications.

Strauss R. G. (1983). Granulocyte transfusion therapy. *Clinical Oncology*, **2**, 635.

Wickramasinghe S. M. (1986). *Blood and bone marrow*. London: Churchill Livingstone.

Chapter 12

NORMAL LYMPHOCYTES AND THEIR BENIGN DISORDERS

M. K. BRENNER AND A. V. HOFFBRAND

INTRODUCTION

Lymphocytes form up to 45% of blood leucocytes in humans. They are the main cellular constituent of lymph nodes, spleen, thymus and Peyer's patches and are distributed diffusely and in small follicles throughout other tissues such as bone marrow and intestinal mucosa. Collectively, they make up 0.5–1% of the body weight.

Lymphocytes divide into two main subgroups on the basis of function, cell markers (Table 12.1) and response to various antigens and mitogens. T lymphocytes play a major role in cell immunity and are responsible for defence against particular pathogens (viruses and fungi), delayed hypersensitivity and rejection of allografts, including graft-versus-host disease. They interact with B lymphocytes to induce them to differentiate. Plasma cells derived from B cells are responsible for the secretion of soluble antibody.

Modern theories of lymphocyte function and interaction are based on two concepts: (1) that individual cells have specific receptors which allow them to be selected for proliferation and differentiation by particular antigens (clonal selection); and (2) that each particular effector function (e.g. cytotoxicity, antibody production) is associated with a definable and distinctive cell phenotype.

While both concepts are undoubtedly correct, it is becoming apparent that antigen non-specific mechanisms are also important in cell proliferation and differentiation and that the function of a given cell may often depend on the precise context in which it is acting.

Morphology

The majority of lymphocytes in the blood are small cells (diameter 10 μm) (Fig. 12.1). In fresh preparations they are actively motile. In fixed preparations the cell nucleus is round or sometimes slightly indented; it stains deeply and shows dense aggregates of chromatin. Nucleoli are not usually seen but may be revealed with specialized staining techniques. The cytoplasm is sky-blue and usually scanty; it may form only a thin rim around the nucleus although in some cells, notably those seen in chronic lymphocytic leukaemia, even this may be difficult to detect. Cytoplasmic granules are not characteristic but occasionally a few azurophilic ones are seen. About 10% of circulating lymphocytes are larger cells (12–16 μm); their nucleus may resemble that of the small lymphocyte but the cytoplasm is much more abundant and more frequently contains granules (large granular lymphocytes).

Lymphocytes are normally formed in the lymphoid tissue of the bone marrow, thymus, spleen and lymph nodes; other aggregations of lymphoid tissue (e.g. Peyer's patches, tonsils) may participate in lymphocyte production but their exact contribution is obscure. It is likely that the B lymphocyte precursor in the bone marrow is a terminal deoxynucleotidyl transferase (TdT) positive cell, which is also HLA class II positive. Some TdT$^+$ marrow cells also contain intracytoplasmic immunoglobulin (pre-B cells). Cortical thymocytes are TdT$^+$ but HLA class II negative (see below).

Examination of the small lymphocyte by electron

Table 12.1

Cluster of differentiation (CD) antibodies recognizing human leucocyte antigens (compiled from the third International Workshop, 1986)

Cluster	Example	Molecular weight (kD)	Main distribution	Other comments
CD1a	NA1/34	49	Thymocytes	Langerhans' cells
CD1b	NU-T2	45	Thymocytes	
CD1c	M241	43	Thymocytes	
CD2	T11	50	Pan T cell	SRBC receptor
CD3	T3	28, 22, 20	Pan T cell	TCR complex
CD4	T4	60	T helper subset	Macrophages
CD5	T1	67	Pan T cell	B-CLL
CD6	T2, 3A1	40	Pan T cell	
CD7	3A1	40	Pan T cell	FcμR
CD8	T8	32, 30	T suppressor cell	Nerves, splenic sinusoids
CD9	BA-2	24	Pre-B cells	Monocytes, platelets
CD10	J5	100	Pre-B, cALL	Kidney, intestine
CD11a	LFA-1	180 (95)	Leucocytes	
CD11b	Mac 1	160 (95)	Monocytes, PMN	Share β-chain CD18
CD11c	3.9	150 (95)	Monocytes, PMN	
CD13	MY7, MCS3	150	Monocytes, PMN	Skin, kidney + others
CD14	UCHM1	55	Monocytes (PMN)	FDC
CD15	Leu M1		Pan (monocytes)	X-hapten
CD16	MC38	50–60	PMN	FcR-low affinity
CD17	(G)035		PMN, monocytes, platelets	Lactoceramide
CD18	60.3	95	Leucocytes	Common CD11 chain
CD19	B4	90	B cells	FDC
CD20	B1	35	B cells	FDC
CD21	B2	180	B cells	FDC, C3dR
CD22	HD39	135	B cells	
CD23	MHM6	45	Activated B cell	FDC, low affinity IgE FcR
CD24	BA-1	45, 55, 65	B cells, PMN	
CD25	Tac	55	T cells, B cells, macrophages	
CDW26	TI19-4-7	130	Activated T cells	
CD27	VIT14	120–155	T cells, plasma cells	
CD28	9.3	44	T cytotoxic subset	
CDW29	4B4	135	T helper inducer	PMN, B cells
CD30	Kil		Activated T & B cells	H-RS cell
CD31	SG134	130–140	Monocytes, PMN, platelets	gpIIa?
CDW32	2E1	40	Monocytes, PMN, platelets	FcR-high affinity
CD33	MY9	67	Myeloid leukaemia	
CD34	MY10	115	Myeloid and lymphoblastic leukaemia	
CD35	TO5	220	PMN, monocytes, FDC	CR1—kidney
CD36	4C7	85	Monocytes, platelets	gpIV
CD37	BL14	40–45	Pan B cells	FDC
CD38		45	Multiple lineages	
CD39	G28-10	80	B cells, macrophages	Blood vessels
CDW40	G28.5	50	B cells, IDC	Carcinomas
CDW41	J15		Platelets	gpIIb/IIIa
CDW42	HPL14		Platelets	gpIb

Table 12.1 (*Continued*)

Cluster	Example	Molecular weight (kD)	Main distribution	Other comments
CD43	G10-2	95	Leucocytes	Brain
CD44	F10-44-2	64–85	Leucocytes	Brain
CD45	T200	200, 205, 190	Leucocytes	LCA
CD45R	2H4	200, 205	Leucocyte subsets	Restricted LCA

B–CLL, B cell chronic lymphocyte leukaemia; C3dR, receptor for complement C3d; CRI, receptor for complement; FcR, receptor for Fc fragment; FcμR, receptor for the Fcμ fragment of IGM; FDC, follicular dendritic cell; gp, glycoprotein; H–RS, Hodgkin's Reed–Sternberg cells; IDC, interdigitating dendritic cells; LCA, common leucocyte antigen; LFA, leucocyte function antigen; PMN, polymorph (neutrophil); SRBC, sheep red blood cells; TCR, T cell receptor.

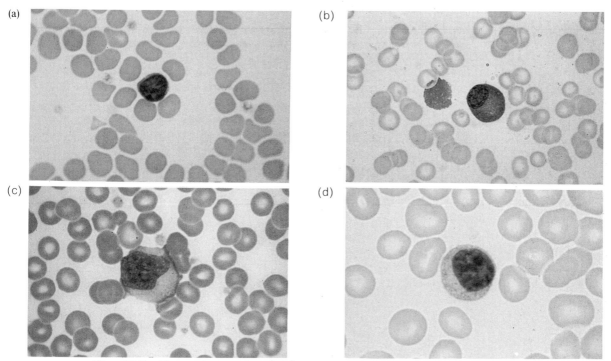

Fig. 12.1. *Photomicrographs of (a) a small lymphocyte, (b) plasma cell, (c) 'atypical' lymphocyte, (d) large granular lymphocyte.*

microscopy reveals features of a 'resting' or 'inactive' cell which is making only negligible quantities of nucleic acids and protein. Electron-dense heterochromatin forms heavy clumps throughout the nucleus and is believed to be metabolically relatively inert; the nucleolus is small and inconspicuous. In the cytoplasm the Golgi apparatus is also small, and centriolar budding is absent; ribosomes are not clumped but scattered singly throughout; mitochondria are few. Leukaemic lymphoblasts, in contrast, have more prominent nuclear euchroma-

tin and conspicuous nucleoli; their cytoplasm shows ribosomes clumped and attached to endoplasmic reticulum and the Golgi zone is larger than that of the 'inactive' cell.

LYMPHOCYTE CIRCULATION

The structures of the bone marrow and spleen are described in Chapter 1. The lymph node has a collagenous capsule beneath which is a marginal sinus lined by phagocytes (Fig. 12.2). The cortex contains numerous follicles which are aggregates of B cells with a mixture of dendritic cells of macrophage origin and occasional CD4$^+$ T cells. The follicles often contain a centre of actively proliferating B cells (germinal follicles), with a less actively proliferating mantle zone of B cells. Around the follicles are paracortical T cells (CD4$^+$ or CD8$^+$) with interdigitating cells (antigen-presenting cells). The medulla is the site of entry of arteries and veins and contains a mixture of B and T lymphocytes, plasma cells and macrophages.

The thymus is bilobed and each lobe contains many lobules, separated by connective tissue, the lobules themselves being divided into an outer cortical and inner medullary region. The cortex contains immature TdT$^+$ thymocytes, including a rim of the earliest cortical blast cells, while in the medulla are the more mature TdT$^-$ T cells. Both areas also contain thymic epithelial cells and interdigitating cells, part of the monocyte–macrophage system. Hassall's corpuscles, consisting of degenerate epithelial cells, are in the medulla. About half the lymphocytes belong to a pool that continuously recirculates between the blood and lymphatic system. Lymphocytes in the bloodstream are carried by arteries to the lymphoid tissues; in the paracortical regions of the lymph nodes they leave the vascular lumen by passing directly through the cytoplasm of highly specialized endothelial cells

forming the wall of post-capillary venules. Lymphocytes also enter the node via afferent lymphatics into the sinus. They then pass into the substance of the lymph node where they remain for a time. In due course they leave the node by way of the efferent lymphatics from the medulla which lead eventually to the thoracic duct; the latter empties into the venous circulation and the cycle is then repeated.

T AND B CELLS: DEVELOPMENT AND FUNCTION

Ontogeny of Lymphocytes

All lymphocytes originate from stem cells in the fetal yolk sac, migrating (in humans) to the liver, spleen and then bone marrow and thymus between the 8th and 16th week of fetal life. During later fetal life and after birth, lymphocyte generation gradually moves away from the liver and spleen and ultimately, in humans, primary lymphocyte generation occurs in the bone marrow and thymus with secondary generation in spleen, lymph nodes and the other collections of lymphoid tissue.

T Cell Ontogeny

Bone marrow lymphocytes follow two discrete paths of maturation. One set of cells leaves the bone

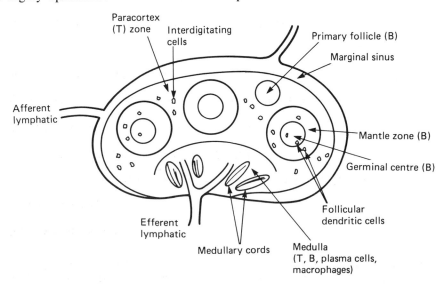

Fig. 12.2. *The structure of a lymph node; the B and T cell areas are indicated.*

marrow and travels in the blood to the thymus, where the cells undergo a sequence of maturation from cortex to medulla and emerge as mature thymus-derived lymphocytes (T cells). The exact characteristics of the bone marrow lymphoid precursor prothymocyte destined to become a T cell in humans remains unclear. The CD7 antigen is the first recognizable T cell marker and it may be that a very rare normal CD7$^+$, TdT$^+$ cell in marrow is the prothymocyte. The process of thymic maturation is associated with major phenotypic changes (Fig. 12.3) and equally major functional alterations which are described below. The earliest thymic cortical 'blast' cell expresses TdT and is CD7$^+$ and probably intracytoplasmic CD3$^+$. While being processed in the thymus, T cells are in intimate contact with thymic epithelial cells and with marrow-derived antigen-presenting cells. Both cells have an important role in inducing maturation and in selecting which T lymphocytes survive thymic 'education', for the great majority of thymus lymphocytes never emerge into the periphery but die in situ. Having left the thymus, T cells circulate in peripheral blood and localize in the T-dependent paracortex and interfollicular areas of lymph nodes and spleen. Recirculation between nodes and bloodstream occurs, and cells also pass through vascular endothelium to enter tissue spaces before returning to lymph nodes via afferent lymphatic channels, or to the bloodstream by the thoracic duct. Mature T cells are long lived (up to 10 years) and production of new cells declines as age increases.

Phenotypic and Functional Distinctions Between T Cells: CD4 and CD8 Cells

T cells are a central component of the immune system. Helper T cells are responsible both for generating the signals that recruit B cells to produce antibodies against most antigens and for the induction of other T lymphocytes with cytotoxic activity against target cells, for example cells infected with virus or cells of aberrant phenotype. T cells are also responsible for down regulating the immune response (T suppressor cells). Helper and cytotoxic T

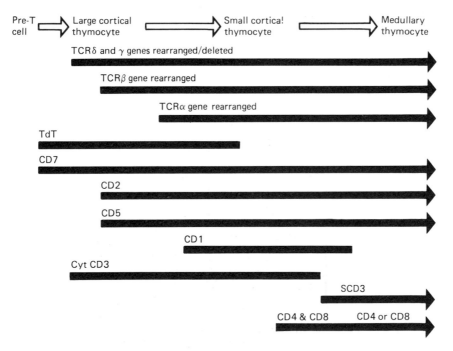

Fig. 12.3. *The sequence of events during early T cell development. The earliest events appear to be the expression of surface CD7, intranuclear TdT and intracytoplasmic CD3 followed by T cell receptor (TCR) gene rearrangement.*

cells can be distinguished phenotypically on the basis of expression of the CD4 (helper-associated) or CD8 (cytotoxic-associated) antigens. CD4 cells predominate in normal adult peripheral blood in the ratio of 2:1 whereas this ratio is reversed in bone marrow. Suppressor cells are also CD8 positive; whether they can be further phenotypically distinguished from cytotoxic T cells or whether the distinction is purely functional is controversial.

Although the existence of T cells which act functionally to suppress the immune system is not in doubt, their existence as a phenotypically discrete subset is uncertain. It has been suggested that suppressor cells are effectively cytotoxic T cells which have cells of the immune system as their target (see section on idiotypes). This problem remains to be resolved.

CD4 and CD8 antigens are not simply convenient identification labels for helper or cytotoxic cells. Instead they have an important role in determining the nature of the antigen T cells recognize and the context in which these cells will act.

T Cell Receptors and Major Histocompatibility Complex Restriction

All T cells possess antigen-specific receptors. These receptors are complex (Fig. 12.4): the antigen-binding portion consists of an alpha and a beta chain linked by disulphide bonds. The way in which the genes coding for this component undergo rearrangement and generate diversity of antigen recognition and the sequence of rearrangement in relation to antigen expression are described in Fig. 12.3. These α and β chains are assembled on the T cell surface in association with another molecule, CD3, which consists of three invariant chains, γ, δ and ε. This molecule acts as a signal transduction mechanism from the receptor to the cell interior. The antigen receptor on T cells does not generally recognize molecules free in solution and instead interacts with antigens on the surface of other cells. Helper T cells interact with specialized antigen-presenting cells in lymph nodes and spleen which present processed antigen in physical association

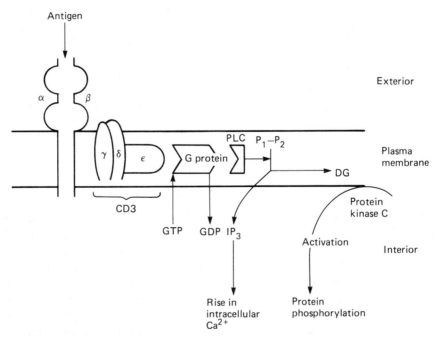

Fig. 12.4. *The mechanism by which antigen binding to the T cell antigen receptor causes a protein phosphorylation signal and rise in intracellular calcium ion concentration. It is likely that another lipid breakdown compound, IP_4, causes entry of calcium from the exterior. (For abbreviations see text.) (PLC, phospholipase C.)*

with class II molecules of the major histocompatibility complex (MHC; Fig. 12.5). Class II MHC molecules are usually only expressed on cells of the immune system (Fig. 12.6) and T cells from one individual will only recognize antigens if these are presented on cells bearing the same class II allotype as the T cell. This phenomenon of MHC restriction is a consequence of a selection process by MHC-expressing thymic epithelial and antigen-presenting cells, in which the only lymphocytes to leave the thymus are those with low affinity binding to self MHC molecules. Lymphocytes with high affinity binding are deleted as are those which do not bind at all.

Generation of CD8$^+$ cytotoxic effector cells requires interaction with CD4$^+$ helper T cells and is also class II MHC restricted, but once these cytotoxic T cells have been induced, they recognize antigen in association with class I molecules of the

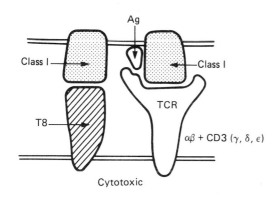

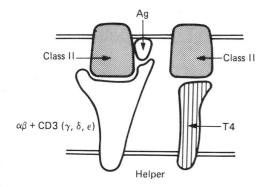

Fig. 12.5 *A model for T cell–target, e.g. antigen-presenting T or B cell interaction. Class I-restricted (cytoxic, suppressor) T cells bear the CD8 antigen while class II-restricted T cells (helper) bear the CD4 antigen.*

MHC on almost any cell—a necessary requirement if these cytotoxic effector cells are to destroy target cells outside the immune system (see Fig. 12.6). It is not certain if CD4 and CD8 molecules actually form part of the antigen-specific T cell receptor itself or if these molecules determine whether the T cell recognizes class I or class II MHC molecules, but it seems likely that CD4 and CD8 both play an important role in determining the recognition pattern of the T cell (see Fig. 12.5).

T Cell Activation

Activation generally occurs when antigen has been bound to the specific receptor complex, and is followed by a sequence of events which induces activation of a GTP-binding protein and breakdown of a membrane lipid by a phospholipase with release of two second messengers, inositol triphosphate (IP3) and diacylglycerol (DG). There is calcium entry, release within the cell of calcium ions, and activation of a cascade of phosphorylation events ultimately resulting in cell DNA synthesis and mitosis (see Fig. 12.4). Activation also causes expression of receptors for the T cell growth factor interleukin-2 (IL-2). T cells can also be activated in vitro by stimulation of another cell surface molecule, CD2; although this structure is known operationally to bind sheep red blood cells (a fact which has been used to separate T cells from non-T-cells), the physiological importance of the CD2 molecule and its natural ligand (LFA3) are not yet known.

B Cell Ontogeny

In birds, B lymphocytes develop in a specialized gut-associated tissue, the bursa of Fabricius. In some mammals, such as sheep, gut-associated lymphoid tissue is also a major source of these cells throughout life, but in postnatal primates, B cells predominantly originate and develop in the bone marrow. There, they undergo a sequence of phenotypic and genotypic changes (Fig. 12.7). The earliest recognizable progenitor is a TdT$^+$, CD10$^+$, HLA-DR$^+$ cell resembling a small or intermediate-sized lymphocyte. Commitment to the B cell lineage is heralded by rearrangement of the immunoglobulin heavy chain gene; subsequently, the light chain

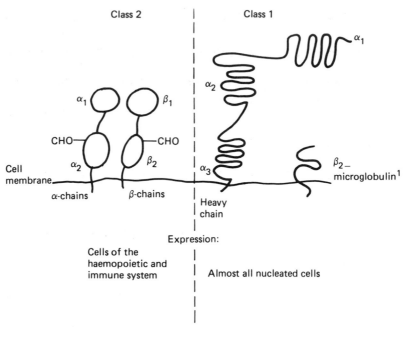

¹Not coded by chromosome 6

Fig. 12.6. *Structure and distribution of the major histocompatibility (MHC) antigens. These molecules combine with antigen for presentation to cells of the immune system.*

genes rearrange (Fig. 12.7). When the cell expresses intracytoplasmic immunoglobulin (IcIg), it has been called a pre-B cell and at this stage TdT expression diminishes. Immunoglobulin is then expressed on the B cell surface as the antigen-specific receptor, which is identical to the antibody that the B cell will secrete (see below). As well as surface immunoglobulin, B cells have receptors for the C3 component of complement and for the Fc fragment of immunoglobulin. The B cells then migrate from the marrow to the germinal centres of lymph nodes and spleen.

DNA Rearrangements in B and T Cell Ontogeny

The chromosome localizations of the immunoglobulin and T cell receptor genes are shown in Table 12.2. These genes remain in their germ-line configuration in all body cells, with two exceptions: immunoglobulin genes are rearranged in B cells and the T cell receptor genes in T cells.

Immunoglobulin Gene Rearrangements

In the germ-line state, the kappa (κ) and lambda (λ) light chain genes each exists as a number of variable (V) and joining (J) segments and a constant (C) region. During B cell formation, one of the V regions is juxtaposed to one of the J regions with excision of the intervening DNA (Fig. 12.8a). The rearranged VJ segment, together with the C region and the intervening DNA, is transcribed; RNA sequences derived from intervening DNA are spliced out and an immunoglobulin light chain protein is produced from the processed messenger. Both alleles may rearrange but, due to an ill-understood process of allelic exclusion, only one is productive. It may be that in normal B development a productive first rearrangement ensures that the other allele remains in the germ-line configuration.

Heavy chain (H) gene rearrangement is more complicated since a number of diversity (D) segments exist between the V and J regions (Fig. 12.8b).

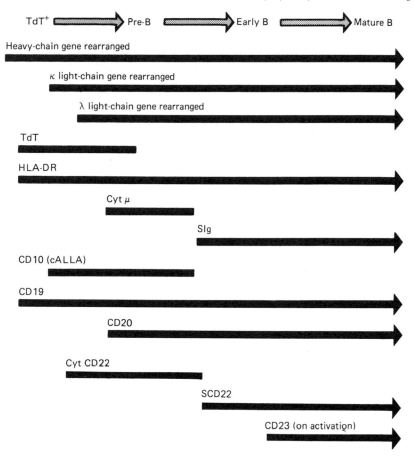

Fig. 12.7. *The sequence of events during early B cell development. (S, surface; Cyt, cytoplasmic.)*

Table 12.2

The chromosomal localization of the T cell receptor and immunoglobulin genes

	Chromosome	
T cell receptor	Number	Band
δ	14	q11
γ	7	p14–15
β	7	q35
α	14	q11
Immunoglobulin chain		
Heavy	14	q32
Kappa	2	p12
Lambda	22	q11

DJ joining takes place first before C-DJ joining. Moreover, the heavy chain constant gene cluster includes nine different genes corresponding to the different Ig subtypes. Class switching involves a rearrangement within this H chain gene cluster to bring a new constant gene into the position normally occupied by the $C\mu$ gene with excision of the intervening DNA so that the same antigen specificity is preserved but the class of immunoglobulin secreted changes. The nature of the CH segment joined to the VDJ region determines the class of immunoglobulin secreted.

The sequence of Ig gene rearrangements is H, κ then λ, so a λ-secreting B cell will have rearrangement of all three genes, although the κ gene is nonproductive. Variability among B cells (and among cortical thymocytes) is produced not only by

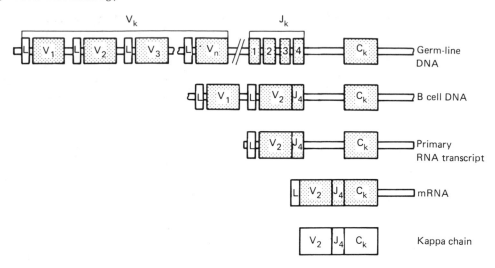

Fig. 12.8a. *Light chain gene (kappa) rearrangement. During differentiation of the pre-B cell, one of several V_K genes is recombined with a V_K segment. The B cell transcribes a segment of DNA into a primary RNA transcript from which the segments between the J and C_K sequences are spliced out to form mRNA.*

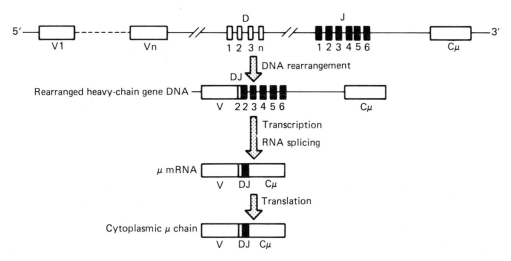

Fig. 12.8b. *Rearrangement of a heavy chain Ig gene. One of the V segments is brought into contact with a D, a J and a C (in this case $C\mu$) segment, forming an active transcriptional gene from which a primary RNA transcript is produced and after splicing out intervening segments, an active mRNA. DJ joining precedes VDJ joining. The other eight constant regions ($\delta, \gamma 1$–$4, \varepsilon, \alpha 1, 2$) occur downstream from $C\mu$.*

combinations of different V, D, J and C segments but also by frameshifts, since new DNA bases may be added by the enzyme terminal deoxynucleotidyl transferase (TdT) which is expressed in early B lymphoid cells at the time of VDJ joining. These frameshifts may also lead to non-productive rearrangements with probable death of the B or T cell.

T Cell Receptor Gene Rearrangements

The T cell receptor (TCR) is a 90 kDa heterodimer consisting of 40 kDa and 50 kDa α and β subunits. Two gene complexes are involved: the TCR α and β genes code for the α and β chains of the receptor. A second, more primitive receptor coded for TCR γ and TCR δ genes occurs in the earliest thymocytes. Both the γ and β genes contain two tandemly arranged constant regions and each is associated with D and J regions. There is a single set of variable segments.

During T cell ontogeny a Dβ segment juxtaposes with a Jβ segment and then a Vβ region to assemble a complete variable region gene. One of the constant regions is brought into juxtaposition, with splicing of the intervening sequences at the mRNA level. The TCRα gene consists of at least 13 families of V genes, and 50 or more J gene segments 5' to the single Cα gene. These rearrange subsequent to β rearrangements whereas TCRγ and TCR δ rearrangement occurs prior to that of β, at least in a subset of thymic cells. The TCR δ gene occurs within the TCR α gene and is excised when the TCR α gene rearranges.

Clonal Gene Rearrangements

The DNA recombinations in the immunoglobulin and TCR genes produce changes in the location of restriction endonuclease sites that can be used in Southern blot analysis to distinguish the rearranged from the germ-line forms of the gene. Thus it is possible to determine clonality, lineage and stage of maturation of lymphoid malignancies by analysing the genes encoding immunoglobulins and the TCR (see Table 14.8). Tumours derived from mature B cells (e.g. myeloma, many non-Hodgkin's lymphomas, B-CLL, B-ALL and hairy cell leukaemia) show monoclonal rearrangements of Ig genes, implying these tumours arise as a clone from a single malignant B cell which has fully rearranged its Ig genes. c-ALL and null-ALL show rearrangement of at least one Ig heavy chain gene (and, in some cases, also of light chain genes), implying B cell commitment. Tumours of mature T cells (e.g. Sézary's syndrome, T-CLL, T cell lymphomas) show clonal rearrangement of TCR β, δ and γ genes, as do most immature T cell tumours, (e.g. T-ALL). The TCRα gene is too complex to be used easily as a marker of clonality. The explanation for cross-lineage rearrangements which have been found in some cases of ALL and, less frequently, in more mature lymphoid malignancies, remains uncertain. It could be due to immortalization by the malignant process of a rare normal cell with cross-lineage rearrangement destined to die, or it could be due to scrambling of the normal sequence of rearrangements by the leukaemic process. It may also be that the cells immortalized at an early stage lack the signals present in more mature cells which terminate gene rearrangements. The same enzymes (recombinases) are responsible for Ig and TCR gene rearrangements and they may remain active until they are switched off by mature Ig or TCR molecules or their corresponding mRNAs. The recombinases recognize certain heptamer or nonamer sequences at the 3' end of V and D and at the 5' end of D and J sequences. Base pairing between these sequences joins the two exons together under the action of enzymes similar to those involved in DNA repair (DNA ligases). Malignant transformation of these early cells in B and T cell ontogeny may allow a prolonged 'window' for action of the recombinases and also lead to dual arrangements.

Antibody Production

This generally depends on collaboration between B cells and specific T helper (Th) cells in linked recognition in which a Th cell recognizes one determinant (epitope) on an antigen and a B cell recognizes a second epitope on the same molecule (Fig. 12.9). Helper signals pass from the T cell to B cell to induce activation, which is followed by proliferation and differentiation and the production of antibody with specificity against the epitope stimulating the B cells. As a consequence of these processes, B cells may become terminally differentiated plasma cells secreting Ig. Alternatively they may become centrocytes or centroblasts which probably represent B memory cells capable of responding to antigen restimulation with high titre, high affinity antibody production. The exact nature of the T helper signals is unknown but they consist in part of soluble factors which promote the growth and differentiation of any B cell in the appropriate

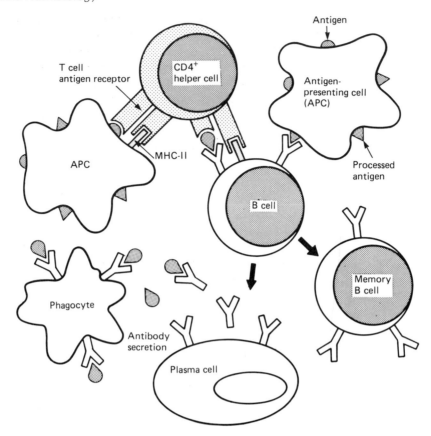

Fig. 12.9. *The immune response: there is interaction between an APC and a CD4⁺ (helper) T cell, with MHC-II and antigen–T cell receptor recognition. Both cells interact with a B cell, with recognition between its surface immunoglobulin and the antigen. T cells and B cells interact with different epitopes of the antigen. As a result, clones of T cells and B cells are stimulated to proliferate, the B cells becoming either plasma cells, secreting antibody to the antigen, or memory B cells. A phagocyte takes up the antigen–antibody complex.*

state of activation. Antibody responses begin as IgM but then mature to IgG (or IgA when the antigenic stimulus is at a mucosal surface). This maturation and antibody class switch is associated with gene rearrangements but it is unknown if T cells induce the changes or simply select those cells which have randomly undergone class switching (see earlier). It must be emphasized that this class switch affects only the IgH constant region of the immunoglobulin heavy chain so that the antigenic specificity of the cell and of its products is unaltered.

Some B cells are independent of helper T cells and can produce Ig on exposure to antigen alone. These cells are phenotypically distinct from Th-dependent B cells and make an IgM response to a limited antigen repertoire which consists predominantly of polysaccharides with repeating subunit structure. It is suggested that antigens with repeating subunits can cross-link the B cell receptor and, in some way, provide the same membrane-triggering stimulus as an antigen-specific T lymphocyte.

Idiotypes and Anti-idiotypes

Every clone of T cells and B cells has receptors with a different primary sequence and hence a different final shape which provides a structure specific for different antigens. These unique receptor structures (idiotypes) are themselves potentially immunogenic.

When a T or B cell clone with a receptor bearing an idiotypic structure reaches a sufficient size to encounter T or B cells capable of recognizing this idiotype, then an anti-idiotype response is triggered. This in turn may induce a further anti-anti-idiotype response, and so on, 'like the ripples after a stone is dropped into a pond'.

Idiotype recognition may be an important way in which immune system responses are up or down regulated. The outcome of idiotype–anti-idiotype interaction probably depends on the nature of the anti-idiotype-recognizing cell (e.g. T helper or T cytotoxic/suppressor) and the nature of the target (e.g. resting B cell or activated B cell). Perturbation of immune networks may underlie many aberrant immune responses and some autoimmune diseases, while the commercial production of anti-idiotypic antibodies able to induce protective antibody responses against a number of viral, bacterial and protozoal pathogens is well advanced (Fig. 12.10).

OTHER CELLS OF THE IMMUNE SYSTEM

Plasma Cells

Plasma cells are terminally differentiated B cells, represent about 0.1–3.5% of nucleated cells in the bone marrow and are the main source of immunoglobulin in humans. They are not found in the peripheral blood in health. The cells are very variable in size (12–20 μm) and round, oval or irregularly shaped in fixed preparations (see Fig. 12.1). The nucleus is round and typically placed at the periphery of the cell, almost in contact with the cytoplasmic membrane. The nuclear chromatin is arranged in dense masses. The cytoplasm appears dark blue when stained by Romanowsky methods and often contains small granules. There is a well-defined paranuclear clear zone.

Immunofluorescence methods have revealed the presence of immunoglobulins IgG, IgA, IgM and IgD within plasma cells of bone marrow, but the cells lack surface immunoglobulin and many of the other markers present on less 'terminal' B cells. In general, only one immunoglobulin of specified heavy and light chain types can be demonstrated within a single plasma cell, but exceptions to this rule have been identified. Electron microscopy has confirmed the localization of antibodies in plasma cells and immunoglobulin has been identified within the tubules or dilated cisternae of the cell's prominent endoplasmic reticulum.

Apparently immature plasma cells with less dense cytoplasm and very prominent nucleoli may be present in the marrow in some cases of multiple myeloma (see Chapter 17) and are often referred to as plasmablasts. It is possible that the normal plasma cell resembled these plasmablasts at some stage during its development from a B cell, but this remains unproven.

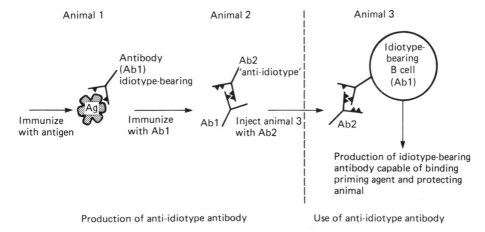

Fig. 12.10. *Anti-idiotypic antibodies for the induction of immune responses to pathogens.*

Antigen-presenting Cells

Once antigen enters the body, it encounters cells which are responsible for processing the material and presenting it to other cells of the immune system. These specialized cells are called by the generic term antigen-presenting cells (APC). They are found in lymphoid organs, blood and skin, and vary in their surface markers, their capacity to phagocytose antigen and in the cells to which they present. In general the cells have a large cytoplasmic:nuclear ratio and form prominent cytoplasmic veils or dendritic processes, to which lymphocytes attach and receive activation and maturation signals (e.g. IL-1). It is likely that phagocytic cells ingest antigen, process it and either re-present it *themselves* on their own surface or release it for capture by non-phagocytic APC. Most APC have a high density of class II MHC antigen on their surface, allowing them to present antigen to MHC-restricted T cells. However, follicular dendritic cells, which present to B cells in lymph nodes, lack class II antigens, implying that interaction between B cells and these APC is MHC unrestricted. Because different APC appear to present antigen to different cell types within the immune system, the route of entry of an antigen, the APC it encounters and the way in which the antigen is processed may therefore modify the immune response elicited—for example, help or suppression, neutralizing IgG antibody or IgE antibody inducing anaphylaxis.

Natural Killer Cells

These cells were defined originally on a functional basis as cells which kill targets to which they have not previously been exposed, in an MHC-unrestricted manner. In humans, they usually have a large granular lymphocyte morphology (see Fig. 12.1) and the acidophilic granules probably represent part of their killing mechanism. There has been considerable dispute as to whether they are of lymphoid or myeloid origin, as they may carry antigens associated with either T cell (CD2, SRBC receptor and CD8, suppressor/cytotoxic T cell) or myeloid lineages (CD16, Fc receptor). Typical phenotypes include $CD16^+$, $CD2^+$, $CD8^-$, $CD3^-$; or $CD8^+$, $CD2^+$ $CD16^-$, $CD3^-$; or $MAC-1^+$,

$CD2^+$ $CD3^-$. Most natural killer (NK) cells express IL-2 receptors on activation and some NK cell clones have rearranged T cell receptor γ and β chain genes, though the complete, antigen-specific, T cell receptor is not expressed. It therefore seems that NK cells fall into two distinct groups: those which are part of the pool of prethymic T cells, and those which form an entirely separate lineage of development. Whatever their origin, NK cells can recognize targets bearing activation antigens, altered cell surface carbohydrate patterns or certain polymorphic alloantigens, and appear to have a significant role in elimination of malignant or virally infected target cells. NK cells may be particularly important following bone marrow transplantation, as *host* NK cells are partly responsible for graft rejection, while *donor* NK cells provide the most rapidly recovering component of the regenerating immune system. Exposure of peripheral blood lymphocytes to cytokines such as IL-2 induced lymphokine-activated killer (LAK) cells, some of which develop from NK cells, and some of which are simply activated T cells. These LAK cells have enhanced cytotoxicity, killing more efficiently and with a broader spectrum than fresh NK cells. Considerable effort has been devoted to a study of the therapeutic benefits of these cells in treatment of malignant disease, but the effects to date have been limited.

CYTOKINES

We have emphasized that one of the key features of the immune system is its specificity, which is a consequence of the presence of specific antigen receptors. However, following antigen-directed interactions, there is release of 'non-specific' growth and differentiation factors; these recruit any immune system cell provided it is in a state of development or activation that enables it to express receptors and respond to the factors (or cytokines) produced. Some of these cytokines act on cells outside the immune system and their overall effects depend on the site in which they are released, their concentration and the sequence and duration of their production (Fig. 12.11). Identification of these cytokines and analysis of their function have only really become possible with advances in gene cloning technology, which have allowed production of

Table 12.3

Cytokines and their origin

Cytokine	Alternative names	Cell of origin (chromosome)	Molecular weight (kD)
IL-1 α and β	See Fig. 12.14	Monocytes, B cells, endothelial cells, glial cells, fibroblasts (2 q 14 for β IL-1)	17
TNF	TNFα	Macrophages, NK cells (chromosome 6)	17
Lymphotoxin	TNFβ	T cells (chromosome 6) (close to TNF & MHC)	20
γIFN		T cells (chromosome 12)	17
IL-2	T cell growth factor		17
IL-4	B-cell-stimulating factor 1	T cells, monocytes ? Other cells	18
IL-5	T cell replacing factor, BCGFII	T cells	30–60
IL-6	B cell differentiation factor	Fibroblasts, T cells, cardiac myxomas, bladder epithelium	26
IL-7	? Pre-B cell growth factor		

IFN, interferon; TNF, tumour-necrosis factor; IL, interleukin. A growth factor for pre-β cells has recently been termed IL-7.

large quantities of pure factors and the assignment of function to defined molecules (Table 12.3).

Interleukin-1

Interleukin-1 (IL-1) is one of the most 'promiscuous' of all immune system cytokines. Two forms of this molecule are produced by activated macrophages and B cells, alpha and beta which have 45% homology between nucleotide sequences. Both are biologically active, but ten times as much of the IL-1 beta form is produced. Cells outside the immune system have also been shown to produce IL-1 alpha and beta, including endothelial cells, astrocytes and fibroblasts. The widespread activities of IL-1 are illustrated in Figure 12.12, and can be summarized by saying that IL-1 is a major mediator for the recruitment and activation of cells involved in the inflammatory response and in wound healing. Within the immune system, IL-1 induces lymphokine secretion and expression of IL-2 receptors on T cells and maturation of pre-B cells. IL-1 was previously thought to cause bone resorption (osteoclast activating factor, OAF) but this is now known to be lymphotoxin. IL-1 is also important in stimulating bone marrow stromal cells to secrete colony-stimulating factors GM–CSF, M–CSF and G–CSF.

Interleukin-2

Interleukin-2 (IL-2) is perhaps the keystone among lymphokines. Human IL-2 is a glycosylated protein with a molecular weight of about 17 000. In the absence of IL-2, T lymphocyte growth is not maintained and T cells no longer release growth factors for the rest of the immune system (see Fig. 12.11). In addition, IL-2 promotes the cytotoxic effector function of LAK cells. IL-2 is also released by activated large granular lymphocytes and may play a role in B cell growth and differentiation (see below). In other words, this cytokine, initially called T cell growth factor, is not exclusively produced by or active upon T lymphocytes. IL-2 acts via specific receptors. The high-affinity IL-2 receptor has been identified as a two-chain heterodimer expressed on mitogen- or antigen-activated T cells, some B cells and monocytes. Lower affinity monomeric struc-

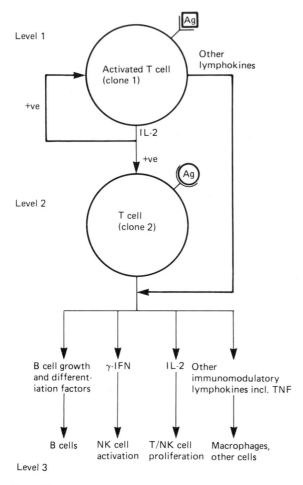

Fig. 12.11. *Lymphokines in the immune system: three levels of action.*

tures may be present on these cells before activation. The receptor is detected by specific monoclonal antibodies belonging to the CD25 group, the best known being anti-Tac which reacts with the low affinity 55 kDa chain. The IL-2 receptor is also expressed on the neoplastic cells in hairy cell leukaemia, adult T cell leukaemia, B-CLL, Hodgkin's disease and some cases of ALL.

B Cell Growth and Differentiation Factors

The dissection of the different stages of B cell activation and differentiation and the understanding of the different factors involved in these processes have only recently begun to be possible. Three active growth factors have now been identified and cloned. These appear to work in a continuum over the stages of B cell development so that there is no clearly defined point where one factor stops working and another starts. The three factors described are as follows.

(1) B-cell-stimulating factor-1 (BSF-1, IL-4). This factor is produced by T cells and induces resting B cells to express class II MHC antigens. It also drives B cells that have been activated (for example by binding anti-IgM) into proliferation. IL-4 also modifies the growth and function of T cells.

(2) B cell differentiation factor (BCDF; IL-6) is now known to be the same molecule as beta-2 interferon—an interferon with extremely feeble antiviral activity. BCDF induces B cells to differentiate into immunoglobulin-secreting cells but, again, only after appropriate pre-activation. The molecule also stimulates the growth and proliferation of mast cell lines and may well have an important role in modulating growth and differentiation of other cells outside the immune system, including haemopoietic progenitors.

(3) T-cell-replacing factor (B cell growth factor-2; IL-5) is thought to act on B cells in a later stage of activation and differentiation than those responding to BCDF and in mice induces specific antibody production from antigen-stimulated B cells even in the absence of T cells. In humans, activity of IL-5 on B cells has not yet been demonstrated and this molecule appears mainly to be acting as an eosinophil growth factor.

IL-2 may also act as a T-cell-replacing factor in humans, but its importance in this role remains to be established. Recently IL-7 had been cloned and sequenced, and initial data indicate that this cytokine can act as a pre-B cell growth factor. Finally, it must be repeated that IL-1 has a major role in the initial activation and stimulation of B cells (Fig. 12.12).

Gamma Interferon

Gamma interferon (IFN), like beta-2 interferon/BCDF, is an interferon with comparatively weak antiviral activities but with potent capacity to modulate the function and differentiation of cells both within and outside the immune system. Gamma interferon is a dimeric glycoprotein, molecular weight 45 000, with variable glycosylation. It is produced by activated T cells and production is

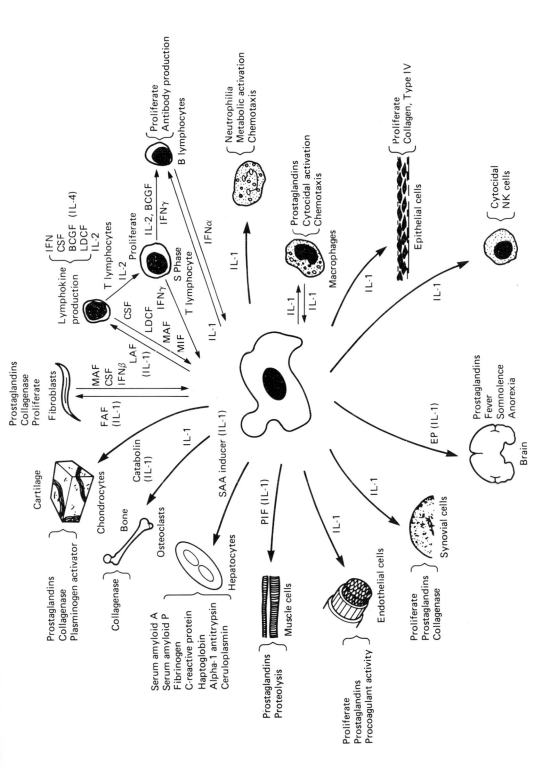

Fig. 12.12. *The effects of IL-1 on target cells and tissues. (IFN, interferon; CSF, colony-stimulating factor; BCGF, B cell growth factor; LDCF, lymphocyte-derived chemotactic factor; SAA, serum amyloid A; PIF, proteolysis-inducing factor; EP, endogenous pyrogen; FAF, fibroblast-activating factor; MAF, macrophage-activating factor; MIF, migration inhibition factor.) (From Oppenheim et al. (1986), with permission.)*

increased by IL-1 and IL-2. Released gamma interferon has a number of effects. (1) It increases the number of IL-2 receptors on T cells and increases the cytotoxic efficacy of T cells and NK cells. (2) It activates macrophages which more readily phagocytose micro-organisms, and develop greater resistance to viral invasion. In addition they generate increased quantities of hydrogen peroxide and superoxide. Gamma-IFN-stimulated macrophages also secrete more IL-1, which participates in the positive feedback loop for the production of more gamma interferon. (3) Class II antigen expression is promoted on B cells, T cells and antigen-presenting cells, so facilitating cell interactions. Class II antigen expression is also induced on cells outside the immune system, for example endothelial cells, astrocytes and thyroid epithelium, an effect which may in part be responsible for the induction and maintenance of autoimmune diseases directed against these target organs. (4) Finally, gamma interferon has potent growth inhibitory properties and it is these that have attracted the most attention in clinical use. Trials of gamma IFN have been conducted in haematological and non-haematological malignancy in an attempt to induce or maintain remission. Some successes have been reported in chronic granulocytic leukaemia (CGL), hairy cell leukaemia and renal cell carcinoma, but the capacity of gamma interferon as a single agent to make a substantial impact on these diseases is dubious. The combination of gamma interferon with other cytokines (in particular TNF, with which it has synergistic antiproliferative actions) may prove more promising.

Infusion of gamma interferon produces fever, rigors, malaise and drowsiness. Some of these effects appear to be a direct consequence of the gamma IFN but many may be due to secondary release of other cytokines such as IL-1.

Although not clearly involved in the immune response, two other cytokines of haematological importance are mentioned here for the sake of completeness.

Alpha Interferon

Alpha interferons comprise a family of 12 closely related non-glycosylated proteins with potent antiviral activity and are produced by many cell types. Recently, the main interest in these agents has focused on their antineoplastic activity. Mixtures or single subtypes of alpha interferon derived from leucocytes and lymphoblastoid cell lines have now been extensively tested against a variety of malignancies. They have been shown to have activity in a number of haematological diseases, including hairy cell leukaemia, non-Hodgkin's lymphoma, essential thrombocythaemia and CGL. Tumours of ovary and bladder may also respond. In addition, the antiviral activity of alpha interferon has been exploited in the treatment of chronic viral infections, e.g. hepatitis B (e antigen positive), chronic active hepatitis and recurrent genital warts.

The mechanisms underlying the antineoplastic activity of alpha interferon are uncertain. Induction of the enzyme 2′-5′ oligo-A synthetase, which leads to a rise in cell oligo-A which stimulates breakdown of RNA, may be one pathway. But since tumour sensitivity does not relate either to the presence or to the number of IFN receptors, this direct action, modulating a variety of second messengers which transmit regulatory signals to the nucleus, is almost certainly complemented by additional effects on the release of and response to growth factors for tumour cells. Alpha interferon may also inhibit angioneogenesis. It seems probable that most benefit from alpha IFN therapy will be obtained when it is combined with other cytokines and with traditional chemotherapeutic agents.

Tumour Necrosis Factor

Tumour necrosis factor (TNF) was first obtained from monocytes; a closely related factor—lymphotoxin—comes from lymphocytes. NK cells also produce a molecule called natural killer cytotoxic factor which appears to be almost identical to lymphotoxin. TNF was first characterized as a product from activated macrophages that induced regression of some transplanted tumours in rodents, while having little or no effect on primary cell cultures or normal cell lines. It is now clear that TNF has multiple other functions in addition to its capacity to inhibit tumour growth. Thus, it regulates the growth of many normal cells, including haemopoietic progenitors, by producing reversible suppression of some specific cellular proteins at the level of transcription and by increasing production of others, including GM–CSF, G–CSF and M–CSF from stromal cells. TNF may also have growth-promoting activity, for example on fibroblasts, T cells and B cells, and so may stimulate the growth of some tumour cells. Although many cells express TNF receptors, as with alpha interferon, the number of these receptors does not correlate with the degree of response to the cytokine.

TNF may have a role in treatment of malignant disease, and phase II trials of TNF in a number of solid tumours including ovarian carcinoma are now underway. TNF may have an additional therapeutic role in the treatment of parasitic infections, since it is directly toxic to many parasites and also enhances eosinophil-mediated parasite killing. TNF and gamma interferon may act in synergy, and combinations of these cytokines are now being evaluated in the treatment of neoplasia. Lymphotoxin (TNFβ) has similar activities and also 'OAF' (p. 339) activity.

Network of Cytokines

Physiologically, the cytokines behave as an interactive network with one mediator modulating the release or the response to another. In general, these agents function to mobilize the immune system and non-specific defence mechanisms to increase the rapidity and effectiveness of the response to tissue damage or invasion. The factors described all have positive effects on mobilization of these systems: it

may well be that the short half-lives of the cytokines and of their mRNAs ensure that responses are so shortlived that restoration of homeostasis by inhibitory or down-regulatory cytokines is unnecessary. Our suspicion, however, is that such regulatory cytokines do indeed exist and are awaiting characterization.

IMMUNODEFICIENCY STATES

Congenital or acquired deficits in any of the components of the immune system may lead to an inadequate immune response and increased susceptibility to infection (Table 12.4). Abnormality may occur in cell development or survival, in the microenvironment of the immune system or in the cell interactions which go to make up the immune response. Quite separate defects may produce a broadly similar clinical outcome; nonetheless, detailed laboratory investigation to characterize the nature of the abnormality must always be preceded by history taking and physical examination, which enable these investigations to be appropriately focused.

Abnormalities Affecting the Humoral Immune Response

In general, these deficiencies are manifest by frequent bacterial infections, particularly of sinuses and lungs. Diarrhoea is also common and usually

Table 12.4
Diseases associated with hypogammaglobulinaemia

Organ	Disease	Organisms
Respiratory tract	Sinusitis Bronchitis Bronchiectasis	*Haemophilus influenzae* Pneumococcus
Gastrointestinal tract	Chronic diarrhoea or malabsorption Intestinal lymphangiectasia	Campylobacter Cryptosporidia (*Isospora hominis*)
Central nervous system	Encephalitis Dementia	Echovirus? Retrovirus Poliovirus (live attenuated)
Joints	Scleroderma-like syndrome	Echovirus

has an infective origin. Although these patients do
not generally have an increased susceptibility to
virus infection, echoviruses may produce chronic
encephalitis or a scleroderma-like syndrome (see
Table 12.4).

Congenital Hypogammaglobulinaemia

This is usually a sex-linked recessive defect,
although an autosomal recessive variant has
been described (Table 12.5). It is not clear why
the X chromosome should be so important in
B cell growth and development, but X-linked
hypogammaglobulinaemia is by no means unique
to humans. The infants are usually well for the first
few months of life because they are protected by
transferred maternal IgG, but then infections begin.
Physical examination shows absence of tonsils and
laboratory investigation reveals absent IgA and
IgM with low—and falling—IgG. T cells are present in the peripheral blood but surface immuno-
globulin-bearing B cells are essentially absent.

Some pre-B cells (with cytoplasmic IgM) may be
found. These B cells fail to respond to mitogens or
to B cell growth and differentiation factors.

Some patients have near normal levels of IgM
and IgM-bearing B cells in the peripheral blood,
but the normal sequence of isotype maturation does
not occur in vivo and cannot be induced in vitro.

Common Variable (Acquired) Hypogamma-globulinaemia

As the name implies, this is a heterogeneous group
of diseases characterized by low immunoglobulin
levels usually affecting all isotypes. The onset is
usually later than 6 months after birth and often
first develops in adult life. On examination, patients
may have signs of chronic respiratory disease (e.g.
wheezing, chronic bronchitis or bronchiectasis with
clubbing) or of malabsorption from chronic gut
infection (see Table 12.4). Tonsillar development
appears normal. Investigation shows low IgG, IgM
and IgA, but the measured levels of these isotypes

Table 12.5
Inheritance of primary immunodeficiency

Defect	Inheritance
B cell	
X-linked hypogammaglobulinaemia	X linked
Acquired hypogammaglobulinaemia	Non-inherited
T cell	
DiGeorge syndrome	Non-inherited
Mucocutaneous candidiasis	Autosomal recessive
Purine nucleoside phosphorylase deficiency	Autosomal recessive
NK cell	
Chediak-Higashi syndrome*	Autosomal recessive
Combined	
Adenosine deaminase deficiency	
Bare lymphocyte syndrome	Autosomal recessive
LFA1 deficiency	
Ataxia telangiectasia	
Neutrophil	
Chronic granulomatous disease	X linked—occasionally
Chediak-Higashi*	autosomal recessive

*See Chapter 11 for discussion.

may vary widely with time and between individuals. The patients show a complex and rather confusing pattern of abnormalities in their B cells. Total B cell numbers may be low or normal, although IgD or IgG-bearing cells are almost invariably reduced. These B cells respond poorly to growth and differentiation signals although they can be induced by EBV to synthesize substantial quantities of IgM and sometimes IgG, IgA and IgD as well. Different investigators have found T helper function to be normal or impaired, depending on the test system used. More recently, absence of antigen-presenting cell (APC) subsets has been identified in some of these patients. This observation, coupled with the isolation of HIV-like retroviruses from affected individuals, has led to the suggestion that common variable hypogammaglobulinaemia (CVH) is, in fact, a disease of viral aetiology in which the target cells are the APC required for B cell maturation and maintenance. As yet there is no firm proof for this hypothesis. A small proportion of patients with CVH also have a thymoma, and in these patients T cells are generally present which in vitro can suppress allogeneic mitogen-driven immunoglobulin responses even by normal B cells.

Isotype and Subclass Deficiencies

Some patients may be deficient in single isotypes or subclasses. IgA is the most common single isotype defect and is often entirely asymptomatic and detected on routine screening. Occasionally it is associated with allergy, particularly to IgA in transfused blood products, and with high titre antibodies to food antigens—presumably due to their unobstructed entry from the bowel. Respiratory tract infections usually occur only if there is coexisting IgG_2 subclass deficiency. Individuals may also have isolated IgG subclass deficiencies, and an increased risk of Pseudomonas infection may be associated with IgG_1 defects. These patients all have normal Ig structural genes, and it is not clear why there is failure of class switching.

Treatment

As we do not yet know the nature of the underlying defects in sex linked hypogammaglobulinaemia and CVH, treatment is aimed at preventing infections by replacing the missing immunoglobulins and at prompt antibiotic treatment of those infections that do arise. Ideal immunoglobulin replacement therapy would contain all isotypes including secretory IgA. For practical reasons this is impossible, and patients instead receive the IgG fraction of pooled human serum, generally prepared by cold ethanol and ammonium sulphate precipitation. At first this material was administered intramuscularly at 1–3-weekly intervals. These injections were intensely painful and the limited volume that could be given meant that optimal levels of serum IgG were rarely obtained. The development of aggregate-free intravenous (i.v.) IgG preparations bypassed these difficulties. Early batches of intravenous IgG unfortunately also transmitted non-A, non-B hepatitis virus (and perhaps HIV) but this problem has now been overcome. Although there is no doubt that intravenous preparations have improved the quality of life of affected individuals, the preparations are relatively ineffective at treating established echovirus infections of the CNS or protozoal infestations of the bowel.

Although the availability of recombinant-DNA-derived growth and differentiation factors for B cells offers an additional therapeutic approach, the observation that patients produce these factors in normal quantities but lack appropriately responsive B cells suggests these recombinant agents may be ineffective.

Cell-mediated Defects

DiGeorge Syndrome

If the third and fourth pharyngeal pouches do not develop normally during the first trimester of pregnancy, there is absence of both thymus and parathyroid glands. This, in turn, leads to absence of T cells and to hypocalcaemic tetany. There may also be abnormal development of the great vessels and facial abnormalities (including malformed ears and micrognathia), with mental retardation. The disease presents in varying degrees of severity, usually with infection, fits (due to hypocalcaemia) or cardiac abnormalities. Investigation shows normal B cells and serum Ig levels. $CD3^+$ cells are reduced in number and usually in function too, although $CD16^+$ (NK) cell numbers and cytotoxic effector function may be normal. In the most severely afflicted children, the widespread nature of the defect makes heroic treatment unjustified. When the defects are largely confined to the immune system, transplantation with fetal or infant thymus has worked well. Infusion of thymus-derived hormones has proved of less benefit.

Purine Nucleoside Phosphorylase Deficiency

This disease is inherited as an autosomal recessive. The substrates of purine nucleoside phosphorylase (PNP)—inosine, deoxyinosine, guanosine and deoxyguanosine—accumulate in patient serum and urine. The lymphoid cells are predominantly affected as they contain the enzyme deoxycytidine kinase which phosphorylates deoxyguanosine to dGTP and have little ability to degrade dGTP (Fig. 12.13). The high levels of dGTP inhibit ribonucleotide–reductase-mediated reduction of cytidine diphosphate to deoxycytidine diphosphate so that lymphocyte DNA synthesis is impaired. Although there is considerable evidence to support this explanation, other mechanisms must also be important in determining which cells are affected, for patients with PNP deficiency have relatively normal T helper and B cell function, and present instead with infections associated with defective cytotoxic T cell activity. The affected children may also have neurological abnormalities. Investigation shows lymphopenia, usually poor proliferation to T cell antigens in vitro (mumps, candida), but normal serum immunoglobulins and antibodies. Serum and urine PNP substrate levels are high (see above). Patients are normally treated with antibiotics or by bone marrow transplantation (BMT) (see adenosine deaminase deficiency).

Severe Combined Immunodeficiency (SCID)

Defects in stem cell development or in cell interactions may lead to absence of T cell, B cell and NK cell function with potentially dire results. The nature of many of these defects has not yet been elucidated, and only a minority of children fall into one of the clear-cut aetiological categories we outline. In mice, an abnormality of the gene recombinase enzymes (p. 335) has been described as a cause.

Adenosine Deaminase Deficiency

This disease has an autosomal recessive inheritance. The absence of the enzyme adenosine deaminase (ADA) predominantly affects T and B lymphocytes because the accumulation of deoxyadenosine triphosphate (dATP) interferes with ribonucleotide reductase and prevents DNA synthesis (see Fig. 12.13). dATP may also reduce the response of lymphocytes to growth stimuli by blocking intracellular Ca^{2+} mobilization. There have been many explanations for the death of resting lymphocytes with ADA deficiency (or following ADA inhibition by the drug deoxycoformycin) including inhibition of S-adenosyl-methionine-mediated reactions due to accumulation of S-adenosyl homocysteine, development of double-stranded DNA breaks, NAD depletion, inhibition of processing of polyadenylated RNA and ATP depletion. None is firmly established as the main mechanism.

Unlike children with PNP deficiency, those with ADA deficiency have combined immunodeficiency presenting in the first few weeks of life with candidal infection, diarrhoea and severe chest problems. On examination, tonsils are absent as is the thymus on chest x-ray. Immunological investigations show profound lymphopenia, absence of circulating T cells, low serum Ig and unresponsiveness of lymphocytes in vitro to almost every mitogenic and antigenic stimulus. At present there are two therapeutic strategies available for the treatment of the defect. Detection in utero allows a therapeutic termination to be offered to affected families; alternatively, BMT from an HLA-matched sibling or unrelated HLA-matched donor can be offered. However, very small quantities of ADA can correct the lymphocyte defect so that transient improvement may be obtained simply from transfusing normal (irradiated) blood which, of course, contains the missing enzyme. ADA deficiency may therefore be the first genetic disease to be treated by gene therapy, by reinfusing patient stem cells into which the ADA gene and a suitable promotor have been inserted. Low levels of gene expression would be expected to produce adequate clinical results and the dangers of producing unregulated overexpression seem small. This approach has worked in both murine and non-human primate models.

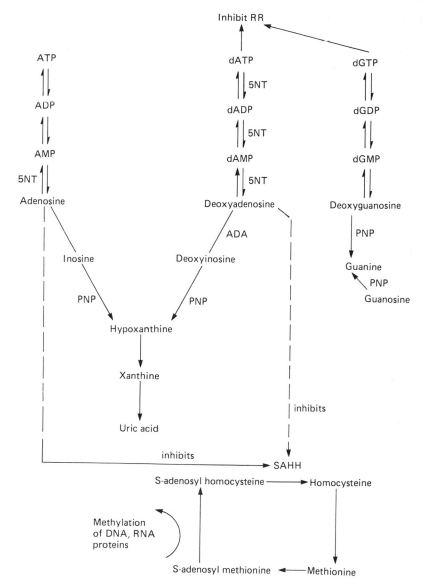

Fig. 12.13. *The roles of adenosine deaminase (ADA), purine nucleoside phos-phorylase (PNP) and 5 nucleotidase (5NT) in purine metabolism. (A, adenosine; G, guanosine; d, deoxyribose; MP, DP, TP mono-, di- and triphosphate; RR, ribonucleotide reductase; SAHH, S-adenosyl homocysteine hydrolase.)*

Failure of Cell Interaction

Lymphocytes co-operate by two major mech-anisms—recognition of antigen in the context of MHC molecules, followed by cell adhesion through lymphocyte-function-associated antigens (e.g. LFA-1) and their ligands. Failure to express either of these groups of molecules leads to pro-found immunodeficiency.

In the bare lymphocyte syndrome, HLA class I antigens are not expressed, usually due to failure to synthesize functional β2 microglobulin. More re-cently, patients lacking class II antigens have also been described. The patients usually have combined immunodeficiency with infections of lung and bowel and profound T-lymphopenia but with near normal B cell numbers. Curiously, however, HLA expression on skin fibroblasts is often normal. HLA expression can be increased with both alpha and gamma IFN but this does not appear to improve the outcome of the disease which, at present, is best treated by BMT.

Lymphocyte-function-associated Antigen Deficiency

Lymphocyte-function-associated antigen-1 (LFA-1) has an alpha chain (CD11a) and beta chain (CD18). Most deficiency syndromes are due to failure to synthesize a stable beta chain, so that other cell surface molecules which show the same β chain (Mac 1, complement receptor 3) are affected. The deficiency affects both lymphocytes and neutrophils, so that patients have a particularly severe combined immunodeficiency with inability to form pus. Again, while alpha IFN may enhance expression of LFA-1, at present BMT is the only curative treatment.

Ataxia Telangiectasia

This condition is inherited as an autosomal recessive (see Table 12.4). Patients usually present in childhood with progressive ataxia and chest infections. Examination shows cerebellar ataxia and telangiectasia in the mouth and conjunctivae. Investigation shows lymphopenia with absence of B cells and low or absent serum IgA. Chest x-ray reveals thymic hypoplasia and may also show evidence of bronchiectasis. Chromosomal analysis and culture of patient lymphocytes in vitro reveal a high frequency of spontaneous chromosomal breaks and rearrangements, particularly translocations and inversions involving chromosomes 7 and 14. These cells are hypersensitive to radiation—exposure to low levels enormously increases the number of breaks. It has therefore been suggested that ataxia telangiectasia represents a failure of DNA repair mechanisms used by cells during maturation and differentiation. In favour of this concept is the observation that patients have high circulating levels of the fetal antigens alphafetoprotein and carcinoembryonic antigen. They are also susceptible to lymphoid malignancy, which is the second commonest cause of death after chest infection. Some patients have been helped by BMT, but the generalized nature of the defect means that the procedure does not resolve all the problems.

Wiskott–Aldrich Syndrome

This disease is of autosomal recessive inheritance. Patients present in childhood with eczema, excessive bruising or spontaneous bleeding and with frequent infection. Investigation reveals lymphopenia, hypogammaglobulinaemia, poor in-vitro response of lymphocytes to mitogens, and low platelet count. Although splenectomy corrects the thrombocytopenia, and immunoglobulin therapy reduces the incidence of chest infection, the defect in T-cell-mediated immunity means that BMT offers the main prospect of cure.

Acquired Immunodeficiency

The acquired immunodeficiencies are considerably more common than the primary immune defects. Nonetheless, the same principles of diagnosis and treatment apply. These secondary defects occur during the course of many different states of disease and abnormal nutrition (Table 12.6), and detailed discussion of these conditions can be found in general medical texts. Viruses have been known to be associated with immunodeficiency states for many years. Although the most widely publicized cause of secondary immunodeficiency is human immunodeficiency virus (HIV), other human viruses may affect immune function. Cytomegalovirus infections may be associated with prolonged impairment of T cell function, even though there is no evidence that the virus can invade lymphocytes directly, and congenital rubella is associated with hypogammaglobulinaemia. Finally, measles and related viruses can reduce both humoral and cell-mediated immunity in humans and animals. However, none of these agents attacks the immune system quite so specifically or so severely as HIV.

Acquired Immunodeficiency Syndrome (AIDS)

Viral Structure

Human immunodeficiency virus (HIV) is a retrovirus of the lentivirus subgroup whose other mem-

Table 12.6
Causes and manifestations of secondary immunodeficiency

Cause	Effects
Malnutrition including vitamin deficiencies	Reduced T cell numbers and function
	Low Ig
	Avoid live attenuated vaccines
Protein-losing states, e.g. nephrotic syndrome, protein-losing enteropathy	Predominant effects on humoral immune system
	Predominant effects on humoral immune system
Burns	Predominantly on T cell function
Uraemia	
Drugs, e.g. cytotoxic agents	T and B cell function suppressed
Radiotherapy	
Tumours	
Chronic lymphocytic leukaemia	Hypogammaglobulinaemia
Hodgkin's disease	T cell paresis
Myeloma	Suppression of normal Ig responses
Disseminated carcinoma	T and B cell suppression
Infections	
Viral (see section on HIV)	T cell function
Bacteria, e.g. leprosy	T cell function
Parasites, e.g. schistosomiasis, malaria	Hypergammaglobulinaemia

bers include the agents causing visna, maedi and caprine arthritis–encephalitis. These viruses contain RNA in two subunits and all have three genes central to their action: gag (group-specific antigen) coding for proteins within the viral particle; pol coding for reverse transcriptase which converts the RNA into DNA within the host cell; and env which codes for envelope glycoproteins. The HIV (Fig. 12.14), in addition, contains two open reading frames (orf), sor and 3′ orf. Although the infected host produces antibodies which react with the 3′ orf product, the function of these last two viral gene products is unknown. Sequence data from different HIV isolates have shown the virus is intensely polymorphic, particularly in the env and 3′ orf regions. This polymorphism is probably a consequence of the high error rate inherent in the HIV reverse transcriptase. Although errors in many parts of the viral genome may be lethal, changes in 3′ orf and in envelope proteins appear to be compatible with survival and may help the virus to keep changing antigenic 'shape' and avoid the effects of the recipient immune system.

Viral Transmission

Although the virus is found in serum, semen, saliva and other body fluids, the number of particles is small and the virus is highly susceptible to dessication. For this reason, transmission usually occurs by sexual contact, blood or blood products. It has been suggested that infected lymphocytes and macrophages are particularly effective at transmission, but the infection of haemophiliacs given contaminated Factor VIII demonstrates that extracellular viruses are potent.

Latency

Although some cells are lysed directly by replicating HIV, the virus remains latent in most and so cannot be recognized by the immune system. Once a

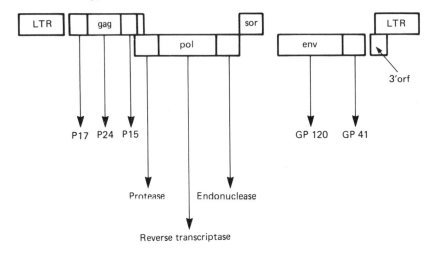

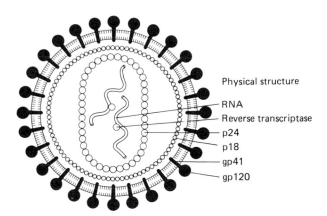

Fig. 12.14. *The structure of the HIV genome and virus.*

latently infected T cell is activated, however, viral replication begins, and cell death follows.

Target Cells

The HIV produces its dominant effects on CD4$^+$ T cells, which are lysed or form syncytia with adjacent CD4$^+$ cells. However, the main site of viral replication may be in CD4$^+$ antigen-presenting cells which can release high titres of active virus. The CD4 antigen appears to be the main receptor for HIV, and CD4 antibodies and free CD4 antigens can block infection. However, CD4$^-$ B cells and T cell lines, brain cells and haemopoietic progenitor cells can also be infected, so alternative receptors can presumably be used by the virus.

Clinical Effects of HIV

The outcome of HIV infection is divided into four stages (or groups) (Centers for Disease Control, 1986; Table 12.6) and it is not yet clear what factors determine whether (or how rapidly) movement from one stage to another occurs. It seems likely that between 30% and 50% of carriers will move into Group 4 from 6 months to 10 years or more from infection.

HIV produces two types of effects: those due to the virus itself (group 1, and the neurological deficits of group 4), and those due to the immune deficiency that follows destruction of components of the immune system. Haematological abnormalities may occur by both mechanisms.

Table 12.7
Modified CDC classification of HIV infection

Group 1: Initial infection
Patients in this group may be designated as symptomatic seroconversion or asymptomatic seroconversion (with or without haematological abnormalities).

Symptomatic infection may include a mononucleosis-like syndrome, aseptic meningitis, rash, musculoskeletal complaints.

Group 2: Chronic asymptomatic infection
Patients in this group have a normal laboratory evaluation or specified laboratory abnormalities: anaemia, leucopenia, lymphopenia, decreased T-helper lymphocyte count, thrombocytopenia, hypergammaglobulin-aemia and cutaneous anergy.

Group 3: Persistent generalized lymphadenopathy
Patients in this group may or not have the laboratory abnormalities (see Group 2).

Group 4: Other diseases
(Medical evaluation must exclude the presence of other intercurrent illnesses that could explain the symptoms.)

   Subgroup 4A: Constitutional disease
   Fever for more than 1 month, involuntary weight loss greater than 10% of baseline body weight, diarrhoea lasting more than 1 month, or any combination of these.

   Subgroup 4B: Neurological disease
   Category 1: CNS disorders   Includes (a) dementia, (b) acute atypical meningitis (occurring after initial infection), and (c) myelopathy. Category 2: Peripheral NS disorders   Includes (a) painful sensory neuropathy, and (b) inflammatory demyelinating polyneuropathy.

   Subgroup 4C: Secondary infectious diseases
   Category 1: *Pneumocystis carinii* pneumonia, chronic cryptosporidiosis, toxoplasmosis, extraintestinal strongyloidiasis, isosporiasis, candidiasis (oesophageal, bronchial or pulmonary), cryptococcosis, disseminated histoplasmosis, mycobacterial infection with *M. avium* complex or *M. kansasii*, disseminated cytomegalovirus infection, chronic mucocutaneous or disseminated herpes simplex virus infection and progressive multifocal leucoencephalopathy. Category 2: Oral hairy leucoplakia, multidermatomal herpes zoster, recurrent salmonella bacteraemia, nocardiosis, tuberculosis or oral candidiasis (thrush).

   Subgroup 4D: Secondary cancers
   Kaposi's sarcoma, non-Hodgkin's lymphoma (small, non-cleaved lymphoma or immunoblastic sarcoma), or primary lymphoma of the brain.

   Subgroup 4E: Other conditions
   Includes patients with clinical findings or diseases, not classifiable above, which may be attributed to HIV infection and/or which may be indicative of a defect in cell-mediated immunity. Patients in this group may be designated on the basis of the types of clinical findings or diseases diagnosed, e.g. chronic lymphoid interstitial pneumonitis.

Haematological Changes

Anaemia, granulocytopenia and thrombocytopenia are more frequent with increasing severity of the clinical picture. The bone marrow is often hyper-cellular, with increase in plasma cells and lympho-cytes and dysplastic features. The cytopenias appear to be due to direct infection of bone marrow progenitors as well as to autoimmune reactions and perhaps to more subtle disturbances of haemopoiesis.

Diagnosis

While the patient may fall into a high-risk category (origin from Central Africa, homosexual, haemophiliac or intravenous drug user), it is probable that such categorization will become obsolete as the virus extends to the community at large. Thus, any patient presenting with suspicious symptoms or signs (see above and Table 12.6) must be investigated for evidence of exposure to HIV. Immunological abnormalities include low numbers of CD4 lymphocytes with reversal of CD4:CD8 ratio (normal 1.2–3.6:1.0) in the presence of normal or often a polyclonal rise in serum Ig. The diagnosis is confirmed by serology or by detection of HIV antigens. Serodiagnosis at present consists of detection of antibody either using antigen to capture serum antibodies directly or by competition of serum with labelled specific antibodies. These tests generally make use of crude antigen extracts and have a high level of false positivity. Although the introduction of rec-DNA-derived antigens may reduce this problem, Western blots of apparently positive sera will still be needed for confirmation. The disadvantage of any antibody test is the lag period between infection and seroconversion, which may be several months and during this time the patient may be particularly infectious. Sensitive and robust tests for circulating HIV antigens, for example p. 24 from gag, are now available.

Prevention

The social and behavioural changes that would reduce the spread of HIV have been exhaustively reviewed. For the physician, the primary concern is to prevent iatrogenic spread by routine screening of blood and blood products and by appropriate sterilization of surgical implements. The extreme polymorphism of the virus envelope means the development of a suitable vaccine is proving problematic as antibodies raised against a vaccine strain would be unlikely to neutralize wild-type virus. It may be possible to identify proteins produced by conserved sequences and construct subunit vaccines, or to use anti-idiotype vaccines.

Treatment

The main focus for attention for pharmacological attack has been the HIV reverse transcriptase — the dominant unique feature of the virus. Azidothymidine (AZT) inhibits the activity of the enzyme but cannot eliminate latent virus from infected cells. Other pharmacological agents are under development, including cloned CD4 molecules which may compete with CD4 receptors on T cells and thereby inactivate virus particles.

LYMPHOCYTOSIS

The term lymphocytosis is applied to an increase above normal in the number of circulating lymphocytes (Table 12.8). It is important to distinguish the raised percentage with normal total numbers of lymphocytes seen when the neutrophil count is low (relative lymphocytosis) from a true lymphocytosis (absolute lymphocytosis) when total numbers exceed $3.5 \times 10^9/l$. Newborns and infants, however, normally have an increased percentage of circulating lymphocytes. Greatly raised numbers of morphologically normal lymphocytes ($25–100 \times 10^9/l$) are seen in infectious lymphocytosis, a rare disease that mainly afflicts children; it usually occurs in small epidemics and may be due to an enterovirus. An absolute lymphocytosis may also be seen in

Table 12.8
Causes of lymphocytosis

Acute infections: infectious mononucleosis, acute infectious lymphocytosis, mumps, rubella, pertussis
Chronic infections: tuberculosis, syphilis, brucellosis, infectious hepatitis
Thyrotoxicosis (usually only relative)
Chronic T lymphocytosis
Chronic lymphocytic leukaemia and various B or T cell lymphomas

infectious mononucleosis and certain other viral infections, when the presence of 'atypical' forms may be helpful in diagnosis. Infants with pertussis may exhibit extreme degrees of lymphocytosis (up to 150×10^9/l). High lymphocyte counts are seen in a variety of chronic infections, especially where chronic granulomas occur. In all these infectious causes of lymphocytosis, the cells usually are large, with abundantly vacuolated cytoplasm and irregular margins. In chronic T lymphocytosis there is often an associated cytopenia. In about two-thirds of cases, the lymphocytosis can be shown to be monoclonal (as in T cell lymphomas) by T cell receptor gene rearrangement studies (see Chapter 15). Finally, the most important cause of a high lymphocyte count in adults is chronic lymphocytic leukaemia or some form of non-Hodgkin's lymphoma, usually—but not invariably—a B cell disorder (Table 12.8). In these diseases, the B cells can be shown to be monoclonal by determining surface light chain expression (i.e. kappa or lambda restriction) or by showing monoclonal rearrangement of immunoglobulin genes.

INFECTIOUS MONONUCLEOSIS

Infectious mononucleosis (IM) is usually an acute illness caused by primary infection with Epstein–Barr virus (EBV). It is characterized by a more or less typical picture of fever, sore throat, lymphadenopathy and splenomegaly, increased numbers of mononuclear cells of atypical morphology in the peripheral blood and the appearance in high titre of serum antibodies that agglutinate sheep erythrocytes. The disease is still sometimes referred to as glandular fever, a term that is historically inaccurate and now obsolete.

The disease may occur in epidemic or sporadic form. The former used to attack young children and adults in institutions and the armed forces, but no epidemic has been reported in recent years. The peak incidence of the disease is now between the ages of 15 and 25 and it becomes increasingly rare thereafter. It probably has a worldwide distribution and its apparent rarity in some regions and some racial groups may be due to milder infection at a younger age and consequent lack of recognition.

The epidemic form appeared to be highly contagious, but the sporadic form does not spread within a patient's family or his close associates; since individuals who contract IM continue to secrete EB virus (see below) in their saliva for months or years after primary infection, it is probable that the disease may be acquired by intimate oral contact, such as occurs in kissing. It can presumably also be transmitted in other ways, including transfusion of blood products.

Aetiology

Infectious mononucleosis is caused by a virus first described in 1964 by Epstein and Barr and now designated EB virus (EBV). By electron microscopy, these workers identified particles with the morphological characteristics of a herpes group virus in cells cultured from Burkitt's lymphoma biopsy material. Antibody to this virus was subsequently identified in the sera of approximately 90% of normal adult males; only persons without such antibody were susceptible to IM, and when they contracted the disease they developed anti-EBV antibody that persisted indefinitely in the serum. This and other evidence means that the EBV isolated originally from Burkitt's lymphoma in Africa is the causal agent of IM.

The haematological and immunological changes associated with IM are best explained as follows. Only B lymphocytes have EBV receptors on their membranes (CD21) and EBV is thought initially to infect these lymphocytes, which then begin to proliferate and are altered antigenically, evoking a massive proliferative response in the patient's T lymphocyte population, which is not infected by EBV. Thus most of the 'atypical' mononuclear cells in the circulation during the acute phase of the disease are T lymphocytes, the majority containing tartrate-resistant acid phosphatase and bearing cytotoxic/suppressor markers, e.g. CD8, while about 10% are B lymphocytes. The transformed T cells are cytotoxic for the EBV-infected B lymphocytes and the majority of the latter are gradually destroyed. The destruction of these B cells may cause release of autoantigens which stimulate the autoantibodies that are characteristic of the disease. The antigenic counterpart of the heterophile antibody is, however, unknown.

Although EBV causes classical IM, a similar clinical syndrome, often with negative serology, can probably be caused by other agents, including *Toxoplasma gondii* and cytomegalovirus. The latter is the main agent of the infectious mononucleosis-like syndrome that may follow the perfusion of donor blood during open heart surgery.

Clinical Picture

The incubation period is not established and may be as long as 5–8 weeks. The illness begins with malaise; fever, pharyngitis and lymphadenopathy appear after a few days. The fever has no characteristic pattern: it may be mild and transient, but in a few cases it may reach 40.0 °C or even higher. Occasionally fever is absent altogether. The pharyngeal involvement is marked by inflamed pharynx and fauces with hypertrophy of the tonsillar and adenoidal lymphoid tissues. The whole of the pharynx, including soft palate and uvula, may show oedema, with a gelatinous appearance or a patchy grey exudate. Pinhead-sized spots may appear at the junction of the soft and hard palates. Lymphadenopathy is almost invariable and is usually bilateral and symmetrical; nodes in the cervical and supraclavicular regions are swollen and tender; enlargement of the axillary and inguinal nodes is frequent. Occasionally, asymmetrical adenopathy gives rise to diagnostic difficulty. Splenomegaly is detected in 50–70% of cases clinically but the enlargement is usually only mild or moderate. On rare occasions the organ descends more than 8 cm below the left costal margin, and splenic rupture, sometimes fatal, is a well recognized if very rare complication of the disease.

Less common manifestations of the disease include rashes, jaundice, haemorrhagic complications and nervous system involvement. The rash may be a faint cutaneous erythema or sometimes a fine macular rash resembling rubella. Hepatic involvement is common if serum enzymes are the criterion, and the liver is palpable in about one-third of cases. Jaundice, however, is seen in only about 10% of cases and is usually mild. Bleeding manifestations include epistaxis, bleeding gums, haemoptysis and occasional gastrointestinal blood loss. Purpura may occur in the absence or presence of only mild thrombocytopenia and is presumably due to a vascular defect.

Central nervous system involvement appears to occur in 1–2% of cases, but the incidence varies widely in different series. Headache and blurred vision are the most common symptoms and all manner of neurological signs may be present, suggesting cerebral, cranial nerve or spinal cord involvement or a combination of these. On occasion the Guillain–Barré syndrome has been seen, and deaths from encephalitis or respiratory paralysis have been reported.

Gastrointestinal symptoms including nausea, vomiting and abdominal pain sometimes occur. Periocular oedema is not uncommon. Much less frequent are electrocardiographic changes suggesting myocardial damage, enlargement of mediastinal lymph nodes, pulmonary parenchymal infiltrates and pleural effusions.

The duration of the illness is unpredictable but the fever usually persists for 1–3 weeks. Subjective symptoms have usually disappeared after 4 weeks but in some cases persist for 6 months or more. The adenopathy, splenomegaly and changes in leucocyte morphology may, however, persist for months. The continuing presence of serum antibody to EBV and the ability to detect EBV in leucocytes cultured from apparently normal persons show that EBV may persist indefinitely in the body.

Blood Picture

The total peripheral leucocyte count is typically between 12.0 and 18.0 × 10⁹/l, although it may be normal (about 30% of cases), below normal or occasionally very high (above 40 × 10⁹/l). Generally, the white cell count tends to be lower during the first week and its rise thereafter parallels the course of the disease. The main increase is in mononuclear cells; in addition to morphologically normal lymphocytes and monocytes, large numbers of 'atypical' lymphocytes are present (see Fig. 12.1). Such cells are seen in lesser numbers in other virus diseases (such as varicella, mumps, infectious hepatitis), in some bacterial infections (such as brucellosis), in drug reactions and sometimes in malignant disease. The 'atypical' cells are appreciably larger than the small lymphocyte from which they are probably derived. They seem to be in a proliferative phase and actively synthesize nucleic acids. In the fixed preparation they have oval, reniform or slightly lobulated nuclei. In some the nuclear chromatin forms coarse strands or masses; in others the chromatin may show a diffuse sieve-like arrangement and one or two nucleoli may be present. The cell cytoplasm is frequently abundant and may be vacuolated or foamy in appearance. The peripheral cytoplasm often stains a more intense blue with Romanowsky stains than the perinuclear areas; the cytoplasmic border may be irregular and there is a notable tendency for it to appear to be indented by one or more adjacent red cells. As mentioned earlier, these 'atypical' mononuclear cells are predominantly activated CD8 T lymphocytes.

A peripheral neutrophilia may be seen early in the disease but a neutropenia is equally common and immature cells of the granulocyte series may circulate in the peripheral blood. Eosinophilia is not unusual, especially during convalescence. Thrombocytopenia may occur and is occasionally severe. Anaemia is rare and then usually haemolytic due to anti-i autoantibodies. The presence of an anaemia of non-haemolytic origin should cast doubt on the original diagnosis of IM.

The bone marrow, which may be examined for the exclusion of other diseases, shows only non-specific changes. There may be some hyperplasia in the granulocytic series and eosinophilia may be prominent. Small epithelioid granulomata, seen also in other conditions including brucellosis and Hodgkin's disease, may be identified.

Serology

A variety of antibodies appear in the serum during the course of the disease that are not present at other times. These may be categorized as: (1) virus specific, (2) heterophile, and (3) autoimmune. The viral-specific antibodies are at first IgM and later of IgG class directed against an EBV-associated 'early antigen' and an EB viral capsid antigen (VCA). The development of IgM antibodies to VCA is good evidence for primary infection with EBV. IgG antibody to VCA persists throughout life.

In 1932, Paul and Bunnell reported that patients with IM have serum agglutinins directed against sheep erythrocytes. Such antibody that appears to react with antigen seemingly unrelated to the antigen that stimulated its production is known as heterophile antibody, and a serum titre of anti-sheep erythrocyte agglutinins in excess of 1:112 is highly suggestive of IM. High titres of heterophile antibody are, however, seen in certain other conditions including leukaemia, lymphoma, polycythaemia, serum sickness and after immunization with blood group substances. Antibodies that agglutinate sheep red cells are also present in low titre in the sera of healthy persons; these are of 'Forssman' type and react against an antigen present in many other animal tissues, including guinea-pig kidney. For these reasons, a differential test was developed by Davidsohn that depends on the fact that the heterophile antibodies of IM are absorbed only partially or not at all by guinea-pig kidney but completely by the antigen found in beef erythrocyctes.

Formalin-treated horse erythrocytes appear to be agglutinated exclusively by the heterophile antibody of IM. Perhaps the simplest of all tests is the widely used 'monospot' test of Lee and Davidsohn. In this test, sera are mixed first with either guinea-pig kidney suspension or beef erythrocyte stromata: the mixtures are then reacted with a suspension of horse erythrocytes in sodium citrate; the presence or absence of agglutination is recorded at 2 minutes. The results are interpreted as with the classical differential test using sheep erythrocytes. The diagnostic accuracy of this rapid 'monospot' test appears to be extremely high and it has generally replaced the classical Paul–Bunnell reaction.

Total serum γ-globulin levels increase about 4 weeks after the onset of symptoms and raised values may persist for months. Immunoelectrophoresis shows that the greatest proportional increase is in IgM (which includes the heterophile antibody) but IgG may also be raised. In addition to the anti-sheep erythrocyte antibody, a variety of autoantibodies with other specificities may be detected in the serum. Cold agglutinins appear not infrequently and are generally IgM of anti-i specificity, but agglutinins with anti-I specificity and of IgG and IgA class are occasionally present. Rarely, the serological test for syphilis is positive (less than 1% of cases) and rheumatoid factor may be found.

In contrast to the variety of serum antibodies produced, cell-mediated immunity is uniformly depressed during the early weeks of the disease. There is cutaneous anergy to most antigens, and lymphocyte responsiveness to a variety of mitogens and antigens in vitro is diminished.

Differential Diagnosis

Because of its protean manifestations, the list of diseases to be considered in the differential diagnosis of IM is long (Table 12.9). The appropriate cultures may exclude a bacterial cause. The liver is usually more tender in infectious hepatitis and the jaundice more impressive. Atypical lymphocytes may be seen in other viral infections. In such cases, tests for heterophile antibody are negative but not infrequently the virus is unidentified. On occasion, the blood picture may raise the suspicion of acute monocytic or lymphoblastic leukaemia: in such cases examination of the bone marrow and heterophile antibody test will help. Tests for specific IgM and IgG anti-EBV antibodies can be carried out and high rising titres suggest active EBV infection.

There may sometimes be difficulty in ascertaining the cause of asymptomatic lymphadenopathy. Significant lymph node enlargement that persists beyond a few weeks suggests the need for diagnostic biopsy. In this regard it is worth remembering that the 'monospot' test is occasionally falsely positive in lymphoma.

Treatment

No specific therapy is available, and antibiotics do not alter the course of the disease but may cause a rash. When fever or prostration is considerable, corticosteroids may produce improvement. Corticosteroids are also indicated in severe liver disease, neurological complications, acute haemolysis and thrombocytopenic purpura or other haemorrhage. They are not indicated in the average uncomplicated case.

Unusual Manifestations of EBV Infection

Primary EBV infection in older patients may present in an atypical manner. Patients between the ages of 40 and 70 may develop fever without conspicuous pharyngitis or lymphadenopathy. Liver involvement may, however, be prominent, with raised bilirubin and abnormal aspartate transaminase values. The diagnosis may not be obvious, particularly when patients give a history consistent with infectious mononucleosis in the past, and such patients are sometimes subjected to needless investigations. Heterophile antibody is usually, but

Table 12.9
Differential diagnosis of infectious mononucleosis

Disorders with a similar clinical picture	Disorders with a similar blood picture
Acute infections	Acute leukaemia
Influenza	Toxoplasmosis
Brucellosis	Cytomegalovirus infection
Typhoid, etc.	Acute infectious lymphocytosis
	Serum sickness
Pharyngitis	Infectious hepatitis and other viral diseases
Streptococcal, etc.	
Diphtheria	
Agranulocytosis	
Infectious hepatitis	
Toxoplasmosis	
Lymphoma	
Hodgkin's disease	
Lymphoblastic lymphoma	
Cat scratch disease	

not always, detected in the serum; the finding of IgM antibody to VCA confirms the diagnosis.

Duncan's syndrome is a rare condition in which patients have an apparently specific inability to combat infection with EBV. The condition is inherited in an X-linked recessive manner. Patients may die as a result of primary infection with EBV and the progressive and generalized effects of IM, or they may develop agammaglobulinaemia, aplastic anaemia, agranulocytosis or B cell lymphoma.

Patients immunosuppressed following renal transplantation who are carriers for EBV may develop lymphoma-like polyclonal proliferations of B lymphocytes that carry the EBV genome. In some cases the disease progresses to a fatal monoclonal lymphoma. The same sequence of events has occurred occasionally after allogeneic bone marrow transplantation for leukaemia or aplastic anaemia and is a well-recognized complication of the acquired immunodeficiency syndrome (AIDS). After marrow transplantation, the lymphoma usually involves B lymphocytes of donor origin, and EBV DNA can be demonstrated in the malignant B lymphocytes.

SELECTED BIBLIOGRAPHY

Balkwill F. R., Smyth J. F. (1987). Interferons in cancer therapy: a reappraisal. *Lancet*, **ii**, 317.

Brenner M. K. (1988). Tumour necrosis factor. *British Journal of Haematology*, **69**, 149–52.

Gordon J., Guy G. R. (1987). The molecules controlling B lymphocytes. *Immunology Today*, **8**, 339.

Hood L. R. *et al.* (1984). *Immunology*, 2nd edn. New York: Benjamin-Cummings.

Groopman J. E. (1988). Acquired immunodeficiency syndrome. In *Recent advances in haematology*, Vol. 5, pp. 291–304. (Ed. A. V. Hoffbrand). Edinburgh: Churchill Livingstone.

Immunology Today. Amsterdam: Elsevier. (Has regular, short and up-to-date reviews of many of the topics covered in this chapter.)

Janossy G. (Ed.) (1982). The lymphocyte. *Clinics in Haematology*, **3**, (2).

McMichael A. J. *et al.* (Eds.) (1987). *Leucocyte typing III*. Oxford: Oxford University Press.

Oppenheim J. J., Kovacs E. J., Matsushima K., Durum S. K. (1986). There is more than one interleukin 1. *Immunology Today*, **7**, 45.

Pinching A. J. (Ed.) (1986). AIDS and HIV infection. *Clinics in Immunology and Allergy*, **6**, (3).

Reis M. D., Griesser H., Mak T. W. (1988). Gene rearrangements in leukemias and lymphomas. In *Recent advances in haematology*, Vol. 5, pp. 99–120. (Ed. A. V. Hoffbrand). Edinburgh: Churchill Livingstone.

Roitt I. M. (1988). *Essential immunology*, 6th edn. Oxford: Blackwell Scientific Publications.

Roitt I. M., Brostoff J., Male D. K. (1985). *Immunology*. London: Gower Medical.

Toy J. L. (1983). The interferons. *Clinical and Experimental Immunology*, **54**, 1.

Vossen J., Griscelli C. (Eds.) (1984 and 1986). *Progress in immunodeficiency research and therapy*, Vols. 1 and 2. Amsterdam: Elsevier/Excerpta Medica.

Zanetti M., Sercarz E., Salk J. (1987). The immunology of new generation vaccines. *Immunology Today*, **8**, 18–26.

Chapter 13

CYTOGENETICS AND LEUKAEMOGENESIS

L.M. SECKER-WALKER AND J.M. GOLDMAN

For many years chromosomal abnormalities have been regarded as valuable in the diagnosis of different types of leukaemia. The identification of chromosomally abnormal cells from the leukaemic tissue in patients whose constitutional chromosomal make-up is normal, has provided evidence of the clonal nature of leukaemia and for the origin of the clone in a single chromosomally altered cell. However, until recently their role in the pathogenesis of leukaemia or lymphoma has not been clear. In the last decade it has been shown that certain RNA viruses capable of causing leukaemia and other tumours in experimental animals (termed retroviruses) contain 'transforming sequences' coded for by RNA bearing a high level of homology with DNA sequences located in different parts of the normal human genome. The RNA sequences coding for these transforming proteins are known as viral oncogenes (v-oncs), while the homologous genes in the human genome are called proto-oncogenes or cellular oncogenes (c-oncs). It is now clear that various acquired genetic alterations, including point mutations, chromosomal deletions and translocations, may lead to inappropriate activation of these cellular oncogenes, which is associated with and may play a central role in the malignant process. These observations have confirmed the concept of malignancy as an acquired genetic disorder in a particular cell type. In this chapter, cytogenetic nomenclature and techniques for studying chromosomes in haematological malignancies are dealt with first. Then follows a description of the cytogenetic abnormalities associated with different haematological disorders, and their diagnostic or prognostic importance. The last part of the chapter covers the general mechanisms

of leukaemogenesis, including the structure and action of retroviruses and the mechanisms of oncogene activation and their association with specific chromosomal translocations.

CYTOGENETICS

The purpose of a cytogenetic investigation in a haematological disorder is to determine whether the karyotype (chromosomal make-up) of the affected cells is abnormal and if so in what way. Chromosome findings at diagnosis are important for the classification and diagnosis of the disorder. In the acute leukaemias the karyotype may be an important and independent prognostic factor in predicting remission achievement and the length of remission and in distinguishing long-term survivors from those likely to fail on standard therapy. Cytogenetic investigation during the course of an indolent leukaemia may be used to predict transformation to a more aggressive phase. The outcome of bone marrow transplantation, when donor and recipient are of opposite sex or have distinct chromosomal polymorphisms detectable with special staining techniques, can be determined cytogenetically to distinguish successful engraftment from regeneration of host cells and impending relapse.

Constitutional Karyotype

A number of constitutional chromosome disorders predispose to leukaemia. These include whole chromosome disorders such as Down's syndrome (trisomy 21) or the sex chromosome abnormality in males, Klinefelter's syndrome (XXY). There is some evidence that individuals with a balanced translocation without apparent phenotypic effect may be at increased risk of malignancy. Other predisposing conditions are the recessively transmitted chromosome breakage syndromes, Bloom's syndrome, ataxia telangiectasia and Fanconi's anaemia. The constitutional karyotype of a patient is best established from lymphocytes stimulated to divide with phytohaemagglutinin (PHA).

Techniques

Chromosomes are visible only in the condensed form which they adopt at metaphase during cell division (mitosis). Populations of dividing cells occur normally in the bone marrow and, in malignant conditions, are also found among blasts which have spilled over into the peripheral blood. Contrary to what might be supposed, malignant blasts are frequently more inert in culture than their normal counterparts. In order to ensure a dividing population of malignant cells, a variety of culture times and mitotic stimulants may be necessary. Marrow is always preferable to blood for cytogenetic study but the chance of detecting an abnormal clone is greatest if both marrow and blood with blasts are studied simultaneously.

Chromosomes are arrested at metaphase by the spindle poison colcemid. They are stained by so-called banding techniques developed during the 1970s to produce a specific banding pattern in which darkly staining portions of the chromatin alternate with lighter staining regions. The two standard banding techniques are Giemsa (or G) banding and quinacrine (or Q) banding. G banding produces a permanent stain which can be seen under a light microscope. Quinacrine is a fluorescent dye which requires a fluorescence microscope attachment. Q banding fades rapidly. The banding pattern of each chromosome pair is unique, allowing positive identification of every chromosome. At mid-metaphase a total of 240–330 bands can be seen over the whole karyotype. If the cells are examined at prometaphase, the number of bands visible may be increased to 850 or more. To increase the number of cells at prometaphase, an agent such as methotrexate, which blocks DNA synthesis, is introduced into the cell culture medium. Subsequent removal of the blocking agent and exposure of the cells to a thymidine-enriched culture medium yields a population of cells at prometaphase as they re-enter mitosis. The technique is particularly useful in acute myeloid leukaemia. Problems of the technique encountered in other leukaemias are related to the toxicity of methotrexate for some leukaemic cells and to variations in cell cycle time following release from the blocking agent.

Terminology

Normal human somatic cells contain a diploid set of 46 chromosomes in 23 pairs made up of 22 pairs of autosomes numbered 1–22 and a pair of sex chromosomes XX (female) or XY (male). Chromosomes are derived equally from the haploid set of 23 chromosomes in each parental germ cell.

Each chromosome has a long (or q) arm and a short (or p) arm separated by a primary constriction, the centromere. Each chromosome arm is divided into regions and subregions based on the bands and numbered from the centromere out towards the ends (telomeres). Thus 11q23 is on the long arm of chromosome 11, region 2, subregion 3.

Chromosome abnormalities in individual cells may be numerical or structural. Numerical change is the gain or loss of one or more chromosomes. The gain of any single individual chromosome results in trisomy for that chromosome (indicated by the prefix +). The loss of a single chromosome results in monosomy for that chromosome (indicated by the prefix −). Structural change includes deletions (del) when part of one of the chromosome's arms is missing, e.g. del (11) (q23) is loss of material distal to 11q23, or translocations (t), when chromosomal material is repositioned on another chromosome. All translocations are assumed to be reciprocal; they usually result in shortening of one chromosome and lengthening of the other. The terms p− or q− and p+ or q+ (with the − or + as a suffix) describe the resulting derived chromosomes. A reciprocal translocation may be between two chromosomes (simple) or between three or more chromosomes (complex). Inversion (inv) describes the inversion of the segment lying between two bands.

Chromosome abnormalities may result in a change of ploidy from the normal diploid complement. Cells with fewer than 46 chromosomes are described as hypodiploid; cells with more than 46 chromosomes are hyperdiploid; and cells with 46 chromosomes with structural change or chromosome gain matched by chromosome loss, are pseudodiploid.

Chromosome abnormalities may be random or clonal. Random change describes one or more abnormal cells, each with a different abnormality, in a population of otherwise normal cells. Random chromosome loss may be a technical artifact which results from the rupture of fragile cells during chromosome preparation. Gaps or breaks may be induced in a random fashion by environmental carcinogens or by treatment.

Clonal abnormalities are defined as at least two cells with the same extra chromosome or structural rearrangement or three cells with the same missing chromosome. For purposes of chromosomal classification, only clonal abnormalities are considered.

Fragile Sites

There exists in the human genome a number of chromosomal sites called fragile sites. These are specific points on a chromosome which appear as non-staining gaps of variable width that usually involve both chromatids. Fragile sites are heritable (can be demonstrated in other family members) or constitutive (are not passed from one generation to the next).

There are at least 17 heritable fragile sites which are inherited in a Mendelian dominant fashion (Fig. 13.1). Most of these are expressed spontaneously in a proportion of cells but their expression is enhanced by, and may be dependent on, culture of lymphocytes in medium which lacks folic acid and thymidine (folate sensitive). Others are inducible by culture with distamycin A. One is induced by culture with bromo-deoxyuridine. The true incidence of heritable fragile sites is unknown because no large surveys aimed at their detection have been undertaken. One survey detected a folate-sensitive fragile site in 1 in 700 infants in a sample of 3090 infants. There are 23 constitutive fragile sites which may be induced under certain culture conditions

(low folate levels and added aphidicolin) in a large number of individuals.

The role of fragile sites in the non-random chromosome abnormalities seen in leukaemia and lymphoma is not always clear. At least nine fragile sites are situated at one of the breakpoints found in chromosome abnormalities in cancer or leukaemia. The presence of a heritable fragile site at 16q22 has been found in patients with acute myelomonocytic leukaemia in whom the leukaemic cells have an abnormality involving a breakpoint at 16q22.

Homogeneously Staining Regions and Double Minutes

Homogeneously staining regions (HSR) and double minutes (DM) are chromosome abnormalities which may contain multiple copies of specific structural genes. They are associated with drug resistance. An HSR is an abnormally long, uniformly stained chromosomal band; HSRs have been identified on various chromosomes. Double minutes are small, paired chromatin bodies without centromeres whose number varies from cell to cell. It has been suggested that DMs may derive from the breakdown of an HSR. HSRs and DMs have been found in a number of tumours and established tumour cell lines; they are rare in haematological malignancies.

The following section deals with the cytogenetic abnormalities found in leukaemias and lymphomas. A later section deals with the roles these abnormalities may have in the pathogenesis of the disease by causing inappropriate activity of certain cellular genes (oncogenes).

Chronic Myeloid Leukaemia

The most consistent chromosome abnormality associated with a haematological malignancy is the Philadelphia (Ph[1]) chromosome, first described by Nowell and Hungerford in 1960. The Ph[1] is a chromosome number 22 from which the long arms are deleted (22q−). It is part of a reciprocal translocation in which the second chromosome is commonly number 9 (92% of cases) — t(9;22)(q34;q11) or 9q+, 22q−. Approximately 4% of cases have a 'variant' translocation in which the second chromosome is other than number 9. The remaining 4% of

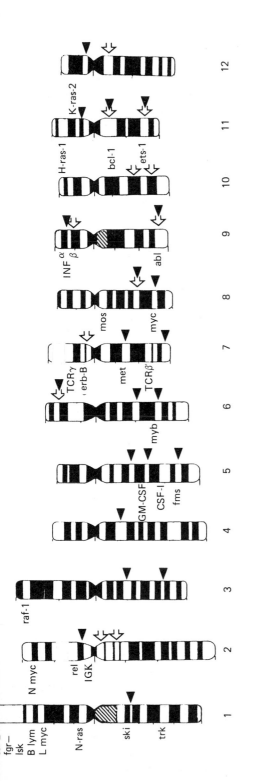

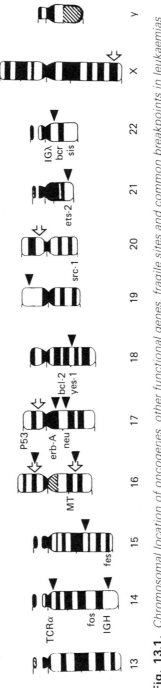

Fig. 13.1. *Chromosomal location of oncogenes, other functional genes, fragile sites and common breakpoints in leukaemias and lymphomas. Genes are listed on left of chromosome, fragile sites and breakpoints on right. Genes for erythropoietin and G-CSF occur on chromosomes 7q and 17q respectively.*

Key

▼   = cancer breakpoint

⇐   = heritable fragile site

lower case   = c-oncogene

IGκ   = immunoglobulin kappa light chain gene

IGλ   = immunoglobulin lambda light chain gene

IGH   = immunoglobulin heavy chain gene

GM-CSF   = granulocyte–macrophage colony-stimulating
            factor (IL-3 gene closely associated)

CSF-1   = monocyte–macrophage colony-stimulating factor

TCRα   = T-cell antigen receptor α chain

TCRβ   = T-cell antigen receptor β chain

TCRγ   = T-cell antigen receptor γ chain

INFα   = interferon α gene

INFβ   = interferon β gene

MT   = metallothionein gene cluster

cases have a complex translocation involving numbers 22 and 9 and one or more additional chromosomes (Table 13.1).

It is not possible to demonstrate cytogenetically that chromosome 22 has received a part of chromosome 9 as the portion received is so small. Submicroscopic portions of DNA can now be detected using somatic cell hybrids with enzyme studies or with recombinant DNA technology. Individual genes can be visualized on the chromosomes by in situ hybridization.

The Philadelphia translocation occurs in about 90% of patients with chronic myeloid leukaemia (CML). In about 5–10% of Ph[1]-positive cases, additional chromosome abnormalities are present in the chronic phase (see Table 13.1). When patients enter the terminal acute phase, about 80% acquire or have acquired additional abnormalities.

The significance of additional change at diagnosis in CML is not clear. Additional change detected by serial chromosome studies after diagnosis generally heralds the accelerated phase or acute transformation.

Acute Myeloid Leukaemia

Chromosome abnormalities have been reported in at least 50% of patients with acute myeloid leukaemia (AML). However, recent results from specialist laboratories suggest that the true figure may be much higher (>80%). Abnormal clones are best detected in marrow cultured for 24–72 hours rather than processed directly. Examination of prophase chromosomes is necessary to detect minor abnormalities. The FAB classification for AML consists of seven main groups (M1–M7) with two subtypes, M3V (variant) and M4Eo (with increased or abnormal eosinophils) (see Chapter 14). The relationship between chromosomal abnormalities and clinical or blast cell features is of three kinds:

(1) those strongly associated with a particular FAB type;
(2) those associated with morphological features of the marrow which do not contribute to the FAB classification (Table 13.2);
(3) those which are found throughout AML (Table 13.3).

t(8;21)(q22;q22)

This is found predominantly in FAB-type M2 (acute myeloid leukaemia with granulocytic maturation at or beyond promyelocyte stage) and has also been reported in M4 (myelomonocytic leukaemia). The translation is frequently accompanied by the loss of a sex chromosome (−Y in males, −X in females); a chromosomally normal cell line is often also present. The translocation is found in all age groups but is commonest under the age of 40 years. M2 cases with t(8;21) have a much better remission rate than do other M2 cases; in spite of this, the median survival of 8;21 cases is not significantly improved.

Table 13.1

Chromosome abnormalities in Philadelphia (Ph[1]) positive chronic myeloid leukaemia

	Chromosome abnormality	Incidence (%)
	t(9;22)(q34;q11)	92
	Variant translocation t(n;22)	4
	Complex translocation t(9;22;n;n;)	4
Additional change	+Ph[1]	
	+8	
	i(17q)	
	+19	

n = chromosome other than 9.

Table 13.2

Acute myeloid leukaemia chromosome abnormalities associated with a particular FAB type or specific marrow morphology

Chromosome abnormalities	FAB type	Morphology
t(8;21)(q22;q22)	M2	Myeloblasts
−X (68%)	18% of M2	Monocytes
−Y (85%)		
t(15;17)(q22;q12 or q21)	M3	Promyelocytes
	M3 variant	and with microgranules
	70% of M3	
inv(16)(p13q22)	M4	Abnormal eosinophils
del (16)(q22)		
del or t(11)(q23)	M5	Monoblastic
t(11)(q13)		Monocytoid
t(9;11)(p22;q23)		
t(6;9)(p23;q34)	Not specific	Increased basophils
inv(3)(q21;q26)		Thrombocytosis
t(3;3)(q21;q26)		Abnormal megakaryocytopoiesis

Table 13.3

Cytogenetic abnormalities not specific for a FAB type or other blast cell features in AML

−5 or 5q−
−7 or 7q−
5 and 7 abnormalities
+8
t/del 12p
+21

t(15;17)

This is specific for acute promyelocytic leukaemia (APL) M3 and the M3 variant; breakpoints are at 15q22 and at 17q12 or q21. Chromosomally normal cells accompany the clone in half the reported cases. t(15;17) is commonest in patients under 35 years at presentation. With optimal treatment, remission achievement is good.

inv16, 16q− and t(16; 16)

These are found in M4 and are notable for their association with abnormal eosinophilia. Abnormalities of chromosome 16 are associated with a good prognosis.

del/t (11) (q23)

Abnormalities of 11q23 are most common in FAB type M5, especially in children aged under 2 years.

t(6; 9) (p23; q34)

Bone marrow basophilia has been reported in some but not all patients with this translocation. The age at presentation is commonly under 30 years. Although reported remission rates are good, survival in these patients is fairly short (mean 8.5 months).

inv (3) (q21;q26), t(3;3) (q21;q26)

Classification of these cases within the FAB system may be difficult. A notable feature of this group is an unusually high platelet count and abnormal thrombocytopoiesis.

del/t (12) (p11–p13)

This abnormality is frequently found in association with other chromosome disorders; it occurs in M2 and M4 cases. FAB classification of these cases may be difficult owing to malignant involvement of several haemopoietic cell lineages, particularly basophils and eosinophils.

Other Changes

Finally, there are chromosomal changes which are found in all FAB types except M3 (Table 13.3). These occur in patients with a median age at presentation of over 55 years. 5q— comes in three different sizes, according to the length of the missing portion. The proximal breakpoint may be at q 11/12, q14/15 or q 22, the distal breakpoint is always between q 32 and q 34. The region q 22–q 23

is consistently lost. Additional abnormalities are frequent in these clones. Trisomy 8 is the commonest abnormality in AML (Fig. 13.2); it frequently accompanies one of the other chromosome changes. Abnormalities of chromosomes 5 and 7, monosomy or partial arm deletion are associated with a low remission rate and poor survival. The prognostic status of other chromosomal groups is as yet unknown.

The significance of a totally normal (NN), totally abnormal (AA) or mixed (AN) population of cells in de novo AML is no longer clear. In many earlier studies the absence of an abnormal clone was associated with a favourable outcome. Recently, it has been appreciated that it is the kind and extent of abnormalities present which influence prognosis. Some simple changes—t(8;21) and inv(16)—carry a relatively good prognosis, while others (of chromo-

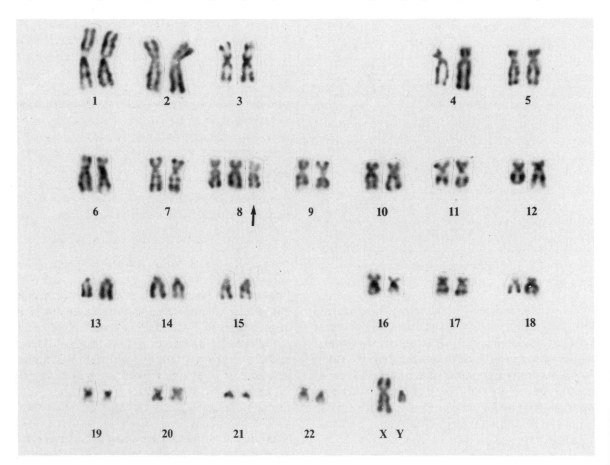

Fig. 13.2. *Karyotype to show trisomy 8 in the bone marrow cells of a patient with acute myeloid leukaemia, 47, XY, +8.*

some 5 or 7) carry a poor prognosis. Complex chromosome change, particularly with four or more abnormalities in the same clone, is always associated with a particularly poor response to treatment.

Secondary Leukaemia

Chromosome abnormalities have been described in at least 80% of cases in AML following cytotoxic treatment and arising as a second malignancy. A similar incidence of abnormalities is found in patients with AML who have been exposed to environmental genetic agents. The chromosomes most often involved are numbers 5 and 7. Clones tend to be complex, with a number of different chromosomal changes superimposed. These cases have a poor response to treatment.

Myelodysplastic Syndromes

Between 40% and 60% of patients with primary myelodysplastic syndromes (MDS) have clonal abnormalities. In secondary MDS the incidence is over 90%. Many of the karyotypic changes are similar to those found in AML and additional to Ph[1] in CML, namely +8, +19, +21. The most common single abnormalities are 5q− and monosomy 7. Multiple karyotypic abnormalities in a clone are more common than are single changes. A complex karyotype carries a higher incidence of progression to leukaemia and signifies a particularly grave prognosis. More than half the MDS patients presenting with a single chromosome abnormality progress to leukaemia, but overall survival of this subgroup is little different from that of MDS patients with a karyotypically normal bone marrow.

The 5q− Syndrome

Deletion of a portion of the long arm of chromosome 5 is found in a wide spectrum of haematological disorders, including de novo AML, secondary leukaemias and myeloproliferative disorders. However, the term 5q− syndrome refers specifically to a condition first described by Van den Berghe and his colleagues (1974) in which a clone with 5q− as the sole chromosomal abnormality coexists with chromosomally normal cells in the bone marrow. The extent of the long-arm deletion is variable.

Most affected patients are elderly females with severe refractory anaemia without an excess of blasts, with no underlying haematological disorder and no significant history of exposure to drugs or toxins. The median duration of survival of this subset of patients is 28 months. Only one in eight develops AML. Additional chromosomal abnormalities which may be present and influence survival adversely include 7q−, −7, +8, +11, −17 and +21.

Myeloproliferative Disorders

This group of disorders includes polycythaemia rubra vera, myelofibrosis, undifferentiated myeloproliferative disorder and essential thrombocythaemia (see Chapter 20).

Overall prognosis in this group is better than for patients with MDS, but the grave prognostic significance of a clone with multiple chromosome abnormalities is also apparent in these patients; frequencies of progression to leukaemia are generally paralleled by survival data. The most common abnormalities, in decreasing order of frequency, are 20q−, +8, +9, 13q− and partial trisomy 1q. A clone with a single karyotypic abnormality, with the exception of monosomy 7 (a poor risk finding), does not appear to be different in terms of overall survival or of progression to leukaemia than in myeloproliferative disorders (MPS) without chromosome abnormalities.

Acute Lymphoblastic Leukaemia

Clonal abnormalities are found in about 70% of cases of acute lymphoblastic leukaemia (ALL). With improved techniques, this figure may rise to over 90% of cases. Clones are nearly always accompanied by a chromosomally normal cell line. There are a number of factors which make cytogenetic studies in ALL particularly difficult. In some cases the leukaemic blasts are inert in culture; in others, chromosome morphology and response to band staining are poor. In childhood ALL, chromosome analysis is particularly difficult but chromosomal classification is important. The kind of abnormality helps to distinguish long-term survivors from those who appear certain to fare badly even with intensive therapy.

Chromosomal abnormalities which define subgroups in ALL are listed in Table 13.4. Particular abnormalities are commonly associated with the

Table 13.4

Structural chromosome abnormalities in acute lymphoblastic leukaemia (ALL)

c-ALLA +ve	t(9;22)(q34;q11)
L1 or L2	t/del 12p12
	del(6)(q21–23)
pre B-ALL	
(CIg +ve)	t(1;19)(q23;p13)
null-ALL	
TdT +ve or TdT −ve	t(4;11)(q21;q23)
Excess of L2:L1	
T-ALL	inv(14)(q11q32)
	t(14)(q11-q13)
	t(11;14)(p13;q13)
B-ALL	
L3	t(8;14)(q24;q32)
	t(2;8)(p12;q24)
	t(8;22)(q24;q11)

phenotypes listed, but exceptions are found in most groups. Abnormalities of 8q24 are found almost exclusively in B-ALL L3. Philadelphia-positive ALL is much commoner in adults (where it accounts for up to 20% of cases) than in children (where it is found in 2–3% of cases). Each of the other subgroups accounts for about 5% of cases in children and adults. t(4;11) is a particularly well-defined subgroup with a number of associated high-risk features: leucocyte counts above $50 \times 10^9/l$ and frequently above $100 \times 10^9/l$; FAB-type L2 blasts are more common than L1 and they may express myeloid features. It is common in infants and is found more frequently in girls than in boys. Abnormalities with a breakpoint at 14q11 are found in T-cell ALL. Partial karyotypes of translocations found in ALL are given in Figure 13.3.

The presence of a particular translocation carries a poor prognosis, and has been demonstrated for the subgroups t(4;11), t(8;14), t(9;22) and t(1;19). The prognostic importance of other translocations or of a partial arm deletion, such as 6q−, is not clear.

Ploidy classification is also important to prognosis (Table 13.5). Patients with more than 50

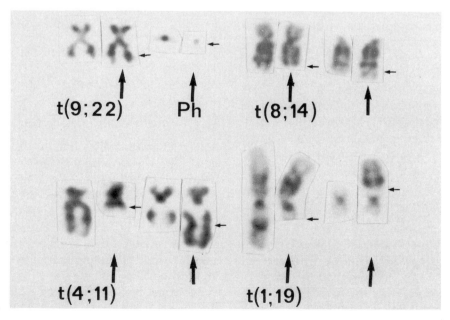

Fig. 13.3. *Partial karyotypes from marrow cells of patients with acute lymphoblastic leukaemia, each showing a reciprocal translocation associated with a poor prognosis. The normal chromosome of each pair is on the left, the translocated (abnormal) chromosome on the right (large arrows). The breakpoints are indicated by the small arrows.*

Table 13.5
Ploidy classification of acute lymphoblastic leukaemia (ALL)

Ploidy	Children (%)	Adults (%)
High hyperdiploidy (> 50 chromosomes)	25	5
Low hyperdiploidy (47–50 chromosomes)	12	17
Pseudodiploidy (46 with rearranged chromosomes)	22	30
Hypodiploidy (< 46 chromosomes)	5	10
Normal	36	38

chromosomes do best and those with pseudo-diploidy do worst. Hypodiploidy generally constitutes a poor-risk group, and near-haploidy (a rare finding of 23–30 chromosomes) is associated with particularly intractable cases of leukaemia. It is therefore of interest that high hyperdiploidy is the most frequent abnormal finding in children and is a rare finding in adults. Certain translocations carry an equally bad prognosis, whether they are found as the only karyotypic change in a pseudodiploid clone or whether, as occurs more rarely, they are accompanied by numerical change in clones of 47–50 or > 50 chromosomes. It is important to exclude the presence of one of the poor-risk translocations in a hyperdiploid clone before designating the patient as a good-risk case.

Chronic Lymphoproliferative Disorders

This group of disorders is characterized by the malignant proliferation of mature lymphocytic cells in the bone marrow and in the blood. Chronic lymphocytic leukaemia (CLL) and prolymphocytic leukaemia (PLL) are predominantly (95%) B cell disorders. T cell disorders account for only 5% of cases. Both B and T cells are particularly inert in culture and have to be stimulated to mitosis with mitogens. Because it is impossible to know to which mitogen the cells will respond, it is necessary to do multiple cultures in each case. In addition to PHA and pokeweed mitogen, concanavalin A (conA), EB virus, lipopolysaccharide W from *Escherichia coli* (LPS), protein A (ProtA) from *Staphylococcus aureus*, and tetradecanoyl phorbol acetate (TPA) may also be used. Due to the diverse methods of processing samples, it is difficult to estimate the frequency of clonal abnormalities in T and B cell CLL.

The major cytogenetic changes are listed in Table 13.6. In the B-cell CLL, the commonest abnormalities, in decreasing order of frequency, are trisomy 12, t(14), t/del (12) (p12–13), del (3) (p13). T-cell cases may have inv(14)(q11q32) and t or del (14)(q11).

In adult T-cell leukaemia endemic in Japan and in the Caribbean, breakpoints are seen at 14q11 and 14q32. Trisomy 7 and del(6)(q) are common findings. A feature of T-cell neoplasms appears to be high frequency of random chromosome change in untreated patients. Independent clones within a single case indicate the rare occurrence in these patients of polyclonal disease.

Malignant Lymphomas

Non-Hodgkin's Lymphomas

Chromosome analysis of lymph nodes in the non-Hodgkin's lymphomas (NHLs) reveals 80–90% with karyotypic abnormalities in patients with bone marrow involvement. The same abnormalities are frequently found in the bone marrow and peripheral blood cells.

The most consistent cytogenetic abnormalities in NHL are listed in Table 13.6. Follicular lymphoma, a B lineage tumour also called small cleaved-cell malignant lymphoma, is consistently (85%) associated with t(14;18) (q32;q21). t(11;14) (q13;q32) is commonly found in small cell lymphocytic lymphoma. Burkitt's lymphoma (BL) has one of the three translocations listed in Table 13.6 in nearly every case reported. The t(8;14) is found in 75–85% of cases; the remaining cases have one of the variant translocations t(2;8) or t(8;22). Additional chromo-

Table 13.6

Chromosome abnormalities in chronic lymphoproliferative disorders and non-Hodgkin's lymphomas

	Breakpoints or translocations
Chronic B-cell leukaemia/lymphoma (B-CLL)	$+12$ t(14)(q32) t(11;14)(q13;q32) $+8$ 6q$-$
Chronic T-cell leukaemia/lymphoma (T-CLL)	14q11 14q32
Adult T-cell leukaemia	14q11 $+7$ 6q$-$
Non-Hodgkin's lymphoma	
Small cleaved-cell lymphoma, follicular lymphoma	t(14;18)(q32;q21)
Small cell lymphocytic lymphoma	t(11;14)(q13;q32)
Burkitt's lymphoma	t(8;14)(q24;q32) t(2;8)(p12;q24) t(8;22)(q24;q11)

some abnormalities frequently accompany each of these BL translocations.

LEUKAEMOGENESIS

There is considerable, if circumstantial, evidence that cancer arises from genetic damage of different kinds, recessive and dominant mutations, large rearrangements of DNA, and point mutations, all leading to alterations of the expression or biochemical function of genes.

Contributions to understanding the aetiological and pathogenetic mechanisms of cancer in humans have come from three major sources: (i) the identification of some new, powerful carcinogens and a few viruses of supposed aetiological significance; (ii) the identification of proto-oncogenes and their role in carcinogenesis; and (iii) the chromosomal localization of proto-oncogenes and other structural genes and the recognition of chromosomal translocations

in leukaemias and lymphomas result in the reorganization of these genes in the genome.

Retroviruses

Cancer or leukaemia in animals can result from the introduction of oncogenes into cells when they become infected by certain viruses known as retroviruses. The life cycle of retroviruses provides clues as to how cellular genes might take part in tumorigenesis. Like all viruses, retroviruses consist of a core of nucleic acid surrounded by a coat of protein. The retroviral nucleic acid is a single-stranded RNA and the viruses contain a few molecules of the enzyme reverse transcriptase. Once a retrovirus enters a cell, the protein coat is digested and the RNA is then used as a template for the synthesis of a complementary single strand of DNA under the influence of the reverse transcriptase, so called because the usual flow of genetic information is from DNA to RNA. The single-stranded DNA serves as a template for the synthesis of a complementary strand of DNA and the resulting double-stranded virally coded DNA eventually becomes incorporated into one of the host's chromosomes. A cell infected by a retrovirus thus ends up with an extra sequence of DNA in its genetic programme.

After the retroviral DNA has been incorporated into the chromosome, it is usually transcribed into RNA by the enzymes of the host cell. Two different categories of RNA are synthesized. First, several different mRNA molecules are synthesized, spliced and then translated to produce viral proteins, including the coat and the reverse transcriptase. Second, the entire genetic programme of the retrovirus is transcribed into one long stretch of RNA, which is packaged together with protein molecules and reverse transcriptase and surrounded by viral coat proteins, thus producing a new retrovirus particle. On their release from the host cell, the new retroviruses are ready to begin the infection cycle again.

Retroviruses can cause cancer in two different ways. Weakly oncogenic retroviruses induce cancers after a long latent period lasting for many months. In this case (insertional mutagenesis) the DNA encoded by the viral RNA is inserted into the chromosome. Integration of viral DNA is potentially mutagenic, it can damage cellular genes directly and it can influence their expression by bringing them under the control of the viral genome (promoter insertion). It is believed that the transcription of the virally derived DNA causes a nearby proto-oncogene to be transcribed at a higher rate than normal—the building of the regulatory protein coded for by the proto-oncogene resulting in the transformation of the infected cells.

Highly oncogenic retroviruses cause animals to develop cancer a few weeks after infection. The DNA added to the genetic programme in this case contains a viral proto-oncogene or v-oncogene, which adds to the host genome an extra copy of a proto-oncogene, an oncogene which is transcribed every time the virus replicates. The consequent accumulation of a normal or abnormal replicatory protein pushes the host cell towards cancer.

Human T-Cell Lymphotropic Viruses

The only naturally occurring retroviruses known to cause disease in humans are the members of the HTLV family. The first isolates of HTLV came from T-cell lines established from two American patients and a Japanese patient with adult T-cell leukaemia/lymphoma (ATLL) (see Chapter 19). Subsequently, additional isolates of virus as well as serological evidence of infection were obtained from patients in the United States, Japan, the Caribbean islands and in Caribbean and African immigrants to Europe. This virus was later designated HTLV-I when a second virus, related to but distinct from HTLV-I, was isolated from a T-cell line that had been established 4 years earlier from the spleen of a patient with hairy cell leukaemia. This virus was designated HTLV-II.

The concept that HTLV-I causes or is a necessary cofactor in the aetiology of ATLL is based on the following observations: (1) epidemiological evidence shows that the areas of high incidence of ATLL correspond to those of high prevalence of HTLV-I infection; (2) patients with ATLL all have evidence of HTLV-I infection; (3) all the ATLL tumour cells carry the HTLV-I provirus while non-malignant cells from the same patients may or may not carry the provirus; and (4) HTLV-I can transform human and animal T cells in vitro.

A third human retrovirus was isolated from a patient with persistent generalized lymphadenopathy, a condition considered to be a prodrome of the acquired immunodeficiency syndrome (AIDS). This virus was named lymphadenopathy-associated virus (LAV). Subsequently, it was shown that antibodies to this new virus cross-reacted with HTLV-I and HTLV-II antigens and there was at least some homology between the genomes of the three viruses. It was therefore renamed HTLV-III. The virus that causes AIDS is now termed human immunodeficiency virus (HIV) (see Chapter 12).

Like all retroviruses, the genome of HTLV-I consists of two 35S polyadenylated subunits that serve as template for reverse transcription into DNA. The gag, pol and env genes are arranged in the usual order. Three gag proteins of molecular weight 24 kD, 19 kD and 15 kD have been characterized. The pol gene codes for a polymerase with a molecular weight of about 95 kD, which seems antigenically distinct from reverse transcriptase in animal retroviruses. The env gene codes for at least three protein products, of which a glycoprotein of molecular weight 46 kD is thought to be the major virion envelope antigen. An unusual feature of the HTLV-I genome is the presence of a long sequence, designated X, between the env gene and the 3′ long terminal repeat (LTR). It is worth noting the HTLV-I carries no viral oncogene and does not appear to insert near to a particular cellular oncogene. Within any particular case of ATLL, its site of insertion in different cells is consistent, but among different cases the insertion site appears to be random. Thus, the manner in which it exerts its oncogenic potential is unknown but a protein coded for by the X gene could play some role in inducing transformation.

Human Oncogenes

A number of genes have been identified in the normal human genome that could be critical links in the chain that causes malignant disease in humans. In general, such oncogenes have been identified in one of two ways. One group of oncogenes was recognized as a result of the characterization of the transforming sequences in selected oncogenic viruses: such RNA sequences, designated viral- or v-oncs, proved to have considerable homology with corresponding genes in the normal human genome, designated cellular- or c-oncs or proto-oncogenes. It was thought originally that the c-onc in the human genome had originated from the corresponding retrovirus, but the reverse sequence now seems more likely, namely, that the retrovirus acquired the oncogene from the human genome at some time in its evolution. Other oncogenes were identified first by their capacity to cause morphologically recognizable changes in an unique mouse fibroblast cell line, NIH-3T3, cultured in vitro. In this assay, high molecular weight DNA is extracted from tumours or from cell lines and introduced into the NIH-3T3 cells by transfection. Transforming activity is then assayed by measuring the ability of DNA to induce foci of morphologically overgrown or transformed cells against the background of the non-transformed NIH-3T3 monolayer. The precise DNA sequence responsible for inducing this transformation can then be characterized.

The majority of the oncogenes associated with retroviruses code for proteins whose functions have

Table 13.7

Proto-oncogenes whose functions have been partially characterized

Family	Principal properties	Examples
Tyrosine-specific protein kinase	Kinase reactivity specific for tyrosine Some proteins are receptors	c-*erb-B* (EGF receptor) c-*fms* (CSF-1 receptor) c-*abl* c-*src*
Serine–threonine kinase	Kinase activity with specificity for serine or threonine	c-*mos* c-*raf*
Homology to oestrogen receptor	Proteins without known kinase activity	c-*erb-A* (thyroid hormone receptor)
GTP-binding proteins	Bind guanine nucleotides and hydrolyse GTP	c-Ha-*ras* c-Ki-*ras* c-N-*ras*
Growth factors	B-chain of platelet-derived growth factor	c-*sis*
Nuclear proteins	Generally shorter half-life and rapid inducibility, Bind DNA	c-*myb* c-*myc* c-*fos* p53 ski

not been fully determined; some of these proteins, however, have the capacity to phosphorylate other proteins on tyrosine or, less commonly, on serine or threonine residues. The relevance of kinase activity is unclear but it could be necessary for activating proteins in the sequence that leads to malignant transformation.

Oncogenes Identified by Homology with Known Retroviruses

One of the most instructive oncogenes is the c-*myc* oncogene, homologous with the transforming sequence (v-*myc*) of the avian myelocytomatosis virus. Translocations that involve c-*myc* may be involved in the pathogenesis of Burkitt's lymphoma (see below). Two oncogenes are of especial interest in the myeloproliferative disorders, namely c-*abl* and c-*sis*. The Abelson strain of Moloney murine leukaemia virus (MLV) was isolated from a prednisolone-treated mouse infected with MLV and retains some homology with the Moloney MLV. It appears that about 3.6 kilobase pairs (kb) of the Moloney MLV genome have been replaced by Abelson (v-*abl*) specific sequences. The Abelson MLV induces pre-B cell lymphoma in mice and transforms some fibroblast lines and lymphoid cells in culture. The cellular homologue of v-*abl*— c-*abl*— is located on chromosome 9 in normal human cells. Its translocation to chromosome 22 may be critical in the pathogenesis of chronic myeloid leukaemia (CML, see below). The simian sarcoma virus (SSV) was isolated from a pet woolly monkey with a spontaneous sarcoma and is the only transforming virus yet isolated from primates. The transforming sequence is designated v-*sis*. The gene product of c-*sis* is known; it codes for the B subunit of the platelet-derived growth factor, a well-defined protein derived from alpha-granules of platelets and megakaryocytes that has the capacity to stimulate fibroblastic proliferation in vitro and probably has a fundamental role in control of cell proliferation in vivo.

Oncogenes Identified by Use of the Transfection Assay

The Kirsten and Harvey murine sarcoma viruses (Ki-MSV and Ha-MSV) are closely related but independent isolates obtained from sarcomas that developed in rats after inoculation with Kirsten or Moloney strains of murine leukaemia virus. Both isolates contained related oncogene sequences (*ras*) acquired during serial passage in the rats. They can induce sarcomas and erythroleukaemia in mice and can transform mouse cells in culture, but have genomes very different from that of the Moloney sarcoma virus. A specific sequence of the Ha-MSV has been characterized and is thought to encode a 21kD protein that can transform target cells in culture.

Studies over the last 5 years have shown that DNA from a variety of sources can cause transformation of NIH-3T3 cells in culture, including DNA from rat neuroblastomas and haemopoietic tumours. Normal human DNA, however, has no transforming ability. It transpired that the molecular nature of these transforming DNAs was remarkably consistent. Almost all of the transforming sequences were found to be members of the *ras* family, homologous with Ki-*ras* or Ha-*ras*. A third member of the family—N-*ras*—was found in active form in the DNAs of a variety of haemopoietic tumours, including acute promyelocytic leukaemia, acute lymphoblastic leukaemia, chronic myeloid leukaemia and Burkitt's lymphoma.

Like other cellular oncogenes, the *ras* oncogenes isolated from malignant cells arise as altered versions of corresponding proto-oncogenes. In all cases described to date, the mutated oncogene differs from its normal allelic counterpart at a single critical nucleotide. This alteration, or point mutation, is invariably found in the portion of the oncogene responsible for encoding the p21 protein. These p21 proteins are located on the inner surface of the plasma membrane and bind the nucleotides guanosine diphosphate (GDP) and guanosine triphosphate (GTP) and are able to hydrolyse GTP to GDP by a GTPase portion of the protein. It seems likely that the *ras*-encoded proteins take part in transduction of growth signals from outside the cell through the membrane to the nucleus (see below).

The functions of a number of oncogenes have been partially characterized as listed in Table 13.7. Oncogene products localized in the cytoplasm or cell membrane are likely to be growth factors, growth factor receptors or kinases which may interact with growth factors or their receptors and/or be concerned in signal transduction from cell membrane to nucleus. For example, sequences on c-*sis* and c-*erbB* show homology with sequences of platelet-derived growth factor (PDGF) and epidermal growth factor (EGF), respectively. c-*fms* is thought to code for the macrophage colony-stimulating factor (CSF-1) receptor. Kinase activity or structural homology to kinases has been demonstrated for the oncogenes *src, fes/fps, yes, ras, abl, erbB, mos, raf, met* and *syn,* although in a number of cases the substrate for phosphorylation is unknown.

The products of some oncogenes are localized in the cell nucleus and are thought to play a role in the regulation of gene transcription. These oncogenes include c-*myc*, N-*myc*, c-*myb*, c-*ski*, c-*fos* and p53. The mechanisms of activation of these genes result in the deregulation of the level of their protein products.

Oncogene Activation by Point Mutation

Activation of the N-*ras* gene has been found in the acute myeloid leukaemias. The mechanism of activation of the *ras* gene family is thought to be due to a single point mutation resulting in a single amino acid change. Hot spots for mutations resulting in potential oncogene activity have been identified in amino acid positions 12 and 61 in the *ras* gene family. Mutations in positions 13, 59–63 are also active. *Ras* gene proteins act normally as transducers, conveying signals from membrane receptors to cell nucleus. They have the capacity to bind GTP (which activates the protein) and hydrolyse it to GDP. Following point mutations, the resulting proteins have transforming ability and reduced GTPase activity.

Oncogene Activation by Chromosomal Translocation

The chromosome locations of many human proto-oncogenes are now known. A number of these are sited at the breakpoints of consistent chromosome change in leukaemias and lymphomas (see Fig. 13.1). The remarkable specificity of certain chromosome changes may be associated with proliferative advantage in a particular cell lineage and only at a particular stage of differentiation. The gene situated at the other breakpoint of a translocation is likely to be a gene of functional importance in the affected cell type. As the result of a translocation, genes which are normally on separate chromosomes are brought together, and will therefore be subject to control by their new, rather than their normal, neighbours (Table 13.8).

The molecular characteristics and biological consequences of translocations have been most investigated in B-cell and T-cell leukaemias and lymphomas, and in Ph^1-positive cases of chronic myeloid and acute lymphoblastic leukaemia. Molecular probes derived from normal genes have been used to demonstrate DNA rearrangements related to the translocations. Subsequently, genomic libraries have been constructed from these malignancies and molecular clones of the rearranged segments isolated and analysed. A number of translocations have been studied in details and their genetic consequences worked out.

Burkitt's Lymphoma and B-cell Acute Lymphoblastic Leukaemia

In all Burkitt's lymphomas and in some B-cell ALLs, one of three translocations is found: t(8;14)(q24;q32) (approx. 80%), t(2;8)(p12;q24) (6%), or t(8;22)(q24;q11) (14%). Chromosomes 14, 2 and 22 carry the genes coding for the immunoglobulin (Ig) heavy chain (H), and kappa (κ) and lambda (λ) light chain genes respectively. The oncogene c-*myc* is normally located at chromosome 8q24. As a result of each translocation, the coding regions for the c-*myc* gene are brought into close proximity with one of the Ig genes (Fig. 13.4). Immunoglobulin genes in B cells undergo a series of rearrangements and recombinations. The enhanced expression of c-*myc* demonstrated in BL cells is therefore believed to result from c-*myc* coming under the control of these highly active genes and being inappropriately switched on. The result is an uncontrolled expansion of a malignant B-cell clone. The translocation appears cytogenetically identical in African Burkitt's lymphoma (which occurs endemically in equatorial Africa and is associated with the presence of Epstein–Barr virus (EBV) in more than 90% of cases) and in sporadic cases (found in Europe and North America, in the ab-

Table 13.8
Genes located to breakpoints in haematological malignancies

Oncogene	Lineage-specific gene		Translocation or breakpoints	Diagnosis
5q31	c-*fms*		del(5)(q15q33)	MDS, AML
5q23	GM-CSF		del(5)(q22q33)	AML
6q15–23	c-*myb*	?	del(6)(q21/q23)	c-ALL, CLL
8q24	#c-*myc*	2p12 Igκ	t(2;8)(p12;q24)	BL, B-ALL
8q24	c-*myc*	14q32 IgH	t(8;14)(q24;q32)	
8q24	#c-*myc*	22q11 Igλ	t(8;22)(q24;q11)	
8q24	c-*myc*	14q11 TCRα	t(8;14)(q24;q11)	T-ALL, T-CLL
9q34	c-*abl*	22q11 bcr	t(9;22)(q34;q11)	CML, c-ALL
9q34	#c-*abl*	6p23?	t(6;9)(p23;q34)	AML
11q23	c-*ets*-1	4q21?	t(4;11)(q21;q23)	null-ALL
11q23	c-*ets*-1	9p22 # IFNαβ_1	t(9;11)(p22;q23)	AML
11p13	?H-*ras*	14q11 TCRα	t(11;14)(p13;q13)	T-ALL, T-CLL
11q13	bcl-1	14q32 IgH	t(11;14)(q13;q32)	B-CLL, C-ALL
12p11–13	κ-*ras*-2	?	del or t(12)(p11/p13)	c-ALL, AML, MDS
17q21–q22	c-*erb-A*	15q22?	t(15;17)(q22;q21)	AML M3
18q21	bcl-2	14q32 IgH	t(14;18)(q32;q21)	FL
21q22	c-*ets*-2	#8q?	t(8;21)(q22;q22)	AML M2
16p13	?	16q22 MT	del(16)(q22) inv(16)(p13 q22)	AML M4

Key
bcr, bcl-1, bcl-2 = genes of unknown function.
# = does not translocate.
TCR = T-cell antigen receptor.
NIF = interferon.
Ig = immunoglobulin.
H = heavy chain.
κ = kappa light chain.
λ = lambda light chain.
MT = metallothionein gene cluster.

null = c-ALL negative, terminal deoxynucleo-
tidyl transferase positive.
MDS = myelodysplastic syndromes.
AML = acute myeloid leukaemia.
ALL = acute lymphoblastic leukaemia.
CLL = chronic lymphocytic leukaemia.
BL = Burkitt's lymphoma.
B = B cell.
T = T cell.
c = common ALL antigen positive.
FL = follicular lymphoma.

sence of viral infection). A difference is seen at the molecular level. By analysing the DNA from tumours carrying the t(8;14) by Southern blotting, using probes from the c-*myc* gene, one of two results is obtained. In sporadic cases, DNA rearrangements are found, indicating that c-*myc* is structurally altered as a result of the translocation. In most endemic African Burkitt's lymphomas, no rearrangement of c-*myc* can be found.

T-Cell Tumours

A similar effect has been demonstrated for T-cell malignancies. The genes for the α, β and γ chains of the T-cell receptor (TCR) have been mapped to 14q11, 7q32–36 and 7p15 (see Fig. 13.1). 14q11 is frequently involved in T-cell malignancies, for example inv(14q11q32) splits the α-chain gene and results in a site-specific recombination of an Ig segment from 14q32 with a TCR Jα segment at 14q11. In T-cell leukaemias with t(8;14)(q24;q11), the cα locus from chromosome 14 was found to be fused 3′ of the c-*myc* third exon.

B-Cell Chronic Lymphatic Leukaemia and B-Cell Lymphomas

In other B-lymphocyte-derived malignancies, two putative oncogenes—bcl-1 and bcl-2—have

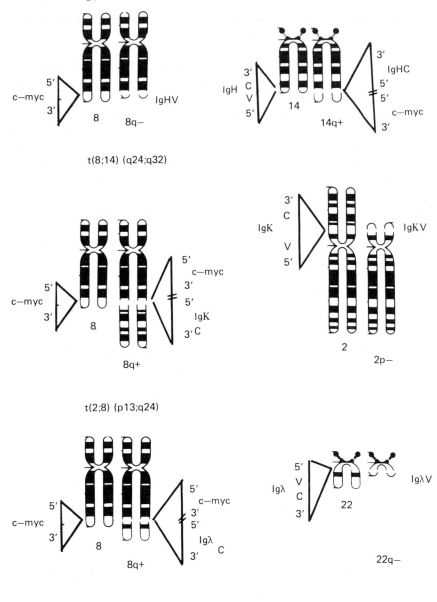

Fig. 13.4. *Diagram to show the genetic events of the three translocations found in Burkitt's lymphoma and B acute lymphoblastic leukaemia.*

been located on 11q13 and 18q21 respectively. In B-CLL and in some cases of diffuse small cell and diffuse large cell lymphomas, the translocation t(11;14)(q13;q32) is found. The breakpoint on 14 is found within the J_H segment of the IgH gene, the breakpoints on 11 are clustered to within eight

nucleotides, in the region termed *bcl*-1 (Fig. 13.5a). In most follicular lymphomas, the most common B-cell malignancy, the translocation t(14;18)(q32;q21) is found. The breakpoint on chromosome 14 occurs at the Ig heavy chain locus within or directly adjacent to a J_H segment. The breakpoints on chromosome 18 cluster within a 5.4 kb region flanking a transcriptionally active locus termed *bcl-2*—a putative oncogene (Fig. 13.5b). Nucleotide sequence analyses have shown that the 6-kb *bcl-2* mRNA potentially encodes a 26 kd protein that is homologous to a predicted EBV protein. As a result of the t(14;18) hybrid *bcl-2*/immunoglobulin heavy-chain transcripts are produced that consist of the 5' half of the *bcl-2* mRNA fused to a decapitated immunoglobulin heavy chain mRNA. The hybrid transcripts encode a normal *bcl-2* protein. It seems therefore that t(14;18) alters the expression of the *bcl-2* gene both by transcriptional activation and by abnormal post-transcriptional regulation of *bcl-2* mRNA.

Chronic Myeloid Leukaemia

The genomic breakpoint on chromosome 22 associated with the 9; 22 translocation in different patients with chronic myeloid leukaemia (CML) occurs at different points within a relatively short sequence (5.8 kb) of DNA that has been termed the 'breakpoint cluster region' (*bcr*), such that the 5' portion of *bcr* remains on the Ph chromosome and the 3' portion is translocated to chromosome 9q. This *bcr* 'region' (also known as the major break-point cluster region M-BCR) forms part of a large gene known as the *bcr* (or *phl*) gene. Since the breakpoint on chromosome 9 occurs near the 5' end of the *c-abl* oncogene, the t(9;22) results in the

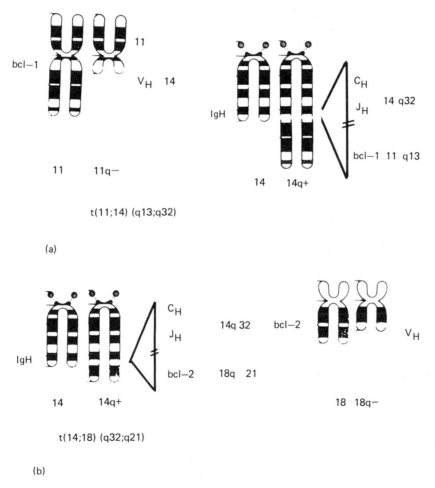

Fig. 13.5. *Diagrams to show the genetic events of the two translocations in mature B-cell lymphomas and leukaemias: (a) t(11;14)(q13;q32), (b) t(14;18)(q32;q21).*

formation on the Ph[1] chromosome of a chimeric gene consisting of the 5' portion of the *bcr* fused in frame to the major part of the *c-abl* coding sequences (see Figs. 13.6 and 16.2). This *bcr–abl* chimeric gene produces a larger mRNA (8.5 kb) than that produced by the normal *c-abl* (6.0 or 7.0 kb) and has a larger (210 kd) than normal (145 kd) protein product. The P210*bcr–abl* has increased tyrosine kinase activity. The normal functions of the *bcr* and *c-abl* genes are unknown. Rearrangement of the *bcr* region has been detected by Southern blotting in almost all cases of Ph[1]-positive CML, which is circumstantial evidence for its central role in the pathogenesis of CML.

Molecular investigations of variant Ph translocations, of cases of Ph[1]-negative CML and of Ph[1]-positive acute leukaemias have revealed a number of additional facts about the role of the chimeric *bcr–abl* gene. In complex and variant translocations (in variant translocations, chromosome 9 appears not to be involved), *c-abl* has been found to be translocated to chromosome 22q11. In a number of Ph[1]-negative cases of CML, the *c-abl* gene is translocated to chromosome 22 as in Ph[1]-positive disease but there is no reciprocal movement of the 3' portion of the *bcr* gene. In Ph[1]-positive ALL, the molecular consequences of the t(9;22) are of two kinds. In about half the cases studied, there is rearrangement in the *bcr* region as in Ph[1]-positive CML, with formation of a 8.5 kb mRNA and a P210*bcr–abl*. In the remaining cases the breakpoint occurs upstream of the *bcr* region in the large first intron of the *bcr* gene (see Fig. 16.2), with formation of a smaller *bcr–abl* chimeric gene distinct from that characteristic of CML. This new chimeric gene is transcribed as a novel mRNA and produces a

protein of molecular weight 190 kd (P190), with enhanced tyrosine kinase activity similar to that of the P210. Indeed, the only difference between the P190 and the P210 is the omission of the peptides encoded by the majority of the 5' exons of the *bcr* gene. Similar molecular changes with either P190 or P210 formation are seen in the rare cases of Ph[1]-positive AML. These two molecular variants of Ph[1]-positive acute leukaemia do not apparently correlate with different clinical features.

There are a number of other translocations in the acute leukaemias with breakpoints close to a cellular oncogene (see Fig. 13.1 and Table 13.8). In some of these, movement of the oncogene has been demonstrated (e.g. t(4;11) and *c-ets*-1, t(8;22) and *c-ets*-2) but the molecular consequences of these translocations are not known.

For other rearrangements, one of the breakpoints has been mapped in terms of the neighbouring genes, but it is not clear what role, if any, these genes have in the pathogenesis of the leukaemia. Thus inv(16)(p13q22) splits the metallothionein gene cluster normally at 16q22, with the result that part of the gene cluster is resituated on the short arm. The breakpoint on chromosome 17 in t(15;17) has been mapped distal to the c-oncogene *erb*-A. No alteration in the structure of c-*erb*-A has been found.

Recessive Genes, Translocations and Leukaemogenesis

Leukaemias associated with total or partial chromosome loss suggest that malignancy can result from the unmasking of a recessive malignant

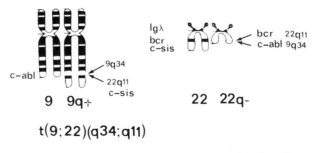

Fig. 13.6. *Diagram of the Philadelphia translocation in chronic myeloid leukaemia to show the movement of genes brought about by the translocation.*

gene by the loss of a normal allele, 5q−, found in refractory anaemia and in AML, particularly that induced by cytotoxic treatment, may be an example of this mechanism. Genes which encode proteins involved in the regulation of myeloid cells are situated on chromosome 5q. Thus genes for both GM-CSF (which stimulates the proliferation of cells from the granulocytes, and macrophage lineages) and CSF-1 (which stimulates cells of the macrophage lineage) as well as the proto-oncogene *fms* (believed to encode the receptor for CSF-1) are all situated on 5q. Some or all of the genes have been shown to be lost with the missing portion of 5q. It is speculated that the loss of these wild-type genes may allow the expression of a recessive mutant in these cases.

Partial or total trisomies would also be expected to perturb gene dosage. Thus, the frequency with which trisomy 12 is seen in CLL suggests the possible involvement of c-Ki-*ras*, the cellular counterpart of the Kirsten rat sarcoma oncogene, located on chromosome 12. There are as yet no reports of its amplification or altered expression in B-CLL.

Increase in the number of copies of a given proto-oncogene per cell might result in malignant transformation. Amplification of proto-oncogenes has been demonstrated in association with double minutes and homogeneously staining regions. Increased expression of c-*myc* has been found in acute promyelocytic leukaemia; c-*myb* expression is increased in some cases of acute myeloblastic leukaemia.

In conclusion, the normal human genome includes a class of genes, the proto-oncogenes, which, following genetic changes, code for malignant transformation; genetic changes in proto-oncogenes resulting from chromosomal aberrations or mutations can be demonstrated in malignant tissue. The normal function of proto-oncogenes suggests that the underlying lesion in neoplasms might be an alteration in the expression of proto-oncogenes resulting in a permanent stimulation of cell growth.

Leukaemogenesis is now widely regarded as a multistep process. The transition from preleukaemia to acute myeloid leukaemia and from chronic phase to blast crisis in CML usually involves two or more chromosomal abnormalities. It is known that the co-operation of two different oncogenes, or the increased expression of an already mutated oncogene, is required to achieve full malignant potential. In some cases of Burkitt's lymphoma, activation of c-*myc* has been found, together with mutation of the proto-oncogene N-*ras*.

In many of the haematological malignancies, genetic damage has not as yet been detected. There is now sufficient evidence from cytogenetics and molecular genetics to suggest that, in time, many more genes involved in malignant transformation will be sequenced. Other mechanisms of malignant transformation will be uncovered and the biochemical mechanisms of leukaemogenesis more fully understood.

SELECTED BIBLIOGRAPHY

Bishop M. J. (1987). The molecular genetics of cancer. *Science*, **235**, 305–311.

Bloomfield C. D., de la Chapelle A. (1987). Chromosome abnormalities in acute non-lymphocytis leukemia: clinical and biological significance. *Seminars in Oncology*, **14**, 372–383.

Bunn H. F. (1986). The 5q− syndrome. *Clinics in Haematology*, **15**, 1023–1035.

Butturini A., Gale R. P. (1988). Oncogenes and human leukaemias. *International Journal of Cell Cloning*, **6**, 2–24.

Cleary M. L., Smith S. D., Sklar J. (1986). Cloning and structural analysis of c-DNAs for BCLZ and a hybrid BCL 2/immunoglobulin transcript resulting from the t(14;18) translocation. *Cell*, **47**, 19–28.

Croce C. M., Nowell P. P. (1985). Molecular basis of human B cell neoplasia. *Blood*, **65**, 1–7.

Gale R. P., Cannani E. (1985). The molecular biology of chronic myelogenous leukaemia. *British Journal of Haematology*, **60**, 385–408.

Haluska F. G., Tsujimoto Y., Croce C. M. (1987). Mechanisms of chromosome translocation in B and T-cell neoplasia. *Trends in Genetics*, **3**, 11–15.

Heim S., Mitelman F. (1987). *Cancer cytogenetics.* New York: Alan R. Liss.

Mitelman F. (1988). *Catalog of chromosome aberrations in cancer.* New York: Alan R. Liss.

Nowell P. C., Hungerford D. A. (1960). A minute chromosome in human granulocytic leukemia. *Science*, **132**, 1497.

Nowell P. C., Besa C. E., Stelmach T., Finan B. S. (1986). Chromosome studies in preleukemic states. *Cancer*, **58**, 2571–2575.

Pedersen-Bjergaard J., Andersson P., Philip P. (1986).

Possible pathogenetic significance of specific chromosome abnormalities and activated protooncogenes in malignant diseases of man. *Scandinavian Journal of Haematology*, **36**, 127–137.

Rooney D. E., Czepulkowski B. H. (1986). *Human cytogenetics. A practical approach.* Oxford: IRL Press.

Rowley J. D. (1984). Biological implications of consistent chromosome rearrangements in leukemia and lymphoma. *Cancer Research*, **44**, 3159–3168.

Russo G., Haluska F. G., Isobe M., Groce C. M. (1988). Molecular basis of B- and T-cell neoplasia. In *Recent advances in haematology*, Vol. 5, pp. 121–130. (Ed. A. V. Hoffbrand). Edinburgh: Churchill Livingstone.

Sandberg A. A. (1980). *The chromosomes in human cancer and leukemia.* New York: Elsevier.

Sandberg A. A. (1986). The chromosomes in human leukemia. *Seminars in Hematology*, **23**, 201–217.

Secker-Walker L. M. (1984). The prognostic implications of chromosomal findings in acute lymphoblastic leukemia. *Cancer Genetics and Cytogenetics*, **11**, 233–248.

Shikano T., Kaneko Y., Takazawa M., Veno N., Ohkawa M., Fujimoto T. (1986). Balanced and unbalanced 1;19 translocation-associated acute lymphoblastic leukemias. *Cancer*, **58**, 2239–2243.

Sutherland G. R., Hecht F. (1985). *Fragile sites on human chromosomes.* Oxford Monographs on Medical Genetics. Oxford: Oxford University Press.

Thomson B. J., Dalgleish A. G. (1988). Human retroviruses. *Blood Reviews*, **2**, 211–212.

Van den Berghe H., Cassiman J. J., David G., Fryns J. P., Sokal G. (1974). Distinct haematological disorder with deletion of long arm of No.5 chromosome. *Nature*, **251**, 437–438.

Weinberg R. A., (1985). The action of oncogenes in the cytoplasm and nucleus. *Science*, **230**, 770–776.

Yunis J. J., Brunning R. D. (1986). Prognostic significance of chromosomal abnormalitites in acute leukaemias and myelodysplastic syndromes. *Clinics in Haematology*, **15**, 597–620.

Yunis J. J. *et al.* (1978). The characterisation of high resolution G-banded chromosomes of man. *Chromosoma*, **67**, 293–307.

Chapter 14

ACUTE LEUKAEMIA

D. CATOVSKY AND A. V. HOFFBRAND

The terms 'acute' and 'chronic' used to define and classify human leukaemia reflect an historical concept derived from the time when no treatment was available for these conditions. In fact it is still true that without therapy patients with any kind of acute leukaemia would die in a matter of weeks, whereas those with chronic leukaemia may remain alive untreated for a period of months to many years as in the case of chronic lymphocytic leukaemia (CLL). Since the advent of antileukaemic agents this outlook has changed in so far as in some forms of acute leukaemia, e.g. childhood acute lymphoblastic leukaemia (ALL), more than half of the patients have a probability of cure whereas this is rarely the case in the chronic leukaemias, in particular chronic myeloid leukaemia (CML) for which the overall survival has not changed in the last 20 years, except for the few cases which may be cured by bone marrow transplantation (BMT).

The acute leukaemias are better described pathologically as blast cell leukaemias or malignancies of immature haemopoietic cells. Although in many instances the different types of blast cells, representing progenitors of myeloid and lymphoid cells, may be recognized by simple morphological and cytochemical stains, in others it is necessary to employ immunological reagents, e.g. monoclonal antibodies (McAb), or, less frequently, electron microscopy or molecular biological techniques such as gene rearrangement studies, to identify their particular differentiation features. This is important as the natural history and response to therapy may vary according to the type of blast involved in the leukaemic process.

For several good reasons it is customary to divide the acute leukaemias according to two main age groups: childhood (<15 years) and adult (≥ 15 years). This age limit varies slightly in different countries according to local practice: sometimes it is 14 years and sometimes 20 years. Recently a third group has been separated, that of adults aged ≥ 50 years, because their response to current treatment protocols, both for ALL and acute myeloid leukaemia (AML), is inferior and because these patients are not included for the more radical approaches using autologous or allogeneic BMT.

The main difference between leukaemia in children and adults is that ALL constitutes over 80% of childhood cases whilst AML constitutes around 80% of adult cases. This different incidence of ALL and AML according to age clearly reflects the susceptibility of different haemopoietic precursor cells and/or the influence of as yet undefined leukaemogenic events in the pathogenesis of human acute leukaemias. In practice, the clinical and management problems are similar in AML regardless of age, whereas there are differences between adults and children with ALL and therefore these two forms will be described separately.

EPIDEMIOLOGY

Apart from the age differences referred to above, there have not been major differences in incidence according to geography or between urban industrialized and rural areas. Nevertheless, some sociocultural factors have been noted to influence the incidence of the common form of ALL (cALL), which is relatively less frequent in African countries and in poorer sections of the community in the USA, e.g. black or Spanish. In the Gaza Strip it was noted that the relative incidence of cALL increased to the levels seen in Israel generally when major urban developments took place.

A number of environmental agents have been implicated in the induction of certain types of leukaemia, chiefly ionizing radiation and chemical carcinogens, mainly alkylating agents used to treat other malignancies. Other environmental factors have also been implicated but as yet without firm evidence. A number of surveys in the UK have shown a clustering of cases of childhood ALL in the vicinity of nuclear power installations, but this association is still currently being investigated.

In addition to the above, acute leukaemia may evolve as a result of host susceptibility, e.g. in genetic disorders (Table 14.1), and may supervene as blast transformation or blast crisis in pre-existing myeloproliferative or myelodysplastic disorders (Table 14.1). There is no good evidence at present for a role of oncogenic viruses in the causation of human acute leukaemias, although one such agent, HTLV-I, is directly implicated in adult T-cell leukaemia/lymphoma (see p. 443).

Ionizing Radiation

X-rays and other ionizing rays were the first identifiable agents associated with the induction of leukaemia. This became apparent in the survivors of the atomic bomb explosions in Hiroshima and Nagasaki, and the latter has been the single most important source of information on radiation leukaemogenesis in humans. It has shown, for example, that people exposed at a younger age or closer to the hypocentre of the bomb had the shorter latent period of risk for the development of leukaemia. AML and chronic myeloid leukaemia (CML) were the predominant types, although ALL was also reported, particularly in younger individuals. There are abundant case reports of patients treated by irradiation for other malignancies (Hodgkin's disease, carcinoma of the breast, etc.) and developing AML, in many cases preceded by myelodysplasia. The combination of irradiation and alkylating agents results in a higher incidence of 'secondary' leukaemia. Evidence for a leukaemogenic effect of low-dose irradiation (e.g. exposure to diagnostic x-rays or radioisotopes at diagnostic levels) has not been substantiated.

Chemicals

Two types of chemicals have been involved or are strongly suspected of being leukaemogenic: (1) benzene and other petroleum derivatives, and (2) alkylating agents. Benzene has been known for many years to be aetiologically related to the high incidence of leukaemia and aplastic anaemia in people occupationally exposed to it, e.g. shoemakers in Italy and Turkey. Whether this is also the reason for the apparently higher incidence (33%) of AML among childhood leukaemias in Turkey is not yet clear; one-third of them present with chloroma-like deposits in the eye and orbit. Some studies have suggested that occupational exposure to petroleum products (e.g. handling of petrol-driven motors such as buses or trucks) may be important as a causal agent for AML in the 35–50-year age group. Non-industrial exposure, such as from using plastic glues with a high benzene content in poorly ventilated rooms for years, may also be important. Benzene, which constitutes 6–8% of the content of petrol and up to 30% of some liquid lacquers, is known to produce chromosome abnormalities.

In an increasing number of reports alkylating agents have been directly implicated in the induction of secondary AML. The resulting leukaemia sometimes evolves slowly with myelodysplastic changes and has a lesser degree of leukaemic infiltration and a significantly higher incidence of chromosome abnormalities than de-novo AML, particularly involving chromosomes 5 and 7, e.g. 5q− and monosomy 5 and/or 7. Secondary AML has been well documented in myelomatosis (following melphalan but not cyclophosphamide), lung and ovarian cancers (following busulphan) and Hodgkin's disease. In the last-mentioned condition the cumulative dose of alkylating agents and patient age were found to be the main independent factors for developing AML. The main drugs implicated are nitrogen mustard, lomustine and chlorambucil. The risk increases from 1 year after the start of treatment and rises steeply in the first 1–2 years, levelling off at 7 years, and reaching in one study 13% at 10 years (Pedersen-Bjergaard *et al.*, 1987).

Table 14.1
Conditions predisposing to acute leukaemia*

Genetic or constitutional	Down's syndrome	{Transient {Persistent (ALL or AML)
	Bloom's syndrome	
	Fanconi's anaemia (AML)	
	Ataxia telangiectasia (ALL, lymphoma)	
Acquired	Myelodysplasia (AML)	
	Chemotherapy ± radiotherapy (MDS → AML)	
	Chronic myeloproliferative disorders: CGL, PRV, myelofibrosis (AML)	
	Aplastic anaemia (ALL)	
	Paroxysmal nocturnal haemoglobinuria (AML, rarely ALL)	

*Predominant type of leukaemia in parentheses.
ALL, acute lymphoblastic leukaemia; AML, acute myeloblastic leukaemia; MDS, myelodysplastic syndrome; CGL, chronic granulocytic leukaemia; PRV, polycythaemia rubra vera.

Chromosome and Oncogene Abnormalities

The cytogenetic abnormalities found in AML and ALL and the abnormalities of oncogenes that have been identified so far are dealt with in Chapter 13.

DIAGNOSIS

The diagnosis of acute leukaemia is made by careful examination of well-prepared blood and bone marrow films stained with appropriate Romanowsky dyes. In cases with a high WBC (e.g. $> 50 \times 10^9/l$) the diagnosis is self-evident from the peripheral blood. A bone marrow aspirate is necessary to confirm the diagnosis and for the precise classification (see below). Bone marrow trephines are not yet routine but they are essential to demonstrate blast cell infiltration when aspirates are inadequate due to dense cellular infiltration (rarely) and/or increased reticulin fibrosis (commonly). Bone marrow trephines are important to follow the effect of treatment, particularly in AML, and to distinguish a poor aspirate due to hypocellularity from one with persistent leukaemia. Difficulties in diagnosis are encountered in cases presenting with low WBC,

e.g. in aleukaemic ALL with a packed hypercellular marrow or in promyelocytic leukaemia where aspirates may yield a dry tap due to quick clot formation. The recognition of aleukaemic forms, particularly of ALL, is important because it represents a group with very good prognosis and treatment should not be delayed. Bone marrow trephine may be needed to exclude an alternative diagnosis of aplastic anaemia. Such patients are sometimes referred for BMT with an incorrect diagnosis of aplastic anaemia based on a poor aspirate.

Cases of AML presenting with a low WBC and relatively low percentage of bone marrow blasts may present diagnostic difficulties. The FAB group has published revised proposals for the classification of AML that take into account the percentage of bone marrow blasts out of all nucleated cells and, in some circumstances, considering separately this percentage out of the non-erythroid cells (excluding identifiable erythroblasts). This may be important to distinguish erythroleukaemia (M6) from myelodysplastic syndrome (MDS). If the percentage of bone marrow blasts is greater that 30%, the diagnosis is always AML. If the percentage is 30% or less, the diagnosis may be MDS or M6 and this will depend on the erythropoietic component. If the percentage of erythroblasts is greater than 50%, the count of blasts is calculated out of the non-erythroid cells, and if greater than 30% the diagnosis will be M6, if less it will be MDS. The reason behind this proposal is twofold. First, although the erythroid component may be part of the leukaemia, this may be difficult to prove by morphology only; and second, the erythroid component is often subject to variations, e.g. following a blood transfusion (where it may decrease significantly), and thus may not be a reliable indicator of the underlying process. It is understood that even with these relatively simple guidelines, the diagnosis of borderline cases may be difficult and sometimes more than one bone marrow examination may be necessary. In few situations this may affect the treatment decision as the treatment of young (< 50 years) patients with MDS is similar in some centres to that of primary AML.

The recognition of MDS features, even in cases presenting as de-novo AML (with greater than 30% blasts), may be important to identify a particular subgroup of AML (up to 15% of cases) designated AML with trilineage myelodysplasia (Brito-Babapulle *et al.*, 1987a), which may or may not have evolved from an underlying MDS. This group of patients responds less well to induction treatment and even if they do, may relapse with pure MDS. Features for the recognition of this group of AML are summarized in Table 14.2.

Eosinophilia and ALL

The association of a high eosinophil count before, during or after the diagnosis of ALL has been recognized and there have been several reports, particularly in childhood ALL. The blasts have either a cALL phenotype (see below) or, more frequently, T-cell features. In general it has been considered that the eosinophils are 'reactive' to some factor or lymphokine released by the lymphoblasts. However, a recent study based on cytogenetic data suggested that in some circumstances the eosinophils may be part of the leukaemia (Keene *et al.*, 1987).

CLASSIFICATION

There are several ways to classify the acute leukaemias. The most simple, and available to all haematologists, is based on the morphology of the blast cells (Table 14.3). This in itself may be inadequate for the cases in which the blasts do not show cytological features of differentiation, which include all cases of ALL of L2 type (see below) and some of L1 type, and also immature forms of AML, e.g. M1 and M5 (see below). The original proposal of the FAB group (Bennett *et al.*, 1976) stressed the need

Table 14.2

Features of AML with trilineage myelodysplasia

Qualitative changes	Dyserythropoiesis (as in MDS) in ≥ 25% erythroblasts
	Hypogranular, agranular and/or Pelger-like neutrophils
	Dysplastic megakaryocytes, mononuclear, hypersegmented etc.
Quantitative changes*	Blood-blast cell count < 20%
	Low WBC < 11 × 10^9/l
	Bone marrow blasts 30–40% (≤ 60%)
	Hb < 6 g/dl
	Erythroblasts in peripheral blood

*Compared with de-novo AML, without myelodysplasia. (Reproduced from Brito-Babapulle *et al.* (1987a), with permission.)

Table 14.3

The morphological classification of the acute leukaemias

Lymphoblastic (ALL)

L1:   small, monomorphic, high N:C ratio (scores 0, 1 or 2)*

L2:   large, heterogeneous, nucleolated, low N:C ratio (scores −1, −2, −3)*

L3:   Burkitt-cell type, basophilic, vacuolated

Myeloid (AML)

MO: undifferentiated myeloblastic†

M1:   myeloblastic without maturation

M2:   myeloblastic with maturation

M2-Baso: M2 with basophil-blasts

M3:   hypergranular promyelocytic

M3-variant: micro- or hypogranular bilobed promyelocytes

M4:   myelomonocytic, with both granulocytic and monocytic differentiation

M4-Eo: M4 with bone marrow eosinophilia

M5:   monocytic; monoblastic (M5a) and promonocytic-monocytic (M5b)

M6:   erythroleukaemia, with > 50% erythroblasts and ≤ 30% or > 30% blasts

M7:   megakaryoblastic‡

---

*See text; also Bennett *et al.* (1981).

†Identified by myeloid McAb and/or ultrastructural peroxidase (Matutes *et al*., 1988; Oliveira *et al.*, 1988).

‡Identified by McAb against platelet glycoproteins and/or ultrastructural platelet peroxidase (Bennett *et al.*, 1985a).

for cytochemical techniques to distinguish ALL from AML where morphology alone (as in the case of L2) may be inadequate for that purpose.

Lately it has also become apparent that there is considerable heterogeneity within ALL, and this can only be recognized by membrane marker studies, in particular McAb, which allow a clear separation between B-lineage and T-lineage ALL, and which, with the exception of the relatively uncommon L3-type, do not correlate with the morphological classification. In addition, immunological techniques have become necessary to identify infrequent types of AML, such as MO (undifferentiated myeloblastic leukaemia) and M7 (megakaryoblastic leukaemia).

There is a need therefore to integrate all these elements in the classification of acute leukaemia,

which will thus become more precise, have greater reproducibility and be clinically more relevant. A further integration, with the karyotype of the neoplastic cells, has recently been proposed for ALL and AML (the MIC classification, 1987 and 1988). This is based on the demonstration of highly specific chromosome translocations in AML cases defined by morphology and cytochemistry and ALL cases defined by cell markers (see also Chapter 13).

Morphology

ALL

The FAB classification has evolved with minor improvements over the last 12 years (Bennett *et al.*, 1976, 1980, 1981, 1982, 1985a and 1985b). The two main groups of ALL and AML are clinically relevant as the treatment programmes for adults and children are different in both types of disorder.

As stated above, the morphological classification of ALL needs to be supplemented by the immunological classification. Reasons for retaining the morphological criteria are· threefold. Firstly, the L1 group is the most common type in children (approximately 80%) and represents half the adult cases and can be recognized with adequate preparations by morphology alone in most instances. Secondly, the L2 type, which represents 50% of the adult cases and approximately 20% of childhood cases, is the one in which additional cytochemistry and marker studies are essential; Furthermore, a number of studies have shown that L2 morphology is a bad prognostic feature in childhood ALL. Thirdly, the Burkitt-type or L3 type, which is rare (1–2%) in children and adults, should be identified primarily by morphology, secondly by markers (membrane immunoglobulin-positive blasts) and thirdly by karyotype (t(8;14)). L3 cases represent the worst prognostic category within ALL and are one of the few undisputed indications for BMT in ALL.

The morphological identification of L1 and L2 has been facilitated by relatively simple criteria, or 'ALL score' (Bennett *et al.*, 1981), which takes into account: nucleo:cytoplasmic (N:C) ratio (high in L1), the presence of a prominent nucleolus in >25% of blasts (criterion for L2), the irregularity of the nuclear membrane (criterion for L2), and cell size (if more than 50% of blasts are large, L2 is indicated). The sum of the score—positive for L1 (0 to 2) and negative for L2 (−1 to −3)—based on examination of the bone marrow, not the peripheral blood film, facilitates the diagnosis of L1 (Fig. 14.1) or L2 (Fig. 14.2). L3 cells (Fig. 14.3) are homogeneous and larger than L1 cells, with a loose arrangement of the nuclear chromatin and an inconspicuous nucleolus. In common with the cells of Burkitt's lymphoma (as seen in imprints, not on haematoxylin and eosin (HE) stained sections), L3 cells have a deeply stained basophilic cytoplasm which is often vacuolated (due to neutral fat inclusions which stain positively with oil-red O). Numerous mitotic figures are often seen in the bone marrow of L3 cases; this is rare in L1 and L2. Almost all cases of L3 correspond to SmIg+ blasts;

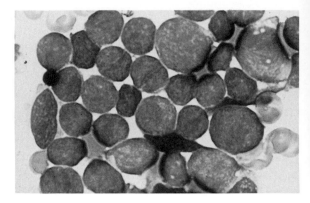

Fig. 14.1. *Childhood ALL, L1 type. Note high N:C ratio and lack of visible nucleolus; common ALL phenotype (bone marrow, × 1400).*

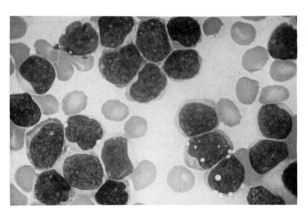

Fig. 14.2. *Adult ALL, L2 type. Note more abundant cytoplasm than the blasts in Fig. 14.1 and slightly more irregular nuclear shape; null-ALL phenotype (bone marrow, × 1300).*

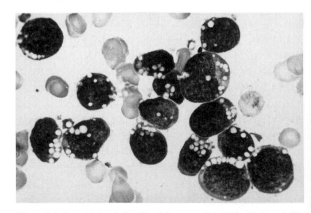

Fig. 14.3. *ALL, L3 (Burkitt type) with basophilic cytoplasm and cytoplasmic vacuolation; mature B-markers (SmIg+) (bone marrow, × 1300).*

rarely, L2 blasts positive for SmIg are seen in adults (Fig. 14.4). These latter cases probably do not represent true ALL but are examples of B-cell lymphomas which rarely manifest with initial bone marrow involvement and L2 type blasts. Another correspondence between morphology and markers can be found when L2 blasts have nuclear convolutions and correspond to T-lineage lymphoblasts (Fig. 14.5). Although this criterion often correlates with T-blasts, the reverse is not the case, as T-lymphoblasts may have regular nuclear outline and resemble L1 or L2 cells. The acid phosphatase with a strong localized paranuclear reaction is seen,

within ALL, almost exclusively in T-blasts (Fig. 14.6). However, as discussed below, blasts in M6 and M7 types of AML may show a similar localized pattern with this cytochemical reaction (Oliveira *et al.*, 1987).

AML

As stated above, most forms of AML can be recognized morphologically. MO is a type not included in the FAB classification and represents cases of myeloblastic leukaemia with negative cytochemistry (for AML) at light microscopy (see below). M1 and M5a often require cytochemical evidence (Table 14.4), although the presence of Auer rods in M1 or abundant greyish cytoplasm in M5a may be suggestive. In M1, 90% or more of the blasts have no granules (type 1 blasts) (Fig. 14.7) or have few azurophil granules (type 2 blasts) (Bennett *et al.*, 1982), or a single Auer rod. M2 cases show clear myeloblastic–promyelocytic differentiation and, often, also cells beyond the promyelocyte stage. A proportion of M2 cases have promyelocytes with coarse granules and frequent Auer rods. These cases often carry the translocation t(8;21) characteristic of M2 (see Chapter 13). Peroxidase and Sudan black B are always positive (Fig. 14.8). In rare cases of M2 there is evidence of basophilic differentiation shown by increased numbers of basophils and, by electron microscopy, of blasts with typical basophil granules; these cases are provisionally designated as M2-Baso.

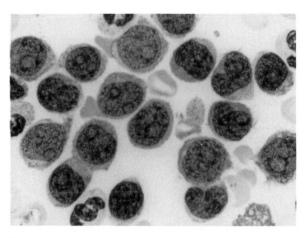

Fig. 14.4. *ALL, L2 type in an adult of 60 years. This case was unusual in having a mature phenotype (SmIg +); this suggests that it was a B-cell lymphoma in leukaemic phase (bone marrow, × 1300).*

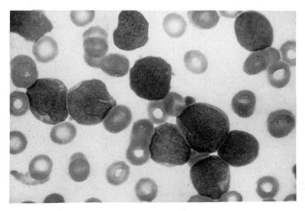

Fig. 14.5. *Convoluted blasts (L2) of a case of T-ALL (bone marrow, × 1300).*

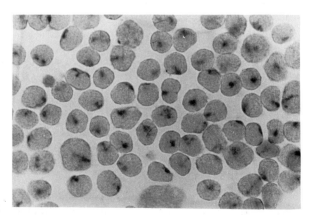

Fig. 14.6. *Acid phosphatase localized reaction in the paranuclear zone in a case of T-ALL (cytocentrifuge slide, × 1200).*

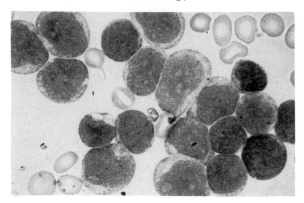

Fig. 14.7. *AML, M1 type. These blasts are morphologically similar to L2 cells except for the fact that the peroxidase and Sudan black B reactions are positive in M1 and negative in L2 (bone marrow, × 1400).*

M3 represents 5–7% of all AML and should always be recognized in Romanowsky-stained slides: heavily granulated promyelocytes with multiple Auer rods arranged in bundles (or 'faggot' cells) and bilobed nucleus (Fig. 14.9). The M3-variant (approximately 15% of M3 cases) may present difficulties for its recognition as the cells are not obviously granular and have a deceptive monocytoid appearance (Fig. 14.10). In fact, the nucleus is typically bilobed and occasional faggot cells and more granular ones may be seen in the bone marrow (Fig. 14.11). M3-variant cases, in contrast with typical M3, present with elevated WBC. The correct interpretation of peripheral blood films is essential for the diagnosis of these cases. Both M3 and M3-variant cases carry the t(15;17) translocation which is not seen in other types of acute leukaemia (see Chapter 13).

M4 may resemble M2 if only the bone marrow is examined; the monocytic component is more apparent in the peripheral blood, which has usually $> 1 \times 10^9$/l monocytes (Figs. 14.12 and 14.3). When the monocytic component is less apparent, cytochemical methods for demonstrating monocytic differentiation are required and/or sometimes evidence of increased serum or urinary lysozyme is necessary (Bennett *et al.*, 1986). M4 should be distinguished from chronic myelomonocytic leukaemia (CMML) by the evidence (in M4) or more than 30% of type 1 or 2 blasts in the bone marrow. These blasts are usually less than 5% in the bone marrow of CMML. Some cases of M4 have a prominent eosinophil component only in the bone marrow. These eosinophils have immature granules (prominent and basophilic) together with the specific eosinophil granules. This variant of M4 (M4-Eo) is often associated with abnormalities of the long arm of chromosome 16, 16q− or inv(16) (see Chapter 13).

In M5, particularly M5b, the monocytic differentiation is self-evident. This represents the type formerly described as Schilling type of monocytic leukaemia. The M5a (monoblastic) type (Fig. 14.14) is frequent in children below the age of 2 years and is

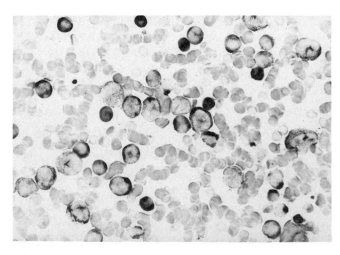

Fig. 14.8. *Strong peroxidase reaction in a case of AML, M2 type (bone marrow, × 1000).*

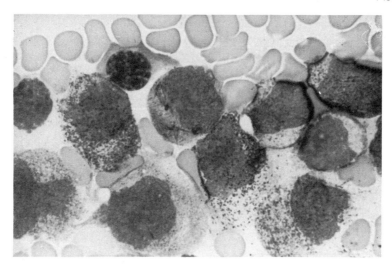

Fig. 14.9. *AML, M3 (hypergranular promyelocytic); the blasts have variable numbers of azurophil granules and one has bundles of Auer rods 'faggots' (bone marrow, ×1500).*

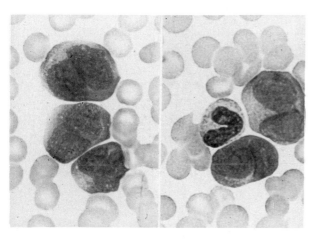

Fig. 14.10. *AML, M3-variant (micro- or hypogranular variant) showing blasts with bilobed nucleus (peripheral blood, ×1400).*

also seen in adults. In common with other type of AML, it is also associated with chromosome abnormalities (Chapter 13).

M6, as discussed above, is the only type in which a diagnosis of AML can be made with less than 30% blasts in the bone marrow. The blast cell component is generally myeloid (more often myeloblasts) but in rare cases the blast cells may be erythroid precursor cells (Fig. 14.15). In the latter case they are negative with cytochemical reactions for myeloblasts or monoblasts and may show instead an erythroid pattern (see below) and some of them may react with specific McAb, e.g. against glycophorin-A. Morphologically the erythroid component is often bizarre and shows megaloblastic features and bi- or trinucleated forms. Circulating erythroblasts are a common feature of M6; similarly, most cases show evidence of trilineage MDS, as shown by granulocyte and megakaryocyte abnormalities in addition to dyserythropoiesis.

The blasts in megakaryoblastic (M7) AML are morphologically undifferentiated; they often resemble either L1 or L2 cells. They can be small and round with dense chromatin or large with several nucleoli. Often they show cytoplasmic blebs; occasionally platelets are seen shedding from the cytoplasm or may appear as bare nuclei. Bone marrow aspirates are difficult to obtain and often characterization of the blasts is only possible on peripheral blood samples. Bone marrow biopsies are essential for the diagnosis of M7. They will show blasts and sometimes marked megakaryocytic differentiation (Fig. 14.16). Marked reticulin fibrosis is a constant feature. A high proportion of cases present as 'acute' myelofibrosis, but it should be borne in mind that less frequently other types of AML, M6, MDS, or even ALL may present with similar degrees of bone marrow fibrosis.

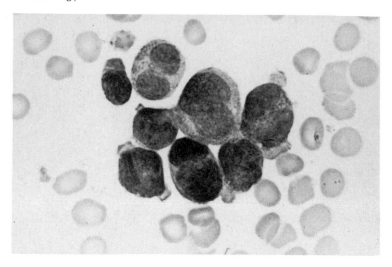

Fig. 14.11. *AML, M3-variant (bone marrow, × 1400).*

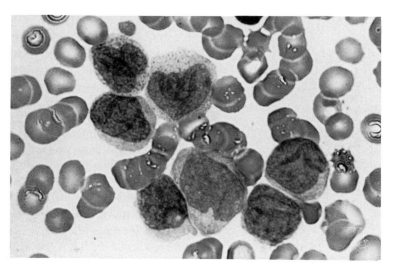

Fig. 14.12. *AML, M4 with blasts of monocytic morphology (peripheral blood, × 1400).*

Cytochemistry

There are two types of cytochemical tests which are essential for the diagnosis and precise classification of AML: (a) the peroxidase and Sudan black B (SBB) reactions, either of which is contributory to the diagnosis of four types of AML—M1, M2, M3 and M4 (see Table 14.4); and (b) a non-specific esterase reaction, commonly the alpha-naphthyl acetate esterase (ANAE) or alpha-naphthyl butyr-ate esterase (ANBE), or the naphthol-AS acetate esterase (NASA), all of which give a characteristically strong diffuse reaction in monocytic leukaemias, M4 and M5; ANAE also gives a strong localized pattern in M6 and M7 (Oliveira *et al.*, 1987). All these esterase reactions are sensitive to inhibition by sodium fluoride (see Table 14.4).

Other cytochemical methods add useful information: naphthol-AS chloracetate esterase, reactive with myeloblastic leukaemias, M1, M2 and M3;

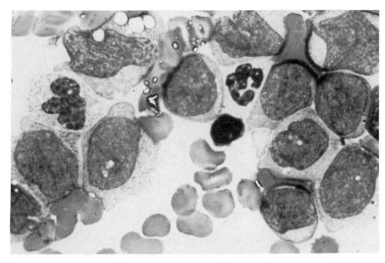

Fig. 14.13. *AML, M4 type. Note some blasts with granulocytic and others with monocytic differentiation (bone marrow, × 1400).*

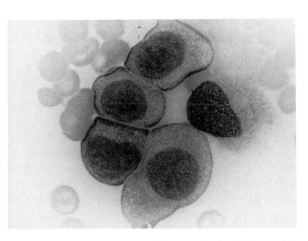

Fig. 14.14. *AML, M5a (monoblastic leukaemia). Blasts are large and have abundant cytoplasm (bone marrow, × 1200).*

acid phosphatase which has a distinct localized pattern in T-ALL, and also in M6 and M7 blasts and a diffuse reaction in M5 (Oliveira *et al.*, 1987); the PAS reaction which has a granular pattern, usually as a single block of positivity in ALL; and the cytobacterial test for lysozyme, which is positive in M4 and M5 cells, but may be negative in the monoblasts of M5a. This test for lysozyme correlates with the result of serum estimations. An elevated level is useful to define a monocytic component, particularly in cases of M4 with low monocyte

counts and bone marrow aspirates which may be interpreted as M2. These cytochemical methods, excluding those for SBB or peroxidase and ANAE or NASA, are not performed routinely in many laboratories since the advent of McAb, which are more helpful for the immunological classification of ALL (thus making the use of the PAS and acid phosphatase reactions less essential in ALL) and also in some types of AML (e.g. MO). The chloracetate esterase rarely provides more information than the SBB, although it gives a characteristic positive reaction in the eosinophils of M4-Eo which is not observed in normal eosinophils. Lysozyme is rarely positive (or high) in cases of M5a. Peroxidase, SBB and chloracetate esterase are much more sensitive for the identification of Auer rods than the Romanowsky stains, particularly in cases of M1, M2 and M3. In the latter, it helps to identify faggot cells. In addition these reactions allow the recognition of mature neutrophils with absent primary granules and which are therefore peroxidase and SBB negative. This phenomenon is seen particularly in cases of M2, M4, M6 and in MDS.

The most important application of cytochemistry is in the separation of AML—in which the most common types (M1, M2, M3, M4 and some M5) show always some degree of positivity with SBB or similar tests (see Table 14.4), and others (M5, M6 and M7) show a characteristic reactivity with

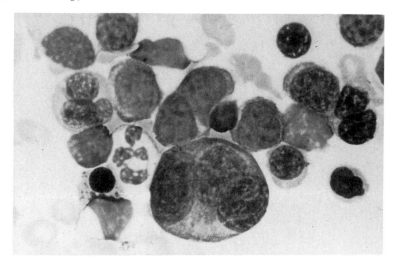

Fig. 14.15. *AML, M6 (erythroleukaemia) showing a mixture of bizarre erythroid precursors and myeloblasts (bone marrow, × 1400).*

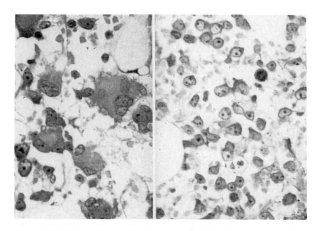

Fig. 14.16. *AML, M7 (megakaryoblastic leukaemia). Two areas of a bone marrow trephine biopsy, one showing undifferentiated blasts and the other clusters of megakaryocytes (× 600).*

ANAE—from ALL, particularly from cases with L2 morphology which are more commonly seen in adult patients. There is a minority of such cases (approximately 5%) which are negative with most cytochemical tests or do not show any of the patterns characteristic of M1 to M7, which we have designated MO (Oliveira *et al.*, 1988). Although some of the MO cases (up to 40%) may be TdT positive (Parreira *et al.*, 1988), they lack reactivity

with any of the specific McAb for B or T lineage ALL and they react with at least one of the specific anti-myeloid McAb and show peroxidase activity at ultrastructural level (see below).

Electron Microscopy

Electron microscopy (EM) permits more detailed examination of blast cells and the recognition of some structures which may not be apparent by light microscopy (LM). This may help in the classification of a particular cell type, but it cannot be used to establish a diagnosis of leukaemia. Characteristically, blast cells show very little nuclear chromatin condensation and have a variable nuclear shape. Myeloblasts and promyelocytes have primary (electron dense) granules which are usually larger than those seen in promonocytes. The latter cells have a monocytoid nuclear configuration and small cytoplasmic projections.

Auer rods can be recognized by their characteristic periodic structure. Undifferentiated blasts, including those of ALL, are difficult to distinguish from each other on morphological grounds alone. Lymphoblasts, as distinct from myeloblasts, have few or no electron dense granules. L2 blasts are large, lack chromatin condensation and have, in general, an irregular nucleus and a prominent nucleolus. L1 blasts have a round or slightly indented

Table 14.4
Cytochemical findings in AML and ALL*

Reaction	M0	M1	M2/M3	M4	M5	M6/M7	ALL
Peroxidase Sudan black-B Chloracetate	−	+	++	+	−/+	−ᵃ	−
ANAEᵇ NASA	−	−	−/++	++	++	+	−/±
			(diffuse)			(localized)	
Acid phosphatase	−	−	+	+	++	+	−/+ᶜ
			(diffuse)			(localized)	
PAS	N.D.	−	+	+	++	+	+ᵈ
			(diffuse)		(diffuse and granular)	(blocks)	
Lysozyme (cyto-bacterial or serum)	−	−	−	+	++/−	−	−

* Refers to findings in the predominant blast cell population.
ᵃ Positive only if myeloblastic component is present.
ᵇ Mostly NaF sensitive.
ᶜ In T-ALL (including pre-T-ALL with negative E-rosettes).
ᵈ Not in T-ALL; mainly in cALL and more frequently in children than in adults.
N.D. = No data.

nucleus, an inconspicuous nucleolus, some peripheral chromatin condensation with clumps of heterochromatin inside the nucleus. L3 cells lack nuclear maturation (as L2) but they have abundant polyribosomes and fat globules in the cytoplasm. Cells in T-ALL have L1 or L2 morphology and frequently a highly convoluted nucleus. Erythroid precursors may show ferritin particles and tropheocytosis. Rare cases of AML (M2-Baso), as well as some blast crises of CML, have blasts with typical basophil granules.

Peroxidase and acid phosphatase reactions can also be studied at EM level. Peroxidase is positive in the primary granules in blasts of the granulocytic series. Commonly the proportion of peroxidase-positive blasts identified by EM is about twice as high as seen by LM. This is especially so in AML-MO where the granules may be small and sparse or may show only the reaction product in the nuclear membrane, endoplasmic reticulum and Golgi region using unfixed preparations (Matutes *et al.*, 1988). This pattern of reaction may be similar to that seen in megakaryoblasts, except that in the latter neither granules nor Golgi membranes show peroxidase (platelet–peroxidase) activity. The acid phosphatase reaction is also positive in the primary granules of myeloid cells. In monoblasts, numerous small granules which are acid phosphatase positive and peroxidase negative are a characteristic feature of early differentiation. In T-ALL a strong reaction is seen in the membranous structures of the Golgi zone and in the cytoplasmic granules of T-lymphoblasts.

Cell Markers

Advances in immunological techniques in the last decade have made possible the identification of specific receptors, antigens and other molecules on the membrane and/or the cytoplasm of lymphoid cells (see Chapter 12). For both ALL and AML these markers show that the blast cells resemble very closely rare cells in normal bone marrow, or for T-ALL the thymus, and from which the leukaemias appear to be derived by clonal expansion. The major progress followed the development of the hybridoma technology which guarantees the production of pure and specific reagents in unlimited amounts for clinical use. The early tests were rosetting methods using erythrocytes from various species, sheep for T-cells (E-rosettes), mouse for a subset of B-cells (M-rosettes). The E-rosette test is still used as a reliable T-cell marker. The receptor for sheep erythocytes appears on the membrane of T-lymphocytes during thymic differentiation, and although it is not the earliest feature of T-cell maturation, most normal and leukaemic T-lymphocytes are positive with the exception of the very early T-lymphoblasts (pre-T-ALL) (Table 14.5). The binding of sheep erythrocytes takes place at 4°C; at 37°C the erythrocytes are released from the binding on mature T-cells but not on thymic cells or T-lymphoblasts. Nowadays, e.g. McAb CD2 (OKT11) can be used, instead of sheep erythrocytes, to demonstrate this receptor.

Before the discovery of McAb, another important marker used for the typing of ALL cells was the anti-ALL serum raised by Greaves and colleagues (1975) in rabbits by injecting lymphoblasts which were E-rosette and SmIg negative and were previously incubated with an anti-lymphocyte serum to coat common antigenic sites. This polyclonal antibody was used extensively for the typing of leukaemic blasts and was crucial for the identification of the common type of ALL in children, cALL. The cALL antigen, a glycoprotein of 100 kD, is currently detected by several McAb clustered in the CD10 group (Table 14.5).

The Immunological Classification of ALL

Because lymphoblasts are poorly differentiated cells with little morphological evidence of heterogeneity or maturation features, the current approach is to use a panel or reagents, chiefly McAb, which help

Table 14.5
Immunological classification of ALL

| Type of reagent | Marker* | B-lineage† | | | | T-lineage‡ | |
		Null	cALL	pre-B	B-ALL	pre-T	T-ALL
Against precursor cells	HLA-Dr	+	+	+	+	−/±	−
	TdT	+	+	+	−/±	+	+
	CD34(3C5)	+	+	+	−	−	−
Against B-cell antigens	CD19 (B4)	+	+	+	+	−	−
	CD22 (Cyt)	+	+	+	+	−	−
	CD10 (J5)	−	+	+	−/±	−/±	−
	CD20 (B1)	−	−/+	+	+	−	−
	Cyt μ chain	−	−	+	+	−	−
	SmIg	−	−	−	+	−	−
Against T-cell antigens	CD7 (3A1)	−	−	−	−	+	+
	CD3 (Cyt)	−	−	−	−	+	+
	CD5 (UCHT2)	−	−	−	−	−/+	+
	E-rosettes (CD2)	−	−	−	−	−	+
	CD1 (OKT6)	−	−	−	−	−	−/+

*Given according to cluster of differentiation (CD) number and, in brackets, the corresponding McAb used in the laboratory of one of the authors (DC). The McAb are listed according to the sequential order in which they are first expressed in cells of the B- and T-cell lineage.
†All cases show rearrangement of the Ig heavy chain gene.
‡All cases show rearrangement of the T-cell receptor β and/or γ and/or δ chain genes.
Abbreviations: Cyt: cytoplasmic expression; TdT: terminal deoxynucleotidyl transferase; E: sheep RBC cells; SmIg: membrane-bound Ig.

identify early B-cells, early T-cells and/or other precursor cells (see Table 14.5).

One of the most important early markers of lymphoblasts is the enzyme terminal deoxynucleotidyl transferase (TdT), a remarkable DNA polymerase which was originally found in high concentrations in the thymus. After the initial work with biochemical assays, TdT is now routinely demonstrated in the nucleus of B and T lineage lymphoblasts by means of a polyclonal antibody, using immunofluorescence or immunoperoxidase. Although TdT may also be expressed in some early leukaemic myeloblasts (Table 14.6; Bradstock *et al.*, 1981; Jani *et al.*, 1983; Parreira *et al.*, 1988), it is still a valuable reagent for the diagnosis of ALL as well as of lymphoblastic crisis of CGL.

There are two major lymphoid lineages: B and T. Leukaemias derived from early or more mature lymphoid precursors can be identified objectively by the reactivity with one or more McAb and some polyclonal reagents (see Table 14.5). The specificity of these reagents is confirmed by the fact that McAb against T-cells do not react with B-lineage lymphoblasts, and, with few exceptions, McAb against B-cell antigens are not positive in T-lymphoblasts. The expression of these antigens correlates in B-cells with the rearrangement of the immunoglobulin heavy chain gene and in T-cells with the reorganiz-ation of the T-cell receptor (TCR) α, β, γ, and δ genes (Table 14.7; see also Chapter 12).

The incidence of the various immunological type of ALL varies according to age groups. In children (aged 2–5 years), cALL is the most common (70–75%) including pre-B ALL; 5% have null-ALL, 15–20% T-ALL (including 5% with pre-T ALL) and less than 1% B-ALL (with SmIg+). In infants (less than 2 years) null-ALL is the most common. In adults (more than 15 years of age) 70% are cALL, including pre-B ALL, 10% null-ALL, 15% T-ALL and 5% B-ALL. The last-mentioned may include, in addition to the Burkitt type, or L3 ALL (see Fig. 14.3), some cases of undifferentiated B-cell NHL which may present as an acute leukaemia (see Fig. 14.4). Except for B-ALL, there is no correlation between the immunologically and morphologically defined FAB subtypes of ALL. There is, on the other hand, a good correspondence between some of the immunologically defined subtypes of B- and T-lineage ALL and specific chromosome abnormalities, as described by the First MIC Cooperative Study Group (1987) (see also Chapter 13).

The Immunological Classification of AML

Numerous McAb are now available which help identify specific types of AML. In general, these

Table 14.6
Cell markers in AML

McAb	MO*	M1	M2/M3	M4/M5	M6	M7
CD34 (3C5)	+	+	±/−	±/−	−	±
CD13 (MCS2)[†]	+	+	+	+	+	+
CD33 (MY9)	±	+	+	+	±	+
CD11b (OKM1)	−	−	+	±	−	−
CD14 (FMC17)	−	−	−	+	−	−
Glycophorin	−	−	−	−	+	−
CDw41/42	−	−	−	−	−	+
TdT[‡]	−/+	−/+	−	−	−	−

*Undifferentiated myeloblastic leukaemia with negative light microscopy cytochemistry for AML; absence of lymphoid antigens; and positive peroxidase by electron microscopy.

[†]More sensitive when tested on fixed cells (cytoplasmic expression) (Oliveira *et al.*, 1988).

[‡]Positive in up to 50% of MO/M1 cases, and in less than 10% of other types of AML (M2 to M7) (Parreira *et al.*, 1988).

Table 14.7

T cell receptors and immunoglobulin gene rearrangements in AML, ALL and lymphoproliferative diseases[a]. (Adapted from T. Mak (1988). Personal communication.)

IgH	−	+	+	+[c]	+[c]	+[c]	+[c]	+[c]	+[c]	+	−	−	−
IgL	−	+	+	−	−	−	−	−	−	−	−	−	−
TcRγ	−	−	+	−	+	−	+	−	−	+	+	+	+
TcRβ	−	−	+[c]	−	+[c]	−	−	+	−	+	−	+	+
TcRδ[b]	−	−	−	−	−	+	+	+	+	+	−	−	+
Leukaemias													
T-ALL	0	0	0	0	0	0	0	0	0	10	0	45	45
B-ALL	0	70	30	0	0	0	0	0	0	0	0	0	0
non-T non-B	0	0	0	10	0	10	20	10	20	30	0	0	0
ATL	0	0	0	0	0	0	0	0	0	0	0	0	100
AML	70	0	0	0	0	0	0	0	0	5	5	5	15
Lymphomas													
T	0	0	0	0	0	0	0	0	0	0	0	60	40
B	0	60	40	0	0	0	0	0	0	0	0	0	0

[a] Germ-line (−) and rearranged (+) structures of these genes are denoted. The distributions of the individual types of disorders with a specific pattern of rearrangement are expressed as percentages (approximate) of the total number of cases examined.
[b] Analyses included both rearrangement and deletion of the δ chain genes.
[c] Patterns most likely representing only DJ rearrangements.
Abbreviations: Ig, immunoglobulin; TcR, T cell receptor.

reagents do not react with ALL and have a variable expression in the various types of AML (Table 14.6). Some, e.g. CD13 and CD33, are good overall markers for AML. Using both types of McAb it is possible to recognize 90% or more of AML cases (Oliveira *et al.*, 1988). Some McAb react with differentiation antigens, e.g. to CD15 (not shown in Table 14.6) which reacts with granulocytic cells, whilst CD14 McAb reacts with monocytes. Other reagents are specific for erythroid cells (e.g. anti-glycophorin-A) or react with platelet glycoproteins which are also expressed on megakaryoblasts.

The immunological profile of myeloid blasts defined by McAb shows some correspondence with the morphological and cytochemical pattern of differentiation, as defined by the FAB group (Bennett *et al.*, 1976 and 1985b). AML subtypes correspond, on the other hand, with some precision to karyotypic abnormalities as compounded by the MIC classification (Second MIC Cooperative Study Group, 1988) (see also Chapter 13).

Biphenotypic and Mixed Leukaemias

The increasing use of McAb has disclosed a degree of 'promiscuity' in the expression of certain antigens on blasts cells (Greaves *et al.*, 1986). In some studies, a relatively high frequency of myeloid antigens in childhood (Stass and Mirro, 1986) and in adult-ALL has been reported (Sobol *et al.*, 1987). Furthermore, 'a phenotypic switch' from ALL to AML, or vice versa, after complete remission has been well documented. Often too the expression of TdT identifies AML cases in which lymphoid antigens (or rearrangement of Ig or TCR genes) are also present (Hoffbrand *et al.*, 1988; Parreira *et al.*, 1988; Table 14.7). Although the significance of these findings is not yet completely understood, it is important to document and describe precisely such cases with all available techniques, including ultrastructural cytochemistry and DNA analysis.

Three types of unusual cases can be found. (1) Cases of undifferentiated leukaemia in which specific lymphoid markers are negative, TdT may or may not be expressed, and in which the evidence by light microscopy of morphology and cytochemistry is not sufficient for a diagnosis of AML. The predominant cells resemble L2 blasts and do not show any of the typical cytochemical patterns seen in AML (see Table 14.4). Blasts of such cases, which are wrongly described as adult-ALL (Sobol *et al.*, 1987), are usually positive with CD13 and/or CD33 (Oliveira *et al.*, 1988) and show peroxidase activity at ultrastructural level (Matutes *et al.*, 1988) and are therefore designated AML-MO (see above). (2) Cases in which the blasts are, by most criteria, either typical lymphoblasts or myeloblasts, and which, unexpectedly, express one or more antigens of the opposite lineage. These cases have been designated biphenotypic or hybrid (expression of myeloid and lymphoid antigens on the same cell) and may represent a misprogramming of differentiation or immortalization by the leukaemic process of a normally rare precursor with mixed features (perhaps normally destined to die), reflecting the 'promiscuity' of early haemopoietic cells (Greaves *et al.*, 1986) (see also Chapter 12). In adult-ALL these mixed cases are associated with a poor prognosis (Sobol *et al.*, 1987). (3) Cases which show separate populations of blasts with myeloid or lymphoid features. These cases, designated mixed or bilinear acute leukaemia, differ from the biphenotypic cases in that they allow a clear separation of two types of blasts. They represent the proliferation of early haemopoietic cells with cells undergoing separate maturation along myeloid and lymphoid pathways. There is no evidence that two separate clones are present. It is likely that the published examples of 'phenotypic switches' originate from such cases. It is envisaged that in such situations the effect of specific therapy, either anti-lymphoid or anti-myeloid, will induce a remission in one of the particular lineages, thus allowing the switch to become more apparent.

CLINICAL MANAGEMENT OF THE ACUTE LEUKAEMIAS

There are major differences in age incidence, drug sensitivity, therapeutic strategy and overall prognosis which justify a different therapeutic approach in AML and ALL. Furthermore, a number of clinical and laboratory features suggest that the management of adult ALL also requires to be different from that of childhood ALL.

Childhood ALL

The disease has a peak incidence between the ages of 4 and 5 years and presents usually with a short history, rarely of more than 2 or 3 months. The symptoms may be due to anaemia, thrombocytopenia and/or joint or bone involvement. Joint involvement with associated inflammation is not a rare presenting symptom, and often leads to an initial investigation for rheumatoid arthritis or rheumatic fever. Bone pain is present in 50% of cases, and may be associated with radiological changes, although the two do not necessarily correlate. Characteristic x-ray changes are: transverse metaphyseal bands of decreased density in the long bones, diffuse demineralization and solitary osteolytic lesions or periosteal reaction. A few cases present with aplastic anaemia which is transient. Physical signs may be absent or there may be lymphadenopathy in 50% of cases and/or hepatosplenomegaly in 65%. Enlarged mediastinal nodes or, more frequently, an anterior mediastinal mass are demonstrated on a chest x-ray in 5% of cases. In T-ALL, widening of the mediastinum can be seen in 40–50% of cases. These and a number of other features suggest that T-ALL may start outside the bone marrow.

Prognostic Features

There are listed in Table 14.8. The most important bad prognostic feature is a high WBC, which is more common in T-ALL than in B-lineage ALL. Both high WBC and an anterior mediastinal mass

Table 14.8
Prognostic factors in ALL*

Feature†	Bad	Good
WBC ($\times 10^9$/l)	> 50	< 10
Age (years)	< 2; ≥ 15; > 50	2–10
Sex	Male	Female
Chromosomes	Translocations t(8; 14); t(4; 11); t(9; 22); hypodiploidy	Hyperploidy > 50 chromosomes
Morphology (FAB)	L3; L2	L1
Cell markers	B(SmIg +); ?T	cALL (cD10)
Others	CNS leukaemia; organomegaly	remission in 4 weeks

* For both children and adults, although some factors have more weight in childhood series.
† In order of importance as independent variables (at clinical presentation, before treatment) to predict mainly disease-free survival.

are so closely associated with T-ALL that it is difficult to separate whether these features or the T-cell nature per se is the factor which confers a worse prognosis. Given intensive therapy, patients with T-ALL without these adverse features may not have a particularly bad prognosis.

The worse prognosis for boys, highlighted by the incidence of testicular disease, is still apparent in modern studies in which the overall results have improved. In studies with less intensive regimens during the last decade the worse outcome for boys was very striking. Cell morphology correlates with age and prognosis. Adults more frequently than children have blasts with L2 morphology. This feature seems to influence the incidence of remission induction (which is better with L1), particularly in adults. In children, L1 morphology seems to be a useful predictor of long-term disease-free survival (Lilleyman *et al.*, 1986). L2 is also associated with a higher incidence of aneuploidy than L1. L3, as indicated above, is associated with the worse type of ALL, B-ALL (SmIg positive).

Several structural chromosome abnormalities have also been shown to be strong predictors of short survival (Table 14.8). On the other hand, patients with hyperdiploid karyotypes (> 47 chromosomes), particularly those with > 50 chromo-

somes, have the best prognosis, with 70% remaining in first remission for over 5 years, as demonstrated by data from the Third International Workshop (Bloomfield *et al.*, 1986).

It is important to realize that the value of these prognostic factors depends on the intensity and quality of treatment. As stated above for sex, the clinical significance of other features which in the past were clearly associated with poor prognosis has been modified with the advent of improved treatments.

Principles of Therapy

Progress has continued in the treatment of childhood ALL, notably by the use of more intensive regimens and by efforts to 'tailor' protocols according to prognostic risks. The overall principles for therapy of this disease are outlined in Table 14.9. Although the items listed have not changed much over the last decade, the details of each stage have altered considerably. The concept of 'total therapy' of the Memphis group has remained, the role of L-asparaginase during the induction phase is well established, and so is the use of periodic reinduction courses with vincristine and prednisolone during maintenance. With such protocols the figures for

Table 14.9
Principles of therapy in ALL

---

1. *Remission induction*
   Vincristine (weekly for 4 weeks)
   Prednisolone (4 weeks)
   Daunorubicin (for 2 days)
   L-asparaginase (for 3 weeks)

2. *Consolidation*
   For example a combination of vincristine, daunorubicin, prednisolone, cytosine arabinoside, etoposide and thioguanine (for 5 days)

3. *Consideration of BMT* (allogeneic or autologous)
   For high risk cases only

4. *CNS prophylaxis*
   Cranial irradiation: 1800 cGy (children), 2400 cGy (adults), and intrathecal methotrexate (6 injections)

5. *Late intensification*
   For example as consolidation or using other agents (cyclophosphamide, intermediate or high dose methotrexate, etc.)

6. *Maintenance (for 2 years)*
   A common regimen consists of methotrexate (weekly), 6-mercaptopurine (daily), vincristine (monthly) and prednisolone (monthly for 5 days)

N.B. More intensive alternative regimens are needed in SmIg + B-ALL.

disease-free survival currently obtained in children range from 50% to 75%, depending on the prognostic category. Some aspects are still being debated, for example the optimal consolidation regimen, the ideal regimen for CNS prophylaxis which will prevent meningeal leukaemia with the minimum of late toxicity, and the role of intermediate doses of methotrexate (Mtx), e.g. 500 mg/m^2 given as a 24-hour infusion, to overcome drug resistance and cross the blood–CNS barrier.

The drugs used for the treatment of ALL are active at different phases of the cell cycle, thus their combination and sequential use make them very effective in the various stages of treatment.

Remission Induction

Complete remission (CR) can be easily achieved without myelotoxicity in over 90% of cases using vincristine and prednisolone. The addition of other drugs, e.g. daunorubicin and L-asparaginase (see Table 14.9) produces even higher CR rates (95–98%) and it is intended to improve the long-term results by increasing the initial cell kill. One minor drawback of adding extra drugs during induction is that it may delay regeneration and cause some toxicity, e.g. mucositis. For that reason, daunorubicin should be used instead of doxorubicin (Adriamycin) at this early stage. Details of the mode of action and toxicities of the agents used for the treatment of acute leukaemia (as well as other cytotoxic drugs) are given in Table 14.10. A CR can be obtained in the first 4–6 weeks of induction therapy with normalization of blood counts.

Consolidation

This phase should include alternative drugs to those used during induction. It is an intensification phase

Table 14.10

The mode of action and side-effects of drugs used in leukaemia therapy. (N.B. Nearly all cause nausea, vomiting and marrow toxicity)

Drug	Action	Main side-effects
Alkylating agents		
Cyclophosphamide	Cross-link double-stranded DNA; inhibit RNA formation	Alopecia, haemorrhagic cystitis, cardiac toxicity, water retention
Chlorambucil		Hepatic toxicity, dermatitis
Busulphan Melphalan		Marrow aplasia, pulmonary wasting syndrome, hyperpigmentation
Corticosteroids	Steroid–receptor complex affects gene expression; reduced prostaglandin and leukotriene formation; direct membrane damage	Peptic ulcer, obesity, hypertension, osteoporosis, diabetes, psychosis, hypokalaemia
M-amsacrine	as daunorubicin	Mucositis, hypokalaemia
α-Interferon γ-Interferon	Induce 2-5 oligo-A-synthetase, activate RNA breakdown	Flu-like symptoms, fever, thrombocytopenia, leucopenia, cardiac and neurological (at high doses)
Antimetabolites		
Methotrexate	Inhibits dihydrofolate reductase	All these antimetabolites: gastrointestinal toxicity, mouth ulcers, myelotoxicity with megaloblastic marrow changes, hepatic toxicity (with long-term therapy)
6-Mercaptopurine	Inhibits de-novo purine synthesis and purine interconversions	
6-Thioguanine	Incorporated into DNA with strand breaks	
Cytosine arabinoside	Incorporated into DNA with termination of DNA synthesis	Cerebellar damage, conjunctivitis with high doses
Hydroxyurea	Inhibits ribonucleotide reductase	Skin atrophy
5-Azacytidine	Inhibits de-novo pyrimidine synthesis; incorporated into DNA and RNA	

Table 14.10 (*Continued*)

Drug	Action	Main side-effects
Vinca alkaloids	Bind tubulin, inhibit microtubule polymeriz-ation needed for spindle formation	
Vincristine (a)	Mitotic inhibition	Neurotoxicity (peripheral, paralytic ileus, bladder dysfunction) (a) > (b) > (c)
Vindesine (b)		Alopecia
Vinblastine (c)		Myelotoxicity (c) > (b) > (a)
Anthracyclines		
Daunorubicin	Inhibition of topoisomerase 2; free radical generation; DNA intercalators	Mucositis
Hydroxodaunorubicin (doxorubicin, Adriamycin)		Cardiac damage
Mitoxantrone		
Enzyme inhibitors		
Deoxycoformycin	Inhibits adenosine deaminase with dATP accumulation and inhibition of ribonucleo-tide reductase; also double-stranded DNA breaks, NAD depletion	Fenal, ocular, neurotoxicity at high doses; haemolytic anaemia; neutropenia
L-Asparaginase	Hydrolyses L-asparagine and inhibits protein synthesis	Hypersensitivity and anaphylaxis, liver dysfunction, pancreatitis, hyperglycaemia, encephalopathy, low albumin and coagulation factors
Epipodophyllotoxins		
VP 16 (etoposide)	Inhibit topoisomerase II and cause double-stranded DNA breaks	Alopecia, mouth ulcers, gut toxicity
VM 26 (teniposide)		

which takes advantage of the improved clinical and haematological state of the patient and aims at ensuring a greater leukaemic cell kill. In the current UK ALL trial the agents listed in Table 14.8 are being used. In other countries, and particularly for high-risk patients, alternative protocols are employed. For example, the West German studies (Riehm *et al.*, 1987) use a 4-week intensification with cyclophosphamide, 6-mercaptopurine (6-MP), cytosine arabinoside (ara-C), 6-thioguanine, vincristine, dexamethasone and doxorubicin. Others use intermediate doses of Mtx or threefold higher doses of prednisolone, or cyclophosphamide, or a combination of teniposide (VM-26) and ara-C for those presenting with high WBC (Dahl *et al.*, 1987). For patients with T-ALL, radiation to areas of bulky disease has also been used at this stage. Whilst a consolidation phase is nowadays an essential component of the treatment strategy, the need for a late (e.g. 3 months after remission) intensification is still debated and, for example, this is currently being tested both in children and adults with ALL in the UK ALL Xth trials. It should be borne in mind that increase in the intensity of treatment is associated with greater morbidity and even mortality of patients.

CNS Prophylaxis

Historically, meningeal leukaemia occurred in over 50% of cases during haematological remission in the first 3 years of the disease. The CNS is considered a sanctuary site not normally reached by the drugs used in ALL. The classic established method for preventing this complication is cranial irradiation and six injections of Mtx given intrathecally, two before and four during the period of irradiation. Other methods for CNS prophylaxis have also been used, some without the use of irradiation. Because of the delayed effects of irradiation (neuropsychological sequelae and CT scan changes) the original dose which was found to be effective, 2400 cGy, has been reduced to 1800 cGy for children with a low risk of CNS disease. The cranial radiation is usually given in fractions of 200 cGy over 3 weeks. In addition to the long-term effects, a short-term syndrome of somnolence and lethargy occurs in some patients after cranial irradiation.

Treatment involving intermediate doses of Mtx or regular intrathecal injections without irradiation may also be effective but there is no conclusive evidence that this is better than the method listed in Table 14.9. The dose of intrathecal Mtx should not be calculated by body size but by age and CNS volume: e.g. 5 mg are used for less than 1 year of age; 7.5 mg for 1–2 years; 10 mg for 2–3 years, 12.5 for 3–15 years and 15 mg in adults. Despite prophylaxis, CNS leukaemia still occurs in about 5% of cases.

A more severe form of CNS toxicity has been documented: a subacute necrotizing demyelinating leucoenocephalopathy, characterized by progressive neurological deterioration, dementia, ataxia and coma. This complication has occurred in two instances: (1) when cranial irradiation was followed by repeated courses of intrathecal Mtx as part of the treatment of established CNS disease; and (2) when cranial irradiation, used for prophylaxis, was followed by a high dose (over 40 mg/m^2) of Mtx given weekly intravenously. Because meningeal leukaemia is now less common, and because high-dose systemic or intrathecal Mtx is avoided after cranial irradiation, it is likely that the occurrence of this problem will be extremely rare.

Maintenance Therapy

It is generally agreed that the best results in childhood ALL have been obtained when remission was maintained with continuous therapy for 2 or 3 years, and that the best two agents for this purpose are 6-MP and Mtx. The object of maintenance therapy is to eradicate progressively any remaining leukaemic cells. This can be achieved by two cell-cycle phase specific agents (both active only during S phase) if residual blast cells enter regularly into the cell cycle after remaining in Stage G_0 or G_1 for variable periods. This form of therapy, with periodic reinductions with vincristine and prednisolone every 4–6 weeks, is given for 2 years and will contribute to the continuation of remission in 60% or more of the cases.

Close attention to the dosage used and patient compliance is an important factor in the success of the maintenance treatment in childhood ALL. For 6-MP, used at a dose of 75 mg/m^2, it has been suggested that myelosuppression should be the limiting factor as patients may absorb and metabolize this drug (and also Mtx) in different ways. With the current intensive protocols, the WBC in patients on maintenance drugs should be maintained between 2.5 and $3.5 \times 10^9/1$ (granulocytes $> 1.0 \times 10^9 l$). Chronic underdosage of may result in early relapse.

Mtx is one of the first and most effective drugs for maintenance treatment of ALL. Like its related analogues (pyrimethamine and trimethoprim), it inhibits the enzyme dihydrofolate reductase, which converts dihydrofolate (produced during the thymidylate synthetase reaction) to tetrahydrofolate. Tetrahydrofolate coenzymes are essential for thymidylate synthesis and two reactions in purine synthesis (see Chapter 3). For maintenance therapy, Mtx (e.g. $20 \, mg/m^2$) is usually given orally, like 6-MP, before breakfast. Because of differences in absorption, some centres recommend that it should be given intramuscularly. One way to titrate the dose of weekly Mtx is to give the highest dose that does not cause mouth ulcers. If a patient is receiving 25 mg/week and ulcers appear, the dose should be reduced to 22.5 mg and continued provided no new regular mouth ulceration occurs. If this happens only at infrequent intervals, the dose need not necessarily be reduced.

Regular blood counts and tests of liver function (every 2–4 weeks) are necessary to monitor the dosage of the maintenance drugs and to control their side-effects. As in the management of most haematological malignacies, the follow-up of the blood counts and of other changes during therapies is best done by using appropriate haematological charts. It has been customary in the recent past to carry out a bone marrow test every 12 weeks to confirm the continuation of CR. Recently, several studies have shown that this is not necessary and there is no survival advantage in recognizing a relapse slightly earlier by means of a bone marrow test. In practice, a relapse can be suspected when the blood counts change unexpectedly, e.g. a drop of platelets below $100 \times 10^9/l$. A drop in Hb concentrations may not necessarily indicate relapse as some patients experience marked megaloblastic changes with the weekly doses of Mtx and daily 6-MP.

Relapse in Childhood ALL

The three major forms in which a relapse may manifest itself in ALL are: (1) bone marrow or haematological relapse, (2) meningeal leukaemia, and (3) testicular infiltration. It goes without saying that the aim of treatment should be to prevent a relapse and that a long period of 'disease-free' survival is the only guarantee of a clinical cure. Thus, relapse is always a major setback which reduces considerably the chances of cure. However, the significance of a relapse depends very much on its timing. When this occurs in the first 2–3 years, particularly during maintenance, the prognosis is very poor as it always indicates resistant disease and can probably only be cured by bone marrow transplantation (BMT). Late relapses are less frequent, but if they occur 2 or 3 years after treatment has been discontinued, they do not preclude the possibility of achieving a new CR, although the chances of a cure with chemotherapy alone will remain very low. If the primary site of relapse is in the CNS or the testis, which probably reflects inadequate early treatment, the chance of a cure with more effective agents is still open.

Bone Marrow Relapse

The chances of a second CR after relapse are high (88%) if the treatment has been discontinued for some time. However, the duration a of a second CR is short. A careful analysis of the initial treatment may give some clues about the protocols which offer more chances of a prolonged remission. A minority of late relapses (18 months or longer off all therapy) can sometimes be rescued by intensive therapy including some new agents and/or combinations. Bone marrow relapse is indeed one of the indications for bone marrow transplantation if a suitable HLA-compatible donor is available (see below). However, the outcome after BMT in such patients depends, as for the chemotherapy regimens, on the features of the disease, e.g. low cure rate for early relapses and good for late relapses. In cases of high-risk ALL the probability of disease-free survival after BMT in a second CR is of the order of 20%.

Meningeal Leukaemia

Anatomically, the involvement of the meninges seems to follow early infiltration of blasts in the walls of veins of the arachnoid tissues. Clinically this is manifested by headaches, vomiting, meningeal signs and bilateral papilloedema due to increased intracranial pressure. Unilateral papilloedema may be due to infiltration of the optic nerve. Facial palsy is another not uncommon initial manifestation of neuroleukaemia.

The diagnosis is made through the examination of the CSF: the WBC is usually high, more than 20×10^6 cells/l; glucose is low and protein is increased. Careful examination of the cells, preferably on slides made in a cytocentrifuge, is of the utmost importance, particularly for the differential diagnosis from viral conditions, not uncommon in children with ALL in remission who may present with similar symptomatology and show an increased WBC in the CSF. Cytocentrifuge-prepared slides tend to exaggerate the nuclear indentation of the cells. However, the monomorphic infiltration with blasts is quite characteristic. The appearance of the preparation in viral infections is usually more pleomorphic, with a predominance of small lymphocytes, some transformed, and the presence of a small proportion of monocyte–macrophage forms. In case of doubt, and particularly if the surface phenotype of the ALL is known, the cells should be tested for surface markers as described above. A positive ALL antigen (CD10) will point to a CNS relapse in cALL. A high percentage of T markers in a case known to be of B-lineage ALL will favour a reactive lymphocytosis. The presence of TdT which is absent from mature B or T lymphocytes, will always favour a relapse, whether found in isolation or in combination with B- or T-cell markers.

There is no satisfactory treatment for meningeal leukaemia but long-term remissions can be obtained with craniospinal irradiation alone (2400 cGy to the cranium and 1000 cGy in the spine) or long-term courses of intrathecal injections, either rotating Mtx and ara-C or combining both with hydrocortisone, a method more favoured lately. Initial control of the symptoms and signs can be achieved quickly with intrathecal injections of Mtx given initially twice a week, and later weekly until the WBC falls below 10×10^6 cells/l and no blasts are recognized by cytology.

Subsequently the main problem is to decide which approach will produce the longest remission, or even eradicate the leukaemia from the CNS. Long-term remission of the CNS leukaemia can be obtained in two-thirds of cases in their first relapse by craniospinal irradiation. A convenient method of administering intrathecal drugs on a long-term basis is through an Ommaya reservoir. Because bone marrow relapse often occurs at the time of, or just before, CNS relapse, it is always recommended that reinduction therapy should be administered at the time of initiating control of the CNS disease.

Testicular Relapse

One of the reasons for the worse prognosis of boys is the high incidence, in earlier studies, of testicular infiltration. This complication may occur early or late. Testicular relapse during maintenance therapy (early) is rare, affecting less than 2% of boys with high-risk factors. This is as a rule bilateral and reflects poor control of the leukaemia. Late relapse occurs off therapy and does not necessarily carry the bad prognosis of early relapse. This complication is seen in cases of low-risk ALL after all treatment has stopped and is manifested by unilateral testicular swelling. This should be treated by local irradiation (2400 cGy), systemic reinduction and maintenance treatment for another 2 years.

Because testicular swelling is a relatively late feature, some trials have recommended routine bilateral testicular biopsies on completion of maintenance therapy before it is discontinued. However, the value of this procedure has been questioned as the pick-up rate of relapses is low while a negative biopsy does not preclude a subsequent overt testicular relapse. Involvement of the testes is shown histologically by peritubular, rarely tubular, leukaemic infiltration. The diagnosis of small leukaemic foci may be difficult and the immunohistochemical determination of TdT in testicular biopsies does not appear to improve the precision or to provide an early diagnosis of testicular relapse (Chessells *et al.*, 1986).

There is no agreement about the best way of preventing this complication. The use of prophylactic testicular irradiation, postulated if one considers the testis as a sanctuary site, has now few advocates. It is apparent that the testes usually represent the 'tip of the iceberg' and often reflect inadequate overall control of the disease. This concept, rather than that of a sanctuary site, implies that improved systemic therapy, including perhaps agents which may cross the putative blood–testicular barrier (e.g.

Mtx given at intermediate doses in 24 hours' infusion), will be the best prevention of a testicular relapse. Current results with improved protocols support this assumption.

B-ALL

This disease carries such a poor prognosis, even with intensive regimens used for other types of ALL, that many centres are now using alternative intensive chemotherapy similar to that used in poor prognosis lymphomas. The 'MACHO' protocol, for example, incorporates high-dose cyclophosphamide, doxorubicin, and vincristine, followed by courses of high-dose methotrexate and high-dose ara-C, as well as intrathecal methotrexate. It is followed by allogeneic or autologous BMT.

Infections in Childhood ALL

In contrast to AML, bacterial infections are uncommon during remission induction of ALL. Usually a rapid haematological response is obtained without a period of sustained neutropenia. On the other hand, neutropenia is now seen later, after the first consolidation regimen (see Table 14.9) which results in granulocyte counts below $0.5 \times 10^9/l$ for 1 or 2 weeks. Non-bacterial infections are a more common cause of morbidity and mortality and these occur during periods of CR, when lymphopenia rather than neutropenia is the rule. They account for up to 5% of deaths in remission during the first 2 years of therapy. This is one reason to avoid 'overtreating' good prognostic cases, as the unnecessary intensification of therapy will result in more deaths due to infections. Most problems are due to the viral infections which are common in childhood, namely measles and varicella zoster.

Measles in children with ALL may be associated with severe complications of giant-cell pneumonia and atypical forms of encephalitis, both with high mortality. The most common fatal infections in ALL are interstitial pneumonitis and 40% of them are caused by measles. The best prophylaxis is to use γ-globulin with a high antibody titre within 48 hours after contact with a known infected child has been documented.

Varicella zoster (chickenpox) may also follow a severe course with visceral dissemination, pneumonia and encephalitis. To avoid this infection zoster-immune globulin must be given within 72 hours of exposure. Treatment of established infection should be given with intravenous acyclovir at high doses (10 mg/kg).

Cytomegalovirus (CMV) infection probably results from the reactivation of an existent infection acquired early in life or from blood products. Its frequency is high after allogeneic BMT, when it is one of the main causes of morbidity and mortality (see Chapter 10). The clinical features of fever, hepatitis, lung infiltrates, splenomegaly, skin rash and pancytopenia may mimic a relapse.

Pneumocystis carinii pneumonitis is also a serious complication in immunosuppressed patients. Until recently this has been the main cause of death in childhood ALL in the USA. In its most severe form the disease is fatal, so that an accurate diagnosis is important. This can be done by visualizing the organism in living material obtained by needle aspiration or bronchial washings. The use of co-trimoxazole for the prevention and treatment of this infection may overcome the need for potentially dangerous diagnostic procedures. A widely adopted regimen for prophylaxis (Hughes *et al.*, 1987) is to give co-trimoxazole on 3 alternate days each week for the whole duration of the ALL treatment. This regimen was shown in randomized trials effectively to prevent pneumocystis and not to predispose to fungal infections, as do daily doses. The incidence of other bacterial infections also seems to decrease with agent. On the other hand, adverse effects of co-trimoxazole are skin rashes and a tendency for granulocytopenia.

Infections caused by other common viruses— rhino-, adeno- and enteroviruses—usually have a normal clinical course. The management and prevention of viral complications require a great deal of alertness by paediatricians regarding contacts at home and at school. Mumps meningoencephalitis also occurs, but its course is not particularly severe. Defective responses to DNA viruses may result in a severe haemophagocytic syndrome which has in the past been wrongly considered as a transformation of the ALL.

ALL in Adults

Patients aged 15 or over with ALL seem to constitute a group which should be separated from childhood ALL and from AML for several reasons. Two are of practical importance: (1) the heterogeneity of the group which is greater than in childhood ALL; and (2) the overall poor remission rate and survival. It is difficult to identify clear prognostic subcategories in this group or to understand easily the reasons for their poorer prognosis. However, it is evident that Ph$^+$ ALL, which is more frequent in adults, T-ALL and B-ALL have a bad prognosis in adults. T-ALL cases have similar clinical and haematological features as in children, and in some studies fare significantly worse than common-ALL or null-ALL, although the newer more intensive regimens have modified that outcome. Age and WBC remain the most important prognostic factors. Patients aged 50 years or over, usually associated with L2 morphology and null-ALL phenotype, have a particularly poor prognosis. Younger patients with a low WBC and cALL phenotype fare better, provided they have no chromosome translocations. The presence of myeloid antigens on the blasts from adult ALL may also indicate a worse prognosis (Sobol *et al.*, 1987).

Ph$^+$, irrespective of its pathogenesis in relation to the *bcr* gene has, overall, a very bad prognosis. About one-third of Ph$^+$ ALL cases have a rearrangement of the *bcr* gene and express a p210 protein as gene product. These patients are almost always adults and may, in some cases, represent CGL presenting in lymphoblastic crisis. Some of them present with a very large spleen and high WBC and a few revert to a chronic phase CGL after CR has been achieved. Two-thirds of Ph$^+$ ALL do not rearrange the *bcr* gene and express a p190 protein; less than half of these cases are children and the rest are adults. There is no evidence so far for any clinical differences between *bcr* + or *bcr* − Ph$^+$ cases (Secker-Walker *et al.*, 1988). All have a low remission rate (approximately 50%) and a high relapse rate. As a consequence the median survival is short (14 months for children and adults).

Treatment

One reason why adult ALL should be distinguished from AML is that the incidence of CNS leukaemia is as high as in childhood ALL, unless CNS prophylaxis is performed routinely. Most series reported so far describe remission rates of the order of 65–80%.

The early addition of powerful agents such as daunorubicin or doxorubicin, as used in AML, is essential to achieve the best possible response. A CR can also be achieved by a regimen devised primarily for AML, e.g. DAT × 10, without vincristine or prednisolone. The current view is that an aggressive approach to therapy in these patients is necessary and this should include 'anti-AML' and 'anti-ALL' agents. The outline given in Table 14.8 could be suitable for adult ALL. However, results in adults with such regimens are not as good as in children as the nature of the disease is different. For CNS prophylaxis the dose of 2400 cGy is recommended in adult patients. Regimens for adult-ALL have reported median remission duration of 18–24 months and an overall cure rate of 35%. More intensive treatments (reviewed by Hoelzer and Gale, 1987) have improved such prospects but mainly for low-risk cases. Although adult ALL corresponds to cases with bad prognosis, the incidence of testicular involvement, at least at the present time, seems to be lower than in children. It is not clear whether this is because they often relapse before the completion of the maintenance programme or because of the preferential leukaemic infiltration of the pre-pubertal testis.

BMT, either allogeneic or autologous is now being performed for poor prognosis adult ALL in first remission. The approximate long-term disease-free survival with either technique is 45–50%.

Clinical Management of AML

The management of AML is usually more complex and laborious than that of ALL. This results from the following facts: (1) the patients are older; (2) the drugs used in the treatment of AML appear to have less selectivity against the leukaemic cells than those used in ALL; and (3) to achieve a complete remission (CR) appears to require, as a prerequisite, inducement of a profound, albeit transient, bone marrow hypoplasia. Nonetheless, there are now several chemotherapeutic agents—daunorubicin (DNR), ara-C, etoposide, 6-thioguanine, amsacrine and mitoxantrone—which have improved the remission rates, from 10% before their introduction in 1968 to 80–85% at the present time, for patients less than 50 years of age.

As there are several factors which are critical for the successful management of AML, it has been difficult to identify clear-cut prognostic criteria which are generally acceptable for clinical use. As treatment results improve, it will become more apparent in the near future if some types of AML are worse than others. This point is illustrated by hypergranular promyelocytic leukaemia (M3), a form of AML which used to have a bad prognosis in the past, but which, as a result of improvements in its early management (e.g. control of the bleeding process), is now one of the forms with the best long-term prognosis, provided CR is achieved. On the other hand, monoblastic leukaemia (M5a) patients have a good and rapid CR but tend to have a high relapse rate and few long-term survivors.

The following features have been said to indicate a poor prognosis in AML: age over 60 years, a high WBC and thrombocytopenia ($< 25 \times 10^9$/l) at presentation, some chromosome abnormalities, a documented preleukaemic phase and/or morphological features of trilineage MDS (Brito-Babapulle *et al.*, 1987a). Age seems to be the most important for remission induction: older patients are more vulnerable during the early stages of treatment; this does not relate to a different susceptibility of the leukaemic cells to the cytotoxic agents. In early MRC AML trials (1970–1974), the median survival of patients over the age of 60 was less than 7 weeks, whilst in those below the age of 30 it was 40 weeks. This difference was largely accounted for by the high death rate in the older patients during the period of neutropenia in the first 6 weeks of treatment. The age difference disappears after the patients achieve remission, suggesting that age may not carry a bad prognosis if supportive care can reduce the risk in the early stages. In more recent trials in the 1980s, the CR rate has improved in all age groups, but still those over 60 years fare worse than younger patients. In the recent AML 9th trial (1984–1988) the CR rate for those aged 60 or over was 41%, for those between 40 and 59 years it was 68%, and for those aged less than 40 years it was 83%. The presence of blasts in peripheral blood during the recovery period after induction, even with a bone marrow consistent with CR, correlates with a high chance of relapse.

Special Forms of AML

Some types of AML, such as M3, M5 and M7, are associated with clinical and laboratory features which are important from a diagnostic and therapeutic point of view.

Hypergranular Promyelocytic Leukaemia (M3)

The main features of this type of leukaemia are: incidence of 3–7% of all AML cases, young age (often less than 40 years, mean 25 years), characteristic morphology (see above), pancytopenia at presentation with low WBC (except for the M3 variant), a high incidence of haemorrhagic phenomena due to disseminated intravascular coagulation (DIC) in 85% of cases, a unique chromosome abnormality, t(15;17), and in some series a prolonged survival. DIC is usually present at diagnosis or is precipitated shortly after therapy is started, and is caused by procoagulant activity of the leukaemic promyelocyte, particularly its granular fraction. The bleeding manifestations of purpura, gum bleeding, epistaxis, haematuria etc., often precede the diagnosis of leukaemia by 2–8 weeks. Because of the DIC, thrombocytopenia is disproportionately severe in relation to the degree of bone marrow infiltration. Bone marrow aspirates tend to clot rapidly and may often result in a dry tap. M3 constitutes one of the few medical emergencies during the treatment of AML. It is essential that supportive measures and the chemotherapeutic treatment (see below) should start almost immediately after diagnosis is made.

Monocytic Leukaemia (M5)

Monocytic leukaemia is less rare than is generally thought; the monoblastic type is common in young children. The clinical manifestations which are most characteristic are related to monocytic differentiation and are therefore more common in cases with well differentiated morphology. Several of these features are also seen in M4 (myelomonocytic) leukaemia. These are: lymphadenopathy, gum hypertrophy, skin infiltrates, high WBC ($> 50 \times 10^9$/l) and elevated concentrations of lysozyme in serum urine. In addition to its diagnostic value, the high lysozyme level may cause renal tubular dysfunction and hypokalaemia at clinical presentation.

Megakaryoblastic Leukaemia (M7)

This disorder has now been well characterized by clinical and laboratory studies (Den Ottolander *et al.*, 1979; Bain *et al.*, 1981; Bennett *et al.*, 1985a; Oliveira *et al.*, 1987). This disease can be confused with ALL (see above) but does not respond to anti-ALL therapy. Bone marrow fibrosis and low WBC at presentation are features of M7 which cause diagnostic difficulties. The CR rate is probably lower than in other forms of AML, but the data are conflicting.

Principles of Therapy

These are summarized in Table 14.11. The combinations of drugs used in AML follow in general the principles resulting from cell kinetic studies by using agents which are active at different phases of the cell cycle. Details of the mode of action and main toxicities of the drugs used were given in Table 14.10.

Remission Induction

The achievement of CR is the first most important objective of the treatment of all but the oldest and most infirm patient with AML, as remitting patients survive significantly longer than non-remitters. Failure to remit is not only a measure of the effectiveness of the drugs used, but also of the successful management of the resulting complications. A survival curve of AML shows three major dips: (1) The initial dip is due to early mortality during remission induction: with adequate supportive care the early figure of 20–30% mortality at this stage has now been reduced to 5–10%; this mortality also includes 5–10% of primary resistant cases. (2) A second dip during the first 12 months reflects the occurrence of early relapse in 15–20% of cases and 5–10% of patients who die during intensive consolidation courses, after CR; a second CR is difficult to achieve in the early relapses, which reflects drug resistance. (3) The final dip occurs after the first year and is due to late relapses. More than 50% of cases are now expected

Table 14.11
Principles of therapy in AML

1. *Remission induction*
   Combination of 3 drugs: DAT or DAE (10 days), e.g.
       daunorubicin (days 1, 3, 5)
       cytosine arabinoside (ara-C) (days 1–10)
       thioguanine (days 1–10) or
       etoposide (days 1–5)
   (1 or 2 courses necessary to complete remission)

2. *Consolidation*
   As for (1) with DAT or DAE (for 8 days) followed by another 3-drug combination, e.g.
       MAZE or MACE (5 days)
       M-Amsa (amsacrine), azacytidine or
       ara-C and etoposide (all for 5 days)

3. *Consideration of BMT*
   Autologous ($\pm$ BM purging) or
       allogeneic (HLA-matched sibling)

   or

   Further intensification
   e.g. 2-drug combination:
       mitoxantrone (days 1–5)
       moderately high dose ara-C (days 1–3)

to live more than 1 year, and in these the chances of a late relapse seem to decrease gradually with time. In some series, this part of the survival curve appears to reach a 'plateau' suggestive of cure, at least for some patients. Long survivals in AML, which were rare in the past, are now beginning to be seen with greater frequency: 15–20% of all cases and 30–35% of complete remitters may have a prolonged disease-free survival which is equivalent to a clinical cure. The most common regimens currently used in the UK for remission induction are shown in Table 14.11. The MRC AML 9th trial compared DAT × 10 days (3 + 10) with DAT × 5 days (1 + 5) and showed that the stronger regimen (3 + 10) was more effective in achieving CR in all age groups, the CR was obtained quicker and required less supportive care and may be responsible for longer remissions. Daunorubicin and ara-C are the single most important agents for the treatment of AML. Daunorubicin has, in addition to its myelotoxic effect, a late dose-related cardiomyopathy which tends to occur with doses greater than 500 mg/m^2. This is rarely reached in current protocols unless the patient experiences a relapse. Ara-C is best given as a continuous intravenous infusion because of its selective effect during S phase. The conventional dose for remission induction is 100 mg/m^2 per 24 hours. Higher doses, from 0.5 g to 2 g/m^2, appear to increase the anti-leukaemic effect. Moderate doses of 1 g/m^2 given over 4 hours in twice-daily infusions appear to improve the long-term prospects. The role of 6-thioguanine in the DAT regimen is controversial. In the past this drug was shown to potentiate the effect of ara-C. The current (10th) MRC AML trial will compare DAT with daunorubicin, ara-C, etoposide (DAE), using etoposide (E), a semi-synthetic podophyllotoxin, as the third agent instead of 6-thioguanine.

Assessment of CR may not be easy, and delayed responses with little haemopoietic recovery require careful examination of BM aspirates and trephine biopsies. It is well known that a similar degree of pancytopenia can be caused by a hypocellular or a heavily infiltrated BM.

Blood counts and bone marrow tests should be performed regularly in order to monitor the induction therapy. In addition the following tests should be checked periodically: ECG, plasma electrolytes, liver function and renal function tests, chest x-ray, control of urine output, coagulation screening to detect DIC, etc. Problems which can arise are hyperuricaemia due to rapid destruction of leukaemic cells, hyper- or hypokalaemia, liver function changes due to the cytotoxic drugs, renal failure due to antibiotic and antifungal therapy, ototoxicity and neurotoxicity etc. Regular control of the patient's temperature (every 4 hours) and measures associated with the management of infection will be detailed below.

Consolidation Therapy

The concept of consolidation in acute leukaemia assumes correctly in the vast majority of patients that after CR has been reached there are still leukaemic cells in the bone marrow and/or other sanctuary sites and that if no further therapy is given a relapse will follow. Once patients are in CR they tolerate better further intensive courses of treatment and experience a more rapid recovery of blood counts. Current practice is to give consolidation courses of the same intensity as the induction therapy. In fact, experience has shown that a DAT × 8 days is better than a repeat of DAT × 10 days because the latter may be associated with marked gut toxicity and resulting Gram-negative sepsis. It is logical that the first consolidation course should consist of the same drugs used successfully for remission induction. Subsequently a different combination is recommended to avoid the emergence of resistant clones; for this, MAZE or MACE, with ara-C instead of 5-azacytidine (Table 14.11) can be used.

Because the main problem facing AML patients in CR is the possibility of a relapse, consolidation therapy is followed in many units by further intensification, using for example a combination of moderately high-dose ara-C (1 g/m^2 every 12 hours, given over 2 hours, for 3 days) and mitozantrone (Mtz, 10 mg/m^2 daily × 5 days), which has been used successfully to treat relapse AML (Brito-Babapulle *et al.*, 1987). This moderately high dose of ara-C is significantly less neurotoxic than the high doses used in other studies (3 g/m^2) and may be equally effective in overcoming resistance due to the impaired transport of ara-C across the cell membrane. Several studies have shown that consolidation or intensification courses using high-dose ara-C may increase the number of patients who become long-term disease-free survivors. Further intensification requires rescue procedures by means of autologous or allogeneic BMT (see below).

The current MRC AML 10th trial will compare precisely these options: the value of autologous or allogeneic BMT in first CR (after four courses of chemotherapy, total body irradiation and high-dose cyclophosphamide) against the use of auto-logous BMT later in those patients who relapse at least 6 months after the BM harvest (which is performed after the third course of chemotherapy).

Remission Maintenance

There is no agreement as to whether long-term maintenance with drugs given continuously, as in ALL, or with intermittent courses of, for example, ara-C and 6-thioguanine, is important to improve the outcome in AML. Such an hypothesis was tested in the MRC AML 9th trial but the final results are still not available. Other studies have shown that maintenance may prolong the duration of CR by delaying the time to relapse, but the eventual outcome is the same. Therefore the cure rate does not appear to change significantly with this approach. Most emphasis is given currently to the intensification of therapy rather than to the long-term maintenance. Courses of late intensification after 1 year in CR have shown some advantage, particularly when using different drugs from those used early on. There is, however, an element of selection here, as whenever AML series are analysed those patients that remain in remission for the first 6–12 months, and are thus treated by BMT (autologous or allogeneic) or late intensification courses, may have already been selected out by the exclusion of those patients who relapse within the first 6 months and who have, naturally, a worse prognosis.

Treatment of Relapse

Most efforts should be directed towards preventing rather than treating relapse. If this occurs, the recommendation for therapy would depend on what treatment the patient has received already. In ALL, early relapses reflect drug resistance and are unlikely to be rescued by chemotherapy. Patients who undergo late relapses, after 1 or 2 years in CR, particularly if the relapse occurs off therapy, have a chance of a second CR and, rarely, even a chance of cure provided that the new treatment programme is more intensive and effective than the original one. The MRC AML 10th trial may answer the question of the value of late autologous BMT as a rescue procedure. The same applies to allogeneic BMT which in some studies has shown to salvage up to 30% of patients in second CR. If this figure is added to the 30% of remitters who do not relapse, it could theoretically increase the cure rate of AML to about 50%, well above the present figures using chemotherapy alone. The decision as to when is the optimal time to use the more radical procedures of BMT (autologous or allogeneic) is difficult considering that they are still associated with a significant morbidity and mortality. The older the patient, the more chemotherapy (until relapse) becomes the preferred option.

CNS Prophylaxis

There is no overall agreement about the need for prophylaxis in AML as the incidence of meningeal leukaemia has varied in different studies. The impression is that using regimens which include prolonged infusions or high doses of ara-C, the incidence of CNS relapse is low in AML and may be limited to patients presenting with high WBC ($\geq 100 \times 10^9$/l), those with monocytic leukaemia (M5) and myelomonocytic leukaemia with BM eosinophilia (M4Eo). The last disorder is associated with abnormalities of chromosome 16, inv(16), a high CR rate and the occurrence of intracerebral leukaemic deposits (Second MIC Cooperative Study Group, 1988). CNS relapse is also more common in children. If considered, CNS prophylaxis as used in ALL (see above) should be given. Alternatively, some studies have used courses of intrathecal injections, e.g. alternating Mtx and ara-C, with each course of therapy (between five and six injections). It is possible that if the exact incidence of this complication and the types of AML in which it occurs are better defined, more precise protocols for the selective group of patients with high risk for CNS leukaemia will evolve.

Treatment of Promyelocytic Leukaemia (M3)

As stated above, patients with M3 AML may have a high cure rate provided that their initial management is optimized to prevent fatal bleeding complications. It is agreed that DIC with intracranial haemorrhage, particularly after treatment is started, is the main cause of the high mortality. The use of heparin has been gradually introduced in the last 20 years but the value of this therapy remained disputed. Some authors considered that adequate support with platelets, fresh frozen plasma and cryoprecipitate may suffice. A non-randomized but probably definitive retrospective analysis of 115 patients with M3 treated in MRC trials between 1976 and 1986 has just been published (Hoyle *et al.*, 1988). This study showed conclusively that the CR rate was higher (86% as opposed to 49% in the control group) in patients for whom heparin was used as part of the induction therapy. In fact, from the clinical history it would appear that heparin was used in patients with a higher risk of bleeding complications. The survival of the group treated with heparin was also significantly prolonged. The doses used varied but most cases were treated with 12 000–24 000 i.u. per day, usually given as a continuous infusion at a rate of 500–1000 i.u. per hour, with appropriate controls of clotting time and PTTK; the optimal dose is usually between 15 000 and 20 000 i.u. per day.

Another interesting observation of the management of M3 was published by Stone *et al.* (1988). These authors recorded that, in contrast with other forms of AML, a period of BM hypoplasia is not regularly documented in M3. Bone marrow samples remain cellular and often with an obvious persistence of abnormal-looking promyelocytes even after a second course of chemotherapy. This observation was also made by one of us (DC) in several patients with M3 AML who, as in the cases of Stone *et al.*, had a long disease-free survival. In the report of Stone *et al.* 40% of patients who achieved CR (74% in their study) remained alive and in remission at the time of reporting. The implication is that therapy in promyelocytic leukaemia may act by differentiation rather than by pure cytotoxicity as in other types. Against that is the fact that the structural chromosome abnormality associated with M3, t(15;17), would

theoretically persist if only a differentiation effect is obtained and this is unlikely to be associated with a relatively high cure rate.

AML in the Elderly

As mentioned earlier, if complete remission is achieved, patients aged over 60 years may have as prolonged remission as younger subjects. The decision to give intensive therapy may, however, be difficult, particularly for patients in poor general health presenting with low peripheral blood blast counts and who can be maintained on blood transfusions and platelet support alone, possibly for many months. The decision to give intensive therapy will depend on the general physical state of the patient, the presenting complications and the rate of progression of the disease. Some workers reduce the intensity of the first course, e.g. to $1 + 5$ or $2 + 7$ instead of $3 + 10$, balancing the risk of not achieving remission against that of prolonged hypoplasia. If remission is achieved, the number or intensity of consolidation therapies may be reduced. Low doses of ara-C or alternative combinations with newer drugs, e.g. mitoxantrone, are being investigated but have not yet been established as preferable.

Supportive Care in AML

Measures to support the patients during the periods of drug-induced cytopenia are an essential component of the management of AML. This is more critical during the first 4–6 weeks, before a CR is achieved, and slightly less so after the intensification courses. The quality of support can be measured by the mortality due to haemorrhage, infections and metabolic complications in a particular study. It is possible, with optimal care, to reduce the mortality due to these causes to less than 10% during induction and to less than 5% during consolidation courses, in patients aged less than 50 years. Supportive care measures can be divided into three main types: (1) blood products, (2) prevention and treatment of infections, and (3) management of metabolic complications. Additional special measures are necessary for patients undergoing BMT, particularly from allogeneic or matched unrelated donors.

Blood Products

The aim is to replace the blood elements according to the patients' needs. Transfusion of whole blood, even when fresh, is only useful to replace loss of blood. Although patients should not be exposed to prolonged periods of anaemia, particularly over the age of 50, blood transfusions have a lower priority than platelet transfusions, unless there is active blood loss. Three important points should be remembered when indicating a blood transfusion of RBC. (1) For patients presenting with high WBC, particularly over $100 \times 10^9/l$, blood should not be given before the WBC is substantially reduced because of the risk of sudden death due to cerebral leucostasis which is associated with a high plasma viscosity due to the high WBC and a Hb over 10 g/dl. (2) For patients on intravenous drips, particularly those of Na-retaining antibiotics, and receiving other blood products, there is a risk of precipitating left ventricular failure with pulmonary oedema; diuretics will be required to cover the transfusion. (3) In thrombocytopenic patients the transfusion of large volumes of blood will result in a substantial drop in the platelet count due to a dilution effect. Platelets should always be given first to cover this contingency.

The following rules may help to decide when platelet transfusions are useful. (a) A platelet count below normal (e.g. $<50 \times 10^9/l$) may be an indication if there is evidence of purpura or other haemorrhagic manifestations. (b) A platelet count below $20 \times 10^9/l$ in a patient undergoing active treatment can usually predict that the value will drop further. Platelet prophylaxis should be given in these instances even in the absence of bleeding. (c) For patients with a stable low platelet count for whom therapy has stopped for over 2 weeks, there is no need for prophylactic transfusion even with counts close to $20 \times 10^9/l$. A sudden and/or persistent drop in counts is more ominous than a persistently low count in a patient with no evidence of bleeding. Exceptions to this rule are patients with M3 AML, to whom massive platelet transfusions (10–20 units a day) should be given together with heparin infusions, fresh frozen plasma and the specific anti-leukaemia treatment.

Granulocyte transfusions are less popular nowadays than when their use was established 15 years ago. One of the reasons is the improvement in antibiotics and the more frequent use of antifungal agents at an early phase. Still, some units use repeated granulocyte transfusions (e.g. buffy coats or cells harvested from patients with CGL) when severely neutropenic patients ($<0.2 \times 10^9/l$) are receiving the appropriate antibiotics for a documented serious infection and when the fever fails to respond adequately or there is clinical deterioration.

Infections in AML

In febrile neutropenic AML patients undergoing therapy the most common pathogenic organisms are the Gram-negative ones, *Klebsiella* and *Enterobacter* species, *Pseudomonas aeruginosa*, *Escherichia coli* and *Proteus*, which usually originate from the patient's own gut bacterial flora. Hence the documented benefit of gut decontamination protocols. The increasing use, in recent years, of long-term indwelling catheters, including Hickman catheters, has seen a shift in the patterns of infection, which now includes Gram-positive cocci, chiefly *Staphylococcus epidermidis*, *Staph. aureus* and *Streptococcus*, which form part of the normal flora of skin and mucous membranes. Prolonged periods of neutropenia and second febrile episodes are frequently caused by fungal infections, mainly *Candida albicans* and *Aspergillosis*. These are often, but not always, associated with lung shadows visible in chest x-rays. Some of these febrile episodes respond to antifungal agents without a documented fungal infection. Occasionally such episodes are associated with changes seen by ultrasound examination of the liver which disclose multiple hypoechoic areas which, after fine needle aspiration, may show fungal hyphae. The high incidence of fungal infections provides a rationale for prolonged oral prophylaxis with various absorbable and non-absorbable agents. Viral infections are relatively rare in the setting of AML and are more common in the context of BMT, particularly *cytomegalovirus*, *herpes simplex* and others. Two aspects should be considered separately: (1) measures for the prophylaxis of infection, and (2) the treatment of established infections.

Prophylaxis of Infection

A number of measures are effective for this purpose.

(1) Protective isolation in the form of single rooms with varying degrees of reverse barrier nursing. These measures aim at protecting the patient from airborne infections. Some degree of protective isolation is useful for the treatment of AML. The most elaborate isolation methods are important for patients undergoing more intensive treatments and who are expected to have prolonged periods of neutropenia, and BMT.

(2) Gut decontamination with non-absorbable antibiotics helps to reduce the rate of infection by reducing the number of Gram-negative organisms which are of intestinal origin. A typical regimen combines colistin, neomycin, nystatin and ketoconazole with amphotericin syrup and betadine mouthwashes. In the last 10 years an absorbable antibiotic, co-trimoxazole (Septrin), has been incorporated as a mildly decontaminating agent to reduce and/or delay the incidence of infections in neutropenic patients. Monitoring of the gut flora may disclose Septrin-resistant organisms and this is an indication for adding oral colistin and neomycin as these organisms are likely to colonize and infect the patient once the neutrophil count falls below 0.1 $\times 10^9/l$. Study of the prevalent gut flora could give an early warning of an impending sepsis which is often preceded by diarrhoea, abdominal pain and a drop in blood pressure.

(3) Other measures help reduce the number of pathogenic organisms in the skin (e.g. by using solutions or creams of chlorhexidine and antiseptic soaps), and include oral hygiene for dental and gingival sepsis and decontamination and hygiene of the throat, clean food, avoiding fresh salads, fresh fruit etc.

(4) Antifungal agents: oral amphotericin, nystatin, in tablets, suspension and lozenges, and some absorbable oral agents such as ketaconazole or itriconazole.

Treatment of Infection

This section could also be described as 'The management of fever in AML'. Some facts are well established. (1) About one-third of the time a patient spends in hospital he or she is febrile. (2) Two-thirds or more of the fevers are due to infections (septicaemia, pneumonia or others). (3) Often the fever is associated with no other useful clinical signs suggestive of infection. (4) Bacteriological proof of the fever being caused by infection is obtained in less than 50% of febrile episodes. (5) The majority of severe infections are caused by a few Gram-negative organisms; pseudomonal infections are particularly dangerous; fungal infections are also not rare and have a higher fatality rate and should be suspected in cases not responding to first-line antibiotics, particularly if there are gastrointestinal signs (e.g. dysphagia, oesophagitis, etc.) or atypical lung shadows. Fungal infections are often the cause of second fevers, e.g. after the patient has responded to an infection and while still on antibiotics. It should also be remembered that fever is not a feature of infection in patients on corticosteroid therapy. Other signs are useful here: diarrhoea, hypotension, tachycardia, sudden deterioration, etc. Perianal lesions are less frequent with regimens of gut decontamination; still they should be taken into account as a major cause of Gram-negative sepsis. The fever chart of a neutropenic patient should be kept under very close scrutiny; any consistent elevation to 38°C or over and not directly explained by the prior administration of a blood product requires immediate blood cultures (from at least two venepuncture sites or from one site and the indwelling catheter) and immediate institution of a wide spectrum systemic intravenous antibiotic regimen ('fever regimen'). The antibiotics used should primarily be aimed at covering the organisms commonly associated with infection in these patients and should relate to known local experience. Two situations could arise following the institution of the fever regimen. (1) The fever responds and the patient improves: in these circumstances it is important to avoid the temptation to stop the antibiotics prematurely. If the patient remains neutropenic, it is often useful to continue the antibiotics until there is evidence of a rising neutrophil count, although periods longer than 10 days are probably not advisable. (2) The fever does not respond to the initial antibiotics: in these cases the antifungal agent amphotericin-B is usually needed. The indications for this are: any antibiotic-resistant fever; a previously documented, deep-sited fungal infection; persistent *Candida* colonization;

and/or new infiltrates on the chest x-ray or epistaxis and evidence of sinus tenderness. If there is evidence of an infection or inflammation in the sites close to the indwelling catheters and the patient is not clinically seriously ill, vancomycin may be used first, at least for 24 or 48 hours before deciding that there is a response. Usually courses of 5–7 days of vancomycin may suffice when dealing with coagulase-negative cocci. Close monitoring of blood urea, creatinine and potassium levels should be carried out for patients treated with amphotericin-B. If viral infections are suspected, e.g. by the presence of herpetic vesicles, a 7–10-day course of intravenous acyclovir should be given.

The initial fever regimen in febrile neutropenic patients should consist mainly of one or more antibiotics with known anti-Gram-negative activity. The aminoglycosides, e.g. gentamicin, netilmicin, amikacin, tobramycin, sisomycin, are effective in neutropenic patients. The beta-lactam group of antibiotics is also very efficacious for this purpose. The beta-lactams include: (1) the cephalosporins, of which ceftazidime is an excellent third generation agent; (2) the penicillins of extended spectrum, e.g. piperacillin or azlocillin; (3) the carbapenems, e.g. imipenem; and (4) monobactams, e.g. aztreonam. In some studies the combination of ceftazidime and an aminoglycoside, e.g. amikacin or netilmicin, or the combination of an aminoglycoside with piperacillin or azlocillin was preferred. The new agents with anti-Gram-negative activity, particularly against *Pseudomonas aeruginosa*, are aztreanam, imipenem and ciprofloxacin of the new group of the quinolones, which is also available in oral form. Most of the above agents have little anti-Gram-positive activity and in some centres the initial combination may include, for example, ceftazidime, aztreonam or ciprofloxacin plus vancomycin, or the combination of amikacin and azlocillin, leaving open the addition of amphotericin-B or other appropriate antibiotics if there is no response to fever.

Metabolic Abnormalities

A number of metabolic abnormalities can occur during the initial treatment of AML. They are often due to the disease itself, the specific treatment, or result from the clinical complications and/or their treatment. They can be divided into two main categories.

1. *Electrolyte and renal abnormalities*. Hypokalaemia and hyponatraemia are the most common. A low K may be seen at presentation, in particular in M4 or M5 due to high lysozyme levels causing proximal tubular dysfunction. In addition, the fever regimen and amphotericin regularly cause hypokalaemia. Renal failure may be due to hyperuricaemia if adequate allopurinol and hydration are not achieved during initial induction. Also, many of the antibiotics, particularly amphotericin, the aminoglycosides and vancomycin, are nephrotoxic to the renal tubules and combinations of these agents should be monitored very closely.

2. *Liver function abnormalities*. Although some changes in the liver profile may be present at diagnosis, more often (20% of cases) they occur during treatment. The frequency depends on the regimen used. Commonly this is manifested by episodes of jaundice and a consistent elevation of the transaminases and sometimes, also, of the alkaline phosphatase. These changes are not associated with ascites or the development of portal hypertension. This is seen, on the other hand, in a serious complication of BMT: veno-occlusive disease of the liver, which has often a fatal outcome. Some drugs could also produce some degree of cholestasis (e.g. ara-C and 5-thioguanine). Other recognized causes of liver abnormalities are viral hepatitis and cytomegalovirus infection, both associated with blood products given early in the therapy. Although these liver function changes rarely progress or give major symptoms, they should be taken into account when prescribing drugs metabolized through the liver, as their blood concentration may rise excessively due to liver dysfunction.

BONE MARROW TRANSPLANTATION FOR ACUTE LEUKAEMIA

The general principles and problems associated with BMT are described in Chapter 4. We concentrate here on the particular techniques used and the results of BMT for acute leukaemia.

Acute Myeloblastic Leukaemia

Allogeneic transplantation from a fully matching (HLA A, B, C and DR), mixed lymphocyte culture (MLC), unreactive sibling offers the possibility of long-term disease-free survival in about 50% of children or young adults (i.e. less than 40 years old) with AML in first remission (Table 14.12). The results are less good in adults over the age of 40. A variety of regimens are used for conditioning the recipient, usually involving high-dose chemotherapy combined with total body irradiation (TBI). Cyclophosphamide 60 mg/kg for 2 days (with MESNA to protect the bladder), followed by fractionated TBI (6 or 7 × 200 Gy fractions) is the most widely used regimen but some groups use high doses of other chemotherapeutic agents, e.g. busulphan, cytosine arabinoside, melphalan or VP 16 with or instead of cyclophosphamide. TBI is omitted completely in some protocols while in others it is given in more or fewer fractions or as a single dose. A few units give TBI before instead of after chemotherapy. This preparation is given to immunosuppress the recipient to allow engraftment of donor marrow stem cells and is also aimed at eliminating residual leukaemia. The fact that re-

lapse rates are of the order of 60% following identical twin (syngeneic) transplants (rather than 20–25% as in allogeneic transplants) suggests that at least 50% of the 'cure' of AML by allogeneic BMT derives from a graft-versus-leukaemia effect; these are absent in identical twin BMT where the conditioning alone is presumed to kill remaining leukaemic cells.

Immediate post-transplant mortality in AML and ALL in first CR is as high as 10–15% in most centres. Infections, including bacterial, fungal and viral, are a major complication. Cytomegalovirus may produce a fatal pneumonitis which may be predisposed to by irradiation of the lungs and by GvHD. Acute grade 3 or 4 GvHD with widespread skin, and serious liver, and gastrointestinal involvement is also a significant cause of mortality. Venoocclusive disease of the liver, cardiac failure and haemorrhage are additional less frequent fatal complications. Graft failure is another grave situation which is best treated by reinfusing the patient's own pre-transplant remission marrow if this has been stored. In the longer term, after 3 months, relapse of AML, chronic GvHD and continuing susceptibility to infections are the main causes of death.

GvHD is more frequent if there is any degree of

Table 14.12

Current results of HLA-identical allogeneic BMT for acute leukaemia and chronic myeloid leukaemia

	Relapse rate	*Actuarial survival (% at 5 years)*
AML		
First CR	20–25	45–50
Second CR	50–60	30
Advanced disease	65	20
ALL		
First CR	30	40–50
Second CR	50–60	30–40
Advanced disease	60	20
CML		
CP	10–15	50–60
AP	40	20–30
Second CP	65	30

CR, complete remission; CP, chronic phase; AP, accelerated phase.

HLA mismatch between donor and recipient and also in older subjects. Methotrexate and/or cyclosporin A may be given post-transplantation to prevent GvHD or to reduce its severity. GvHD may be more effectively reduced in incidence and severity by T-cell depletion of donor marrow in vitro (e.g. by monoclonal antibodies and complement). However, in some but not all centres, T-cell depletion has increased the risk of graft failure and of leukaemic relapse. Adequate conditioning reduces the incidence of these problems but as yet no clear survival benefit is apparent whether or not T-cell depletion is carried out in acute leukaemic transplants.

Allogeneic BMT may be delayed until second CR in AML or performed in early relapse. The cure rate with such transplants is less than in first CR. Sufficiently rapid availability of a transplant centre may also be a problem. For children and adults at least up to the age of 30 years, where immediate transplant mortality is low, it seems preferable to perform allogeneic BMT for AML in first CR.

For patients with AML, without a suitable fully matching sibling donor, trials of autologous BMT in first CR are being carried out. It is usual to transplant marrow harvested after two or three courses of intensive chemotherapy and reinfuse this after the patient has received further chemotherapy and with preparation of the patient as for allogeneic BMT. Some, but not all, chemotherapy regimens have given results as good as those using TBI. Some centres attempt to purge the marrow of residual leukaemia in vitro, e.g. with cyclophosphamide derivatives such as 4-hydroxy-cyclophosphamide, but as yet no benefit has been proven. Autologous BMT in the first CR of AML gives an approximately 50% 3-year disease-free survival, but controlled trials are needed to establish its value compared with further intensive chemotherapy or indeed allogeneic BMT. Autologous BMT for AML in second remission has given variable results but usually worse than for first CR. Autologous BMT in relapse gives very few, if any, long-term survivors.

The use of HLA A, B and DR matching unrelated donors for AML, e.g. in second CR, is being explored in a number of centres. Graft rejection and GvHD are more common than with matched sibling BMT. The value of additional immunosuppression of the recipient by, for example, in-vivo monoclonal antibodies or total lymphoid irradi-ation is being explored. BMT from siblings with more than one HLA locus mismatch gives less good results than fully matched allogeneic BMT. Haplo-identical BMT gives very poor results.

Acute Lymphoblastic Leukaemia

The decision to recommend allogeneic BMT for ALL in first remission for a patient with a fully matched sibling donor depends largely on the correct assessment of the patient's prognosis with the best conventional chemotherapy. In most children it is usual to attempt to cure with induction, consolidation, intrathecal methotrexate and cranial radiotherapy, and maintenance chemotherapy, alone. For B-ALL and for patients with cALL, null-ALL or T-ALL with a very high presenting WBC, or other bad prognostic features such as the t(4;11) or t(9;22) cytogenetic abnormalities, allogeneic BMT in first CR is considered for those with a suitable donor. For adult patients less than 40 years of age with ALL and poor prognostic features (see Table 14.7), BMT may also be preferred in first CR. Otherwise allogeneic BMT is reserved for second CR when it is the best chance of a cure. For patients in first full CR with a poor prognosis but lacking a matching sibling, autologous BMT after intensive consolidation is considered and long-term survival of up to 50% may then be achieved. The marrow is harvested after recovery from consolidation therapy and it is usually 'purged' of residual leukaemic cells by monoclonal antibodies with complement or linked to immunotoxins, magnetic beads or to an immunoabsorbent column. The antibodies should be directed against the patient's original blast cells. The value of this purging is, however, not yet established, nor are the long-term results of autologous BMT for ALL in first or subsequent remission. Autologous BMT for ALL in relapse gives poor results because of the very high incidence of subsequent relapse.

SELECTED BIBLIOGRAPHY

Appelbaum F. R., Thomas E. D. (1985). Treatment of acute leukemia in adults with chemoradiotherapy and bone marrow transplantation. *Cancer*, **55** (Suppl. 9), 2202–2209.

Baker M. A. (1987). The management of leukaemia in the elderly. In *Clinical haematology* (Ed. T. J. Hamblin), pp. 427–448. London: Baillière Tindall.

Bennett J. M., Catovsky D., Daniel M-T., Flandrin G., Galton D. A. G., Gralnick H. R., Sultan C. (FAB Co-operative Group) (1976). Proposals for the classification of the acute leukaemias. *British Journal of Haematology*, **33**, 451–458.

Bennett J. M., Catovsky D., Daniel M-T., Flandrin G., Galton D. Λ. G., Gralnick H. R., Sultan C. (ΓAB Co-operative Group) (1980). A variant of hypergranular promyelocytic leukaemia (M3). *British Journal of Haematology*, **44**, 169–170.

Bennett J. M., Catovsky D., Daniel M-T., Flandrin G., Galton D. A. G., Gralnick H. R., Sultan C. (FAB Co-operative Group) (1981). The morphological classification of acute lymphoblastic leukaemia: concordance among observers and clinical correlations. *British Journal of Haematology*, **47**, 553–561.

Bennett J. M., Catovsky D., Daniel M-T., Flandrin G., Galton D. A. G., Gralnick H. R., Sultan C. (1982). Proposals for the classification of the myelodysplastic syndromes. *British Journal of Haematology*, **51**, 189–199.

Bennett J. M., Catovsky D., Daniel M-T., Flandrin G., Galton D. A. G., Gralnick H. R., Sultan C. (1985a). Criteria for the diagnosis of acute leukemia of megakaryocytic lineage (M7): A report of the French–American–British Cooperative Group. *Annals of Internal Medicine*, **103**, 460–462.

Bennett J. M., Catovsky D., Daniel M-T., Flandrin G., Galton D. A. G., Gralnick H. R., Sultan C. (1985b). Proposed revised criteria for the classification of acute myeloid leukemia: A report of the French–American–British Cooperative Group. *Annals of Internal Medicine*, **103**, 620–629.

Bloomfield C. D., Goldman A. I., Alimena G. et al. (1986). Chromosomal abnormalities identify high-risk and low-risk patients with acute lymphoblastic leukemia. *Blood*, **67**, 415–420.

Blune K. G., Forman S. J., Snyder D. S., et al. (1987). Allogeneic bone marrow transplantation for acute lymphoblastic leukemia during first complete remission. *Transplantation*, **43**, 389–392.

Bradstock K. F., Hoffbrand A. V., Ganeshaguru K., Llewellin P., Patterson K., Wonke B., Prentice A. G., Bennett M., Pissolo G., Bollum F. J., Janossy G. (1981). Terminal deoxynucleotidyl transferase expression in acute non-lymphoid leukaemia: an analysis by immunofluorescence. *British Journal of Haematology*, **47**, 133–143.

Breton-Gorius J., Gourdin M. F., Reyes F. (1981). Ultrastructure of the leukemic cell. In *The leukemic cell* (Ed. D. Catovsky), pp. 87–128. Edinburgh: Churchill Livingstone.

Brito-Babapulle F., Catovsky D., Galton D. A. G. (1987a). Clinical and laboratory features of de novo acute myeloid leukaemia with trilineage myelodysplasia. *British Journal of Haematology*, **66**, 445–450.

Brito-Babapulle F., Catovsky D., Slocombe G., Newland A. C. Marcus R. E., Goldman J. M., Galton D. A. G. (1987b). Phase II study of mitoxantrone and cytarabine in acute myeloid leukemia. *Cancer Treatment Reports*, **71**, 161–163.

Brito-Babapulle F., Catovsky D., Galton D. A. G. (1988). Myelodysplastic relapse of de novo acute myeloid leukaemia with trilineage myelodysplasia: a previously unrecognized correlation. *British Journal of Haematology*, **68**, 411–415.

Catovsky D., Melo, J. V. M., Matutes E. (1985). Biological markers in lymphoproliferative disorders. In *Chronic and acute leukaemias in adults*. (Ed. C. D. Bloomfield) pp. 69–112. Boston: Martinus Nijhoff.

Champlin R. E., Gale R. P. (1987). Bone marrow transplantation for acute leukaemia: Recent advances and comparison with alternative therapies. *Seminars in Haematology*, **24**, 55–67.

Chessells J. M., Pincott J. R., Daniels-Lake W. (1986). Terminal transferase positive cells in testicular biopsy specimens from boys with acute lymphoblastic leukaemia. *Journal of Clinical Pathology*, **39**, 1236–1240.

Clift R. A., Buckner C. D., Thomas E. D. et al. (1987). The treatment of acute non-lymphoblastic leukemia by allogeneic marrow transplantation. *Bone Marrow Transplantation*, **2**, 243–258.

Creutzig U., Ritter J., Riehm H., Budde M., Schellong G. (1987). The childhood AML studies BFM-78 and -83: Treatment results and risk factor analysis. In *Acute leukemias. Prognostic factors and treatment strategies* (Eds. T. Buchner, G. Schellong, W. Hiddemann, D. Urbanitz, J. Ritter), pp. 71–75. Berlin: Springer.

Dahl G. V., Rivera G. K., Look A. T., Hustu H. O., Kalwinsky D. K., Abromowitch M., Mirro J., Ochs J., Murphy S. B., Dodge R. K., Pui C-H. (1987). Teniposide plus cytarabine improves outcome in childhood acute lymphoblastic leukemia presenting with a leukocyte count $\geqslant 100 \times 10^9/l$. *Journal of Clinical Oncology*, **5**, 1015–1021.

Dharmasena F., Galton D. A. G. (1986). Circulating blasts in acute myeloid leukaemia in remission. *British Journal of Haematology*, **63**, 211–213.

Fefer A. (1986). Current status of syngeneic marrow transplantation and its relevance to autografting. *Clinics in Haematology*, **15**, (1), 49–65.

First MIC Cooperative Study Group (1987). Morphologic, immunologic and cytogenetic (MIC) working classification of acute lymphoblastic leukemias. *Cancer Genetics and Cytogenetics*, **23**, 189–197.

Gale R P., Hoffbrand A. V. (Eds.) (1986). Acute leukaemia. *Clinics in Haematology*, **15**, 3.

Goldstone A. H. (Ed.) (1986). Autologous bone marrow transplantation. *Clinics in Haematology*, **15**, 1.

Gratwohl A., Hermans J., Lyklema A., Zwaan F. E. (1987). Bone marrow transplantation for leukemia in Europe. Report form the leukemia working party. *Bone Marrow Transplantation*, **2** (Suppl. 1), 15–18.

Greaves M. F., Brown G., Rapson T., Lister T. A. (1975). Antisera to acute lymphoblastic leukaemia cells. *Clinical Immunology and Immunopathology*, **4**, 67–84.

Greaves M. F., Chan. L. C., Furley A. J. W., Watt S. M., Molgaard H. V. (1986). Lineage promiscuity in hemopoietic differentiation and leukemia. *Blood*, **67**, 1–11.

Grier H. E., Gelber R. D., Camitta B. M., Dealorey M. J., Link M. P., Price K. N., Leavitt P. R., Weinstein H. J. (1987). Prognostic factors in childhood acute myelogenous leukemia. *Journal of Clinical Oncology*, **5**, 1026–1032.

Hoelzer D., Gale R. P. (1987). Acute lymphoblastic leukemia in adults: Recent progress, future directions. *Seminars in Hematology*, **24**, 27–39.

Hoffbrand A. V., Leber B. F., Browett P. J., Norton J. D. (1988). Mixed acute leukaemias. *Blood Reviews*, **2**, 9–15.

Hoyle C. F., Swirsky D. M., Freedman L., Hayhoe F. G. J. (1988). Beneficial effect of heparin in the management of patients with APL. *British Journal of Haematology*, **68**, 283–289.

Hughes W. T., Rivera G. K., Schell M. J., Thornton D., Lott L. (1987). Successful intermittent chemoprophylaxis for *Pneumocystis carinii* pneumonitis. *New England Journal of Medicine*, **316**, 1627–1632.

International Committee for Standardization in Haematology (ICSH) (1983). Recommended methods for cytological procedures in haematology. *Clinical and Laboratory Haematology*, **7**, 55–74.

Jani P., Verbi W., Greaves M. F., Bevan D., Bollum F. (1983). Terminal deoxynucleotidyl transferase in acute myeloid leukemia. *Leukemia Research*, **7**, 17–29.

Janossy G., Coustan-Smith E., Campana D. (1988). The reliability of cytoplasmic CD3 and CD22 antigen expression in the immunodiagnosis of acute leukaemia–a study of 500 cases. *Leukaemia*, (in press).

Keene B., Mendelow B., Pinto M. R., Beezwoda W., MacDougall L., Falkson G., Rugg P., Bernstein R. (1987). Abnormalities of chromosome 12p13 and malignant proliferation of eosinophils: a nonrandom association. *British Journal of Haematology*, **57**, 25–31.

Kersey J. H., Wesdorf D., Nesbit M. E. *et al.* (1987). Comparison of autologous and allogeneic bone marrow transplantation for treatment of high risk refractory acute lymphoblastic leukemia. *New England Journal of Medicine*, **317**, 461–467.

Lilleyman J. S., Hann I. M., Stevens R. F., Eden O. B., Richards S. M. (1986). French American British (FAB) morphological classification of childhood lymphoblastic leukaemia and its clinical importance. *Journal of Clinical Pathology*, **39**, 998–1002.

Martin P. J., Hansen J. A., Storb R., Thomas E. D. (1987). Human bone marrow transplantation. An immunological perspective. *Advances in Immunology*, **40**, 379–438.

Matutes E., de Oliveira M. P., Foroni L., Morilla R., Catovsky D. (1988). The role of ultrastructural cytochemistry and monoclonal antibodies to clarify the nature of undifferentiated cells in acute leukaemia. *British Journal of Haematology*, **69** (in press).

Oliveira M. S. P. de, Gregory C., Matutes E., Parreira A., Catovsky D. (1987). The cytochemical profile of megakaryoblastic leukaemia. A study with cytochemical methods, monoclonal antibodies and ultrastructural cytochemistry. *Journal of Clinical Pathology*, **40**, 663–669.

Oliveira M. S. P. de, Matutes E., Rani S., Morilla R., Catovsky D. (1988). Early expression of MCS2 (CD13) in the cytoplasm of blast cells from acute myeloid leukaemia. *Acta Haematologica*, **80**, 61–4.

Parreira A., Oliveira M. S. P. de, Matutes E., Foroni L., Morilla R., Catovsky D. (1988). Terminal deoxynucleotidyl transferase positive acute myeloid leukaemia. An association with immature myeloblastic leukaemia. *British Journal of Haematology*, **68** (in press).

Pedersen-Bjergaard J., Specht L., Larsen S. O., Ersboll J., Struck J., Hansen M. M., Hansen H. H., Nissen N. I. (1987). Risk of therapy-related leukaemia and pre-leukaemia after Hodgkin's disease. *Lancet*, **ii**, 83–88.

Prentice H. G., Brenner M. K. (1988). Bone marrow transplantation for acute leukaemia. *Recent advances in haematology*, Vol. 5, pp. 153–178. (Ed. A. V. Hoffbrand). Edinburgh: Churchill Livingstone.

Reis M. D., Griesser H., Mak T. W. (1988). Gene rearrangements in leukemias and lymphomas. In *Recent advances in haematology*, Vol. 5, pp. 99–120. (Ed. A. V. Hoffbrand). Edinburgh: Churchill Livingstone.

Riehm H., Feickert H. J., Schrappe M. (1987). Therapy results in five ALL-BFM studies since 1970: Implications of risk factors for prognosis. *Haematology Blood Transfusion*, **30**, 139–146.

Secker-Walker L. M., Cooke H. M. G., Browett P. J., Shippey C. A., Norton J. D., Coustan-Smith E., Hoffbrand A. V. (1988). Variable Philadelphia break points and potential lineage restriction of *bcr* rearrangement in acute lymphoblastic leukemia. *Blood*, **72**, 784–91.

Second MIC Cooperative Study Group (1988). Morphologic, immunologic, and cytogenetic (MIC) working classification of acute myeloid leukemias. *Cancer Genetics and Cytogenetics*, **30**, 1–15.

Seremetis S. V., Pelicci P-G., Fabilio A., Ubriaco A., Gringnani F., Cuttner J., Winchester R. J., Knowles D. M., II, Dalla-Favera R. (1987). High frequency of clonal immunoglobulin of T cell receptor gene rearrangements in acute myelogenous leukemia expressing terminal deoxyribonucleotidyl transferase. *Journal of Experimental Medicine*, **165**, 1703–1712.

Simone J. V. (1976). Factors that influence haematological remission duration in acute lymphocytic leukaemia. *British Journal of Haematology*, **32**, 465–472.

Slavin S., Kedar E. (1988). Current problems and future goals in clinical bone marrow transplantation. *Blood Reviews*, **2**, 259–269.

Sobol R. E., Mick R., Royston I., Davey F. R., Ellison R. R., Newman R., Cuttner J., Griffin J. D., Collins H., Nelson D. A., Bloomfield C. D. (1987). Clinical importance of myeloid antigen expression in adult acute lymphoblastic leukemia. *New England Journal of Medicine*, **316**, 1111–1117.

Stass S. A., Mirro J. (1986). Lineage heterogeneity in acute leukaemia. *Clinics in Haematology*, **15**, 811–828.

Stone R. M., Maguire M., Goldberg M. A., Antin J. H., Rosenthal D. S., Mayer R. J. (1988). Complete remission in acute promyelocytic leukemia despite persistence of abnormal bone marrow promyelocytes during induction therapy: experience in 34 patients. *Blood*, **71**, 690–696.

Chapter 15

CHRONIC LYMPHOID LEUKAEMIAS

D. CATOVSKY

Neoplastic proliferations of mature-looking lymphoid cells constitute the heterogeneous group of lymphoproliferative disorders. Here, we are concerned mainly with diseases which involve the blood and bone marrow, and are therefore defined as lymphoid leukaemias. Their course is, in general, chronic and they include a number of non-Hodgkin lymphomas (NHL) with frequent blood and bone marrow involvement (leukaemia/lymphoma syndromes) which often present problems of differential diagnosis with the more pure leukaemic processes. The chronic lymphoid leukaemias are distinguished from acute lymphoblastic leukaemia (ALL) by the morphology of the cells and their degree of maturation. The malignant cells in ALL are blasts which are immunologically immature. In addition, the chronic leukaemias affect mainly adults over the age of 30 years, whereas in ALL the majority of patients are children or young adults.

The methodology for the study of lymphoid leukaemias has been enriched in the last few years with the advent of monoclonal antibodies (McAb) which define antigenic determinants which are specific for the B- and T-cell lineages. The study of lymphoid malignancies is now not possible without the use of McAb and/or other membrane markers which define the cell lineage and often the maturation stage of the leukaemic cell. Lately, DNA analysis for the detection of immunoglobulin and T-cell receptor gene rearrangements has been incorporated as another diagnostic test for cell lineage and clonality (see also Chapter 12).

METHODS OF STUDY

There are five methods for the study of lymphoproliferative disorders which involve: (1) morphology, (2) membrane markers, (3) cytochemistry, (4) histopathology, and (5) DNA analysis.

Morphology

The morphological examination of leukaemic cells in well-prepared peripheral blood and bone marrow films stained with Romanovsky dyes is the first and most important diagnostic procedure. Occasionally the cytology of lymph node cells from aspirates or imprints may also be useful. Details which are often helpful in the analysis of cell types are: cell size, nucleo:cytoplasmic (N:C) ratio, regularity or irregularity of the nuclear outline, the characteristics of the cytoplasm such as the presence and length of any villous formations and the presence or absence of azurophil granules, the degree of nuclear chromatin condensation and its pattern, and the prominence, frequency and localization of the nucleolus.

In some instances, additional techniques are useful to improve the cytologic diagnosis, for example cell volume estimations could give precision to the assessment of cell size. Transmission electron microscopy (TEM) is important to establish the precise nuclear morphology, particularly when the cells are small. It is very useful to confirm a diagnosis of small cell Sezary syndrome, T-prolymphocytic leukaemia (PLL) or, rarely, follicular lymphoma.

Membrane Markers

Although it is possible to 'guess' the nature of the cell lineage involved in several of the lymphoid leukaemias, e.g. when dealing with cases of typical chronic lymphocytic leukaemia (CLL), hairy cell leukaemia (HCL) or some T-cell leukaemias, it is often safe to establish with the methodology currently available whether the leukaemic cells have a B or T membrane phenotype. For this a small battery of reagents is necessary. The number of tests may increase according to particular needs or to solve subtle diagnostic points as within the B and T cell leukaemias the composite pattern of certain markers has diagnostic value. The list of tests useful for this purpose is given in Table 15.1.

Cytochemistry

Cytochemical tests for two acid hydrolases — acid phosphatase (with and without inhibition by tartaric acid) and alpha-naphthyl acetate esterase (ANAE), and, less frequently, others such as, β-glucuronidase, β-glucosaminidase and dipeptidylaminopeptidase IV (DAPIV) — are still contribu-

tory to the diagnosis and characterization of B and T cell disorders. A tartrate-resistant acid phosphatase (TRAP) is found almost exclusively in hairy cells. With the exception of HCL and myeloma, most reactions for acid hydrolases are weak or negative in B cell disorders and strong in T cell disorders. In the latter, ANAE has a distinct localized pattern in T cell PLL and acid phosphatase is strong in T cell CLL.

Histopathology

When considering the possibility of a diagnosis of NHL, it is essential to utilize tissue histology to confirm this suspicion and facilitate the classification of the lymphoproliferative disorder. Lymph node biopsies are also required when the WBC count is low (below 10×10^9/l), even when a diag-

Table 15.1
Reagents for the diagnosis of lymphoid leukaemias

Test	Reagent/CD number	Other names	Specificity
SmIg/CyIg*	Anti-human Ig		B lymphocytes
M-rosettes	Mouse erythrocytes		B-CLL
E-rosettes	Sheep erythrocytes (CD2)		T lymphocytes
McAb	CD5	Leu1, UCHT2	T cells (strong) and B-CLL cells (weak)
McAb	CD10	J5, OKB-CALLA	Early B cells (common ALL) and follicular lymphoma
McAb	CD11C	Leu M5	Hairy cells; monocytes
McAb	CD19/CD20/CD24	B4/B1/BA1	Most B lymphocytes
McAb	CD22	Leu14, T015	B cells†
McAb	FMC7		Late B cells, B prolymphocytes and hairy cells
McAb	CD25	anti-Tac	Activated B and T cells; hairy cells
McAb	CD38	OKT10	Activated B and T cells; plasma cells
McAb	HC2		Hairy cells; activated B cells
McAb	Anti-class II MHC antigens	HLA-Dr, OKIa	Most B cells; activated T cells
McAb	CD3‡	OKT3, UCHT1	Mature T cells
McAb	CD4	OKT4, Leu3	Helper/inducer T cells
McAb	CD8	OKT8, Leu2	Cytotoxic/suppressor T cells
McAb	Leu7		Large granular lymphocytes with cytotoxic function; mainly T cells

*When tested on cell suspensions it detects membrane-bound immunoglobulins (SmIg); on cytospin-made slides it may also detect cytoplasmic immunoglobulins (CyIg). The immunoperoxidase method on fixed cells detects both SmIg and CyIg.
†When tested on cytospin-made slides (fixed cells) it detects most B lymphocytes; when tested on cell suspensions (by immunofluorescence) it detects mainly late B cells, including B prolymphocytes and hairy cells.
‡This antigen is expressed early in the cytoplasm of T cells (lymphoblasts of T-ALL) but it appears on the membrane at the late or post-thymic stage where it is also expressed in the cytoplasm.

nosis of CLL is entertained. When the WBC is high (e.g. above $50 \times 10^9/l$) and the blood film shows an unequivocal diagnosis of CLL or PLL, lymph node histology may not be necessary.

Bone marrow trephine biopsies, on the other hand, are always required as they provide important diagnostic and prognostic information. The pattern of bone marrow infiltration—paratrabecular, diffuse, nodular or interstitial—the cell morphology, the status of the normal haemopoietic elements, the presence of fibrosis etc. are all features which can help to confirm a diagnosis of leukaemia or NHL, provide indication about the mechanism of anaemia or thrombocytopenia and help predict the outcome of splenectomy (in HCL). The pattern and degree of lymphocytic infiltration in CLL have been considered an important prognostic variable independent of the clinical stage. For disorders with an enlarged spleen, e.g. B-PLL, HCL, splenic lymphoma with villous lymphocytes (SLVL), splenic forms of B-CLL, or of some NHL, the histology of the spleen is often of diagnostic value in defining whether the main cellular involvement is in the white or red pulps or in both. Also, the spleen histology may demonstrate features which are typical for some disorders, e.g. the characteristic pseudosinuses and red cell lakes in HCL.

DNA Analysis

Techniques for the demonstration of immunoglobulin (Ig) and T-cell receptor genes with appropriate probes and Southern blotting are outlined in Chapter 12. As mentioned above, the most important application in the study of lymphoproliferative disorders is the possibility of demonstrating clonality in cases of apparently 'benign' T-cell proliferations. The light chain restriction in the B-cell leukaemias makes it less imperative to perform DNA analysis in such cases. However, the applications of this technique are likely to extend beyond the demonstration of clonality and cell lineage (when marker studies are not possible or unavailable). For example, DNA analysis is essential for sequential studies in cases of relapse or transformation. Some cases of Richter syndrome, transformation from B-CLL, have been found to represent new clones rather than a transformation from the pre-existing clone. Rare cases of B-PLL, HCL-

variant and follicular lymphoma (FL) have non-demonstrable SmIg but have been shown with appropriate probes to have a rearrangement of the heavy and light chain Ig genes. Finally, cases of biclonal proliferation and cases with small tissue samples (e.g. in cutaneous T-cell lymphomas) may be shown to be clonal, and possibly malignant by this technique.

Diagnosis of Lymphocytosis

Frequently, in asymptomatic patients with only moderately raised lymphocyte counts (e.g. between $5 \times 10^9/l$ and $10 \times 10^9/l$), the question arises whether the lymphocytosis is a transient reactive phenomenon or represents the early manifestation of a lymphoid leukaemia. Attention to the morphology may provide some guidance about the nature of the process. Cell markers are essential to establish whether the pattern is that seen in normal blood, with a predominance of T cells, or whether B cells predominate. Reactive B cell lymphocytosis is extremely rare. By testing for surface membrane Ig (SmIg) with anti-light-chain reagents, it is possible to establish readily whether the majority of circulating lymphocytes (e.g. over 50%) stain only for kappa or lambda light chains or whether the normal kappa:lambda ratio (3:1) is altered significantly. This would indicate that a monoclonal B cell disorder is the likely cause of the lymphocytosis.

When T cells are the predominant type, it is often more difficult to establish the clonal nature of the T lymphocytosis, firstly because the values have to be significantly different from normal and, secondly, because reactive T cell lymphocytosis to viral agents or other pathological processes is not uncommon. Three features may be helpful: (i) whether the T lymphocytosis has no obvious clinical cause, (ii) whether the latter persists for 3 months or longer, and (iii) whether the lymphocytes appear of uniform morphology, e.g. granular or with irregular nuclear outline. Marker studies may also indicate whether a particular cell phenotype, not seen in normal individuals, or representing a significant increase (e.g. 100-fold) of a cell rarely seen in normal blood, e.g. CD8+, CD11b+ or CD4+, Leu7+, etc., is now the prevalent cell type. Conclusive evidence for T cell clonality in these circumstances is provided by chromosome analysis or by the analysis of the rearrangement of the T cell receptor genes (β and/or γ and δ chains) (see p. 335).

CLASSIFICATION

With the methods outlined above it is possible to classify the heterogeneous group of lymphoproliferative disorders. In many instances this also has a bearing on the patients' management. The main subdivision is between the B-cell disorders, which are by far the most common in Western countries, and the T-cell leukaemias, which, although less frequent, are of great interest with respect to aetiopathogenesis and epidemiology.

B-Lymphoid Leukaemias

Two major groups are considered: the leukaemias proper and the leukaemic phase of NHL (Table 15.2). Marker studies may be very similar in many of these disorders, thus the morphological and histological analyses are the key diagnostic tests. As B-cell leukaemias represent clonal proliferations of B cells at different stages of maturation, the pattern of membrane markers may be of diagnostic value. Of all these disorders, B-CLL

Table 15.2
Classification of B-lymphoproliferative disorders

Leukaemias
B-chronic lymphocytic leukaemia
  common-type (B-CLL)
  with > 10% prolymphocytes (CLL/PL)
B-prolymphocytic leukaemia (B-PLL)
  (> 55% prolymphocytes)
Hairy cell leukaemia
  classic form (HCL)
  variant form (HCL-V)
Plasma cell leukaemia (PCL)
  lymphoplasmacytic
  differentiated form

Lymphoma/leukaemia syndromes
Splenic lymphoma with villous lymphocytes (SLVL)
Waldenström's macroglobulinaemia
Follicular centre cell lymphoma (FL)
Intermediate (diffuse centrocytic) NHL
Large cell NHL

---

has a membrane phenotype which is different from that of the other B-cell disorders (Table 15.3). The B-CLL lymphocytes represent a slightly immature (but immunocompetent) B-cell type with weak expression of SmIg, consistent expression of the p67 antigen detected by McAb of the CD5 group, and high affinity for binding mouse erythrocytes. Cells expressing p67 (CD5) and membrane IgM have been found in the vicinity of the mantle zone in normal lymph nodes.

In addition to the markers summarized in Tables 15.2 and 15.3, other McAb may add information of diagnostic value. For example, LeuM5 is a McAb which reacts with monocytes and macrophages and, within B-cells, reacts strongly mainly with HCL and some HCL-variants. Also, the McAb HC2 reacts with most HCL cases but not with the other B-cell disorders, including HCL-variant. Thus, hairy cells, which are late B-cells, have a number of unique membrane features which, in combination, are diagnostic for this disease: SmIg +, CD5 −, CD25 +, HC2 + and LeuM5 +.

Chromosome Abnormalities in B-cell Leukaemias

The advent of polyclonal B-cell activators such as EBV, TPA (phorbol ester), lipopolysaccharide (LPS), pokeweed mitogen (PWM), has made it possible to elicit metaphases from seemingly slowly dividing cells from the peripheral blood of the chronic B-cell leukaemias. In addition, dividing cells can also be obtained from direct sampling and short-term culture from lymph nodes, spleen and, sometimes, also bone marrow in NHL. There are some features in common in the chromosome abnormalities of B-cell malignancies. Chromosome 14 is frequently affected, with a breakpoint at 14q32 which is the location of the immunoglobulin heavy chain gene. However, translocations involving this segment are not the same in all B-cell disorders. The marker 14q + is rare in early or uncomplicated B-CLL whilst it is seen more frequently in advanced B-CLL and in cases with an increased proportion of prolymphocytes (CLL/PL). It is even more frequent in B-PLL, where 15 out of 23 cases in our series had this marker. In five of them the abnormality involved a reciprocal translocation—t(11; 14) (q13; q32)—which has also been observed in plasma cell leukaemia. The breakpoint 11q13 in-

Table 15.3

Membrane markers in chronic B-cell leukaemias and NHL in leukaemic phase

Markers	CLL	PLL	HCL	SLVL	FL	PCL
SmIg*	±	++	++	++	++	−
CyIg	−	−/+	−/++	−/++	−	++
M-rosettes	++	−	−	−	−/+	−
CD5(p67)	+	−/+	−	−	−	−
FMC7/CD22†	−/+	++	++	++	++	−
CD19/20/24 and class II	++	++	++	++	++	−
CD10	−	−/+	−	−	+	−/+
CD25	−/+	−/+	++	−/+	−/+	−
CD38	−	−	−	−	−	++

*The Ig heavy chain classes in CLL, PLL, FL and SLVL are IgM and IgD. In HCl, several heavy chain isotypes are often expressed, IgM, IgD, IgA and IgG; in HCL-V it is almost always IgG only.
†Membrane immunofluorescence only (on cell suspension); despite the similar distribution, these two McAb do not detect the same antigen.

volved in the translocation includes the oncogene *bcl*-1. Another abnormality involving chromosome 14 is characteristic of follicular (centroblastic/centrocytic) lymphoma, resulting from the reciprocal translocation t(14; 18). The breakpoint in 18q also involves the oncogene *bc*1-2.

Analysable metaphases can be obtained in most B-PLL cases, and in half of those with CLL/PL and B-CLL. Whilst most mitotic figures are abnormal in PLL and CLL/PL, at least half may be normal in CLL, more frequently in early disease, reflecting the mitoses of residual normal T cells. Of CLL cases with cytogenetic abnormalities, an extra chromosome 12 (trisomy 12) is found in one-third of cases. Trisomy 12 is also found in CLL/PL and is infrequent (2 of 23) in B-PLL. Progression of the disease and/or the appearance of prolymphocytic changes is associated with the presence of the marker 14q + and a worse prognosis in CLL patients. It is debated whether the presence of trisomy 12 alone confers a worse prognosis in CLL, although in some studies patients with that abnormality appear to have required more active treatment.

T-Lymphoid Leukaemias

These disorders are often more difficult to recognize due to their lower frequency and because they often present with atypical features. The diagnostic elements discussed above (markers, morphology,

cytochemistry and histopathology) should all be taken into account. In addition, it is now important to carry out serological assays to define the cases of adult T-cell leukaemia/lymphoma (ATLL) which are associated with the infection by human T-cell leukaemia virus I (HTLV-I), the first recognized human retrovirus, which seems to cause this T-cell malignancy. The classification of mature T-cell malignancies is listed in Table 15.4. Geographical and epidemiological factors, linked to the incidence of HTLV-I, should also be taken into account in this classification. The presence of serum antibodies to HTLV-I can be assessed by radioimmunoassays. More detailed analysis is possible by means of McAb against the major viral proteins (tested on the infected cells after 1 week of culture) and by molecular probes by Southern blot analysis. As discussed above, to distinguish relatively benign T-CLL cases from reactive or non-neoplastic T-cell

Table 15.4

Classification of T-cell lymphoproliferative disorders

T-chronic lymphocytic leukaemia (T-CLL) or large granular lymphocyte (LGL) leukaemia
T-prolymphocytic leukaemia (T-PLL)
Adult T-cell leukaemia/lymphoma (ATLL)
Sezary's syndrome (SS)
T-cell NHL (HTLV-I negative)

lymphocytes may also require the use of molecular probes to detect rearrangements of the T-cell receptor genes.

Table 15.5 summarizes the main findings with a battery of McAb and other immunological reagents. The chronic T-cell leukaemias are also described as mature because their membrane phenotype corresponds to that of post-thymic lymphocytes (TdT and CDI are both always negative in these cells). It should be noted that the only two consistently positive pan-T markers in these cases are CD2 (or E-rosettes) and OKT17 (this McAb is not frequently used). Others, like CD3 (which is negative on cell suspensions in 20% of T-PLL and 10% of SS and ATLL) or CD5 (negative in T-CLL) or CD7 (often negative in ATLL and SS), do not react as expected in normal mature (peripheral blood) T lymphocytes. It should also be noted that the results in Table 15.5, which are a summary of our experience in 100 cases with these disorders, may be oversimplified as cases with phenotypes different from those listed are seen, particularly in the heterogeneous group of T-CLL. Overall, nevertheless, most cases of T-CLL (or LGL-leukaemia) are CD8+, Leu7+ proliferations, whilst the other diseases are mainly CD4+ malignancies. Despite this, differences within the last group are apparent

(Table 15.5). For example, CD7 is expressed in all cases of T-PLL and not in ATLL or SS; CD25 (reacting against the receptor for interleukin-2) is positive in most ATLL cases and much less frequently (and in a lower percentage of cells) in T-PLL and SS. In addition to these differences it has been established that CD4-positive cells in T-PLL and SS may act, in functional assays, as helper cells, whilst CD4-positive ATLL are shown to act in vitro as suppressors of B-cell differentiation.

Chromosome Abnormalities in T-cell Leukaemias

Abnormal metaphases are obtained with T-cell mitogens (phytohaemagglutinin, PHA) in most cases of T-PLL, ATLL and SS. Mitoses are more difficult to elicit in CD8-positive T-CLL, but when these are obtained they are found to be abnormal. The most consistent findings are in T-PLL, where an inversion of chromosome 14—inv(14) (q11q32)—was observed by us in 9 of 15 cases. The breakpoints in this abnormality, which results in a marker 14q+ chromosome, involve the T-cell receptor alpha-chain gene region (14q11) and the immunoglobulin heavy chain region (14q32). A

Table 15.5
Membrane markers in mature T-cell leukaemias

Markers	T-CLL	T-PLL	ATLL	SS
TdT*	−	−	−	−
CD1(T6)	−	−	−	−
CD2(T11) or E-rosettes	+	+	+	+
CD3(T3)‡	+	+/−	+	+
CD4(T4)	−	+/−†	+	+
CD5(T1)	−	+	+	+
CD7(3A1)	−/+	+ +	−	−
CD8(T8)	+	−/+†	−	−
OKT17	+	+	+	+
CD25(Tac)	−	−/+	+ +	−/+

*Terminal deoxynucleotidyl transferase, nuclear enzyme demonstrated in T lymphoblasts by means of a polyclonal antibody.
†CD4 and CD8 are coexpressed in 16% of T-PLL, in very rare SS and ATLL, and some T-NHL.
‡CD3 is expressed on the membrane as well as in the cytoplasm at this stage of T-cell maturation.

breakpoint at 14q11, as part of a t(11; 14) (p13; q11), has also been found in T-ALL.

Other abnormalities in T-PLL and some SS cases involve the long arm (q) of chromosome 8 in trisomy or multisomy. Similarly, trisomy or partial trisomy for 7q, often involving band 7q35, in which the gene for the beta chain of the T-cell receptor is located, is also found in T-PLL and in ATLL. Japanese authors have also described a marker 14q + in the latter condition.

B-CELL LEUKAEMIAS

Chronic Lymphocytic Leukaemia

Chronic lymphocytic leukaemia (B-CLL) accounts for about 25% of all leukaemias. In adults over the age of 50 years it is the most common form, particularly in the West. In the Far East its incidence is low. It is also the most common of the lymphoproliferative disorders.

Chronic lymphocytic leukaemia affects twice as many males as females, with a peak incidence between 60 and 80 years. In the MRC CLL 1 trial, 71% of cases entered were aged over 60 years, only 6% were less than 50 years, and 5.5% were 80 years or over. There is a tendency for older patients to present with less advanced disease. B-CLL is rarely diagnosed below the age of 40 years and is even more rare below 30 years. In such cases a diagnosis of follicular lymphoma should be carefully excluded. A greater understanding of the pattern of B-cell maturation and the available reagents for immunological phenotyping have helped to define the features of the B-CLL more precisely and to clarify the diagnostic criteria. In the past, many of the other disorders described in this chapter were included under the diagnosis of CLL. Of all the leukaemias, B-CLL has the highest familial incidence, which can be documented in 1% or 2% of patients. Evidence of another malignancy is also often disclosed in CLL patients.

Pioneering work by Dameshek (1967) and Galton (1966) introduced the concept of CLL as a progressive accumulation of monoclonal B lymphocytes, starting in lymph nodes and/or the bone marrow, and gradually expanding to most haemopoietic organs. This concept of slow progression was the basis of the clinical staging system proposed by Rai *et al.* (1975). Advanced involvement will bring about abnormalities in the normal function of the immune system and result in hypogammaglobulinaemia and, less frequently, autoimmune complications. The bone marrow, viewed by detailed histological studies, also reflects the progression of CLL from early interstitial nodular infiltration to late diffuse lymphocytic replacement of normal haemopoietic elements.

Clinical and Laboratory Features

In 25% of patients the disease is diagnosed by chance following a blood examination. In others, the presentation is prompted by symptoms of anaemia or by the discovery of painless lymph node enlargement. Systemic symptoms such as pyrexia, sweating or weight loss are rare. Not infrequently, a severe chest infection or pneumonia is the first manifestation of CLL.

Lymph node enlargement is symmetrical and involves the neck, axillae and inguinal regions. Splenomegaly of variable degree is present in two-thirds of cases. Significant hepatomegaly is less frequent. It is possible to document lymph node enlargement in the hilar regions on routine x-rays, or in the retroperitoneal regions by ultrasound or CT scanning procedures. In general, these areas are not routinely investigated as they have not been found to give additional prognostic information.

The diagnosis of CLL presupposes by convention that there is a persistent lymphocytosis of at least $10 \times 10^9/l$ and lymphocytic infiltration in the bone marrow of at least 40%. With immunological methods, particularly the detection of monoclonal B-cell populations by light chain restriction, it is possible to diagnose the disease with lymphocyte counts between $5 \times 10^9/l$ and $10 \times 10^9/l$. Morphologically (Fig. 15.1), the lymphocytes in blood films are small, show scanty cytoplasm and a characteristic pattern of nuclear chromatin clumping; the nucleolus is inconspicuous, and azurophil granules are seen in a minority of cells (they correspond to the normal T-cell population). The presence of smear cells, which correlates with the level of WBC, is often of diagnostic value.

As stated above (Table 15.3), a combination of membrane markers is often diagnostic of B-CLL,

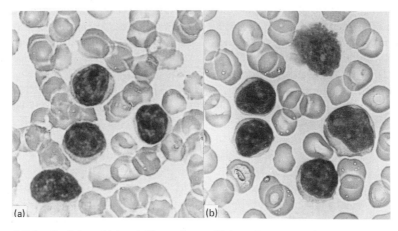

Fig. 15.1. *Peripheral blood films of two CLL patients showing condensed and clumped nuclear chromatin. Note in (b) a larger cell and a cell smudge (× 1200).*

not only for distinguishing it from T-cell disorders but also from other B-lymphoproliferative disorders. The disease which is often confused with B-CLL is follicular lymphoma, which may present with moderate lymphocytosis, usually up to $30 \times 10^9/l$ but occasionally above $50 \times 10^9/l$.

Anaemia and thrombocytopenia are the most important prognostic features in CLL. In advanced disease these result from bone marrow failure, with the trephine biopsy showing heavy replacement of fat spaces and haemopoieitc cells by lymphocytes. However, in an ageing population it is important always to exclude nutritional deficiencies (iron, folate), which can be easily corrected by appropriate supplements. The possible causes of anaemia in B-CLL are listed in Table 15.6. The current staging systems do not distinguish the causes of anaemia as having different prognostic significance. This is probably because marrow failure is by far the most common cause and there is an assumption that

Table 15.6
Causes of anaemia in B-CLL and their management

Cause	Diagnostic method	Treatment	Significance
BM failure	BM aspirate and trephine biopsy	Corticosteroids and other anti-CLL agents	Advanced disease, Stage III (Rai); C (International)
Fe or folate deficiency	Indices, Fe and folate levels, BM aspirate; dietary history	Appropriate supplements	None; restage patient when anaemia is corrected
Hypersplenism	Splenomegaly; BM aspirate and trephine biopsy show residual haemopoiesis	Treatment for CLL; consider splenectomy	If isolated, it will correct by splenectomy; good prognosis
IHA	Direct antiglobulin test; spherocytosis	Corticosteroids; rarely, splenectomy	If corrected, prognosis according to residual stage

BM, bone marrow; Fe, iron; IHA, immune haemolytic anaemia.

most haematologists will spot the nutritional deficiencies. There is evidence, however, that auto-immune complications (anaemia or thrombocytopenia) which are rare at presentation (*c.* 5% of cases), if adequately treated, do not confer a bad prognosis. It is therefore important always to carry out the direct antiglobulin test at diagnosis in each patient. In a proportion of cases the immune complications follow the initiation of therapy with alkylating agents or radiotherapy, as classically described by Lewis *et al.* (1966). As seen in Table 15.6, a bone marrow biopsy is a key investigation to sort out the mechanism of the anaemia or thrombocytopenia. If the platelets are low due to antibodies or hypersplenism, the core biopsy will show a normal or increased number of megakaryocytes in an otherwise moderately infiltrated bone marrow.

Biochemical analysis may show a rise in uric acid levels which often correlate with the height of the WBC and the overall tumour mass. Renal and liver function abnormalities are rare, but a nephrotic syndrome is well documented in a minority of cases. Serum immunoglobulin levels are low and tend to decrease further with disease progression. This decline, which often starts with low IgA levels, is rarely corrected, even with successful treatment. Marked hypogammaglobulinaemia is the rule in advanced CLL and is responsible for the high incidence of upper respiratory infections. Small monoclonal (M) bands, often IgM, are seen in less than 10% of cases. The appearance of an M band during the evolution of the disease or the discovery of free light chains in the urine (Bence–Jones proteinuria) may indicate transformation of the disease to a more refractory state.

Differential Diagnosis

As discussed in the introductory section, good morphological criteria and a small battery of membrane markers may suffice for the diagnosis of CLL. Bone marrow examination is important in cases of minimal lymphocytosis to satisfy the criterion of 40% infiltration, and the trephine biopsy is essential to consider the alternative diagnosis of NHL, to indicate the degree of involvement in relation to prognosis, and to clarify the cause of anaemia (Table 15.6). In my experience, careful examination

of well-prepared peripheral blood films is the single most important diagnostic step in CLL (and often too in the other B-cell leukaemias). One source of confusion may be the existence of cases with over 10% of prolymphocytes in which an alternative, or refined, diagnosis of CLL/PL is considered (to be discussed below). In cases with low counts an alternative diagnosis of NHL—usually follicular lymphoma (FL) or splenic lymphoma (SLVL)—should be considered. If possible, a lymph node biopsy and the extent of lymph node involvement should be assessed in FL, and spleen histology and bone marrow status should help the diagnosis of SLVL. In both these conditions, marker studies may be suggestive when showing strong SmIg expression, membrane positivity in over 50% of cells with FMC7 and CD22, and negative CD5 expression. Whenever the marker studies are not consistent with typical B-CLL (see Table 15.3), the above diagnostic procedures are mandatory.

Staging Systems

The two widely accepted systems are that of Rai and the more recent one from the International Workshop on CLL, which followed work by Binet *et al.* (1981) in Paris. Rai's staging system takes the view that CLL cells accumulate first in the blood and bone marrow, then in lymph nodes, spleen and, finally, there is bone marrow failure. The chances of a patient surviving, assuming he is not treated or the treatment does not work, will depend largely on the stage in which he presents to the physician's attention. The Rai system has five stages: O, no anaemia, thrombocytopenia or physical signs; I, lymphadenopathy only; II, splenomegaly and/or hepatomegaly, with or without lymph node enlargement and without anaemia or thrombocytopenia; III, anaemia, initially below 11.0 g/dl, lately modified to 10.0 g/dl by some groups, irrespective of physical signs; IV, thrombocytopenia below 100 × 10^9/l, with or without any of the above features. Binet modified this system following extensive multivariate analysis from two French studies. This proposal was later accepted by an International Workshop on CLL, which included Rai as one of the coauthors. The new system is simpler, has only three stages and is probably more accurate with respect to the prognosis for patients with Rai stages I and II. The Rai system does not distinguish patients with stage I with one or several lymph node areas involved, nor, in stage II, patients with just splenomegaly or with splenomegaly plus involvement of one or more lymph node areas. For patients with Rai stages I and II, a subdivision according to the number of involved sites (as in Binet's staging) shows prognostic advantages over the subdivision in I and II. The International (Binet) system groups together patients with anaemia (Hb < 100 g/l) and thrombocytopenia (platelets < 100×10^9/l), or Rai stages III or IV, as Group C. The remainder of patients are staged according to the number of lymphoid organs involved, considering as one each of the following areas whether the involvement is unilateral or (more often) bilateral: neck, axilla and inguinal regions, spleen and liver. Group A patients have no organ enlargement or up to two areas; group B patients have three to five involved areas. The International Workshop proposed to retain the Rai stages as substages for Group A, as A(O), A(I) and A(II), mainly with the view of preserving the identification of the most benign group of Rai stage O. From several studies, including the MRC trial No. 1, it appears that there is a distinct trend favouring A(O) compared with A(I) and A(II), but the difference is not highly significant.

In practice, the idea of staging is to be able to predict prognosis, make decisions about which patients need treatment, and to facilitate allocation in randomized trials. There is no argument that stage C patients need therapy and also those in stage B, the majority of whom show features of disease progression—upward trend in the WBC, greater lymph node enlargement leading to symptoms of sweating and weight loss if the disease becomes bulky.

The distribution of patients in the various stages, although variable, depending on whether from a retrospective study or a prospective randomized trial, is as follows: A, 50%; B, 30%; and C, 20%. It is of interest that in the MRC CLL 1 trial the proportion of males with stages B and C was significantly higher than that of females, whilst for stage A the proportion of males was slightly lower than expected. For both sexes the proportion of stage A patients increased with age, with the highest proportion recorded over the age of 70 years.

Prognostic Factors

In a disease with such a variable pattern of survival it is important to examine critically the factors which determine survival. Most studies have shown that the best prognostic feature is the stage of the disease by either system (slightly better with the simpler ABC system). Individual features such as Hb, platelets, spleen size and number of lymph nodes enlarged are all important but are incorporated already in the stages. Two other categories of factors seem to add important prognostic information in addition to staging: (1) laboratory, and (2) biological features (Table 15.7). A number of studies have shown that some of these prognostic factors are independent of staging. Of the laboratory features, the size of the WBC, the degree of prolymphocytoid change, and the pattern of bone marrow involvement have been shown to be important by several groups. Similarly, response to treatment seems to be an important independent feature. Although patients with early disease respond better than those with late disease, within each stage those who respond better will have a longer survival. Age is relevant in as much as in the CLL age group, causes of death other than the disease itself are also very important. The influence of age is greater in the early stages of the disease. In the MRC CLL 1 trial, one-third of patients died of causes other than CLL, such as other neoplasms or cardiovascular accidents, and these were significantly influenced by age.

Table 15.7
Factors of poor prognosis in B-CLL in addition to staging*

Laboratory features
Lymphocyte count (> 50×10^9/l)
Lymphocyte doubling time (< 12 months)
Prolymphocytes (> 10%; > 15×10^9/l)
Bone marrow histology (diffuse involvement)
Karyotype (marker 14q + ; complex abnormalities)

Biological features
Age (> 70 years)
Sex (males)
Response to treatment (poor response)

*Including features taken into account for staging, e.g. Hb, lymph nodes, spleen, etc. (also see text).

Transformation of B-CLL

Two types of transformation are recognized in CLL: (1) prolymphocytoid or CLL with increased proportion of prolymphocytes (CLL/PL), and (2) immunoblastic. The first change is probably more common than hitherto recognized, is subtle and is associated with features of disease progression and refractoriness to treatment. The second is more dramatic and represents a transformation in the true sense of the word.

Detailed analysis of over 300 patients by Melo *et al.* (1986) has defined a group of patients with intermediate clinical and laboratory features between B-CLL and B-PLL, which is designated CLL/PL. This group is heterogeneous. Some cases clearly present with features of CLL and gradually, over some years, progress with an increased proportion of prolymphocytes (these cells are often more pleomorphic than B-PLL cells), and represent what was originally described by Enno *et al.* (1979) as prolymphocytoid transformation (Fig. 15.2). Some patients may just represent the extreme of the spectrum of either B-CLL or B-PLL, and present with an increased proportion of prolymphocytes which may, in turn, influence their prognosis. Finally, some patients with CLL/PL may indeed represent those with an intermediate disease. This is manifested also by the higher predominance of splenomegaly and of some cases with intermediate

markers (one-third of CLL/PL cases have only one or two of the expected marker profiles for B-CLL, the remaining cases have the expected three to four positive markers as typical B-CLL, see Table 15.3), and a slightly higher proportion of cases with karyotypic abnormality. At the present time, evidence for an increased proportion of prolymphocytes represents in general a clinically more aggressive form of CLL with a lower response rate to conventional therapy than the typical cases.

'Immunoblastic' transformation or Richter's syndrome is well recognized in CLL. The change occurs usually in one or several lymph nodes which, when examined histologically, show the features of large-cell lymphoma (sometimes in the past confused with Hodgkin's disease). Richter's syndrome is often associated with systemic symptoms (fever and weight loss) and with unexpected unilateral lymph node enlargement, not rarely in the retroperitoneal area. Richter's syndrome occurs in 3–5% of CLL cases, but the incidence may be found to be higher if lymph node biopsies are always performed when clinical changes with systemic symptoms develop in a patient with previously well-controlled disease. In rare cases, this transformation occurs in the bone marrow, and therefore is seen in trephine biopsies, and may have significant 'spill-over' to the blood. In such cases, the morphology resembles that of an acute leukaemia, with rather large blasts which are positive for SmIg and some of the other

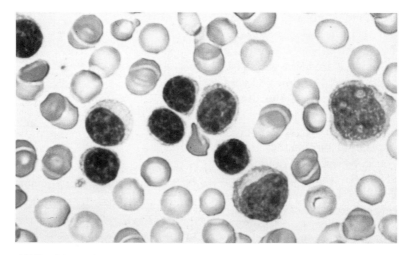

Fig. 15.2. *Blood film of a case of CLL/PL showing a double cell population: small typical CLL lymphocytes and two prolymphocytes, one of them almost a blast (× 1200).*

markers of CLL. Richter's syndrome is often associated with monoclonal spikes in the serum or free light chains in the urine.

Management

The indications for active treatment depend on the stage of the disease. For patients with stage A (Rai stages O, I and II), a period of observation may be necessary to decide whether the pattern of the disease is stable or progressive. Most patients with stage B and two-thirds of those with Rai stage II will show progression within the first year or two after diagnosis. This is manifested by further organ enlargement, a downward trend in the Hb and/or platelets, and a slowly rising WBC. As responses are better in early disease, some trials (e.g. the MRC CLL 2 trial) are comparing early therapy versus delayed therapy (if disease progresses) to see whether survival may be improved. Similar French trials have so far shown no advantage of early treatment (this is given usually until a good response is obtained but never for longer that 1 year). In the context of CLL, good responses are the technical definition of complete remission, with normalization of blood and bone marrow, or partial remission which means the regression of at least 50% of physical signs, lymphocyte counts less than $15 \times 10^9/l$ and normal Hb and platelet counts.

The various treatment modalities used for B-CLL are listed in Table 15.8. The role of corticosteroids as initial treatment for stage C patients is generally accepted in the UK. Platelets rise within 4–6 weeks; the Hb also rises; the WBC follows a characteristic curve, rising after 3 or 4 weeks, sometimes doubling the initial count, and then gradually coming down. This is nearly always accompanied by a decrease in size and a softening of lymph nodes and spleen. This beneficial effect facilitates the subsequent measures which employ agents having an effect on normal haemopoietic cells. There is no evidence that chlorambucil given monthly in higher doses is more effective than a low dose administered continuously. However, the intermittent dose achieves the same effect with a smaller amount of the alkylating agent. The CLL lymphocytes are very sensitive to low-dose irradiation, splenic irradiation has been used successfully in the MRC trials. It is clear that radiation to the spleen has a general effect which is sometimes manifested by a reduction in peripheral lymphadenopathy. The spleen size often regresses to become unpalpable and there is a dramatic fall in the WBC.

There have been several trials comparing chlorambucil versus the combination cyclophosphamide, oncovin and prednisolone (COP); none showed an advantage for COP. It is apparent that the antimitotic agent oncovin (vincristine) has no positive role in CLL, nor in other similarly slowly progressive diseases such as HCL. The value of

Table 15.8
Treatment modalities in B-CLL

Corticosteroids	i) 4-week course as initial therapy to stage C patients (30 mg/m²)
	ii) combined with monthly courses of chlorambucil or as part of COP
	iii) prolonged courses for the treatment of autoimmune complications
Chlorambucil	i) high dose intermittently every month (20 mg/m² × 3 days)
	ii) continuous low dose (4–6 mg daily)
COP	Cyclophosphamide 250 mg/m² × 5 days, oncovin 2 mg × l day, prednisolone 40 mg/m² × 5 days, monthly courses
CHOP	COP plus doxorubicin 25 mg/m² monthly
Splenic irradiation Splenectomy	100 cGy a week for 10 weeks

prednisolone given in monthly courses, in COP or with chlorambucil, is being tested at the present time. Cyclophosphamide has no advantage over chlorambucil in the treatment of CLL and it is obvious that either agent may be shown to be superior to the other depending on the doses employed in a particular study. In general, the higher the doses of alkylating agent used, the better are the responses. And, as mentioned above, good responses are advantageous for survival. It is generally useful to continue a particularly successful treatment for as long as possible until the maximum response is obtained. Patients achieving complete remission can often look forward to 2 or 3 years without the need for any further therapy. By the same token, it is not advisable to continue a particular line of therapy when, after a trial period of 3–4 months, it has not led to any measurable response. CHOP (Table 15.8) is a useful combination for some patients with progressive disease failing to respond to chlorambucil and prednisolone.

Low-dose total body irradiation, 5–10 cGy given two or three times a week, has been used in CLL but has shown no appreciable advantage over the more conventional regimens. In patients with bone marrow failure it can lead to unacceptable toxicity. Splenectomy is indicated for patients presenting with a large spleen and in whom the treatment given achieves only a moderate reduction of the spleen size (Fig. 15.3). Patients with splenic forms and manifested features of hypersplenism (as judged by blood counts and bone marrow findings) may benefit from splenectomy. Splenectomy is also indicated for patients with autoimmune thrombocytopenia or haemolytic anaemia refractory to corticosteroids. Provided patients are given long-term penicillin therapy after splenectomy, this operation often has a beneficial effect on the disease, even if only as part of a debulking procedure. In our hands this procedure has been associated with no mortality and seems to have been of positive benefit to patients with a large spleen and blood counts consistent with stage C disease.

As the treatment for CLL is not radical and the main objective is to prolong survival with a good quality of life, care should be taken to prevent and/or treat promptly any complications arising

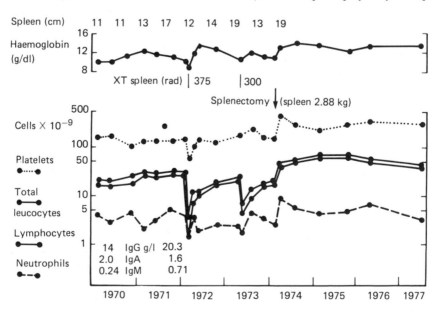

Fig. 15.3. *Male, 54 years, with chronic lymphocytic leukaemia Stage IIIS (see text) treated by two courses of splenic irradiation and splenectomy. The chart shows the distance of the lower pole of the spleen from the left costal margin, the treatments, the haemoglobin concentration, the platelet, leucocyte, neutrophil, and lymphocyte counts, and the serum immunoglobulin concentrations, over an 8-year period. (XT spleen: splenic irradiation.)*

from the immunodeficiency associated with B-CLL. Thus, prompt antibiotic treatment for seemingly benign upper respiratory infection and antiviral measures to prevent the spread of herpetic infections are as important as the specific treatment for the disease. Patients with repeated infections and very low gammaglobulin levels may benefit from courses of intramuscular or intravenous gammaglobulin injections. Studies to assess the prophylactic value of such measures have recently confirmed their value. Additional measures, such as the administration of allopurinol when starting therapy with a $WBC > 50 \times 10^9/l$, oral amphotericin and ranitidine when using corticosteroids, should always be part of the treatment of CLL patients.

Prolymphocytic Leukaemia

Prolymphocytic leukaemia (B-PLL) was considered a variant of CLL since its description by Galton *et al.* in 1974. In the last decade it has become apparent that there are important clinical and laboratory differences between these disorders which, despite the existence of the group with CLL/PL discussed above, suggest that B-PLL is a distinct disorder. This is supported by differences in the morphology and cell markers from CLL cells, the physical signs (almost exclusively splenomegaly in PLL), clinical evolution and spleen histology.

The key for the diagnosis of PLL is the recognition in well-prepared peripheral blood films of the prolymphocyte as the predominant cell. Without membrane markers, it is not always easy to distinguish B from T cases, thus the name PLL has been retained for both disorders, although they have nothing else in common. B-PLL is three times more common that T-PLL, and both together constitute less than 10% of the chronic lymphoid leukaemias. In fact, within the mature T-cell leukaemias (all of them rare), T-PLL is, in our experience, the most frequent. The mean age of patients presenting with B-PLL is 70 years, which is 5 years older than that of B-CLL.

Clinical and Laboratory Findings

The main features of B-PLL are splenomegaly (mean size 10 cm below the costal margin in our series) without lymphadenopathy, and a rising WBC, usually over $100 \times 10^9/l$ at the time of presentation. Anaemia and thrombocytopenia (as for stage C B-CLL) are seen in at least 50% of cases, twice the incidence of B-CLL. Other laboratory findings are no different from high-count CLL: increased uric acid, low serum immunoglobulins, although the incidence of a monoclonal band is close to 30%, much higher than in CLL.

Differential Diagnosis

The main diagnostic criterion is the identification of prolymphocytes as the predominant population in blood films. It is essential that these should be carefully prepared and that observations should be made in areas where the cells are well, but not too much, spread. In the study by Melo *et al.* (1986), 55% of prolymphocytes was the figure that best discriminated the clinical and laboratory features of B-PLL from those in B-CLL and the CLL/PL cases; the mean percentage of prolymphocytes in B-PLL was 74%. The prolymphocyte is larger (usually twice the size of a small CLL lymphocyte), has moderately condensed nuclear chromatin, a prominent central nucleolus and a lower nucleo:cytoplasmic ratio than CLL cells (Fig. 15.4). The B prolymphocytes are more uniform and have a more regular nuclear outline than those of CLL/PLL. They are larger and have a more clear cytoplasm and lower nucleo:cytoplasmic ratio than T prolymphocytes (Fig. 15.5). Electron microscopy is not necessary for the diagnosis of B-PLL, but may be necessary for T-PLL cases with small-size prolymphocytes where the nucleolus is masked by the nuclear chromatin under light microscopy examination.

Problems of differential diagnosis may occur with other B-cell disorders, B-CLL, CLL/PL, and the variant of HCL which has clinical features and laboratory features resembling B-PLL, such as anaemia, splenomegaly, high WBC and prominent nucleolus. The distinction from the HCL variant is mainly based on the appearances of the cytoplasm, which in HCL-variant cells is more abundant and distinctly villous (Fig. 15.6), whilst in B-PLL it is in general smooth. Marker studies are different from those of classic B-CLL and from two-thirds of cases of CLL/PL. No single case of B-PLL in our series

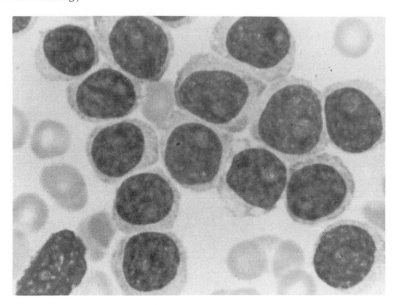

Fig. 15.4. *Peripheral blood film of B-PLL, showing a uniform picture of large nucleolated prolymphocytes (×1300).*

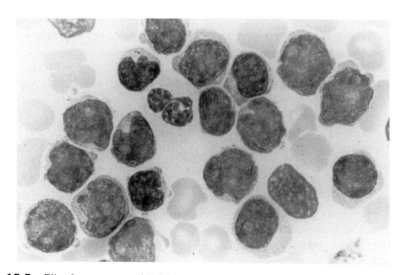

Fig. 15.5. *Film from a case of T-PLL. In contrast to B-PLL (see Fig. 15.4), these cells are slightly smaller, have a higher nuclear to cytoplasmic ratio, are more pleomorphic and the nucleolus is not always visible in all the cells (×1300).*

had the characteristic phenotype of B-CLL (high M-rosettes, weak SmIg, over 50% CD5 positive and less than 30% FMC7-positive cells, see Table 15.3); one-third of them (as one-third of CLL/PL) may have one or two markers the same as those of B-CLL, such as CD5 positivity and M-rosettes over 30% although rarely over 50%. The mean percentage of M-rosettes apparent using neuraminidase-treated lymphocytes is 60% in B-CLL, 52% in CLL/PL and 15% in B-PLL. SmIg staining is uniformly strong and FMC7 is positive in over 50% of cells in nearly all B-PLL cases. The distinction

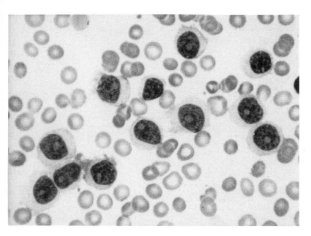

Fig. 15.6. *Blood film from a case of HCL variant. Note the prominent nucleolus and abundant cytoplasm with irregular (hairy) cytoplasmic outline (× 800).*

between CLL/PL and B-PLL may be semantic because when the absolute prolymphocyte count is high in either disease, the prognosis is equally poor. CLL/PL cases have two morphologically distinct cell populations: small lymphocytes (as in typical CLL) and prolymphocytes (as in PLL). Cell volume measurements may help define these populations; in B-PLL, a more uniform population is the rule.

Histopathology is rarely required for a diagnosis of B-PLL. The bone marrow infiltration is diffuse, as in advanced CLL or mixed interstitial nodular and mainly occupies the intertrabecular space. Lymph node biopsies are rarely available. Spleen histology shows extensive white and red pulp involvement, with large proliferative nodules with a characteristic bizonal appearance. These features were not seen in the cases of HCL-variant that we have studied; in HCL-variant the red pulp is predominantly involved, as in typical HCL.

Treatment

Conventional chemotherapy regimens as for CLL, e.g. chlorambucil or COP, are of little value in the management of B-PLL. Response rates (partial responses and few complete remissions) to splenic irradiation (as given for CLL) and/or the combination cyclophosphamide, doxorubicin, oncovin and prednisone (CHOP) have been recorded in 25–30% of cases. Additional measures are also necessary to manage this relentlessly progressive disease. Splenctomy is often useful to remove a major proliferative focus which represents a considerable part of the tumour mass in this disease, to relieve hypersplenism and to facilitate further therapy. In patients with disease resistant to irradiation, splenectomy followed by regular leukapheresis or the experimental agent 2′ deoxycoformycin has allowed prolongation of survival. Even in good responders, splenectomy has improved the prospects of long-term survival. Considering the older age group affected by B-PLL, splenectomy may not be possible in a proportion of patients.

Hairy Cell Leukaemia

Hairy cell leukaemia (HCL) is now a well-recognized clinicopathological entity which affects males more frequenetly than females (M:F ratio 4:1), usually over the age of 45 years. The disease has always elicited great interest, for different reasons: first, in the 1960s, in order to establish clearly the diagnostic features of the newly described entity, and subsequently, in parallel with advances in immunology, to identify the nature and tissue origin of the hairy cell. This has now resolved conclusively with the use of McAb and other marker techniques, and the unequivocal demonstration of rearrangement of the heavy and light chain immunoglobulin genes. Lately, HCL has attracted considerable attention because of the significant advances in its treatment with new agents—alpha-interferon (IFN-alpha), and 2′deoxycoformycin (DCF).

Clinical and Laboratory Findings

The main presentation features are a consequence of pancytopenia affecting these patients. Often they present with symptoms of anaemia, sometimes with bleeding manifestations and, not infrequently, with an infective episode which does not run its normal course. HCL patients are moderately neutropenic and severely monocytopenic; thus, bacterial and opportunistic infections do occur. There is evidence that the incidence of typical and atypical mycobacterial infections is increased. The main physical signs are splenomegaly (85–90% of cases) and hepatomegaly (50%). The spleen may be moderately to massively enlarged. Lymphadenopathy is very rare but it may occur as a late event. Most patients are pancytopenic at presentation. The anaemia results from reduced bone marrow production and splenic pooling. Haemolysis is exceptional. Isotope studies for spleen and bone marrow function may help clarify the mechanism of anaemia in these patients. The total WBC may be low, normal or high (although rarely above 20×10^9/l), but neutropenia and monocytopenia are common. The remainder of the WBC is comprised of variable proportions of hairy cells. A minority of patients have no detectable hairy cells on blood films; two-thirds of cases have 10–50% hairy cells, and some have more than 50%. Patients with low WBC and few or no circulating hairy cells present diagnostic problems. Platelet counts are below 100×10^9/l in 80% of cases.

There are few biochemical abnormalities associated with this disease. Liver function tests may be moderately abnormal, reflecting the degree of hairy cell infiltration in hepatic sinuses and portal tracts. Serum immunoglobulins are normal and monoclonal bands are rare.

Diagnosis

The recognition of typical hairy cells in peripheral blood films is extremely useful for establishing or suggesting this diagnosis. Hairy cells are large—twice the size of a normal lymphocyte—and have abundant cytoplasm (low N:C ratio) which is characteristically villous in its outline (Fig. 15.7). The nucleus is round, oval or slightly indented, and occasionally is frankly bilobed. Not all villous lymphocytes are hairy cells; for this reason, the smooth nuclear chromatin, absence of a visible nucleolus and low N:C ratio are landmarks of typical hairy cells. Cells from the rare HCL variant have similar cytoplasmic features but have a round nucleus with a more condensed chromatin pattern and a distinct nucleolus (resembling in this respect prolymphocytes, see Fig. 15.6).

Even when the appearance of blood films is very suggestive, it is important to confirm the diagnosis by additional techniques, the most important of which is a bone marrow biopsy, followed by cytochemistry and membrane markers.

Bone marrow aspirates are as a rule unsuccessful as no fragments and few cells are obtained. There-

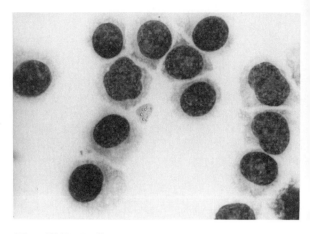

Fig. 15.7. *Buffy coat preparation from a typical HCL. Note the absence of visible nucleolus in contrast to the HCL-V (see Fig. 15.6) and the rather blunt nucleus and hairy cytoplasm (× 1300).*

fore, a trephine biopsy is essential. This shows diffuse infiltration of variable degree. A typical feature is the arrangement of the cellular infiltrate which is loose, leaving plenty of space between cells, often with a clear zone around each cell which is rather unique to this condition. This contrasts with the more dense infiltration in CLL, PLL, or the paratrabecular involvement in NHL.

Lymph node biopsies are not indicated in HCL. Spleen histology, when available, shows distinct diagnostic features: infiltration by mononuclear cells with a blunt nucleus in the red pulp with little residual white pulp, and formation of pseudosinuses filled with erythrocytes ('red cell lakes'). Tartrate-resistant acid phosphatase (TRAP) demonstrated on hairy cells (on blood buffy coats, cytospin preparations, spleen or bone marrow imprints and/or sections) corresponds to a unique isoenzyme 5 and is quite specific for HCL, although in some cases the proportion of TRAP-positive cells is low; TRAP is usually absent from the HCL-variant cells and is rarely seen in other disorders, e.g. B-PLL or T-CLL, although it may be apparent in a minority of cells. Electron microscopy may be of diagnostic value in difficult cases. In addition to the cytoplasmic villi, ultrastructural analysis may reveal ribosome–lamella complexes on one-third to half of the cases. Rarely, this intracytoplasmic inclusion can be seen in isolated cells from other B-cell disorders.

Membrane markers (see Table 15.3) show a distinct membrane phenotype for hairy cells. On this basis, hairy cells are now considered to be activated B cells, with features of late maturation stages. SmIg is usually strong and characteristically shows several heavy chain isotypes, often including IgA and IgG, and sharing a single heavy chain. The cells of most cases of HCL variant express IgG as a single heavy chain. As in B-PLL, HCL cells are FMC7 and CD22 positive, but, in contrast to other B-cell disorders, they consistently express CD25 (demonstrated by anti-Tac), RFB1 (as B-CLL but with stronger staining), HC2 and LeuM5 (antigen shared with monocytes and macrophages). In contrast to B-CLL, hairy cells are always CD5 negative; only the residual normal T cells are positive. The immunophenotyping of hairy cells can be performed selectively by means of flow cytometers which allow their separation from other lymphoid cells on the basis of their large volume. Because of high-affinity Fc receptors on the membrane of hairy cells, care should be taken in the immunological analysis to avoid false positive results.

Hairy Cell Leukaemia Variant

A minority of patients with HCL, usually presenting with high WBC 50–80 × 10^9/l) and splenomegaly show cells with a prominent nucleolus, lacking HC2 and Tac antigens, and with IgG or no immunoglobulin on the membrane. TRAP is absent and the patients respond less well to IFN-alpha or deoxycoformycin.

Differential Diagnosis

Conditions which should be taken into account for the differential diagnosis are: B-CLL with isolated splenomegaly, splenic lymphoma with villous lymphocytes, B-PLL (with the HCL variant) and, rarely, primary myelofibrosis. In these situations all the results of the investigative procedures should be taken into account. Again, the careful analysis of peripheral blood films and interpretation of bone marrow trephine biopsies are most important. Rare patients with HCL seem to have a predominantly splenic form of the disease with little or no bone marrow involvement. These cases are diagnosed mainly after splenectomy; here, it is the spleen histology which is the key diagnostic test.

Treatment

Many modalities have been tried in the past to improve the bone marrow function of HCL. The prime objective of the treatment should be the normalization of the blood counts since pancytopenia is the main source of complications. There are now three modalities which alone or used in succession can achieve that aim with very little toxicity. More aggressive treatments, used in the past with moderate success, such as low-dose chlorambucil, splenic irradiation or anthracyclines, are no longer indicated for the majority of patients, but may help those for whom the main treatments currently used are not available or contraindicated. The current treatments for HCL are: splenectomy, interferon-alpha (IFN-alpha) and 2′deoxycoformycin (DCF or pentostatin).

A few patients with HCL may not require treatment. The majority have symptoms and abnormal blood counts at presentation and therefore will require some form of treatment. As all the above three modalities have been shown to be effective, the question arises as to how to select and which to use in order of preference. Splenectomy is a well-established treatment and has been shown to improve the quality of life and prolong survival in this disease. However, if the spleen is small (less than 5 cm at rest below the costal margin) or non-palpable, the benefits of splenectomy are minimal, if any, and therefore this operation is not indicated. In the remaining patients, the long-term results depend on the degree of normalization of counts after splenectomy. If they become normal with few or no hairy cells in the blood films, then this good response may be prolonged. In about 20% of successfully splenectomized patients, the counts remain normal for many years and no other therapy is thus indicated. The results of splenectomy not only depend on the spleen size but, perhaps more importantly, on the degree of involvement of the bone marrow. If 80% or more of the bone marrow is infiltrated by hairy cells, the effect of splenectomy will be negligible or short lasting. Therefore, in the majority of patients, alternative treatment is necessary. Of these, DCF is still moderately experimental and is only available for special protocols. On the other hand, IFN-alpha is widely available and there has been considerable experience with its use accumulated over the last 3 years in the UK and elsewhere.

Although the exact mechanism of action of IFN-alpha in HCL is not known, this agent seems to act directly upon the hairy cells via specific receptors on the cell surface and not through the indirect mechanism of stimulating natural killer cell activity as previously suspected. IFN-alpha given in daily injections of 3 megaunits or in 3-weekly injections, induces a gradual and remarkable normalization of blood counts within the first 6 months of treatment, including: increase in Hb and platelets, rapid reduction of hairy cells in blood and gradually from the bone marrow, return of monocytes, and improvement of neutropenia. Neutrophils, however, may remain slightly subnormal in some patients whilst on therapy because of a known effect of IFN-alpha on granulopoiesis. In fact, this effect is currently being exploited in the treatment of CGL. The effect of IFN in HCL can be summarized as follows: complete responses in the blood counts obtained in at least 90% of patients; partial remission in the bone marrow in the majority (more than 50% reduction in the infiltration by hairy cells) and complete remission (no visible hairy cells) in 25–30% of cases; the degree of response and its durability depend on the duration of treatment—when this is prolonged (over 1 year and close to 2 years), the proportion of bone marrow complete remission is greater than 50%.

It is of interest that despite a complete remission, normal aspirates are not easy to obtain, at least for the first year. The duration of response once IFN-alpha is discontinued is variable, but blood counts may remain normal for well over a year in many patients. The tendency once therapy has ceased is to relapse slowly; retreatment is often possible. No evidence of resistance has been documented and few, if any, patients relapse during long-term maintenance with one or two injections a week.

Purified forms of IFN have been shown to be as effective as the original partially purified type. The three types of IFN-alpha currently available are human lymphoblastoid (Wellferon), recombinant IFN-alpha 2b (Intron), and recombinant IFN-alpha 2a (Roferon). Patients with a large spleen respond to IFN with regression of splenomegaly. However, the time to achieve an optimal response in these patients is, in our experience, significantly longer. Unless there is a contraindication to surgery, splenectomy should be the first line of attack, followed closely by IFN-alpha as soon as the blood parameters indicate progression. Age may be a contraindication to both splenectomy and IFN. It is possible, nevertheless, to obtain good responses with half or a third of the currently recommended doses of IFN, and also the metabolic and cerebral side-effects likely to affect the elderly can be minimized.

Just as the full benefits of IFN-alpha were beginning to be enjoyed by most patients, DCF, a drug previously used for T-ALL and other forms of T-cell leukaemia, was shown by Spiers *et al.* to have a remarkable effect in HCL. DCF is a potent inhibitor of adenosine deaminase (ADA), an enzyme of the purine metabolism. Early work used this drug to treat leukaemia with high levels of ADA. This required relatively high doses with consequent renal toxicity. Recent work has shown that DCF can be equally, or even more, effective when the cellular ADA concentrations are low. For this, lower doses (e.g. $4 \, mg/m^2$ weekly, intravenously) are sufficient and the toxicity is minimal. The responses to DCF appear as good or even better than those obtained with IFN-alpha. However, the side-effects and infective complications may be higher. Response rates as high as 91%, with over half being complete remissions (with aspirable bone marrow), have been reported and are obtained over 3–4 months, and, in the preliminary data available, may last well over 1 year unmaintained. In contrast to IFN-alpha, DCF seems to be moderately myelo- and immunosuppressive and the doses required for an optimal response with minimal toxicity have not been established. The initial treatment aggravates the cytopenia in the first 2 or 3 weeks and this may precipitate serious infection complications. Despite the good responses, five (15%) of the patients treated by Spiers *et al.* died of infectious complications, two others died of other causes, and three had life-threatening infections or related respiratory problems. This contrasts with the safety of IFN-alpha which, in my experience, can be given even in the presence of active infections.

It is likely that all the elements for an optimal strategy to treat HCL are now available. The optimal treatment will probably use the available three components to the patient's advantage. Splenectomy will still be an important debulking procedure. IFN-alpha will reduce the leukaemic mass and encourage normal haemopoiesis. DCF will complete the strategy by eliminating, with safety, the residual tumour mass.

Plasma Cell Leukaemia

Plasma cell leukaemia (PCL) is a rare but serious disease whose nosologic position in any classification is difficult. Morphological and immunological criteria indicate that the cells are at the end-stage of the B-cell maturation pathway. Clinically the disease is acute, with the combined problems of bone marrow failure and organomegaly plus the manifestations of myelomatosis—renal failure, hypercalcaemia and bone involvement. The diagnosis is often not easy to make and problems of recognition may delay treatment, followed by clinical deterioration.

Clinical and Laboratory Features

By definition, PCL is diagnosed when the number of identifiable plasma cells in the peripheral blood is greater than $2 \times 10^9/l$. In our series, the WBC counts ranged from $9 \times 10^9/l$ to $150 \times 10^9/$(median $56 \times 10^9/l$), with 50% or more of the circulating cells being of the plasma cell series. PCL occurs chiefly as a primary disease but sometimes as a terminal event of multiple myeloma (in less than 5% of cases).

Anaemia, thrombocytopenia and rising WBC are the main haematological features. The physical signs include hepatosplenomegaly; bone pain may be present but not frequently, and osteolytic lesions are not widespread. Laboratory features of myeloma are present in most cases—monoclonal band in the serum and/or free light chains in the urine. This is often associated with hypercalcaemia and high levels of serum creatinine and blood urea. Renal function is impaired as a result of the hypercalcaemia or the Bence–Jones proteinuria, or both. These clinical and laboratory features, sometimes aggravated by an intercurrent infection, make it essential to reach a diagnosis rapidly and to institute the appropriate therapy.

Diagnostic Criteria

Again, the clue for the diagnosis lies in the correct identification of the circulating cells as plasma cells in blood films. Three types of morphological appearances may be encountered: (i) lymphoplasmacytic cells, (ii) plasma cells, and (iii) plasmablasts.

Lymphoplasmacytic cells may deceptively resemble small lymphocytes and can only be recognized by a slight excess of basophilic cytoplasm and a moderately eccentric mature nucleus. Some of the cells have a prominent nucleolus, thus resembling prolymphocytes. Of the ten cases of primary PCL that we have studied in the last 5 years, two had the morphology and the markers (see below) of B-lymphocytes in transition to plasma cells. The rarity of this presentation and the fact that the main immunological markers of plasma cells were present justify their inclusion in the group of PCL.

Presentation with predominantly plasma cells is the most common (7/10 cases). However, these cells are not typical plasma cells; they tend to be smaller than bone marrow plasma cells and often present a range of features, from small lymphocytes and lymphoplasmacytic cells to typical plasma cells. Few are nucleolated; not rarely, the nucleus shows marked irregularity; binucleated cells are not rare either. The irregular nucleus, basophilic cytoplasm and moderate-size nucleolus may lead to confusion of these cells with the small cells of T-PLL. Care should be taken in interpreting the results of the marker studies as these plasma cells, like their normal counterparts, lack class II MHC antigens (Ia) in the membrane, most of the commonly tested B-cell antigens (CD 19, 20, 21), and also have negative SmIg (see Table 15.3). The typical combination of positive markers in PCL is: CD38(OKT10)+, CytIg+ (kappa or lambda) and reactivity with some recently recognized plasma-cell-associated antigens: PCA-1, BU11, Ri-3, etc. Some of the cases with lymphoplasmacytic cells may still retain some of the late B-markers, like FMC7 or SmIg, but are always CD38+, the main antigen of plasma cells.

A rare form of PCL (1/10) resembles an acute leukaemia; the cells are blasts and may or may not have some plasma cell characteristic recognized by light microscopy (plasmablasts). These cases may present major diagnostic problems as all the markers for blasts—(a) B lymphoblasts, Ia, CD19(B4), CD10, TdT; (b) T lymphoblasts, CD2, CD5, CD7, TdT; and (c) myeloid blasts, Ia, CD13(MY7), CD11b(OKM1), CD33(MY9), CD34(3C5, MY10)—are negative, except for CD38(OKT10) and CytIg, as stated above. Electron microscopy may be essential to clarify the diagnosis in some of these cases, particularly those with lymphoplasmacytic or plasmablastic features. This analysis will show the characteristic concentric arrays of rough endoplasmic reticulum, sometimes with dilated sacs containing immunoglobulin, and well-developed Golgi apparatus with early development of electron-dense lysosomal granules in its vicinity.

Bone marrow aspirates and trephine biopsies may be extremely useful because often they show more clearly than peripheral blood films the features of plasma cell differentiation.

Treatment

Management of PCL should be considered an emergency, as in cases of promyelocytic leukaemia. The problems of marrow and renal failure need urgent attention and do not improve until cytotoxic therapy is instituted. The poor outcome of PCL is largely related to treatment delays. Some patients do in fact respond promptly and extremely well to combination chemotherapy, e.g. CHOP (cyclophosphamide, doxorubicin, oncovin and prednisone), or other intensive protocols used in myelomatosis, e.g. ABCM (doxorubicin, BCNU, cyclophosphamide and melphalan) rather than to more conventional myeloma therapy with melphalan and prednisone. Some good prolonged responses have been reported with high-dose melphalan given as single agent intravenously ($140 \ mg/m^2$). Although some prolonged remissions (3–5 years) have been reported, PCL tends to relapse and become resistant. Obviously a curative approach may involve more intensive regimens, perhaps with rescue by bone marrow transplantation.

Follicular Lymphoma in Leukaemic Phase

The majority of patients with follicular lymphoma (FL) present with some degree of bone marrow involvement, which can be best recognized on trephine biopsies. A proportion of them present with lymphocytosis which often ranges from $5 \times 10^9/l$ to $20 \times 10^9/l$. Careful immunological markers, in particular the kappa:lambda ratio, could establish the existence of this clonal (leukaemic) lymphocytosis even when the WBC is normal or slightly raised. By extrapolation, one can argue that if frequently FL involves blood and bone marrow, the term follicular centre cell leukaemia could also be applicable. This would probably be confusing, as we know that FL is one of the most common NHLs, and the disease starts in the follicular centres of the affected lymph nodes. The term FL 'in leukaemic phase' is probably more adequate. The term leukaemia could be used with reservations to distinguish the less common cases which present with very high WBC, e.g. over $50 \times 10^9/l$.

Spiro *et al.* (1975) described the leukaemic phase of FL in a series of patients all of whom were well characterized histologically by Lennert. They distinguished two phenomena. The presentation of FL was associated with a lymphocytosis ($\geq 5 \times 10^9/l$) which superficially resembled CLL in 22.6% of cases, the highest WBC in the series being $30 \times 10^9/l$, and the less common terminal event in which cells resembling blasts (presumably centroblasts) are present with a clinical picture of disease progression, resembling an acute leukaemia. The moderate lymphocytosis, now well recognized in FL, is not necessarily associated with a poor prognosis, whereas the blastic phase is. More recently, we were able to identify a group of 10 patients also with a diagnosis of FL (centroblastic/centrocytic) but with presenting WBC of $40 \times 10^9/l$ or over (the highest was $220 \times 10^9/l$). These patients had florid disease, hepatosplenomegaly, generalized lymphadenopathy, marked bone marrow involvement and anaemia. This group probably represents the extreme leukaemic end of the clinical spectrum of FL. If one is not aware of this presentation, with very high WBC in FL, it can be mistakenly diagnosed as, for example, CLL or atypical lymphoid leukaemia.

Diagnostic Features

The morphology of the peripheral blood cells described by Galton as notched nuclei cells and by Lukes as small cleaved cells, can, in the majority of cases, be distinguished from B-CLL. Five cytological features need to be remembered: (i) the cells are of very small size, often smaller than normal blood lymphocytes; (ii) there is almost no visible cytoplasm and the N:C is high; (iii) the nuclear chromatin is smooth without clumps of heterochromatin (as in B-CLL) and without a visible or prominent nucleolus; (iv) the nuclear outline is not regular and has an angular shape; and (v) a high proportion of the lymphocytes have a deep and narrow nuclear indentation or cleft (Fig. 15.8), which, although it may not be easily visible in all cells by light microscopy, can be seen clearly under the electron microscope. Another difference between FL and B-CLL blood films is that smudge cells are not a feature of FL in leukaemic phase, nor of B-PLL.

Membrane marker studies are helpful in distinguishing the phenotype of these cells from that of B-CLL (see Table 15.3). Even in rare cases where the morphology of the peripheral blood or bone marrow is not typical (as described above), the membrane markers often show a B-cell proliferation very distinct from that of B-CLL: SmIg is strong, FMC7 and CD10 (CALLA) are often positive, and CD5 is, as a rule, negative; the number of M-rosettes is usually low and, even in the rare cases when these are positive, the percentage of rosettes rarely reaches 50%.

In addition to the above features, bone marrow histology may show a more predominant paratrabecular involvement, although this may not always be so in cases with WBC over $50 \times 10^9/l$. Lymph node histology is an essential investigation (Fig. 15.9): in low WBC cases and in those in which there is a clonal B-cell population in the peripheral blood, it allows the establishment of a definitive diagnosis. In high count cases or in those with markers suggestive of FL but without typical morphology (not many) lymph node histology can be used to confirm that the underlying disease is FL and not another B-cell tumour.

Treatment

The management of FL in leukaemic phase is no different from the primary treatment of this NHL. However, the disease appears to be more aggressive in those cases presenting with a high WBC. Thus, the conventional approach, with courses of the combination of COP (cyclophosphamide, oncovin and prednisolone) or chlorambucil and prednisolone, may not be sufficient. It is always worth starting with this approach and escalating further with the addition of doxorubicin (as in CHOP), intermediate or high doses of methotrexate, and bleomycin (as in M-BACOD).

Splenic B-cell Lymphoma with Circulating 'Villous' Lymphocytes

This NHL (SLVL), which is primarily a splenic lymphoma, evolves with a variable degree of peri-

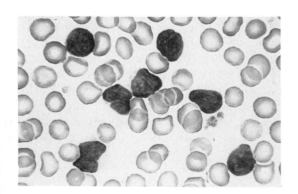

Fig. 15.8. *Peripheral blood film from a FL showing small lymphocytes with a deep nuclear cleft and almost complete absence of visible cytoplasm (× 1300).*

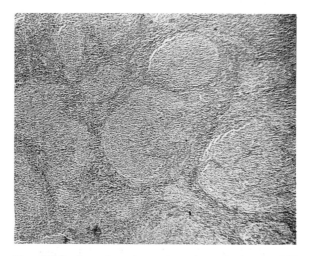

Fig. 15.9. *Lymph node section of a typical case of FL showing the marked ('giant') proliferation of follicular centres (× 60).*

pheral blood lymphocytosis and has now been recognized as a distinct disease entity. A number of reports in the last 10 years have called attention to a disorder which was frequently misdiagnosed as HCL but for which close examination showed that the circulating cells were not typical hairy cells, that the patients often had monoclonal spikes in the serum and, more importantly, that when splenic tissue was examined, it lacked the features considered typical of HCL (see above). We have recently analysed a series of 22 patients with SLVL (Melo, Hegde *et al.*, 1987) and have been able to define more precisely the features of this disease, which is probably more common than previously realized. SLVL has previously been described as 'spleno-megalic immunocytoma with circulating hairy cells', 'malignant lymphoma', and 'chronic lympho-proliferative disorder resembling leukaemic reticuloendotheliosis or HCL'.

Clinical and Laboratory Features

Patients are elderly (range 57–88 years, mean 72) and sometimes are diagnosed by chance on investigation for another complaint. The spleen is enlarged in the majority and is often massive (up to 27 cm below the costal margin). Lymphadenopathy, superficial or abdominal, is extremely rare. One-third of patients are anaemic (Hb below 110 g/l), but thrombocytopenia (less than 100 $\times$ 10^9/l) is even less common (4 of 20). Peripheral blood lymphocytosis is a constant feature; the WBC is often above 10 $\times$ 10^9/l (rarely, above 25 $\times$ 10^9/l), with over 50% lymphocytes in the majority of cases. The highest lymphocyte count in our series was 35 $\times$ 10^9/l. Two-thirds of patients have a monoclonal band in the serum (usually IgM, sometimes IgG), only in the urine as free light chains, or in both serum and urine. The serum band is always below 20 g/l, and this is important to distinguish SLVL from Waldenström's macroglobulinaemia which is a disorder within the same spectrum of lymphoplasmacytic NHL, or immunocytomas.

Diagnostic Criteria

The defining feature is the presence in blood films of a population of lymphocytes which are slightly larger than those of B-CLL, with a slightly high N:C ratio and an irregular plasma membrane outline with thin and short villi, usually confined to one pole of the cell (Fig. 15.10). The nucleus is often ovoid, has clumped chromatin and a visible nucleolus in half the cases. A small proportion of cells have more abundant cytoplasm and slightly longer cytoplasmic villi; these cells, if seen in isolation, resemble hairy cells. In addition, 5–10% of lymphocytes have more marked cytoplasmic basophilia, suggestive of lymphoplasmacytic differentiation. We have found no convincing evidence of TRAP positivity in these cases. However, some of the reports of SLVL in the literature suggest that TRAP-positive cells may be found in some.

Bone marrow is an important investigation, largely because it provides one of the main diagnostic tools to distinguish SLVL from HCL. Firstly, with few exceptions, it is nearly always possible to aspirate bone marrow fragments of good cellularity. Secondly, in half of the cases the films of this aspirate do not show an increase in lymphoid cells; in some of these, however, the bone marrow biopsy shows a nodular infiltrate but no infiltration in the others. An increase in lymphocytes of the same morphology as in the peripheral blood is shown in some of the aspirates. The core biopsy may show diffuse or patchy infiltration or a moderately nodular one. Lymph nodes are rarely available for diagnosis. On the other hand, spleen histology shows the main difference from HCL: as in other B-cell lymphoproliferative disorders, except HCL and HCL-variant, it shows variable white and red

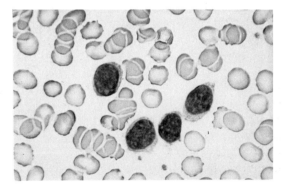

Fig. 15.10. *Blood film from a case of SLVL. The cells are smaller than hairy cells, and have less cytoplasm, which is slightly polarized and shows short villi (×1300).*

pulp involvement, with evidence of lymphoplasmacytic differentiation. In fact, in half of our cases, the white pulp was shown to be mainly involved and this corresponds to the other reports of SLVL cited in the literature.

Membrane marker studies, carried out on peripheral blood cell suspensions, show, as in other disorders of mature B-cells, strong SmIg stain, low M-rosettes, reactivity with McAb against Ia and B-cell antigens including CD19, 20, 22 as well as FMC7 (see Table 15.3). In some cases the plasmacytic differentiation is confirmed by the expression of CytIg as well as the CD38 antigen.

Differential Diagnosis

This should be considered in the context of other B-cell disorders with splenomegaly. Almost half of the cases referred to us had a presumptive diagnosis of HCL made by the referring physician; the other diagnosis considered in one-third of cases was B-CLL. This reflects the appearances of the circulating lymphocytes: when the 'villous' features are stressed, the first thought is HCL; when the villi are not so apparent, nor the condensed nuclear chromatin and the overall cell size, one can suspect the diagnosis of CLL. We have recently reclassified a case from atypical B-PLL to SLVL. The distinction from HCL is made by the cytology of blood films. Overall, the villi in SLVL are shorter, polarized and less marked; another very important difference is the N:C ratio, which is greater in SLVL. In addition, the lack of TRAP positivity, the histology of the bone marrow and some markers (negative CD25 and HC2) contribute to distinguish SLVL from HCL. The separation from HCL variant is a bit more difficult sometimes because the membrane phenotype is identical and the nucleolus may be prominent in the cells of some SLVL cases. The separation from B-CLL and B-PLL is made on clinical grounds, bone marrow histology, morphology, and markers (for B-CLL, not B-PLL). In addition, rarely, CLL lymphocytes and prolymphocytes show a significant degree of plasmamembrane irregularities or villi.

Natural History and Treatment

SLVL has a benign clinical course. No therapy may be required in a minority of patients for prolonged periods of time. When symptoms make treatment necessary, measures directed against the spleen seem to be beneficial, namely splenectomy or splenic irradiation. Low-dose continuous chlorambucil (4 mg/m² a day) or a high dose administered intermittently (60 mg/m² monthly, given over 3 days) may also be effective, although we have seen several patients in which this modality was ineffective. Treatment response can be monitored by the spleen size, blood counts and the size of the monoclonal band (if present).

T-CELL LEUKAEMIAS

The incidence of the various types of mature (post-thymic) T-cell leukaemias probably reflects the incidence of the different T-cell subsets in blood and haemopoietic tissues. For example, the most common phenotype encountered is CD4 +, which is the predominant subpopulation in the blood. On the other hand, very rare phenotypes, as seen in some examples of LGL-leukaemias, correspond to rare cell types. In fact, on occasion the discovery of such unusual leukaemias has helped to identify subsequently that particular T-cell subset in normal tissues. With the exception of most cases of LGL-leukaemia (or T-CLL) with the phenotype CD4 −, CD8 +, all other types of T-cell leukaemia have a relatively aggressive clinical course and represent a major challenge to find adequate treatment modalities.

T-Prolymphocytic Leukaemia

As soon as the early membrane markers became known in the 1970s, it became apparent that a significant minority (1 in 4) of cases presenting with high WBC, splenomegaly and prolymphocyte morphology, lacked SmIg and were instead forming rosettes with sheep erythrocytes (E-rosettes). In the last 10 years we have studied 42 cases of T-prolymphocytic leukaemia (T-PLL), which is probably the most common form of mature T-cell leukaemia. This is not generally acknowledged in the literature, partly because there is no uniform classification for these disorders and partly because T-PLL has some degree of heterogeneity when examined with cell markers and, despite its apparent uniform morphology, it has also enough variation in morphology to present some problems for diagnosis and classification. In close to 50% of cases, T prolymphocytes tend to resemble B prolymphocytes and are therefore easy to recognize in well-prepared blood films by their regular and round nuclear outline and a prominent nucleolus. In the other half of the cases, the T prolymphocytes tend to have an irregular shape (see Fig. 15.5). Furthermore, in 25% of cases the cells are small and the nucleolus may not be readily visible by light microscopy. Despite this variation, the disease tends to have a uniformly aggressive course and consistent clinical manifestations.

Clinical and Laboratory Features

T-PLL patients always present with a variety of symptoms of short duration. The main findings are splenomegaly (72%), hepatomegaly (42%) and generalized lymphadenopathy (55%). The last-mentioned plus the presence of skin lesions (but no erythroderma) (25%) and of serous effusions (20%), contrast with findings in B-PLL where these features are seen in less than 5% of patients.

Half of the patients are anaemic and thrombocytopenic at presentation. The majority have WBC over $100 \times 10^9/l$, which in two-thirds is over $200 \times 10^9/l$. The median WBC in our series was $230 \times 10^9/l$, ranging from $28 \times 10^9/l$ to $1000 \times 10^9/l$. Over 90% of the cells in the peripheral blood films have uniform morphology and correspond to prolymphocytes, which (as stated above) may show some variation from case to case. Serum immunoglobulins are normal.

Membrane markers are useful, primarily to establish the diagnosis of a T-cell rather than a B-cell malignancy. In 75% of cases, the phenotype is CD4+, CD8− (see Table 15.5). A distinct group of 16% of cases coexpressing CD4 and CD8 is seen almost uniquely in this disease. Different from the cells in T-lymphoblastic lymphoma, which may also be CD4+, CD8+, T prolymphocytes have a post-thymic phenotype—CD1−, TdT−. As noted above, the expression of other T-cell antigens is different in T-PLL than in the other CD4+ proliferations: namely, CD7(McAb 3A1, Leu9 or OKT16) is strongly positive in all cases (but rarely in ATLL and SS), and membrane CD3(OKT3,

UCHT1) is negative in 20% of cases (this is also important to bear in mind so as not to rely on this single marker to define T-cell nature).

Irrespective of the expression of membrane antigens, T-PLL cells are always, in our experience, strongly ANAE positive, with a distinct pattern of one or two large blocks of reaction product; DAPIV is positive except for the rare cases (6%) which are CD4−, CD8+.

Other investigations may be necessary according to the clinical features of the patient. Skin biopsy will show dense cellular infiltrates but without involving the epidermis, as in SS. The spleen histology shows red pulp or red and white pulp infiltration. In lymph nodes the neoplastic cells predominate in paracortical areas.

Differential Diagnosis

Morphologically, T-PLL should be distinguished from B-PLL, SS, ATLL and T-CLL. Without markers available, the cytochemical profile of strong reactions for acid hydrolases is suggestive of T rather than B-PLL. Some subtle morphological differences may also be apparent in Romanovsky-stained films: T prolymphocytes tend to be smaller, have a higher N:C ratio and more marked cytoplasmic basophilia than B prolymphocytes. The last-mentioned feature could be so marked in some cases that morphologically they may resemble PCL. In addition, the nucleolus may not be visible in all cases (and therefore requires ultrastructural confirmation) and the nuclear outline may be very irregular. In the latter instance, the possibility of ATLL or SS could arise. Other clinical features, some data of the markers, HTLV-I serology, skin histology, and ultimately electron microscopy may clarify the diagnosis of a particularly difficult case.

Rarely, T prolymphocytes may be interpreted as T lymphoblasts. In addition to age and other clinical features, the maturity of the phenotype is very important here.

Treatment

There is no well-established therapy for T-PLL. The disease runs a progressive course which, in the absence of a good response to therapy, leads to survival of less than 1 year. The median survival in our series is 6 months, no different from that of ATLL (5 months). However, it is apparent that the short survival results from an overall poor response to treatment in this disease, and therefore the emphasis is on searching for new treatment modalities. Some patients respond to courses of CHOP and may have a better outlook. Lately, we have observed partial and complete responses with DCF (Pentostatin) used in low doses of 4 mg/m^2 every week. Of interest is that the responses in these cases, as in other mature T-cell leukaemias, do not seem to correlate with high levels of ADA or morphology, but with membrane markers. Good responses have only been observed in cases with CD4+, CD8− phenotype.

Adult T-cell Leukaemia/Lymphoma

Independent discoveries by Gallo of the human T-cell leukaemia virus type I (HTLV-I), by Takatsuki *et al.* (1977), who first described adult T-cell leukaemia/lymphoma (ATLL, designated ATL), and by Hinuma *et al.* (1981) and Miyoshi *et al.* (1983) of C-type particles from an ATLL cell line, were key events in associating this T-cell malignant disease with its causative agent, HTLV-I. The disease was thought originally to be confined to Japan, where B-CLL and other B-cell disorders are uncommon, but it was later realized that Blacks of Caribbean origin, living in the islands of the Caribbean basin, or immigrants to Europe (UK, The Netherlands, etc.) have a disease identical to that prevalent in Japan. Virological and sero-epidemiological studies confirmed later the identity of the retrovirus in both geographical regions. The disease has now been reported in some areas of the USA (also mainly in people of Caribbean or African descent) and some countries of the north of South America. With one single exception, all cases recognized in the UK were in individuals born in the Caribbean basin, and who had been residents in this country for many years.

The disease has now been well characterized at clinical, histopathological, immunological and molecular biology level, and therefore it is a distinct and unique entity with a well-characterized aetiological agent. The neoplastic ATLL lymphocytes display a remarkable pleomorphism in size and nuclear shape, with a consistent CD4+ membrane pheno-

type (see Table 15.5). It is interesting that these CD4 + lymphocytes appear to have unique 'suppressor' properties and lack helper function in a pokeweed-induced system.

Clinical and Laboratory Features

ATLL has a spectrum of manifestation; the most common is classical or acute ATLL (65% of cases), the other components of the spectrum being smouldering ATLL (10% of cases), with minimal symptoms and signs, stable blood picture and some abnormal lymphocytes in the peripheral blood, and lymphoma-type of ATLL (25% of cases) with features of NHL but no obvious blood or bone marrow involvement. Patients with all these forms of ATLL have serum antibodies to HTLV-I, and monoclonal integration of HTLV-I proviral-DNA in the malignant T cells. The site of integration is, however, different between different cases. There are many more individuals in the affected regions with serum antibodies but no clinical abnormalities than there are patients with ATLL. This suggests that although the initial event is the infection by the retrovirus, a second or third event is necessary to cause the malignancy. This process of multistage leukaemogenesis is supported by the existence of a group of seropositive individuals (intermediate state of Yamaguchi) who have non-specific complaints and have a low, but detectable, proportion of circulating ATLL cells and show polyclonal integration of HTLV-I proviral DNA. Healthy carriers have fewer ATLL cells but polyclonal integration is not demonstrable (due to the small numbers). CD4+ ATLL-like cells can also be found in normal seronegative individuals by special immunoelectron microscopy. These cells may be the target for HTLV-I.

Features of acute ATLL are: lymphadenopathy (90%), hepatosplenomegaly (45%), skin lesions (35%), hypercalcaemia (70%), leukaemic blood picture ($> 10 \times 10^9/l$ abnormal lymphocytes, range $6–197 \times 10^9/l$; median $30 \times 10^9/l$) (80%). Patients present with acute symptoms and they are often very ill, with symptoms of severe hypercalcaemia. The latter seem to result from the activation of osteoclasts by a lymphokine secreted by ATLL cells, as suggested by studies of the bone marrow biopsy (and at post-mortem) which show disproportionate osteoclastic proliferation and bone absorption with little or no direct infiltration by ATLL cells.

Other findings are abnormal liver function tests (due to hepatic infiltration) in 50%, and anaemia and thrombocytopenia in only 30% (reflecting an extramedullary origin for the disease). Renal failure is rare and is secondary to the hypercalcaemia.

Diagnostic Criteria

The diagnosis of ATLL requires to take into account the clinical and laboratory features mentioned above as well as evidence of infection with HTLV-I (serum antibodies, or evidence for HTLV-I related proteins on the neoplastic cells or evidence of integration of HTLV-I proviral DNA; although

the latter is not a routine method). The morphology of the abnormal peripheral blood cells is characteristically multilobed, small to medium-sized lymphoid cells, with different shapes and degrees of nuclear irregularity (Fig. 15.11). The nuclear lobes have clear spaces between them which are visible by light microscopy. In Sezary cells the so-called cerebriform nucleus has deep nuclear indentations which are so narrow they are seen as clear spaces only by electron microscopy. ATLL cells have no visible azurophil granules and may or may not have a visible nucleolus. There are also larger, blastic-looking cells with basophilic cytoplasm, resembling transformed lymphocytes (Fig. 15.11c).

Marker studies (see Table 15.5) are helpful in defining the characteristics of ATLL cells. The main consistent difference between these and other neo-

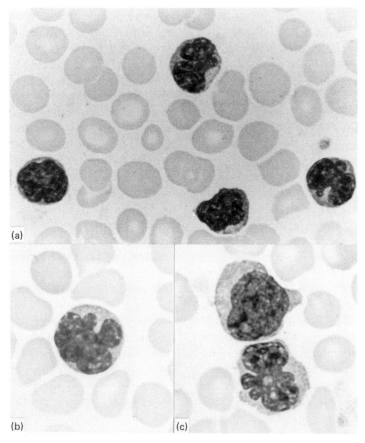

Fig. 15.11. *Composite of cells from three patients with ATLL (ABC). Cells in (a) are smaller and have more condensed chromatin. In (b) and (c) they are larger, and blastic in (b) (× 1200).*

plastic T cells is the expression of the receptor for interleukin-2, shown by the McAb anti-Tac (CD25) and the absence of the p40 antigen detected by McAb of the CD7 group (similar to SS cells). Marker studies may be performed on peripheral blood cells or on cryostat sections of affected lymph nodes. Lymph node histology is suggestive of a diagnosis of ATLL showing features of pleomorphic diffuse (mixed small and large cell) NHL, characteristics suggesting T-cells include proliferation of post-capillary venules. The histology of some cases may show a predominance of large cells and immunoblasts, thus resembling a large-cell NHL. In such cases, as in those showing changes resembling angioimmunoblastic lymphadenopathy, the lymph node histology alone is not diagnostic.

All these elements may be necessary to distinguish some atypical cases from T-PLL (the WBC in ATLL is rarely > 100×10^9/l), Sezary syndrome (ATLL has no erythroderma but occasionally the skin deposits may show epidermotropism), and other T-cell NHL (HTLV-I negative).

Treatment

Control and normalization of hypercalcaemia are only possible with combination chemotherapy which reduces the tumour bulk in ATLL. The overall treatment for ATLL has remained unsatisfactory and survival is short. Patients with smouldering ATLL or the rare chronic forms may remain static for some years and usually terminate in acute transformation. Combination chemotherapy (e.g. CHOP, M-BACOD) has claimed remissions, but these are short lived. DCF has achieved some complete remissions in one-third of patients, but no long follow-up data are available. Opportunistic infections, sometimes with bizarre organisms, are common in ATLL, and may affect patients with active disease or even in remission. ATLL is a good example of a well-characterized disease, even to the level of the aetiological agent where so far this knowledge has not helped in finding a cure.

Sezary Syndrome

Patients with Sezary syndrome (SS) present with exfoliate erythroderma and lymphomatous infil-

tration in the epidermis and upper dermis, affecting mainly the face, palms and soles. The presence of the characteristic cerebriform Sezary cells in peripheral blood films is a distinctive feature of this disease. Lymphadenopathy and splenomegaly may also be found. The closely related form of cutaneous T-cell lymphoma, mycosis fungoides, has cells of similar morphology in the skin lesions, which here constitute large plaques and multiple tumours.

Diagnostic Criteria

The key for the diagnosis is the identification of the typical Sezary cells. This may be difficult by light microscopy analysis and frequently requires electron microscopy for confirmation. Sezary cells have a highly convoluted nucleus with deep and narrow indentations. The ratio between the length of the longest indentation and that of the maximal nuclear diameter should be greater than 0.66 in at least 30% of cells (by ultrastructural analysis). Small-size Sezary cells seem to be more common than large SS cells. There are some overlapping features with ATLL cells, and therefore HTLV-I serology and the clinical and epidemiological features should be taken into account in the differential diagnosis. The skin biopsy shows infiltration in the epidermis with typical epidermotropism and the not infrequent feature of Pautrier microabscesses. These features are not seen in the skin deposits of T-PLL but may occasionally be seen in ATLL.

Bone marrow biopsy is not helpful for diagnosis except to show that it is not involved in the early phases of the disease. Infiltration by Sezary cells can be seen in advanced stages.

Treatment

Many forms of treatment have been used, including chemotherapy, local radiotherapy, electron therapy, DCF and the use of a photo-activable drug (8-methoxypsoralen) in combination with ultraviolet A light (PUVA). The last-mentioned has lately been applied by means of the extracorporeal activation of lymphocyte fractions outside the circulation (extracorporeal photopheresis) with encouraging results. It is not certain yet whether these new approaches will improve the prognosis of patients with SS.

T Chronic Lymphocytic Leukaemia

This designation refers to cases with persistent T lymphocytosis and neutropenia; some patients have an aggressive clinical course and these correspond to cases with cells of unusual or rare membrane phenotype. The defining feature of T chronic lymphocytic leukaemia (T-CLL) is the presence in the peripheral blood of increased numbers of mature lymphocytes with azurophil granules resembling large granular lymphocytes (LGL), as pointed out in the first report in 1975 by Brouet and colleagues from the Hospital Saint Louis. An alternative good designation, LGL-leukaemia, underlies (as in HCL and PLL) the morphology of the leukaemic cells. Other names given to this disease in the literature, such as chronic T-cell lymphocytosis, Tγ-lymphoproliferative syndrome, T-suppressor cell leukaemia or natural killer (NK) cell leukaemia, are less satisfactory, largely because they do not take into account the consistent feature of the cell morphology; the phenotype and function (very rarely of true NK cells) are, on the other hand, variable. Some of the above terms were used when the clonal nature of this disorder was in doubt because of the very benign and chronic evolution of the majority of cases. Lately, the techniques of molecular biology have shown that the T-cell receptor β-chain and/or γ-chain are rearranged in genuine cases of T-CLL. As discussed earlier, it is important that not all cases of T lymphocytosis should be considered as T-CLL.

Clinical and Haematological Features

A common feature of most cases is the presence of a persistent lymphocytosis without an obvious clinical cause. The WBC is only moderately raised ($5–25 \times 10^9$/l), with lymphocytes constituting 60–99% of the cells in the differential count. Rarely, the WBC is low and the T lymphocytosis with LGL only becomes manifest following the removal of a large spleen. Neutropenia (neutrophils $< 1.0 \times 10^9$/l) is a feature in 85% of cases; other patients also have moderate anaemia (Hb 90–110 g/l) and a few, thrombocytopenia. The Hb level is very low (50–80 g/l) in cases with pure red cell aplasia. The cytopenia usually affects mainly one of the bone marrow series.

The mean age of T-CLL patients is 50 years but the range is very wide; in our series (Newland et al., 1984), it was from 4 to 78 years. On the whole, very young patients are rare. The clinical presentation relates to which bone marrow lineage is affected. Neutropenia, the most common, is associated with malaise, fever and recurrent infections, although these are rarely severe; mouth ulcers are a manifestation in some patients. The anaemia, when marked, is aregenerative with low reticulocyte counts and very few erythroid precursors in the bone marrow. The direct antiglobulin test is often negative and there is no evidence of platelet antibodies, although cases with antibodies against erythrocytes or platelets have been reported. Antibodies against granulocytes have also been reported in some patients but this has not been the general experience.

The bone marrow findings are often non-diagnostic; in general, there is a moderate degree of lymphocyte infiltration (between 40% and 50%) which tends to progress slowly over the years. The biopsies show diffuse or focal infiltration. Despite the cytopenia, there is active haemopoiesis with 'maturation arrest'; erythroid precursors are absent in the cases of erythroaplasia. Megakaryocyte numbers are normal or increased in cases of thrombocytopenia.

There is a variable degree of splenomegaly in well over half of the cases; in some, the spleen may become very large (greater than 10 cm below the costal margin). There is no laboratory evidence of hypersplenism. This is further supported by the lack of response to splenectomy. Hepatomegaly is found in some and abnormal liver function tests are seen in 20% of cases relating to the degree of hepatic cell infiltration.

One-third of cases in our series had serological and clinical evidence for rheumatoid arthritis, i.e. bilateral small joint polyarthritis and positive rheumatoid factor, respectively. This has been also recorded by others (Loughran et al., 1985). The incidence of this association is close to 25%. Several of these patients have been diagnosed as suffering from Felty's syndrome because of the combination of splenomegaly, neutropenia and positive rheumatoid factor. In classic Felty's syndrome the neutropenia follows many years of rheumatoid arthritis and there is no increase in LGL. In this atypical form of Felty's syndrome associated with T-CLL, both features tend to appear at the same time. In addition to rheumatoid factor, evidence for other circulating immune complexes, antinuclear antibodies and increased Clq binding has been documented in a number of patients. Exceptionally, there is hypogammaglobulinaemia and the pathogenesis of this, as that of the cytopenias, relates to the inherent function of the expanded clone of T lymphocytes.

In a minority of patients the disease has a more aggressive course, with rising WBC counts and organomegaly; this corresponds to cases with a rare membrane phenotype (see below) and it is likely that the disease in this group is clinically and biologically quite different from that in those with the common T-CLL phenotype.

Membrane Phenotype

The proliferating cells of T-CLL correspond to T lymphocytes with Fc receptors for IgG (Tγ-lymphocytes) and cytotoxic potential (antibody-dependent cytotoxicity or killer cell function). Despite the relatively uniform morphology (in over 90% of cases) and function (in 60–70% of cases), the membrane phenotype of T-CLL cells is heterogeneous, reflecting both the existence of different types of LGL Tγ-cells and, perhaps, the cells at different stages of maturation.

The most common phenotype (see Table 15.5) is CD2+, CD3+, CD4−, CD8+, also frequently Leu7+ and CD5−; class II MHC antigens (Ia) may be occasionally expressed in these CD4−, CD8+ lymphocytes of T-CLL. Markers of mature natural killer (NK) function (cytotoxicity not mediated by antibodies), CD11b(OKM1) and CD16 (Leu11), are not expressed in cases with the common phenotype and this correlates well with the lack of NK function by these cells. Interestingly, in the cases with unusual phenotypes and expression of CD11b or CD16, NK function is also often negative. NK function has only been demonstrated in a few cases in which the only T characteristic of the T-CLL cells was the expression of receptors for sheep erythrocytes (CD2+), with all other T antigens, including CD3, not expressed.

Two types of unusual phenotypes are seen: those expressing CD4 and others expressing CD8. These usually represent the expansion of corresponding rare normal T subsets, such as CD4+, CD8−, CD11b+, CD16+, Leu7−, or CD4+, CD8−, CD11b−, CD16−, Leu7+, or CD4−, CD8+, CD11b+, CD16−. Recently we have seen a case with CD4+, CD8+, CD11b+, CD16−, Leu7+, lymphocytes.

The majority of cases with the common and unusual phenotypes have been shown to be clonal proliferations of T cells. This has been demonstrated in some by the presence of karyotypic abnormalities and in the majority by the demonstration of rearrangement of the T-cell receptor β and γ chain genes. The failure to demonstrate rearrangement of the β-chains is not sufficient evidence to rule out clonality as we have shown recently in a case with CD3+, CD4−, CD8+ cells in which the T-cell receptor γ and δ chain genes, but not the β chain genes, were shown to be rearranged. These cells seem to correspond to a normal T-cell subset which, despite the expression of the CD3 antigen, does not rearrange the gene for the β-chains of the T-cell receptor.

Differential Diagnosis

The main problem is linking the T lymphocytosis with the patient's cytopenia(s). Close examination of blood films will disclose the uniform population of LGL with eccentric mature nucleus, low N:C ratio, prominent Golgi zone and the presence of abundant azurophil granules in the cytoplasm. Often these granules are coarse. In most cases they correspond to lysosomal granules and to distinct structures known as parallel tubular arrays (PTA). These are also seen in normal Tγ-lymphocytes with a similar phenotype to T-CLL cells. In only two of the cases we have studied, which corresponded to rare phenotypes, the cells had granular structures but not PTA at ultrastructural level.

The bone marrow examination may help exclude other causes of cytopenia with splenomegaly. Sometimes the T lymphocytosis becomes more manifest after splenectomy. The key to the diagnosis is the identification of the LGL as the cause of the cytopenia. The lymphocytosis needs to be persistent ($\geq 5 \times 10^9$/l for at least 3 months and preferably 6 months) and to have cells of uniform phenotype. Reactive T lymphocytosis, including those cases seen non-specifically after splenectomy, may have a relative increase in CD8+ cells; however, there are usually numerous other lymphoid cells (e.g. CD4+) which make the diagnosis of T-CLL unlikely. Splenectomy rarely corrects the neutropenia, thus hypersplenism can be excluded by this procedure. Examination of the spleen histology shows moderate to marked lymphocytic infiltration of the red pulp with prominent germinal centres and some epithelioid granuloma. Liver biopsy (in cases with abnormal function tests) show portal tract and sinusoidal lymphocytic infiltration as well as granuloma formation.

Pathogenesis of the Cytopenia

This problem has attracted the attention of several groups. Despite the splenomegaly, hypersplenism has no major role in causing the cytopenia in T-CLL. Two main lines of evidence have emerged. One, not supported by many studies, relates the selective neutropenia to the existence of antibodies against neutrophils or other blood components. The bone marrow is never sufficiently heavily infiltrated to account for the low peripheral blood counts. Rarely, antibodies to platelet or to erythrocytes (direct antiglobulin test in one case with haemolysis) are thought to be the cause of the cytopenia. Stronger evidence, although not always supported by experimental results, suggests that the neoplastic T cells cause suppression of erythropoiesis (in cases with red cell hypoplasia) or granulopoiesis (inhibition of CFU–GM growth shown in some cases) and that the main pathogenetic mechanism of the cytopenia is the cell-mediated suppression of normal haemopoiesis.

Treatment

Although the course is benign in two-thirds of cases, the presence of neutropenia or anaemia makes it necessary to correct this abnormality. Splenectomy has been carried out in patients with an enlarged spleen with only moderate benefit. Corticosteroids alone or in combination with alkylating agents (cyclophosphamide or chlorambucil) or methotrexate have achieved prolonged complete remissions in some patients. These measures will not suffice for cases with aggressive forms of T-CLL. Other forms

of more intensive therapy may be required; in our hands, CHOP has not been very successful. One case with the phenotype CD4+, CD8−, CD11b+ responded twice with prolonged remissions to DCF, but this therapy did not affect the course of a case with CD4−, CD8+, CD11b+ cells.

CONCLUSIONS

It is apparent that the chronic lymphoid leukaemias and their related leukaemia/lymphoma syndromes constitute a heterogeneous group of distinct clinicopathological entities. Careful use of simple laboratory methods, in particular the morphology of the circulating lymphoid cells, detailed clinical history and physical examination, and the use of some selective specialized investigations, will allow the recognition of the most common of these disorders and lead to a suspicion of the rare ones. Bone marrow aspirates and trephine biopsies play an essential part in the investigative procedures. A precise diagnosis and the correct disease classification are likely to improve the results of treatment and will facilitate the analysis of new therapeutic modalities which may be more effective in some diseases than in others. The recently discovered therapeutic agents of IFN-alpha and DCF are good examples of the advantage of an accurate pathological and immunological characterization of the lymphoid neoplasias.

SELECTED BIBLIOGRAPHY

Binet J. L., Auquier A., Dighiero G., Chastang C., Piguer H., Goasguen J. *et al.* (1981). A new prognostic classification of chronic lymphocytic leukemia derived from a multivariate survival analysis. *Cancer*, **48**, 198–206.

Brito-Babapulle V., Pittman S., Melo J. V., Pomfret M., Catovsky D. (1987). Cytogenetic studies on prolymphocytic leukemia. I. B cell prolymphocytic leukemia. *Hematologic Pathology*, **1**, 27–33.

Brouet J-C., Flandrin G., Sasportes M., Preud'Homme J. L., Seligmann M. (1975). Chronic lymphocytic leukaemia of T-cell origin; an immunological and clinical evaluation of eleven patients. *Lancet*, **ii**, 890–893.

Catovsky D. (1977). Hairy cell leukaemia and prolymphocytic leukaemia. *Clinics in Haematology*, **6**, 245–268.

Catovsky D. (1987). Cytogenetic studies on prolymphocytic leukemia I.B. cell prolymphocytic leukemia. *Hematologic Pathology*, **1**, 27–33.

Catovsky D., Greaves M. F., Rose M., Galton D. A. G., Goolden A. W. G., McCluskey D. R. *et al.* (1982). Adult T-cell lymphoma–leukaemia in blacks from the West Indies. *Lancet*, **i**, 639–643.

Catovsky D., Melo J. V., Matutes E. (1985). Biological markers in lymphoproliferative disorders. In *Chronic and acute leukemias in adults*, pp. 69–112 (Ed. C. D. Bloomfield). Boston: Martinus Nijhoff.

Dameshek W. (1967). Chronic lymphocytic leukemia— an accumulative disease of immunologically incompetent lymphocytes. *Blood*, **29**, 556–584.

Enno A., Catovsky D., O'Brien M., Cherchi M., Kumaran T. O., Galton D. A. G. (1979). 'Prolymphocytoid' transformation of chronic lymphocytic leukaemia. *British Journal of Haematology*, **41**, 9–18.

Foon K., Gale R. P. (1988). Chronic lymphocyte leukaemia. In: *Recent advances in haematology*, Vol. 5, (Ed. A. V. Hoffbrand). Edinburgh: Churchill Livingstone.

Gallo R. C. (1986). The first human retrovirus. *Scientific American*, **255**, 78–88.

Galton D. A. G. (1966). The pathogenesis of chronic lymphocytic leukemia. *Canadian Medical Association Journal*, **94**, 1005–1010.

Galton D. A. G., Goldman J. M., Wiltshaw E., Catovsky D., Henry K., Goldenberg J. (1974) Prolymphocytic leukaemia. *British Journal of Haematology*, **27**, 7–23.

Greaves M. F., Verbi W., Tilley R., Lister T. A., Habeshaw J., Guo H-G. *et al.* (1984). Human T-cell leukaemia virus (HTLV) in the United Kingdom. *International Journal of Cancer*, **33**, 795–806.

Hinuma Y. *et al.* (1981). Adult T-cell leukaemia antigen in an ATL cell line and detection of antibody to the antigen in human sera. *Proceedings of the National Academy of Sciences*, **78**, 6476–6480.

International Workshop on CLL (1981). Chronic lymphocytic leukaemia: proposals for a revised prognostic staging system. *British Journal of Haematology*, **48**, 365–367.

Lewis F. B., Schwartz R. S., Dameshek W. (1966). X-radiation and alkylating agents as possible 'trigger' mechanisms in the autoimmune complications of malignant lymphoproliferative disease. *Clinical and Experimental Immunology*, **i**, 3–11.

Loughran T. P. Jr, Kadin M. E., Starkebaum G., Abkowitz J. L., Clark E. A., Disteche C. *et al.* (1985). Leukemia of large granular lymphocytes: association with clonal chromosomal abnormalities and autoimmune neutropenia, thrombocytopenia, and hemolytic anemia. *Annals of Internal Medicine*, **102**, 169–175.

Matutes E., Garcia Talavera J., O'Brien M., Catovsky D. (1986). The morphological spectrum of T-prolymphocytic leukaemia. *British Journal of Haematology*, **64**, 111–123.

Melo J. V., Catovsky D., Galton D. A. G. (1986). The relationship between chronic lymphocytic leukaemia and prolymphocytic leukaemia. I. Clinical and laboratory features of 300 patients and characterisation of an intermediate group. *British Journal of Haematology*, **63**, 377–387.

Melo J. V., Catovsky D., Gregory W. M., Galton D. A. G. (1987). The relationship between chronic lymphocytic leukaemia and prolymphocytic leukaemia. IV. Analysis of survival and prognostic features. *British Journal of Haematology*, **65**, 23–29.

Melo J. V., Hegde U., Parreira A., Thompson I., Lampert I. A., Catovsky D. (1987). Splenic B-cell lymphoma with circulating 'villous' lymphocytes: differential diagnosis of B-cell leukaemias with a large spleen. *Journal of Clinical Pathology*, **40**, 642–651.

Melo J. V., Wardle J., Chetty M., England J., Lewis S. M., Galton D. A. G. *et al.* (1986). The relationship between chronic lymphocytic leukaemia and prolymphocytic leukaemia. III. Evaluation of cell size by morphology and volume measurements. *British Journal of Haematology*, **64**, 469–478.

Miyoshi I. *et al.* (1983). Transmission of Japanese monkey type C virus to human lymphocytes. *Lancet*, **ii**, 166–167.

Montserrat E., Sanchez–Bison O. J., Vinolas N., Rozman C. (1986). Lymphocyte doubling time in chronic lymphocytic leukaemia: analysis of its prognostic significance. *British Journal of Haematology*, **62**, 567–575.

Newland A. C., Catovsky D., Linch D., Cawley J. C., Beverley P., San Miguel J. F. *et al.* (1984). Chronic T cell lymphocytosis: A review of 21 cases. *British Journal of Haematology*, **58**, 433–446.

Nowell P. C., Vonderheid E. C., Besa E., Hoxie J. A., Moreau L., Finan J. B. (1986). The most common chromosome change in 86 chronic B cell or T cell tumours: A 14q32 translocation. *Cancer Genetics and Cytogenetics*, **19**, 219–227.

Parreira A., Robinson D. S. F., Melo J. V., Ayliffe M., Ball S., Hegde U. *et al.* (1985). Primary plasma cell leukaemia: immunological and ultrastructural studies in 6 cases. *Scandinavian Journal of Haematology*, **35**, 570–578.

Pittman S., Catovsky D. (1984). Prognostic significance of chromosome abnormalities in chronic lymphocytic leukaemia. *British Journal of Haematology*, **58**, 649–660.

Rai K. R., Sawitsky A., Cronkite E. P., Chanana A. D., Levy R. N., Pasternack B. S. (1975). Clinical staging of chronic lymphocytic leukemia. *Blood*, **46**, 219–234.

Rozan C., Monsterrat E., Rodriguez–Fernandez J. M., Aytas R., Vallespi T., Parody R. *et al.* (1984). Bone marrow histologic pattern—the best single prognostic parameter in chronic lymphocytic leukemia: A multivariate survival analysis of 329 cases. *Blood*, **64**, 642–648.

Spiers A. S. D. *et al.* (1987). Remissions in hairy-cell leukemia with Pentostatin (2'-deoxycoformycin). *New England Journal of Medicine*, **316**, 825.

Spiro S., Galton D. A. G., Wiltshaw E., Lohmann R. C. (1975). Follicular lymphoma: A survey of 75 cases with special reference to the syndrome resembling chronic lymphocytic leukaemia. *British Journal of Cancer*, **31**, Suppl. II, 60–72.

Takatsuki K., Uchiyama J., Sagawa K., Yodoi J. (1977). Adult T-cell leukaemia in Japan. In *Topics in haematology*, pp. 73–77 (Eds. S. Seno, F. Takaku, S. Imino). Amsterdam: Excerpta Medica.

The T- and B-cell Malignancy Study Group (1985). Statistical analyses of clinico-pathological, virological and epidemiological data on lymphoid malignancies with special reference to adult T-cell leukemia/lymphoma: A report of the second nationwide study of Japan. *Japanese Journal of Clinical Oncology*, **15**, 517–535.

Uchiyama T. (1988). Adult T-cell leukemia. *Blood Reviews*, **2**, 232–238.

Uchiyama T., Yodoi J., Sagawa K., Takatsuki K., Uchino H. (1977). Adult-T-cell leukemia: clinical and hematological features of 16 cases. *Blood*, **50**, 481–491.

Chapter 16

CHRONIC MYELOID LEUKAEMIA

J. M. GOLDMAN

DEFINITIONS

The term chronic myeloid leukaemia (CML), usually used interchangeably with the terms chronic granulocytic leukaemia, chronic myelogenous leukaemia and chronic myelocytic leukaemia, describes a relatively well-defined disease characterized in most cases by insidious onset of ill-health in association with increasing splenomegaly and leucocytosis that leads inexorably in most cases to death after a number of years. Standard treatment is usually effective in alleviating symptoms but does not prolong life. It has been proposed that the term chronic granulocytic leukaemia should be reserved for patients with clinically and haematologically typical disease whose myeloid cells have a Philadelphia chromosome, and that the term chronic myeloid leukaemia be used generically to include the classical and the atypical forms of the disease. However, this proposal has not yet gained general acceptance. Other forms of CML are listed in Table 16.1.

CHRONIC MYELOID LEUKAEMIA

Epidemiology

Chronic myeloid leukaemia (CML) occurs with an annual incidence of about 1 case per 100 000 of the population. This incidence appears to be constant worldwide. Males are affected slightly more often than females (ratio 1.4:1). The diagnosis is made most commonly in patients in the fifth and sixth decades of life, but CML can occur at both extremes of life, in neonates and in very old persons. In most

Table 16.1
Classification of the chronic myeloid leukaemias

Chronic myeloid leukaemia (Ph positive)
Chronic myeloid leukaemia (Ph negative)
Juvenile chronic myeloid leukaemia
Chronic neutrophilic leukaemia
Eosinophilic leukaemia
Chronic myelomonocytic leukaemia

cases there are no known predisposing causes. The incidence of CML was significantly increased in those who survived following exposure to radiation from the atomic bomb explosions at Hiroshima and Nagasaki, but for most patients radiation plays no definite role in causation. Likewise, toxic chemicals implicated in the aetiology of other forms of leukaemia do not apparently predispose to CML. No viruses have been associated with CML, although the apparent role of the *ABL* oncogene isolated originally from a murine leukaemia virus will be discussed below.

Pathogenesis

What is known of the pathogenesis of CML can be considered most conveniently in chronological sequence (see Chapter 13). In 1960, Nowell and Hungerford, working in Philadelphia, reported that myeloid cells from patients with CML showed a deletion of portions of the long arms of one member of the G group of chromosomes. This was subsequently shown to involve the G group pair other than the pair implicated in Down's syndrome (trisomy 21) and was thus designated 22. The abnormal chromosome was called the Philadelphia, or Ph[1], chromosome. In 1973, Janet Rowley examined banded preparations of chromosomes from CML patients and noted that cells with the Ph[1] chromosome had elongation of the long arms of one member of the number 9 pair of chromosomes. Later it became clear that the Ph[1] chromosome was the result of reciprocal translocation of genetic material between chromosomes 9 and 22, an event designated t(9;22). Until recently it was still uncertain whether the Ph[1] chromosome played an important role in the pathogenesis of CML or whether it was merely a convenient marker for the leukaemic cell. Very recently it has been suggested that the superscript '1' should be dropped and the chromosomal abnormality designated simply 'Ph'.

It has become clear that the exchange of genetic material between chromosomes 9 and 22 involves reciprocal translocations of the proto-oncogenes *ABL* (from number 9 to number 22) and *SIS* (from number 22 to number 9) (see Chapter 13). The *SIS* oncogene is situated a considerable distance away from the breakpoint on chromosome 22 and there is no evidence of altered *SIS* expression in CML cells. In contrast, *ABL* on the Ph chromosome comes into close juxtaposition with the 5' portion of the *BCR* gene and a hybrid gene consisting partly of *BCR* and partly of *ABL* sequences is expressed in leukaemic cells from patients with CML (Fig. 16.1). The precise function of the *BCR–ABL* gene product, a P210 with tyrosine kinase activity, is not known, but one may speculate that it is capable in some way of perturbing the mechanisms that control the proliferation of haemopoietic stem cells. If this is so, it would be strong evidence that the Ph chromosome and the translocation of *ABL* play a central role in the pathogenesis of CML.

Chronic myeloid leukaemia is commonly re-

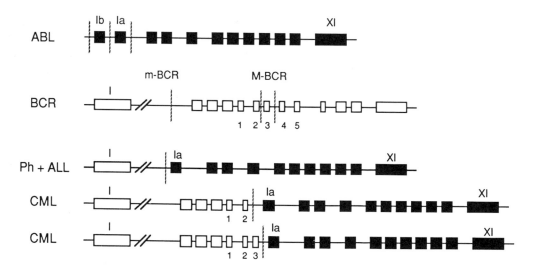

Fig. 16.1. *Schematic representation of the BCR and ABL genes showing known exons (indicated as boxes); introns are shown as lines. Either exon Ib or exon Ia of ABL gene is spliced to the second ABL exon. The arabic numerals below the BCR gene identify the exons within the classical breakpoint cluster region. Representative positions for the breakpoints in CML and Ph-positive ALL are shown as vertical dashed lines. In the current nomenclature the breakpoint cluster region involved in CML is known as the major breakpoint cluster region (M–BCR) and the region of the first intron on the BCR gene involved in Ph-positive ALL is known as the minor breakpoint cluster region (m–BCR). The breakpoint in m–BCR gives rise to the fused gene Ph+ ALL (below), and the two different breakpoints in M–BCR give rise to the two genes with slightly different linkages characteristic of CML.*

garded as a clonal disease arising in a single pluri-potential haemopoietic stem cell which acquires a growth advantage that permits its progeny to pro-liferate steadily and to usurp normal 'non-clonal' haemopoiesis. The evidence in favour of this con-cept is derived mainly from consideration of the distribution of the Ph chromosome and enzymatic markers and is thus only circumstantial, but is compelling nonetheless. Thus, the Ph chromosome is found not only in cells of the granulocytic lineage but also in monocytes and in erythroid and mega-karyocytic progenitors that can be cultured in vitro. Some B lymphocytes also carry a Ph chromosome, as do probably a minority population of T lympho-cytes. These findings suggest that the target cell for the critical leukaemic transformation is a stem cell. Study of black female patients heterozygous for the two X-linked isoenzymes of glucose-6-phosphate dehydrogenase provides additional support. The normal somatic cells from such patients all express either isoenzyme A or isoenzyme B as a result of random X-chromosome inactivation in embryo-genesis. However, their leukaemic cells prove all to be either of one or the other isoenzyme type but never of both, again implying that the leukaemia originated in a single cell. Other evidence, however, suggests that the development of CML may involve a multistep process, in which the acquisition of the Ph chromosome may not necessarily be the first event.

At diagnosis, a patient's total circulating granulo-cyte count is typically increased by a factor of 5 to 50. This reflects an increase in the body's total granulocyte mass that may range from 5- to 30-fold. The numbers of myeloid progenitor cells (CFU–GM, BFU–E, CFU–Mk and CFU–mix) are also very greatly increased in comparison with normal in the peripheral blood and to a lesser extent in the marrow. All the progenitor cells carry the Ph chromosome. At the cytokinetic level it seems that CML develops as a result of a pheno-typic change acquired by the stem cell that then replicates excessively and produces vast numbers of more differentiated progeny. This expanding leuk-aemic cell population apparently has the ability to suppress haemopoiesis by residual normal leuk-aemic stem cells, for few if any Ph-negative meta-phases can be detected in the marrow of newly diagnosed patients; however, such cells must still be present in G_0 and can in certain circumstances be induced to proliferate.

Clinical Features

In most patients, CML is a biphasic or triphasic disease. The initial chronic phase may last for some years without change, but ultimately it either changes abruptly to an acute or blastic transform-ation or, more commonly, it evolves slowly into a phase of acceleration that in turn progresses to transformation. The patient in chronic phase typic-ally presents with lethargy and other symptoms of anaemia or may have noted increasing abdominal discomfort due to splenomegaly. Increased sweat-ing and moderate weight loss are common, but fever as a presenting feature for patients in chronic phase is rarer. Occasionally, spontaneous bleeding or bruising without obvious trauma is the first feature that leads to a diagnosis of CML. Rarer symptoms include non-specific visual disturbances due to hy-perviscosity, deafness or priapism. In developed countries where blood tests are carried out rou-tinely for many purposes, including for regular medical examinations, before blood donation and during pregnancy, 20–30% of patients are totally without symptoms when the diagnosis is made.

The principal physical sign at diagnosis is spleno-megaly (Fig. 16.2). About 10–15% of patients have impalpable spleens, but in the remainder the spleen may range from being just palpable below the left costal margin to being so enormous as to occupy the bulk of the abdomen anteriorly. The lower border may then be palpable in the right iliac fossa. The liver is enlarged in about 50% of cases but its lower edge is usually smooth. A small proportion of patients at diagnosis have generalized lymphadeno-pathy, which does not necessarily indicate that the disease has already transformed.

Patients frequently ask the haematologist how long their leukaemia was present before diagnosis. This question is essentially unanswerable since the point at which the disease begins cannot be defined. However, recent studies have suggested that a routine blood test performed 3–9 months before the actual diagnosis would have established the diag-nosis of CML in about half the patients; conversely, patients who are asymptomatic at diagnosis may develop symptoms within 3–12 months if untreated.

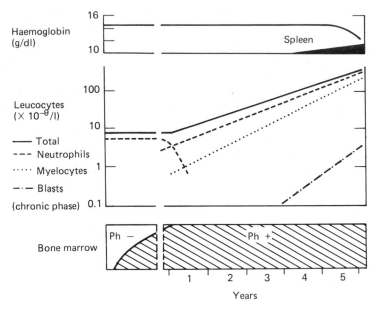

Fig. 16.2. *Schematic representation of the evolution from initial event to estab-lished chronic phase in a patient with Ph-positive chronic myeloid leukaemia. The scheme shows the insidious replacement of the marrow by the Ph-positive clone, gradually rising leucocyte count, onset of splenic enlargement, and eventual fall in the haemoglobin level.*

Course of Disease

The median duration of chronic phase disease is 3.5 years but the range is wide, varying in individual patients from 1 to more than 10 years. It might be logical to imagine that appropriate treatment that reduces the patient's leucocyte count would pro-long survival, but in practice no form of treatment (other than bone marrow transplantation) has any effect on the duration of survival. A number of attempts have been made to establish criteria that might predict the duration of survival in individual patients (Table 16.2). In general, patients with large spleens, high leucocyte counts or low haemoglobin concentrations at diagnosis may fare somewhat less well than patients with impalpable spleens, rela-

Table 16.2
Prognostic features assessed at diagnosis, based on retrospective analysis of groups of patients with Ph-positive chronic myeloid leukaemia

Series	Patient numbers	Sex	Clinical grade	Spleen size	Liver size	WBC	Plate-lets	Haemo-globin	Blast cell numbers
Italian	255	−	−	+	+	+	+	−	+
UK	169	−	+	+	−	+	−	+	−
Spanish	107	−	−	+	+	−	−	−	+
International	625	+	−	+	−	−	+	+	+

Ph-negative patients were included in the Italian series but excluded from the other series.
+ indicates that this feature assessed at diagnosis was considered to influence prognosis, while − means that for this feature no influence on prognosis was discernible.

tively low leucocyte counts or normal haemoglobin values, but the actual differences are not great; thus, patients classified in a good prognosis category may have a median survival of 5.5 years and those in a poor prognosis category may have a median survival of only 2.5 years. Another possibly useful index that may correlate with survival is the tempo of the disease as measured by the response to treatment. Thus patients who have a low requirement for cytotoxic drugs, illustrated, for example, by the fact that their leucocyte count remains within the normal range for some months or even years after a single course of busulphan, may survive longer than those who need continuous treatment for control of symptoms and leucocyte counts.

The patient may or may not have symptoms when the disease begins to accelerate. The accelerated phase defies precise definition, but some of the criteria that may lead the clinician to conclude that the patient is no longer in the uncomplicated chronic phase of the disease but not yet in frank transformation are listed in Table 16.3. With appropriate treatment a patient may remain in the accelerated phase without symptoms for a number of months and occasionally for more than a year. Sooner or later, however, a blastic phase or life-threatening marrow failure supervenes.

An acute transformation or blastic phase of CML can occur precipitously in a patient who was until days earlier undoubtedly in the chronic phase. More commonly, the evolution from chronic phase to acute transformation proceeds over weeks or months and the point of transition cannot be specified precisely. Nevertheless, blast transformation is often arbitrarily defined by the presence of more than 30% of blast cells or blasts plus promyelocytes in the blood or marrow. At this stage the patient may or may not be unwell. Symptoms when present include fever, sweats, weight loss, bone pain that may be generalized or localized to one or two sites, and pain in the splenic area, which may be pleuritic. The patient may show an increased bleeding tendency or have symptoms attributable mainly to the effects of anaemia. Occasionally patients have multiple subcutaneous nodules or generalized lymphadenopathy. Symptoms of hyperviscosity due to intracerebral or intrapulmonary leucostasis are sometimes present. Very occasionally, patients may present in blastic transformation with symptoms of disease in the central nervous system, including features of raised intracranial pressure or focal neurological signs. More commonly, such features develop after temporarily successful efforts to control a lymphoid medullary transformation.

Haematology and Other Laboratory Investigations

The leucocyte count when CML is diagnosed is typically between $100 \times 10^9/l$ and $300 \times 10^9/l$ but the possibility of CML may be entertained in asymptomatic patients with leucocyte counts in the range $20–40 \times 10^9/l$, while occasional patients present with counts in the range $500–1000 \times 10^9/l$. The leucocyte differential shows a full spectrum of immature and mature granulocytes with 'peaks' of

---

Table 16.3

Features that may be used to recognize the accelerated phase of chronic myeloid leukaemia

---

Leucocyte count resistant to control with busulphan or hydroxyurea
Very rapid leucocyte doubling time
More than 12% blasts in blood
More than 20% blasts plus promyelocytes in marrow
More than 20% basophils plus eosinophils in blood
Anaemia or thrombocytopenia despite adequate chemotherapy
Thrombocytosis above $1 \times 10^{10}/l$ (in the absence of splenectomy)
The acquisition of new chromosomal abnormalities (in addition to the Ph chromosome)
Splenomegaly persisting or increasing when the leucocyte count is normal or near normal
Development of marrow failure associated with myelofibrosis

The blast phase is arbitrarily defined when the proportion of blasts plus promyelocytes in the marrow and/or blood equals or exceeds 30%.

blasts, myelocytes and mature neutrophils (Fig. 16.1). Blast cells may constitute up to 12% of the differential; their percentage (as well as their absolute number) rises in parallel with the total leucocyte count. The bulk of the leucocytes comprise mature neutrophils, but the percentages of eosinophils and basophils are usually also increased. Absolute lymphocyte numbers are normal and relative monocyte numbers are usually reduced. The morphology of the mature neutrophils is normal. The amount of alkaline phosphatase in the neutrophil cytoplasm is greatly reduced or absent in comparison with neutrophils from normal individuals. This may be the result of low ambient levels of GM–CSF. Haemoglobin values are often normal if CML is diagnosed when the leucocyte count is only moderately raised; conversely, patients with leucocyte counts above $150 \times 10^9/l$ are almost always anaemic, and occasionally patients present with haemoglobin concentrations below 50 g/l in association with very large spleens and very high leucocyte counts. The platelet count is usually moderately elevated, in the range $300–700 \times 10^9/l$, but may occasionally be over $1 \times 10^{12}/l$ at diagnosis. The number of very small platelets is larger than normal. Occasional normoblasts are present in the peripheral blood film.

Haemopoietically active bone marrow expands in CML to fill the cavities of all the major bones in the body. The marrow becomes densely hypercellular with loss of most, or usually all, of the normal fat spaces between the haemopoietic elements. Marrow aspiration frequently fails to reveal fragments but shows instead a dense population of myeloid cells at all levels of differentiation and increased numbers of megakaryocytes with low numbers of nuclei and relatively sparse cytoplasm. Erythroid activity is increased much less than that of the granulocyte series. Bone marrow biopsy confirms the absence of fat spaces and frequently reveals increased quantities of reticulin and sometimes diffuse fibrosis. Rarely, fibrosis at diagnosis is extensive, in which case attempts to aspirate marrow fail. Examination of a patient's bone marrow is not strictly necessary to establish a diagnosis, but adequate cytogenetic preparations are more reliably obtained from the marrow than from peripheral blood and it is useful to document the degree of marrow fibrosis present at diagnosis.

The enlargement of the spleen is due principally to infiltration with myeloid tissue. Histological examination reveals massive expansion of the red pulp which is occupied by cells of the granulocytic series at all levels of differentiation together with megakaryocytes and erythroid precursors. The liver likewise shows infiltration of myeloid cells in the periportal tracts, but the scale of involvement is much less than in the spleen. In both these organs the amount of myeloid infiltration is very greatly reduced by effective chemotherapy, in contrast to the marrow, the appearances of which do not greatly alter after the patient's leucocyte count has been restored to normal.

There are distinctive changes in other laboratory investigations at diagnosis. The serum vitamin B_{12} and B_{12}-binding proteins are greatly increased as a consequence of increased production of transcobalamin I by myeloid cells. The serum alkaline phosphatase and uric acid are also moderately increased. All these values tend to return to normal when the patient is treated.

Various haematological changes occur during the evolution of the chronic phase of CML such that the distinction between chronic phase and accelerated phase is necessarily rather arbitrary. Thus, in some cases the platelet count rises steadily in spite of treatment, while in other cases the degree of eosinophilia or basophilia progresses. The degree of marrow fibrosis may also increase from year to year. In the latter cases the peripheral blood may come to resemble the picture of primary myelofibrosis with increased numbers of blast cells, thrombocytopenia and erythroid poikilocytosis with tear-drop forms and normoblasts. The marrow then becomes inaspirable and the biopsy picture is identical to that of primary myelofibrosis.

Blastic transformation, also referred to as acute transformation or blast cell crisis, is usually defined by the percentage of blasts or blast plus promyelocytes in the blood or marrow. The leucocyte count may be unexpectedly increased with blast cells predominating, or, less commonly, the absolute number of leucocytes may be normal or subnormal. Sometimes the changes appear to involve only immature blast cells, while at other times the full spectrum of immature granulocytes is involved in the clonal evolution. In about 70% of cases of blastic transformation the blast cells have morphological and cell marker characteristics of myeloid cells—that is, they resemble myeloblasts, monoblasts or erythroblasts or occasionally immature eosinophils, basophils or mast cells. In about 20% of cases the predominating blast cell is lymphoid with pre-B markers very similar to that of acute lymphoblastic leukaemia—surface membrane positivity for c-ALL and Ia antigens and nuclear positivity for the enzyme terminal deoxynucleotidyl transferase. Very occasional lymphoid transformations with blast cells with T-cell markers have been reported. About 5–10% of transformations have blast cells with mixed myeloid and lymphoid features.

Treatment

Management of the Chronic Phase

Once the diagnosis of CML is established, the first obligation of the haematologist is to discuss the problem with the patient and his or her family. There will be circumstances in which it is deemed expedient not to reveal essential details of the diagnosis or of the disease to an individual patient, but in most cases honesty in relation to diagnosis is the best policy and the prognosis can be given as a range, say survival for 2 to 10 years, without undue distortion of the facts. For younger patients, questions of fertility and the side-effects of cytotoxic drugs should be discussed at this stage. Inevitably the patient or a relation will enquire about the role of bone marrow transplantation, if the haematologist has not already introduced the subject, and an appropriate policy should be presented.

There is no evidence that conventional methods for control of the leucocyte count in the chronic phase of CML prolongs survival. The object of all treatment (other than bone marrow transplantation and possibly alpha-interferon) is therefore to reverse or to prevent the onset of symptoms. Thus, in the asymptomatic patients the haematologist may opt to delay treatment with cytotoxic drugs, but of course the patient must be aware of the rationale. Some patients undoubtedly feel happier if their leucocyte count is normal or near normal and, for these, treatment may reasonably be initiated even in the absence of symptoms.

The two drugs used most commonly in the management of CML in chronic phase are busulphan and hydroxyurea. Busulphan is usually administered at an initial daily dose of 6 mg or 8 mg. The blood count must be monitored closely (at intervals no greater than weekly for the first 8 weeks) because the occasional patient manifests idiosyncratic hypersensitivity to the drug and will experience a rapid and precipitous reduction in leucocyte count. Usually the count falls more slowly, such that it reaches $20–30 \times 10^9/l$ within 3 to 6 weeks of starting treatment. Busulphan should be discontinued or the dose greatly reduced before the leucocyte count has reached normal values because the count will continue to fall for 2–3 weeks thereafter. Once the count has reached normal or near-normal levels, there are two options: to withhold further treatment until the leucocyte count has risen again to $50–100 \times 10^9/l$ or to attempt to define a busulphan dosage (usually 0.5–2 mg/day) that will keep the leucocyte count steadily in the normal range. Neither approach is clearly superior. The use of busulphan is associated with a number of predictable or possible side-effects. In younger women who receive the drug, menstruation usually ceases within a few months and they may become permanently infertile; males are rendered oligospermic or azoospermic, with little prospect of recovery. After some years of treatment with busulphan, most patients become gradually pigmented—their face and body assumes a brown coloration such that in extreme cases their racial origin may appear different from that of their relations. A clinical syndrome resembling Addison's disease, but lacking the biochemical features, has been described as a complication of treatment with busulphan. A pulmonary complication characterized by fever, cough, dyspnoea with progressive ventilatory deterioration and death has been designated 'busulphan lung'. Histological examination of biopsy or autopsy material in these cases shows extensive interstitial and intra-alveolar fibrosis. Very rarely, the development of cataracts has been attributed to busulphan.

The precise mode of action of hydroxyurea is unknown but it probably acts by inhibiting ribonucleotide reductase, an enzyme required for de-novo synthesis of deoxynucleotides. It thus blocks DNA synthesis and causes cells to accumulate in the S-phase of the cell cycle. It can be administered to a patient with a high leucocyte count as a starting daily dose of 1.5 g or 2.0 g. Thereafter the leucocyte count can be monitored at weekly or 2-weekly intervals until it is in the normal range. The dosage of hydroxyurea can then be halved, but treatment (eg. with 0.5 g or 1.0 g daily) will have to be continued indefinitely to control the leucocyte count. At relatively high dosage the drug causes nausea and occasionally vomiting. Headaches may also be attributable to hydroxyurea. The marrow is rendered moderately megaloblastic by hydroxyurea. In general the drug is well tolerated for a number of years and the principal objection to its use is the necessity for the patient to take two or three tablets on a permanent basis.

Various other drugs have been used successfully in the treatment of the chronic phase of CML. Dibromomannitol is effective in controlling the leucocyte count in patients in the chronic phase but offers no advantage over the use of busulphan. Other alkylating agents, such as cyclophosphamide and melphalan, will control the leucocyte count. Antimetabolites such as 6-mercaptopurine and 6-thioguanine are also useful. Either of these may be used in combination with busulphan to produce rapid reduction of the leucocyte count and to reduce the amount of busulphan required for maintenance. Recently a number of specialist centres have explored the use of alpha- interferon for CML. Preliminary results show that lymphoblastoid-cell-derived and recombinant alpha-interferons are both highly effective in reversing symptoms and controlling the leucocyte count; about one-third of patients show re-establishment, at least temporarily, of Ph-negative (presumably normal) haemopoiesis, an occurrence that is exceedingly rare with conventional treatment. Toxicity included somnolence, depression, memory defects and some weight loss and myalgias, all eventually reversible. It is not yet clear whether treatment with interferon can prolong the duration of chronic phase, which would constitute a major benefit for the patient, but undoubtedly controlled studies should continue.

Management of the Accelerated Phase

No precise guidelines can be specified for management of the patient whose disease has entered an accelerated phase. If busulphan is no longer effective in controlling the leucocyte count, a switch to use of hydroxyurea may prove valuable. Conversely, a switch from hydroxyurea to busulphan may also control features of the disease no longer controlled by hydroxyurea. There are at least three good reasons for considering splenectomy for a patient in accelerated phase. If the spleen is enlarging at a time when the leucocyte count is normal or only slightly raised, splenectomy may permit the administration of lower doses of cytotoxic drugs. Splenectomy may also facilitate treatment of the patient in whom thrombocytopenia limits the amount of busulphan or hydroxyurea that can safely be administered. It may also be valuable for patients with progressive splenomegaly with myelofibrosis. Alternatively, supportive therapy including the use of red cell and platelet transfusions may be the mainstay of treatment for some months or even years for the patient whose principal manifestations of acceleration involve increasing myelofibrosis and associated marrow failure.

Management of the Blastic Transformation

Although the correlation between phenotypic features of the predominating blast cell and response to appropriate therapy is not perfect, it is still reasonable to treat the patient initially in accordance with the results of blast cell typing. Thus patients with myeloid transformations may be treated with any of the combinations of cytotoxic drugs used in the management of acute myeloid leukaemia. For example, some combination of an anthracycline with cytosine arabinoside with or without 6-thioguanine is a reasonable choice. Other possible approaches include the use of high-dose cytosine arabinoside or mitozantrone. In general the results of treating myeloid transformation of CML are disappointing. Initially the numbers of blast cells in the blood and marrow almost always fall, often precipitously, and the response seems gratifying. Severe pancytopenia then ensues and only rarely does the patient recover haemopoiesis typical of chronic phase disease. More commonly, blast cells reappear in the blood after a variable number of weeks and their numbers rise inexorably thereafter. Alternatively, the severe pancytopenia may be prolonged and may lead to the patient's death from haemorrhage or infection.

There is no universally agreed protocol for the management of patients with lymphoid transformation of CML, but the majority will respond to cytotoxic drugs that are usually effective in the management of acute lymphoblastic leukaemia. Thus treatment may reasonably begin with vincristine, corticosteroids and possibly an anthracycline. The addition to the protocol of L-asparaginase is optional, but one should bear in mind that the capacity of the marrow of patients with CML to regenerate after intensive chemotherapy may be reduced in comparison with that of a newly diagnosed patient with acute lymphoblastic leukaemia (ALL). In most cases, chemotherapy will reduce the numbers of blast cells in the blood and marrow and restore the patient to a haematological picture consistent with chronic phase disease. In almost all cases the haemopoiesis remains entirely Ph positive.

When the patient with lymphoid transformation has been successfully restored to 'second' chronic phase, the best approach to further treatment probably involves the use of a 'maintenance' protocol appropriate for 'adult' or 'poor prognosis' ALL. This will typically include 6-mercaptopurine and intermittent methotrexate with 'timed' reinductions with an anthracycline, vincristine and corticosteroids. Because patients with treated lymphoid transformations have a substantial risk of developing leukaemic infiltration of the central nervous system, some approach to 'neuroprophylaxis' is also desirable. Six intrathecal injections of methotrexate may suffice; if the patient is otherwise in good health, the use of cranial irradiation should also be considered.

Bone Marrow Transplantation

Initial efforts to treat and indeed to cure patients with CML by bone marrow transplantation were carried out in the 1970s. It soon became clear that, even for younger patients with HLA-identical sibling donors, bone marrow transplantation performed in the accelerated or blastic phase was almost universally unsuccessful. Conversely, bone marrow transplantation using identical twin donors for patients still in the chronic phase of the disease resulted in long-term remission with Ph-negative haemopoiesis. Most of the patients in the latter category were probably cured. In the early 1980s, a number of specialist centres started to

transplant patients under the age of 40 with marrow from HLA-identical siblings while the disease remained in the chronic phase. The preliminary results of the studies can be summarized as follows: there is a transplant-related mortality of about 30%; about 10% of patients who survive the transplant will relapse within 2 years and will eventually die of leukaemia, though their survival may be longer than it would have been with conventional therapy; about 50–60% of patients will become long-term disease-free survivors and the great majority of these are almost certainly cured. In contrast, the probability of long-term disease-free survival for patients transplanted in accelerated phase or blastic transformation is about 10–15%.

These results mean that bone marrow transplantation can cure eligible patients but must be restricted at present to younger patients with suitable donors, who probably constitute only 10% of newly diagnosed patients with CML. One must hope that in the next few years there will be improvement in the technical aspects of bone marrow transplantation that will permit successful treatment of older patients and successful use of donors other than those genetically HLA-identical with the patient.

Ph-POSITIVE ACUTE LYMPHOBLASTIC LEUKAEMIA

About 20% of adults and 2–3% of children who present with acute lymphoblastic leukaemia have blast cells with a Ph chromosome due to t(9;22) indistinguishable on cytogenetic grounds from patients with Ph-positive CML. In general, these patients have relatively small spleens and no other haematological features suggestive of CML. The prognosis for patients with Ph-positive ALL seems worse than that of comparable patients lacking cytogenetic abnormalities. Studies at the molecular level show that some of the patients have breakpoints within the *bcr* region (M-*BCR*) while others have breakpoints that are located 5′ (upstream) in the first intron of the *BCR* gene (see Fig. 16.1). The latter patients have an abnormal *ABL*-related mRNA and a P185 distinct from the mRNA and P210 characteristic of CML.

Patients with Ph-positive ALL are usually treated with drugs appropriate to poor prognosis children's or adult ALL, and remission is usually achieved. These patients should receive standard neuroprophylaxis with cranial irradiation and intrathecal methotrexate or BMT (see Chapter 14). In remission the majority of these patients have morphologically and cytogenetically normal marrow, but in a minority partially or completely Ph-positive haemopoiesis analogous to CML in chronic phase is revealed.

Ph-NEGATIVE CHRONIC MYELOID LEUKAEMIA

Between 5% and 10% of patients with clinical and haematological features similar or identical to Ph-positive CML lack a Ph chromosome in their leukaemic cells. Usually in these cases the karyotype is normal, but a variety of cytogenetic abnormalities not involving 22q has been described. These patients present with clinical features very similar to those with Ph-positive disease. Occasionally the spleen is smaller than might be expected at a given leucocyte count.

The haematological features may be entirely characteristic of Ph-positive CML; in other cases there are subtle clues that suggest Ph negativity. These include a low platelet count ($< 100 \times 10^9$/l) at presentation, the absence of the typical predominance of myelocytes in the leucocyte differential count, and absence of eosinophilia and basophilia. Some of the neutrophils may show dysplastic changes. Conversely, the presence of significant numbers of monocytes in the peripheral blood also suggests a diagnosis of Ph-negative CML. The bone marrow is typically hypercellular and usually has no features that clearly exclude the possibility of Ph positivity. On molecular analysis some of these patients have the same abnormal *BCR–ABL* gene with associated mRNA and P210 as is found in Ph-positive disease, while in others no characteristic genomic abnormalities have yet been defined. Thus, in some ways, Ph-negative CML is a more heterogeneous condition than Ph-positive disease.

The older literature suggests that patients with Ph-negative disease have a median survival of 1–2 years, which is considerably shorter than that of those with Ph-positive disease. More recent series, from which patients with highly atypical forms of CML and chronic myelomonocytic leukaemia have been excluded, suggest that for the patient with a form of leukaemia very close to classical CML that differs only in that the Ph chromosome is absent, the prognosis is similar to that of a patient with Ph-positive CML. It is therefore reasonable to start treatment with busulphan or hydroxyurea. If the response is poor, then the addition of 6-thioguanine or the use of drug combinations effective for AML may be valuable.

JUVENILE CHRONIC MYELOID LEUKAEMIA

Juvenile chronic myeloid leukaemia is a rare disorder seen in young children. The child presents with sweats, fever, weight loss or a variety of septic lesions. The spleen and liver are considerably enlarged and lymphadenopathy is prominent. There may be a variety of rashes. The degree of leucocytosis is variable but the blood film is not usually confused with that of Ph-positive CML. There are immature granulocytes and blasts but there is no undue prominence of myelocytes, and eosinophilia and basophilia are lacking. Monocytes may be conspicuous; platelets may be low. The neutrophil alkaline phosphatase score is normal or raised, and the level of fetal haemoglobin is typically raised. Cytogenetic examination of the leukaemic cells usually shows a strictly normal karyotype.

These patients respond poorly to treatment with cytotoxic drugs though the disease may be controlled for months or sometimes years with drug combinations that are effective in AML. They should be considered for treatment by bone marrow transplantation if a suitable donor can be identified.

EOSINOPHILIC LEUKAEMIA

Eosinophilic leukaemia is a very rare and poorly defined entity which may present with a variety of symptoms including sweats, weight loss, non-specific rashes or cardiac abnormalities. Patients may or may not have splenomegaly. The cardiac lesions include various dysrhythmias and disturbances of valvular function, probably due to the direct toxic action of eosinophil cationic proteins and other enzymes on the endomyocardium. The blood film shows a considerable increase in the number of eosinophils, some of which appear partially degranulated or vacuolated. Occasional immature eosinophils and blast cells may also be present in the circulation. The leukaemic cells may have normal karyotypes but various cytogenetic abnormalities have been described including trisomy for C group chromosomes and an isochromosome 17. The finding of a Ph chromosome suggests that the correct diagnosis is, instead, eosinophilic transformation of Ph-positive CML.

Eosinophilic leukaemia must be distinguished from the more common (but still rare) condition designated hypereosinophilic syndrome (HES; see Chapter 11). In the latter syndrome, peripheral blood eosinophilia may be pronounced, but immature cells are usually absent. Cytogenetic study of the marrow is always normal in HES. There are no established rules for treating patients with eosinophilic leukaemia; they may respond to a variety of cytotoxic drugs, and hydroxyurea, vincristine and prednisolone should all be used, separately or in an appropriate combination. The clinical status of patients with eosinophilic leukaemia may remain unchanged for some years but eventually the disease undergoes transformation to a blastic phase which responds poorly to all forms of treatment.

CHRONIC NEUTROPHILIC LEUKAEMIA

Chronic neutrophilic leukaemia (CNL) is an exceedingly rare condition in which the patient is found to have a raised neutrophil count. This is usually an incidental finding but may occur in the course of investigations for other reasons. The patient may have modest splenomegaly or a spleen of normal size. Immature cells are absent from the peripheral blood. There is no increase in eosinophil or basophil numbers. The neutrophils may show toxic granulation and the neutrophil alkaline phosphatase score is normal or high. The marrow is cytogenetically normal.

Most patients with initially unexplained neutrophil leucocytosis have occult infection or malignant disease which manifests itself after appropriate investigation or after some weeks or months of follow-up. The diagnosis of CNL can only be accepted when all primary causes of a neutrophil leucocytosis have been excluded with reasonable certainty. In the absence of symptoms, treatment is not necessarily required.

CHRONIC MYELOMONOCYTIC LEUKAEMIA

Chronic myelomonocytic leukaemia may be classified either as a rare subtype of chronic myeloid leukaemia or as one form of the myelodysplastic syndrome (see Chapter 17). The disease is diagnosed principally in older men, who may present with weight loss or symptoms of anaemia. The spleen may be enlarged and minor or moderate lymphadenopathy may be present. The diagnostic feature of the blood film is the presence of large numbers of mature monocytes associated with increased numbers of band forms and mature neutrophils. Various dysplastic changes, including hypogranular neutrophils, Pelger forms, dyserythropoiesis with ringed sideroblasts and micromegakaryocytes, may be present. Serum lysozyme levels are greatly elevated and hypokalaemia is sometimes seen. The marrow is usually hypercellular and contains mature and immature monocytes in excess. The Ph chromosome is not detected.

The disease often runs an indolent course and treatment other than blood transfusion may not initially be required for months or years. At some stage the disease usually transforms to a more acute phase with promonocytes and blast cells proliferating in the marrow and blood. Treatment may be initiated with drug combinations appropriate for AML, but remissions are rarely achieved.

SELECTED BIBLIOGRAPHY

Champlin R. E. (1986). Chronic leukemias: oncogenes, chromosomes and advances in therapy. *Annals of Internal Medicine*, **104**, 671–688.

Champlin R. E., Golde D. W. (1985). Chronic myelogenous leukemia: recent advances. *Blood*, **65**, 1039–1047.

Dreazen O., Canaani E., Gale R. P. (1988). Molecular biology of chronic myelogenous leukaemia. *Seminars in Hematology*, **25**, 35–49.

Gale R. P., Cannani E. (1985). The molecular biology of chronic myelogenous leukaemia. *British Journal of Haematology*, **60**, 395–408.

Galton D. A. G. (Ed.) (1977). The chronic leukaemias. *Clinics in Haematology*, **6**, 1–274.

Goldman J. M. (1986). Management of chronic myeloid leukaemia. *Scandinavian Journal of Haematology*, **37**, 269–279.

Goldman J. M. (Ed.) (1988). Chronic myeloid leukaemia. In *Clinical haematology*, Vol. 1(4). London: Bailliere Tindall.

Goldman J. M. (Ed.) (1988). Chronic myeloid leukaemia: pathogenesis and management. In *Recent advances in haematology*, Vol. 5, pp. 131–152. (Ed. A. V. Hoffbrand). Edinburgh: Churchill Livingstone.

Koeffler H. P., Golde D. W. (1981). Chronic myelogenous leukemia—new approaches. *New England Journal of Medicine*, **304**, 1201–1209, 1269–1274.

Kurzrock R., Gutterman J. U., Talpaz M. (1988). The molecular genetics of Philadelphia chromosone-positive leukemias. *New England Journal of Medicine*, **319**, 990–8.

Nowell P. O., Hungerford D. A. (1960). A minute chromosome in human chronic granulocytic leukemia. *Science*, **132**, 1497.

Shaw M. T. (Ed.) (1982). *Chronic granulocytic leukaemia*, pp. 1–251. Eastbourne: Praeger.

Talpaz M., Kantarjian H. M., McCredie K. B., *et al.* (1986). Chronic myelogenous leukemia; hematologic remissions and cytogenetic improvements induced by recombinant alpha A interferon. *New England Journal of Medicine*, **314**, 1065–1068.

Chapter 17

THE MYELODYSPLASTIC SYNDROMES

D. A. G. GALTON

The term myelodysplastic syndrome (MDS) is applied to a group of acquired conditions characterized by progressive bone marrow failure associated with normocellular or hypercellular bone marrow that cannot be attributed to nutritional deficiency, chronic infection, or other chronic systemic illness, and cannot be reversed by the successful treatment of those conditions. The patients usually present with symptoms resulting from anaemia, neutropenia, or thrombocytopenia, or from combinations of these. The cytopenias progress and are the commonest cause of death. In a proportion of cases acute leukaemia, almost always acute myeloid leukaemia, develops. Although, in the majority of cases, MDS cannot be linked with any environmental feature, a minority, now unfortunately increasing in frequency, arise as a consequence of prolonged exposure to cytotoxic drugs, most commonly alkylating agents. Whereas these cases of secondary MDS occur at all ages, primary MDS is essentially a disease of the elderly, though no age group is exempt.

THE RANGE OF MYELODYSPLASTIC SYNDROMES

In the past 15 years it has become recognized that two groups of conditions, formerly not regarded as related, are biologically similar, and represent the extreme manifestations of a spectrum of disorders arising as a result of a heritable defect involving a pluripotential haemopoietic stem cell. The MDS are therefore fundamentally neoplastic conditions, but the severity of the underlying defect, the extent of involvement of the different haemopoietic cell lineages, the rate of progression, and the magnitude of the risk of transformation to overt acute leukaemia vary greatly from the relatively stable almost benign forms to those in which the distinction from overt acute leukaemia remains a matter of arbitrary definition.

The more benign group includes the refractory anaemias (RA), intensively studied since the 1930s, when it became clear that nutritional replacement therapy was not effective in all cases of anaemia not resulting from blood loss, red-cell destruction, or reduced production. In the 1950s, a subgroup of acquired refractory anaemia, acquired idiopathic sideroblastic anaemia (AISA), was characterized by the presence of ringed sideroblasts in the bone marrow and defective haem synthesis. The risk of death from leukaemia was appreciated in the early descriptions of refractory anaemias, and later, features that seemed to indicate a high risk of progression to leukaemia led to the description of a 'preleukaemic syndrome'.

The less benign group includes a range of conditions described from the 1950s onwards as preleukaemia, low-percentage leukaemia, oligoblastic leukaemia, smouldering leukaemia, the Di Guglielmo syndrome, chronic erythraemic myelosis, and refractory anaemia with excess of myeloblasts. Cytopenias of one or more haemopoietic cell lineage characterize all of these conditions and the refractory anaemias, but since 1974, for reasons described below, chronic myelomonocytic leukaemia (CMML) has been included in the MDS.

FAB CLASSIFICATION OF THE MYELODYSPLASTIC SYNDROMES

The multiplicity of terms and definitions frustrated attempts to compare published descriptions in the effort to assemble information on the pathogenesis, natural history, biology, complications, and survival patterns of the conditions now grouped as components of the MDS.

The French–American–British (FAB) cooperative group proposed semi-quantitative arbitrary guidelines for subdividing the intergrading conditions that range from refractory anaemia to overt acute leukaemia (Table 17.1). The basis of the classification is the percentage of blast cells in the bone marrow: <5% for the refractory anaemias, 5–20% for 'refractory anaemia with excess of blasts' (RAEB), and 21–29% for 'RAEB in transformation' (RAEB-t). However, in the presence of >5% of blast cells in the peripheral blood or of Auer rods in the blast cells, the diagnosis becomes RAEB-t regardless of the percentage of blasts in the bone marrow; further, a diagnosis of CMML is made when the absolute blood monocyte count is $\geq 1 \times 10^9$/l, regardless of the percentage of blasts in the bone marrow. Note that RA, an unsatisfactory but long-used term, includes cases (about 5%) of solitary neutropenia or, rarely, thrombocytopenia, and no anaemia (haemoglobin less than 130 g/l for men, 120 g/l for women).

In recent years, large series of cases classified according to the FAB recommendations have been studied and it is now clear that the arbitrary cut-off points between the named conditions do indeed separate groups with differing prognosis. The prospect for survival for patients with the refractory anaemias is markedly better than that for those with RAEB, while RAEB-t has the shortest median duration of survival. In nearly all series, the group with the highest proportion of long-term survivors is refractory anaemia with sideroblasts (RAS), identical to idiopathic acquired sideroblastic anaemia except that the lower limit for the proportion of bone marrow normoblasts that are ringed sideroblasts in the bone marrow is 15%, compared to 10% for AISA. A representative set of survival curves is shown in Figure 17.1.

The FAB classification provides a valuable reference framework for comparative studies that are still in progress, and for planning clinical trials of different treatments, while its use by many groups has led to the recognition of additional features with prognostic significance, discussed below.

PATHOLOGY

Pathogenesis

The feature common to all groups of MDS is the association of cytopenias with bone marrow of

Table 17.1

The French–American–British (FAB) classification of the myelodysplastic syndromes

Bone-marrow blast-cell count (% of nucleated cells) <5		≥5	
Ringed sideroblasts (% of nucleated red cells)		5–20	21–29
≤15	>15	RA with excess of blasts	RAEB in transformation
Refractory anaemia RA	RA with sideroblasts RAS	RAEB	RAEB-t

N.B. In all categories the diagnosis is RAEB-t if:
   (i) blast cells in the peripheral blood are ≥5%, or
   (ii) Auer rods are present in bone marrow or peripheral blood blasts.
The diagnosis is chronic myelomonocytic leukaemia (CMML) if the peripheral blood monocyte count is $\geq 1 \times 10^9$/l.

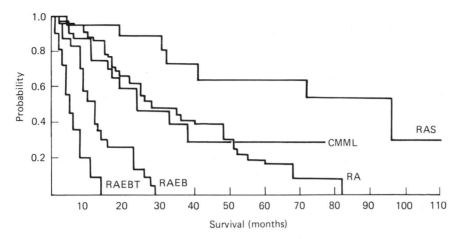

Fig. 17.1. *Survival according to the FAB classification of the myelodysplastic syndrome (see text) of 141 patients. RAS: refractory anaemia with ringed sideroblasts (21 patients); median survival 76 months. RA: refractory anaemia (53 patients); median survival 32 months. RAEB: RA with excess of blasts (25 patients); median survival 10.5 months. RAEB-t: RAEB in transformation (11 patients); median survival 5 months. (From Mufti et al. (1985), with permission.)*

normal or, more often, increased cellularity. Rarely, the bone marrow is hypocellular and the distinction from aplastic anaemia is made on the presence of characteristic dysplastic features in the haemopoietic cells (see below). Occasionally the presence of reticulin prevents the aspiration of bone marrow fragments. Active or even excessive haemopoiesis fails to maintain adequate numbers of circulating red cells, platelets or granulocytes. It seems probable that this ineffective haemopoiesis results from the replacement of the normal haemopoietic stem cells by abnormal ones whose differentiated descendents in one or more cell lineages give rise to defective, short-lived progeny. The absence of normal stem cells is shown best by karyotypic analysis in secondary MDS, in almost every case of which all countable metaphases are abnormal, and usually clonal; the findings are similar in rather less than one-half of the cases of primary RAEB and RAEB-t. The replacement of the normal haemopoietic stem cells by an abnormal clone indicates that the latter has a growth advantage of neoplastic nature over the normal haemopoietic stem cells. The severity of the stem cell defect in the different groups of MDS determines the extent to which the different cell lines are involved, the severity of the cytopenias, the rate of progression, and the extent to which the

abnormal clone supplants the normal stem cells. In some cases of RAS, anaemia may be the only functional abnormality for many years, while in RAEB with pancytopenia, the condition may remain relatively stable for some years, or may progress in a few months. The interrelationship of all the conditions is shown by the observation of individual cases of RA and of RAS, in which progression through RAEB and RAEB-t to acute myeloid leukaemia (AML) has been observed. Nevertheless, it is not known whether RAEB and RAEB-t are always preceded by a phase of unrecognized RA or RAS. In the latter conditions, the stem cell defect may be expressed only in the erythroid lineage, though present in the other lineages, until an additional change or mutation leads to their functional involvement, whereas in RAEB the defect may be expressed in all lineages from its inception. It is likely that the progression to acute leukaemia involves a further stem cell mutation leading to the appearance of a clonogenic cell with its capacity for replication and self-renewal intact but with little or no capacity for differentiation and subsequent maturation. In the great majority of cases the leukaemia that develops is AML, but the fact that acute lymphoblastic leukaemia (ALL) has occasionally been recorded, even in RAS, indicates a pluripotential cell as the target for myelodysplasia. In one case, in which the patient was a woman heterozygous for glucose-6-phosphate dehydrogenase (G6PD), one set of B lymphocytes which expressed a single immunoglobulin light chain, as well as all myeloid cells (red cells, platelets, granulocytes, and marrow nucleated cells), showed only one allotype of G6PD, suggesting descent from a common stem-cell precursor. The myeloid cells, but not the cultured monoclone of B lymphocytes, were karyotypically abnormal, suggesting that chromosome abnormalities in MDS arise as a result of a second event in an already transformed clone.

Morphological and Functional Abnormalities

For the haematologist, the most impressive demonstration of the interrelationship between the groups of MDS is the presence, in varying degree, of striking and characteristic morphological abnormalities in all three cell lineages. None of these abnormalities is specific for the MDS, but considered in the context of active or hyperactive but ineffective haemopoiesis and cytopenias, they are highly characteristic, and they provide important diagnostic clues as well as prognostic information. They are seen in well-stained Romanowsky films of blood and bone marrow (Fig. 17.2), and are described below (Table 17.2).

Dyserythropoiesis

Some degree of dyserythropoiesis is so common in haematological disorders that it is probably the least significant of the dysplastic features found in the MDS, especially when it is relatively minor and not accompanied by dysgranulopoiesis, dysmegakaryocytopoiesis, or both. The presence in the bone marrow of ringed sideroblasts in significant numbers ($\geq 15\%$) may be suspected from the dimorphic appearance of the red cells on the blood films, with a mixture of normochromic cells and of hypochromic, often large, cells. In the Romanowsky-stained bone marrow, conspicuous non-haemoglobinized areas of pallor are seen in the cytoplasm of late and intermediate normoblasts, and their frequency is often proportional to the frequency of ringed sideroblasts as seen in the Perls-stained preparation. Smaller vacuoles may be seen in early erythroblasts that often appear megaloblastic. In the Perls-stained films the siderotic granules of ringed sideroblasts are grouped round the nucleus, and transmission electron microscopy shows the iron to be located within mitochondria, whereas in physiological sideroblasts the iron is in the form of ferritin in the cytoplasm. Other dyserythropoietic features seen in the MDS include bilobed, trefoil or tetrafoil nuclei, usually in late erythroblasts, sometimes in earlier forms, double or triple nuclei, internuclear bridging, and the presence of one to many nuclear fragments. In the peripheral blood, macrocytosis and a high mean corpuscular volume (MCV) are commonly found, and normoblasts, frequently dyserythropoietic, are not rare.

Dysgranulopoiesis

The main cytoplasmic abnormality in peripheral blood films is hypogranularity or agranularity, but excellent Romanowsky staining is essential. In well-stained May–Grünwald–Giemsa preparations, the agranular neutrophil has a transparent, almost colourless, empty cytoplasm while hypogranular cells have scanty, often vary small, granules. Döhle bodies are sometimes present in the clear cytoplasm. The common nuclear abnormality is the acquired Pelger–Huët defect: the nucleus is round or bilobed and has mature-type chromatin condensation. Multisegmented nuclei, not resembling those found in megaloblastosis, are not uncommon, and occasionally multiple chromatin extrusions lacking the features of Barr bodies are seen. Nuclear and cytoplasmic abnormalities may occur in the same cell. Abnormal neutrophils are sometimes found in the bone marrow but not in the peripheral blood, perhaps reflecting a defect in the release mechanism, while in the bone marrow secondary granules may be deficient or absent in myelocytes and metamyelocytes as well as in neutrophils. Primary granulation may be deficient or absent in promyelocytes, and occasionally the primary granules coalesce into irregular bodies of varying size. Cells from the myelocyte stage onwards, with cytoplasmic and nuclear features of both granulocytic and monocytic lineages, are often difficult to identify, and some can be shown, by the use of a dual esterase stain, to have positivity for both granulocytic and monocytic enzymes.

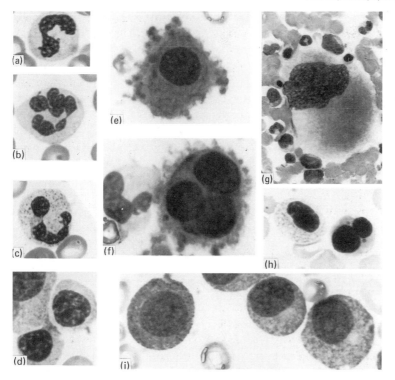

Fig. 17.2. *May–Grünwald–Giemsa-stained blood film (a, b and c) and bone-marrow films. (a). Agranular neutrophil × 1500. (b) Hypersegmented agranular neutrophil × 1500. (c) Normal neutrophil from same blood film as (a) and (b) × 1500. (d) Agranular metamyelocyte and agranular mononuclear (Pelger–Huët) neutrophil × 1500. (e) Small mononuclear megakaryocyte (micromegakaryocyte) × 1500. (f) Polynuclear megakaryocyte and agranular neutrophil × 1500. (g) Large mononuclear megakaryocyte × 600. (h) Large bilobed late normoblast with chromatin projections and a hypogranular metamyelocyte × 1500. (i) Normal promyelocyte, myelocyte lacking secondary (specific) granules and promyelocyte lacking primary (azurophilic) granules × 1500. (The photomicrographs were taken by Mr W. Hinkes at the Royal Postgraduate Medical School.)*

Dysmegakaryocytopoiesis

Megakaryocyte abnormalities are the most significant morphological features of the MDS but are often missed, especially when few megakaryocytes are present in the bone marrow films. They may be left behind when increased amounts of reticulin are present and are then better seen in trephine sections. Bone marrow films must be systematically searched from end to end to find every megakaryocyte. A wide variety of abnormalities may be seen, but three are especially characteristic of the MDS. The micromegakaryocyte, often overlooked, is about the size of a monocyte, or smaller, has a single small, round central nucleus and characteristic megakaryocyte cytoplasm at different stages of platelet maturation. The polynuclear megakaryocyte has two to twelve or more small, round, separate nuclei. The micromegakaryocyte and the small binucleate form resemble the megakaryocytes seen in fetal bone marrow up to the 23rd week of gestation; they are the forms most commonly found in the '5q − syndrome' (see below), but generally occur in the MDS in association with the other polynuclear forms and the large mononuclear form, that has a single, large, round or ovoid nucleus. The three

Table 17.2

Qualitative abnormalities in the myelodysplastic syndromes

Lineage	Peripheral blood	Bone marrow
Erythroid	Macrocytes, dimorphism, polychromatic cells, punctate basophilia, normoblasts (often dyserythropoietic)	Ring sideroblasts, vacuolated cytoplasm, megaloblasts, nuclear fragmentation, irregular shape, bi-, tri-, tetralobed forms, nuclear bridging, cytoplasmic bridging, multiple nuclei, giant forms
Megakaryocytic	Giant platelets, megakaryocyte fragments	Small mono- or binucleate, large mononuclear, polynuclear forms; large multisegmented forms with many round, ovoid or irregular segments and nuclear fragments of unequal size
Granulocytic	Hypo- and agranular neutrophils, Pelger–Huët cells with round or bilobed nuclei, grossly hypersegmented or polyploid neutrophils	Promyelocytes with few or no azurophilic granules; partial or complete loss of secondary granulation in myelocytes, metamyelocytes and neutrophils, 'Pelger–Huët' neutrophils
Monocytic	Nuclei may be sausage shaped or trilobed; promonocytes (fine azurophilic granulation)	Promonocytes may be present, but monocytic lineage often conspicuously absent
Blasts	Mainly small round blasts with scanty agranular cytoplasm (type I) or sparsely granular (type II)	

classical forms of dysplastic megakaryocytes are rarely found in conditions other than MDS, though very occasional abnormal cells may be seen in otherwise 'normal' bone marrow films. However, the classical dysplastic forms are seen in over one-half of all cases of chronic granulocytic leukaemia. In the peripheral blood, giant platelets are almost always present, and megakaryocyte fragments occasionally, especially when the bone marrow reticulin is increased.

The Blast-Cell Component

In the refractory anaemias, by definition, blast cells account for fewer than 5% of the bone marrow nucleated cells; in the majority of cases their numbers are well below 5%. In some cases of CMML, too, the blast-cell count may be <5%. In the FAB classification, two types of cells are counted as blasts: the type I blast has uncondensed chromatin, prominent nucleoli and agranular cytoplasm. In some cases the cytoplasm is scanty in a majority. The type II blast usually has more cytoplasm, and always a few azurophilic granules. It must not be confused with the promyelocyte, which is usually considerably larger, has a clearly visible Golgi apparatus near the excentric nucleus and facing the centre of the cell, a nucleolus and some chromatin condensation, and voluminous cytoplasm with numerous azurophilic granules (which, however, may be absent or weakly staining in some cells).

In decalcified 2-μm trephine sections prepared from bone marrow cores embedded in methylmethacrylate, and stained with Gallamine-blue Giemsa or May–Grünwald–Giemsa, small clusters and aggregates of small blast cells in the intertrabecular spaces have been claimed to be characteristic of MDS. This 'abnormal localization of immature precursors' (ALIP) is of special significance in the refractory anaemias, because it appears to identify those patients at risk of undergoing transformation to AML. ALIP cannot be identified in most routinely prepared trephine sections.

Functional Defects

Numerous functional defects have been described in the MDS. Red cell abnormalities include altered function of glycolytic enzymes, increased concentration of Hb-F, and altered expression of blood-group antigens. Granulocyte abnormalities include defective adhesion, chemotaxis, phagocytosis, and killing capacity against bacteria and yeasts. Platelet abnormalities include defective aggregation, adhesion to glass, and reduced thromboxane A_2 activity. In-vitro culture of MDS bone marrows has shown a variety of abnormalities that appear to indicate the loss of normal colony-forming stem cells, the failure of the abnormal stem cells to form normal colonies, and aberrant production of colony-stimulating activity. So far, tests for these abnormalities have not been incorporated into the routine investigation of the MDS.

Chromosomal Abnormalities

As mentioned above, chromosomal abnormalities are found in almost all cases of secondary MDS, but in less than 50% in primary MDS. The abnormalities, usually clonal as in AML, tend to be non-random, and the most common involve partial or total loss of 5 or 7, and trisomy 8, which are also common in AML. However, two characteristic abnormalities found in AML, namely t(8;21) and t(15;17), are hardly ever found in MDS, and the Ph^1 chromosome has been found only once. An interstitial deletion of the long arm of chromosome 5 has been associated with a particular clinical and haematological pattern, the 5q− syndrome. This affects elderly women with RA whose platelet counts are often initially high; in the bone marrow, erythropoietic cells are few, and micromegakaryocytes and small binucleated megakaryocytes are prominent. The prognosis is good, the risk of transformation to AML low, but repeated transfusions lead to iron overload. In general, the presence of chromosomal abnormalities is not of prognostic significance, but there is a trend towards shorter survival when complex abnormalities are present, and additional abnormalities may appear when transformation to AML takes place.

Ras Oncogene Mutations

Point mutations in codons 12, 13, 59 or 61 in the N-ras, K-ras or H-ras oncogenes have been described in a minority of patients with MDS.

CLINICAL FEATURES

About one-half of the patients with primary MDS are over the age of 70, while more than half of the remainder are aged over 50. Those who have only anaemia tend to present with a low haemoglobin concentration, often with relatively mild symptoms indicating that they have adapted well over a long period of time to a slowly falling Hb. MDS is therefore sometimes discovered by chance during admission for other reasons, such as a fractured femoral neck. Slow evolution is also suggested by finding a low Hb in otherwise symptomless patients who present with an acute infection resulting from neutropenia, or with bruising of recent onset resulting from thrombocytopenia. On examination, the findings are non-specific. Fewer than one in five of the patients have a palpable spleen, a sign more likely to be found in CMML than in the other MDS. The slow evolution of MDS is well seen in secondary MDS. The patients, often young persons, have been treated with cytotoxic drugs and often with radiotherapy for malignant or non-malignant conditions, and are seen at regular intervals as part of their routine follow-up. Nevertheless, the MDS is often well advanced before it is diagnosed. Dysplastic features are prominent, even when the bone-marrow blast-cell count is <5%. The clinical features are as non-specific as those of primary MDS. The drugs responsible for secondary MDS include melphalan, chlorambucil, treosulphan, procarbazine, cyclophosphamide, busulphan, razoxane, and the nitrosoureas.

The frequency of secondary MDS may vary according to the age of the patient, the condition for which the drug was administered, the drug used, the dosage schedule and the duration of exposure to it.

In general, the risk is higher in older patients and is proportional to the duration of exposure. MDS usually develops between 3 and 6 years from the end of treatment, but may not become manifest for as long as 16 years. In the first two Medical Research Council trials in myelomatosis, in which the efficacy of cyclophosphamide administered at low daily dosage indefinitely was compared with that of melphalan administered in the same way (first trial) or at higher dosage intermittently (second trial), 12 patients out of 648 entered died from MDS (3 also had overt AML). All had been allocated to one of the melphalan arms, and cyclophosphamide was not found to be oncogenic in the conditions in which it was used in those trials, though it is certainly oncogenic in other circumstances. The risk of MDS following melphalan in myelomatosis patients was estimated by J. Cuzick to be about 3% for each year of administration, with patients receiving the drug for 5 years having a risk of developing MDS 5 years later of about 20%.

Diagnosis

The diagnosis rests on the finding of anaemia, thrombocytopenia, and neutropenia, alone or in different combinations, in association with a cellular, usually hypercellular, bone marrow and, almost always, at least some of the morphological abnormalities described above. Even in the absence of other abnormalities, the abundance of ringed sideroblasts is diagnostic in RAS, but in those cases of RA in elderly subjects with low blast-cell counts and minimal dysplasia, nutritional deficiency should be excluded, even when normal concentrations of serum folate and vitamin B_{12} are found, by a therapeutic trial of these vitamins and also of pyridoxine. Difficulties arise, too, when increased bone marrow reticulin prevents aspiration or yields unrepresentative samples. Dysplastic megakaryocytes can be readily identified in routine trephine sections, which are, however, rarely suitable for recognizing dyserythropoiesis and dysgranulopoiesis. Nevertheless, the recognition of dysplastic megakaryocytes in sections is reliable only when the majority of cells are dysplastic. This is because the normal megakaryocyte is a very large cell, and a 2–5-μm tangential section through one or two nuclear lobes may be mistaken for a dysplastic

form. MDS occurs occasionally when the bone marrow is hypocellular, and the condition can be distinguished from aplastic anaemia only by the identification of positive and unequivocal features of MDS as already described.

The diagnosis of CMML depends on a monocyte count of $\geqslant 1 \times 10^9/l$ and cannot usually be made from the bone marrow, which merely permits a diagnosis of RA, RAS, RAEB or RAEB-t because so few monocytic cells are present. In many cases, neutrophilia is present as well as monocytosis, and the absolute neutrophil counts may exceed the monocyte counts; the monocytes are mature, or may include some with fine azurophilic granules, while some or all of the neutrophils may be hypo- or agranular. In CMML, immature granulocytes account for <5% of the blood nucleated cells; with higher counts, the diagnosis of atypical chronic myeloid leukaemia should be considered, especially when the immature granulocyte count is $\geqslant 15\%$. As already mentioned, splenomegaly, sometimes considerable, is more often found in CMML than in the other forms of MDS, and the liver may be enlarged also. Rare patients have rashes which prove on biopsy to be due to monocytic infiltrates, while others have hypertrophied gums, or serous effusions; unexpectedly, these manifestations do not necessarily indicate that transformation to AML has occurred.

Secondary MDS may resemble primary MDS but the frequency of increased bone marrow reticulin is higher, aspirated marrow fragments may be fatty and hypocellular, and cytogenetic abnormalities, often multiple, are almost always found.

Prognosis

Figure 17.1 shows the survival of groups of MDS patients, seen in Bournemouth, classified according to the FAB criteria. The median durations of survival were 76 months for RAS, with about 65% surviving beyond 5 years, 32 months for RA, 10.5 months for RAEB, and only 5 months for RAEB-t. The median survival of CMML in all groups was 22 months. The findings in other series are similar. The bone-marrow blast-cell count appears to be the single most important determinant of the prognosis, the duration of survival being markedly worse when the blast-cell count is $\geqslant 5\%$. This perhaps reflects the severity of the ineffective haemopoiesis and also the increased risk of progression to overt AML. The severity of the cytopenias has prognostic relevance also, and the Bournemouth workers devised a simple score based on this and the bone-marrow blast-cell count from which three groups of good, poor and intermediate prognosis could be derived. The severity of dysplastic changes in the megakaryocytes and the granulocytes also has prognostic significance. The most clinically relevant prognostic indicators would be those that helped the identification of good-risk and poor-risk disease in the group of refractory anaemias with or without ringed sideroblasts, and it is in these cases particularly (all, by definition, with a marrow blast-cell count of < 5%) that the adverse prognostic significance associated with severe cytopenias, severe dysmegakaryopoiesis, severe dysgranulopoiesis, the presence of ALIP, and spontaneous colony-stimulating activity in bone marrow culture is likely to have clinical value.

In all series, the group of RAEB-t has the worst prognosis, with a median survival of less than 6 months. Most of the patients in this group appear to be those whose MDS has already progressed to overt AML but have been diagnosed before their blast cell counts have reached the arbitrary 30% of the FAB classification because of the symptoms arising from their cytopenias. However, some RAEB-t patients probably have genuine 'smouldering leukaemia', and may survive with stable blast cell counts of 20–29% for many months.

Overt AML with MDS

Since most cases of RAEB-t already have AML, it is not surprising that some patients will not come to medical attention until their disease is slightly more advanced and their bone-marrow blast-cell count is ≥ 30%. They will then be diagnosed as AML, and the question arises as to the proportion of cases of apparently de novo AML in which the disease has arisen from a pre-existing but symptomless MDS.

In AML, symptoms usually arise because of cytopenias. In de novo AML, these are a result of marrow failure caused by replacement of the haemopoietic cells by leukaemia cells; however, the cytopenias do not become serious enough to cause

symptoms until the haemopoietic cells have been reduced to the order of 10–20% of their normal numbers, when the required output of red cells, platelets, and neutrophils can no longer be sustained. In MDS, in contrast, the marrow fails because haemopoiesis from the MDS clone is ineffective, and this clone gradually replaces the normal haemopoietic cells whether leukaemic blasts are present or not. Therefore, when a leukaemic clone does arise it is unlikely to expand very far before the cytopenias have become severe enough to lead to the appearance of symptoms. The evolution of AML from MDS is most readily observed in cases of secondary MDS during the course of regular follow-up, but there can be no doubt that apparently de novo AML, seen for the first time, evolves in about 15% of cases in the same way. It is easy to recognize when the blast cell count is just on the 'leukaemic' side of the RAEB-t/AML boundary (usually 30–50%), when a clone of blast cells is seen alongside haemopoietic cells showing the morphological abnormalities of severe trilineage myelodysplasia. In the case of M6, which appears always to arise from a pre-existing MDS, the FAB criteria require ≥ 50% of all the nucleated bone marrow cells to be erythroblasts (usually severely dysplastic), with ≥ 30% of the non-erythroblastic cells being blasts. In a series of 160 cases of apparently de novo AML, the haemopoietic cells of the bone marrow in 24 cases showed severe trilineage myelodysplasia; in 60% of these cases the blast cell counts were < 60%, whereas in the bone marrow of the 136 cases without evidence of trilineage myelodysplasia, the blast cell counts were < 60% in only 11%. Note that in M2 and M4 AML, however, dysgranulopoiesis is part of the leukaemic process, and can lead to the onset of neutropenia or infections in the presence of normal counts of presumably nonfunctional neutrophils when the marrow blast-cell count is still relatively low. In these cases the megakaryocytes are morphologically normal and dyserythropoiesis is absent or minimal. It is true that in cases of AML with blast-cell counts exceeding 85% the number of residual haemopoietic cells may be insufficient to permit the recognition of trilineage myelodysplasia, but, for the reasons given, it is improbable that blast-cell replacement of a dysplastic bone marrow could progress so far without symptoms arising. Thus it seems likely that about 15% of cases of apparently de novo AML arise on a pre-existing symptomless MDS.

TREATMENT

Low-grade MDS

RAS and RA are not ordinarily life-threatening in the short term, and are managed conservatively with filtered blood transfusions and platelet transfusions as required. In the long term, iron overload may become a problem, while in a minority of cases of RAS the spleen has enlarged progressively, occasionally to an enormous size with the development of a fibrotic bone marrow, the onset of other cytopenias, and an accompanying increase in the transfusion requirement. Splenectomy has been helpful in some of these cases in the short term but is hazardous in the presence of thrombocytopenia. Between 5% and 10% of patients with RAS and RA may be expected to develop AML. It is possible that in the future the development of acceptable guides for identifying the poor-risk cases will justify trials of some of the forms of treatment that at present are confined to high-grade MDS. Neutropenic patients are susceptible to infections that can be lethal, and they require prompt treatment with the appropriate antibiotics, as used in the management of acute leukaemia.

High-grade MDS

The following forms of treatment are now under trial for treating the high-grade syndromes, RAEB and RAEB-t.

1. Putative stem-cell differentiating agents, especially cytosine arabinoside at low dosage.
2. Intensive chemotherapy as used for AML.
3. Marrow-ablative treatment followed by allogeneic bone marrow transplantation.

It must be emphasized that none of these treatments yet has an accepted place in the management of MDS, and it is possible that more effective methods will be developed before the full value of any of them has been worked out. Some general comments are nevertheless appropriate. Marrow-ablative treatment is generally restricted to patients below the age of 40 who have a histocompatible sib as the bone marrow donor. However, the majority of such patients with RAEB or RAEB-t will be cases of secondary MDS; many will have received irradiation for their primary neoplasm at a dosage that precludes the possibility of administering whole-body irradiation as part of the marrow-ablation therapy and conditioning to prevent graft rejection. Thus, unless major changes in transplantation technology are developed, the number of patients treated will remain small. For those who can be treated the success rate is likely to be similar to that for de novo AML, with rather more than one-half of the patients cured.

Intensive chemotherapy, as used for treating de novo AML, is justified for RAEB or RAEB-t patients below the age of 50 because their prospects for survival if treated only by supportive measures are so poor. However, the remission rate and pattern of survival will not be known until larger numbers of patients have been treated. The risks of treatment are greater than in AML, because the marrow of some patients remains hypoplastic after intensive chemotherapy and fails to regenerate. A reliable test for the presence of residual normal stem cells would permit the exclusion of patients who have few or none from a trial of intensive chemotherapy. In some cases the bone marrow that regenerates after the first course of treatment contains only dysplastic cells, in others some normal cells reappear, or the majority of cells are normal. The most favourable cases are those in which the proportion of dysplastic cells drops after each successive course of treatment until few or none can be seen. The risks of treatment are even greater in secondary MDS than in primary MDS.

An indication of the type of response to be expected is provided by the results of treating patients who present with apparently de novo AML and severe trilineage myelodysplasia as described above. The bone-marrow blast-cell count may be reduced to about 1% after the first course of intensive chemotherapy, but dysplastic cells in all lineages may persist, though in declining proportions, until four or five courses have been administered. However, if sufficient normal stem cells remain, normal blood counts will be restored after each course of treatment. Subsequently, complete remission may continue for long periods, or MDS alone returns after a few months but sometimes not for some years, while in other cases AML blasts reappear independently of the MDS. The occurrence of some long remissions justifies the use of intensive chemotherapy for younger selected patients with RAEB or RAEB-t with severe symptoms and for those whose MDS has already progressed to overt AML.

The use of putative differentiating agents was based on the experimental finding that leukaemia cell populations could be reduced by exposing them to agents that induced the blast cells to enter a differentiation pathway and so lose their self-replicating capacity. Cytosine arabinoside (Ara-C) was one such agent, and the effect was demonstrated at very low dosage that was not cytotoxic. In the treatment of MDS, however, Ara-C at doses of the order of 10–20 mg/m^2 b.d. subcutaneously has proved to be cytotoxic and will cause bone marrow hypoplasia. It is therefore not a 'safe' treatment, and patients must be followed with the same care and full support as those receiving intensive therapy. But the treatment is well tolerated and is acceptable to elderly patients, who make up the majority of all cases of RAEB and RAEB-t. Ara-C is usually given for 14 to 21 days, courses being repeated 4- or 6-weekly. The majority of favourable responses occur after one or two courses, and subsequently 7-day courses are administered each month. Complete remissions are unusual, but about one-third of the patients derive some benefit insofar as their transfusion requirement lessens and their platelet and neutrophil counts rise to less dangerous or even adequate levels for some months at least.

The retinoid cis-retinoic acid (CRA) has also induced shortlived benefit in cases of MDS but, as with Ara-C, there is insufficient information to define precisely its role in management. The Medical Research Council's Working Party on Leukaemia in Adults has started a multicentre trial in which the effect of Ara-C at low dosage (5 mg/m^2 b.d.) will be compared with that of Ara-C in combination with CRA (40 mg/m^2 daily).

Chronic Myelomonocytic Leukaemia

Patients with an enlarged spleen, high monocyte counts, anaemia or thrombocytopenia sometimes benefit from cytoreductive therapy with hydroxy-urea, mercaptopurine, etoposide, razoxane, or Ara-C at low dosage, and prednisolone as the sole agent is sometimes effective but has usually been administered in combination with one or more of the other drugs. The spleen shrinks, the monocyte count falls and the haemoglobin rises. Treatment may be continuous or intermittent, with dosage adjusted according to the blood count trends as in the treatment of chronic granulocytic leukaemia; good control may be achieved for months, occasionally years. CMML is rare and there have been no satisfactory formal trials of the agents mentioned; it is inadvisable to attempt specific recommendations.

When CMML undergoes blastic transformation, the ensuing downhill and fatal course usually progresses rapidly. A 5-day course of mitozantrone, a recently introduced anthracenedione administered intravenously at 10 mg/m^2, in combination with 2-hour intravenous infusions of Ara-C at 1 g/m^2 12-hourly for six doses, each infused for 4 hours, has induced prolonged remission, but this treatment induces profound marrow hypoplasia, requires the full supportive care appropriate to the management of AML, and is dangerous in the elderly patients who make up the majority of cases of CMML.

SELECTED BIBLIOGRAPHY

Bloomfield C. D. (1986). Chromosome abnormalities in secondary myelodysplastic syndromes. *Scandinavian Journal of Haematology*, **36(45)**, 82–90.

Francis G. E., Hoffbrand A. V. (1985). The myelodysplastic syndromes and preleukaemia. In *Recent advances in haematology*, Vol. 4, pp. 239–267 (Ed. A. V. Hoffbrand). Edinburgh: Churchill Livingstone.

Galton D. A. G. (1984). The myelodysplastic syndromes. *Clinical and Laboratory Haematology*, **6**, 99–112.

Griffin J. D. (Ed.) (1986). The myelodysplastic syndromes. *Clinics in haematology*, Vol. 15, No. 4. London: W. B. Saunders.

Mufti G. J. *et al.* (1985). Myelodysplastic syndromes: a scoring system with prognostic significance. *British Journal of Haematology*, **59**, 425–433.

Pedersen-Bjergaard J., Larsen S. O. (1982). Incidence of acute non-lymphocytic leukaemia, preleukaemia and acute myeloproliferative syndrome up to 10 years after treatment of Hodgkin's disease. *New England Journal of Medicine*, **307**, 965–971.

Ruutu T. (Ed.) (1986). The myelodysplastic syndromes. *Scandinavian Journal of Haematology*, **36**, Suppl. 45.

Chapter 18

MYELOMATOSIS

D. A. G. GALTON

Myelomatosis (MM) is one of the lymphoproliferative disorders affecting the B-lymphocyte system. Unlike chronic lymphocytic leukaemia (CLL), which is considered to arise by the proliferation of a clone of 'virgin' B lymphocytes at an early stage of immunological maturation before contact with antigen has been made, MM involves a clone of immunoglobulin-secreting cells. Normally, such cells proliferate as a result of stimulation by antigen, but it is not known whether myeloma clones arise in this way, though there is suggestive evidence that they might, at least in some cases. Other monoclonal proliferative conditions involving immunoglobulin-secreting plasma cells include the following: (a) monoclonal gammopathy of undetermined significance (MGUS); (b) equivocal myelomatosis (EMM); (c) solitary myeloma of bone (SMB); (d) extramedullary plasmacytoma (EMP); (e) immunoproliferative small-intestinal disease (IPSID, α-chain disease and other 'heavy-chain' diseases); (f) plasma-cell leukaemia (PCL). Waldenström's macroglobulinaemia (WM) is a monoclonal proliferation of B lymphocytes at a more advanced stage of immunological maturation than those of CLL, but less so than those of the above-named conditions. In WM, a range of cell types is found, including lymphocytes bearing surface immunoglobulins M and D, or M only, plasmacytoid lymphocytes containing cytoplasmic IgM, and IgM-secretory plasma cells. In rare cases resembling WM clinically, cytologically and histologically, the paraprotein found is IgG or IgA. Although in classical WM the clinical manifestations are the result of the continuous production over a period of years of large amounts of monoclonal macroglobulin, there is a continuous spectrum of clinical presentations between those with the classical manifestations and those with frank malignant lymphoma.

MM differs from the other plasma-cell tumours, except PCL, in that it is disseminated from the earliest recognizable stage, and, with the exception of the rare patients known to have had an SMB up to 20 years before, no primary focus can be found. In clinical practice it is important to distinguish MGUS and EMM from MM because treatment is indicated only for MM.

EPIDEMIOLOGY AND AETIOLOGY

Myelomatosis is not a disease of recent times, for bones showing the typical lesions have been found at archaeological sites. However, national mortality trends that suggest rapid increases in the past 40 years must be interpreted with caution because MM was underdiagnosed before the general use of modern diagnostic techniques, particularly bone-marrow puncture and the identification of paraproteins, which were introduced gradually and at different times in different countries. However, in American blacks the incidence in all age groups is considerably higher than in whites; the incidence in Japan is lower than in Europe; and it is generally lower in rural than in urban communities. These differences are not entirely explained by differences in access to medical care, and part of the general recorded increase may be genuine; in the past 30 years, for example, the increase for males has slightly exceeded that for females, while cohort data for England and Wales suggest that, for persons born in 1880, the death rate doubled about every 10 years whereas for those born between 1905 and 1915, it doubled about every 5 years from age 45–49 when it was about 1 per 100 000. Thus MM is predominantly a disease of the elderly. Everywhere there is a slight excess among males. Rarely, MM occurs in sibs or in parent and child; there is one record of a pair of identical twins, but none yet of an affected spouse. As in some other malignant diseases, a few myeloma-prone families have been reported with several affected first- and second-degree relatives.

There are few aetiological leads. Mineral oils injected intraperitoneally in mice induce granulomas in which plasmacytomas often develop. They produce paraproteins, some of which have antibody activity against antigenic determinants of the murine gut flora. However, plasmacytomas do not develop in mineral-oil granulomas induced in 'germ-free' mice, although poorly differentiated lymphomas do. Thus the mineral oils are oncogenic, but the differentiation and maturation of the target cell are influenced by other environmental factors, in this case chronic antigenic stimulation. Antibody activity has only rarely been demonstrated by human paraproteins in spite of extensive search. However, the number of antigenic determinants so far tested represents an infinitesimally small proportion of possible stimulators.

A small minority of M-proteins in human MM react specifically with α-staphylolysin, streptococcal hyaluronidase, and other bacterial antigens. In rare cases, the antibody specificity of these M-proteins is against antigens to which the patients had been exposed many years earlier, for example antistreptolysin activity in a patient who had had repeated attacks of rheumatic fever, or antihorse $α_2$-macroglobulin activity in a patient who had, on two occasions 6 months apart, received horse serum injections 30 years before. It is conceivable, though unproved, that all M-components have specific reactivity with unknown antigenic determinants. If so, the malignant clone of myeloma cells would represent a mutation in a previously normal monoclone, itself selected in the course of long-continued reaction against a particular antigen. However, only in rare cases is it possible to obtain a clinical history of long-standing chronic infection that could provide the conditions for the evolution of a normal antibody-producing monoclone and the

subsequent mutation to malignant growth. Furthermore, MM would be expected to arise most commonly in the tissue containing the greatest concentration of plasma cells under the continuous stimulus of antigenic stress. This tissue is the lamina propria of the bowel, one of the most common sites of origin of extramedullary plasmacytoma, but, so far as is known, never a primary focus of MM. Moreover, if the lamina propria were a common site for the development of MM, a high proportion of cases would be associated with an IgA paraprotein, but the distribution of the immunoglobulin classes in MM suggests a random origin determined only by the relative frequencies of the plasma-cell precursors responsible for the production of immunoglobulins of each class. Nevertheless, in IgA MM compared with cases of other Ig classes, a higher proportion of patients appear to have a history of long-standing chronic gastrointestinal or biliary-tract disease.

The long latency period in the cases cited above is of interest in relation to ionizing radiation as a possible cause of MM, because the available evidence from, for instance, the survivors of the atomic bomb explosions of 1945 indicates a period beyond 15 years between exposure and diagnosis.

Whatever the cause of the expansion of the monoclone, the paraproteins produced by the cells are normal immunoglobulins distinguished only by the identity, in any one case, of all the molecules in respect of every known structural feature. In a small minority of cases, MM is oligoclonal, usually biclonal; when combinations such as IgGK and IgAL occur, it is not possible to infer the origin of one clone from the other as a result of mutation. When a light chain is shared, analysis of the immunoglobulin gene rearrangement would show whether it is indeed the same protein, and whether the $γ$ and $α$ chains arose from the same gene by class switching.

PATHOGENESIS

The current concept of the pathogenesis of MM has been greatly influenced by the recent discoveries about the nature and origin of the immunoglobulins in humans and in experimental animals, summarized in Chapters 8 and 12. In MM, the paraprotein serves as a cell marker, its homogeneity indicating that all the cells synthesizing it are related by descent from a single precursor and, therefore, represent a clone. The site of origin of the precursor cell is unknown, and by the time the disease is detectable it is usually widely disseminated throughout the red bone marrow of the axial skeleton.

In immunological reactions involving antibody production, the antibody-secreting plasma cells are end cells produced by the division and maturation of antigen-stimulated B lymphocytes, but they do not themselves proliferate. The lesions of MM appear histologically to be composed almost entirely of plasma cells; it is not possible to recognize a developmental sequence between lymphocytes and plasma cells, and this is true also of Romanowsky-stained bone marrow films. Binucleate, or even tetranucleate, cells are usually a feature, as they sometimes are in reactive plasmacytosis, but it is rare to be able to identify a mitotic cell as a plasma cell. Nevertheless, the common appearance of multiple spherical lesions widely disseminated in the skeleton suggests the growth of colonies of cells from single bloodborne precursor cells. Indeed, the blood lymphocytes in MM include, in varying proportions, monoclones bearing surface immunoglobulins identical in all respects, including idiotypic specificity, with the monoclonal Ig secreted by the myeloma cells, and these circulating cells also show the same immunoglobulin gene rearrangement pattern. Perhaps circulating lymphocytes are the source of the plasma-cell infiltrates and discrete lytic lesions of MM, and it has been suggested that the clonogenic cell is a small non-secretory lymphocyte bearing the C-ALL antigen (CD10) but not containing terminal deoxynucleotidyl transferase (TdT). However, it is not clear whether a continuous supply of lymphocytes is necessary to perpetuate the infiltration or whether the lesions, once established in a favourable environment, are self-perpetuating. Possibly the spherical tumour nodules that in serial x-rays over a number of years may be observed to increase in diameter, are self-perpetuating tumours, while the diffusely infiltrating plasma cells interspersed among the haemopoietic cells may be end cells.

Recently, myeloma cells from human bone marrow taken from patients with MM have been successfully cultured in vitro and the clonogenic cells have the morphology of plasmablasts.

Growth Rate in Myelomatosis

The development of MM has been observed in many untreated patients in whom the diagnosis was made early by chance, or was uncertain when the paraprotein was first detected in the serum. In most cases, the serum levels of paraprotein increased exponentially over the period of observation, up to 8 years before treatment was begun. In the IgG disease, the serum concentration of paraprotein was shown by Hobbs (1969) to double every 10.1 months on average, in IgA disease every 6.3 months, and in Bence Jones protein disease the urinary output doubled every 3.4 months. The average serum concentration of IgA paraprotein at the time of clinical presentation in one series was between 25 g/l and 30 g/l, representing a daily production of about 15 g of paraprotein. The corresponding figure for IgG myeloma was 13 g. If the estimate for the daily production of paraprotein of 14 mg per gram of plasma cells were correct, the average total mass of tumour cells at clinical presentation would be about 1 kg, corresponding to about 4.6×10^{11} cells. Direct estimates by Salmon and Smith (1970) of the rate of paraprotein synthesis by myeloma cells in fresh marrow samples by means of radioimmunoassay capable of measuring nanogram amounts, showed that single cells produced an average of 12 pg of paraprotein per day, and their estimate of the total tumour mass in the body at the time of clinical presentation was of the order of 3 kg, corresponding to between 0.3×10^{12} and 3.0×10^{12} myeloma cells. These estimates are close to the order of magnitude estimated for acute leukaemia in the subterminal stage, and the median survival in untreated MM from the time of clinical presentation is probably of the order of 1 year or less.

The lowest detectable serum concentrations of paraproteins correspond to between 20 g and 50 g of tumour, and the lowest detectable concentration of Bence Jones protein in concentrated urine (about 100 mg/l of unconcentrated urine) corresponds to about 5 g of tumour, and between 10^9 and 10^{10} cells. Assuming that the growth rate of the myeloma cells and their rate of paraprotein production remain unchanged from the inception of the malignant transformation of the first myeloma cell, Hobbs extrapolated the curve backwards by plotting the total number of tumour cells (calculated from the observed paraprotein concentrations) against the time interval between the first detection of paraprotein and the onset of clinical MM, and estimated the total duration of IgG MM as of the order of 33 years, of the IgA disease as 21 years, and of the Bence Jones disease as 11 years. These estimates are consistent with the fact that, in patients presenting below age 50, there is an increasing proportion of Bence Jones MM in successively younger age groups. However, there is evidence that growth slows in the terminal stage. The retardation of growth rate with increase in the total number of tumour cells is well known in the case of solid tumours in experimental animals and is described mathematically by the Gompertzian expression which includes a constant defining the rate of retardation. Salmon found that the observed growth rate in MM is better described by the Gompertzian than by the uncorrected exponential function. Hobbs' estimates would therefore be far too long. In some cases of MGUS in which the paraprotein concentration has remained stable for many years, a rapid increase occurs in 1 or 2 years with the development of overt MM.

Features of Growth and Spread

The harmful effects of MM are the result of two main events: first, the cellular proliferation itself, and secondly, the excessive production of paraprotein, especially Bence Jones protein.

The cellular proliferation is at first largely confined to red bone marrow which, as the disease advances until more and more haemopoietic tissue becomes replaced by myeloma-cell infiltration, extends into the fatty marrow of the long bones, which in turn becomes infiltrated with myeloma cells. The replacement of haemopoietic tissue leads first to impairment of bone marrow function and finally to failure.

The infiltration takes two main forms: there is diffuse infiltration in which the myeloma cells are intimately admixed with the haemopoietic cells, and there are tumour nodules composed entirely of myeloma cells which displace the haemopoietic tissue in which they develop. The arrangement of the myeloma cells and their relationship to the haemopoietic cells in the two forms of infiltration can be appreciated only in histological sections of bone marrow, but films made from randomly aspirated samples usually show fragments of bone marrow of normal structure and the trails contain a mixture of haemopoietic cells and myeloma cells. Myelomatous nodules are sometimes entered in an attempt at routine aspiration which proves difficult; a core of whitish tissue is found at the end of the needle which spreads with difficulty on slides, but proves to consist almost entirely of myeloma cells.

Bone Lesions

Radiological examination (Fig. 18.1) shows the nodules as round, sharply circumscribed lucent areas, usually less than 1 cm in diameter, with no evidence of surrounding tissue reaction indicating new bone formation. In cancellous bone the fine trabeculae are completely destroyed in the region occupied by the nodules. Where the nodules encroach on cortical bone, the same sharply circumscribed destruction occurs, giving the characteristic punched-out appearance. Patients with lytic lesions practically always have diffuse infiltration also, and there is often generalized osteoporosis, involving the long bones as well as the axial skeleton. About 20% of patients have diffuse bone marrow infiltration but few or no lytic lesions, and show no radiological abnormality.

Because of the concentration of the disease in the axial skeleton in the earlier stages, the main effects of the osteoporosis and of the lytic lesions are in the vertebrae, pelvis, ribs and sternum. Wedging and gross collapse of vertebral bodies, especially in the mid-dorsal, lower dorsal and upper lumbar vertebrae, are common. Later, pathological fractures of the long bones, especially the femora, ribs and sternum, occur. It is difficult to relate the occurrence of bone pain to the degree of skeletal involvement assessed radiologically, apart from that associated with the wedging and collapse of vertebral bodies, or gross destruction of bone in a particular region. Some patients with extensive skeletal involvement have little or no pain, others with much pain have no radiologically detectable lesions. The vault of the skull is often peppered with myriads of lytic lesions when other bones contain few. The skull lesions scarcely ever give rise to pain, whereas patients with lesions of similar radiological appearance resulting from metastatic cancer often have pain. The radiological lesions of MM, though highly characteristic, are sometimes closely mim-

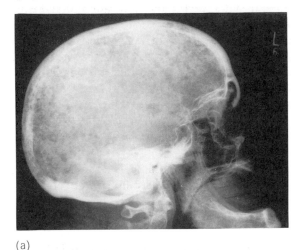

(a)

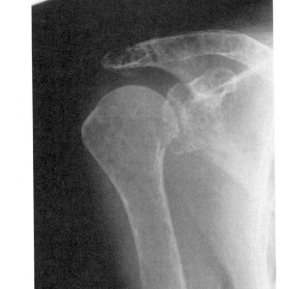

(b)

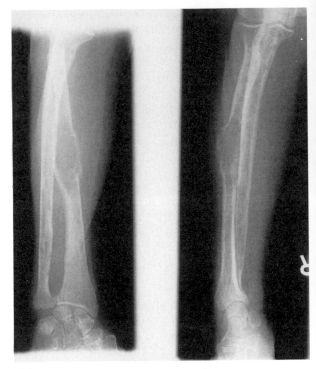

(c)

Fig. 18.1. *X-ray appearance of (a) skull, and (b) and (c) long bones in myelomatosis.*

icked by metastatic malignant disease of varied origin. A very rare form of MM usually affecting patients below age 40 and often associated with peripheral neuropathy gives rise to sclerotic bone lesions.

At presentation, about 60% of all patients with MM have recognizable lytic lesions, with or without osteoporosis, wedging or collapse of vertebral bodies, and pathological fractures; about 20% of patients have only osteoporosis, and the remainder have no relevant radiological abnormality. About one-half of patients with IgG MM and four-fifths of those with only Bence Jones protein have extensive lytic lesions at presentation, the frequency in IgA disease being intermediate. In a group of cases of IgG MM, Salmon found that the degree of skeletal involvement was correlated with the total estimated myeloma-cell mass.

The osteolytic action of the myeloma cells causes continuing loss of calcium from the skeleton. At presentation, nearly one-quarter of all the patients have a serum calcium concentration above the upper limit of normal, 2.5 mmol/l, the frequency being highest in Bence Jones protein MM (more than one-third), in which a higher proportion of patients have extensive lytic lesions at presentation. There is little attempt at bone repair in or around the lytic lesions, though callus formation and the laying down of new bone do occur in those parts of the bone ends in pathological fractures not wholly replaced by tumour. Thus the serum alkaline phosphatase level remains normal except in the presence of healing fractures. Episodes of acute hypercalcaemia leading to severe dehydration and uraemia may be life threatening. Sharply defined sickle-shaped white deposits of metastatic calcification at the corneal limbus are easily visible in many cases, but gross deposits elsewhere, especially in the kidneys, are rare.

The lytic effect of myelomatous deposits is due to the action of osteoclasts, and there is evidence that they are stimulated by a product of plasma cells. Culture medium in which myeloma cells have been growing has been shown to have osteolytic activity and it has been possible to estimate the amount of osteoclast-activating factor (OAF) produced by single myeloma cells in short-term cultures. Recent work suggests that osteoclasts are activated by the leucocyte-activating factor interleukin-1 and by tumour-necrosis factor β, but other substances may be active also.

Acute hypercalcaemia is most frequent in patients with generalized osteoporosis and extensive lytic lesions, but occurs occasionally when the tumour-cell mass is still below the size at which a formal diagnosis of MM is possible; such a patient presenting in acute hypercalcaemia may therefore be found on investigation to have the features of EMM. In these cases the myeloma cells presumably secrete unusually large amounts of OAF.

Soft-tissue Involvement

In a minority of cases of MM, the spleen, liver or lymph nodes are enlarged at presentation, and involvement of these organs is found in about 15% of cases *post mortem*. The blood films of these patients often show small numbers of myeloma cells. The myeloma cells tend to get carried to the end of the film when it is being spread and should be

sought there. The frequency of soft-tissue involvement of this type is apparently high in the rare IgD MM. Considerably more common, however, is the extension of individual deposits of tumour into the tissues outside the bone as a result of complete erosion of the cortex and infiltration of and extension beyond the periosteum. When this occurs from a vertebral body into the spinal theca, a thick cuff of tumour may spread extradurally or may erode the pia-arachnoid causing spinal compression. (This type of extension is discussed further in the section on treatment.) Rarely, deposits occur in other tissues such as the skin, but the majority of cases of skin and subcutaneous involvement by plasma-cell tumours are examples of metastases from extramedullary plasmacytoma, a condition distinct in most respects from MM (see below).

Hyperproteinaemia and Proteinuria

The continued production of paraprotein has several consequences. By far the most serious is the synthesis of Bence Jones protein (BJP), the persistent production of which leads to functional and structural damage to the kidneys, irreversible beyond a critical point. This substance consists of monoclonal light chains in a monomeric (molecular weight approximately 22 000) or dimeric (molecular weight approximately 44 000) form, and enters the renal tubule with the glomerular filtrate. Enormous quantities, of the order of 50 g, may enter the urine every 24 hours, but in most cases the amount excreted daily is less than 15 g. The mechanism whereby the passage of BJP damages the renal tubular epithelium is largely unknown. The visible manifestation of damage as seen *post mortem* in some but not all patients who have died in renal failure is the so-called myeloma kidney. The BJP is precipitated as a viscous mass in the collecting tubules and the distal convoluted tubules, causing obstruction. Proximal to the obstruction the tubule dilates, the epithelial cells atrophy, and macrophages cluster round the deposits of BJP. No doubt large numbers of glomerulotubular units are destroyed in this way, and BJP may impair tubular function. It has been shown to inhibit the transport of p-amino hippurate; this may be caused by inhibition of the active transport enzyme oubainsensitive Na-K-ATPase. BJP also influences the capacity of the tubule for reabsorbing low-molecular-weight proteins. In the urine of normal persons, traces of immunoglobulin light chains are present in the proportions in which they are present in the serum immunoglobulins, two-thirds being κ chains, one third λ. In experimental animals the rate of disappearance of injected radioiodine-labelled BJP from the serum has been shown to be greatly retarded by nephrectomy, but not by ligation of the ureters. Evidently, most of the light chains in the normal glomerular filtrate are reabsorbed by the renal epithelium and are catabolized there, but the capacity for doing so is limited.

The myeloma cells of about 15% of MM patients secrete only BJP, while the cells of about 70% of the remainder secrete BJP as well as a complete Ig, ranging from trace amounts to large quantities. The mean concentration in the urine is markedly higher in IgGL and IgAL cases than in IgGK and IgAK cases, but markedly lower than in pure BJP disease in which the concentration in type L cases is nearly twice that in type K cases. In untreated patients whose cells secrete both complete Ig and BJP, the concentrations of both increase in parallel, suggesting an imbalance in the rate of synthesis and assembly of light and heavy chains. In a minority of patients whose urine does not contain detectable BJP at presentation, the protein appears later in the course of the disease, and is of the same light-chain class as that in the complete serum Ig; in these cases a further mutation may have led to the emergence of a subclone no longer capable of synthesizing heavy chains. Note that isoelectric focusing is a far more sensitive method for detecting trace amounts of BJP than conventional immunoelectrophoresis, but is still not widely used.

Renal Failure

About one-quarter of MM patients are azotaemic (blood urea concentration (BUC) ≥ 10 mmol/l) at presentation. In a minority of these the BUC will fall to normal levels after 48 hours of hydration therapy, but raised levels persist in the remainder. If untreated, the risk of dying is high: about 70% of those with a BUC > 15 mmol/l or a serum creatinine concentration of > 200 μmol/1 die within 100 days.

The cause of acute renal failure in MM is not clear. It is strongly associated with Bence Jones proteinuria which causes selective tubular damage as shown by failure to reabsorb α_1 microglobulin and α_1 acid glycoprotein but with retention of the capacity to reabsorb other low-molecular-weight proteins, including retinol-binding protein and β_2 microglobulin. This tubular dysfunction is not by itself sufficient to initiate acute renal failure for it is present in patients with a normal or moderately raised BUC who have Bence Jones proteinuria. Precipitating factors include dehydration, hypercalcaemia, cast formation, and pyogenic infection. A minority of patients excrete large amounts of BJP for long periods without going into renal failure but it has not been possible to show that some light chain molecules are more nephrotoxic than others. The 'myeloma kidney' is the commonest renal lesion associated with renal failure, and other lesions such as those of pyelonephritis, renal vein thrombosis, amyloid deposition, κ-light chain deposition, and plasma-cell infiltration are uncommon.

Though Bence Jones proteinuria is the most dangerous consequence of paraprotein production by the myeloma cells, other effects contribute in varying degree to the morbidity and to the mortality. Thus, paraprotein production is strongly associated with *low serum concentrations of the normal immunoglobulins*. In about two-thirds of the cases of IgG MM at presentation, the serum concentrations of the normal immunoglobulins are less than 20% of the mean normal levels; this is the case in about one-third of the cases of IgA MM, and about one-fifth of BJP MM. Equally severe depletion is found in the rare cases in which no paraprotein is detectable in the serum or in the urine. The relationship between paraprotein production and the reduction in the serum concentration of the normal immunoglobulins is complex. Normal levels are rarely seen following conventional chemotherapy, even when the concentrations of serum paraproteins, initially high, fall to undetectable levels, but are always observed following 'high-dose melphalan' therapy (see below), which induces complete remission. The low serum concentrations of the normal immunoglobulins are thought to reflect decreased synthesis because cells producing them are difficult to demonstrate in bone marrow films by immunofluorescence staining. However, in the presence of serum paraprotein at high concentration, the catabolic rate is increased, and this may account in part for the high frequency of low serum concentrations of the normal immunoglobulins in IgG MM in which the mean serum levels of paraprotein are higher (> 40 g/l) than in IgA MM (< 30 g/l). However, the lower mean serum concentration of IgA paraprotein itself reflects its high fractional catabolic rate.

The reduction in the serum levels of the normal immunoglobulins is associated with impaired capacity to respond to antigenic stimulation and with an increased incidence of respiratory tract infection. It is of interest to note, however, that the overall risk of infection is less in MM than in CLL in which comparably low serum levels of the normal immunoglobulins are found. This is because cell-mediated immunity, impaired in CLL, remains intact in MM. Hence, attacks of severe herpes zoster are common in CLL but rare in MM. Nevertheless, about one-fifth of all patients with MM give a history of respiratory infection during the year preceding the diagnosis, and life-threatening pyogenic infections are a substantial risk throughout the disease.

Rectal biopsy samples from λ-secreting MM patients show greatly reduced numbers of plasma cells in the lamina propria, especially affecting λ cells, but in cases of κ-secreting MM, the numbers of both κ- and λ-bearing plasma cells are reduced.

At high serum concentrations, paraproteins coat the surface of platelets and of leucocytes, and in-vitro tests show impairment of function, for example in the phagocytic capacity of neutrophils.

Two rare consequences of excessive paraprotein production are the hyperviscosity syndrome and the clinical effect of cryoglobulinaemia. The hyperviscosity syndrome occurs in MM only when the serum paraprotein levels are very high (usually over 80 g/l), usually in IgA MM. In IgA MM the whole blood viscosity is usually above the normal range and increases proportionally with increase in the proportion of paraprotein that is dimerized; however, the hyperviscosity syndrome is uncommon and sometimes results from protein aggregation. The effect on viscosity of the molecular shape, size, chemical configuration of the molecular surface,

and the serum concentration of paraprotein is complex. There is variation among the four subclasses of IgG paraproteins in this regard: with IgG, there is a linear relationship between the serum concentration and the viscosity, but at the lower concentrations, IgG_3 is associated with higher viscosity, and over part of the range the viscosity increases rapidly with small increases in concentration, as in the case of IgM which is associated with even higher viscosity at the lower serum concentrations. Therefore, the hyperviscosity syndrome is relatively more frequent in Waldenström's macroglobulinaemia than in MM.

The relationship between the properties of cryoglobulins and the production of clinical effects is complex. Cryoglobulins are found in the laboratory in the serum of patients who have no clinical disabilities that can be attributed to them, whereas other patients with clinical disability have cryoglobulins at lower concentrations that precipitate in the same thermal range. The physicochemical features responsible for cryoprecipitating properties are unknown, although IgG cryoproteins are more often IgG_3 paraproteins, which account for only 10% of IgG proteins. The protein precipitates in the microcirculation in the coldest parts of the skin, especially on the outer aspects of the feet, heels, legs, thighs, buttocks, arms and forearms. The clinical manifestations are varied, and include purpura, Raynaud's phenomenon and, in severe cases, areas of microinfarction with the production of extremely painful areas of necrosis in the affected skin. Microscopic haematuria with progressive impairment of renal function has been reported. About half the patients have perforations of the anterior part of the nasal septum resulting from tissue necrosis. The cryoprecipitating properties of the protein lead to the production of symptoms, whereas at the same or higher concentrations proteins without these properties would remain undetected. MM in which the paraprotein is a cryoprotein presents at an unusually early stage for this reason and the diagnosis is often missed because the very small numbers of myeloma cells in the bone marrow are likely to be overlooked, and radiologically detectable lesions are unlikely to have developed. Occasionally, the paraprotein forms immune complexes with one of the normal immunoglobulins, and the complex behaves as a cryoprotein.

Amyloidosis is found during life in less than 5% of all cases of MM, but, *post mortem*, is present in about 10%. It is associated with Bence Jones proteinuria and is more common in BJP and IgA MM but does occur rarely in the IgG disease. Evidence of amyloidosis may appear during the course of the disease, or may precede the discovery of MM. In some cases of primary amyloidosis, in most of which at least traces of BJP are found in the urine, the most careful investigation during life and *post mortem* fails to show the presence of MM. The precise relationship between primary amyloidosis and MM is still disputed. In association with MM, the common presentations of amyloidosis are the carpal tunnel syndrome, congestive cardiac failure, macroglossia, and lesions of the skin, subcutaneous tissues, tendon sheaths and fasciae, whereas in primary amyloidosis other presentations, rare in association with MM, also occur, the nephrotic syndrome being the most common. Skeletal involvement is uncommon and the percentage of plasma cells in the bone marrow rarely exceeds 10%. However, the relationship with MM is shown by the presence of a variable proportion of highly abnormal plasma cells, especially when a paraprotein at high concentration is also present. The progression of renal amyloidosis may be arrested by the treatments used to control MM, whereas the other manifestations of amyloidosis, whether primary or in association with MM, are not affected by treatment. Amyloidosis often involves the liver and heart simultaneously, and may be suspected clinically if hepatic enlargement is out of proportion to the degree of cardiac failure.

Amyloid is an insoluble complex deposit with a characteristic fibrillary ultrastructure. In both primary amyloidosis and in amyloidosis associated with MM (AL amyloid), its major component is a sequence of amino acids belonging to the variable portion of the monoclonal immunoglobulin light chain, usually lambda. As in some cases of MM with cryoglobulinaemia, clinical manifestations occur when the total plasma-cell mass is small, because of the special properties of the paraprotein, in this case those of the amyloid material. Occasionally, amyloid deposits gradually replace cellular myelomatous infiltrates, leaving few or no traces of the original cellular lesion; lytic lesions in the skeleton diagnosed radiologically as myelo-matous may prove to be amyloid deposits *post mortem*, and extensive amyloidosis may also be found in other tissues not at any time infiltrated by tumour cells, such as ligaments, tendon sheaths, fasciae, synovial membranes, muscles and nerves.

Although, biologically, primary amyloidosis is clearly a variant of MM in that it arises as a result of the activity of a monoclone of plasma cells, the clinical manifestations and course of the disease are so different from those of MM that it is better considered as a separate entity.

Light-Chain Deposition Disease

Light-chain deposition disease (LCDD) is a recently characterized entity analogous to amyloidosis in that it involves the deposition in various organs of an amorphous substance derived from immunoglobulin light chains. In contrast to amyloid and other deposit nephropathies, the material deposited in LCDD comes mostly from κ chains and includes part of the constant region. Deposits occur in the liver, heart and central nervous system where they rarely give rise to clinical manifestations, whereas renal deposition is highly dangerous. The extent of deposition is not correlated with the amount of κ chains in the urine, which may even be undetectable. The deposits are easily demonstrated by immunofluorescence with labelled antilight chain antiserum. In the kidney the deposition is on tubular basement membrane and irregularly in the glomerular basement membrane and mesangium where it eventually leads to nodular glomerulosclerosis, and end-stage renal failure. In most cases the patients present with proteinuria and sometimes also in renal failure. As in amyloidosis, the source of the light chains may be difficult to find. Occasionally a plasmacytoma is found. Cytotoxic chemotherapy has been effective in preventing further deposition of light chains and, when the kidney has not been irreversibly damaged, the proteinuria may cease and normal renal function may be restored; thus, in a case of a large retroperitoneal plasmacytoma, the tumour regressed following treatment with five monthly courses of melphalan, doxorubicin, cyclohexylnitrosourea and prednisolone and the nephrotic syndrome resolved completely.

PRESENTING FEATURES

Clinical

The onset of MM is usually insidious and therefore several symptoms have often appeared by the time the most insistent of them compels the patient to seek medical advice. Bone pain is the major symptom in about 60% of all cases. Symptoms resulting from anaemia and uraemia, often associated, account for 20% of cases in which bone pain is absent or a minor complaint. In 10% of cases an infection, most commonly pneumonia, is the presenting feature. In the remaining 10% of cases, the less common presentations include the carpal tunnel syndrome and other manifestations of amyloidosis, compression paraplegia and other syndromes arising from extraosseous extension, oliguric renal failure, neuropathies, thromboembolic disease, acute hypercalcaemia and hyperviscosity.

Major Laboratory Findings

Biochemical

The distribution of the M-protein types among 1608 patients in the first four MRC trials is shown in Table 18.1 and is representative. Note that the frequency of λ light chains is disproportionately high in IgA, IgD, and Bence Jones protein cases. Other findings are summarized in Table 18.2.

Haematological

Almost always the anaemia is normochromic and normocytic, and results from inadequate erythro-poiesis. Megaloblastosis, apparent in bone marrow films in about 10% of cases, is usually associated with low serum folate levels. Very rarely, the anaemia is hypochromic, and ringed sideroblasts or other features of the myelodysplastic syndrome are found in the bone marrow.

The depression in the neutrophil and platelet counts reflects the extent of the myeloma-cell infiltration in the marrow and varies from minor reduction to profound pancytopenia. Very rarely, the disease presents with a leukaemoid picture simulating chronic granulocytic leukaemia. A leuco-erythroblastic picture, sometimes with myeloma cells in the peripheral blood, occurs in about 10% of cases.

The myeloma-cell infiltrate in the bone marrow varies from case to case. The myeloma cells vary in their maturity: at least some are unusually large, have large nuclei with less well-condensed chromatin than the average normal plasma cell, and contain single nucleoli of varying size and prominence, while the voluminous cytoplasm is densely baso-philic, often with a floccular or ground-glass appearance, and the juxtanuclear pallor of the Golgi region may be scarcely visible (Fig. 18.2). In reactive states, the Golgi region is usually prominent in cells resembling myeloma cells in other respects. Nuclear or cytoplasmic inclusions of many kinds, and bi-, tri-, or tetranucleated cells, however, are found in reactive states as well as in MM. In general, myeloma cells are readily distinguishable from the normal plasma cells seen in rheumatoid arthritis, chronic liver disease, Hodgkin's disease and carcinoma, in which up to 20% of all the marrow cells may be plasma cells. But it is uncertain whether

Table 18.1

Distribution of paraprotein types in 1608 cases of myelomatosis (Medical Research Council's trials 1 to 4)

	γ	α	δ	μ	Light chain only	No paraprotein	All light chains
κ	562	246	3	2	126	—	939
λ	316	180	21	1	109	—	627
$\kappa + \lambda$	2	0	0	0	1	—	3
No light chain	—	—	—	—	—	18	18
Light chain not known	17	3	0	1	—	—	21
Total	897	429	24	4	236	18	1608

Table 18.2
Some laboratory findings in myelomatosis (MM)

Prognostic group	Serum concentration of						Polyclonal Ig < 20% of mean normal	Free monoclonal light chains (BJP) in urine
	Hb (g/l)	Urea (mmol/l)	Creatinine (μmol/l)	Albumin (g/l)	Calcium (μmol/l)	β₂ microglobulin (mg/l)		
Good risk	<75	<8	<130	Usually within normal range	Minimally raised in <50%	<4	In 65% of IgG 30% of IgA cases	Higher excretion in BJP disease (15% of all cases) $\lambda > \kappa$
Poor risk	≥100	>10	≥200	Often <35	>2.5 in >50%, especially in BJP disease	>6	20% of BJP MM	Larger amounts in IgAL and IgGL than in IgAK and IgGK

BJP, Bence Jones protein.

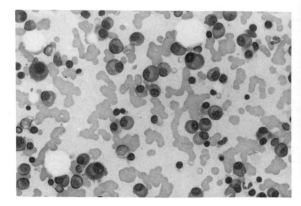

Fig. 18.2. *Film of bone marrow aspirate in myelomatosis. May-Grünwald-Giemsa stain. (By courtesy of Dr E. Wiltshaw.)*

myeloma cells can always be distinguished from the large plasma cells found in reactive states. The difficulty is greatest when the percentage of plasma cells is low and the cells, mostly mature, vary in size, shape and extent of cytoplasmic basophilia. A careful search will often be rewarded by the finding of at least a few cells sufficiently abnormal to suggest MM; if none is found, a confident diagnosis cannot be made, though the patient may indeed have MM; on subsequent review of the films, abnormal cells previously overlooked may be found.

Marrow films stained with monospecific anti-human immunoglobulin antisera prepared in rabbits and conjugated with fluorescein-isothio-cyanate, rhodamine and similar compounds confirm that all the myeloma cells synthesize monoclonal immunoglobulins of the same heavy-chain and light-chain classes.

In some cases the myeloma cells may be deeply basophilic ovoid forms with regular outlines and well-demarcated borders. In others, many cells have greyer cytoplasm, becoming deeply eosinophilic towards the periphery, with ill-demarcated borders and projections or wisps of eosinophilic material protruding from the border. These features are not associated with particular immunoglobulin classes. The majority of myeloma cells in any one case may be mature forms, while in others they may be so poorly differentiated as to be scarcely recognizable as plasma cells. Several types of cytoplasmic inclusions including bizarre elongated crystalline bodies are seen in almost every myeloma cell in rare cases. In the rare non-secretory forms, electron microscopy shows greatly distended sacs of endoplasmic reticulum in which immunoglobulin is retained.

Diagnostic Criteria

There is little difficulty in arriving at a diagnosis of MM when a patient complaining of skeletal pain is found to have: (1) the characteristic radiological appearances, (2) a monoclonal paraprotein in the serum, urine or both, and (3) myeloma cells in the bone marrow. Problems arise when the only abnormality found is an M-component in the serum, or a moderate increase in plasma cells of essentially normal morphology in bone marrow films. Suggestive radiological appearances in the absence of an M-component or of marrow infiltration are unlikely to be due to MM. It is rarely possible to diagnose MM unless two of the three major features are present, and even then it is important in doubtful cases to err on the side of caution and to repeat the investigations at intervals. Thus, a middle-aged woman with chronic low-back pain but no radiological abnormality, a normal bone marrow on several occasions, no Bence Jones protein detectable in the concentrated urine on several occasions, but a monoclonal paraprotein at a concentration of 30 g/l in the serum over an observation period of 7 years, during which the normal serum immunoglobulins remain at normal concentrations, is unlikely to have MM. The interpretation of the bone marrow in such a case when a small percentage of normal plasma cells is found has been considered elsewhere.

Monoclonal Gammopathy of Undetermined Significance

In the general population, some 3% of persons over 70 years have in their serum a monoclonal IgG, IgA or IgM (M-component), of no apparent pathological significance. The characteristic features of these benign conditions are: (1) the serum concentration remains unchanged over many years or may decline; (2) the concentration is usually less than 25 g/l; (3) the polyclonal immunoglobulins are almost always present at normal concentrations; (4) Bence Jones protein is absent or detectable in concentrated urine in trace amounts only in a minority of cases; (5) the bone marrow plasma cells are < 10% of the nucleated cells unless there is an associated cause of reactive plasmacytosis; and (6) the serum β_2 microglobulin is usually < 2 mg/l. This condition is not confined to elderly subjects, though its frequency in younger age groups is lower. It must be emphasized that such a benign monoclonal gammopathy may be suspected but cannot be diagnosed from the result of a single investigation. In most cases the condition remains unchanged, but some patients in fact have early MM and will show progressive increase in the paraprotein concentration for many years until overt MM is obvious, while in other cases the paraprotein concentration after several years of stability increases to high levels in the ensuing year or two, accompanied by the appearance of other features of MM. At presentation, therefore, it is wiser to classify these patients as having monoclonal gammopathy of undetermined significance (MGUS) because the true diagnosis can be established only after prolonged follow-up. In population-based studies the great majority prove to be benign, but in hospital practice about one in three cases shows progression to MM, or, in the case of IgM paraproteins, to WM after 15 years.

Equivocal myelomatosis (EMM) is a useful term for cases in which the findings are outside the range usual for MGUS, and may suggest MM but the patient is asymptomatic and the distinction between early progressive MM and 'smouldering' or 'non-progressive' MM cannot be made without regular follow-up. The category EMM offers the opportunity for prolonged observation before deciding whether and when treatment should be started.

In EMM, the serum paraprotein concentration may exceed 25 g/l, there may be some reduction in the concentration of polyclonal Ig, the bone marrow plasma cells may be up to 25% of the nucleated cells in the absence of an associated cause for reactive plasmacytosis, but urinary BJP if present will be minimal (less than 1 g/g of urinary creatine), the serum β_2 microglobulin (see p. 486) will be < 4 mg/l, there will be no impairment of bone marrow function, no more than one non-symptomatic osteolytic lesion, no impairment of renal function, and no evidence of progressive MM.

Very occasionally, an M-component appears transiently in the serum following an infectious disease, usually viral, and is probably an antibody. The same is probably true of M-components appearing and disappearing over the course of a year or more in a variety of chronic diseases. More stable M-components occasionally accompany malignant diseases other than the lymphomas, in which they are not uncommon. The nature of these M-components is controversial, but they have been considered as antibodies with specificity against tumour antigens, and in some cases immunofluorescent-antibody staining of sections of the tumour has shown positivity in some of the plasma cells concentrated in the neighbourhood of the tumours. However, the M-component usually persists after removal of the tumour when metastases are not known to be present. In some cases the M-component is due to coexisting MM, and in others is unrelated to the tumour and properly classified as MGUS; its nature may be clarified only by repeated investigation over a long period of time. The interpretation of bone marrow films requires special care because the proportion of plasma cells is often increased in many forms of malignant disease. The plasma cells show the same variation in size and shape as is usual in reactive states, and bi-nucleate cells and cells containing a variety of cytoplasmic inclusions are not uncommon, but the gross abnormalities usually found in MM are not seen, and the proportion of immature cells is usually low. Fortunately the practical management hinges on the treatment of the malignant disease already diagnosed, and coexisting MGUS or EMM should not necessitate any alteration in the planned treatment.

Symptomless primary amyloidosis may underlie the chance finding of an M-component, and the appropriate investigations are indicated. At some stage, BJP is likely to appear in the urine.

PRESENTING FEATURES INFLUENCING PROGNOSIS

Many features recorded at presentation have been examined singly and by multivariate analysis for possible prognostic significance, and several prognostic groupings and staging systems have been devised. In the staging system of Salmon and Durie, the features found to be of prognostic significance were selected after they had been shown to be correlated with estimates of the total tumour cell mass derived from quantitative assays of the rate of secretion of paraprotein by myeloma cells in short-term culture. In Cuzick's prognostic groupings the features of prognostic importance were found empirically by examining many features recorded at presentation in relation to the duration of survival of 485 patients entered into the Medical Research Council's Third MM trial. In the Salmon–Durie system the size of the total tumour mass can be inferred as low ($< 0.6 \times 10^{12}$ cells/m^2), intermediate or high ($> 1.2 \times 10^{12}$ cells/m^2) from the concentrations of Hb, calcium, paraprotein, the 24-hour BJP excretion and a numerical rating for the extent of skeletal involvement. The prognosis was found to be better in patients with a low tumour cell mass, and worse in those with a high tumour cell mass. In Cuzick's system the three most powerful independent determinants of prognosis were found to be the Hb, probably reflecting the total tumour cell mass, the blood urea concentration, reflecting renal function, and the performance status; these values were used to construct three groups of patients with good, intermediate and poor prognosis.

More recently, the serum concentration of β_2 microglobulin (β_2M) has been shown to be the most powerful single determinant of prognosis. β_2M, a polypeptide of 100 amino acids, is the light chain of the HLA class I antigens, and on the cell surface it is the extrinsic hydrophilic part of the complex. Its serum concentration increases with age but normally does not exceed 2 mg/l. It is excreted by the kidneys and the serum concentration increases as renal function deteriorates. In MM, the β_2M concentration therefore reflects renal function, itself a major prognostic determinant, but it also has independent prognostic value. However, it is the uncorrected β_2M serum concentration that provides the best prognostic guide, with one-half of the patients whose β_2M concentration is < 4 mg/l surviving beyond 3 years, compared with less than one-fifth of those with concentration > 20 mg/l. Moreover, the β_2M concentration has prognostic significance in treated patients who have reached the plateau phase when the paraprotein concentration has fallen to undetectable levels (about 10% of patients) or has remained stable at a low level. It is not understood why β_2M has prognostic significance independently of its role as an indicator of renal function. Indeed, its prognostic value, when examined in the Medical Research Council's fourth myelomatosis trial, though apparent in all three Cuzick prognostic groups, was greatest in the 'good' and 'intermediate' groups in which early death from renal failure was uncommon when compared with the 'poor prognosis' group. Most deaths from renal failure occur within 1 year, and when the predictive values of various presenting features were compared in all patients who survived 1 year after entry to the fourth trial, serum $\beta_2 M$ and haemoglobin were still the most important predictors. A special analysis involving a stepwise proportional hazards model showed that $\beta_2 M$ alone gave the most useful prognostic information, and haemoglobin added little.

The serum $\beta_2 M$ appears to bear some relation to the total tumour mass, because the concentration tends to fall during treatment that has brought down the serum paraprotein concentration, to remain stable during the 'plateau' phase, and to increase during the terminal phase of progression.

The bone-marrow plasma-cell labelling index (LI) has also been claimed to have prognostic value. A sample of aspirated bone marrow is exposed to ^{3}H-thymidine for 1 hour and the uptake recorded by high-speed scintillation autoradiography. Plasma cells actively synthesizing DNA are labelled by five or more black silver grains over the nucleus, and the number of labelled cells in 1000 counted is determined. A broad correlation between LI and survival has been found, and it is independent of the total tumour cell mass. Thus, among 'high-tumour-mass' (Salmon–Durie) patients, those with a low LI ($<1\%$) had a median duration of survival of 30.5 months, compared with only 5.3 months for those with a high LI ($>3\%$). The LI probably reflects the growth rate of the tumour.

TREATMENT

Theoretical Considerations

Survival curves for MM, unlike those for the acute leukaemias, Hodgkin's disease, and some types of non-Hodgkin lymphoma, show a continuous downward trend with no suggestion of a plateau of long survivors. Thus the aims of conventional treatment are to relieve symptoms and to bring about regression of the myeloma cell proliferation or at least to arrest or slow down its progression. The chief methods of treatment are: (1) chemotherapy with the alkylating agent melphalan or cyclophosphamide, and with prednisolone, and (2) radiotherapy for the relief of local bone pain. Ancillary methods include the administration of prednisolone, inorganic phosphate, mithramycin, or calcitonin for the immediate relief of acute hypercalcaemia, blood transfusion for the relief of anaemia, plasmapheresis for the immediate relief of symptoms arising from hyperviscosity of the blood due to the presence of paraprotein at high concentration or in a polymerized state, and the administration of diphosphonates to lessen the drain of calcium from the the skeleton.

We have seen that the evolution of the disease is slow, is in a preterminal stage when symptoms appear, and only slightly less advanced when the diagnosis is made by the chance discovery of a paraprotein in the serum. The situation is analogous to that for lymphoblastic leukaemia but there is an important difference. In the case of lymphoblastic leukaemia, there is no theoretical obstacle to the declared aim of radical therapy, and all the pathological effects of widespread blast cell infiltration are potentially reversible. In contrast, much of the damage caused by MM is irreversible, the most life-threatening injury being that to the kidneys. Major skeletal deformities, destructive bone lesions, and pathological fractures are also permanent, though orthopaedic surgery can do much to alleviate their effects. The analogy with lymphoblastic leukaemia stands in two respects: first, treatment successfully reduces the plasma cell infiltration in the bone marrow and so permits the regeneration of the haemopoietic cells and the recovery of bone-marrow function; and, second, the reduction in the total plasma cell number necessary to achieve this has been estimated as between 90% and 99% of the approximate number present at the start of treatment (the order of 10^{12}). Three inferences from these considerations are: (a) that the possibility of successful treatment is limited by the amount of irreversible damage already done; (b) that when the amount of irreversible damage is still small, treatment should be continued after all reversible manifestations have been eliminated; and

(c) that the prospects of curing the disease by new methods of treatment are likely to be greatest when the diagnosis is made by chance, because the total number of myeloma cells to be destroyed would be smaller than that present in more advanced disease.

Treatment Prospects Limited by Extent of Irreversible Damage

In MM the blood urea and creatinine concentrations, when not elevated as a result of hypercalcaemia and extrarenal causes, are reliable guides to the extent of renal damage. When the amount of surviving functional renal tissue is too small to sustain life, even the total destruction of all the tumour cells would be of no avail for the patient would die from renal failure. The quality of the treatment is irrelevant, for remedies far more effective against MM than any now available could not improve the results in this group of patients unless renal function could be restored. A transplanted kidney could sustain renal function as long as the MM was controlled but would fail to do so during relapse when, like the patient's own kidneys, it would be affected by the disease.

Irreversible skeletal damage is not directly life threatening, but its effects can be highly deleterious. Enforced immobility resulting from unrelieved compression paraplegia aggravates the loss of calcium from the skeleton and damages the kidneys. The gross kyphosis resulting from the collapse of many dorsal vertebral bodies leads to greatly impaired chest expansion and increases the risk, already higher than normal, of chest infections in elderly subjects. Pathological fractures of the femur should be pinned at the earliest opportunity because immobility is dangerous.

Amyloid once deposited appears to be permanent, but it seems possible that treatment may reduce the rate of deposition. Cardiac and renal damage already done may be regarded as irreversible, and is likely to persist during otherwise effective treatment. Humoral immunity is deficient in MM, and this is reflected in the low serum levels of the polyclonal immunoglobulins. When remission has been induced and paraprotein is no longer detectable in the serum or the urine, the concentration of the normal immunoglobulins rises only in a minority of cases, and normal levels are hardly ever achieved. The patients therefore remain unduly susceptible to infections while in remission, though, having regard to their high average age, intercurrent infection is perhaps less frequent than might be expected in relation to the low serum levels of immunoglobulin. Thus in every case, the prospects of what treatment may be expected to achieve must be considered in relation to the irreversible damage already done.

Necessity for Long-continued Treatment in Good-risk Cases

It is necessary to reduce the total body burden of myeloma cells to between 10^9 and 10^{10} in order to permit some recovery of bone marrow function, and, with continued treatment, further improvement occurs; in about 10% of cases, optimal clinical and biochemical conditions may not be achieved for as long as 2 years after the start of treatment. However, in most cases no further lowering of the serum or urinary Ig concentration occurs after 1 year, even when the initial treatment is continued. In practice, it is recommended that treatment should be continued for no more than 6 months after the establishment of a 'plateau' in the serum paraprotein concentration or after the disappearance of the paraprotein from the serum in the 10% of cases in which this happens.

Treatment of the Symptomless Patient

If effective treatment for MM were available, it would be logical to treat symptomless patients diagnosed by chance. Some clinicians already do so with the alkylating agents melphalan or cyclophosphamide. However, this practice is inadvisable even if MGUS and EMM are excluded. There are still a few symptomless patients with the criteria of definite MM whose disease is non-progressive and whose treatment may reasonably be deferred. Probably all patients who respond to melphalan or cyclophosphamide, and who do not succumb to unrelated diseases, become resistant to these alkylating agents. Resistance may not develop for as long as 7 years, but more often appears within 5 years and occasionally within 1 year. Thus, symptomless patients who have received prolonged treatment are likely to have become totally resistant to treatment by the time symptoms appear, which is the very time when they most need medical help. Meanwhile they would have been subjected to anxiety and inconvenience while receiving treatment, by no means innocuous, for a disease which had never troubled them and which the treatment failed to cure. There is also a small risk of the development of the myelodysplastic syndrome or of acute myeloid leukaemia in patients who have received long-term alkylating agent therapy. At present, therefore, and with a special reservation to be considered shortly, the treatment of the symptomless patient would seem not to be justified.

The conservative policy is advocated only because of the inevitability of the development of resistance to the treatments now available, and the certainty of this must be weighed against the probability of the development of irreversible renal damage. The regular estimation of the BUC is the best method of detecting early renal damage, and the examination of the urine for the presence of even a trace of BJP offers early warning of a trend which, if allowed to continue, is likely to damage the kidneys. Three-monthly estimations of the serum albumin, immunoglobulin, paraprotein, and calcium concentrations, of the blood urea, creatinine, and haemoglobin concentrations, platelet, total leucocyte and differential leucocyte counts, and examination of the urine for red cells, leucocytes, casts, protein and BJP should serve to permit the early recognition of deterioration on which the decision to start treatment is based. Bone marrow examination and radiological survey of the skeleton are of little value in deciding whether treatment should be started, but they are helpful as guides in following the progress of the disease and should be performed yearly.

Before the general use of melphalan, most MM patients died within 1 year, though a few survived beyond 10 years. Radiotherapy remains the quickest way of relieving localized bone pain but it does not influence the progress of the disease and for this chemotherapy is necessary. In the 1970s the standard treatment was melphalan and prednisolone in combination, but two successive Medical Research Council trials failed to show any evidence that prednisolone had any additional effect on survival; the addition of vincristine was also shown not to confer extra benefit. Melphalan treatment relieves bone pain, reduces the total plasma cell mass sufficiently to cause striking falls in the concentration of paraprotein in the serum and urine, and clears enough plasma cells from the bone marrow to permit the return of haemopoietic activity and the restoration of normal blood counts.

Melphalan, p-di-2-chloroethylamino-L-phenylalanine, is a bifunctional aromatic alkylating agent. In standard therapy it is administered orally in 4-day courses, with an interval of 21 days between the first days of successive courses, at a daily dose of 7 mg/m^2. If the serum creatinine concentration is > 200 μmol/1, the daily dose is reduced to 5 mg/m^2. Melphalan is myelosuppressive and patients who are already neutropenic or thrombocytopenic as a result of loss of haemopoietic tissue from plasma cell infiltration of the bone marrow cannot tolerate it. These patients and the few who do not absorb melphalan well are better treated with cyclophosphamide until their bone marrow function is restored, as are patients who have started treatment with melphalan but are unable to continue because of drug-induced thrombocytopenia or neutropenia. Cyclophosphamide is given weekly as a single intravenous dose of 300 mg/m^2. At this dosage it is well tolerated and is less myelosuppressive than melphalan. However, long-continued administration carries a risk of urothelial damage which can lead to persistent and occasionally uncontrollable haematuria. This is caused by acrolein, a metabolite of cyclophosphamide, which can be counteracted by giving mesna with each dose. Treatment with melphalan may be resumed when the total tumour cell mass has been reduced enough to restore haemopoiesis.

The beneficial effects of chemotherapy are the relief of bone pain and of anaemia, and the objective evidence of response is the favourable change in the blood counts, the serum and urine paraprotein concentrations, the β_2M concentration, and the bone marrow appearance. The improvement takes place gradually, is usually apparent within 6 months, but optimal control may be achieved only after 1 year or more of treatment. In spite of the partial or complete relief of bone pain, the skeletal lesions do not usually show any radiological evidence of resolution or calcification, and the subnormal serum concentrations of polyclonal immunoglobulins rarely increase to the normal ranges.

In patients who respond to treatment the rate of fall in the paraprotein concentration varies, and there is evidence that the prognosis is better when the rate of fall is slow (6 months to a year or more). In 85% to 90% of responders, the fall eventually ends and the paraprotein concentration becomes stabilized at a lower level. This is the plateau phase, and when there is clear evidence that the plateau phase is established, as shown by three successive estimations in a 6-month period, the treatment should be discontinued because there is no evidence that further treatment prolongs survival. After stopping the treatment, the duration of the stable phase varies from a few months to several years. Patients whose disease progresses soon after the end of treatment are less likely to respond when the treatment is resumed than those who relapse after a long period of stability, and subsequent responses are seldom as good as the first; in the later stages of the disease, bone pain becomes increasingly difficult to control, and pathological fractures, compression paraplegia, episodes of hypercalcaemia, bone marrow failure, intercurrent infections and renal failure are common.

In the first few months of treatment it is difficult to predict the outcome except when the disease advances rapidly, because of the varying and sometimes slow speed of response. In addition, some patients with localized bone pain that responds to radiotherapy remain well for long periods without showing any significant reduction in their paraprotein concentrations. In the past, chemotherapy was sometimes continued for years in these cases because of the possibility that it was retarding the progress of the disease. Nowadays it would be more usual to try a 'second-line' treatment after a trial of the first for 12 to 18 months. Unfortunately, the benefits of second-line treatments are usually short-lived and often obtained at the cost of unacceptable toxicity. For elderly patients particularly, it is important to avoid inflicting toxic treatments that do not bring benefits that they appreciate, even though a temporary fall in the paraprotein level allows the result to be recorded as a response. Even if it could be shown that second-line treatment could prolong life by a few months, such treatment would not be justified if it led to poor quality of life. There is now

clear evidence from the MRC fifth trial that the proportion of patients who reach plateau is higher, while the duration of the plateau phase before relapse and the duration of survival are longer when the treatment is with the four-drug schedule ABCM administered in 6-weekly cycles to a maximum of 12 than with the standard melphalan schedule. Each ABCM cycle consists of intravenous doxorubicin 30 mg/m^2 i.v., followed by carmustine (BCNU) at the same dose, both on day 1; on day 22, a 4-day course of melphalan at a daily dose of 6 mg/m^2 and of cyclophosphamide at a daily dose of 100 mg/m^2 are given. Appropriate dose reductions of melphalan and cyclophosphamide are made for azotaemic patients and of daunorubicin for patients with impaired liver function. ABCM is more toxic than the standard melphalan schedule, but is generally well tolerated and should now be accepted as the treatment of choice. Patients who are neutropenic or thrombocytopenic may be treated first with weekly cyclophosphamide as described above and with ABCM when the bone marrow function has improved.

In spite of the superiority of ABCM, the aim of the treatment is good palliation, and if ABCM is judged unacceptable to a patient, the standard melphalan schedule should be used.

Ancillary Treatment

Management of Renal Failure

Until recently, the high fatality of patients presenting in renal failure dominated the mortality statistics of MM. It was believed that renal failure was a direct consequence of light-chain-induced tubular damage and that it would be necessary to reduce light-chain excretion drastically to restore renal function; this was the rationale for the unsuccessful trial of intensive chemotherapy in the MRC third trial in MM. Seventy per cent of the patients who presented with a BUC of > 15 mmol/l had died within the first 100 days. In the fourth trial, patients whose BUC was still > 15 mmol/l or whose serum creatinine was > 200 μmol/l after 48 hours of hydration therapy continued to receive 3 litres of fluid daily for at least 3 months. Following this simple treatment, the fatality in the first 100 days fell to 40%, while the serum creatinine returned to normal in one-third of the survivors, and improved in most of the remainder. After the first 100 days the survival of the azotaemic patients was not markedly different from that of the remainder. There was no evidence that the administration of sufficient bicarbonate to render the urine neutral, in the hope that this would reduce the precipitation of BJP as casts, was beneficial.

Clearly, renal failure is not as lethal or as irreversible as it was formerly thought to be, but after an initial period of intravenous hydration therapy it is important to convince patients of the necessity of maintaining a fluid intake of 3 litres per day for at least 3 months. A minority of patients, for example those in cardiac failure, will be unable to tolerate this and may require short periods on dialysis. It should be noted that a favourable response to hydration therapy, with a fall in the serum creatinine and BUC, is not necessarily accompanied by a parallel fall in the BJP excretion, indicating that BJP alone is not the cause of renal failure.

Treatment of Acute Hypercalcaemia

Patients who develop acute hypercalcaemia rapidly become thirsty, mentally confused or drowsy, and vomiting starts a vicious cycle, while the deposition of calcium phosphate reduces the sensitivity of the renal tubules to antidiuretic hormone, thus increasing the dehydration and precipitating renal failure. They require carefully supervised hydration with intravenous fluids regulated by loop diuretics such as frusemide, and nearly always respond rapidly to steroids which after the first few hours can be taken orally as prednisolone at a daily dose of 30 mg. Buffered phosphate mixtures that deliver 1 g of inorganic phosphate intravenously or orally in 24 hours will lower the serum calcium concentration rapidly but are rarely necessary and should be used only if renal function is normal and the serum phosphate concentration low. In refractory cases, an intravenous 4-hour infusion of mithramycin at 15 μg/kg is often effective and may be repeated daily up to 4 days. Calcitonin is also transiently effective at an intravenous dose of 100–200 u. Steroids and calcitonin probably act by inhibiting OAF, either indirectly or directly. Aminohydroxypropylidene diphosphonate (APD) also inhibits osteoclast activity and is effective in relieving acute hypercalcaemia,

though little response occurs within 48 hours. APD is administered as a single intravenous infusion of 1 mg/kg over 24 hours.

Possible Use of Diphosphonates

The diphosphonates are pyrophosphate analogues that are resistant to endogenous phosphatases. They depress the activity of osteoclasts and so reduce bone resorption. In MM, osteoporosis, involving the widespread loss of trabecular bone, is irreversible because new trabecular bone can be laid down only on pre-existing surfaces. Dichloromethylene diphosphonate (DMDP) has been shown to reduce the urinary loss of calcium and hydroxyproline in MM, and also to reduce the number of osteoclasts, suggesting the reduction of bone resorption. It is possible that the long-term use of DMDP in MM might reduce the incidence of hypercalcaemia, the frequency of pathological fractures, and even the amount of bone pain as has been reported for bone metastases from breast cancer. The value of DMDP will be examined in the MRC sixth MM trial, but the drug is not yet generally available. The commonly available diphosphonate, ethanehydroxydiphosphonate (EHDP) is not suitable for long-term use because it inhibits the entry of calcium into bone and therefore leads to demineralization and osteomalacia.

Intercurrent Infection

Myelomatosis patients are vulnerable to intercurrent infection. About one in five patients acquires pyogenic chest infections in the first year of treatment. It is important to alert the patient and the general practitioner to the potential danger of apparently trivial infections and to ensure that febrile illnesses are treated vigorously and without delay. Patients should keep a supply of cotrimoxazole or amoxicillin.

Place of Radiotherapy

Chemotherapy sometimes relieves generalized bone pains within a few weeks, but in other cases the pains are not completely relieved for many months. In others, severe bone pain at a particular site is the major presenting feature, or develops during the early months of chemotherapy in spite of improvement in other respects. Local irradiation usually relieves severe bone pain, often within a week. Radiotherapy to the spine should also be started as soon as possible after surgical decompression for paraplegia of rapid onset. In all these situations the volumes of tissue irradiated are relatively small, and the extent of bone marrow depression resulting from irradiation only rarely necessitates interruption of chemotherapy. New patients with severe local pain, however, should receive radiotherapy first to secure relief of pain as quickly as possible; the vulnerability of their bone marrow (discussed already) contraindicates simultaneous chemotherapy and radiotherapy, and the low neutrophil and platelet counts after chemotherapy necessitate the postponement of radiotherapy longer than is justified. For the relief of pain, a dose of 1000 cGy is usually sufficient, and may be conveniently administered in a single exposure. Note that a few patients with well-preserved haematological function who require local radiotherapy for pain relief may be symptom-free for several years thereafter, although they show no response to chemotherapy in terms of reduction in their paraprotein levels, while others who appear to be responding to chemotherapy develop bone pain which requires radiotherapy but does not necessarily indicate an adverse change in the character of the disease heralding more rapid progression, and there is no immediate need to change the chemotherapy.

In the terminal stage of MM, severe bone pain has been relieved by half-body irradiation at low dosage. The best results have been obtained when a second course to the other half of the body was given 6–8 weeks after the first. The treatment is myelosuppressive and has caused radiation pneumonitis, especially when the dose rate was above 25 cGy/minute. The treatment cannot be repeated, and subsequent cytotoxic chemotherapy may be poorly tolerated. Nevertheless, some patients have survived beyond 2 years with good quality of life, and the method deserves to be used more often than it has been.

Follow-up Procedure

The recording of the progress of the disease, the details of the treatment, the response to it, and the early detection of resistance to treatment and of relapse require the methodical entry of a large number of observations in a readily retrievable form. The charting method, as commonly used in the management of leukaemia patients, is most valuable (Fig. 18.3). The following observations should be entered for each date on which they are made.

At Presentation

Clinical

Indicate the degree of disability by a simple grading system: grade I, no disability, minimal symptoms and signs; grade II, moderate disability, reduced capacity for work or general activity; grade III, considerable disability, unfit for work, but ambulant; grade IV, seriously disabled, bedridden.

Radiological

Indicate the sites x-rayed on the appropriate dates (at presentation, a full skeletal survey including the long bones of the extremities should be made). It is not practical to record the detailed radiological findings on the chart, but major abnormalities may be indicated by a coding system on the following lines: GO = generalized osteoporosis; WT10, L5 = wedging of bodies of 10th thoracic and 5th lumbar vertebrae; L SK, 2F = lytic lesions in skull and both femora.

Biochemical

Record the serum concentrations of albumin, globulin, paraprotein, β_2 microglobulin, normal polyclonal immunoglobulins, calcium, alkaline phosphatase, and the BUC, the total urinary protein, and amount of BJP (if present), expressed as amount excreted in 24 hours.

Haematological

Plot the haemoglobin concentration, the platelet, total leucocyte, and absolute neutrophil counts. Note major features of the blood film, for example the presence of myeloma cells, or of leucoerythroblastosis. Indicate in abbreviated form the main bone marrow findings against the appropriate date.

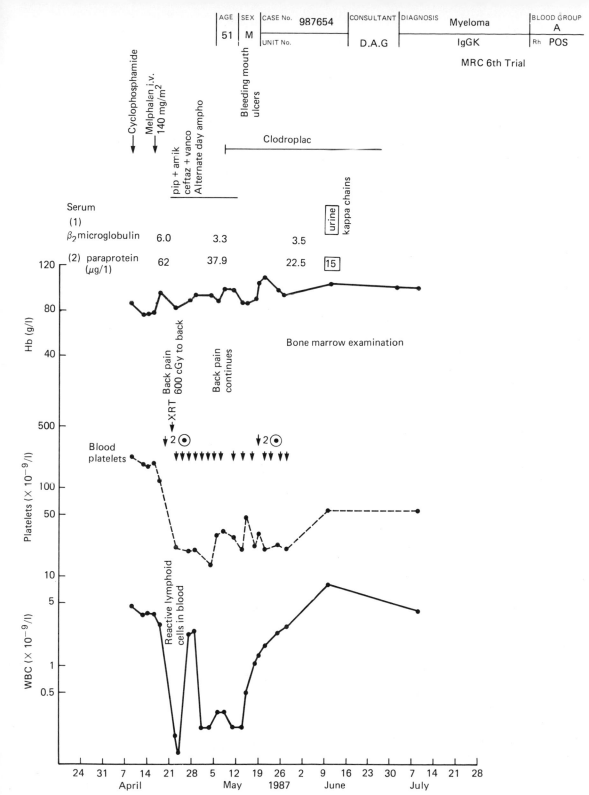

Fig. 18.3. *Haematological chart of patient with myelomatosis. 2⊙, 2 units of blood transfused; pip + amik, piperacillin + amikacin; ceftaz + vanco, ceftazidime + vancomycin; alternate day ampho, amphotericin administered intravenously on alternate days.*

Therapeutic

Enter the dates of starting and discontinuing drugs, and indicate the daily doses of each. Enter the corresponding radiotherapeutic data and the site irradiated.

Follow-up Data

The frequency of many of the above observations is determined by the needs of day-to-day management, but the following should be repeated at regular intervals: skeletal survey after 6 months and yearly thereafter; all biochemical investigations after 1 month and 3-monthly thereafter. It is useful, as a reminder, to mark arrows in pencil against the dates on which these investigations are due.

Indications of Relapse

Any of the adverse changes now to be described, appearing alone or in various combinations, may occur during the period of clinical remission. They may progress imperceptibly over a period of years during which the patient remains well, or rapidly in a few months accompanied by clinical deterioration. The changes are due to renewed activity of the disease which has now become resistant to the treatment.

The commonest indications of relapse are impairment of bone marrow function resulting from the accumulation of myeloma cells throughout the bone marrow and the reappearance of and gradual increase in the concentration of the same paraprotein as was originally present in the serum or urine. Impaired marrow function is indicated by the downward trend of the platelet count, the haemoglobin concentration, and the neutrophil count, often in that order. Inspection of the haematological chart shows that the trends are independent of the courses of treatment.

In some cases the relapse takes different forms, indicative of the evolution of a new cell line with different and often more malignant growth characteristics. In many of these cases, the appearance of the new cell line may be detected biochemically during a period of clinical and haematological stability. Bence Jones protein may appear in the urine where none had been found at presentation, and it may consist of light chains of the same or of a different class from that of the original paraprotein. When the protein is of the same class it may nevertheless differ from the original protein in the electrophoretic mobility, or a paraprotein indistinguishable from that originally identified may reappear but its concentration may increase at a higher rate, suggesting that the clone of cells producing it is proliferating at a higher rate than that of the cells of the population from which it arose. In another pattern of relapse, a paraprotein appears differing from the original in its heavy-chain class, or in its heavy and light-chain classes. It is reasonable to infer that in all these cases the new paraprotein is produced by a clone of cells that arose during a period in which the proliferation of the parent population of cells was still controlled by the treatment. The new clone is thus resistant to the treatment and has escaped from its control.

An analogous process is likely in those cases in which locally aggressive tumours appear during a period of clinical and haematological stability. These tumours usually arise in pre-existing bony lesions, but they erode the cortex of the bone and encroach on and destroy the neighbouring soft tissues. For example, lesions in the base of the skull will cause cranial nerve lesions, and may grow large enough to produce palpable or visible swellings in the temporal and orbital regions; lesions in the ribs may cause palpable or visible swellings on the chest wall, and those in the sacrum may cause large masses bulging into the pelvis. In all situations mentioned, the invasion of peripheral nerve sheaths causes pain and impairment or loss of sensory and motor function. In some of these cases, histological examination of the tumours shows a marked change in appearance, with features characteristic of malignant growths, namely cellular pleomorphism, a high proportion of undifferentiated cells, frequent mitotic figures and the presence of tumour giant cells. Occasionally the cells are so poorly differentiated that they are no longer identifiable as plasma cells by light microscopy. The clonal nature of these aggressive tumours seems highly probable from the circumstances in which they arise and from their altered growth characteristics and histological appearance, and is supported by the occasional appearance of a new paraprotein of one of the types discussed. In most cases, however, the tumours are probably too undifferentiated to be capable of synthesizing an immunoglobulin, though para-proteins have not been sufficiently sought by modern techniques.

Second-line Treatments

Most second-line treatments consist of combinations of drugs including doxorubicin, a nitrosourea, vincristine, steroids and other drugs. Good results are reported for the VAD regimen (vincristine, adriamycin (doxorubicin) and dexamethasone), the attraction of which is that all patients likely to benefit will respond after the first course. If a response is not obtained, the treatment is at once abandoned. Vincristine and doxorubicin are administered by continuous intravenous infusion over 4 days at a daily dose of 0.4 mg and 9 mg/m², and the patient also receives 4-day courses of high-dose steroid as dexamethasone, 40 mg, starting on days 1, 9, and 17 of alternate cycles, the second two being omitted in the other cycles. The rationale for the infusions was that the very slowly dividing tumour cells would have a greater chance of being killed by continuous exposure to the drugs than by rapid exposure to the same total dose Precautions appropriate to high-dose steroid therapy are essential, and there is a high risk of serious infection. The response to VAD is usually shortlived. Surprisingly, about one-third of patients with refractory disease respond to weekly cyclophosphamide injections at 300 mg/m² in combination with prednisolone at standard dosage. This regimen is well tolerated, far less hazardous than VAD and other intensive treatments, and good control may be possible for as long as 2 years; efficacy is difficult to explain.

Interferons (IF), derived from human leucocytes, lymphoblastoid cell lines, or by genetic engineering, have some activity in about one-quarter of the cases of refractory MM. The IF is administered intramuscularly, daily for a month or more and several times weekly thereafter. In the early phase it induces influenza-like symptoms. It has not yet found a place in the routine management of MM, but trials are in progress of its use in induction or plateau phase.

An inhibitor of adenosine deaminase, 2'-deoxy-coformycin has been shown to reduce paraprotein concentrations and the size of soft tissue masses in a proportion of cases of refractory MM. Plasma cells contain adenosine deaminase that can be inhibited in vitro by deoxycoformycin. The drug is nephrotoxic and contraindicated for azotaemic patients. It has been given intravenously in 3-day courses every 2 weeks. It causes anorexia, nausea, vomiting, and sometimes confusion, disorientation, and poor memory. Although there is clearly room for further trials of IF and deoxycoformycin, these drugs appear to be markedly less effective in MM than in hairy-cell leukaemia.

Secondary Myelodysplasia and Acute Myeloid Leukaemia

The association of MM with the myelodysplastic syndrome (MDS), though rare, occurs more often than would be expected by chance. Melphalan-treated patients are at risk of developing MDS sometimes followed by acute myeloid leukaemia. The risk increases to a cumulative maximum of about 3%, 3–6 years after 1 year of treatment, with an additional 3% for each additional year of treatment. There were 12 cases of MDS/AML among the 648 patients entered into the MRC randomized comparison of melphalan and cyclophosphamide (trials 1 and 2), all of which occurred in patients randomized to receive melphalan. Since the results became known, melphalan administration has been limited to 1 year, when the benefit far outweighs the risk of inducing MDS/AML.

Possible Future Approaches

It has been estimated that conventional chemotherapy reduces the total tumour cell mass by no more than 2 log amounts at best. It may be supposed that more intensive therapy would kill more cells and so defer relapse and prolong survival. However, this has been difficult to demonstrate, though in the Medical Research Council's fifth MM trial, as described above, the four-drug combination of melphalan, cyclophosphamide, doxorubicin, and 1,3-*bis*-chloro(2-chloroethyl)-1-nitrosourea (BCNU) has proved superior to the standard melphalan schedule.

Another promising form of intensive therapy appears to be that of McElwain and colleagues, who administer a single dose of melphalan alone at very high dosage (up to 140 mg/m²). This treatment causes prolonged myelosuppression, shortlived nausea, vomiting and diarrhoea, mucositis of the mouth, throat, and oesophagus, and alopecia. It therefore requires prolonged hospital admission and exacting supportive care of the type used in the treatment of acute myeloid leukaemia. It is not suitable for older patients or those with any complication that might increase their vulnerability to the consequences of bone marrow failure. The full potential of the method remains to be worked out, but it is already clear that the best responses obtained are of a different order from those resulting from any other treatment and suggest that the proportion of tumour cells killed is very much higher. The paraprotein becomes undetectable, the polyclonal immunoglobulins return to normal concentrations, lytic lesions recalcify. Unfortunately, most patients relapse within 2 years, but the quality of life is excellent during this period and the treatment has been repeated in some cases. At present, studies are underway to see whether high-dose steroid therapy will add to the effect of high-dose melphalan (HDM). HDM will be compared with a multidrug regimen used alone or in combination with intermediate-dose steroid in the Medical Research Council's sixth MM trial. It is possible, too, that patients in complete remission following HDM might benefit from further chemotherapy and whole-body irradiation followed by an autograft of bone marrow collected after the bone marrow has regenerated from the HDM treatment. Ways might be found for treating the marrow before reinfusion to remove any residual myeloma cells. A few patients have been treated by high-dose cyclophosphamide and whole-body irradiation followed by bone marrow transplantation, and it seems likely that the proportion of myeloma cells destroyed is greater than for any other treatment, but unlikely that any patient has yet been 'cured'. In short, the time is now ripe for moving forward from the current palliative approach to MM towards putative curative treatment, but for many years these efforts will necessarily be confined to special centres.

OTHER PLASMA CELL TUMOURS

Solitary Myeloma of Bone

Solitary myeloma of bone (SMB) is a rare condition that usually presents as a locally painful lesion.

Very rarely, several lesions are found. Radiologically, the lesions have a characteristic trabeculated or soap-bubble appearance quite different from the lytic lesions of MM (Fig. 18.4). Surgical exploration and biopsy examination show the lesion to be composed of well-differentiated plasma cells, but a radiological survey of the skeleton fails to reveal any other sites of involvement. Bone marrow examination shows 1–2% of well-differentiated plasma cells of normal morphology such as are found in most samples of normal marrow; these must not be interpreted as pathological simply because of the presence of a solitary myeloma. Immunofluorescence studies with antibodies against individual light and heavy chains show them to be polyclonal. The serum immunoglobulins are normal and BJP cannot be demonstrated in the

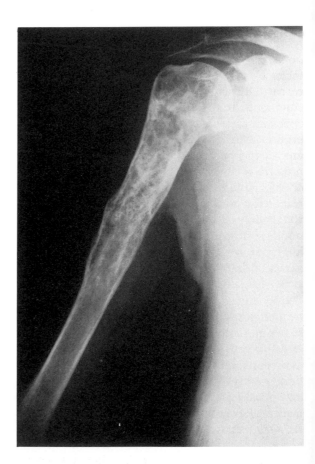

Fig. 18.4. *X-ray of humerus showing solitary myeloma of bone. (By courtesy of Dr E. Wiltshaw.)*

urine. Solitary myeloma of bone responds well to radiotherapy and may never recur. However, regular follow-up is essential, and yearly estimation of the serum immunoglobulins and examination of the urine for BJP should be carried out, because MM may develop and become apparent after as long as 20 years. Patients with multiple solitary myelomas also have indolent disease; pain at several sites is best treated by chemotherapy. Most patients with SMB relapse with MM within 5 years.

Extramedullary Plasmacytoma

Extramedullary plasmacytoma (EMP) is a rare tumour, histologically indistinguishable from SMB and MM, that arises most commonly from the tissues underlying the mucous membrane of the upper respiratory passages, but can arise also from the gastrointestinal tract, the breast, the gonads, lymph nodes and other tissues. EMP arising in the upper air passages is more likely to be localized than EMP arising in the gastrointestinal tract where the primary tumours are often bulky and metastasis has already taken place. Unlike MM, which hardly ever occurs below the age of 20, EMP occurs occasionally in childhood, though the modal age range is in the sixth decade. At the primary site the tumour is often multicentric. After excision or radiotherapy, the tumour may not recur, may recur locally, again responding to surgery or radiotherapy, or may metastasize to local lymph nodes. Later, single or multiple metastases may appear in soft tissues, commonly in the skin and subcutaneous tissues, or in bone where, in contrast to MM, EMP shows no preference for haemopoietic bone marrow, and metastases occur at random throughout the skeleton. Metastases tend to occur singly, but even when multiple metastases are present, random samples of bone marrow are often entirely normal, in marked contrast to MM.

Extramedullary plasmacytoma is very rare, and few biochemical studies have been made. Paraproteins have sometimes been found; in a few cases they have disappeared when the tumour has been excised, to return with the growth of metastases. The production of a paraprotein may not depend only on the presence of a critical mass of tumour as in MM; paraprotein has not been found in several cases of EMP in which large masses of tumour were present, perhaps because the tumour cells did not synthesize immunoglobulin. Nephrotic syndrome resulting from light-chain deposition on glomerular basement membrane may occur in the absence of detectable Bence Jones proteinuria. The EMP responds to the alkylating agents melphalan and cyclophosphamide. Because bone marrow function remains unimpaired, single large doses may be administered and repeated at 3–6-weekly intervals, a regimen that would rarely be tolerated in MM. Dramatic regressions of the tumours occur, and remissions may last for several years. The treatment should probably be continued for 1 year after all evidence of disease has disappeared, though no systematic study has yet been made. The value of multiple-drug therapy or HDM remains to be determined.

Plasma-Cell Leukaemia

Plasma-cell leukaemia (PCL), another excessively rare condition, presents as an acute leukaemia with symptoms resulting from bone marrow failure. The clinical and laboratory features are described in Chapter 15. On physical examination the spleen is almost always considerably larger than would be expected in any of the common types of acute leukaemia. The true nature of the disease is apparent from the morphology of the blast cells in the peripheral blood and bone marrow, except when the cells are very poorly differentiated. The presence of rouleaux and background protein staining in the blood films supports the diagnosis, and biochemical examination shows the presence of a paraprotein in the serum, of BJP in the urine, or both. Radiological survey of the skeleton, however, is likely to disclose no abnormality. PCL is less likely to respond to the type of treatment ordinarily used for the acute leukaemias than to the drug schedules used in the treatment of MM, with the provisos as to dosage in the presence of bone marrow or renal failure as described above. The response is usually temporary, and resistance to further treatment rapidly acquired. Rarely, meningeal PCL occurs. PCL should not be confused with the spillover of plasma cells into the peripheral blood in established MM.

WALDENSTRÖM'S MACROGLOBULINAEMIA

The lymphoplasmacytic lymphomas (LPL) constitute an uncommon group of slowly progressive B-lymphoproliferative disorders, rare below the age of 40 and increasing in frequency with advancing age, in which the cells are intermediate in immunological maturation between those of the small-cell lymphomas and the plasma cell dyscrasias. The cells that accumulate in the bone marrow, in lymph nodes, and in the spleen include small lymphocytes, plasmacytoid lymphocytes, and plasma cells in varying proportions. Many cells synthesize a monoclonal immunoglobulin, cytoplasmic or on the surface membrane, and the same Ig is exported into the serum. In the majority of cases the heavy chain is μ, and at high concentration in the serum this is responsible for the clinical and biochemical features of Waldenström's macroglobulinaemia (WM). Rarely, the heavy chain is α or γ. Histologically the infiltrate is at first non-destructive, and in lymph nodes the architecture is preserved. Amorphous deposits of paraprotein may be seen and PAS staining shows the presence of intranuclear and cytoplasmic inclusions in some cells. Mast cells are usually conspicuous, and should be sought in the fragments of conventional marrow films as well as in the trails. In all infiltrates macrophages are also conspicuous.

In classical WM the clinical manifestations are dominated by the large amounts of IgM secreted by tumours of small bulk which may be clinically undetectable. Occasionally high serum concentrations occur in the absence of physical signs and little or no bone marrow infiltration. Even when numerous lymph nodes are enlarged and the bone marrow is heavily infiltrated, bone marrow function may be well preserved and the lymphomatous element of the condition may remain essentially static for several years. In LPL generally, plasmacytoid lymphocytes may appear in the peripheral blood in small numbers, or there may be enough to suggest an initial diagnosis of a chronic lymphoid leukaemia. In elderly patients with a static lymphomatous element, the whole course of the disease may be characterized by the clinical effects of the macroglobulinaemia, while in those with a progressive lymphoma the course is determined more by tumour growth and by increasing marrow infiltration with eventual marrow failure. New patients with a lymphomatous presentation and an IgM paraprotein at serum concentrations too low to give rise to symptoms (< 25 g/l) are better classified as having LPL with macroglobulinaemia than WM. At some stage, monoclonal light chains appear in the urine in LPL, often only just detectable in concentrated urine. As in other B-lymphoproliferative conditions, amyloidosis may arise during the course of the disease or its manifestations may precede the recognition of LPL. In LPL, as in other B-lymphoproliferative conditions, there is an increased risk of other forms of malignant disease. Macroglobulinaemia may also occur during the course of B-lymphoproliferative conditions that do not have the polymorphic histology of LPL, but the serum concentration is usually below 25 g/l. Rare patients with the clinical, radiological, and haematological features of MM have an IgM paraprotein, and occasional patients with the clinical, haematological, and histological features of WM develop lytic bone deposits. Finally, WM is distinguished from idiopathic cold-antibody disease in which the clinical course is dominated by the antibody activity of the IgM with specificity for the red cell antigen I, and from MGUS.

Some WM paraproteins have been shown to have antibody activity against cytoskeletal elements, especially actin and tubulin.

Effects of Serum Macroglobulin at High Concentration

Immunoglobulin M paraprotein, of molecular weight of approximately 1 million, increases the viscosity of the blood at lower concentrations than IgG or IgA proteins, and the curve relating viscosity to concentration in serum is steeply curvilinear, so that above a concentration of about 30 g/l, small increases lead to rapid increase in the viscosity and, conversely, reduction in the concentration over the same range lowers the viscosity equally rapidly. The removal of the macroglobulin contained in 1 litre of blood usually lowers the viscosity sufficiently to bring about rapid and dramatic relief of symptoms. Because of its high molecular weight, most of the macroglobulin produced is intravascular, so that the lowering of the concentration achieved by plasmapheresis is not rapidly reversed by the entry into the circulation of macroglobulin from the extravascular compartment. Unfortunately, the rate of production of the macroglobulin is often so high that the serum concentration rises to its former level in a few weeks.

The symptoms of hyperviscosity include muscular weakness, lethargy, mental confusion proceeding to coma, purpura, haemorrhages from the gums, nose, gastrointestinal and genitourinary tracts, neuropathies, and visual disturbances. In individual cases the onset and progression of symptoms often follow a regular sequence after plasmapheresis, and for patients treated for several years by plasmapheresis alone, the frequency may sometimes be adjusted according to the onset of the first symptoms. For patients with visual disturbance the frequency should be adjusted to keep the serum viscosity below the level at which blurred vision occurs.

Prognosis and Treatment

As in other low-grade B lymphomas, the necessity for treatment, which at present is only palliative, must be assessed on the stage of advancement and the rate of progress of the disease. Symptomless patients with static disease are best observed without treatment and they may remain well for a decade or more. Symptoms arising from hyperviscosity are rapidly relieved by plasmapheresis, most readily carried out with a cell separator, and some patients may be managed for several years by plasmapheresis alone. This treatment is most appropriate for patients with essentially static lymphoproliferation and well-preserved bone marrow function whose serum viscosity increases to symptomatic levels at a rate which permits control by leucapheresis at intervals of 1–3 months. Patients with progressive lymphomatous disease and declining bone marrow function require chemotherapy designed to reduce the total mass of lymphocytes as in the treatment of other low-grade lymphomas. The alkylating agents chlormabucil, cyclophosphamide or melphalan are most commonly used, alone or in combination with prednisolone. Treatment reduces the bone marrow infiltration and so leads to improvement in bone marrow function, and it reduces the serum concentration of paraprotein. As in the treatment of low-grade lymphoma generally, optimal control may require treatment for 1 year or more. The principles of management are those described for CLL in Chapter 15. In general, courses of treatment should be administered at the lowest frequency consistent with maintenance of optimal conditions.

More rapidly progressive disease, either in new patients or in those who have become refractory to conventional therapy, requires consideration of more intensive therapy with such drugs as doxorubicin, vincristine, and bleomycin in combination with alkylating agents and prednisolone; however, most patients are elderly, and the decision to try more intensive therapy must be based on an assessment of the extent of benefit that might be conferred in relation to the toxicity. The hyperviscosity syndrome in patients who are refractory to chemotherapy may still be controllable by plasmapheresis, but rarely for more than a year.

HEAVY CHAIN DISEASE

The term heavy chain disease(s) has been applied to a clinically heterogeneous group of B-lymphoid cell neoplasms whose principal common denominator is the presence in the serum of a monoclonal protein consisting of a heavy chain (or part of a heavy chain) of the immunoglobulin molecule. Neoplastic diseases in which the monoclonal proliferation involves γ-, α-, μ- and δ-chains have been described but the only disease that represents a reasonably discrete clinical entity is α-(heavy) chain disease.

γ-Heavy Chain Disease

This relatively rare condition occurs more commonly in men than in women and infrequently below the age of 40. The clinical course resembles that of lymphoma rather than MM. The onset is usually gradual with malaise, weakness and sometimes fever; examination shows lymphadenopathy and hepatosplenomegaly. In occasional patients there is erythema and oedema of the palate. The blood shows mild to moderate anaemia, eosinophilia and sometimes atypical lymphocytes. The marrow may show increased numbers of plasma cells, lymphocytes, eosinophils, or may be normal. X-rays of the skeleton are usually normal. The serum paraprotein has a molecular weight from 45 000 to 80 000 daltons and consists of an incomplete portion of the heavy chain (Fc fragment) of the γ-immunoglobulin molecule. Serum levels range from 20 g/l to 40 g/l.

Patients are best treated as if they had a lymphoma of low or intermediate-grade malignancy. Survival has ranged from 4 months to more than 5 years. Cyclophosphamide, melphalan and steroids have been used but such agents should be administered with caution as most patients die of pneumonia, septicaemia or other infectious causes.

α-Heavy Chain Disease

Immunoglobin A heavy chain (α-chain) disease is the commonest type of heavy chain disease. Though originally described as 'Mediterranean-type abdominal lymphoma', it is now clear that it can occur also in individuals of other ethnic and geographical backgrounds. The major clinical features are progressive wasting, malabsorption and chronic diarrhoea unresponsive to treatment with a gluten-free diet. It can occur in relatively young patients. Intestinal biopsy or laparotomy reveals massive infiltration of the lamina propria and abdominal lymph nodes with lymphocytes and plasma cells. The bone marrow may show a moderate increase in plasma cell numbers but in general the disease spares the liver, spleen and other lymphoid organs. Electrophoretic analysis of the serum shows a broad monoclonal peak traversing the β- and α₂-mobility range; immunochemically the monoclonal protein is difficult to characterize—its carbohydrate content is, however, high and it may include the entire Fc component of the α-chain. No portion of the light chain is demonstrable. The serum level of paraprotein is much lower than in other monoclonal conditions.

Treatment with antimicrobial agents, especially tetracycline, has led to complete remission of all clinical features of the disease and restoration to normal of immunoglobulin values. More commonly, the disease progresses in spite of treatment and terminates in death from severe wasting and malabsorption, or from transformation to a malignant plasmacytoma.

μ-Heavy Chain Disease

Very occasional patients have been identified with μ-heavy chain fragments in their serum. Some had a long-standing chronic lymphoid leukaemia characterized by lymphocytes and vacuolated plasma cells in the bone marrow. Rare patients have had clinical features of lymphoma.

δ-Heavy Chain Disease

One patient with δ-chain disease has been reported. The bone marrow showed increased numbers of plasma cells, the skull x-ray showed lytic areas, and he died of renal failure. Clinically the condition was thus indistinguishable from MM.

SELECTED BIBLIOGRAPHY

Azar H., Potter M. (Eds.) (1973). *Multiple myeloma and related disorders*. New York: Harper and Row.

Bersagel D. E. (1983). Progress in the treatment of plasma cell myeloma? Editorial. *Journal of Clinical Oncology*, **1**, 510–512.

Brandes L. J., Israels L. G. (1982). Treatment of advanced plasma cell myeloma with weekly cyclophosphamide and alternate-day prednisone. *Cancer Treatment Reports*, **66**, 1413–1415.

Cuzick J., Copper E. H., MacLennan I.C.M. (1985). The prognostic value of serum β_2 microglobulin compared with other presentation features in myelomatosis (A report to the Medical Research Council's Working Party on Leukaemia in Adults). *British Journal of Cancer*, **52**, 1–6.

Cuzick J., Velez R., Doll R. (1983). International variations and temporal trends in mortality from multiple myeloma. *International Journal of Cancer*, **22**, 13–19.

Durie B. G. M., Salmon S. E. (1975). A clinical staging system for multiple myeloma. *Cancer*, **36**, 842–854.

Durie B. G. M. (1988). Multiple myeloma. In *Recent advances in haematology*, Vol. 5, pp. 305–327. (Ed. A. V. Hoffbrand). Edinburgh: Churchill Livingstone.

Hobbs J. R. (1969). Growth rates and responses to treatment in human myelomatosis. *British Journal of Haematology*, **16**, 607–617.

Kyle R. A. (1984) Treatment of multiple myeloma. A small step forward? *New England Journal of Medicine*, **310**, 1382–1384.

Levine A. M., Lichtenstein A., Gresik M. V., Taylor C. R.,

Feinstein D. I., Lukes R. J. (1980). Clinical and immunologic spectrum of plasmacytoid lymphocytic lymphoma without serum monoclonal IgM. *British Journal of Haematology*, **46**, 225–233.

McElwain T. J., Powles R. L. (1983). High-dose intravenous melphalan for plasma-cell leukaemia and myeloma. *Lancet*, **2**, 822–824.

Medical Research Council (1980). Treatment comparisons in the third myelomatosis trial. *British Journal of Cancer*, **42**, 823–830.

Medical Research Council (1980). Prognostic features in the third myelomatosis trial. *British Journal of Cancer*, **42**, 831–840.

Medical Research Council Working Party on Leukaemia in Adults (1984). Analysis and management of renal failure in the fourth MRC myelomatosis trial. *British Medical Journal*, **288**, 1411–1416.

Medical Research Council Working Party on Leukaemia in Adults (1985). Objective evaluation of the role of vincristine in induction and maintenance therapy for myelomatosis. *British Journal of Cancer*, **52**, 153–158.

Paterson A. D., Kanis J. A., Cameron E. C., Douglas D. L., Beard D. J., Preston F. E., Russell R. G. G. (1983). The use of dichloromethylene diphosphonate for the management of hypercalcaemia in multiple myeloma. *British Journal of Haematology*, **54**, 121–132.

Salmon S. E., Smith B. A. (1970). Immunoglobulin synthesis and total body tumour cell number in IgG multiple myeloma. *Journal of Clinical Investigation* **49**, 1114.

Chapter 19

THE LYMPHOMAS

J. M. GOLDMAN

The term lymphoma embraces a heterogeneous group of disorders, presumed to be malignant, that originate in one or other of the lymph nodes or other lymphatic tissues of the body. The best characterized of the lymphomas is Hodgkin's disease (HD). The remainder constitute a rather motley collection of conditions, ranging from the well-differentiated lymphocytic lymphomas that may prove responsive to therapy and in which prognosis may be measured in years, to the poorly differentiated lymphocytic and true histiocytic lymphomas, with which diagnoses some patients survive only a few months. The phrase non-Hodgkin's lymphoma (NHL) has been coined to cover this latter group of diseases and, though rather unsatisfactory, no better term has yet been proposed.

HODGKIN'S DISEASE

History

In 1832 Thomas Hodgkin read before the Medical–Chirurgical Society in London a paper entitled 'On some morbid appearances of the absorbent glands and spleen'. He described clinical histories and gross post-mortem findings in seven patients who died with lymphadenopathy and splenomegaly and concluded, 'This enlargement of the glands appears to be a primitive [primary] affection of those bodies, rather than the result of an irritation propagated to them from some ulcerated surface or other inflamed texture'. In 1865, Samuel Wilks described a group of similar patients, and designated the condition 'Hodgkin's disease'. In 1872, Langhans described the histological features of the disease and drew attention to the presence of multinucleate giant cells, but Carl Sternberg in 1898 and Dorothy Reed in 1902 are generally credited with the first accurate and thorough descriptions of the histopathology and cytology characteristic of HD. It is interesting that in 1926 Fox was able to examine under the microscope sections which he had prepared from gross specimens of three of Hodgkin's original cases that had been preserved in the Guy's Hospital Pathology Museum. He was able to confirm the diagnosis of HD on histopathological grounds in two of these.

Aetiology

The occurrence of fever, sweating and lymphadenopathy, the last-mentioned sometimes involving nodes lacking features diagnostic of HD, suggests an infectious, possibly viral, aetiology, but extensive searches have failed to reveal any infectious agent consistently present in the tissues of patients with HD. Alternatively, the observation that the clinical picture of HD sometimes resembles that of 'secondary disease' or 'graft-versus-host disease' led to the hypothesis that HD may be due to a 'lymphocyte civil war' resulting from the acquisition by one clone of lymphocytes of a new antigen recognized by other lymphoid tissues as 'foreign'. In practice, HD is usually regarded as a neoplastic process in which the Hodgkin or Sternberg–Reed cell is the characteristic malignant cell. The other cellular constituents of the enlarged lymph node or other affected tissue are then regarded as secondary reactants.

Epidemiology

Hodgkin's disease appears to have increased in frequency during this century. Unlike the other lymphomas in which the incidence increases with increasing age, the age-specific incidence of HD is bimodal with a first early peak in the age range 15–40. It has long been known that HD is more prevalent in males than in females. The male:female sex ratio ranges from 1.4 to 1.9:1. When analysed by age, however, the male:female ratio is much lower in the 15–34 age bracket than after the age of 35, when the male preponderance becomes increasingly marked. The death rate from HD differs in different countries. It appears to be highest in the United States, Canada and Scandinavia (13–18 per million per year) and remarkably low (6 per million per year) in Japan. Both mortality and incidence rates for non-whites (predominantly negroes) are appreciably lower than those for whites. The incidence of HD occurring in two or more members of the same family exceeds what would be expected by chance. An identical twin of the patient has the highest risk of getting HD, sibs of the same sex the next highest risk, followed by sibs of opposite sex. Occasional reports of HD occurring in husband and wife raise the possibility that the association may be familial rather than genetically determined. The suggestion that HD is commoner in individuals whose occupations involve exposure to wood (carpenters, cabinet makers etc.) has not been confirmed. HD may, however, be commoner than expected in patients with epilepsy and the link here may be anticonvulsants of the hydantoin group. Some studies have suggested that infectious mononucleosis is more common in the previous history of patients who subsequently develop HD. Here also the data remain inconclusive.

Clinical Features

The patient with HD most commonly seeks medical attention after having become aware of an unusual lump or mass in the neck. Enlarged lymph nodes are typically neither painful nor tender and they may have reached a considerable size before becoming noticeable. Enlarged nodes may be present in one or both sides of the neck, in the axillae, inguinal or femoral regions. Enlarged epitrochlear nodes are occasionally described. There are well-documented instances of waxing and waning in the size of lymph node masses and, not infrequently, the patient will report apparent diminution in size of lymphadenopathy following treatment with antibiotics. Some patients are febrile at the time of presentation, a feature usually taken to indicate more advanced disease. The fever may be low grade and smouldering in character. The cyclical bouts of high fever described by Pel and Ebstein in 1887, each lasting 1–2 weeks and separated by afebrile periods of similar duration, are now rarely seen except in patients with far advanced untreated disease. Night sweats also characterize advanced HD; when severe these may drench the patient and cause him to wake at night in order to change his night clothes. Weight loss may occur and is thought also to betoken more advanced disease. Pruritus when present is usually generalized in character and may be severe enough to cause the patient to scratch extensively. Occasionally patients will report that the consumption of alcohol leads almost immediately to pain in one or more of their enlarged lymph nodes. The fact that such alcohol-induced pain is very rare in patients with HD, and occurs also in some patients with other neoplastic conditions, limits its diagnostic value. Other symptoms that may lead to a diagnosis of HD include anorexia, generalized weakness and fatigue, back pain, bone pain, or jaundice.

Needle aspiration of an enlarged lymph node can yield material that points to or occasionally clinches a diagnosis of HD, but excision biopsy of an enlarged lymph node or other appropriate tissue is mandatory in any patient where HD is suspected. In patients with localized lymphadenopathy for which no obvious cause exists, a short trial first of antibiotics is reasonable, but biopsy should be carried out if lymphadenopathy persists, at the latest within 4 weeks of original presentation. In patients with generalized lymphadenopathy, the choice of which lymph node to biopsy will depend in part on surgical accessibility, but as a rule lymph nodes in the neck are more likely to yield diagnostic information than those in the axillae, and the histology of inguinal or femoral nodes is sometimes extremely difficult to interpret.

Histopathology

The *sine qua non* for the diagnosis of HD is the identification in properly prepared biopsy material of characteristic Sternberg–Reed cells against a cytoarchitectural background consistent with the disease (Fig. 19.1). Sternberg–Reed cells are large cells with two or more nuclei, each characterized by a single large inclusion-body-like nucleolus that is separated from the nuclear membrane by a clear zone traversed by strands of chromatin. The nuclear membrane itself is often homogeneously thickened. The cytoplasm of the cell is unremarkable and variable in quantity. In some cases, the cytoplasmic membrane appears to have contracted during preparation leaving a clear zone, or lacuna, between the Sternberg–Reed cell and adjacent cells. Such cells are known as lacunar cells and are usually regarded

as diagnostic of the nodular sclerosing type of HD. The origin of Sternberg–Reed cells remains much debated. Gene rearrangement analysis (see p. 332) and monoclonal antibody studies of fresh tissue and cell lines from Sternberg–Reed cells suggest that in some cases they are derived from transformed B lymphocytes; in other cases an origin from T lymphocytes or cells of the monocyte–macrophage series seems likely. The best view at present is that they represent transformed variants of a cell normally present in low numbers in lymph nodes that has not yet been adequately characterized. Though at one time regarded as pathognomonic of HD, it is now apparent that such cells can be found in other conditions, including infectious mononucleosis, recurrent Burkitt's lymphoma and chronic lymphocytic leukaemia. Mononuclear variants of the typical multinucleate Sternberg–Reed cell are

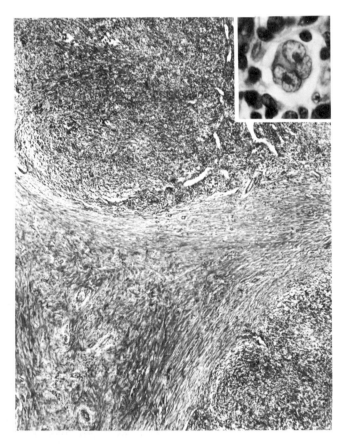

Fig. 19.1. *Section of a lymph node from a patient with nodular sclerosing HD. Note the thick bands of collagen dividing the cellular material into 'nodules'. Inset is a lacunar type of Sternberg–Reed cell.*

frequently recognizable in HD biopsy tissue. These cells are best designated 'Hodgkin cells' and are accepted as proof of HD in the absence of the classical multinucleate variety by some, but by no means all, pathologists.

Jackson and Parker Classification

In 1944 Jackson and Parker proposed that HD could be subdivided into three histopathological categories. In the category *paragranuloma* were placed patients whose normal nodal architecture was virtually completely effaced and replaced by densely packed small mature lymphocytes. Sternberg–Reed cells were usually rather sparse. Patients with paragranulomatous disease usually ran an indolent course with long survival. The category *granuloma* comprised the morphologically classical form of HD in which variable numbers of Sternberg–Reed cells and other types of Hodgkin cells were intermingled with a remarkably variegated and pleomorphic stromal cell population. Such stromal elements usually include lymphocytes, plasma cells, mature neutrophils and eosinophils, normal histiocytes and fibroblasts. Necrosis and fibrosis could be seen in the granuloma form. Prognosis for patients with this histopathological type was less good than that of those with paragranulomatous disease. They gave the name *sarcoma* to that variant of HD likely to run a highly malignant aggressive course. They noted that involved nodes were more likely to occur in deep than in peripheral areas. Microscopically there was an abundance of mononuclear Hodgkin cells with classical Sternberg–Reed cells present in highly variable numbers. The inflammatory stromal cell component was less than that in Hodgkin's granuloma. Of 377 cases reviewed in one series, 344 (91%) were classified as granuloma, 30 (8%) as paragranuloma and 3 (1%) as sarcoma. Thus the principal defect of this classification was its inability to subdivide the majority of patients with HD, and it is now of historical interest only.

The Rye Classification

A revised histopathological classification initially proposed by Lukes in 1963 comprised six categories: (a) lymphocytic and/or histiocytic nodular; (b) lymphocytic and/or histiocytic diffuse; (c) nodular sclerosis; (d) mixed; (e) diffuse fibrosis; (f) reticular. This classification was based on the general observations that there was an inverse relationship between the frequency of lymphocytes and that of abnormal Sternberg–Reed or Hodgkin cells, that two distinctive types of connective tissue proliferation could be observed, and that the lacunar cell characterized one particular type of Hodgkin's disease, namely nodular sclerosis. At a symposium held at Rye, New York, in 1965, this classification was simplified to four categories by combining the nodular and diffuse forms of the lymphocytic and/or histiocytic type and the diffuse fibrosis and reticular types. The Rye classification thus recognizes four subtypes of Hodgkin's disease.

(1) *Lymphocyte predominance*. In this type of HD, the nodal architecture is lost and the principal cell is a homogeneous infiltrate of normal-appearing small lymphocytes. On occasion, normal histiocytes may be the predominant stromal cell type and lymphocytes thereby relatively sparse. Sternberg–Reed cells are seldom numerous. Cellular proliferation may be aggregated into large demarcated nodules or may more usually be diffuse.

(2) *Nodular sclerosis*. Nodular sclerosing HD is characterized by the replacement of part of the lymph node parenchyma by interconnecting bands of collagenous connective tissue encircling nodular areas of abnormal lymphatic tissue (Fig. 19.1). The amount of collagen present in the node is highly variable. At one end of the spectrum an entire lymph node may be virtually obliterated by the sclerotic process, while at the other extreme collagen deposition may be minimal or almost entirely lacking and this condition has been designated the 'cellular phase of nodular sclerosis'. The diagnosis of nodular sclerosis is then based on the presence of the characteristic lacunar variant of the Sternberg–Reed cell.

(3) *Mixed cellularity*. Lymph nodes classified as mixed cellularity have a highly cellular and pleomorphic stroma composed of a mixture of normal histiocytes, neutrophils, eosinophils, plasma cells, lymphocytes and fibroblasts in varying proportions. There may be variable degrees of fibrosis but collagen is absent. Sternberg–Reed and Hodgkin cells are more numerous than in the lymphocytic predominant or nodular sclerosing

types of HD. In a sense there are no features that characterize mixed cellularity disease, which rather categorizes cases remaining when lymphocytic predominance, nodular sclerosis and lymphocytic depletion cases have been recognized and removed.

(4) *Lymphocyte depletion.* This category brings together the diffuse fibrosis and reticular types of HD. In diffuse fibrosis a disorderly distribution of reticulin fibres is seen in association with an amorphous non-cellular material. There is no collagen. Lymphocytes may be sparse and Sternberg–Reed cells may be difficult to find. In the rcticular form of lymphocytic depletion, the node is much more cellular and the fibrosis is less disorderly. Sternberg–Reed cells may be numerous but lymphocytes are infrequent.

Undoubtedly cases of HD exist which cannot be assigned to a specific histological subtype. It is permissible to regard such patients as 'unclassifiable'. The relative frequency of the various subtypes differs substantially in different series and in the opinions of different histopathologists. In most series, nodular sclerosis remains the most common.

Haematology

The peripheral blood picture in patients with untreated HD is frequently normal. Alternatively, patients with early disease may show a mild thrombocytosis. A neutrophil leucocytosis also occurs. Monocyte numbers may be increased and absolute eosinophil numbers may be raised, on rare occasions very considerably. In more advanced disease, lymphocyte numbers may be decreased and the degree of lymphopenia may correlate with the stage of disease. Anaemia may reflect bone marrow involvement, in which case leucoerythroblastic changes may be present, or, more rarely, anaemia results from autoimmune haemolysis. The erythrocyte sedimentation rate (ESR) is usually but not invariably raised in patients with untreated HD. When raised, it should return to normal levels after successful specific treatment. Occasionally patients are seen who throughout their course have a normal ESR.

Immunology

It has been known for many years that patients with HD show loss of delayed hypersensitivity response to tuberculin injected intradermally. It is now recognized that this cutaneous 'anergy' is generalized and involves loss of response to all other delayed hypersensitivity antigens. Patients cannot be sensitized with dinitrochlorobenzene (DNCB) or, if sensitized previously, lose their capacity for secondary response. Blood lymphocyte levels are inversely related to the extent of the disease but immunoglobulin levels are very variable, being raised, normal or depressed at the time of diagnosis.

Diagnostic Evaluation

In most cases, HD appears to have started at a single 'unifocal' site and to have spread thence in an orderly manner involving first adjacent lymph nodes and later more distant lymph node chains. Thereafter, the spleen is invaded and only subsequently does involvement of liver, lungs or bone marrow occur. Because radiotherapy offers a good chance of curing patients with early disease and chemotherapy provides significant palliation and often cure for patients with advanced disease, it is now customary to define as accurately as possible the anatomical extent of a patient's disease at the time of first presentation. For this purpose, a detailed diagnostic evaluation is necessary. It should start with a careful assessment of the patient's history. Particular attention should be paid to eliciting symptoms of fever, night sweats, anorexia, weight loss or possible alcohol-related pain. The possibility of anticonvulsant treatment should be specifically sought, and contact with a variety of infectious diseases, including tuberculosis, enquired about. Physical examination should pay especial attention to all peripherally accessible lymph node areas, and evidence of enlargement of liver or spleen should be searched for. Enlarged para-aortic or iliac nodes are sometimes palpable through the anterior abdominal wall. Patients with back pain should be carefully examined to exclude early involvement of the central nervous system which may presage the onset of paraparesis or paraplegia. Further essential diagnostic studies are shown in Table 19.1.

Mandatory investigations for a newly diagnosed patient include assessment of peripheral blood values. The serum enzymes reflecting liver function are usually measured, though in practice abnormal

Table 19.1

Initial investigations for patients with Hodgkin's disease

Mandatory investigations
Haemoglobin, leucocyte count, differential, platelets, reticulocytes, ESR, direct antiglobulin test, bone marrow aspirate and needle biopsy, urea, electrolytes, uric acid, liver chemistry, serum proteins, immunoglobulins

Chest x-ray
Lymphography
Computerized tomographic (CT) scan of chest and abdomen
Ultrasound examination of abdomen

Optional additional investigations
Examination of post-nasal space

Serum copper
Neutrophil alkaline phosphatase

Tomograms of lung or mediastinum
X-rays of skeleton
Bone scintiscan
Liver and spleen scintiscan
Intravenous urogram

Supplementary node biopsy
'Staging' laparotomy and splenectomy

---

values correlate poorly with histological evidence of liver involvement by HD. A routine chest x-ray will sometimes reveal unsuspected intrathoracic disease. Involvement of para-aortic lymph nodes may be revealed by lymphography, which should be carried out in all patients unless it is specifically contra-indicated. As the compounds used for delineating the lymph nodes contain iodine, patients sensitive to iodine should not be subjected to lymphography. The same prohibition applies to patients with parenchymal lung disease, whether it be due to involvement of lung by HD, to radiation fibrosis or to other causes. Computerized tomography (CT) scanning of the chest and abdomen to assess lymph node, liver and spleen size and to detect any other internal evidence of disease is now carried out routinely.

A number of additional investigations may be carried out at the discretion of the clinician. Involvement of lymph nodes in the upper cervical region or in Waldeyer's ring may suggest the need to examine the post-nasal space. It is sometimes useful to monitor the serum copper level or the neutrophil alkaline phosphatase score as indices of disease activity. An intravenous urogram performed at the same time as the lymphogram may give additional information about para-aortic lymph node enlargement. Routine tomography of the mediastinum or scintiscans of bone and liver are usually unrewarding but may be indicated in certain cases. Examination of the liver, spleen or para-aortic area by ultrasound may, in some cases, reveal involvement by HD that has escaped detection by other means.

Staging

An approach to the anatomical staging of patients with Hodgkin's disease was proposed at the Rye conference in 1965 and modified at the Ann Arbor conference in 1971 (Table 19.2). The Ann Arbor system has gained a wide level of acceptance. The lymph node-bearing regions of the body are arbitrarily divided into a number of separate 'regions' (Fig. 19.2). Stage I disease refers to nodal involvement restricted to one such anatomical region. Stage II defines nodal involvement of two or more regions either all above or all below the diaphragm. Stage III describes nodal involvement above and below the diaphragm. Involvement of the spleen is designated by the subscript S. Stage IV describes disease that appears to have disseminated by the bloodstream to involve lungs, liver, bone marrow or other sites. Localized extension from a lymph node region into another organ does not, however, automatically make a patient stage IV but is designated instead by a subscript E. Patients with one or more of three specified symptoms are designated 'B'. To make a patient 'B' the fever must be otherwise unexplained and rising above 38°C, the night sweats must be of at least moderate severity, or the weight loss must be at least 10% of initial body weight in the 6 months preceding evaluation. Other potentially important symptoms of HD such as fatigue, alcohol-related pain or pruritus are not considered in the staging system.

In recognition of the fact that staging procedures will vary from institution to institution, the eventual

Table 19.2

Ann Arbor staging classification for Hodgkin's disease

Stage	Definition
I	Involvement of a single lymph node region (I) or of a single extralymphatic organ or site (I_E)
II	Involvement of two or more lymph node regions on the same side of the diaphragm (II) or localized involvement of an extralymphatic organ or site and of one or more lymph node regions on the same side of the diaphragm (II_E)
III	Involvement of lymph node regions on both sides of the diaphragm (III), which may also be accompanied by involvement of the spleen (III_S) or by localized involvement of an extralymphatic organ or site (III_E), or both (III_{SE})
IV	Diffuse or disseminated involvement of one or more extralymphatic organs or tissues, with or without associated lymph node involvement

The absence or presence of fever, night sweats, and/or unexplained loss of 10% or more of body weight in the 6 months preceding admission are to be denoted in all cases by the suffix letters A or B, respectively.

Adopted at the Workshop on the Staging of Hodgkin's Disease held at Ann Arbor, Michigan, in April 1971.

stage may be designated in one of two ways. The clinical stage describes the results of full investigation of a patient by non-invasive techniques. If a patient has been investigated by laparotomy with splenectomy or additional attempts have been made to biopsy every organ thought possibly to be involved by HD, the result is described as the pathological stage. Such pathological stage may then be written with individual symbols subscripted + or − according to the result of the biopsy. The recommended abbreviations are: N for other nodes, H for liver, S for spleen, L for lung, M for marrow, P for pleura, O for bone and D for skin. Thus, for example, a patient thought on initial evaluation (clinical stage, CS) to have IIA disease but found after staging laparotomy to have also involvement of the spleen and para-aortic lymph nodes but negative liver and bone marrow (pathological stage, PS), may be designated CSIIA PSIII$_{S+N+H-M-}$.

Two important areas which may be involved are the central nervous system (e.g. extradural and meningeal) and the gastrointestinal tract, in some cases as the sole initial site of involvement but more commonly as part of more generalized disease.

Staging Laparotomy

During the 1970s, specialist centres made increasing use of surgical exploration of the abdomen for complete staging of patients with HD. The usual surgical technique was to explore the abdomen through a paramedian or transverse incision. The spleen was first mobilized and removed. If coeliac or para-aortic lymph nodes were enlarged, one or more of these was excised. Some surgeons routinely biopsied a specified number of apparently normal lymph nodes. One or more needle and wedge biopsies of the liver was then obtained. The spleen was weighed in the operating theatre and then sliced with a sharp knife at 2- or 3-mm intervals. Further sections of the spleen could be made after adequate fixation. The results of staging a large number of newly diagnosed patients by laparotomy have shown that: (1) about one-third of normal size spleens show unsuspected histological evidence of HD; conversely, about one-third of enlarged spleens have no histological evidence of HD; (2) lymphographic assessment of para-aortic nodal disease is quite commonly inaccurate: unsuspected disease

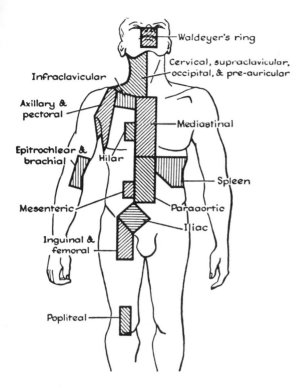

Labels on figure:
- Waldeyer's ring
- Cervical, supraclavicular, occipital, & pre-auricular
- Infraclavicular
- Axillary & pectoral
- Mediastinal
- Epitrochlear & brachial
- Hilar
- Spleen
- Mesenteric
- Paraaortic
- Iliac
- Inguinal & femoral
- Popliteal

Fig. 19.2. *Diagram of the separate lymph node regions defined for staging purposes at the Rye symposium on Hodgkin's disease. Reproduced with permission from a paper by Kaplan and Rosenberg (1966).*

may be identified, particularly in the upper para-aortic regions, and, conversely, occasionally 'positive' lymphograms thought to represent nodal disease cannot be confirmed at surgery; and (3) liver biopsies are frequently normal despite abnormal liver function tests; on the other hand, histological evidence of liver HD is occasionally present in the face of normal liver chemistry. At other times, granulomas in the liver are identified without histological evidence of HD.

Thus, staging laparotomy will often reveal unsuspected intra-abdominal disease. The increased availability of CT scanning and ultrasound since the 1970s has, however, reduced the popularity of laparotomy as a staging procedure. It can now best be justified if the demonstration of unsuspected additional disease would lead to a change in therapeutic strategy. If, for example, it has already been decided to treat a patient with IIIB disease by

chemotherapy, then nothing will be gained by demonstrating that such a patient also has liver disease. If, on the other hand, a patient with clinical IIA disease is scheduled to receive a radiotherapy 'mantle', the demonstration by staging laparotomy that he has in fact IIIA or IVA disease by virtue of spleen or liver involvement will crucially change the therapeutic plan and thereby the patient's prognosis. The decision therefore to undertake staging laparotomy must be linked with a consideration of the way in which results are likely to change the therapeutic strategy. It should not as a general rule be carried out in patients already known to have IIIB or IVB disease, in elderly patients or in those whose clinical condition makes them otherwise unfit.

Patients subjected to splenectomy as part of a staging procedure for HD are unduly susceptible to overwhelming post-splenectomy infection (OPSI) with pneumococcal or *Haemophilus* organisms, as are patients splenectomized for other reasons. They are therefore candidates for pneumococcal vaccination and long-term prophylaxis with oral antibiotics such as penicillin or co-trimoxazole.

Primary Treatment

It is now conventional practice to treat patients with early HD by radiotherapy alone; conversely, patients with advanced HD are usually treated first with chemotherapy. Patients with stage III disease may be treated initially by radiotherapy alone, chemotherapy alone, or by use of both modalities in either sequence (Table 19.3). There is little doubt that substantial numbers of patients with HD can be cured by the correct application of primary therapy.

Radiotherapy

The first reported use of radiotherapy to treat patients with HD was that of Pusey in 1902. Since that time, advances in three major areas—improvements in apparatus and techniques of radiotherapy, increased understanding of the importance of fractionation, and clearer definition of the optimal total radiotherapeutic dose—have contributed to the excellent results that can now be achieved with radiotherapy. The introduction of megavoltage

Table 19.3

Choice of primary therapy for newly diagnosed Hodgkin's disease

Stage I or IIA	Mantle or inverted-Y radiotherapy
Stage IIIA, spleen negative	Total nodal irradiation
Stage I, II or IIIB } Stage IIIA, spleen involved }	Combination chemotherapy followed if necessary by irradiation to areas of previous 'bulk' disease
Stage IVA or B	Combination chemotherapy

techniques, using either a linear accelerator or a ^{60}Co source of suitable power, now allows a number of lymph node regions to be irradiated in a single patient 'in continuity', thereby avoiding the risk of overdosage where adjacent smaller fields overlap. Moreover, the definition of field edge using this modern equipment is sufficiently precise to allow vulnerable tissues not involved by HD to be protected. Another advantage of modern equipment is the relatively trivial skin reactions induced in comparison with the older 'orthovoltage' machines. It has been clearly demonstrated that the risk of a patient developing tumour recurrence within a treated area is inversely related to the dose of radiotherapy delivered to that area. Equally it has now been shown that a given dose of radiotherapy is relatively less effective in preventing local tumour recurrence if it is fractionated over a longer rather than shorter period of time. The conclusion is that radiotherapy using supervoltage techniques intended to cure HD must involve the administration of 3600–4400 cGy in divided doses over a 4-week period.

For stage IA or IIA disease above the diaphragm, the optimal approach now consists of a radiotherapy 'mantle', a field of treatment that includes both cervical regions, both axillary regions and the mediastinum down to the level of L3 (Fig. 19.3). The best results are obtained in centres where the dimensions of this mantle field are tailored to suit each patient individually and where alterations in the fields of radiotherapy can be introduced during the course of treatment. For patients so treated, relapse-free survivals at 5 years exceed 90% and the majority of such patients can anticipate cure. For

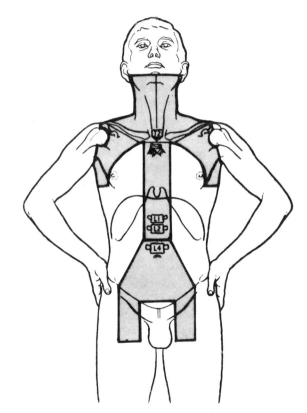

Fig. 19.3. *Typical radiation fields for treatment of a patient with stage IIIA HD. The shaded area above the level of L4 corresponds to a 'mantle' field. The shaded area below the level of L4 is usually described as an 'inverted-Y' field. When both areas are irradiated in sequence, usually first the mantle field and then the inverted-Y field after a 4–6-week interval, the treatment is referred to (somewhat inaccurately) as 'total nodal irradiation'. Note that no splenic field is included as staging for this hypothetical patient has included laparotomy and splenectomy.*

patients staged without laparotomy but still presumed to be IA or IIA, extension of the radiotherapeutic field below the diaphragm to include the upper para-aortic region and spleen is mandatory. For patients with IIIA disease without splenic involvement, the usual first approach is total nodal irradiation involving a mantle field followed after a 4–6-week rest by an 'inverted-Y' that covers para-aortic, iliac, inguinal and femoral lymph node regions (Fig. 19.3). Alternatively, treatment for patients with IIIA disease may be determined on the basis of splenic findings at laparotomy—those with histologically negative spleens receive total nodal irradiation (TNI) while those with III$_s$A disease may be better treated with combination chemotherapy.

Patients with stage I or IIA disease who have a large mediastinal mass are generally thought to constitute a group with an especially poor prognosis. Their treatment, however, is controversial. Some centres recommend the use of radiotherapy as for other cases of early stage disease but with sequential reduction of the radiation field as the mediastinal tumour shrinks. Other centres recommend initial treatment with chemotherapy followed by 'radical' radiotherapy. The clinical results of these different approaches are similar.

Complications of radiotherapy may be very troublesome but are seldom incapacitating. They are related to the volume of tissue irradiated. Patients treated by mantle fields frequently experience transient dryness of the mouth and a cough. Bone marrow suppression is regular but reversible. The long-term side-effects may include (rarely) hypothyroidism, pulmonary fibrosis and pericardial effusion. Patients treated by total nodal irradiation sustain more severe bone marrow depression. The abdominal field frequently produces a feeling of nausea. Radiotherapy to the pelvis of women in whom menstruation is established may lead to amenorrhoea and infertility.

Chemotherapy

The modern era of chemotherapy was ushered in by the recognition in 1946 that nitrogen mustard had activity in the control of HD. Since then, a large number of polyfunctional alkylating agents has been developed and agents in two other classes, the vinca alkaloids and procarbazine, have been shown to have significant activity against HD. In addition, a number of other agents (Table 19.4) are effective to a lesser extent in treating HD. Until the early 1970s the usual chemotherapeutic treatment for HD involved the selection of one agent, such as nitrogen mustard, to treat a patient until resistance developed. The clinician then chose a second agent, such as vinblastine, and continued this drug until the patient demonstrated resistance. Thereafter procarbazine was usually tried and as a last resort some of the 'second-line' agents were administered. There is little doubt that the administration of single drugs in sequence had worthwhile palliative effects but there is no evidence that any patients were cured by this approach.

The use of single agents in sequence has now been entirely superseded by the era of combination chemotherapy. In 1964, De Vita, at the National Cancer Institute (USA), initiated a study in which patients were treated for six 4-week periods with nitrogen mustard, vincristine, procarbazine and prednisone (Table 19.5). Of the original 43 patients with advanced HD so treated, 35 (81%) achieved complete remission and 16 of these were free of disease 5 years after ending therapy. It is probable that some of these patients have been cured of their HD. Subsequently this MOPP combination has been used in many centres throughout the world and complete remission incidences for previously untreated patients with advanced disease have been confirmed at 65–80%. Patients treated previously with radiotherapy have achieved equally good results, but patients whose previous treatment has also included chemotherapy show an inferior rate of response to MOPP. A large number of minor changes have been introduced into the MOPP combination in an attempt to improve its effectiveness. For example, the British National Lymphoma Investigation (BNLI) added bleomycin to the four-drug combination and an American co-operative group incorporated adriamycin into initial treatment. So far, no regimen producing results superior to those of MOPP has been identified. Two variations do, however, deserve mention: at St Bartholomew's Hospital in London, a combination using vinblastine rather than vincristine (MVPP) has been studied and gave results equivalent to those of MOPP with somewhat less neurotoxicity;

Table 19.4
The use of single agents in Hodgkin's disease

Drug	Response rate (%)	Complete remission (%)
Alkylating agents		
Nitrogen mustard	64	13
Cyclophosphamide	54	12
Chlorambucil	60	16
Vinca alkaloids		
Vinblastine	68	30
Vincristine	58	36
Antibiotics		
Actinomycin D	50	0
Adriamycin	41	4
Bleomycin	43	7
Nitrosoureas		
BCNU (Carmustine)	50	5
CCNU (Lomustine)	74	21
Streptozotocin	44	0
Steroids		
Prednisone	61	0
Miscellaneous		
Procarbazine	69	38
Teniposide (VM-26)	39	0
Imidazole carboxamide Dacarbazine	56	6

Response is arbitrarily defined as reduction in tumour mass of 50% or more.
Complete remission usually means eradication of all evidence of disease lasting for a minimum period of 3 (sometimes only 1) months.
(Table modified from Bonadonna *et al.* (1975), with permission.)

alternatively, the substitution of chlorambucil for nitrogen mustard in the MVPP combination (yielding ChlVPP) has given results as good as MVPP and spares patients the severe vomiting associated with nitrogen mustard administration. The use of chlorambucil in place of nitrogen mustard in the MOPP combination (yielding LOPP) has proved to be equally successful. About 40% of patients with advanced HD treated with MOPP or an equivalent combination can expect to be cured of their disease. About 20% will fail to achieve complete remission on primary treatment, and a further 40% will relapse after completing a course of MOPP. Those of the 40% who relapse within 6 months of completing a course can arbitrarily be defined as

having MOPP-resistant disease; those who relapse at a later stage may be expected to respond again to the re-introduction of MOPP.

Maintenance chemotherapy at low dosage after the initial six cycles of MOPP may delay the onset of recurrent disease in patients destined to relapse but there is no evidence that it increases the incidence of cure. For this reason, most centres now recommend somewhat more prolonged initial therapy than that originally envisaged by De Vita—the BNLI recommends a total of six cycles or an additional three cycles after the achievement of complete remission, whichever is the greater number. Other attempts to improve the remission and cure rates with combination chemotherapy have

Table 19.5

Combination chemotherapy for Hodgkin's disease

The MOPP combination

Nitrogen mustard	6 mg/m² i.v. days 1 & 8
Vincristine (Oncovin)	1.4 mg/m² (max. 2.0 mg) i.v. days 1 & 8
Procarbazine	100 mg/m² orally days 1–14
Prednisone	40 mg/m² orally days 1–14

Notes

(a) Each cycle lasts 28 days. The next cycle begins on day 29.

(b) Procarbazine is usually limited to a maximum of 150 mg/day for 10 days only.

(c) The prednisone is given only in cycles 1 and 4 of the six cycles.

The MVPP combination

Nitrogen mustard	6 mg/m² i.v. days 1 & 8
Vinblastine	6 mg/m² i.v. days 1 & 8
Procarbazine	100 mg/m² orally days 1–14
Prednisone	40 mg orally days 1–14

Note

(a) Each cycle lasts 28 days. The next cycle begins on day 29.

The LOPP combination

Chlorambuçil (Leukeran)	10 mg orally days 1–10
Vincristine (Oncovin)	1.4 mg/m² (max. 2.0 mg) i.v. days 1 & 8
Procarbazine	100 mg/m² orally days 1–10
Prednisone	25 mg/m² orally days 1–14

The ChlVPP combination

Chlorambucil	6 mg/m² orally days 1–14
Vinblastine	6 mg/m² i.v. days 1 & 8
Procarbazine	100 mg/m² orally days 1–14
Prednisolone	40 mg orally days 1–14

The LOPP/EVAP combination

Etoposide (VP 16 213)	150 mg/m² orally days 1, 2 & 3, alternating each cycle with the LOPP combination
Vinblastine	6 mg/m² i.v. days 1 & 8
Adriamycin (doxorubicin)	25 mg/m² i.v. days 1 & 8
Prednisone/prednisolone	25 mg/m² orally days 1–14

(The EVAP combination above alternates with cycles of the LOPP combination)

The ABVD combination

Adriamycin	25 mg/m² i.v. days 1 & 8
Bleomycin	10 mg/m² i.v. days 1 & 8
Vincristine	1.4 mg/m² (max. 2.0 mg) i.v. days 1 & 8
DTIC (Dacarbazine)	1.0–1.5 g i.v. day 1

Note. All the drug dosages above are for general guidance only. Precise details of treatment in a given patient must be decided by an experienced oncologist or haematologist.

included the use of MOPP in combination with low-dose radiotherapy and the use of alternating non-cross-resistant regimens such as MOPP in conjunction with ABVD (adriamycin, bleomycin, vinblastine and imidazole carboxamide) for a total of 12 courses (6 of each) in some centres. The BNLI is currently evaluating a treatment schedule in which patients are randomized to receive either LOPP (Table 19.5) for a minimum of eight courses or LOPP for a minimum of four courses alternating with EVAP (Table 19.5) for a minimum of four courses. Preliminary results suggest that the latter combination, though more toxic, is superior.

Chemotherapy with the MOPP combination is rather unpleasant for the patient. The nitrogen mustard regularly causes vomiting which tends to become more severe with successive courses. Vincristine can cause a peripheral neuropathy which may necessitate dose reduction. Constipation and a minor degree of alopecia also occur. The procarbazine can cause nausea and gastrointestinal discomfort. The administration of steroids rarely causes major problems but patients may feel unwell for 2 or 3 days after stopping them. Bone marrow depression occurs regularly after each course of MOPP and tends to be progressively more severe. Male patients usually become sterile and semen storage should be offered to young men before initiation of chemotherapy, even though patients with B symptoms are frequently oligospermic at presentation. In women, combination chemotherapy usually but not always leads to interruption of menstruation, but this may resume 2 or 3 years after the end of treatment. Women may lose their libido and be rendered infertile; the probability that sexual function is irreversibly impaired is related to patient age. Younger women treated with combination chemotherapy who recover menstruation may have normal pregnancies and normal babies. The possibilities for cryopreservation of ova or fertilized embryos should at least be discussed with all women of child-bearing age for whom chemotherapy is planned.

Advanced Resistant Disease

Patients who achieve complete remission after primary treatment for HD should be followed regularly in the out-patient clinic. If relapse is suspected in a previously irradiated patient, an attempt to confirm this histologically is mandatory. Once confirmed, restaging should be undertaken using all appropriate investigational techniques described for primary disease other than a second staging laparotomy. As a general rule, lymph node disease occurring in and restricted to one or more previously unirradiated sites may still be manageable by further radiotherapy. If nodal disease recurs in a previously irradiated area, or is generalized, or the patient is now stage IV, the use of chemotherapy is advisable.

In patients previously treated by chemotherapy, such as the MOPP combination, a further remission may be achieved by use of the MOPP combination again if the interval between initial therapy and relapse is sufficiently long. If this interval is 6 months or less, then success with MOPP is improbable. Resort to an alternative combination is then desirable. The use of a combination incorporating ABVD and of a combination of CCNU, vinblastine and bleomycin have both proved promising. It is probable that some patients who relapse after initial treatment with MOPP can still be cured.

A small number of studies have been reported in which patients with relapsed HD were treated by high-dose chemotherapy and marrow autografting or by allogeneic transplantation with bone marrow from an HLA-identical sibling donor. In most cases the patients have died either from complications of the treatment or from disease, relapsing within a year of transplant. A few patients have become long-term survivors and such transplant techniques will probably play a role of increasing importance in the management of the patient with resistant disease.

Long-term Complications of Treatment

Some of the complications of radiotherapy and chemotherapy have been referred to above. It was recognized in the late 1960s that patients treated for HD had an increased risk of developing acute leukaemia. Subsequently it became clear that second malignancies in general were more common in patients treated for HD than in comparable members of the general population. Recently it has been calculated that the risk of a patient treated for HD developing acute leukaemia may be 1% or higher and applies especially to patients whose treatment has included both radiotherapy and chemotherapy (which includes alkylating agents). The acute myeloid leukaemia (peak incidence 3–5 years post-therapy) is frequently difficult to characterize and may resemble an aberrant form of myelodysplastic syndrome. The prodromal period may be long and characterized by pancytopenia, often with nucleated red cells in the blood film. The marrow may show an excess of myeloblasts, and morphological abnormalities in the developing granulocyte series, the erythroid series and in the megakaryocytes may be prominent. Chromosomal abnormalities in the myeloid series are almost universal, unlike cases of acute myeloid leukaemia developing de novo. The disease responds very poorly to standard therapy and survival is usually measured in months. Occasional patients have been cured by allogeneic bone marrow transplantation and this approach should always be considered in younger patients (aged less than 50 years). The occurrence of second tumours, including acute myeloid leukaemia, in patients apparently cured of HD emphasizes the need to treat patients with the minimum amount of treatment compatible with cure in each case.

NON-HODGKIN'S LYMPHOMA

Aetiology

As little is known of the aetiology of NHL as is known of the cause of HD. The observation that cytoplasmic RNA viruses, classified as C-type particles, can cause leukaemia or lymphoma in various experimental animals has suggested that they may be the cause of lymphoma in humans also, but no convincing proof exists. Though it is probable that the Epstein–Barr virus (EBV) causes infectious mononucleosis and it is known that EBV can induce sustained proliferation of normal human lymphoid cells in vitro, EBV has not yet been shown conclusively to cause Burkitt's lymphoma in Africa but is probably a crucial co-factor. Similarly, serological and epidemiological evidence incriminates HTLV-I as an essential co-factor in adult T-cell leukaemia/lymphoma in Japan and the Caribbean. However, for most human lymphomas the viral aetiology remains in doubt.

Chromosomal abnormalities occur commonly in malignant lymphomas but the changes have been found to be less consistent than, for example, the t(9;22) characteristic of chronic myeloid leukaemia. Patients with Burkitt's lymphoma have often shown a translocation t(8;14) (q24;q32) and this may be identified also in diffuse large-cell lymphomas and small non-cleaved cell lymphomas of non-Burkitt type. This translocation brings the *MYC* proto-oncogene under controlling influences involved in immunoglobulin gene expression (see Chapter 13). The translocation t(14;18) (q32;q21) is found with variable frequency in nodular lymphomas. The breakpoint on chromosome 18 appears to involve an oncogene designated *BCL*-2, and other translocations occur in T-lymphomas (see Chapter 13).

Attempts to demonstrate a predisposition to malignant lymphoma in patients with a specific HLA genotype have been largely unrewarding. In contrast, it is apparent that immunosuppression can, in certain circumstances, predispose to lymphoma. For example, lymphoma is unusually common in recipients of renal transplants and occurs with undue frequency in patients subjected to bone marrow transplantation. A particular aggressive form of NHL which responds poorly to therapy occurs relatively commonly in patients with AIDS (see Chapter 12). Moreover, the hydantoin group of drugs, especially diphenylhydantoin used in the prevention of epilepsy, can induce both a reversible lymphoma-like syndrome (pseudolymphoma) and on occasion a true malignant lymphoma.

Epidemiology

All attempts to characterize the epidemiology of the NHL are marred by vagaries of classification, and results obtained from different centres have only recently become comparable. Bearing in mind these reservations, it appears that the median age at the time of diagnosis of NHL is about 50 and patients under the age of 35 or over 65 are statistically more likely to have diffuse rather than nodular disease. Diffuse lymphomas affect males twice as often as females but the sexes are equally distributed amongst nodular lymphomas.

The NHL are found worldwide but distinctive differences are related to geography. In one Italian series, two-thirds of extranodal lymphomas were in oropharyngeal sites. In the Middle East the commonest site for extranodal lymphoma is the gastrointestinal tract. Kaposi's sarcoma, a lymphoma-like condition of unknown aetiology, is rarely seen in Western countries but is prevalent in some parts of Africa. Similarly African lymphoma, originally described by Burkitt, occurs mainly in Africa in areas of holoendemic malaria. Similar cases occur in other parts of the world, including North America, but their comparability with African Burkitt's lymphoma is disputed and they are very rare. Adult T-cell leukaemia/lymphoma was identified first in the south island (Kyushu) of Japan but cases have now been identified in black patients who have lived in or been associated with the Caribbean islands (see Chapter 15).

Clinical Features

A patient with NHL may present with localized or generalized peripheral adenopathy indistinguishable on clinical grounds from HD, but major constitutional symptoms such as fever, night sweats or weight loss occur less commonly in NHL than in HD. Patients with NHL also commonly present with features of disease outside the lymphatic system, a further point of distinction from HD. Intrathoracic disease may be manifested by hilar or mediastinal adenopathy, superior vena caval obstruction or pulmonary parenchymal involvement. Unilateral or bilateral pleural effusions are not uncommon at the time of presentation. Involvement of Waldeyer's ring is a relatively common presenting feature. Primary involvement of the gastrointestinal tract occurs and may be prognostically favourable if the disease remains localized. Rarely, primary lymphoma develops at a number of other sites, including the central nervous system, thyroid, lung, kidney, ovary, testis, skin or bone.

Histopathology

In contrast to HD, histological subclassification of NHL is probably of greater prognostic significance than accurate staging. However, the relatively clear-cut histological categories of the 1940s and 1950s, incorporating such terms as 'lymphosarcoma', 'reticulum cell sarcoma' and 'giant follicular lym-

phoma' are now obsolete and have given way to a bewildering number of newer classifications. In the last 25 years six different schemes, each subsequently subjected to its own modifications, have been proposed (Table 19.6). The seventh attempt, a so-called Working Formulation, is based on morphological features of the lymphoma and is an attempt to unify the existing classifications. It is inappropriate here to consider the relative merits of each classification but some familiarity with the more popular of them is essential. Thus the essential features of the Rappaport, Lukes/Collins and Kiel classifications will be described and the Working Formulation will be set out.

Rappaport Classification

The Rappaport classification is based on separate analysis of the predominant neoplastic cell and of the cytoarchitectural features of the enlarged lymph node or other involved organ (Table 19.7). Thus the predominant cell if small is designated 'lymphocytic, well-differentiated', if intermediate in size is designated 'lymphocytic, poorly differentiated' and if large 'histiocytic'. If the nodal cytoarchitecture shows division of the lymphomatous tissue into separate spherical foci or 'nodules', the lymphoma is termed nodular; other lymphomas are termed diffuse. From inspection of Table 19.7 it is clear that the Rappaport classification allows a very broad division of all lymphomas into 'good' or 'bad' prognostic categories; nodular disease (other than histiocytic) and well-differentiated diffuse lymphomas carry relatively favourable prognoses while nodular histiocytic and all diffuse lymphomas (other than lymphocytic, well differentiated) have poor prognoses.

The Rappaport classification has a number of defects. For example it fails to take account of the observation that the predominant lymphomatous cell in the nodular lymphomas always has the characteristics of a B cell and the nodules may therefore really be lymphomatous *follicles*. Thus British pathologists prefer the term 'follicular lymphoma' to cover the examples of NHL classified as 'nodular' in the Rappaport scheme. Some justification for this view derives from the unifying clinical features of the follicular lymphomas: patients are more likely to be middle-aged than those with

Table 19.6

Proposed schemes for classifying non-Hodgkin's lymphoma

Authors	Organization or institute	City of origin	Basis for the classification
Rappaport	—	Chicago	Cell morphology and nodal architecture
Lukes–Collins	—	Los Angeles	Membrane marker characteristics
Dorfman	—	San Francisco	Morphology
Bennett–Henry	BNLI	London	Morphology
Mathe	WHO	Paris	Morphology
Lennert	—	Kiel	Morphology
Berard *et al.*	Working Formulation (NCI)	Washington DC	Morphology

BNLI, British National Lymphoma Investigation; WHO, World Health Organization; NCI, National Cancer Institute (USA).

Table 19.7

Relationship of the Rappaport histopathological classification of non-Hodgkin's lymphoma to patient survival

Cytology	Nodal architecture			
	Nodular		Diffuse	
	Number of patients	Median survival (years)	Number of patients	Median survival (years)
Lymphocytic, well differentiated	6	5	10	5
Lymphocytic, poorly differentiated	69	7.5	44	1.8
Mixed lymphocytic–histiocytic	74	7.0	43	1.6
Histiocytic	29	2.9	116	1.1
Undifferentiated	0	—	14	0.5

Data compiled at Stanford University by Jones *et al.* (1973) and reproduced with permission.

diffuse disease, and the disease is more likely to run a benign course for many years but more likely nonetheless to undergo abrupt changes in its natural history. Thus indolent follicular lymphomas can suddenly 'transform' in a number of ways: they may become diffuse and more aggressive, they may form large localized tumours or they may suddenly enter a progressive leukaemic phase with a cellular morphology distinct from that of the original tumour.

Another drawback of the Rappaport classification is the inaccurate use of the term 'histiocytic'. To Rappaport it implied a tumour characterized by a large cell of non-lymphoid origin that presumably shared ancestry with the tissue histiocyte or macrophage. It is now known that the characteristic cell in most 'histiocytic' lymphomas has B-cell features and cannot therefore be regarded as histiocytic. Rare true histiocytic lymphomas do, however, occur.

Lukes and Collins Classification

The Lukes and Collins classification is based on the assumption that malignant lymphomas are neoplasms of the immune system and the lymphoma cells are defective B or T cells resembling to a greater or lesser extent their normal counterparts in site of origin, migration and function. The nodular lymphomas (Rappaport) are believed to derive from lymphomatous follicles composed of follicular centre cells with B-cell features, and thus each morphological type of follicular lymphoma cell corresponds with a different stage in the physiological transformation of the normal follicular centre cell. Conversely, T-cell lymphomas are thought to derive from normal T-cell counterparts and can often be recognized on morphological grounds by their typical convoluted nuclear morphology. Tumours with immunoblastic features may be of B- or T-cell origin. This 'functional' classification of Lukes and Collins is shown in Table 19.8.

The Lukes and Collins classification provides a partial answer to the problem of subclassifying the lymphomas termed 'histiocytic' by Rappaport. This group can now be subdivided according to cellular characteristics into five categories, characterized by: (1) large cleaved follicular centre cells, (2) large non-cleaved follicular centre cells, (3) immunoblastic sarcoma of B type, (4) immunoblastic sarcoma of T type, and (5) true histiocytic. Recognition of the last type, true histiocytic, depends on the presence in the 'lymphoma' cell of a specific histiocytic marker, either α-naphthyl butyrate in tissue imprints or a positive immunoperoxidase stain for lysozyme. Perhaps the term lymphoma should not be applied to the rare true histiocytic tumour.

The Working Formulation for Clinical Usage

In 1980 a group of histopathologists from North America, Europe and Japan met to attempt to bring some order to the confused field of NHL classific-

Table 19.8

Functional histopathological classification of non-Hodgkin's lymphoma (Lukes and Collins)

U cell (undefined)

T cell
Small lymphocyte
Convoluted lymphocyte
Sezary—mycosis fungoides
Immunoblastic sarcoma of T cells

B cell
Small lymphocyte
Plasmacytoid lymphocyte
Follicular centre cell
  (Follicular or diffuse architecture)
  Small cleaved
  Large cleaved
  Small non-cleaved (transformed)
  Large non-cleaved (transformed)
Immunoblastic sarcoma of B cells
Hairy cell leukaemia

Histiocytic

---

ation. The result was a formulation dividing NHL into three basic prognostic categories to which cases already categorized in other systems could be related to a greater or lesser extent (Table 19.9).

Kiel Classification

This system, widely used in Europe, attempts to relate the clonal cell in non-Hodgkin's lymphoma to certain cells in the lymph node from which they are supposed to arise (Table 19.10; Fig. 19.4). Its merit lies in the fact that it combines an immunological and morphological approach and has value in predicting prognosis.

Membrane Marker Characteristics and Evidence for Clonality

In many cases the cells that constitute a given lymphoma appear to be clonally derived. In other words, the use of appropriate techniques provides evidence that all cells in a given population are derived from a single common ancestor. This is

Table 19.9

Working formulation of non-Hodgkin's lymphoma intended for clinical usage

---

Low grade
Malignant lymphoma, small lymphocytic
Malignant lymphoma, follicular, predominantly small cleaved cell
Malignant lymphoma, follicular, mixed small cleaved and large cell

Intermediate grade
Malignant lymphoma, follicular, predominantly large cell
Malignant lymphoma, diffuse, small cleaved cell
Malignant lymphoma, diffuse, mixed small and large cell
Malignant lymphoma, diffuse, large cell

High grade
Malignant lymphoma, large cell, immunoblastic
Malignant lymphoma, lymphoblastic
Malignant lymphoma, small non-cleaved cell

Miscellaneous
Composite malignant lymphoma
Mycosis fungoides
Extramedullary plasmacytoma
Unclassified
Other

---

evidence for, although not proof of, their malignant character. The techniques used to infer clonality include enzymological, membrane marker, genetic and cytogenetic analyses.

Study of lymphomas arising in females heterozygous for G6PD shows that the malignant cells are universally either of one or other isoenzyme type but never of both. This implies that there may have been at some stage in the evolution of the lymphoma a single susceptible target cell. It does not exclude the alternative possibility that multiple cells of one isoenzyme type were collectively affected by the 'lymphomagenic' factor or factors.

Techniques for characterizing the membrane glycoproteins of leukaemic cells have been applied to cells obtained from pathological nodes and other tissues from patients with lymphoma. In almost all cases of nodular lymphoma the predominant neoplastic cell has proved to have characteristics of a B lymphocyte. For example, the cell membrane has antigen determinants reacting with monoclonal antibodies that recognize B cells and the cell expresses either kappa or lambda light chains (but not

both). Study of DNA derived from the nodular lymphoma cells, using Southern technology with appropriate restriction enzymes and immunoglobulin heavy and/or light chain probes, shows abnormal bands consistent with the existence of new restriction fragments distinct from those of germ-line origin. These findings must mean that the lymphoma under study took origin from a single cell that had already undergone a very specific heavy chain or heavy and light chain immunoglobulin gene rearrangement. The majority of diffuse lymphomas resemble the nodular lymphomas in that the predominating malignant cell has B-lymphocyte characteristics as defined by study of surface membrane determinants and Ig gene rearrangements (see p. 332).

A minority of diffuse tumours, perhaps 10%, have cells with the membrane features of a T lymphocyte. They react with monoclonal antibodies that define T-lymphocyte antigens, such as CD3, and some of these tumours have monoclonal rearrangements of the delta, gamma and/or beta chains of the T-cell receptor (TCR). A small pro-

Table 19.10

The Kiel classification of non-Hodgkin's lymphomas
(modified from Lennert *et al.*, 1983)

Low grade
Lymphocytic
 CLL of B-cell type
 CLL of T-cell type
 Hairy-cell leukaemia
 Mycosis fungoides and Sezary syndrome
 T-zone lymphoma

Lymphoplasmacytic/lymphoplasmacytoid
 Plasmacytic
 Centrocytic
 Centrocytic/centroblastic
 Unclassified low grade

High grade
Centroblastic
Lymphoblastic
 B lymphoblastic, Burkitt type, etc.
 T lymphoblastic, convoluted cell type, etc.
 Unclassified

Immunoblastic
 with plasmablastic/plasmacytic differentiation
  (B immunoblastic)
 with plasmablastic/plasmacytic differentiation
  (T immunoblastic)
Unclassified high grade

---

portion of lymphoid tumours have neither B- nor T-cell surface markers and have therefore been designated 'null cell'. Some of these tumours show Ig or TCR gene rearrangements, so they can now be categorized more precisely.

The prognostic value of lymphoma cell surface characteristics is not yet fully established. In general, patients with B-cell nodular lymphomas will survive longer than those with B-cell diffuse tumours (when well-differentiated lymphomas are excluded from the latter group). Within the diffuse category, patients with T-cell or null-cell tumours appear to have prognoses inferior to those with B-cell lymphomas.

Diagnostic Evaluation and Staging

Like the patient with HD, the newly diagnosed patient with NHL should be investigated with a view to establishing the extent of disease. However, because the unifocal origin and subsequent 'orderly spread' are less well established in NHL than in HD, detailed anatomical staging is somewhat less important in NHL. Nevertheless, if the disease is first diagnosed at a nodal site, careful physical examination should be directed at all other node-bearing areas. The post-nasal space should be examined in patients with nodal disease above the diaphragm. Especial attention should be paid to Waldeyer's ring of lymphoid tissue in the lingual and pharyngeal areas. Supplementary biopsies may be necessary to confirm suspected disease. Assessment of the size of liver and spleen is important.

In the absence of lymphoma cells in the peripheral blood, examination of the blood shows fewer abnormalities than in HD. Anaemia may reflect bone marrow failure due to infiltration or autoimmune haemolytic anaemia. Lymphocyte numbers are usually normal but their kappa:lambda ratio may be disturbed in a direction reflecting the light chain determinant characteristic of the lymphoma. There may be neutropenia or thrombocytopenia. Monocytosis, neutrophilia and eosinophilia are unusual. The ESR is not usually helpful in monitoring the progress of patients with nodular lymphoma but may occasionally be useful when initially raised in patients with diffuse disease. The serum alkaline phosphatase may be raised as a result of liver infiltration or extensive bone disease. The serum β_2 microglobulin level also may be raised. Serum protein values may be normal in localized disease but serum albumin may be low if the liver is infiltrated. Serum immunoglobulins are frequently normal but a proportion of patients with well-differentiated diffuse lymphoma have reduced immunoglobulin levels at diagnosis similar to the pattern seen in CLL. About 3% of patients with diffuse lymphoma have a monoclonal paraprotein in their serum at diagnosis or develop one during the course of their disease.

In patients who appear on clinical grounds to have localized disease, further investigations should be carried out. Lymphography may reveal unsuspected involvement of para-aortic lymph nodes and this is particularly true of patients with nodular lymphoma. CT scanning or ultrasound examination of the abdomen or thorax may reveal unsuspected nodal disease. Needle aspiration and

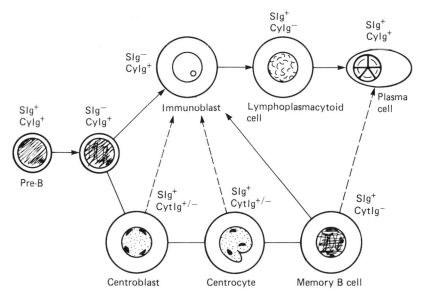

Fig. 19.4. *Suggested maturation of B cells leaving marrow and entering peripheral lymphoid tissue (after Lennert).*

trephine biopsy of bone marrow from the iliac crest may show evidence of marrow involvement by lymphoma. In cases of well-differentiated diffuse lymphoma the proportion of morphologically normal lymphocytes in the marrow may be increased; in other cases lymphocytes may show abnormalities such as clefting or prominent nucleoli. Neoplastic lymphoid cells in the bone marrow frequently form aggregates that are found first in the paratrabecular regions.

In the absence of thrombocytopenia or other contraindication, a patient with apparently localized disease should have a needle biopsy of liver to exclude infiltration. Involvement of the liver in NHL may be focal but in general diffuse involvement starting in the portal tracts is commoner than in HD and thereby more likely to be identified by 'blind' needle biopsy.

Although formally designed for use with HD, the Ann Arbor staging classification is used widely for the staging of NHL also. Fever, however, is relatively uncommon as a systemic manifestation of NHL and sweats and weight loss lack the especial prognostic significance that they appear to have in HD. Consequently NHL patients are usually staged I to IV but the reference to specific constitutional symptoms (A or B) is omitted.

Between 20% and 40% of patients in an unselected series will appear to have localized disease (i.e. stage I or II) at diagnosis. However, examination of results of lymphography, bone marrow and liver biopsies will reveal that many of these patients do indeed have disseminated disease and only those that remain (10–20%) have truly localized disease. Staging laparotomy as used in HD has been explored as an adjunct to staging in NHL but in most cases little additional diagnostic information is provided and the risks of the surgical procedure are greater in NHL than in HD. For these reasons staging laparotomy is not carried out in NHL.

Treatment

A rational strategy for the treatment of the newly diagnosed patient with NHL depends on the results of staging procedures and histological subclassification. The 10–20% of patients who prove to have truly localized (stages I or II) disease may in some cases be treated by radiotherapy alone. Of those with more advanced (stages III or IV) disease, it is reasonable to use the Rappaport or the Lukes and Collins classification to divide cases into those with 'good' or those with 'poor' prognoses. For patients in the former category there is little evidence that treatment can permanently eradicate disease and the first decision is whether the patient warrants treatment immediately or whether treatment could reasonably be deferred until symptoms require it. For patients in the latter (poor prognosis) category treatment should always be initiated as soon as possible after diagnosis.

Stage I or II Disease

Patients with truly localized disease should be treated by radiotherapy. On the uncertain assumption that such disease may spread in a 'continuous' manner, most patients with true histiocytic lymphoma are best treated with 4500–5000 cGy in 200 cGy fractions to involved areas and adjacent lymph node chains. For patients with non-histiocytic NHL, treatment with 2500–3500 cGy may suffice. Such treatment usually leads to total regression of disease within the treated area. When treatment fails, recurrent disease is usually evident within 2 years. Five years after such treatment 40–60% of patients will remain free of disease. In some centres the possible additional benefit of adjuvant chemotherapy is being tested in patients who have achieved complete remission with radiotherapy, but its real value has not yet been established.

Stage III and IV Disease, Favourable ('Good Prognosis') Histology

Though the mere diagnosis of advanced stage favourable histology NHL should not lead automatically to treatment, the presence of constitutional symptoms or generalized lymphadenopathy that is inconvenient for the patient or cosmetically unattractive are reasons for initiating therapy. So also is the presence of threat of major complications such as superior mediastinal obstruction, lymphatic obstruction, obstructive jaundice or marrow failure. The choice of which treatment to use is more difficult (Table 19.11). An alkylating agent such as chlorambucil may be used as a single agent either at continuous low dosage or in short courses given every 4 or more weeks. The latter approach is probably less immunosuppressive and therefore to be preferred. A number of cytotoxic drug combinations has been tried, including COP (cyclophosphamide, vincristine and prednisolone), COPP (cyclophosphamide, vincristine, prednisolone and procarbazine) and BACOP (cyclophosphamide, vincristine, prednisolone, adriamycin and bleomycin) and these in general give higher remission rates (60–80%) than single agents (Table 19.12). Unfortunately, about 50% of patients who achieve complete remission will have relapsed within 2 years of starting treatment, and no difference in survival can be demonstrated between patients treated with single agents or with drug combinations.

As effective as the use of cytotoxic drugs in this category of patients is total body irradiation. A typical course may comprise 15 cGy administered to the whole patient twice weekly to a total dose of 150 cGy; alternatively, one half of the body (e.g. above the diaphragm) may be irradiated first and then the other half (the lower half) after a suitable rest period. This approach is remarkably free of toxicity, but the finding that the incidence of complete remission is exactly the same as that obtained with cytotoxic drugs has limited its popularity.

Stage III and IV Disease, Unfavourable ('Poor Prognosis') Histology

Patients with diffuse, poorly differentiated lymphocytic lymphoma have in the past been treated with drug combinations such as COP (cyclophosphamide, vincristine and prednisolone) with a complete remission rate of 30–50%. Newer cytotoxic drugs have been added and CHOP (COP plus adriamycin) and m(M)-BACOD (intermediate (high) dose methotrexate, bleomycin, adriamycin, cyclophosphamide, vincristine and dexamethasone) are now generally used in preference. The intermediate or high dose of methotrexate is designed to penetrate into the CSF to give CNS protection. In small series the combinations have given remission rates of 50–80% with disease-free survival of up to 50% at 2 years. Essentially the same combinations have been used with success in patients with advanced stage diffuse large cell lymphoma (working formulation). Approximately 40–60% of patients so treated will achieve complete remission. Of special interest is the observation that between 20% and 40% of those who achieve complete remission will remain free of disease at 2 years; after this time the chance of subsequent relapse is apparently small, so

Table 19.11

The use of single agents in non-Hodgkin's lymphoma

Drug	Response rate (%)	
	'Good prognosis' NHL	'Poor prognosis' NHL
Alkylating agents		
Nitrogen mustard	50–70	40–50
Chlorambucil	50–60	20–30
Cyclophosphamide	50–70	50–70
Vinca alkaloids		
Vinblastine	15–25	20–35
Vincristine	40–65	50–80
Antibiotics		
Adriamycin	35–50	50–65
Bleomycin	30–40	30–40
Nitrosoureas		
BCNU (Carmustine)	20–30	25–35
Streptozotocin	20–30	5–15
Steroids		
Prednisone	60–80	20–30
Miscellaneous		
Procarbazine	40–50	20–35
Methotrexate	15–25	15–25
Cytosine arabinoside	20–25	15–20
Cis-platinum	—	10–20
VM-26 (Teniposide)	50–60	30–35
VP-16 213 (Etoposide)	25–35	10–15
Interferon α	NYD	NYD
Mitoxantrone	NYD	NYD
2'-deoxycoformycin	NYD	NYD

In general, *response* is defined as more than 50% tumour regression. The incidence of *complete remission* (eradication of all clinical evidence of tumour lasting for a minimum period of 3 months) with various single agents is substantially lower than the response rates quoted above. (NYD; not yet fully determined.)

it is quite probable that a proportion of patients with diffuse large cell lymphoma treated with combination chemotherapy can be cured.

A small number of patients with 'poor prognosis' NHL in relapse have been treated with combinations of cytotoxic drugs at high dosage with or without total body irradiation, typically 10 Gy, followed by autografting with marrow cells collected earlier. In general, the use of autografting is only logical for patients without overt marrow involvement. In some studies attempts have been made to 'purge' harvested marrow of small numbers of tumour cells by incubation of the marrow cells in vitro with anti-B or anti-T-cell monoclonal antibodies and complement. The clinical results of these studies are not yet fully evaluable. Some patients obtain second remissions and these are durable on occasion, but it is not yet clear whether or not the

Table 19.12

Combination chemotherapy for non-Hodgkin's lymphoma

The COP combination

Cyclophosphamide	600 mg/m² i.v. days 1 & 8
Vincristine	1.4 mg/m² (max. 2.0 mg) i.v. days 1 & 8
Prednisolone	50 mg/m² orally days 1–8

Notes

  (a) The combination is typically continued for a total of 6–9 courses.

  (b) Moderate or complete hair loss may be expected.

The CHOP combination

Cyclophosphamide	750 mg/m² i.v. days 1 & 8
Adriamycin (Hydroxydaunorubicin)	25 mg/m² i.v. days 1 & 8
Vincristine (Oncovin)	1.4 mg/m² (max. 2.0 mg) i.v. days 1 & 8
Prednisolone	50 mg/m² orally days 1–8

Notes

  (a) Most patients will lose all their hair during CHOP therapy.

  (b) Most patients will develop major neutropenia at these dose levels. The cyclophosphamide and adriamycin may be omitted on day 8 if necessary.

  (c) The cardiac status of patients receiving adriamycin must be monitored carefully. It is conventional to omit adriamycin when the patient's total cumulated dose reaches 500 mg/m².

The m-BACOD combination

Methotrexate (with folinic acid rescue)	200 mg/m² i.v. days 8 & 15
Bleomycin	4 mg/m² i.v. days 1 & 22
Adriamycin	45 mg/m² i.v. days 1 & 22
Cyclophosphamide	600 mg/m² i.v. days 1 & 22
Vincristine	1 mg/m² i.v. days 1 & 22
Dexamethasone	6 mg/m² orally days 1–5 & 22–26

Repeat every 3 weeks, ten times

The ProMACE-MOPP combination

Cyclophosphamide	650 mg/m² i.v. days 1 & 8
Adriamycin	25 mg/m² i.v. days 1 & 8
VP-16 213 (Etoposide)	120 mg/m² i.v. days 1 & 8
Prednisone	60 mg/m² orally days 1–14
Methotrexate (with folinic acid rescue)	1.5 g/m² i.v. day 14

Repeat every 28 days until one cycle after disappearance of clinically evident disease, followed by an equal number of cycles of MOPP.

Notes

  (a) The target is to complete six 4-week cycles of m-BACOD.

  (b) Patients treated with adriamycin must be monitored for possible cardiac toxicity (see note (c) above).

  (c) Bleomycin can cause progressive pulmonary fibrosis at total cumulated doses above 300 mg. Rarely, pulmonary problems are seen at lower total dose levels.

Note. It is very important to note that all the drug dosages given are for general guidance only. Precise details of treatment for a given patient should be decided only by an experienced oncologist or haematologist.

same results would have been achieved with more conventional therapy. An even smaller number of patients has been treated by chemoradiotherapy followed by allografting with marrow from HLA-identical siblings. Again the numbers are too few to permit meaningful analysis. If the problems of graft-versus-host disease and interstitial pneumonitis can be prevented, allogeneic marrow transplantation may assume an important role in the treatment of patients with poor prognosis NHL and marrow involvement.

Involvement of the Central Nervous System

Up to 20% of patients with NHL who come to autopsy have evidence of lymphomatous involvement of the central nervous system. As the efficacy of treatment improves and the number of patients with advanced disease who achieve complete remission increases, it has become clear that a proportion will develop clinical features of meningeal or cranial nerve involvement, while the nodal or systemic disease is apparently controlled. The risk of developing CNS involvement is greatest in patients shown to have marrow involvement at diagnosis or subsequently, but patients with favourable histology disease (especially follicular disease) are not apparently at risk. As a consequence, patients with unfavourable histology NHL who also have marrow involvement at diagnosis should receive one of the systemic regimens designed to give CNS prophylaxis (see above). Other regimens used include proMACE-MOPP, COP-BLAM III, and pro-MACE-cytaBOM. Alternatively, the patient should undergo standard measures for prevention of CNS disease as soon as their systemic disease has been controlled. Once established, disease of the CNS is best treated by intrathecal injection of methotrexate or cytosine arabinoside coupled with cranial or craniospinal irradiation.

NON-HODGKIN'S LYMPHOMA IN CHILDREN

Non-Hodgkin's lymphoma is the third commonest malignancy in children under the age of 15 and accounts for 10% of all childhood cancers. The histopathological classifications devised for adults are not usefully applied to children since almost all NHL in children is of the diffuse type and nodular disease is very rare. Nevertheless, using a classification based on that of Rappaport (Table 19.13), about half of all NHL in children is diffuse lymphoblastic, perhaps 15% histiocytic, and the remainder large lymphoid cell or undifferentiated. The lymphoblastic lymphomas may be subdivided into 'convoluted cell' and 'non-convoluted cell'. In children both types of lymphoblastic lymphoma may be associated with mediastinal masses and some at least of such tumours have T-cell characteristics. NHL in children has a high incidence of 'leukaemic transformation', even when apparently localized at initial presentation. Similarly the risk of CNS involvement is higher in children than in adults with comparable disease.

Because of its special features, NHL in children is customarily treated more like acute lymphoblastic leukaemia than like adult NHL. Combination chemotherapy protocols incorporating vincristine, prednisolone, adriamycin and L-asparaginase (OPAL) or cyclophosphamide, vincristine, prednisolone and high-dose methotrexate (LSA2-L2) can produce complete remission rates in excess of 80%. Children who achieve complete remission should receive standard treatment for prevention of CNS disease (e.g. cranial irradiation and intrathecal methotrexate) and cytotoxic drugs should be continued systemically on a maintenance basis for a total of 2–3 years. Such an approach to the management of NHL in children may produce 3-year disease-free survival of 50–80% and it is reasonable to suppose that some of these patients have been cured.

Table 19.13

Histopathological classification of lymphoma in children

Hodgkin's disease
Non-Hodgkin's lymphoma
  Lymphoblastic
    Convoluted
      Non-convoluted
  Large lymphoid
  Histiocytic
  Burkitt's lymphoma
  Undifferentiated

BURKITT'S LYMPHOMA

In 1958 Denis Burkitt, a British surgeon then working in East Africa, described a tumour of African children with special predilection for involvement of bones in the jaw. Subsequently it became clear that a lymphoma with distinctive characteristics was especially common in central Africa—it occurred almost exclusively in areas of low altitude (less than 1500 m), relatively high annual temperature and high annual rainfall. This geographical distribution was almost identical with the distribution in Africa of holoendemic (non-seasonal) malaria. In 1964 Epstein and his colleagues in London were able to isolate from cells cultured from Burkitt's lymphoma (BL) biopsy material a new herpes group virus, subsequently designated Epstein–Barr virus (EBV). All African patients with BL proved to have high serum antibody titres to EBV, and EBV genome was present in the DNA of cells derived from the lymphoma. Thus it is probable that EBV is at least a co-factor in the development of BL; chronic stimulation of the reticuloendothelial system by holoendemic malaria may be a further contributory factor.

The histopathological appearance of the tumour is characteristic. It consists of a monotonous population of lymphoblast-like cells with little variation in size (10–25 μm) or shape. The cells have a scanty cytoplasm that stains red with methyl-green pyronin and includes vacuoles containing neutral fat. The cell nuclei are round or oval without indentations but have one to five prominent nucleoli. Phagocytic macrophages are distributed uniformly throughout the tumour. In routine histological preparations the cytoplasm of these macrophages stains palely and contrasts with the uniformly dark-blue mass of tumour cell nuclei. The term 'starry-sky' has been applied to this overall appearance, which is typical but not diagnostic of BL. The lymphoblasts of BL have the membrane characteristics of a B cell and the tumour may therefore originate from a follicular centre cell. In the majority of cases the BL cell has a specific chromosomal translocation, t(8;14) (q24;q32). In these cases the *MYC* oncogene, normally located on the 8q, is brought into juxtaposition with sequences in the Ig heavy chain locus on chromosome 14 (see Chapter 13). A small minority of BL patients have variant translocations, t(8;22) (q24;q11) or t(2;8) and (p12;q23). In these cases c-*myc* remains on chromosome 8 and the mechanism of *MYC* activation is less clear.

The clinical features of BL in Africa are well defined. It is predominantly but not exclusively a disease of children, with a peak incidence between 3 and 5 years of age. The disease is often multifocal at diagnosis, with rapidly growing tumours in the maxillary or mandibular bones on one or both sides of the face, the abdominal or pelvic viscera or the long bones; less commonly, the thyroid, salivary glands or central nervous system are involved. Involvement of lymph nodes, bone marrow or a leukaemic phase in the blood is uncommon. Untreated, the disease progresses rapidly to death. Treatment with cyclophosphamide in high dosage or with combinations including cyclophosphamide produces rapid regression of the disease, usually complete remission in those with limited-stage disease, and the overall cure rate is about 40%.

The question of whether BL occurs uniquely in Africa or whether similar cases that occur sporadically in other parts of the world are classifiable as BL has been much debated. Non-African Burkitt's lymphoma differs from BL clinically—the patients tend to be older at diagnosis and are more likely to have nodal or marrow disease; high titres of antibody to EBV are less uniformly found in the serum and response to cyclophosphamide is generally inferior to that observed in African BL. A proportion of patients with sporadic Burkitt's can nonetheless apparently be cured.

ANGIOIMMUNOBLASTIC LYMPH-ADENOPATHY (AILD)

In 1975 Lukes and Tindle reported details of an unusual group of patients in a paper entitled 'Immunoblastic lymphadenopathy: a hyperimmune entity resembling Hodgkin's disease'. In the previous year Frizzera *et al.* had described a group of patients with histologically similar features under the heading 'Angioimmunoblastic lymphadenopathy with dysproteinaemia'. Patients with the disease described by Lukes and Tindle had a tendency to develop a neoplastic condition designated 'immunoblastic sarcoma', while the patients in

Frizzera's series did not so obviously have progression to malignancy. With this and other minor reservations, it appears that both groups of workers were describing essentially the same disease.

The cause of AILD is unknown. The frequency with which patients have been taking drugs before the onset of AILD and the development of different types of rash suggest that the patient may be allergic to an undefined antigen or otherwise 'hyperimmune', but the disease may truly be at the interface between a benign reactive condition and a neoplasm. Histopathologically an involved node has three main characteristics. (1) The node is enlarged and the normal architecture is effaced. There is a pleomorphic cellular infiltrate comprising immunoblasts and plasma cells, polymorph neutrophils and histiocytes. (2) There is considerable proliferation of arborizing small blood vessels, characterized as 'post-capillary venules', with PAS-positive thickened walls. (3) There is a deposit of amorphous interstitial material that may be derived from cellular debris associated with rapid turnover of cells in the node. The absence of typical Sternberg–Reed cells and the presence of the 'immunoreactive cell' proliferation distinguish the histological picture from that of HD. Gene rearrangement studies show a monoclonal population of T cells in the majority of cases. In the patients described by Lukes and Tindle, depletion of normal small lymphocytes was a prominent feature, while in those described by Frizzera and his colleagues, the acidophilic interstitial material was not an essential feature but chronic 'reactive' lymph node follicles were prominent.

Clinically the patients present with an acute or subacute illness characterized by fever, sweating, weight loss, generalized lymphadenopathy and hepatosplenomegaly. A history of drug ingestion is frequent and about one-third of patients have non-specific rashes. The majority of patients have polyclonal increases in serum immunoglobulins, involving especially IgM, a feature in marked contradistinction to the usually normal or depressed immunoglobulin levels in straightforward malignant lymphomas. A cryoglobulin is occasionally present. About half the patients have evidence of haemolysis with a positive direct antiglobulin test. The clinical course of AILD after diagnosis is very variable. About two-thirds of patients have a pro-

gressive disease and die eventually from overt malignancy or infectious complications. In the remainder the disease may spontaneously regress or respond to chemotherapy and thereafter it sometimes requires no further treatment. In general, patients requiring treatment have received steroids, vinblastine or cytotoxic drug combinations such as COP or MOPP with variable results. No special features are recognized that will predict whether a given patient will or will not respond.

T-CELL LEUKAEMIA/LYMPHOMA

A specific form of leukaemia/lymphoma associated with infection with human T-cell leukaemia/lymphoma virus I (HTLV-I) was first described in Kyushu (the south island of Japan) in 1979. The lymphoma is due to malignant proliferation of a T4 subset of lymphocytes with cytotoxic/suppressor characteristics. By light and electron microscopy the malignant cell has a characteristic morphology resembling but distinguishable from a Sezary cell. In cell culture, C-type viral particles can be seen budding from the cytoplasmic membrane. The lymphoma is believed to be initiated by infection with the specific retrovirus HTLV-I.

T-cell leukaemia/lymphoma is common in Kyushu but was subsequently recognized in black patients in the West Indies and in patients of Caribbean origin in the United States, the UK and elsewhere. There is a distinct male predominance. The disease may present with generalized lymphadenopathy and hepatosplenomegaly but various types of skin infiltration are commoner than is seen in conventional lymphomas. A proportion of patients have hypercalcaemia. The disease usually responds initially to combination chemotherapy but remissions are short lived and survival in general is poor. Other aspects of T-cell leukaemia/lymphoma are discussed in Chapter 15.

HYDANTOIN-LINKED LYMPHOMAS

The hydantoin group of drugs, especially diphenylhydantoin used in the prevention of epilepsy, occasionally produce in patients an apparently allergic reaction characterized by fever, rash, generalized lymphadenopathy and often splenomegaly. Lymph node biopsy may be carried out and shows an enlarged node, usually with follicular hyperplasia and an inflammatory cell infiltrate comprising immunoblasts, plasma cells, polymorph neutrophils and particularly eosinophils. There may be atypical or binucleate histiocytes but classical Sternberg–Reed cells are lacking. The histological picture closely resembles that of angioimmunoblastic lymphadenopathy. When treatment with hydantoin drugs is discontinued, the lymphadenopathy and other features subside after some weeks. The condition is regarded as benign and sometimes designated pseudolymphoma.

The association of the hydantoins with lymphadenopathy is complicated by the fact that patients have been described in whom the apparent pseudolymphoma fails to regress after stopping the drug but rather progresses in a malignant fashion and terminates in the death of the patient. In other cases the pseudolymphoma has regressed but then recrudesces without further exposure to hydantoins. The histological picture in these cases of apparently true lymphoma has been both that of HD and of NHL. Whether or not the hydantoin drug has directly caused the lymphoma in these patients remains uncertain, but the association is seen more often than would be expected by chance.

MALIGNANT HISTIOCYTOSIS

In 1939 Scott and Robb-Smith introduced the term 'histiocytic medullary reticulosis' to describe a condition characterized clinically by fever, wasting, generalized lymphadenopathy, hepatosplenomegaly and often jaundice. There was widespread infiltration of tissues by cells resembling histiocytes which were capable of phagocytosing erythrocytes. A characteristic mode of lymph node infiltration suggested the term 'medullary'. In 1966 Rappaport introduced the term 'malignant histiocytosis' to describe a disorder involving 'systemic progressive invasion of morphologically atypical histiocytes and their precursors'. He considered the condition synonymous with histiocytic medullary reticulosis.

As for the lymphomas, the aetiology of the condition is unknown. Histopathologically, a biopsied

lymph node shows replacement of normal architecture to a varying degree by an infiltrate of pleomorphic mononuclear cells that may vary in appearance from that of a typical blast cell with rounded nucleus, dispersed nuclear chromatin and meagre cytoplasm to a large cell with abundant non-pyroninophilic cytoplasm containing phagocytosed nuclear debris and occasionally ingested erythrocytes. Rarely, ingested erythroblasts, polymorphs or platelets are visible in the cytoplasm. The same cell may be present in the bone marrow and at times in the peripheral blood. Cytochemically these cells show positive reactions for naphthol-AS acetate esterase, lysozyme and acid phosphatase and thereby show features of a true histiocyte.

Clinically the disease usually begins with systemic features. The patient has fever, anorexia, weight loss and sweats when first seen. He or she proves on examination to have generalized lymphadenopathy and hepatosplenomegaly. The patient may be anaemic, neutropenic and thrombocytopenic. The serum lysozyme is often raised and the serum cholesterol low. Marrow aspirates show variable infiltration with scattered histiocytes of varying maturity or histiocytic cells aggregated into foci. It is the sustained fever and generalized nature of the disease at diagnosis that allow it to be differentiated on clinical grounds from malignant lymphoma, histiocytic ('true' histiocytic).

Treatment of malignant histiocytosis is in general unsatisfactory. In some patients the disease may run an extremely indolent course and some have benefited from splenectomy alone or splenectomy in association with treatment with single cytotoxic drugs. Recently patients with progressive disease treated with the CHOP combination (cyclophosphamide, vincristine, adriamycin and prednisolone) have achieved durable complete remissions and some of these patients may prove to have been cured.

MYCOSIS FUNGOIDES AND THE SEZARY SYNDROME

Mycosis fungoides is a lymphomatous disease originating in the skin, with a slowly progressive course, forming skin plaques and then involving the lymph nodes and internal organs. The disease usually begins as a chronic contact, eczematous or psoriatic dermatitis. Histologically the skin shows Pautrier abscesses, i.e. discrete intraepidermal foci containing both normal and abnormal lymphocytic and monocytic cells. The lymphoma is of T-cell origin. In the Sezary syndrome, the skin shows erythroderma, there is intense pruritus and the blood shows many abnormal T cells with large convoluted or clefted nuclei and cytoplasm which may stain intensely with PAS (see also Chapter 15).

SELECTED BIBLIOGRAPHY

Advances in cancer chemotherapy: lymphomas and breast cancer (1987). *Seminars in Hematology*, **24** (Suppl. 1), 1–65.

Aisenberg A. C., Wilkes B. M., Jacobson J. O., Harris N. L. (1987). Immunoglobulin gene rearrangements in adult non-Hodgkin's lymphoma. *American Journal of Medicine*, **82**, 738–743.

Bonadonna G., Valagussa P., Santoro A. (1986). Alternating non-cross resistant combination chemotherapy or MOPP in stage IV Hodgkin's disease. *Annals of Internal Medicine*, **104**, 739–746.

Canellos G. P. (Ed.) (1979). *The lymphomas. Clinics in haematology*, Vol. 8, Issue 3. London: W. B. Saunders.

Canellos G. P., Come S. E., Skarin A. J. (1983). Chemotherapy in the treatment of Hodgkin's disease. *Seminars in Hematology*, **20**, 1–24.

Canellos G. P., Propert K., Cooper R., et al. (1988). MOPP vs ABVD vs MOPP alternating with ABVD in advanced Hodgkin's disease: A prospective randomized GALGB trial. *Proceedings of the American Society of Clinical Oncology*, **7**, 230–238.

Colgan J. P., Habermann T. M. (1987). Hodgkin's disease and non-Hodgkin's lymphomas. *Current Hematology and Oncology*, **5**, 77–120.

Cullen M. et al. (1979). Angio-immunoblastic lymphadenopathy: a report of ten cases and a review of the literature. *Quarterly Journal of Medicine*, **48**, 151.

Foroni L. et al. (1987). α, β and γ T-cell receptor gene rearrangements correlate with haematological phenotype in T cell leukaemias. *British Journal of Haematology*, **67**, 307–318.

Frizzera G., Moran E. M., Rappaport H. (1974). Angio-immunoblastic lymphadenopathy with dysproteinaemia. *Lancet*, **ii**, 1070–1073.

Griesser H., Feller A., Lennert K., Minden M., Mak T. W. (1986). Rearrangement of the β chain of the T cell antigen receptor and immunoglobulin genes in lymphoproliperative disorders. *Journal of Clinical Investigation*, **78**, 1179–1184.

Horwich A., Peckham M. (1983). 'Bad risk' non-Hodgkin lymphomas. *Seminars in Hematology*, **20**, 35–56.

Jones S. E., Fuks Z., Bull M. et al. (1973). Non-Hodgkin's lymphoma. IV. Clinicopathologic correlations in 405 cases. *Cancer*, **31**, 806–823.

Kaplan H. (1980). *Hodgkin's disease*, 2nd edn. Cambridge, Mass.: Harvard University Press.

Kaplan H., Rosenberg S. (1966). The treatment of Hodgkin's disease. *Medical Clinics of North America*, **50**, 1591–1610.

Lampert I., Catovsky D., Bergier N. (1978). Malignant histiocytosis: a clinico-pathological study of 12 cases. *British Journal of Haematology*, **40**, 65–77.

Lennert K., Collins R. D., Lukes R. J. (1983). Concordance of the Kiel and Lukes–Collins classifications of the non-Hodgkin's lymphomas. *Histopathology*, **7**, 549–559.

Linch D. C., Vaughan Hudson B. R. (1988). Management of Hodgkin's disease and non-Hodgkin lymphomas. In *Recent advances in haematology*, Vol. 5, pp. 215–242. (Ed. A. V. Hoffbrand). Edinburgh: Churchill Livingstone.

Lukes R. J., Collins R. D. (1975). New approaches to the classification of the lymphomata. *British Journal of Cancer*, **31** (Suppl. II), 1–28.

Lukes R. J., Tindle B. H. (1975). Immunoblastic lymphadenopathy. A hyperimmune entity resembling Hodgkin's disease. *New England Journal of Medicine*, **292**, 1–8.

Malpas J. S. (1983). Lymphomas in children. *Seminars in Hematology*, **19**, 301–314.

McElwain T. J., Lister T. A. (Eds.) (1987). The lymphomas. *Clinics in Haematology*, **16**, 1–269.

National Cancer Institute sponsored study of classifications of non-Hodgkin's lymphoma: Summary and description of a working formulation for clinical usage (1982). *Cancer*, **49**, 2112–2135.

Rosenberg S. A., Kaplan H. S. (Eds.) (1982). *Malignant lymphomas: etiology, immunology, pathology, treatment* London: Academic Press.

Stein H., Mason D. Y. (1985). Immunological analysis of tissue sections in diagnosis of lymphoma. In *Recent advances in haematology*, Vol. 4. (Ed. A. V. Hoffbrand). Edinburgh: Churchill Livingstone.

Williams M. E. et al. (1987) Immunoglobulin and T cell receptor gene rearrangements in human lymphoma and leukemia. *Blood*, **69**, 79–86.

Chapter 20

NON-LEUKAEMIC MYELOPROLIFERATIVE DISORDERS

S. M. LEWIS AND T. C. PEARSON

The term myeloproliferative disorders was proposed in 1951 by Dameshek to describe the interrelationship which appeared to exist between acute and chronic myeloid leukaemia, erythroleukaemia, primary proliferative polycythaemia (polycythaemia rubra vera), primary (essential) thrombocythaemia and myelofibrosis. This concept was based on the assumption that all these conditions were expressions of abnormal proliferation of one or other cell lines all of which were derived from a common haemopoietic cell. It helped to explain the transition which sometimes occurs between these conditions. Over the years it has provided a useful histogenetic classification. In recent years, the leukaemias have become more clearly defined and the different types have been characterized. Furthermore, it is now suggested that the myeloproliferative disorders do not have a common pathogenesis but some may occur as a consequence of a disturbed haemopoietic regulator system, or an abnormal microenvironment, or as a clonal abnormality leading to neoplastic change in a differentiated stem cell. However, it is convenient to continue to include under the general designation of 'myeloproliferative disorders' the three interrelated conditions of primary proliferative polycythaemia (PPP), myelofibrosis and primary thrombocythaemia as well as a miscellaneous group of conditions which appear to overlap these well-defined diseases or to be intermediate between them.

The specific clinical and haematological features of the different conditions are described in detail later in this chapter. Their relationship is briefly reviewed here. In PPP, the PCV is raised with an increased red cell mass. There is, as a rule, mild to moderate splenomegaly and hepatomegaly, the marrow is hyperplastic and there is minimal or no extramedullary erythropoiesis. In primary thrombocythaemia, the outstanding feature is a marked proliferation of megakaryocytes in the bone marrow whilst in the peripheral blood the platelet count is in excess of 600×10^9/l, usually more than 1000×10^9/l. However, the platelet count may also increase to this level in PPP.

In myelofibrosis there is marked splenomegaly; most patients are anaemic and show leucoerythroblastic changes in the peripheral blood. Haemopoiesis is predominately extramedullary; in the bone marrow there is extensive fibroblastic proliferation and reticulin (collagen) formation. Some patients have a syndrome intermediate between PPP and myelofibrosis: moderate to marked splenomegaly, extramedullary haemopoiesis, increased reticulin formation in the bone marrow but, at the same time, an erythrocytosis with increased red cell mass and medullary erythropoiesis. This intermediate state may be an evolution from polycythaemia to myelofibrosis but in many cases these features of 'transitional myeloproliferative disease' remain static, with little change in either clinical features or haematology for at least several years. It probably represents one end of the spectrum of the myeloproliferation seen in PPP.

In its early stage, a myeloproliferative disorder is likely to show the following features.

1. Generalized proliferation of bone marrow, frequently with extension into the long bones of the limbs.

2. Large numbers of megakaryocytes in the bone marrow; they often have abnormal nuclei and occur in clusters.

3. Evidence of platelet dysfunction.

4. Increase in fine fibrillar reticulin which may become prominent; in some cases, there is collagen deposition.

A number of patients present initially with this picture, which cannot be categorized into one or other of the disorders. The diagnosis will usually become apparent in due course, but until then it is convenient to refer to it as a 'myeloproliferative disorder'. There are, however, differences in the behaviour of circulating progenitor cells in culture which may help distinguish the conditions, even at this early stage (see p. 551).

As explained above, it is convenient for practical purposes to exclude the leukaemias from this chapter, but it must not be forgotten that there is a close relationship between chronic myeloid leukaemia (CML), PPP and myelofibrosis with overlapping syndromes and, occasionally, termination of PPP in a leukaemic phase. A modified classification of myeloproliferative disorders has been proposed to include also other entities, such as Ph^1-negative CML, and acute (malignant) myelofibrosis.

THE POLYCYTHAEMIAS

There are a number of conditions which share the finding of a raised PCV. These may be divided into two groups on the basis of the red cell mass (RCM) findings (Table 20.1). In the absolute polycythaemias the RCM is above the normal range. In the apparent polycythaemias, the measured RCM falls in the normal range and the raised PCV is due either to a definitely low plasma volume or a combined effect of opposing changes in the RCM and plasma volume within their normal ranges. The absolute polycythaemias may be separated into three groups: (1) the myeloproliferative disorder, primary proliferative polycythaemia (PPP)—this term is preferred to polycythaemia rubra vera (PRV) since, in its strictest sense, the latter means only a true increase in red cells, and this obviously also occurs in the other forms of absolute polycythaemia; (2) secondary polycythaemias; (3) a group, termed idiopathic erythrocytosis, for which a diagnosis of neither PPP nor secondary polycythaemia can be established.

In the assessement of a patient for the presence of polycythaemia, the PCV is a more reliable indicator than the haemoglobin value, since the presence of iron deficiency in the occasional patient may produce a disproportionately low Hb value. Patients with splenomegaly may be found to have an absolute increase in RCM at rather lower values of PCV than non-splenomegalic patients because of red cell pooling in the enlarged spleen and an associated expanded plasma volume.

Primary Proliferative Polycythaemia

Nature

It has been established that primary proliferative polycythaemia is a clonal stem cell disorder. Studies of women with PPP who are heterozygotes for two identifiably different glucose-6-phosphate dehydrogenase (G6PD) types have shown that the red cells contain predominantly one or other of the G6PD types, rather than approximately equal amounts, as would be expected on the basis of the

Table 20.1
Classification of the polycythaemias

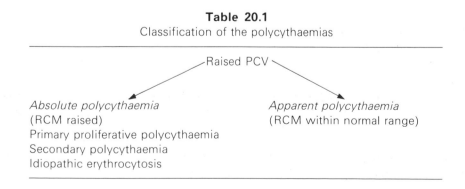

Lyon hypothesis. Further studies have shown that the granulocytes and platelets are derived from the same abnormal clone. This observation, combined with the haematological features of PPP, suggests that there is little disturbance of the differentiation pattern of the stem cells of the clone. The reason that the polycythaemia dominates the clinical picture is that in normal individuals the RCM and PCV are kept within relatively close limits so that any increase in red cell production by the abnormal clone can easily be recognized haematologically or by the clinical manifestations produced by the rise in PCV.

In vivo, the abnormal clone behaves in an autonomous fashion not governed by normal feedback mechanisms. In in-vitro culture of the blood and bone marrow of patients with PPP, it was originally thought that erythroid colonies grew spontaneously from the erythroid progenitors of the abnormal clone, that is, without the addition of erythropoietin. It has now been suggested, however, that since serum is present in the basic culture medium, very small amounts of erythropoietin are present, and that the clonal erythroid progenitors are extremely sensitive to these low levels of erythropoietin. By increasing the erythropoietin concentration, large numbers of colonies are formed. Although the majority are from the abnormal clone, there is a 'background' of normal stem cells, which retain the normal sensitivity to erythropoietin. In vivo, these normal stem cells are suppressed in some way by products of the abnormal clone and decline in numbers as the disease progresses.

Clinical Features

Age and Sex

The predominant age of incidence is between 55 and 60 years, but onset may occur from young adulthood through to old age. There are just a few well-documented cases of PPP in childhood and a similar small number of reports where two individuals in the same family are involved. There is a slight male predominance.

Vascular Complications

These are the most common presenting feature and occur in 30–50% of patients. They are widely distributed, involving arteries and veins approximately equally.

The arterial manifestations may be of a transient ischaemic nature, as in intermittent claudication or cerebral ischaemic attacks, or complete vascular occlusion. Cerebral thrombosis is more common in PPP than coronary thrombosis, whereas the reverse is true in other patients. This suggests that in PPP the cerebral circulation is particularly vulnerable. Patients also complain of non-specific cerebral symptoms, such as headache, impairment of mental function and fullness of the head. Characteristically, these symptoms improve with adequate treatment of the polycythaemia. Other peripheral vessels may also occlude, for example the lower limb, mesenteric and retinal arteries. In a few patients microvascular occlusive lesions occur, particularly involving the toes. These lesions are almost certainly due to local blocking of vessels by platelet aggregates. They are the same as those seen in primary thrombocythaemia (see p. 544).

The following factors are involved in the pathogenesis of the larger arterial vessel complications.

1. Patients are usually at an age when vessel wall disease is common.
2. Generalized blood flow is low due to the increased arterial oxygen-carrying capacity.
3. High PCV and hence blood viscosity adversely influence the outcome of occlusive events.
4. High PCV values increase vessel wall/platelet contact.
5. Some platelet abnormalities of PPP favour thrombus formation, e.g. diminished response to prostaglandin D2.

Venous complications include superficial phlebitis and deep vein thrombosis which is occasionally complicated by pulmonary embolization.

Haemorrhage

There is undoubtedly an increased incidence of haemorrhage in these patients. The cause is almost certainly related to qualitative platelet changes. (This is discussed in more detail on p. 534). Spontaneous bruising is unusual but excessive bruising following trauma occurs more commonly. When there is a peptic ulcer, excessive haemorrhage from the ulceration may lead to some patients presenting with iron deficiency anaemia. Polycyth-aemia only becomes manifest in these patients when there is an excessive rise in the Hb and PCV following healing of the ulcer and adequate iron therapy.

Peptic Ulceration

This was thought to be a common event due either to a high acid secretion by the stomach because of high circulating histamine levels, or to local vessel thrombosis in the mucosal wall. These factors might apply in the occasional patient, but generally the acid secretion is normal, and the incidence of peptic ulceration is probably no greater than normal.

Pruritus

Pruritus occurs in approximately 20–25% of patients and may persist despite adequate treat-ment. It is intermittent and characteristically pre-cipitated by a warm environment or made worse after a hot bath. The mechanism is probably related to histamine levels, which correlate with basophil numbers, but other factors play a part. There is a report of one study in which the pruritus was related to concomitant iron deficiency.

Skin Changes

These include plethoric facies, acne rosacea and prominence of the conjunctival blood vessels. Microvascular lesions of the extremities and livedo reticularis may be found in patients with prominent thrombocythaemia.

Urate Production

Raised serum uric acid levels occur in many patients due to the high nuclear protein turnover. A few patients, perhaps 5%, have gout.

Hypertension

A higher incidence of hypertension in PPP has been suggested. Comparison with age-matched popul-ations, however, reveals that this is probably coinci-dental.

Splenomegaly

Splenomegaly, usually symptomless and modest, is found in approximately half the patients at present-ation. A few patients present with moderate spleno-megaly and these patients appear more likely to develop the features of myelofibrosis at an early stage.

Incidental Finding

Early identification of PPP before symptoms or signs occur is obviously important since the pre-sentation of the patient later with a major vascular occlusion may thus be avoided.

Laboratory Findings

Red Cells

The Hb and PCV are raised and there is absolute polycythaemia. The plasma volume (PV) is normal or slightly reduced, except in patients with signifi-cant splenomegaly, where it is increased and splenic red cell pooling occurs.

Characteristically, at presentation there is normal red cell morphology and lifespan. If the disease progresses into myelofibrosis, the red cells show increasing anisocytosis and poikilocytosis. Some patients present with the red cell changes of iron deficiency. Very rarely, there is macrocytosis due to folate deficiency.

The red cell enzyme activity, surface charge and oxygen dissociation curve are normal. A marked deficiency of glutamate pyruvate transaminase heterozygotes in PPP suggests an irregularity of gene expression by the abnormal clone. Similar abnormal gene expression demonstrated by a change in Rh phenotype has also been reported.

A small percentage of patients show increased levels of HbF. Presumably, this is due to random selection of a clone with high HbF production.

The arterial oxygen saturation is normal, but occasionally at presentation it is in the low-normal range. The saturation rises with treatment. This observation is probably explained by pulmonary ventilation/perfusion abnormalities in the pre-treatment phase.

White Cells

The absolute granulocyte count is increased in two-thirds of the patients, reflecting an enlarged total granulocyte mass. The increased white count is usually moderate, with counts between $12 \times 10^9/l$ and $25 \times 10^9/l$ but occasionally up to $50 \times 10^9/l$. Basophil and occasionally eosinophil numbers may be increased. An occasional metamyelocyte and myelocyte are often present. Neutrophil function is normal.

Neutrophil Alkaline Phosphatase

The neutrophil alkaline phosphatase (NAP) score, which does not correlate with the neutrophil count, is raised in 75% of patients.

Serum B_{12} and B_{12}-binding Capacity

Transcobalamins I and III, which are derived from granulocytes, are higher in PPP than normal, reflecting the increased granulocyte turnover. These transcobalamins have high binding activity, unlike transcobalamin II, and result in a high serum B_{12} level.

Platelets

In 50% of patients the platelet count is raised to between $400 \times 10^9/l$ and $800 \times 10^9/l$, occasionally higher. There are also qualitative changes. These include alterations in morphology characterized by the presence of large forms. In addition, abnormal platelet aggregation and an altered ADP:ATP ratio may occasionally be demonstrated. These changes are similar to those seen in primary thrombocythaemia (see p. 545). Increased platelet turnover has been demonstrated in untreated PPP.

Coagulation Factors

Generally, these are normal, although there may be occasional abnormalities. Increased fibrinogen turnover has been shown. This returns to normal following adequate PCV reduction.

Chromosome Studies

Approximately 15% of patients have an abnormal marrow chromosome karyotype at presentation. The abnormality is usually simple aneuploidy, al-though a translocation can occasionally be demonstrated. Treatment, particularly by ^{32}P, but also by any chemotherapeutic agent, may produce a chromosomal change. There is evidence of better survival in treated patients who maintain a normal marrow karyotype. Recently, an abnormal chromosome, 20q-, has been demonstrated in some patients. This may be present before treatment or sometimes induced by it. The abnormality is not unique to PPP and may be found in other haematological conditions. There has been a single report of the Philadelphia chromosome in acute transformation of PPP, and one report of transition of PPP to Philadelphia-positive chronic myeloid leukaemia.

Marrow

The marrow is hypercellular. Erythropoiesis, granulopoiesis and numbers of megakaryocytes are all variably increased (Fig. 20.1). The changes in erythropoiesis are usually least obvious, although increased erythropoietic activity is well demonstrated by ferrokinetic studies (see p. 15). The marrow appearances are not diagnostic per se. Iron stores are usually absent. Reticulin is of normal pattern initially, increasing as the disease progresses, with coarse bundles of fibres becoming apparent.

CFU–E and BFU–E

Endogenous or spontaneous erythroid colonies may be grown without added erythropoietin from both peripheral blood and marrow samples. Some workers consider this to be a diagnostic feature.

Erythropoietin

Previously, biological measurement of erythropoietin suggested that levels in PPP were zero. More recently sensitive methods, such as the radioimmunoassay, have shown that, as a group, patients with PPP have lower than normal levels, but there is some overlap with the normal range (Fig. 20.2). The levels of erythropoietin do not rise markedly following venesection but stay low following reduction of the Hb and PCV to normal.

Treatment

The treatment of PPP may be divided into the early phase and long-term control. No treatment eradicates the disease.

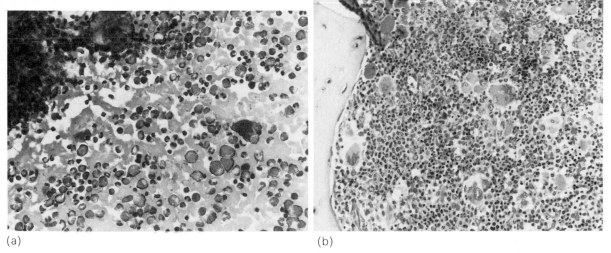

Fig. 20.1. *Bone marrow in primary proliferative polycythaemia. (a) Smear of marrow aspirate showing edge of a hypercellular fragment and a trail of free-lying haemopoietic cells. (b) Iliac crest trephine section: there is increased cellularity (compare with Fig. 1.2, p. 2); megakaryocytes are prominent.*

Early Treatment

Adequate lowering of the PCV is most easily achieved by venesection. Patients with microvascular occlusive disease, or transient ischaemic attacks due to accompanying thrombocythaemia, often benefit from antiplatelet agents which should be stopped once adequate control of the thrombocythaemia is achieved by ^{32}P or chemotherapeutic agents. Erythrocyte, and platelet apheresis where necessary, may be used when local circulatory impairment indicates the necessity for urgent treatment.

Surgery in the untreated patient is hazardous since it is often complicated by thrombosis or haemorrhage; therefore, it is essential to normalize the blood count beforehand. Taking account of the clinical situation, it may be worthwhile to use anticoagulant therapy for a short period while waiting for long-term control to be achieved.

Long-term Control

Adequate control of the peripheral blood count to minimize the risk of vascular occlusion is essential. There is a positive correlation between the PCV level and occlusive risk, and a PCV of less than 0.45 should be the aim. The necessity to control the

platelet count at normal values has been debated, but there are two reasons why the thrombocythaemia should be treated. First, some patients present with symptoms and signs resulting from thrombocythaemia, and second, patients with PPP are usually at an age when vessel disease is present and there is some evidence that high platelet counts increase the incidence of thrombosis.

While venesection achieves the necessary reduction in PCV as a short-term measure, many cases, especially those with a high platelet count, will require myelosuppression. The most convenient method of myelosuppression is to use intravenous ^{32}P in a dose of 2.5–3 mCi/m^2, to a maximum total of 6 mCi. It takes 2–3 months for the blood count to show maximum effect. A single dose is often sufficient to control the blood count and reduce spleen size. Occasionally a further smaller dose is required after 3–4 months. A 'remission' may last from 6 months to 2–3 years. The risk of significant thrombocytopenia or leucopenia is extremely small. Radioactive phosphorus is usually the preferred treatment in patients over the age of 70 years, for logistic reasons.

A number of different chemotherapeutic agents have been used to control the myeloproliferation—particularly busulphan and chlorambucil, but also

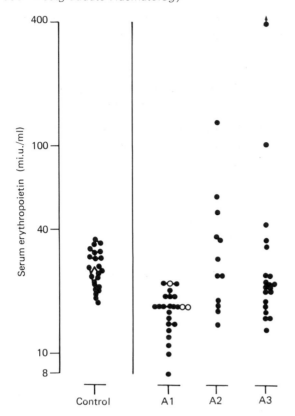

Fig. 20.2. *Serum erythropoietin in the polycythaem-ias, measured by radioimmunoassay. (Al, primary pro-liferative polycythaemia; A2, secondary poly-cythaemia; A3, polycythaemias of unknown aetiology (idiopathic erythrocytosis).) From Cotes et al. (1986), with permission.*

melphalan and thioguanine. In some studies these drugs have been used in an attempt to control the whole proliferative process. The problem with this approach is that fairly high dosages are needed to control erythropoiesis, whereas the control of granulocytic and megakaryocytic proliferation is easier. In one limb of the trial by the Polycythaemia Vera Study Group (PVSG), chlorambucil was used at 10 mg daily for 30 days with a gap of 30 days before the next course. The incidence of acute leukaemia in this group was 13 times greater than that in the venesection-only group. This finding led to the abandonment of chlorambucil treatment. There is also the danger of increased acute leuk-aemia transformation in patients treated with one of the other drugs listed above or with ^{32}P, com-pared with those who have been treated only with venesection. This emphasizes that chemotherapy and radiotherapy should be used judiciously in PPP.

A satisfactory approach to the treatment of PPP is to maintain the PCV at less than 0.45 by venesec-tion and to use low-dose intermittent chemo-therapy, for example busulphan, to control the platelets at less than $400 \times 10^9/l$. The majority of patients need very little chemotherapy. This method gives a median survival of similar duration, if not longer, than other regimens. The incidence of acute leukaemic transformation and other drug side-effects is minimal. The occurrence of vascular occlusive events is also minimized as long as the PCV and platelets are always adequately control-led. The occasional patient has thrombocythaemic symptoms at platelet counts in the order of 400 $\times 10^9/l$ and, in these, the count should be controlled at less than $350 \times 10^9/l$.

A disadvantage of this method of treatment is that it requires hospital attendance about once every 6–8 weeks and adequately accessible veins. Recently the PVSG has reported on the value of continuous hydroxyurea (HU) in a non-random-ized study. The initial response to HU was good, with 80–90% of patients achieving adequate con-trol of PCV and platelet count although only 60% retained satisfactory long-term disease control on continued treatment. Since HU is not an alkylating agent, its mutagenic risk is probably less than with these agents, but long-term assessment is awaited. Hydroxyurea may emerge as the preferred agent for the young patient if treatment other than venesec-tion is indicated.

Nearly all patients treated by regular venesection develop iron deficiency and microcytic hypo-chromic red cell changes. The iron deficiency is not usually attended by the classical symptoms of glos-sitis, dysphagia, etc. However, some patients have otherwise unexplained tiredness. In general, there is no need for iron therapy, but if it is used, careful monitoring of the PCV is needed since the PCV may rise quickly, necessitating more frequent vene-section. Microcytic hypochromic red cells do not give higher blood viscosity values than normo-chromic cells at the same PCV. Blood viscosity can therefore be monitored by measuring the PCV. The microhaematocrit method is preferable to the use of electronic counters, some of which may underestimate the true PCV by up to 10% at low MCH and MCV values.

Other Treatment Measures

Allopurinol should be used prophylactically in patients with a history of an acute attack of gout or who have high uric acid levels. Pruritus is difficult to control but antihistamines, cimetidine, aspirin and cholestyramine have occasionally been found to be of value. Iron therapy has also been reported to alleviate this symptom in some patients with concomitant iron deficiency.

Haematological Course and Prognosis

Fifteen to twenty per cent of cases transform to myelofibrosis with progressive anaemia and increasing splenomegaly due to extramedullary haemopoiesis. This appears to be the natural progression of the disease. Transition may occur from 2 to 25 years after presentation; probably it occurs earlier in patients with significant splenomegaly at presentation. It has not been possible to assess the relative merits of different treatment modalities in preventing the myelofibrotic transition.

An abrupt transition to leukaemia, usually AML, occurs in 2–10% of cases, typically after 6 years, with the lowest incidence in those treated with venesection alone. Characteristically, it is resistant to treatment but there have been reports of a few cases reverting to polycythaemia following remission of the leukaemia.

There have been a few case reports of patients transforming from PPP to a myelodysplastic syndrome. In addition, a number of other haematological conditions, for example myeloma and chronic lymphatic leukaemia, have been described in association with PPP. The relationship is probably coincidental.

The reported median survival of patients with PPP has varied between 8 and 15 years. The PVSG randomized trial showed a median survival of about 9, 12 and 14 years for the chlorambucil, ^{32}P and venesection alone groups respectively. The EORTC randomized trial showed that the 10-year survivals were 70% and 55% in their two limbs of busulphan and ^{32}P, respectively.

Differential Diagnosis of the Absolute Polycythaemias

The PVSG has given the following diagnostic criteria for establishing the diagnosis of primary proliferative polycythaemia.

1. An absolute polycythaemia: RCM males > 36 ml/kg, females > 32 ml/kg.
2. No evidence of a cause of secondary polycythaemia, including an arterial oxygen saturation of $> 92\%$.

(1) and (2) in the presence of splenomegaly confirm PPP. In the absence of splenomegaly, two of the following three features have to be present to confirm PPP.

1. Thrombocytosis: platelet count $> 400 \times 10^9$/l.
2. Leucocytosis: WBC $> 12.0 \times 10^9$/l.
3. Raised neutrophil alkaline phosphatase score (> 100) in the absence of fever or infection; raised serum B_{12} (> 900 ng/l) or unbound B_{12}-binding capacity (> 2200 ng/l).

These criteria may be used to evaluate patients with an absolute polycythaemia, but they do have some limitations. Expression of RCM results in terms of millilitres per kilogram may lead to an incorrect interpretation, particularly in obese patients (this is discussed more fully on p. 11).

Sometimes it is difficult to be certain that one is dealing with a secondary polycythaemia. For example, a solitary renal cyst may be identified but it might just be a coincidental finding. In addition, it must be appreciated that an arterial oxygen saturation of $> 92\%$ during the day does not exclude significant desaturation at night. Reactive thrombocytosis can lead to platelet counts above 400 $\times 10^9$/l. The leucocytosis would be better defined as a granulocytosis $> 10 \times 10^9$/l, with exclusion of reactive neutrophilia.

Splenomegaly is difficult to determine in some patients; splenic scanning techniques are helpful in delineating the spleen (p. 22). An increased splenic red cell pool is another pointer to a diagnosis of PPP.

Serum erythropoietin level is rarely diagnostic but may be helpful. The values in PPP are low but overlap the normal range. The result in secondary polycythaemia is variable: although some are raised as expected, others are in the normal range (Fig. 20.2). Measurement of erythropoietin may also demonstrate autonomous high erythroid production. Culture studies of the peripheral blood and/or marrow may identify patients with a primary myeloproliferative disorder by demonstrating autonomous production of erythroid colonies without added erythropoietin.

The Secondary Polycythaemias

An absolute increase in RCM may arise from a wide variety of causes. These are listed in Table 20.2 and, as shown, they may be divided into three groups.

Hypoxic Secondary Polycythaemia

High Altitude

Ascent to high altitude initially causes fluid retention followed by diuresis. In some, plasma volume (PV) reduction causes relative polycythaemia. This is followed by the gradual development of an absolute polycythaemia.

For the indigenous populations living higher than 1500 metres above sea level, the rise in Hb and PCV values reflects the alveolar oxygen tension. Interestingly, the Sherpas of the Himalayas adapt differently by shifting their oxygen dissociation curve to the left. On the other hand, the American Indians of Peru have high Hb and PCV. Chronic hypoxaemia in these people causes pulmonary hypertension due to persistent pulmonary arterial vasoconstriction. Chronic mountain sickness

Table 20.2
Causes of secondary polycythaemia

Hypoxic (with activation of normal erythropoietin mechanism)
High altitude
Hypoxaemic lung disease (including intrinsic lung disease, hypoventilation, sleep apnoea)
Cyanotic congenital heart disease
High oxygen-affinity haemoglobins
Smoking
Methaemoglobinaemia
Red cell metabolic defect
Cobalt

With 'inappropriate' secretion of erythropoietin
Renal tumour—hypernephroma, nephroblastoma
Renal ischaemia (e.g. cysts, hydronephrosis, renal transplant)
Hepatoma and liver disease
Fibroids
Cerebellar haemangioblastoma
Bronchial carcinoma
Phaeochromocytoma
Bartter's syndrome
Autonomous high erythropoietin production

Miscellaneous causes
Neonatal polycythaemia
Androgen therapy
Cushing's disease
Hypertransfusion

(Monge's disease), manifest by decreased exercise tolerance, headache and somnolence with particularly high Hb and PCV values, occurs in some individuals. It is due to even lower arterial oxygen saturations in these individuals either from co-existent lung disease or due to alveolar hypoventilation resulting from a deficient respiratory drive.

Hypoxaemic Lung Disease

A number of different mechanisms are included under this heading. By far the commonest is chronic obstructive airways disease (COAD), but other intrinsic lung pathology such as pulmonary fibrosis, idiopathic pulmonary arteriovenous aneurysms and lung involvement in hereditary haemorrhagic telangiectasia may lead to significant hypoxaemia. Hypoventilation due to muscle paralysis (e.g. poliomyelitis) or during sleep, particularly in obesity, may also lead to secondary polycythaemia.

In COAD, the degree of PCV elevation and polycythaemia is, in general, inversely proportional to the arterial oxygen saturation. Other factors, however, such as position of the oxygen dissociation curve, carbon monoxide levels in smokers, variable nocturnal hypoventilation, are responsible for considerable individual variation.

Chronic hypoxaemia increases the cardiac output and dilates the peripheral vessels. The pulmonary arteries, however, respond to the hypoxaemia by vasoconstriction resulting in increased pulmonary vascular resistance and pulmonary hypertension, which, in time, may lead to cor pulmonale.

The median survival of these patients is short—in the order of 18 months to 2 years. Not surprisingly, the majority of deaths are from cardiorespiratory causes. Oxygen therapy has been shown to improve the prognosis.

One question in the management of these patients is whether the increased PCV and Hb values, and therefore the increased oxygen-carrying capacity, are a useful compensation to the reduced oxygen saturation, or whether the increased blood viscosity is detrimental. The current evidence suggests that PCV values just above the normal range may be beneficial, but that higher values represent a harmful overcompensation. When the PCV is above 0.55, reduction to 0.50–0.52 leads to an increase in work performance, reduction in pulmonary artery pressure and greater increase in cardiac output on exercise. However, there has been no definitive study examining the effect on survival of controlling the PCV in this way compared with leaving the polycythaemia untreated. The method of PCV reduction used may be by simple venesection, or exchange transfusion with dextran, or erythrapheresis.

As in PPP, repeated venesection causes iron deficiency and may lead to low MCV and MCH values. At any particular PCV value, blood viscosity is not higher at low MCH values, but with a fall in MCH from 30 pg to 20 pg, there is about a 10% drop in Hb, and therefore oxygen-carrying capacity, at a PCV of 0.50. This must be a disadvantage in patients for whom the maximum oxygen-carrying capacity should be maintained to minimize the effects of the reduced oxygen saturation. Iron therapy, however, is usually followed by a rapid rise in PCV, thus necessitating more frequent venesection of the patient to control the PCV. Iron therapy is therefore best avoided except in those cases where there are marked iron-deficient red cell changes.

Cyanotic Congenital Heart Disease

A number of different anatomical defects may lead to right-to-left shunting, significant arterial hypoxaemia and polycythaemia, with very high PCV values (above 0.70) in some patients. Only a few patients with inoperable lesions survive to young adulthood. Post-mortem examination commonly shows pulmonary and cerebral thromboses. The high incidence of thromboses is undoubtedly related to abnormal blood flow which results either from the cardiac defect per se or from this and the raised blood viscosity.

The question of PCV reduction in patients with inoperable lesions is similar to that in patients with arterial hypoxaemia from lung disease. There is no doubt that modest reduction (by 0.08–0.10) of particularly high PCV values (above 0.65) is an advantage, and PCV reduction leads to an increase in stroke volume, systemic blood flow and systemic oxygen transport. The optimal PCV for these patients has not been established; there is probably considerable individual variation.

Venesection should be performed with concomitant fluid replacement to maintain a constant total blood volume. The problem of iron-deficient red cell changes leading to reduced Hb and oxygen-carrying capacity at any given PCV, is the same as in the hypoxaemia of lung disease.

In patients with particularly high PCV values due to cyanotic congenital heart disease, variable combinations of thrombocytopenia and reduced Factors II, V, VII and X have been described. Reduction of the PCV by venesection is followed by an increase in platelet count and coagulation factor levels. Blood loss at surgery is lower in patients who have had prior venesection.

High Oxygen-affinity Haemoglobins

Approximately 30 different α- or β-chain variants have been described (e.g. Hbs Chesapeake, Malmo, San Diego) which cause an increased oxygen affinity of the haemoglobin molecule. Characteristically the oxygen dissociation curve is markedly left-shifted. The electrophoretic mobility of these haemoglobins demonstrated by routine methods is usually the same as that of HbA. A variable increase in cardiac output and/or Hb and PCV occurs in these patients. Only the occasional patient has a PCV value in excess of 0.58.

The risk of vascular occlusion in these patients appears lower than in other forms of secondary polycythaemia or in PPP, but only a small number of patients have been followed. High blood flow has been observed and this possibly reduces the occlusive risk. Myocardial ischaemia and infarction have been observed in some individuals but it is difficult to know whether this is more common than in the normal population.

Lowering of the PCV is not advocated since these individuals are generally symptomless. There have been anecdotal reports of the alleviation of symptoms such as 'light-headedness' and fatigue by modest reduction of the PCV in patients with values above 0.58.

Smoking

Carbon monoxide levels up to 10% can result from smoking 20–30 cigarettes a day, with even higher levels in heavier smokers. The oxygen-carrying capacity of the blood is reduced and the oxygen dissociation curve is shifted to the left. The combined effect is a reduced oxygen delivery with a rise in Hb and PCV.

As a result, smokers have higher Hb and PCV values than non-smokers but the difference in PCV is only in the order of 0.02–0.04, and usually the PCV falls within the normal range. Some patients, however, due to excessive cigarette smoking, coexistent lung disease or to nocturnal hypoventilation, have PCV levels above the normal range. An absolute increase in RCM can be demonstrated in some of these patients although in others the RCM falls within the normal range (apparent polycythaemia; see p. 542). There is some evidence that cigarette smoking can cause a reduction in plasma volume and this might exaggerate the PCV rise.

Methaemoglobinaemia

Congenital methaemoglobinaemia is a very rare disorder due to a deficiency of methaemoglobin reductase (diaphorase). In the homozygous form there is 10–20% methaemoglobin, leading to reduced oxygen-carrying capacity of the blood, increased oxygen affinity of the haemoglobin and higher Hb and PCV values than normal—detailed studies of RCM measurement have not been performed. Large doses of vitamin C or methylene blue reduce the methaemoglobin level.

Red Cell Metabolic Defects

High PCV values have been found in members of a family with reduced red cell 2,3-DPG levels producing a left shift in the oxygen dissociation curve. The defect was thought to be due to the presence of a 2,3-DPG mutase variant with low activity.

Cobalt

Cobaltous chloride produces a respiratory alkalosis with a left shift in the oxygen dissociation curve and hence renal hypoxia with resultant increased erythropoietin production. Some increase in Hb, PCV and RCM has been demonstrated following its administration.

Secondary Polycythaemia with Inappropriate Erythropoietin Secretion

There is a wide range of relatively uncommon but well-recognized disorders which are associated with increased erythropoietin secretion and resultant absolute polycythaemia. The clinical features in these patients are derived from the underlying pathology, but in many an unexplained polycythaemia is the only initial finding. Haematologically there is an increase in Hb, PCV and RCM, and classically no increase in white count or platelet count. However, some tumours are associated with a reactive thrombocytosis and granulocytosis and an incorrect diagnosis of PPP may be made unless appropriate investigations are undertaken.

Renal Pathology

Renal cysts, polycystic kidneys, renal artery stenosis, 'chronic glomerular nephritis' and hydronephrosis have all been associated with an absolute polycythaemia, presumably due to renal ischaemia. Hypernephroma and Wilm's tumour may give rise to polycythaemia in a few of the affected patients. An absolute polycythaemia may occur following renal transplantation, due to increased erythropoietin either from the recipient's own diseased kidneys undergoing cystic change or from the transplanted kidney, possibly due to rejection-related ischaemia. Plasma volume reduction without an absolute polycythaemia may lead to a raised PCV in some post-transplant patients.

Hepatoma and Liver Disease

Hepatoma is uncommon in Europe but is common in the Far East. Polycythaemia occurs in about 12% of cases. In cirrhosis a few patients have raised Hb and PCV values which are due either to reduced degradation of erythropoietin or to arterial hypoxaemia due to pulmonary arteriovenous shunts.

Other Lesions

A number of different tumours (uterine fibromyomata, cerebellar haemangioblastoma, phaechromocytoma and bronchial carcinoma) include ectopic erythropoietin-producing tissue. Hypertrophy of the juxtamedullary apparatus (Bartter's syndrome) may also be associated with polycythaemia.

Autonomous High Erythropoietin Production

A few cases of polycythaemia are due to excessively high erythropoietin levels without any other underlying pathology. Both autosomal dominant and recessive inheritance have been demonstrated. The erythropoietin level may rise or remain unaltered following venesection. Very occasionally these patients have splenomegaly and this may lead to an incorrect diagnosis of PPP unless erythropoietin levels are measured.

Miscellaneous Causes of Secondary Polycythaemia

Neonatal Polycythaemia

In normal newborns, the cord PCV is between 0.42 and 0.62. Neonatal polycythaemia may be defined as a venous PCV exceeding 0.70. The causes of neonatal polycythaemia include placental transfusion (delayed clamping of the cord, twin to twin, mother to fetus) intrauterine hypoxia (placental insufficiency), endocrine disorders (maternal diabetes, neonatal thyrotoxicosis) and congenital anomalies (e.g. Down's syndrome). In some infants with elevated PCV levels, signs of hyperviscosity occur. These include congestive heart failure, respiratory distress, central nervous system disturbance (e.g. irritability and convulsions), diminished renal function and occasionally peripheral gangrene. Thrombocytopenia is commonly found. The pathophysiology involves a reduced cardiac output, increased peripheral resistance, increased pressure in the pulmonary circulation above the systemic circulation leading to right-to-left shunting (through the ductus and foramen ovale), and cyanosis which further increases pulmonary vascular resistance due to pulmonary vasoconstriction. In addition, metabolic changes, hypoglycaemia and hypocalcaemia may also occur and are involved in the cardiac and cerebral changes and signs.

Few paediatricians undertake prophylactic treatment of the newborn to reduce particularly high PCV values. The majority carefully observe for the development of signs, particularly in at-risk babies, and institute venesection with plasma replacement for those with excessively raised PCV values.

Androgen Therapy and Cushing's Disease

Both with androgen therapy and in Cushing's disease, there is increased Hb and PCV and in some an absolute polycythaemia occurs. Androgens increase erythropoietin levels and increase the marrow pool of erythropoietin-responsive cells. Experimentally, hydrocortisone and cortisone have been shown to stimulate red cell production.

Idiopathic Erythrocytosis

Definition

Idiopathic erythrocytosis describes an increased PCV and absolute polycythaemia without, at the time of presentation, other features which would allow classification either as PPP or as some form of secondary polycythaemia. The terms 'benign erythrocytosis and 'pure erythrocytosis' have also been used.

It is likely that this constitutes a heterogeneous group since probably some patients have a secondary polycythaemia but are inadequately investigated and others have PPP but with an absolute erythrocytosis as the only manifestation. Despite adequate investigation, a group of patients remains with an unexplained increase in erythropoietic activity. The precise mechanism or mechanisms in these patients remains to be established.

Clinical Features and Laboratory Findings

The age at presentation is similar to that of PPP. Two of the three published series showed a marked male predominance, but the other showed only a marginally higher male incidence, as in PPP. The most common clinical presentation is with vascular occlusive disease. Others present with non-specific symptoms such as headache and dizziness. Sometimes the high PCV is an incidental finding which leads to further investigation. Clinically, the only findings are plethora in some cases and sometimes evidence of occlusive vascular disease. Haematologically, the Hb, PCV and RCM are raised but typically there are no other features. Isolated findings of a marginally raised white cell count, neutrophil alkaline phosphatase score (NAP) or platelet count are very occasionally present—but obviously not in combination or the patient would be reclassified as PPP.

Course and Treatment

Careful follow-up demonstrates that some of these patients (approximately 20%) develop features of PPP (e.g. splenomegaly, high white cell count, high platelet count) between 1 and 13 years after presentation. In the occasional patient, a lesion associated with secondary polycythaemia becomes manifest, but in the remainder red cell proliferation without any underlying cause remains the only feature.

In the treatment of these patients it is essential to control the PCV adequately to minimize the risk of vascular occlusive episodes. In one series, the incidence of death due to cerebral thrombosis or cerebrovascular accident (CVA) was particularly high in inadequately treated patients. There is a good argument for venesection alone, thus avoiding the risks associated with exposure to ^{32}P or chemotherapy.

Apparent Polycythaemia

Definition and Frequency

The term apparent polycythaemia applies to patients with a raised PCV, but with a measured RCM in the normal range. This occurs much more commonly in men. Apparent polycythaemia is an important condition accounting for approximately half the male patients with PCV values between 0.50 and 0.60.

Other names for this condition include Gaisbock's syndrome, stress, pseudo-, relative and spurious polycythaemia. The definition of apparent polycythaemia by RCM/PV measurement expressed in terms of millilitres per kilogram body weight led to an erroneous impression that the condition occurred particularly in obese individuals and was always due to a very low plasma volume. More accurate expression of RCM/PV measurement related to both height and weight of the individual has shown that although there is a definitely reduced plasma volume (relative polycythaemia) in approximately one-third of patients, in the remainder the rise in

PCV is due to opposite changes in RCM and PV within their normal ranges.

Mechanisms

Physiological controls of PCV and blood volume are described in Chapter 1. Undoubtedly, some of the patients represent the end of the normal physiological range of PCV. In others, pathological changes are present, although in the majority it is difficult to define a single causative mechanism. Suggested mechanisms may be divided into those causing the plasma volume (PV) to fall and those leading to a rise in red cell mass (RCM) but within the normal range.

The possible causes of PV reduction include fluid loss (e.g. burns), diuretic therapy, alcohol, hypertension, stress and smoking. Diuretic therapy at high dosage can certainly significantly reduce the PV and increase the PCV. Continuous diuretic therapy at traditional dosage produces a small reduction, perhaps 5%, in PV which leads to a small rise in PCV (0.02–0.03). This small change may be sufficient to produce an elevated PCV when previously the PCV was at the top of the normal range. Alcohol in sufficient amount can lead to acute fluid loss. Physical stress as a possible cause has also been documented. In some patients with hypertension a small fall in PV occurs. Hypotensive therapy has been shown to reduce the PCV slightly in a few patients. Smoking probably reduces the PV, although the observed changes might in part be a homoeostatic mechanism to maintain a normal blood volume as the RCM rises.

Obviously, all patients who eventually develop an absolute polycythaemia went through a phase when their RCM was elevated for them but still within their predicted normal range—which is very wide; the causes of apparent polycythaemia where the RCM is in the high-normal range include those of an absolute polycythaemia.

Clinical and Laboratory Findings

These include non-specific symptoms, such as headache, fatigue, dizziness, nausea, dyspepsia, and specific symptoms from vascular occlusive events or from a possible causative mechanism, such as chronic lung disease. Sometimes a raised PCV is an incidental finding. Thus, care must be taken not to ascribe the observed symptoms to the raised PCV since they may be totally unrelated.

Typically, physical signs are absent. Hypertension is discovered or already being treated in approximately one-third of the patients.

The haematological features are an increased Hb and PCV with normal WBC, platelet count and NAP score. The RCM/PV findings have been described above. Erythropoietin levels are normal.

Course and Treatment

A few patients progress to an absolute polycythaemia and in some of these an obvious cause is established. Cessation of smoking, and/or alcohol intake, reduction of obesity, treatment of hypertension and discontinuance of diuretic therapy are all factors which have been shown to reduce the PCV in this group. In the majority, however, the PCV remains at its initial level, although in a few there is a spontaneous fall.

An important consideration in this group is the relationship between the elevated PCV and the risk of vascular occlusion. A positive correlation between PCV level and frequency of vascular occlusion has been found in studies of the normal population and in patients with some forms of absolute polycythaemia. Retrospective studies of apparent polycythaemia have suggested an increase in either mortality or morbidity from vascular occlusive episodes. One study suggested that patients with hypertension were at greatest risk and that hypotensive therapy was more important than PCV reduction. The only way to answer the question of whether the reduction of the PCV is an advantage is to undertake a prospective randomized trial of PCV reduction and to examine the incidence of vascular occlusion. Such a study has been initiated under the auspices of the Royal College of Physicians' Research Unit. Patients with both apparent and relative polycythaemia have been included. Patients with PCV values equal to or greater than 0.55 are all venesected to a PCV of less that 0.45 on the grounds that with initial PCV values as high as this there is a significant vascular occlusive risk. Patients with PCV values from 0.51 up to 0.55, whether they have experienced a vascular occlusive episode or not, or have a risk factor such as hypertension, are randomized to observation only or venesection with maintenance of the PCV at less than 0.45. All other treatment is given as indicated. It is hoped that this might provide information about the management of these groups.

While venesection might be considered to be an inappropriate method of PCV control in the relative (low plasma volume) polycythaemia group, it has been shown to be effective in this group. Another suggested approach, namely the use of fludrocortisone, a salt-retaining steroid, at low dose, has been shown to be ineffective. With larger doses of fludrocortisone there is an unacceptable risk of inducing hypertension.

Primary Thrombocythaemia

Nature

Primary thrombocythaemia is one of the chronic myeloproliferative disorders. It is characterized by megakaryocytic proliferation in the marrow and a high number of circulating platelets. Synonyms for the condition include essential or idiopathic thrombocythaemia and primary haemorrhagic thrombocythaemia. As in the other myeloproliferative disorders, this is a clonal disorder involving a multipotential stem cell.

Clinical Features

The mean age at presentation is approximately 60 years, with the majority of patients over 50 years. Very rarely, the condition presents before the age of 20 years and there are a very small number of reports of cases where more than one family member is affected.

A number of patients are asymptomatic at diagnosis, the high platelet count having been found coincidentally. In the symptomatic patients, the presenting features may be broadly divided into haemorrhagic and vascular occlusive; in some patients both are present. Haemorrhage may occur following accidental trauma or surgery leading to massive haematomata or open-wound bleeding. Sometimes excessive subcutaneous bruising following minor trauma is the only symptom. Bleeding

from the gastrointestinal tract is relatively common but the search for a specific bleeding site is usually unrewarding. Bleeding from oesophageal varices due to portal vein thrombosis has been described.

Vascular occlusive symptoms and signs are usually from small vessel obstruction, although larger vessel occlusive events such as myocardial infarction also occur. The initial symptoms/signs include erythromelalgia, particularly of the toes and feet, livedo reticularis, gangrenous or pregangrenous changes of the toes and, very occasionally, the fingers. Typically, the peripheral pulses are present. Cerebral symptoms are usually of a transient ischaemic nature. Transient visual loss (amaurosis fugax) is a common presenting feature. Petit mal and grand mal have also been described. Complete stroke is uncommon. These microvascular occlusive symptoms arise either from spontaneous platelet aggregation in the peripheral small vessels or from peripheral impaction of platelet emboli formed at the site of proximal atheromatous plaques. Splenomegaly (2–3 cm below the costal margin) is present in approximately one-third of patients.

Laboratory Findings

The platelet count is raised, in the range 600–2500 $\times 10^9/l$. The morphology of the platelets in the peripheral blood film is often strikingly abnormal, with many large abnormally staining platelets present (Fig. 20.3). Platelet anisocytosis is reflected in a

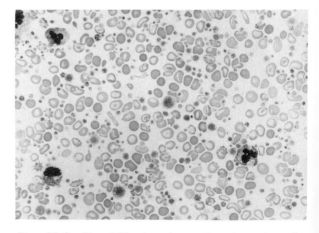

Fig. 20.3. *Blood film in primary thrombocythaemia. The numerous abnormal platelets are a striking feature. There is polymorph leucocytosis; the red cells show features of iron deficiency.*

high platelet distribution width (PDW) but the mean platelet volume (MPV) is often within the normal range.

The Hb and PCV are usually normal, but associated bleeding may lead to iron deficiency with a low MCH and MCV. In these patients, polycythaemia can only be excluded by following the response to iron therapy. The red cell morphology is normal except when iron-deficient changes are present and in the occasional patient with hyposplenic features resulting from splenic atrophy, which may result as a complication of primary thrombocythaemia.

The WBC is above $12 \times 10^9/l$ in about one-third of patients. In the minority of these an absolute eosinophilia and basophilia can be demonstrated and some show the presence of an occasional myelocyte and metamyelocyte. The NAP score is variable—low, normal or high. In patients with very low NAP scores, chronic myeloid leukaemia (CML) must be excluded by chromosome analysis since occasionally CML may present with pronounced thrombocythaemia without any significant leucocytosis.

Marrow aspiration is difficult in many patients. Typically, aspirated material reveals masses of aggregated platelets (Fig. 20.4). Trephine sections show hypercellularity with decreased fat spaces. There is a marked increase in megakaryocytes, which are typically larger than those of reactive

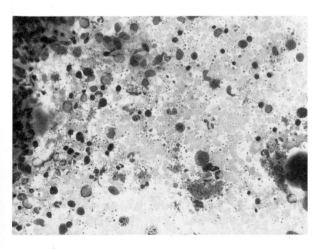

Fig. 20.4. *Smear of bone marrow aspirate in primary thrombocythaemia, showing the presence of megakaryocytes and sheets of platelets. Other haemopoietic cells are normal.*

thrombocytosis. In some patients the content of megakaryocytes in the marrow is so striking that the term 'megakaryocytic myelosis' has been used. There is an increase in reticulin but this is of normal pattern.

Chromosome analyses have shown random abnormalities but no specific markers. By definition, the Philadelphia chromosome is not present. In the untreated patient, the platelet lifespan is decreased and fibrinogen and prothrombin turnover are increased. These coagulation factors return to normal following therapy to reduce the platelet count. A variety of platelet abnormalities have been found in patients with primary thrombocythaemia. These include changes in the platelet morphology and surface membrane, arachidonic acid metabolism and granule content. Platelet aggregation is often decreased in response to adrenaline but a variable response is seen to ADP and collagen. Some patients show spontaneous aggregation in vitro. The bleeding time is either normal or prolonged. There is poor correlation between identified abnormalities and the incidence of clinical manifestations. The question of whether the platelets released from the megakaryocytes are intrinsically abnormal, or whether they only show dysfunctional features having undergone aggregation in vivo and recirculation, is unresolved. Probably both factors are operative.

In-vitro culture studies show abnormal colony formation and involvement of more than one cell lineage. There are sometimes increased numbers of circulating CFU–Mk and CFU–GM. Megakaryocytic colonies derived from the marrow grow without the addition of conditioning medium to the culture. Spontaneous (without added erythropoietin) erythroid colonies can occasionally be grown from the marrow and from the peripheral blood.

Diagnosis

The platelet count is usually higher and the morphology more abnormal in primary thrombocythaemia than in reactive thrombocytosis. In the latter, counts above $1000 \times 10^9/l$ are uncommon. On the other hand, a count as low as $600 \times 10^9/l$ may be associated with symptoms in primary

Table 20.3
Causes of a reactive thrombocytosis

Acute haemorrhage
Malignant disease, e.g. carcinoma, Hodgkin's and non-Hodgkin's lymphoma
Chronic inflammatory disorders, e.g. rheumatoid arthritis, ulcerative colitis, Crohn's disease
Acute inflammation
Postoperative
Splenectomy and hyposplenism
Marrow recovery from drug suppression, or response to haematinic following deficiency
Exercise
Response to certain drugs, e.g. vincristine
Iron deficiency

thrombocythaemia. Causes of secondary thrombocytosis (as listed in Table 20.3) must be carefully excluded. If iron-deficient red cell changes are present, the response to iron therapy must be carefully followed to exclude polycythaemia as the essential diagnosis. Collagen fibrosis of the marrow must be absent when the trephine is examined since this would suggest myelofibrosis. Chromosome analysis of the marrow should be performed to exclude the presence of the Philadelphia chromosome and a diagnosis of chronic myeloid leukaemia. Splenomegaly is not a hallmark of primary thrombocythaemia per se but is a useful sign to distinguish it from reactive thrombocytosis.

Treatment

In principle, treatment is indicated in all patients. However, the risk of complications in the young asymptomatic patient with platelet counts less than $1000 \times 10^9/l$ is probably low, and the necessity for treatment in this group is therefore still a matter of conjecture.

Treatment can be divided into the control of haemorrhage and manifestation of vascular occlusion, and the control of the megakaryocytic proliferation. Acute haemorrhage is sometimes difficult to control, especially in the case of gastrointestinal loss. The problem is to lower the platelet count rapidly and to provide functional platelets. Plateletapheresis has been used effectively in a few patients with very high counts in an emergency situation. Paradoxically, platelet concentrations are then needed to provide normal functional platelets.

There is unconfirmed evidence that hydrocortisone reduces haemorrhage.

Vascular ischaemic or occlusive events indicate the necessity to provide immediate therapy. As mentioned above, plateletapheresis may be very helpful occasionally. Aspirin (300 mg daily) is useful and often provides relief of symptoms before the platelet count is controlled by myelosuppression. The value of adding other antiplatelet drugs such as dipyridamole is debatable. Once the platelet count is lowered by myelosuppression, antiplatelet therapy should not be continued since there is a significant risk of haemorrhage, particularly from the gastrointestinal tract.

A number of agents have proved effective at suppressing platelet production. These include ^{32}P, busulphan, melphalan, hydroxyurea and chlorambucil. The risks are those of causing significant neutropenia or inducing an acute leukaemia. Close supervision is essential to prevent excessive dosage. In view of the mutagenic effect of these drugs, their use should be minimized. ^{32}P is used in doses of 2–3 mCi/m^2 (to a maximum of 5 mCi) intravenously. With this therapy the count begins to fall in a month and reaches its nadir in about 6–8 weeks. High dose intermittent busulphan in doses up to 1 mg/kg (maximum 100 mg) every 2–3 weeks produces rapid lowering of the platelet count and may be the treatment of choice when clinical manifestations indicate the need for urgency. Busulphan given at 4–6 mg/day orally is effective and preferred when there is no such clinical urgency. With continuous busulphan therapy, it usually takes 3–4 weeks for the count to begin to fall. The aim should be to reduce the count to less than $400 \times 10^9/l$. A few patients have ischaemic symptoms with platelet counts between $350 \times 10^9/l$ and $400 \times 10^9/l$ and in these a lower count should be the aim. After the initial therapy the majority of patients go into a prolonged remission and splenomegaly disappears. Experience in the individual patient establishes the closeness of supervision required to maintain the platelet count below $400 \times 10^9/l$. Short low-dose courses of chemotherapy are often then found to be adequate to control the proliferative process.

A recent PVSG report has suggested the use of hydroxyurea, which has probably less mutagenic risk than alkylating agents; the recommended initial dose was 15 mg/kg per day. This usually achieved an adequate haematological response in 4–6 weeks. A lower continuous dose was required to maintain disease control. Macrocytic red cell changes (MCV 100–120 fl) were a consistent harmless side-effect. The long-term effectiveness and safety of HU has still to be assessed but it may be the drug of choice in young patients.

Recently, interferon has been shown to reduce the platelet count in primary thrombocythaemia, and trials of its use in therapy are underway.

Haematological Course and Prognosis

Normally primary thrombocythaemia runs a protracted course with long remissions during which limited or no treatment is required. The median survival is in the order of 8–10 years. The incidence of death due to cardiovascular causes is probably marginally greater than in an age-matched population. Haematological transformations occur in some patients illustrating the close relationship between these myeloproliferative disorders. Polycythaemia occurs in a few patients who are followed for several years. Approximately a quarter of the patients transform to myelofibrosis some 5–10 years after the original diagnosis. Increasing splenomegaly and a diminishing Hb value with a falling platelet count unrelated to therapy would suggest this transition. Acute leukaemic transformation is a rare complication. As in the other myeloproliferative disorders, this risk appears to be a natural feature of the process but the mutagenic effects of drug therapy certainly enhance the possibility.

CHRONIC MYELOFIBROSIS

Chronic myelofibrosis is an important entity in the group of myeloproliferative disorders. In its classic form, chronic myelofibrosis has distinctive clinical and haematological features. It may, however, be difficult in some cases to draw a clear distinction from other myeloproliferative conditions; marrow fibrosis occurs in other myeloproliferative disorders and in some cases may be the dominant feature. It is closely related to primary proliferative polycythaemia and about 20% of patients give a previous history of that disease. It also occurs in lymphoproliferative diseases, non-haematological malignancies, following exposure to benzene, aniline dyes, fluorine, lead and arsenic and in chronic infections, especially tuberculosis and histoplasmosis.

There have been a number of synonyms used to describe chronic (primary) myelofibrosis. The most popular, particularly in the United States, is agnogenic myeloid metaplasia, a term which highlights an essential feature, namely extramedullary haemopoiesis (see below).

Pathogenesis

Despite being called 'primary' myelofibrosis, the fibrosis of bone marrow is almost always a secondary phenomenon. One must, therefore, consider separately the pathogenesis of fibrosis and the pathogenesis of the primary condition.

Marrow Fibrosis

The normal bone marrow has only a few connective tissue fibres and these are found mainly in association with the trabecular bone surfaces and some blood vessels. Proliferation of connective tissue elements within the bone marrow is a constant feature in myelofibrosis. Initially, there is an increase in reticulin fibres and progressive deposition of collagen occurs. Collagen consists of polypeptide chains arranged in a triple helix. The main constituent is glycine, together with proline and hydroxyproline. Depending on the structure of the alpha chains, there are five types of collagen, each with a different tissue distribution. Three types are associated with haematological processes. Types I and

II are normally distributed within the haemopoietic compartment of bone marrow, whereas type IV is localized to the endothelial lining of sinusoids and the blood vessels. In early myelofibrosis, there is an increase in type III, which is a neutral soluble form; as the disease progresses, hydroxylation of the proline residues occurs and the collagen changes to a polymeric form that is more stable, insoluble and cross-linked.

There is no rational basis for distinguishing between collagen fibrosis and reticulin fibrosis. In both cases the fibrous protein deposited in the extracellular space is collagen. The so-called reticulin, which is demonstrated by silver impregnation, appears to be a soluble polysaccharide or glycoprotein associated with fine connective tissue fibres such as fibronectin and basement membrane as well as collagen type III.

Myelofibrosis may or may not be accompanied by new bone formation, either appositional osteoblastic on pre-existing trabeculae or woven intramembranous bone within the marrow spaces. The extent of osseous increase is variable; when it is present, the condition is sometimes referred to as osteomyelosclerosis.

Haemopoietic Microenvironment

The normal haemopoietic microenvironment is disturbed by an increase in connective tissue and by deposition of collagen fibres. This interference with the bone marrow architecture contributes to the haematological abnormalities which are characteristic of myelofibrosis: increase in circulating stem cells, islands of developing haemopoietic cell lines with dysplastic maturation, and intravascular haemopoiesis.

Megakaryocytes

There is increasing evidence that megakaryocytes are involved in the mechanism whereby increased deposition of collagen occurs. The striking presence of megakaryocytes in myelofibrosis was noted in early reviews and their abnormal morphology was commented on, giving rise to speculation that this might be an important aspect of the disease. It has recently been suggested that the essential factor is ineffective megakaryopoiesis with intramedullary death of megakaryocytes and release of platelet-derived growth factor (PDGF). At the same time, platelet factor 4 inhibits collagenase activity, so that excessive production of this factor may also contribute to the pathogenesis of myelofibrosis (Fig. 20.5). Increased numbers of megakaryocytes alone do not necessarily result in myelofibrosis; it is the presence of abnormal amounts of megakaryocyte-derived products from ineffective megakaryocytopoiesis which appears to be the main source of growth factor. It must, however, be remembered that, as myelofibrosis is characterized by abnormality of the entire haemopoietic tissue, other cell types might be responsible for the production of growth factor.

Vitamin D also appears to play a role in the regulation of collagen deposition, either by inhibiting megakaryocyte proliferation or by directly inhibiting collagen synthesis.

Progenitor Cell Defect

There is increasing evidence that the primary defect in myelofibrosis is the occurrence of a neoplastic clone leading to abnormal populations of circulating progenitor cells for megakaryocytes (CFU–Mk) as well as granulocyte macrophages (CFU–GM). The spleen may be a major site for

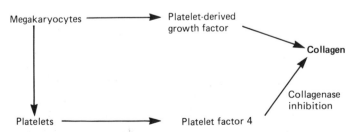

Fig. 20.5. *Megakaryocyte involvement in collagen formation.*

abnormal CFU production in myelofibrosis, although there is contradictory evidence on this. It appears that, at least for some patients, the spleen plays a major role in the abnormal haemopoiesis, and splenectomy for these patients would be expected to reduce the number of circulating progenitors. In other patients, however, significant haemopoiesis takes place also at other extramedullary sites and thus splenectomy would have little or no effect on reducing the circulating progenitor cell numbers.

Clinical Features

The disease occurs especially in the middle-aged and elderly. There may be a preceding history of PPP or primary thrombocythaemia (see p. 530). The onset is insidious, the clinical diagnosis being preceded by a long symptom-free interval which may last for many years. During this period, there is gradually increasing myeloid metaplasia with progressive enlargement of the spleen and sometimes the liver. The patients usually present with symptoms caused by bone marrow failure, splenic enlargement or the metabolic consequences of the underlying myeloproliferative disorder. Complaints of lethargy, weakness and dyspnoea on exertion are common. Splenomegaly may give rise to marked abdominal distension and an inability to take a full meal. With massive splenomegaly, urinary frequency is sometimes a problem. Left hypochondrial pain may reflect splenic infarct or perisplenitis. The metabolic disturbance often results in night sweats, fever, itching, anorexia and weight loss. Hyperuricaemia may lead to gout or renal colic and occasional patients complain of bone pain.

Less than 10% of patients present with serious bleeding diathesis, but skin bruising may occur and on rare occasions gastrointestinal haemorrhage due to an associated portal hypertension may be the presenting symptom.

Physical Examination

In the great majority of patients the dominant finding at diagnosis is splenomegaly; this is usually marked—myelofibrosis is responsible for some of the largest spleens which occur in disease. On the other hand, absence of clinical splenomegaly does not exclude the diagnosis of myelofibrosis but, as the disease progresses, the spleen usually becomes palpable. Rarely, splenic atrophy may follow splenic arterial thrombosis in patients with marked thrombocythaemia. The liver is enlarged in 75% of patients and prominent Riedel's lobe expansion sometimes causes diagnostic confusion. Ascites is usually associated with portal hypertension and parenchymal liver failure and this tends to be a late feature. Lymphadenopathy is unusual but may be involved in extramedullary erythropoiesis. Occasionally unusual clinical presentations may arise when extramedullary haemopoiesis occurs in kidneys, lungs, pleura, peritoneum or gastrointestinal tract. The central nervous system is rarely involved, giving rise to neurological signs.

Radiological Features

The characteristic features are increased bone density due to new bone deposition in the trabeculae, endosteal cortical thickening, obliteration of the corticomedullary junction and narrowing of the medullary spaces of the long bones. In some cases there is only patchy sclerosis, a coarse trabeculation or a mottled appearance of the bones. Sometimes, however, the skeletal system shows no obvious abnormality.

Haematological Features

Morphological changes occur in the blood before the onset of anaemia, and become increasingly abnormal as anaemia develops. The peripheral blood film usually shows leucoerythroblastic changes, sometimes with a large number of nucleated red cells. Polychromasia, anisocytosis and poikilocytosis with tear-drop red cells are typical changes (Fig. 20.6); they occur in 90% of cases but in some they may be relatively inconspicuous. Some macrocytosis is sometimes found as a consequence of dyserythropoiesis, whilst when there is associated folate deficiency, oval macrocytes, megaloblastic normoblasts, and hypersegmented neutrophils will be seen.

The blood count usually shows an anaemia with normal red cell values. The MCV will be high in patients who are folate deficient and low when there is an associated iron deficiency. The reticulocyte

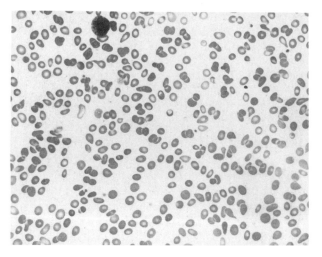

Fig. 20.6. *Blood film in myelofibrosis showing red cell poikilocytosis with characteristic 'tear-drop' cells; there is also a myelocyte.*

count is often elevated, in the range $75-250 \times 10^9/l$. The white cell count may be normal, elevated or decreased. Patients with the most marked myeloproliferation may occasionally present with white cell counts of over $100 \times 10^9/l$; they may be erroneously labelled as having chronic myeloid leukaemia. The platelet count is also variable. In some patients, levels up to $1000 \times 10^9/l$ are found and it may be difficult at first to decide whether to label the disease myelofibrosis or primary thrombocythaemia. In both conditions, platelets in the blood film are bizarre, with giant forms, and circulating megakaryocyte fragments may be seen.

Serum and red cell folate levels are often low and in some patients severe folate deficiency is an important factor in the pathogenesis of the anaemia. Both low dietary intake and increase in turnover of haemopoietic cells may contribute to the folate deficiency.

The neutrophil alkaline phosphatase (NAP) score is typically normal or raised by contrast to the low score found in CML. Total vitamin B_{12}-binding capacity is usually raised, but rarely to the levels found in untreated CML.

Platelet function is defective in up to 50% of patients; abnormalities include diminished response to aggregating agents such as serotonin, adrenaline and adenosine diphosphate. Variable results have been obtained in response to collagen and thrombin. Spontaneous aggregation may occur; this effect can be abolished by small doses of aspirin.

Blood Chemistry

An increased purine turnover results in raised levels of serum uric acid in the majority of cases. Serum levels of hydroxybutyric or lactic acid dehydrogenase show significant and often marked elevations. An increase in white cell turnover is reflected in high levels of serum lysozyme. Patients with portal hypertension may show abnormalities of liver function in the later stages.

Bone Marrow

Attempts at bone marrow aspiration are usually unsuccessful, although occasionally normal or even hyperplastic fragments are obtained. Trephine biopsy is essential for a reliable diagnosis. The characteristic morphological features in the bone marrow can be divided into non-fibrotic and fibrotic. In the former there are qualitative and quantitative changes in all types of cells. These changes are sometimes minimal but in other cases they may be marked. At first there is hyperplasia of all cells, usually with a normal distribution. At a later stage there is a decreasing number of haemopoietic cells and reticulum cells with an increased fat content and this is accompanied by the beginning of fibroblast proliferation. Subsequently, the fibrotic features begin to predominate. There is calcification of the fibrous ground substance, and large and atypical osteocytes appear. Megakaryocytes are prominent and they may appear in cohesive clusters. Increasing fibrosis is paralleled by depletion of haemopoietic cells. In the later stages there is often marrow failure with pancytopenia (Fig. 20.7).

In all cases there is an increase in reticulin fibre density and thickness, demonstrable by silver impregnation. Two patterns of reticulin are seen: (a) an increased amount of fine branching fibres laid out in an essentially normal pattern, and (b) an abnormal design consisting of a coarse mesh of fibres that are thicker than normal and follow a wavy course, aggregating into bundles of parallel fibres with the morphology of collagen. The former pattern is found in association with hypercellularity

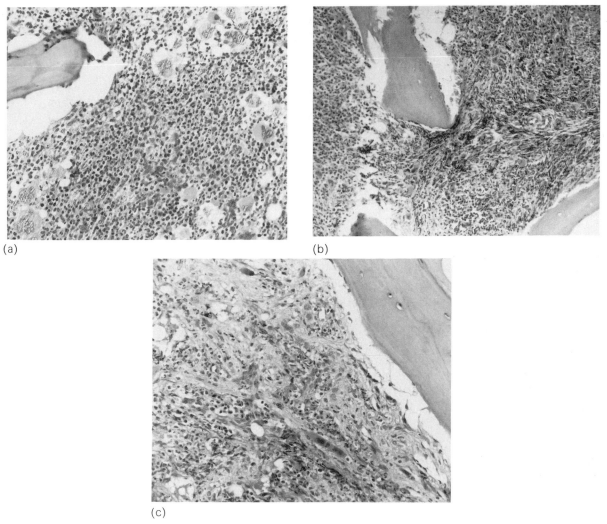

(a)

(b)

(c)

Fig. 20.7. *Iliac crest trephine biopsy sections in myelofibrosis (haematoxylin and eosin stain). (a) Cellular phase showing loss of normal bone marrow architecture with proliferation of haemopoietic tissue, increase in megakaryocytes and some fibroblasts. (b) Fibrotic phase, showing proliferation of fibrous tissue with isolated haemopoietic cells confined to intravascular spaces. (c) Sclerotic phase showing further stage of development of osteomyelosclerosis; there is an increase in trabecular bone and some woven bone adjacent to fibrous tissue. Very few haemopoietic cells are seen.*

per se, whereas the latter type predominates in myelofibrosis (Fig. 20.8). As myelofibrosis advances, there is increasing deposition of collagen. In a small number of patients (less than 10%) osteosclerosis is present (Fig. 20.8). In these patients peritrabecular new bone deposition results in thickened trabeculae, and islands of osteoid are present in the remaining fibrotic intertrabecular space. The histo-

logical course in myelofibrosis is shown in Table 20.4.

Progenitor Cell Assays

As described earlier, there may be increased numbers of circulating CFU–Mk and CFU–GM in myelofibrosis, as demonstrated by in-vitro colony

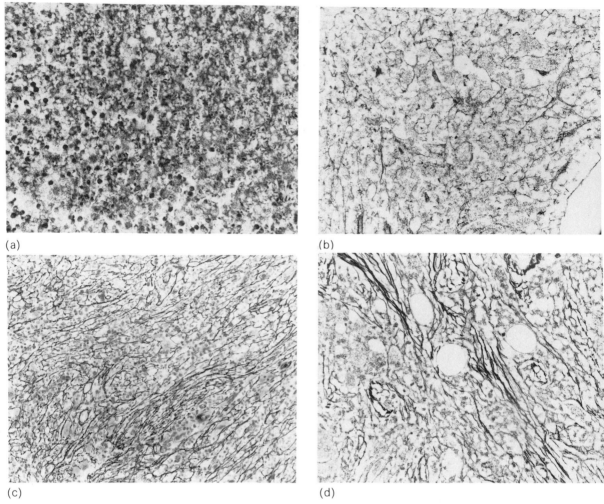

Fig. 20.8. *Iliac crest trephine bone biopsy sections stained by silver impregnation technique. (a) Normal: there are only a few fine reticulin fibres which are widely dispersed. (b) Primary proliferative polycythaemia (see Fig. 20.1b): slight patchy increase in reticulin but individual fibre thickness is not increased. (c) Early myelofibrosis (see Fig. 20.7a): the reticulin is definitely increased in amount, with some coarse fibres. (d) Late myelofibrosis (see Fig. 20.7b): increase in reticulin with coarse, wavy bundles of fibres.*

growth on culture. Whilst this is not specific, the presence especially of a markedly increased number of Mk progenitors is highly suggestive of myelofibrosis. Spontaneous BFU–E are also found in myeloproliferative disorders, especially in PPP, and it has been suggested that in myelofibrosis this is only in cases which have followed on polycythaemia.

Radionuclide Studies

Investigation of blood volume, erythrokinetics and spleen function provides important information for diagnosis and may be useful: (1) to elucidate the mechanism of anaemia, (2) to localize the sites of active erythropoiesis, (3) to evaluate prognosis, and (4) to make therapeutic decisions.

Table 20.4
Histological course in myelofibrosis

Cellular phase
Diffusely hyperplastic; normal maturation of erythropoiesis and granulopoiesis
Megakaryocytes may predominate; some immature forms
Reticulin ± increase

Fibrotic phase
Megakaryocytes still predominant; decreasing numbers of other haemopoietic cells
Altered sinus architecture
Reticulin + +
Collagen +

Sclerotic phase (myelosclerosis)
Grossly disturbed architecture
Markedly reduced haematopoiesis
Megakaryocyte/megakaryoblast clusters
Fibroblasts + + +
Reticulin + + +
Collagen + + +

Osteosclerotic phase (osteomyelosclerosis)
Fibroblasts + + +
Collagen + + +
Osteoblast and osteocyte proliferation with bone formation
Osteocyte proliferation with bone formation

Ferrokinetic Studies

Studies with radioactive iron (^{59}Fe) provide information about the extent and effectiveness of erythropoiesis (see Chapter 1). The injected iron is usually cleared rapidly from the circulation, and the plasma iron turnover is increased in most patients with myelofibrosis. The degree of ineffective erythropoiesis is reflected by a reduction in the maximum red cell iron incorporation. Whilst the majority of patients incorporate 30–70% of the injected ^{59}Fe, in those with either advanced disease or severe folate deficiency there is often marked ineffective erythropoiesis, and figures as low as 15% may be obtained. Surface counting demonstrates the sites of radioactive iron uptake. Radioactivity in the marrow, spleen or liver indicates that erythropoiesis is taking place at these sites. Extramedullary erythropoiesis may be demonstrated in almost all patients—in the spleen in about 80% of patients and in the liver in about 50% (Fig. 20.9). Occasionally, in patients with marrow failure, plasma clearance is slow, plasma iron turnover is not increased, there is a low incorporation of ^{59}Fe into red cells and the surface counting pattern is that of aplastic anaemia, i.e. a slow uptake of ^{59}Fe into the liver only, with little evidence of release from that organ during the 14 days of study. This pattern is usually associated with blastic transformation of myelofibrosis (see p. 556).

Whole-body scanning with cyclotron-produced ^{52}Fe allows a more accurate assessment of the distribution of injected radioiron within the body (p. 15). By this method it is possible to measure the fraction of the injected iron and thus the proportion of erythropoiesis in the liver and the spleen (Fig. 20.10). In many patients with myelosclerosis, more than half the total erythropoiesis occurs in these organs. 111-Indium chloride attached to transferrin has also been used for bone marrow scanning but the distribution of this radionuclide does not always reflect the sites or the amount of

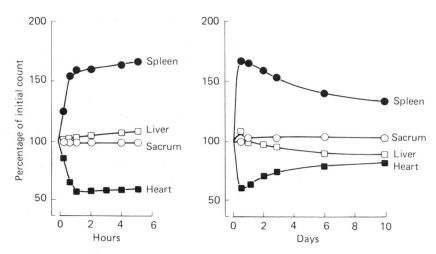

Fig. 20.9. *Ferrokinetic study in myelofibrosis: surface counting pattern follow-ing injection of ^{59}Fe-labelled plasma. Erythropoiesis is taking place mainly in the spleen. Incomplete release of ^{59}Fe from the spleen is due to ineffective erythro-poiesis and also to splenic pooling of red cells subsequent to their entry into the circulating blood.*

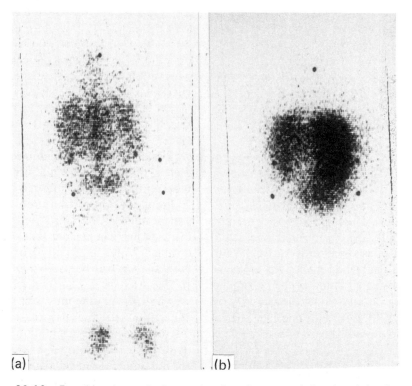

Fig. 20.10. *Ferrokinetic study in myelosclerosis; scans following injection of ^{52}Fe. (a) Uptake of ^{52}Fe by spleen and liver in addition to uptake by the central skeleton. This occurs in the early stages of the disease, and especially in transitional myeloproliferative disease. In this case there were still features of polycythaemia; note iron uptake in the femoral epiphyses. (b) Uptake of ^{52}Fe by spleen and liver with no evidence of skeletal uptake, in a patient with late-stage myelofibrosis. (See also Fig. 1.13, p. 15)*

erythropoiesis, so that the results may be misleading.

Red Cell Survival Studies

Chromium-51(^{51}Cr)-labelled red cell survival studies have shown that the red cell lifespan is moderately shortened in myelofibrosis, usually to 20–40 days. Surface counting and quantitative scanning have shown that the enlarged spleens in myelofibrosis may account for 25–50% of the total red cell destruction.

Measurement of Blood Volume

Splenomegaly is associated with an increased splenic red cell pool and an enlarged plasma volume. In such cases the peripheral blood count does not accurately reflect the total red cell mass, which may be normal despite a low venous PCV. It is important to measure both RCM and PV directly. For red cell mass this is best performed with ^{99}Tc, ^{111}In or ^{113m}In; for plasma volume ^{125}I-labelled albumin is the most suitable. In conjunction with the measurement of red cell mass, the splenic red cell pool can be measured by quantitative scanning of the splenic area.

Platelet Kinetics

In patients with thrombocytopenia, platelet kinetic studies have demonstrated that splenic platelet pooling may be largely responsible for the reduced numbers of platelets in the peripheral blood. In patients with massive splenomegaly, the fraction of platelets in the exchangeable splenic pool may account for up to 75% of the marrow output. Reduction in platelet lifespan has been reported.

Differential Diagnosis

To make a diagnosis of myelofibrosis, it is necessary: (a) to establish that the fibrosis results from intrinsic marrow disease rather than from a systemic disorder, and (b) to distinguish myelofibrosis within the spectrum of chronic myeloproliferative disorders. The American Polycythaemia Vera Study Group has defined myelofibrosis as a clinical illness with the following features.

1. Splenomegaly.
2. Fibrosis involving more than one-third of the sectional area of an adequate bone marrow biopsy.
3. A leucoerythroblastic blood picture.
4. Absence of an increased red cell mass.
5. Absence of the Philadelphia chromosome.
6. Exclusion of systemic disorders.
7. A diagnosis of osteomyelosclerosis requires the presence of sclerotic changes detected radiologically in axial skeleton or long bones.

The systemic disorders in which marrow fibrosis occurs include metastatic carcinoma, non-Hodgkin's lymphoma, irradiation and tuberculosis. Before diagnosing 'primary' myelofibrosis, the likelihood of the presence of one of these conditions should be assessed. Usually, it is relatively easy to distinguish these patients. Greater diagnostic difficulties may arise in distinguishing myelofibrosis from other conditions in the spectrum of myeloproliferative disorders, especially in transitional phases. An overlapping picture is seen most frequently in relation to PPP. Approximately 20% of patients with PPP eventually develop the clinical picture of myelofibrosis with progressive enlargement of the spleen and bone marrow hypofunction with increasing reticulin/collagen fibrosis.

Another form of myeloproliferative disease appears to be intermediate between polycythaemia and myelofibrosis. There are features of the latter disease, including splenic myeloid metaplasia, leucoerythroblastic blood picture, extensive reticulin and even collagen fibrosis in the marrow, but at the same time the blood count is polycythaemic, the patients remain in a remarkably steady state with unchanging features for at least several years. To distinguish this condition from the more common transformation of PPP to myelofibrosis, it has been termed transitional myeloproliferative disorder.

Another syndrome which sometimes gives rise to diagnostic difficulty is a myeloproliferative disorder which appears to be intermediate between CML and myelofibrosis. The peripheral blood shows features of CML but there is bone marrow reticulin and collagen fibrosis which becomes particularly conspicuous at the onset of blastic transformation. The presence of the Philadelphia chromosome and the previous history will indicate the correct diagnosis in such cases.

Prognosis

Median survival is about 3 years from the time of diagnosis, but many patients with benign or slowly progressive disease survive for 10 years or longer. A prognostic index can be derived by analysis of the haemoglobin and reticulocyte count at diagnosis: patients with haemoglobin values below 100 g/l and a reticulocyte count below 2% have the worst prognosis, with a median survival of only 1.7 years; by contrast, patients with haemoglobin levels of more than 100 g/l have median survivals in excess of 6 years. Plasma volume expansion consequent upon splenic enlargement seems to correlate inversely with prognosis; a likely explanation is that patients with the largest plasma volume have the poorest residual marrow function.

The most common causes of death are infection, gastrointestinal haemorrhage, cerebrovascular accident and cardiovascular disease. A small number of patients die of liver or renal failure. Approximately 8% of patients have a terminal transformation to acute myeloid leukaemia. It occurs more frequently in males and usually within 5 years of the original diagnosis of myelofibrosis, but it has been recorded as early as 6 months and as late as 14 years. This condition has a rapidly progressive course and is resistant to usual chemotherapeutic regimens.

Treatment

Treatment is based primarily upon the symptoms that the patient displays. The condition may remain relatively stable for some time, with no more than a moderate degree of anaemia without thrombocytopenia or leucopenia and only very gradual splenic enlargement. There may be few, if any, associated symptoms. These patients require careful observation on a 3–6-monthly basis to detect active progression of the disease but, as a rule, no therapy need be prescribed at this stage.

Patients with a more actively progressive form of myelosclerosis present with symptoms due to anaemia, splenic enlargement, bleeding or the constitutional effects of hypermetabolism. Treatment for these complications is palliative and aimed at the relief of symptoms and maintaining the patient in as comfortable a state as possible for as long as possible.

General Supportive Measures

It has been estimated that 60% of patients with myelofibrosis will become anaemic during their clinical course. For this, blood transfusions should be administered, the aim being to maintain the patient's haemoglobin at a reasonable level. When there is a history of gout and hyperuricaemia, treatment with allopurinol is effective. Other important supportive measures include advice about an adequate diet, iron supplementation for iron-deficient patients, sedatives, analgesics and antipruritics. Some patients develop folate deficiency at some stage during the course of their disease. Provided that vitamin B_{12} deficiency is excluded, anaemic patients with myelofibrosis should be given 5 mg of folic acid daily. However, before diagnosing anaemia, it is important to determine measurement of red cell mass and plasma volume by the extent to which the apparent anaemia is due to an expanded plasma volume.

Androgens

These are indicated in patients with ineffective erythropoiesis, with or without thrombocytopenia. Oxymetholone (200 mg daily) or fluoxymesterone (30 mg daily) may be beneficial. For patients without thrombocytopenia, intramuscular testosterone inanthate may be effective in doses of 400 mg every 3–4 weeks. Response to androgen therapy may be delayed for up to 3–4 months. Thus, treatment should be continued for at least this period of time, with careful monitoring of liver function tests.

In some patients, the improvement is maintained when treatment is stopped, but the majority of patients relapse and maintenance therapy at a reduced dose is required.

Reduction of Splenomegaly

For patients with progressive splenomegaly, the main aim is to reduce the size of the spleen, thus producing relief of symptoms due to pressure and, to a lesser extent, any associated constitutional symptoms. Apart from splenectomy, splenic irradiation and chemotherapy have been used for this purpose.

Splenic Irradiation

Usually only the lower half of the spleen is irradiated; the usual course consists of 25–50 cGy daily for 5 days and a repeated course over 3–4 weeks if necessary. Radiotherapy abolishes haemopoiesis in the treated area. Accordingly, it must be carried out with rigorous haematological control, the blood count being monitored every 2–3 days and, if the white cell or platelet counts show a trend towards dangerously low levels, the course of irradiation should be terminated immediately. Occasionally splenic irradiation is followed by a rise in haemoglobin and PCV, presumably due to a reduction of the splenic red cell pool and expanded plasma volume. As radiotherapy may aggravate the hyperuricaemia, allopurinol should be administered during the courses of therapy.

Chemotherapy

Myelosuppression with busulphan or chlorambucil may be helpful in symptomatic patients with the more proliferative forms of the disease in which the white cell and/or platelet counts are high. Busulphan in a dose of 2–4 mg daily or chlorambucil in a dose of 4–6 mg daily is recommended, but the dose should be adjusted in the light of the response of the individual patient. Treatment must be strictly monitored by regular blood counts with the aim of achieving a reduction in splenic size without giving rise to sufficient myelosuppression to cause the peripheral blood white cell and platelet counts to fall to dangerously low levels. Initial leucopenia or marked thrombocytopenia is a contraindication to this type of therapy.

It has been reported that low doses of hydroxyurea (500–1000 mg per day) may be effective in reducing spleen size and decreasing metabolic activity at the sites of haemopoiesis.

Splenectomy

There is no general agreement on the value and indications for splenectomy. Numerous reports have been published, often with contradictory conclusions. The operation involves definite and grave risks, especially as many of the patients are old and in poor general condition. Moreover the spleen is often grossly enlarged and its removal is technically difficult. Under these circumstances, postoperative mortality and morbidity are high due mainly to bleeding, thromboembolism and infection. In the earlier stages of the disease, especially in patients with normal or high platelet counts, the operation may be followed by thrombocytosis and an increased tendency to thrombosis, as well as by the hazard of postsplenectomy infection. There is also the risk of later liver failure as a result of extramedullary erythropoiesis accumulating in that organ.

Whenever splenectomy is contemplated, it is essential that the patient has an extensive coagulation survey (see Chapter 24).

Indications for Splenectomy

1. *Increasing and excessive transfusion requirements.* Erythrokinetics studies with radionuclides may help to select the suitable patients. In the presence of haemolysis with significant red cell destruction by the spleen, and especially in patients with a marked degree of splenic red cell pooling, splenectomy may reduce or entirely eliminate the need for transfusions. Following splenectomy, the return of the expanded plasma volume to normal is an additional reason why there is often considerable improvement in the degree of anaemia.

2. *Severe thrombocytopenia.* As the spleen may be responsible for sequestering or pooling up to 75% of the marrow platelet output in some cases of myelofibrosis with severe thrombocytopenia, splenectomy may abolish or reduce bleeding and result in an elevation of the platelet count.

3. *Splenic enlargement.* Splenectomy is occasionally indicated when massive enlargement is associated with symptoms which cannot be controlled by chemotherapy or radiotherapy. In approximately two-thirds of patients treated by chemotherapy, the spleen will shrink, but when therapy is stopped, rapid enlargement of the spleen will recur. It is important not to delay surgery until gross splenomegaly creates serious operative problems.

4. *Portal hypertension.* In 6–8% of patients the myelofibrosis may be complicated by portal hypertension. This may occur either as the result of massive increased blood flow from the spleen to the liver or secondary to intrahepatic block as the result of postnecrotic cirrhosis which may follow transfusional hepatitis. Clinically, portal hypertension is characterized by oesophageal varices and/or ascites. When due to increased blood flow, splenectomy will be of benefit; if due to intrahepatic block, splenorenal shunt is the procedure of choice for decompressing the hypertension.

5. *Elimination of abnormal clone.* There is some evidence, albeit controversial, that the spleen is a major site for the production of abnormal progenitor cells in myelofibrosis and that splenic irradiation or splenectomy may result in a significant decrease in the circulating CFU. The effectiveness of splenectomy would depend on the extent to which haemopoiesis is also taking place at other extramedullary sites; there is little evidence to suggest that splenectomy should be performed in every patient as soon as the diagnosis of myelofibrosis is established.

Bone Marrow Transplantation

This has been attempted in a few patients; in at least some of these there has been a good response, with disappearance of fibrosis and regeneration of medullary haemopoiesis. However, the limited number of patients treated by this means is inadequate to assess the possible effect on prognosis.

Malignant (Acute) Myelofibrosis

This term was originally used to distinguish an acute, rapidly progressing illness in patients who showed the histological features of myelofibrosis but with a blood picture suggestive of acute leukaemia, with anaemia, thrombocytopenia and leucopenia with a small proportion of blasts. The marrow showed a remarkable amount of reticulin/collagen and a number of megakaryocyte-like giant cells. Neither spleen nor liver was palpable, but small foci of extramedullary erythropoiesis were demonstrated (at autopsy) in the liver and other organs. Subsequently, there has been confusion caused by the use of this designation to describe other clinical syndromes. The majority of cases which have been described as 'malignant myelofibrosis' have been shown by cytochemistry and electron microscopy to have megakaryoblastic leukaemia (see p. 387). Another condition which should be distinguished is 'acute myelodysplasia with myelofibrosis'. This syndrome is characterized by severe pancytopenia of sudden onset, absence of organomegaly, bone marrow showing reticulin fibrosis, dysmyelopoiesis, and an excess of blast cells of all three myeloid lines, particularly the megakaryocyte series.

SELECTED BIBLIOGRAPHY

Berk P. D., Goldberg J. D., Donovan P. B., Fruchtman S. M., Berlin N. I., Wasserman L.R. (1986). Therapeutic recommendations in polycythemia vera based on Polycythemia Vera Study Group protocols. *Seminars in Hematology*, **23**, 132–143.

Berlin N. I. (Ed.) (1975) Polycythemia 1. *Seminars in Hematology*, **12**, 335–444.

Berlin N. I. (Ed.) (1976). Polycythemia 2. *Seminars in Hematology*, **13**, 1–86.

Castro-Malaspina H., Moore M. A. S. (1982). Pathophysiological mechanisms operating in the development of myelofibrosis: role of megakaryocytes. *Nouvelle Revue Francaise d'Hematologie*, **24**, 221–226.

Cotes P. M., Doré C. J., Liu Yin J. A., Lewis S. M., Messinezy M., Pearson T. C., Reid C. (1986). The use of estimates of serum immunoreactive erythropoietin in the elucidation of polycythemia. *New England Journal of Medicine*, **315**, 283–287.

Dameshek W. (1951). Some speculations on myeloproliferative syndromes. *Blood*, **6**, 372–375.

Frisch B., Lewis S. M., Burkhardt R., Bartl R. (1985). *Biopsy pathology of bone and bone marrow*, pp. 108–145. London: Chapman and Hall.

Jacobson R. J., Salo A., Fialkow P. F. (1978). Agnogenic myeloid metaplasia. A clonal proliferation of haematopoietic stem cells with secondary myelofibrosis. *Blood*, **51**, 189–194.

Lewis S. M. (Ed.) (1985). *Myelofibrosis: Pathophysiology and clinical management.* New York: Marcel Dekker.

Manaharan A. (1988). Myelofibrosis: Prognostic factors and treatment. *British Journal of Haematology* **69**, 295–298.

Njoku O. S., Lewis S. M., Catovsky D., Gordon-Smith E. C. (1983). Anaemia in myelofibrosis: its value in prognosis. *British Journal of Haematology*, **54**, 79–89.

Pettit J. E., Lewis S. M., Nicholas A. W. (1979). Transitional myeloproliferative disorders. *British Journal of Haematology*, **43**, 167–184.

Schafer A. S. (1984). Bleeding and thrombosis in the myeloproliferative disorders. *Blood*, **64**, 1–12.

Van de Pette J. E. W., Prochazka A. V., Pearson T. C., Singh A. K., Dickson E. R., Wetherley-Mein G. (1986). Primary thrombocythaemia treated with busulphan. *British Journal of Haematology*, **62**, 229–237.

Varki A., Lottenberg R., Griffiths R., Reinhard E. (1983). The syndrome of idiopathic myelofibrosis. A clinical review with emphasis on the prognostic variables predicting survival. *Medicine*, **62**, 353–371.

Chapter 21

NORMAL HAEMOSTASIS

R. A. HUTTON

The complexity of the haemostatic mechanism in humans reflects the demands placed upon it by the circulatory system through which metabolic homeostasis is maintained. The high blood pressure generated on the arterial side of the circulation requires an almost instantaneous but strictly localized procoagulant response, in order to minimize blood loss from sites of vascular injury without compromising blood flow generally. Conversely, with the slow or intermittent blood flow in the veins, systemic anticoagulant components are necessary to protect against unwanted thrombus formation. To meet these diverse requirements, a haemostatic system has evolved which contains numerous activating or inhibiting feedback or feed-forward pathways, integrating the blood vessels with the blood platelets and a number of humoral factors, some of which link haemostasis to other components of the body's defence response such as the complement and kinin-generating systems.

Many of the advances of our knowledge about the haemostatic pathways have emerged from studies carried out on patients with congenital or acquired bleeding or thrombotic disorders. These form the basis of the subsequent four chapters, while in the present one, only the fundamental physiological events occurring during the haemostatic response in normal subjects are considered. In order to facilitate comprehension of these complex processes, the chapter is divided into four sections.

1. The roles of the blood vessels and the platelets in the formation of a primary (platelet) haemostatic plug.
2. The interactions between the soluble coagulation factors leading to the formation of a fibrin clot.

3. The roles of the naturally occurring blood coagulation inhibitors in the maintenance of blood fluidity and flow.
4. The role of the fibrinolytic system in the removal of fibrin deposits.

FORMATION OF A PRIMARY HAEMOSTATIC PLUG

Structure and Function of the Blood Vessels

The intimal surface of blood vessels is covered with endothelial cells which rest on a basement membrane of subendothelial microfibrils, these being the only constituents of the capillaries, whose thin walls facilitate exchange of nutrients and waste products. With progressively larger vessels, particularly arteries, increasing amounts of elastin, innervated smooth muscle cells and collagen are found. Elastin affords the vessels a degree of distensibility and accommodates the distortion during body movements or resulting from the pumping action of the heart, as well as contributing to vessel resealing following minor trauma, e.g. venepuncture. The smooth muscle cells influence blood flow since, being arranged in a circular fashion around the vessels, their contraction (due to trauma or to sympathetic nerve stimulation) causes vasoconstriction. Vascular collagen is principally of type II, with smaller amounts of types I and III, all of which appear to be in the correct physical and biochemical configuration to support platelet adhesion and to activate coagulation factor XII (see later). Type III collagen promotes platelet adhesion best and is also critical for the mechanical integrity of the blood vessels, a deficiency such as is seen in Ehlers–Danlos

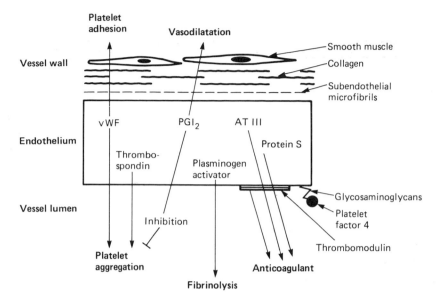

Fig. 21.1. *The endothelial cell.*

syndrome type IV commonly resulting in sudden death due to rupture of a major artery.

The endothelial cells exert a powerful and almost exclusively inhibitory influence on haemostasis by virtue of the factors which they synthesize and release or bind onto their surface (Fig. 21.1). These include tissue plasminogen activators and inhibitors, antithrombin III, heparin-related molecules, platelet factor 4 (PF4), protein S and thrombomodulin, all of which will be discussed in the relevant sections below. Three others which profoundly influence platelet–vessel wall interaction are von Willebrand factor, fibronectin and prostaglandin I_2 (PGI$_2$), sometimes referred to as prostacyclin.

Von Willebrand Factor

Von Willebrand factor (vWF) is a glycoprotein in which galactose residues are essential for its biological activity, probably because these influence its tertiary or quaternary structure. It is synthesized principally by endothelial cells and megakaryocytes and is found in the plasma (concentration 10 μg/ml), in the alpha granules of the blood platelets and in the vessel wall where it is associated with subendothelial microfibrils and collagen. In its basic form, vWF contains 2050 amino acids and has

a molecular weight (mol. wt) of around 300 000, about 20% of which is carbohydrate. When first synthesized (pro-vWF), it contains an additional 'leader' sequence which has a molecular weight of around 60 000 (741 amino acids). A small signal peptide (22 amino acids) is also present initially (pre-pro vWF) and thus the native protein contains 2813 amino acids and after glycosylation has a molecular weight of around 360 000 (309 000 unglycosylated). Apart from glycosylation, post-translational sulphation occurs.

The vWF is coded for by a gene approximately 150 kb long in the p1.2 region of chromosome 12. Cleavage of the signal peptide and leader sequences permits multimers of the subunit to form, the smallest of which is a dimer (mol. wt 450 000) and the largest having a molecular weight in excess of 10×10^6. These are stored in the Weibel–Palade bodies from whence they are slowly released into the plasma. Here, some proteolysis occurs and four main fragments are detectable with subunit molecular weights of 225 000, 189 000, 176 000 and 140 000. Multimers of the smaller fragments may contribute to some extent to the so-called flanking bands which are seen when the multimeric structure is studied in vitro (see Chapter 23).

Stimulated release of vWF from endothelial cells can be induced by thrombin and interleukin-1 and also occurs under the influence of several hormones, of which adrenaline, vasopressin and insulin are the most potent. Vigorous exercise and even simple occlusion are also effective. Raised levels of vWF are also found secondary to many diseases, particularly those involving the liver. Release of the cleaved leader sequence, sometimes referred to as von Willebrand antigen II, occurs in parallel with vWF.

Platelet vWF is stored in the alpha granules (see below) and, during platelet activation, is released into the plasma. Some of the multimers of platelet vWF are of exceptionally high molecular weight and the presence of these in plasma may be a useful indicator of the platelet-release reaction.

In plasma, vWF is found closely associated with coagulation factor VIII and, indeed, it was previously known as factor VIII-related antigen (VIII:Rag). Studies in patients with von Willebrand's disease indicate that the highest molecular weight multimers are essential for platelet adhesion to the subendothelial matrix (see Chapter 23).

Fibronectin

This substance, which is also known as cold-insoluble globulin, is one of the so-called adhesive proteins which include vWF and fibrinogen. It is synthesized chiefly in the liver and has a molecular weight of 440 000. Like fibrinogen, it serves as a substrate for thrombin and factor XIIIa. In the vessel wall it is found cross-linked (factor XIIIa mediated) to collagen, and contributes to fibroblast and platelet adhesion. It also occurs in the plasma (concentration 200–400 μg/ml), where it acts as an opsonin, and in the platelet alpha granules (see later).

Prostaglandin I_2

Prostaglandin I_2 (PGI_2, prostacyclin) is the major prostaglandin synthesized by endothelial cells and is a potent vasodilator which also inhibits platelet aggregation and adhesion. A small amount of PGI_2 is also produced by fibroblasts and smooth muscle cells. The precursor of PGI_2 is arachidonic acid which is liberated from the phospholipids of the endothelial cell membrane by phospholipases.

Arachidonic acid is first converted to prostaglandins G_2 and H_2, the so-called cyclic endoperoxides, by cyclo-oxygenase and thence to PGI_2 under the influence of prostacyclin synthetase. Thrombin generated at the site of injury stimulates the synthesis of PGI_2 by adjacent endothelial cells and this counteracts the platelet-aggregating activity of thrombin and thereby serves to localize platelet plug formation. Elevation of intravascular pressure and trauma, including venepuncture, also increase PGI_2 production, and this may be a source of artefactually high levels observed when bioassays incorporating vascular segments or rings are used. The PGI_2 is rather unstable and largely degrades spontaneously to 6-Keto prostaglandin F_1 alpha (6-keto PGF_1 alpha), with a half-life of only a few minutes in whole blood. 6-Keto PGF_1 alpha is biologically inert, but a variable proportion of PGI_2 may, in some tissues, be enzymatically converted to other prostaglandins such as 6-keto prostaglandin E_1 or di-hydro di-keto prostaglandin F_1 alpha, which retain some platelet-inhibitory activity. Prostaglandin metabolism in endothelial cells and blood platelets is shown in Fig. 21.2.

It was once postulated that PGI_2 was a circulating hormone limiting platelet–platelet interactions within the bloodstream. This theory was based on gross overestimates of the level of 6-keto PGF_1 alpha in the circulating plasma obtained using radioimmunoassays, now shown to be unreliable. When techniques such as gas chromatography and negative ion chemical ionization mass spectrometry are used, the true circulating basal level of PGI_2 has been found to be less than 3 pg/ml, which is at least two orders of magnitude below that needed to inhibit platelet aggregation. Although in some settings, such as following severe trauma, it is possible that markedly raised systemic levels could occur transiently, it is more likely that PGI_2 serves mainly as a local hormone, principally concerned with vascular tone but possibly also inhibiting the extension of the platelet plug beyond the immediate vicinity of any endothelial damage. In this context, the endothelial cells also contain ectoenzymes which degrade adenosine diphosphate (ADP) and 5-hydroxytryptamine (5-HT), both of which are vasoconstrictors and induce platelet aggregation and are likely to be released at points of local injury. These mechanisms may be particularly important

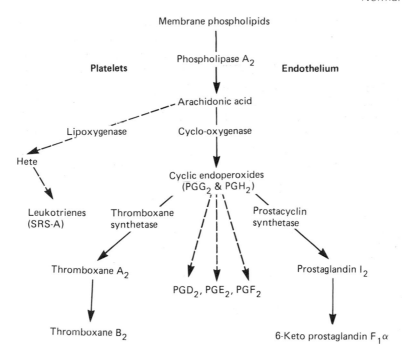

Fig. 21.2. *Prostaglandin metabolism in platelets and endothelial cells.*

in blood vessels which do not produce PGI_2, such as those in the placenta.

THE BLOOD PLATELETS

Formation

The blood platelets are fragments of the cytoplasm of the megakaryocyte, hence they are non-nucleated and formed in the bone marrow. The megakaryocytes are derived from pluripotential stem cells. Under some, as yet undefined, directive, a small proportion of these stem cells become committed to produce platelets and thereafter undergo characteristic differentiation, the first stage of which is the formation of a colony-forming unit–megakaryocyte (CFU–Mk).

At this stage the cell has none of the markers of the megakaryocyte, but under the influence of the colony-stimulating factor–megakaryocyte (CSF–Mk), the earliest recognizable precursor of the megakaryocyte is formed. This is the megakaryoblast, and from this stage onwards the cell ceases to multiply by division and instead under-

goes an unusual form of mitosis in which the nucleus, but not the cell itself, divides. This is called endomitosis, and with each nuclear division there is a burst of membrane formation and increasing maturation of the cytoplasm with the appearance of all of the characteristic features of the platelet itself, e.g. membrane glycoproteins, platelet-specific granules, lysosomes. The increased membrane is accommodated by progressive invagination of the membrane and these invaginations eventually form the demarcation membranes of the individual platelets. The megakaryoblast has a ploidy state of 2–4N and a size ranging from 6 μm to 20 μm. The fully mature megakaryocyte may have a ploidy state as high as 64N, be around 60 μm in diameter and give rise to as many as 3000 platelets.

The maturation of the megakaryoblast appears to be under humoral control, the agent responsible being thrombopoietin, which is itself synthesized in the liver and kidney. There appears to be a negative feedback between thrombopoietin level and the platelet count. In many forms of thrombocytopenia, thrombocytopoiesis is stimulated and the megakaryocyte cytoplasm matures much more rapidly than normal so that octaploid and possibly even some tetraploid cells produce platelets. These platelets tend to be larger, denser and more metabolically active than those in the circulation generally, a finding which has given rise to the theory that newly released platelets are large and haemostatically active and that they decrease in size and functional capacity with age. However, there are dangers in extrapolating results obtained under conditions of 'stressed' platelet production to the normal steady state. Because immature megakaryocytes have less cytoplasm than older ones, they will, if stimulated, produce platelets with less membrane and more granules and this might explain their increased density and haemostatic potential compared to cells produced under normal conditions.

Thus, platelet size and functional activity may not always be directly correlated, and platelet size heterogeneity appears to depend as much on rate of production as on the age of the circulating cells. Together with racial influences, this somewhat confounds the idea that platelet volume determination is a useful marker for certain pathological conditions. Mature megakaryocytes extend pseudopodia through the walls of the marrow sinusoids and either individual platelets or larger fragments of the cytoplasm are broken off, the latter being carried in the bloodstream to the lungs, where the final breakdown to individual platelets is completed mechanically in the pulmonary microcirculation.

Newly released platelets appear to be sequestrated in the spleen for 24–48 hours before reaching the general circulation. The normal spleen contains around 10–20% of the total number of platelets in the body at any one time. By means of some, as yet unidentified, feedback mechanism, but probably involving platelet mass, the platelet count in the peripheral blood is maintained at a fairly constant level which ranges between $150 \times 10^9/l$ and $400 \times 10^9/l$ in normal subjects. A somewhat lower range is seen in the newborn, normal adult levels being achieved by about 3 months. Considerable fluctuation may occur during the course of the menstrual cycle, lowest levels being found at, or just prior to, menstruation. Heavy exercise and adrenergic stimulation tend to increase the platelet count transiently. There are some racial differences in platelet count, for example in Mediterranean races, platelet counts as low as $80 \times 10^9/l$ are sometimes found in normal individuals. However, in these people the mean platelet volume is increased so that the overall platelet mass is unaltered. Apart from this so-called Mediterranean macrothrombocytopenia, no clinically significant age- or sex-related changes in platelet count have been substantiated.

The normal lifespan of platelets ranges between 8 and 14 days, depending mainly on physiological factors but also on the method used for its measurement. Not unexpectedly in view of the instability of the platelets removed from the body, shorter survival times are seen with in-vitro labelling techniques using isotopes such as ^{51}Cr or ^{111}In, whereas longer survival times are generally observed with non-specific in-vivo isotopes such as ^{75}Se-selenomethionine in which errors due to re-utilization of the label may be encountered.

In healthy subjects, the platelet survival curve is linear, indicating that the removal of platelets from the circulation occurs as a consequence of senescence rather than of random utilization (which would give an exponential decay curve), although the latter process might predominate in disorders associated with a hypercoagulable state. Effete platelets are recognized and taken up by the reticuloendothelial system in the liver, spleen and bone marrow.

A non-isotopic method for measuring platelet survival has been described in which the rate of return of prostaglandin synthesis in platelets (as monitored by malondialdehyde production) is determined after this has been blocked by aspirin. Despite the fact that this method does not require the injection of radioisotopes, it has not been widely used. It is possible that the survival of platelets whose function has been inhibited by aspirin might be modified, leading to preferential utilization of cells released after the aspirin has disappeared from the blood.

Structure and Function

Platelets which have been fixed immediately after removal from the body appear under the electron microscope as smooth, biconvex discs with a diameter of 2–4 μm and a volume of 5–8 fl (Fig. 21.3). In terms of their role in haemostasis, a number of the cytoplasmic components of the platelets merit further consideration.

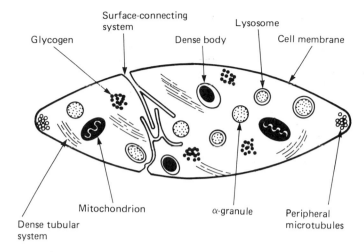

Fig. 21.3. *Diagrammatic representation of a blood platelet.*

Cytoplasmic Granules

Apart from the mitochondria, two other types of granules can be distinguished, the most prolific of which are generally referred to as alpha granules, while the other, far less numerous type, which are extremely electron dense, are known as dense bodies. The contents of these granules, together with their probable function, are shown in Table 21.1. Although the alpha granules are morphologically homogeneous, several types can be distinguished biochemically. Some are lysosomes, others produce catalase and are known as peroxisomes, and still others contain a number of platelet-specific peptides as well as several blood coagulation factors. It is now common practice to restrict the term alpha granule to the last-mentioned group. It is evident from Table 21.1 that the alpha granule contents contribute to platelet function and aggregation, blood coagulation and a variety of non-haemostatic defence mechanisms such as chemotaxis, mitogenesis and vessel repair. Of particular

Table 21.1

Platelet dense body and alpha granule contents and their function

Dense bodies	
ADP	Aggregation, vasconstriction
ATP	Degrades to ADP
5-HT	Vasoconstriction, aggregation
Calcium	?
Pyrophosphate	?
Alpha granules	
Platelet factor 4	Heparinoid neutralization
Betathromboglobulin	? Chemotaxis
Thrombospondin	? Aggregation
Platelet-derived growth factor	Mitogenesis, vessel repair
von Willebrand factor	Adhesion, aggregation
Fibrinogen	Aggregation, coagulation
Factor V	? Prothrombinase activity
Fibronectin	Fibroblast and platelet adhesion
Plasminogen activator inhibitor 1	Inhibition of fibrinolysis

interest in terms of platelet function is the suggestion that thrombospondin, which is also synthesized and released by endothelial cells, may act as an endogenous lectin inducing aggregation by forming bridges between fibrinogen molecules bound to adjacent platelets and promoting adhesion to vessel walls by forming cross-links between platelets and fibronectin bound to collagen fibres. The alpha granules contain two other platelet-specific peptides. These are platelet factor 4 (PF4), which neutralizes heparin and heparin-like molecules (see p. 582–3), and betathromboglobulin, which is thought to be chemotactic for granulocytes.

The dense bodies contain 5-hydroxytryptamine (5-HT) and aggregated complexes of adenine nucleotides with calcium ions. The 5-HT is taken up from the plasma, but there is no known transport mechanism into the dense bodies for adenine nucleotides, which are thought to be incorporated at the time of granule formation in the megakaryocyte. Adenosine triphosphate (ATP) and ADP in the dense bodies, which are referred to as the storage pool, constitute approximately 60% of the total platelet adenine nucleotides, and the ATP:ADP ratio is around 0.6. They do not readily exchange with the adenine nucleotides present in other parts of the platelet (in mitochondria, bound to actin or free in the cytoplasm), which are in a ATP:ADP ratio of around 7.0 and which are referred to as the metabolic pool because they are the major source of the energy required for platelet functions.

Plasma Membrane

This contains a number of specific receptors, often glycoproteins (GPs), through which platelets interact with aggregating agents, inhibitors, coagulation factors and each other. In some instances, the GPs have been isolated and characterized and shown to influence a particular aspect of platelet function (Table 21.2). In other cases, their role remains undefined. The platelet membrane also contains phospholipids which are concerned with prostaglandin synthesis and calcium mobilization within the cell and the generation and localization of procoagulant activity on the outer surface of the platelet (see below).

Surface-connected Canalicular System

This is an extensive system of invaginations of the plasma membrane which serves to increase the surface area across which membrane transport can be effected and through which the products of the release reaction can more rapidly reach the outside of the cell.

Peripheral Band of Microtubules

These structures are generally regarded as the cell skeleton. They are contractile and during aggregation move towards the centre of the cell, entrapping many of the granules. The function of this 'central apposition' is not known, although it is thought that it may facilitate the release reaction.

Cytoplasmic Microfibrils

These are also composed of contractile proteins, some of which are attached to GP receptors which traverse the cell membrane providing a means through which the latter can thus influence intracellular events, such as pseudopod formation and secretion, which follow platelet activation.

Table 21.2
Some important platelet membrane glycoproteins

GP 1a	Collagen adhesion
GP 1b	Subendothelial microfibril adhesion; associated with the P1 E_1 antigen
GP IIb–IIIa	Fibrinogen binding, aggregation; associated with the P1 A_1 antigen
GP IV	Thrombospondin binding
GP V	Thrombin binding, aggregation
GP IX	Platelet adhesion; part of GP–1b complex

Dense Tubular System

This term is synonymous with the endoplasmic reticulum, which is thought to be the site of prostaglandin production and to be concerned with calcium flux within the platelet, both of which are directly involved with the release reaction and platelet aggregation.

Interactions of Platelets with the Vessel Wall

Platelet Adhesion

Platelets do not adhere to endothelial cells and this may be a consequence of the high local concentration of PGI_2, which binds to specific receptors on the platelet membrane, stimulating adenyl cyclase activity and causing a rise of intraplatelet cyclic adenosine monophosphate. This promotes calcium uptake by the dense tubular system and effectively reduces the free calcium concentration, thus inhibiting calcium-dependent functions such as release and aggregation (see below).

Platelets escaping from an injured blood vessel come into contact with and adhere to a number of tissues, in particular collagen and subendothelial microfibrils. The difficulty in obtaining the latter in a purified form and the use of non-vascular collagen for studying platelet adhesion have clouded our understanding of these reactions. However, it appears that although they have some features in common, the two reactions may require different cofactors (Fig. 21.4). Subendothelial microfibrils

bind the larger multimers of vWF and, through these, react with membrane GP Ib, this reaction being calcium ion dependent.

Following this, the platelet membrane GP IIb IIIa complex receptor becomes exposed and forms a secondary binding site with vWF, further promoting adhesion. The GP IIb–IIIa complex also binds fibrinogen through which platelet aggregation may occur. Thrombin binds to GP Ib and also to a closely associated glycoprotein (GP V). However, the former association is not critical, thrombin-induced platelet aggregation being normal in its absence (see Bernard–Soulier syndrome, Chapter 22). Another glycoprotein, GP IX, is also closely linked to GP Ib. It appears to have a stabilizing function and it is also reduced in Bernard–Soulier syndrome.

Adhesion to collagen involves interaction between platelet GP Ia and lysyl groups on the alpha chains of collagen. There is good evidence for an architectural requirement, the minimal structural unit being microfibrillar collagen. The initial process requires little in the way of cofactors, although collagen also contains binding sites for vWF and these may serve to anchor platelets to the collagen in a similar way to that described for subendothelial microfibrils.

Although precise mechanisms have not yet been elucidated, platelet adhesion induces a series of metabolic processes which are thought to initiate the shape change, release reaction and aggregation of platelets. The key response is the activation of

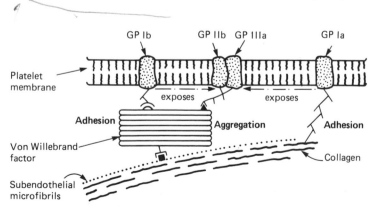

Fig. 21.4. *Platelet adhesion. The binding of GPIb to von Willebrand factor leads to adhesion to the subendothelium and also exposes the GPIIb/IIIa binding site to fibrinogen and von Willebrand factor leading to platelet aggregation (see text). The GPIa binding site permits direct adhesion to collagen.*

phospholipases A_2 (PLA_2) and C (PLC), and other enzymes which together stimulate prostaglandin metabolism and phosphoinositide turnover (see below).

The Platelet Shape Change

Within seconds of their adhesion to vessel wall components or, indeed, to non-physiological surfaces such as glass, platelets undergo a change in shape, becoming more spherical and putting out long, spiny pseudopods, which form the initial points of contact and enhance interaction between adjacent platelets. The shape change is accompanied by reorganization of the internal constituents of the platelet. The peripheral band of microtubules undergoes central apposition which has the effect of forcing the granules towards the plasma membrane, including that of the surface-connected canalicular system, thereby facilitating secretion of their contents. The cytoplasmic microfibrils also appear to depolymerize and then reform within the pseudopods. Later, contraction of these microfibrils may account for the process of clot retraction which helps consolidate the platelet plug.

Platelet Release Reaction

Immediately following their adhesion and shape change, platelets commence a specific release reaction which is sustained for several minutes and the intensity of which varies with the stimulus. Weak inducers, such as low doses of ADP or adrenaline, involve mainly the alpha granule contents, a proportion of which may even leak out from unstimulated platelets in citrated blood. Higher concentrations of ADP or adrenaline and low doses of collagen result in secretion from both alpha granules and dense bodies, while strong stimuli such as thrombin or high doses of collagen, cause release of lysosomal enzymes as well.

The extent to which these events are mirrored in vivo is unknown, although their physiological importance is substantiated by the fact that a deficiency, particularly of the dense bodies or their contents but also, to a minor extent, of the alpha granules, is associated with a clinical bleeding tendency (see Chapter 22). As mentioned above, the release reaction is accompanied by prostaglandin generation and phosphatidyl inositol turnover, both of which also probably contribute to platelet aggregation.

Prostaglandin Metabolism (see Fig. 21.2)

Arachidonic acid liberated by PLA_2 from membrane phospholipids, especially phosphatidyl choline and phosphatidyl ethanolamine, is converted enzymatically, via the cyclic endoperoxides, to thromboxane A_2 (TXA_2). This has a half-life of approximately 2 minutes in plasma and degrades spontaneously to thromboxane B_2 which is biologically inert.

Thromboxane A_2 has powerful vasoconstrictor activity, stimulates further release and induces platelet aggregation. Its importance is indicated by the fact that blocking its production with acetylsalicylic acid (which inhibits the action of cyclooxygenase) also prevents the release reaction. It has been suggested that blocking the action of thromboxane synthetase, with drugs such as hydralazine, might lead to a build-up of cyclic endoperoxides which could leak out of the platelets and thence be utilized by the endothelial cells for PGI_2 synthesis. This 'endoperoxide steal' hypothesis is unlikely to be of great significance since the endoperoxides themselves have aggregating activity and, in any case, can be converted within the platelet to other prostaglandins such as PGD_2, PGE_2 or PGF_2 alpha.

Phosphatidyl Inositol Metabolism

Phosphatidyl inositol (PI) turnover in platelets is stimulated by many of the known platelet agonists and may therefore represent the common pathway for the functional responses of these cells. The precise mechanisms involved are extremely complex and await clarification, but some important contributory events are illustrated in Fig. 21.5. The phosphatidyl inositol diphosphate (PIP_2) in the platelet membrane is cleaved by a specific phosphodiesterase, phospholipase C, yielding diacylglycerol (DG) and inositol triphosphate (IP_3). PIP_2 breakdown is induced by many platelet-aggregating agents including TXA_2 and requires guanosine triphosphate (GTP) whose effects are mediated by GTP-binding proteins (G proteins). Both IP_3 and

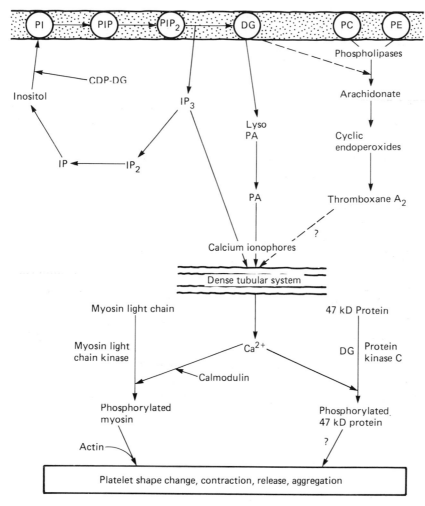

Fig. 21.5. *Some mechanisms involved in platelet activation and release.*

the lysophosphatidic acids (lyso-PA), formed when arachidonate is cleaved from DG and other phospholipids such as phosphatidyl choline (PC) and phosphatidyl ethanolamine (PE), are ionophores which mobilize calcium ions from the dense tubular system that activate myosin light chain kinase. This enzyme phosphorylates the light chain of myosin which then combines with actin to initiate the contractile events involved in the release reaction. Diacylglycerol is also a cofactor for protein kinase C, an enzyme which phosphorylates a 47 000 molecular weight cytoplasmic protein (47 kda protein) whose function is unknown. IP_3 is dephosphorylated to inositol which then combines with cytidine diphosphate-diacylglycerol (CDP-DG) to form phosphatidyl inositol (PI), this being phosphorylated to PIP_2, thus completing the cycle. Platelet activation is accompanied by the influx of calcium ions from the plasma through the calcium channels adjacent to the GP IIb–IIIa receptors and this may sustain or enhance the effects of internally released calcium. Many, if not all, of the effects of calcium ions on these reactions are mediated by the calcium-binding protein calmodulin. This cofactor forms a calcium-containing complex with the enzymes involved and modulates their activity.

There is growing evidence that the products of PI turnover may also participate in non-haemostatic platelet properties such as mitogenesis.

Platelet Aggregation

A wide variety of substances bind to platelets, often via specific receptors, and thereafter induce platelet aggregation or agglutination. Under physiological conditions, only ADP and TXA_2 are likely to reach the concentrations required to induce aggregation, and then only locally and transiently at points of vascular injury. Other agonists such as adrenaline, 5-HT, vasopressin or platelet-activating factor (1.0.alkyl-2 acetyl-sn-glyceryl-3-phosphoryl-choline), may influence aggregation in vivo by acting in an additive or synergistic fashion with ADP. Whatever the agonist, the binding of ADP and fibrinogen to their specific receptors is essential for platelet aggregation. Platelets possess two distinct ADP receptors: one modulates intracellular c-AMP level while the other is closely associated with, and governs the availability of, the fibrinogen receptor (the glycoprotein IIb–IIIa complex).

Although not yet fully defined, the sequence of events leading to platelet aggregation following vascular injury involves the following steps.

1. Release of ADP from damaged cells (including erythrocytes) or from platelets exposed to the sub-endothelium.

2. Binding of ADP to its receptors, resulting in configurational changes in the membrane which expose the GP IIb–IIIa complex, this stage being calcium dependent. Adenyl cyclase is inhibited and so the intracellular c-AMP level falls.

3. Binding of fibrinogen to the GP IIb–IIIa complex via at least three peptides, two on the alpha chain (both of which contain the sequence arg-gly-asp) and the third forming the last 12 amino acids at the carboxy terminal of the gamma chain.

Being a dimer, fibrinogen could thus form direct bridges between adjacent platelets or act as a substrate for the lectin-like protein thrombo-spondin released from activated platelets. In both cases, platelet–platelet interaction ensues, leading to platelet aggregation. Other physiological agonists may act by facilitating ADP binding or, in the case of thrombin, by a proteolytic action either directly on fibrinogen or indirectly on the ADP receptor.

Platelet aggregation causes activation of and release from other platelets and so a self-sustaining cycle of events is set up which results in the formation of a platelet plug at the site of injury.

Platelet Procoagulant Activities

Even after extensive washing, a number of coagulation factors remain associated with the platelets, either within the alpha granules or cytosol or tightly bound to the cell membrane. These include factor XI, factor V, fibrinogen, vWF and factor XIII (subunit a). Intact platelets have little or no intrinsic clot-promoting activity, but within seconds of the onset of aggregation and, to a lesser extent of adhesion, procoagulant activities directed at a number of stages of the coagulation cascade begin to develop on the platelet surface. This close association with the membrane is crucial for the localization of fibrin formation to the platelet plug which forms at the site of vascular injury.

The procoagulant activities of platelets can be classified into two groups: those concerned with contact factor activation and those involving the formation of complexes between coagulation factors and platelet phospholipids.

Platelets and Contact Factors

In the presence of ADP, but without the requirement for aggregation, platelets can activate factor XII directly. This reaction, which is cation independent but which requires kallikrein, is known as contact-product-forming activity. Platelets exposed to collagen, ADP or thrombin can activate factor XI directly, bypassing factor XII. This reaction, which is also cation independent, has been called collagen-induced coagulant activity and is thought to explain why patients with a deficiency of factor XII, prekallikrein or high molecular weight kininogen, do not suffer from a clinical bleeding tendency. In both cases, binding of factor XI to its receptors on the platelet surface ensures that the procoagulant activity remains localized to the platelet plug.

Phospholipid-related Platelet Procoagulant Activities

According to the classical cascade hypothesis of blood coagulation (see Fig. 21.8), there are two points at which complexes between coagulation factors and platelet phospholipids occur. For both, the initial event is an aggregation-evoked reorientation of the platelet membrane, which results in increased surface availability of those phospholipids with greatest clot-promoting activity, especially phosphatidyl serine and phosphatidyl choline. The coagulation cofactors (factors V and VIII) and the vitamin K-dependent coagulation factors interact with these, the former via specific receptors and the latter through calcium bridges between the phospholipids and gamma-carboxylated glutamic acid residues within the proteases (see later). As a result, because of propinquity and possibly also because they are protected from naturally occurring inhibitors such as antithrombin III and protein C (see later), clotting factor interaction is facilitated.

Both of the phospholipid-enhanced coagulation reactions are calcium ion dependent. The first, involving factors IXa, VIII and X, is denoted factor Xa-forming activity. The second, which was previously known as platelet factor 3, but is now more commonly referred to as prothrombinase activity, involves the interaction of factors Xa, V, and II.

FACTORS INVOLVED IN FIBRIN CLOT FORMATION

Of the dozen or so known blood coagulation factors, most have now been purified to homogeneity and in many cases the amino acid sequence has been determined and the gene located and characterized. Studies on the interaction of such purified factors have elucidated many of the biochemical changes occurring during coagulation and have enabled a useful working hypothesis to be formulated, although results obtained must be interpreted with caution since the purification procedures inevitably alter molecular structure. A list of the clotting factors found in humans, together with some of their characteristics, is shown in Table 21.3.

Many clotting enzymes, including all of the vitamin-K-dependent factors (factors II, VII, IX and X) and also factors XI, XII and prekallikrein,

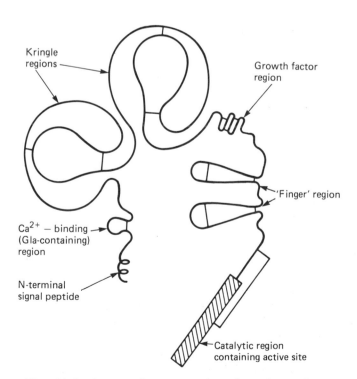

Fig. 21.6. *Structural representation of a serine protease.*

Table 21.3
Some characteristics of clotting factors in humans

Traditional name	Preferred nomenclature	Molecular weight	Plasma concentration (µg/ml)	Half-life (hours)	Gene/product		AAs
					Gene	Chromosome	
Fibrinogen	Factor I	340 000	$2-4 \times 10^3$	90	50 kb,	4	3026
Prothrombin	Factor II	72 000	120	65	21 kb	11p11–q12	579
Tissue factor	Factor III	300 000 +	0	—	—	1p21	263
Calcium	Factor IV	40	100	—	—	—	—
Pro-accelerin	Factor V	330 000	10	15	6.8 (cDNA)	—	2224
Proconvertin	Factor VII	48 000	1	5	12.8	13	406
Antihaemophilic factor	Factor VIII	360 000	0.05	10	190	Xq28	2332
Christmas factor	Factor IX	57 500	4	25	35	Xq26–27.3	415
Stuart–Prower factor	Factor X	55 000	12	40	25	13q34	445
Plasma thromboplastin antecedent	Factor XI	160 000	6	45	23	—	1214
Hageman factor	Factor XII	85 000	40	50	13.5	6	536
Fibrin-stabilizing factor	Factor XIII	320 000	20	200	90	6	2680
Fletcher factor	Prekallikrein	90 000	40	35	—	—	619
Fitzgerald factor*	High molecular weight kininogen	120 000	70	150	27	—	626

* Also known as Williams, Flaujeac and Reid factors.
† Chromosome number.
AAs, number of amino acids.

possess a serine residue at their 'active centre' and are known as serine proteases. They exist in plasma in precursor form and are converted to the active state in a sequential enzyme amplification process which has been called the cascade reaction. Serine proteases, including those of the fibrinolytic system (see later), have a high degree of homology and contain a number of characteristic structural domains (Fig. 21.6), such as the kringles which are concerned with binding to their substrate, or gla residues which bind, via calcium bridges, to phospholipid. Further regions of homology with fibronectin (the finger regions) or epidermal growth factor also occur. Other factors, such as high molecular weight kininogen, factor VIII and factor V, act as non-enzymatic cofactors to the serine proteases.

Synthesis of Coagulation Factors

Although small amounts of some clotting factors are synthesized in platelets, endothelial cells and in the spleen, the major site of production for almost all of them is the liver hepatocyte. The probable exception is factor VIII, which has been located in,

and is possibly synthesized by, the hepatic sinusoidal cells as well as in other organs.

Deficiency of vitamin K, whether caused by inadequate diet, malabsorption or drugs such as warfarin which act as vitamin K antagonists, is associated with a decrease of the functional activity of factors II, VII, IX and X. However, when these proteins are quantitated using gravimetric or immunological techniques, normal levels are found. These non-functional proteins are called 'proteins induced in vitamin K absence' (PIVKA). The conversion of PIVKA factors to their biologically active forms is a post-translational event involving carboxylation of the gamma carbon of a number of glutamic acid residues in the N-terminal region, where these factors show strong sequence homology. The gamma carboxylated glutamic acid, for which the notation gla is conventionally used, binds calcium ions through which it forms a complex with phospholipid. In the process of carboxylation, vitamin K is converted to vitamin K epoxide which is cycled back to the reduced form by reductases. Warfarin (possibly by acting as an alternative substrate for these reductases) prevents reoxidation, thereby leading to a functional vitamin K deficiency

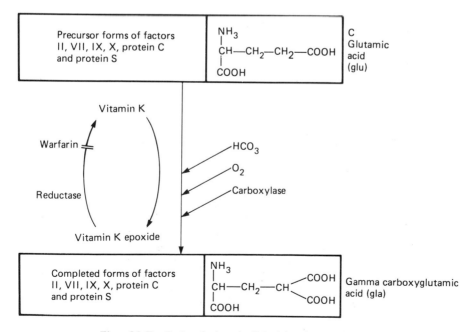

Fig. 21.7. *Role of vitamin K in blood coagulation.*

and subsequent formation of PIVKA factors. A simplified scheme of these reactions is shown in Fig. 21.7.

Factor VIII

Knowledge concerning the structure and function of this molecule was given a boost recently by the production of factor VIII by cloning procedures. It appears to be a single chain protein with a molecular weight of around 360 000 and comprising 2332 amino acids, although with several polymorphisms. Factor VIII is coded for by a 190-kb gene located on the long arm (q2.8 region) of the X chromosome. It circulates bound to vWF which protects it from non-specific proteolysis and may, through the ability of vWF to bind to platelet GP Ib, provide a means by which factor VIII activity can be localized on the platelet surface. Proteolysis of factor VIII by thrombin produces a number of peptides, the combined activity of two of which (mol. wts 93 000 and 80 000) markedly accelerates the activation of factor

X by factor IXa. Factor VIII procoagulant activity is to some extent stabilized by binding to phospholipid, but otherwise rapid decay occurs simultaneously with degradation of the 93 000 fragment caused by thrombin, either directly or via the naturally occurring inhibitor, activated protein C, or through the action of the fibrinolytic enzyme plasmin (see below). The molecular biology and proteolytic processing of factor VIII are examined in greater detail in Chapter 23.

Pathways to Blood Coagulation

An outline of the cascade reaction is shown in Fig. 21.8. Detailed examination of the molecular changes in individual factors is beyond the scope of this review, but some features of the system merit closer consideration.

As shown in Fig. 21.8, there are two pathways for the initiation of coagulation under physiological conditions. These are termed the intrinsic and extrinsic pathways, the latter requiring a tissue factor

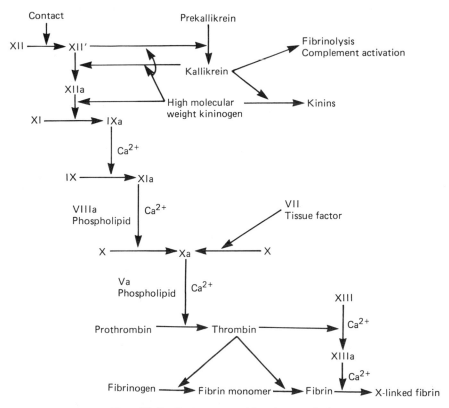

Fig. 21.8. *Pathways to blood coagulation.*

in addition to those in the plasma. Both converge on factor X, from which point they share a common route to fibrin formation. There are several links between the two pathways. The potent tissue factor extracts (such as those derived from brain) used for laboratory testing give a false impression of its physiological role in coagulation. Experiments with dilute preparations of tissue factor indicate that these have a catalytic or priming effect rather than bypassing the intrinsic factors completely. Clearly, since patients with severe deficiencies of factors from either pathway show similar clinical symptoms, both routes are important, and although it might be envisaged that in certain types of injury one or other of the two systems might predominate, there is no good evidence that this is so.

Intrinsic Pathway

The name reflects the notion that only components present in the plasma are involved. However, a major physiological activator of this system is sub-endothelial collagen, and some leucocytes, notably monocytes, contain tissue factor which, if released, may activate the extrinsic pathway. Moreover, it is likely that other extravascular factors enter the bloodstream via the lymphatics, and so the term 'intrinsic' is somewhat misleading.

Studies in vitro have shown the intrinsic pathway to be slow, the generation of factor Xa requiring minutes rather than the few seconds via the extrinsic route. Contributing to this delay are the greater number of procoagulants involved, the slow rate of activation of factors XII and XI, and the time

taken for the clot-promoting platelet phospholipids to become fully available.

Contact Activation

When plasma comes into contact with certain negatively charged foreign surfaces, a series of enzyme cascades is initiated, each contributing to the body's overall defence response to injury. Some of the systems involved are listed in Table 21.4. In each case, the initial stages appear to involve the same three factors, namely factor XII, prekallikrein and high molecular weight kininogen. It must be stated at the outset that it is doubtful whether this route of activation is of physiological significance, since severe congenital deficiency of any of these three factors is clinically asymptomatic with respect both to haemostasis and to the other systems involved. It appears likely that cellular mechanisms, including those mediated by the platelets, e.g. collagen-induced coagulant activity (see platelet section above), are able to compensate for or bypass the plasma deficiencies. Contact activation of blood coagulation involves factor XI in addition to the three factors mentioned above. Most studies on the mechanisms involved have utilized purified components and artificial activators such as kaolin or celite rather than more physiological ones found in the vessel wall. Nevertheless, a working hypothesis of the events involved can be formulated (Fig. 21.9).

Following contact with a foreign surface, factor XII undergoes limited proteolysis, generating modest enzymatic activity (factor XII') which slowly converts prekallikrein to kallikrein and activates factors XI and VII. In the presence of tissue

Table 21.4

Role of contact factors in integrating body defence mechanisms

Pathway involved	Function
Coagulation pathway	Prevention of blood loss
Fibrinolytic pathway	Maintenance of vascular patency
Complement pathway	Contributes to immune response
Kinin-generating pathway	Pain, capillary permeability, cardiovascular effects
Renin–angiotensin system	Blood pressure control
Chemotaxis	Phagocytosis, bacteriocidal activity

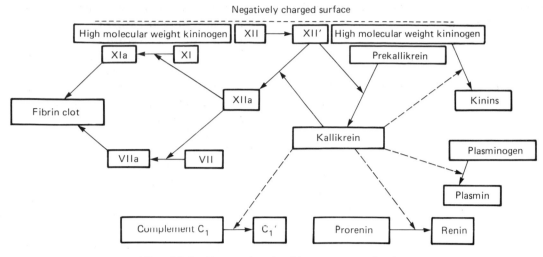

Fig. 21.9. *Factors involved in contact activation.*

factor, the activation of factor VII leads, via the extrinsic pathway (see below), to rapid generation of thrombin in trace amounts but sufficient to activate and increase the potency of factors VIII and V (see below). Kallikrein releases kinins from high molecular weight kininogen, stimulates fibrinolysis by acting as a plasminogen activator and amplifies the intrinsic pathway by reciprocally and fully activating factor XII to XIIa. The catalytic effect of kallikrein on contact activation is clearly demonstrated in the activated partial thromboplastin time of prekallikrein-deficient patients, where the prolongation found with a short (1–2 minutes) period of incubation with kaolin self-corrects with a longer activation time (10 minutes).

High molecular weight kininogen participates as a non-enzymatic accelerator of these reactions, probably through its ability to form a complex with the other contact factors, notably prekallikrein, to which it is found bound in the plasma, thereby drawing them into close spatial relationship and facilitating their interaction. Activated platelets express high affinity receptors for high molecular weight kininogen so that these early events too may be localized to the platelet plug at the site of vascular injury. Of some practical importance is the fact that the enzyme reactions up to the point of activation of factor XI do not require calcium ions and thus occur in citrated plasma, especially in glass containers.

Formation of Factor Xa via the Intrinsic Pathway

Factor IX is a vitamin K-dependent protein containing 12 Gla residues. It is coded for by a 35-kb gene in the q2.6 region of the X chromosome. The activation of factor IX by factor XIa involves two calcium-dependent proteolytic cleavages. Neither surface contact nor platelets promote this reaction although, because factor IX binds to phospholipids via its gla residues, the process is probably localized to the surface of activated platelets. Unlike most other serine protease reactions in the coagulation cascade, no cofactor participation has been identified. It was previously suggested that Passovoy factor may fill this role. However, this explanation now seems most improbable as it has recently been established that the Passovoy defect is due to the presence of a poorly defined coagulation inhibitor in the plasma of the index patient and that Passovoy factor does not exist.

The major substrate for factor IXa is factor X, which is converted to its active form (factor Xa) by cleavage of a single arg–isoleu bond. The reaction rate is physiologically insignificant in the absence of thrombin-activated factor VIII which increases the V_{max} 200 000-fold. The process is further enhanced by the formation of a calcium-dependent complex between factors IXa, VIII and X and the phospholipids exposed on the surface of activated platelets. This complex, which is known as factor Xa-forming activity (see p. 571), reduces the K_m for factor X to its concentration in plasma.

Extrinsic Pathway

The essential components of this pathway for formation of factor Xa are factor VII and tissue factor (factor III).

Factor VII

Uniquely, this factor expresses enzymatic activity in its native form, albeit only 1–2% of that present after its activation to factor VIIa. The innate activity of factor VII as well as that of factor VIIa is atypical in that it is not inhibited by physiological serine protease inhibitors such as antithrombin III (see later). Instead, factor VII activity is controlled by a specific extrinsic pathway inhibitor (mol. wt 35 000) which is associated with the plasma lipoprotein fraction and which, in the presence of calcium ions and factor Xa, reversibly inhibits the tissue factor–factor VII complex. Whether the intrinsic activity of factor VII is attributable to trace amounts of tissue factor in the circulation or whether it is related in any way to the very short half-life of factor VII in vivo is unclear. What is certain is that both factors VII and VIIa are inert in the absence of tissue factor.

As previously mentioned, conversion of factor VII to VIIa is initially brought about by factor XIIa. Once they have been generated, factors IXa, Xa and thrombin also effectively activate factor VII. Factors IX and X are natural substrates for factor VIIa, providing further examples of the reciprocal activation which so commonly amplifies the coagulation cascade.

Tissue Factor

This is an ubiquitous lipoprotein found in especially high concentration in brain, lung and placenta, all of which have been used to monitor the extrinsic pathway in the laboratory. The test used is the prothrombin time, for which most workers prefer to use internationally standardized preparations of rabbit or bovine brain in order to permit inter-laboratory comparison of results. Use of human brain, once widely advocated in the United Kingdom, has now been discontinued because of possible contamination with viruses causing acquired immunodeficiency syndrome or Creutzfeldt–Jacob syndrome.

Endothelial cells and monocytes contain tissue factor but only release significant amounts when pathologically stimulated, e.g. by endotoxin.

The protein component of tissue factor is apoprotein III, a glycoprotein with a molecular weight of around 43 000, which on its own is virtually inactive. Optimal activity is observed when it is combined with phospholipids, especially phosphatidyl ethanolamine-enriched preparations, in a phospholipid : protein weight ratio of around 450 : 1. Tissue factor has no intrinsic enzymatic activity, but it acts as a cofactor, increasing the catalytic activity of factors VII and VIIa which bind to apoprotein III, and complexing via its phospholipid component with factor X, thereby decreasing the K_m of the latter to within its physiological concentration. Both of these properties of tissue factor are calcium ion dependent and are in some ways analogous to that leading to factor X activation in the intrinsic pathway. Indeed, factor VII/VIIa cleaves factor X at the same site as does factor IXa, the product (factor Xa) being identical.

Factor Xa is a two-chain molecule which retains the N-terminal gla domain and hence remains associated with platelet phospholipids.

Final Common Pathway

Factor Xa converts factor II (prothrombin) to IIa (thrombin) in a reaction which has many similarities to that which resulted in its own generation. It is calcium dependent, takes place on the surface of activated platelets and involves an accelerator (factor V), the combination of factors being known as the prothrombinase complex.

Factor V is a large (mol. wt 330 000) single-chain glycoprotein which has little catalytic effect on prothrombin conversion until exposed to thrombin or factor Xa which cleave the molecule into four subunits, two of which are linked by calcium and possess biological (factor Va) activity. Factor Va binds via its heavy chain (mol. wt 105 000) to specific but, as yet, ill-defined receptors on the platelet surface and via its light chain (mol. wt 71 000) to factor Xa and prothrombin, both of which also interact with platelet phospholipids via their gla residues. The formation of this prothrombinase complex leads to a roughly 300 000-fold increase in the rate of thrombin generation.

The central role of thrombin in haemostasis is widely acknowledged. Apart from converting fibrinogen to fibrin and then stimulating factor XIII-mediated cross-linking of the clot, it induces platelet aggregation, activates factors V and VIII and then modulates the inactivation of these two cofactors by protein C. It also acts autocatalytically on prothrombin. The molecular events occurring during the latter reaction have been determined with some precision and indicate the means by which thrombin can control its own generation. The sequence of events is illustrated in Figure 21.10. Prothrombin is split by the Xa–Va complex into two pieces, prethrombin II and fragment 1.2, the

former being further cleaved, again by Xa–Va, into two-chain thrombin. Thrombin itself splits prothrombin between fragments 1 and 2, producing prethrombin I and fragment 1. Since fragment 1 contains the gla residues through which calcium-mediated binding to phospholipid is mediated, conversion of prethrombin I to thrombin is retarded. Factor Va binds to the fragment 2 region of prothrombin and may thus to some extent counteract the decrease in thrombin generation resulting from loss of fragment 1. Lacking the fragments concerned with binding to the prothrombinase complex, thrombin diffuses away and thus becomes more susceptible to neutralization by naturally occurring inhibitors in the plasma, or is free to form a protein C-activating complex with thrombomodulin on the surface of endothelial cells (see below).

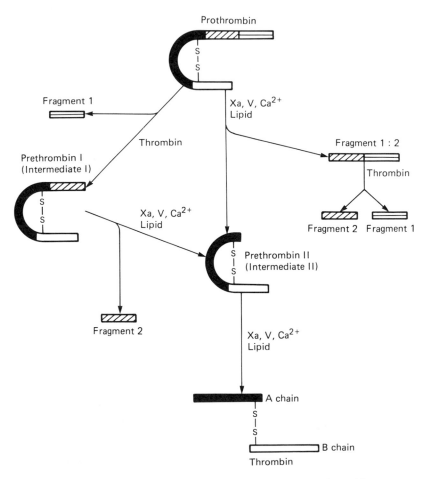

Fig. 21.10. *The conversion of prothrombin to thrombin.*

Structure of Fibrinogen

Fibrinogen is a dimeric glycoprotein with a molecular weight of around 340 000. It is composed of two identical subunits, each containing three dissimilar polypeptide chains denoted Aα, Bβ and γ, joined near the N-terminal by disulphide bonds (Fig. 21.11). The three genes which code for the separate chains occur in a 50-kb segment in the long arm of chromosome 4. The effect of thrombin, and also of the fibrinolytic enzyme plasmin (see below), on its complex structure can be more easily perceived if fibrinogen is viewed as a trinodular molecule, as shown in Figure 21.12.

Thrombin–Fibrinogen Reaction

Thrombin attacks the N-terminal end of fibrinogen and, by cleaving two arginine–glycine bonds, sequentially removes the first 16 amino acids from the

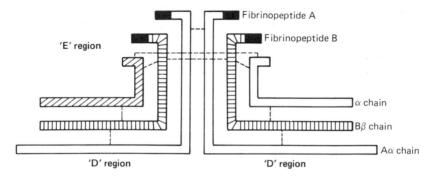

Fig. 21.11. *Simplified diagram of a fibrinogen molecule.*

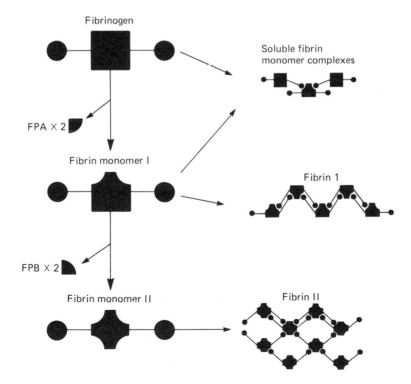

Fig. 21.12. *Polymerization of fibrin.*

α chain and the first 14 amino acids from the β chain, these being known as fibrinopeptides A (FPA) and B (FPB) respectively. Although the fibrinopeptides have a half-life of only a few minutes in vivo, their measurement by radioimmunoassay has been advocated as a sensitive indicator of low-grade intravascular coagulation.

Fibrinogen devoid of FPA is called fibrin monomer I, and removal of FPB as well produces fibrin monomer II. Fibrin monomers combine with each other, the fibrinopeptide-free N-terminal from one interacting with one of the two C-terminal ends of each of two adjacent molecules, and thus the fibrin strands elongate (Fig. 21.12). Provided that both FPA and FPB have been removed, the fibrin strands also grow laterally, increasing in tensile strength and giving the fibrin clot in plasma an opaque appearance. Conversely, if only FPA is removed—as is the case when fibrinogen is attacked by certain snake venom extracts, e.g. ancrod (Arvin)—only limited lateral growth occurs and the fibrin clots formed are friable, functionally ineffective and are translucent in plasma in vitro.

Soluble Fibrin Monomer Complexes

Fibrin monomers will also combine with fibrinogen itself and with small, plasmin-induced fibrinogen degradation products (FDP), forming complexes which, because they cannot polymerize normally, remain soluble in plasma and are known as soluble fibrin monomer complexes (SFMC). In practice, SFMC may be found when fibrin monomers are present but when the ratio of fibrinogen or FDP to fibrin monomers is very high, as can occur in hypercoagulable states. The SFMC can be split by substances such as protamine sulphate or ethanol (which are used to detect SFMC in the laboratory), allowing the monomers to polymerize in the usual way to form fibrin strands.

Stabilization of the Fibrin Clot

Until they have been cross-linked by factor XIIIa, fibrin clots are haemostatically ineffective, being susceptible to degradation by plasmin and other proteases. It can be seen from Figure 21.12 that as the fibrin strands develop, the C-terminal regions of adjacent monomers are brought into close pro-

ximity and it is through these regions that factor XIIIa-mediated cross-linking occurs.

Factor XIII is a tetrameric molecule composed of two similar pairs of non-covalently linked peptide chains, for which the notation a_2b_2 is commonly used. The a chains contain the active site (which is a cysteine rather than a serine) and are found free in platelets, from whence they are released following platelet activation. The b chains (sometimes referred to as S chains) are present in excess in plasma and may act as a carrier for the a chains. Native factor XIII is inert, but following exposure to thrombin, it undergoes a two-stage activation process. A small peptide is released from the a chains producing $a_2^*b_2$, but enzymatic activity does not develop until the a and b chains dissociate, the latter reaction being calcium dependent. In the absence of fibrinogen, the calcium concentration required for dissociation of a and b chains is unphysiologically high and thus the generation of factor XIIIa is limited by the concentration of its major substrate in plasma, i.e. fibrinogen.

Removal of the b chains reveals the a* chains, which have transamidase (factor XIIIa) activity that catalyses the formation of γ glutamyl–ε lysyl bonds between the γ carboxyl group of glutamine and the ε amino group of lysine residues in fibrin, particularly near the C-terminal of the γ chains but also to a lesser extent in the α chains. Cross-linking of fibrin clots imparts resistance to plasmin attack and increases their mechanical strength.

Factor XIIIa might also play an important role in tissue repair since it has been shown to catalyse cross-linking of fibrin to fibronectin and of the latter protein to collagen, a property which might explain the poor wound healing seen in patients with severe factor XIII deficiency.

NATURALLY OCCURRING INHIBITORS OF BLOOD COAGULATION

In common with many other defence mechanisms, such as those resulting in kinin release and complement activation, the blood coagulation process can be activated very rapidly when the need arises. As has been described above, this involves the generation of several proteolytic enzymes which are potentially lethal if their action is not limited in some way. For example, 10 ml of plasma can generate sufficient thrombin to clot all of the fibrinogen in the body in 30 seconds. That it does not normally do so is due in part to the fact that the haemostatic response is most pronounced in the vicinity of the platelet plug at the point of vascular injury, and also to the presence of substances in the blood which exhibit anticoagulant activity.

Classification of Anticoagulant Properties of Blood

In contrast to the procoagulant factors which were identified by Roman numerals only after recognition by an international nomenclature committee, the naturally occurring anticoagulant activities of blood, which were known as antithrombins, were originally classified numerically before their functional and biochemical characterization had been achieved. With the exception of the term 'antithrombin III', this system has fallen into disuse and current practice is to define them in terms of their substrate as either inhibitors of serine proteases or as inhibitors of activated cofactors. All of these inhibitors are effectively brought into play before the process of fibrin deposition has commenced and thus assume great physiological significance.

In addition, there are some other inhibitory mechanisms which do not fit into either of the above categories. Amongst these is the detoxifying property of the liver, which plays an important role in removal of activated clotting factors both directly and after their combination with inhibitors (see below). Furthermore, removal of free thrombin

occurs as a result of its adsorption onto polymerizing fibrin or onto fibrin(ogen) degradation products (FDP) which cannot themselves clot but which may interfere with fibrin polymerization. These last two mechanisms were previously referred to as antithrombins I and VI respectively. They appear to be physiologically important because structural defects of fibrinogen which result in reduced thrombin binding are associated with a thrombotic disorder (see Chapter 24).

Serine Protease Inhibitors

Human plasma contains at least six inhibitors of serine protease coagulation factors (Table 21.5). Though having fairly low specificity, these inhibitors vary in their affinity for different substrates. Only those such as antithrombin III (AT III) and heparin cofactor II, which act predominantly on proteases generated late in the coagulation cascade, i.e. thrombin and factor Xa, assume physiological significance. A deficiency of any of the others, though sometimes giving rise to a clinical disorder due to failure of neutralization of a serine protease not involved in coagulation pathways, is asymptomatic in terms of haemostasis. As mentioned above, AT III has little or no inhibitory action on factor VIIa.

Except when there is severe (pathological) activation of coagulation, these anticoagulants are jointly more than capable of protecting the body against unwanted fibrin deposition. Each millilitre of plasma is able to neutralize 750 i.u. of thrombin,

Table 21.5

Some characteristics of inhibitors of procoagulant serine proteases

Inhibitor	Molecular weight	Plasma concentration (µg/ml)	Half-life (hours)	Major substrate	Other substrates
Antithrombin III	58 000	250	60	IIa, Xa	IXa, XIa, XIIa
Heparin cofactor II	66 000	80	?	IIa	—
Alpha$_1$ antitrypsin	55 000	2500	96	XIa, Xa	Plasmin
C$_1$ esterase inhibitor	105 000	180	40	KK, XIa	XIa
Alpha$_2$ antiplasmin	70 000	70	60	Plasmin	KK, XIIa, XIa
Alpha$_2$ macroglobulin	725 000	2500	240	KK	IIa

KK = kallikrein.

which is more than twice the amount that can be generated in that volume.

Antithrombin III

AT III is a single-chain glycoprotein with a molecular weight of around 61 000, which is synthesized by the liver and by endothelial cells and has a half-life of 2.8 days, this being decreased somewhat (to 2.1 days) in the presence of heparin. The mean level of AT III in plasma is approximately 250 μg/ml. It forms a stable, 1:1 stoichiometric complex with all serine protease coagulation factors except factor VII, whereby the serine at the active centre of the protease cleaves a peptide bond near the carboxy terminal of AT III, revealing an arginine residue which interacts with and, probably by steric hindrance, inhibits the action of the protease. Complex formation is progressive, the half-life of free thrombin being around 35 seconds in vitro. The affinity of AT III for other proteases is lower, the half-life of factor Xa being around 90 seconds and between 10 and 25 minutes for factors XIIa, XIa and IXa in purified systems. In all cases, the inhibitor–protease complex is rapidly removed from the circulation by the liver. The physiological importance of AT III is substantiated by the observation that a modest reduction in the circulating level is associated with an increased risk of venous thrombosis (see Chapter 25).

Heparin, without altering the 1:1 stoichiometry, induces a 2300-fold increase in the rate of thrombin inactivation by AT III such that its action becomes almost instantaneous (half-life = < 1 second). For this reason, AT III is sometimes referred to as heparin cofactor I.

Heparin and Heparin-like Substances in Blood

The heparins belong to the group of sulphated mucopolysaccharides known as glycosaminoglycans. The richest sources of heparin are the mast cells found in bovine lung and hog intestinal mucosa, extracts of which are used for commercial preparations. Only about one-quarter of the subfractions of heparin have any anticoagulant activity. The remaining material may be responsible for some of the side-effects of the molecule, the most important of these being heparin-induced thrombocytopenia which sometimes has an immune aetiol-

ogy and which may occasionally cause arterial thrombosis or lead to a disseminated intravascular coagulation-like syndrome (see Chapter 25).

Heparins exhibit considerable structural and functional heterogeneity. Separation on the basis of molecular weight yields fractions ranging from molecular weight 4000 to 40 000 which differ in their affinity for the plasma factors with which they interact and in the specific serine proteases which they inhibit. These two considerations influence not only anticoagulant activity as monitored by laboratory tests, but also the antithrombotic and haemorrhagic manifestations of heparin. In general, high molecular weight fractions (> 15 000) have a greater effect on thrombin neutralization and carry a higher risk of haemorrhagic complications than low molecular weight fractions (< 10 000) which have predominantly antifactor Xa activity, even when the protease is present as part of the prothrombinase complex. However, antithrombotic effects seem to be related more to antithrombin than to antifactor Xa activity. The clinical use of different heparin fractions is discussed further in Chapter 25.

The molecular weight of heparin also affects its metabolism, the half-life of high molecular weight fractions being about 60 minutes compared to 140 minutes for the low molecular weight group. This can be partly explained by the more effective neutralization of the former by platelet factor 4.

Mechanism of Action of Heparin

By virtue of its strong positive charge, heparin combines non-specifically with a number of cationic proteins such as albumin, but it also reacts in a highly specific way with betalipoproteins, fibrinogen, AT III and heparin cofactor II (see below). Heparin binds to lysyl or tryptophan residues in AT III, inducing a conformational change in the inhibitor as a result of which the reactive arginine residue becomes more readily able to combine with and inhibit the serine active centre of thrombin and other serine protease clotting factors. Following such interactions, heparin dissociates from the complex and may then react with fresh AT III.

With respect to thrombin inhibition, an alternative or additional mode of action for heparin is that it combines directly with the thrombin, rendering it more susceptible to neutralization by AT

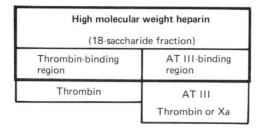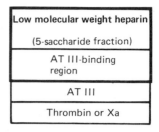

Fig. 21.13. *Interaction of heparin and AT III.*

III. This theory might explain the observation that an 18-saccharide fragment in heparin is needed for maximal thrombin-neutralizing activity, whereas only a pentasaccharide is needed for inhibiting factor Xa. A diagrammatic representation of the anticoagulant action of heparin is shown in Figure 21.13.

Though of significance when considering the clinical use of heparin, the above discussions are of limited relevance to normal haemostasis since there is no detectable heparin in circulating plasma. However, heparin-like molecules (e.g. dermatan sulphate and heparan sulphate) have been found on the surface of endothelial cells and, by enhancing the action of AT III and heparin cofactor II, these would have antithrombotic effects. Such a mechanism seems to be of clinical importance since recurrent thromboses have been reported in association with several dysfunctional AT III molecules which inhibit thrombin normally in the absence of heparin but which do not show enhanced reactivity in its presence, presumably due to defects at the heparin-binding sites.

At points of vascular injury, local accumulation of activated platelets provides a source of heparin-neutralizing activity (PF4) which could overcome the anticoagulant effects of endothelial cell-bound heparinoids and permit normal haemostasis to occur.

Heparin Cofactor II

This is a single-chain glycoprotein, molecular weight 66 000, which is present in plasma in a concentration of around 80 μg/ml. It appears to be a specific inhibitor of thrombin, with which it forms a 1:1 stoichiometric complex, and to have little or no anti-factor Xa activity. The rate of thrombin neutralization by heparin cofactor II is increased approximately 1000-fold by heparin, although this requires five to ten times more heparin than does AT III. Dermatan sulphate, a heparin-like substance found on endothelial cells, also strongly enhances heparin cofactor II activity, as does chondroitin sulphate. The latter, however, is without effect on AT III and can thus be utilized in assays for heparin cofactor II.

That heparin cofactor II has some physiological significance is suggested by the fact that it falls in parallel with AT III in disseminated intravascular coagulation (DIC). However, since AT III is in a threefold molar excess over heparin cofactor II, the latter cannot altogether compensate for a deficiency of AT III, which, as stated above, is associated with a thrombotic tendency. Whether or not a reduction in heparin cofactor II leads to a similar clinical picture remains to be established, since few cases have yet been described and only occasionally has concomitant thrombotic disease been present.

Alpha$_1$-antitrypsin

This is a single-chain glycoprotein whose primary substrates are pancreatic and leucocyte proteases. It is responsible for about 70% and 50% respectively of the factor XIa and Xa neutralizing activity in plasma. However, it has little effect on thrombin inhibition and a deficiency of alpha$_1$-antitrypsin is not associated with hypercoagulability. It has considerable sequence homology with AT III, and an abnormal molecular form of alpha$_1$-antitrypsin, known as antithrombin III Pittsburgh, has been described which has a high affinity for thrombin and which gives rise to a clinical bleeding tendency.

C_1 *Esterase Inhibitor*

The primary substrate of this single-chain glycoprotein is the activated form of the first component of complement. It is also the major inhibitor of kallikrein and factor XIIa and contributes in a minor way to neutralization of factor XIa and plasmin. It forms a 1 : 1 stoichiometric complex with the serine active centre of all of these proteases but its action on the contact factors may be offset somewhat by their prior binding to high molecular weight kininogen. Deficiency of C_1 esterase inhibitor is without effect on the haemostatic system although it causes angioneurotic oedema, the characteristic lesions of which may sometimes be confused with haematomas.

Alpha₂ Antiplasmin

This single-chain glycoprotein is the principal inhibitor of the fibrinolytic enzyme plasmin. It also has weak activity against several coagulation proteases, especially the contact factors. Its mechanism of action and clinical importance are discussed further in the section on fibrinolysis below.

Alpha₂ Macroglobulin

This large glycoprotein (mol. wt 725 000) is composed of four identical chains and is unique in that its effects are not restricted to serine proteases. It binds to coagulation factors (especially thrombin and kallikrein) at a site away from the serine active centre, the interaction involving the formation of a bond between a glutamyl residue in the inhibitor and a lysyl group in the protease. Inhibition is produced by steric hindrance rather than by inactivation and, indeed, the protease retains some esterolytic and amidolytic activity, particularly against small peptides, a fact which should be borne in mind when using chromogenic substrates to assay coagulation inhibitors.

The possibility of thrombotic complications associated with the sustained, low-grade bioactivity of protease–alpha₂ macroglobulin complexes is minimal since these are rapidly removed from the circulation by the liver. Nevertheless, at sites of injury and inflammation, where the acidic conditions (pH < 5.0) enhance their effects, such protease–alpha₂ macroglobulin complexes could represent an important mechanism for retaining procoagulant activity in a controlled fashion, the protease being protected from more potent inhibitors such as AT III.

A deficiency of alpha₂ macroglobulin is not associated with a thrombotic tendency. It is, however, an acute phase reactant and it is possible that, when elevated under conditions of stress, or when the other major antithrombins or antiplasmins are overwhelmed, it might become a significant inhibitor of coagulation or fibrinolysis. Moreover, it has been suggested that the raised level of alpha₂ macroglobulin which exists in children, may compensate for a low level of AT III and explain why thrombotic episodes do not usually occur before puberty in congenitally AT III-deficient patients.

Inhibition of Coagulation Cofactors

The activated forms of coagulation cofactors (factors VIIIa and Va) are potent procoagulants, which enhance the interaction of the serine protease factors in ways which were described earlier. It is not unexpected, therefore, that these cofactors should themselves be subject to some kind of negative feedback mechanism which limits their activity. For many years, this was thought to be due to the direct proteolytic action of thrombin on factors VIIIa and Va, but it is now known to be more complex than was envisaged and to involve a number of additional proteins which together make up the protein C system. The five factors which have thus far been shown to participate in these reactions are protein C, protein S, C4B-binding protein, thrombomodulin and activated protein C inhibitor (Table 21.6). A second inhibitor of activated protein C has also recently been described, although its clinical significance is, as yet, uncertain.

Interactions Between the Components of the Protein C System

There has been intense investigation of the reactions involved in this pathway as a result of the probable association between deficiencies of protein C or S and thrombotic disease (see Chapter 25). However, many studies to date have utilized reagents and experimental conditions which are non-physiological and must therefore be interpreted

Table 21.6
Some characteristics of components of the protein C system

Component	Molecular weight	Plasma concentration (μg/ml)	Half-life (hours)	Further information
Protein C	62 000	4	6	Neutralizes Va and VIIIa, enhances fibrinolysis. Gene on chromosome 2
Thrombomodulin	68 000	0*	?	Potentiates action of thrombin on protein C
Protein S	69 000	35†	?	Promotes protein C binding to platelet phospholipids. Geneon chromosome 3
Activated protein C inhibitor	57 000	5	?	Inhibits protein C
C4B-binding protein	550 000	160	?	Binds protein S in an inactive form

* Thrombomodulin is bound to endothelial cells.
† Includes protein S bound to C4B-binding protein.

cautiously. An outline of the system as it is presently perceived is shown in Figure 21.14.

Protein C

This vitamin-K-dependent serine protease is a two-chain molecule comprising a light chain (mol. wt 22 000) that carries the Gla residues and a heavy chain (mol. wt 40 000) containing the active serine centre. It is so named because it was present in the third of four peaks (peaks A, B and D containing factors IX, II and X respectively) eluted from a chromatography column used to separate the vitamin-K-dependent factors. Like these, protein C can be removed from plasma by adsorption onto

$Al(OH)_3$. In order to exert its anticoagulant and fibrinolytic effects, protein C must first be activated. This is achieved by the action of thrombin which cleaves the heavy chain to reveal the active site serine, a process which is slow in the absence of thrombomodulin. In low concentrations, the light chain of factor Va also accelerates thrombin-induced cleavage of protein C, although high levels are inhibitory.

Thrombomodulin

This factor is found tightly bound to vascular endothelial cells in many body tissues, from which it can be extracted, the usual sources being rabbit

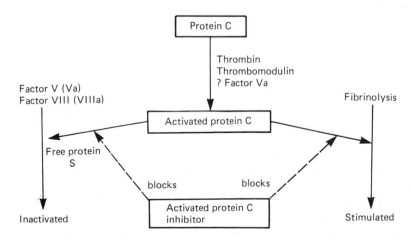

Fig. 21.14. *Protein C pathway.*

lung and human placenta. Although present in the blood vessels supplying the brain, it is uniquely absent from the endothelial cells in the brain itself. Thrombomodulin forms a 1:1 stoichiometric complex with thrombin through which it induces a several thousand-fold increase in the rate of activation of protein C and a concomitant loss of clotting activity. The process is calcium dependent. This change in the substrate specificity of thrombin (from fibrinogen to protein C) means that it effectively becomes an anticoagulant rather than a procoagulant. The factor V and VIII-cleaving and platelet-aggregating properties of thrombin are also lost following its binding to thrombomodulin. Protein C is also activated by a component in the venom of the southern copperhead snake (*Agkistrodon contortrix contortrix*) and this forms the basis of a simple bioassay for protein C.

Activated protein C rapidly degrades the heavy chain of factor V and the biologically active 93 000 molecular weight subunit of factor VIII. The active forms of these cofactors (factors Va and VIIIa) are more susceptible than their native forms to such attack, and the process is enhanced about 15-fold by protein S.

In addition to the above effects, protein C blocks the action, or the release from endothelial cells, of the fast-acting inhibitor of plasminogen activator (PAI-1), the consequences of this being increased plasminogen activator potential and, possibly, enhanced fibrinolysis. Whether this property of activated protein C requires protein S as a cofactor or, indeed, if it has any physiological significance, is uncertain, although evidence is accumulating that a raised level of PAI-1 suppresses fibrinolysis and is sometimes associated with, and may be the cause of, a thrombotic tendency.

Protein S

This single-chain glycoprotein, named after the city of Seattle where it was discovered, is also vitamin K dependent and adsorbed by $Al(OH)_3$, but is not a serine protease. It is chiefly synthesized in the liver but also by endothelial cells. About 40% of the protein S in plasma is in the free form and, though having no direct inhibitory effect on factors VIII and V, this is available to form a calcium-dependent complex with activated protein C on phospholipids exposed on the surface of activated platelets. The remaining 60% of the protein S in plasma is found attached in a 1:1 stoichiometric complex with the C4B-binding protein (which regulates the activity of the C4 component of complement) and cannot react with protein C. The C4B-binding protein is an acute phase reactant and it is likely that raised levels would disturb the equilibrium between free and bound protein S, leading to a fall in the free (biologically active) form, which might result in a thrombotic tendency. Free protein S falls during pregnancy (see Table 21.8) and in females receiving oestrogen supplements, but whether this results from a rise in C4B-binding protein, or if it contributes to the hypercoagulability of pregnancy, is disputed. Total protein S, like other vitamin-K-dependent factors, is reduced in the newborn, levels as low as 20% of adult values being common. However, this is compensated for by a marked reduction in C4B-binding protein (5–20% of adult levels) so that a relatively normal level of functional (free) protein S is maintained.

Activated Protein C Inhibitor

It is logical to suppose that activated protein C, like other serine proteases, should be subject to some form of inhibitor-mediated control. Such an inhibitor has been described. This single-chain glycoprotein has several features in common with AT III, though being immunologically different from it. It progressively blocks the action of its substrates (activated protein C and, to a lesser extent, thrombin and factor Xa), in each case forming a 1:1 inhibitor:protease stoichiometric complex. Its action is enhanced 20-fold by heparin but not by dermatan sulphate, and therefore this observation is unlikely to be of physiological significance. It is not adsorbed by $Al(OH)_3$ and so this manoeuvre can be used as a means of separating protein C from its major inhibitor prior to assay.

The hypothesis that a deficiency of the inhibitor would permit activated protein C to degrade factors V and VIII in an uncontrolled way seemed to be supported initially by finding low levels of activated protein C inhibitor in stored plasma from several unrelated patients with a combined factor V and VIII deficiency. However, this explanation seems unlikely to be wholly, if at all, correct since it is now known that the inhibitor is extremely labile, even in frozen plasma, and that assays must be performed and interpreted with great caution.

FIBRINOLYSIS

It is generally acknowledged that the fibrinolytic system plays an important role in removing fibrin from intravascular and extravascular sites. Moreover, it is becoming increasingly apparent that aberrations of the fibrinolytic response can have catastrophic clinical consequences in terms of both haemorrhagic and thrombotic events (see Chapters 23 and 24). Despite this, fibrinolysis has remained the poor relation of haemostasis in general, with only an occasional attempt being made by clinicians to interfere with the course of nature and few laboratories willing to undertake any but the simplest tests, e.g. fibrin(ogen) degradation product (FDP) assay. The two main reasons for these shortcomings have been, firstly, the difficulty in reconciling the results of time-consuming laboratory tests with the rapidly changing clinical condition of the patient, and, secondly, the lack of safe, effective therapeutic materials with which to treat fibrinolytic disorders. However, simple, rapid assays for components of the fibrinolytic system, based on chromogenic substrates, have now been developed and synthetic t-PA produced by recombinant DNA technology has recently become available. Together with clarification of the physiological and pathological mechanisms involved in fibrin degradation, these advances have enabled clinicians to treat fibrinolytic disorders more effectively, less empirically and with more comprehensive laboratory support than was hitherto the case.

Components of the Fibrinolytic System

These include plasminogen, plasminogen activators, anti-activators and antiplasmins (some characteristics of which are shown in Table 21.7), as well as the products of fibrin degradation. Although enzymes derived from leucocytes (e.g. elastase) contribute in a minor way to clot lysis, by far the most important route is fibrin degradation induced by plasmin, the inactive precursor of which is plasminogen.

Plasminogen and Plasmin

Plasminogen is a single-chain polypeptide, molecular weight 92 000, containing 790 amino acids. Its plasma concentration is around 200 μg/ml (i.e. approximately 2 μmol/l). It contains five homologous, looped structures, known as kringles, four of which have a 'lysine-binding site' through which the molecule interacts with lysine residues in its substrates (e.g. fibrin) and its inhibitors. In its native form (Fig. 21.15) it has a glutamic acid residue at its N-terminal end and is known as glu-plasminogen.

Table 21.7
Some characteristics of components of the fibrinolytic system

Component	Molecular Weight	Plasma concentration (μg/ml) (molarity)		Half-life	Gene	Gene/product Chromosome	AAs
Plasminogen	92 000	200	2 μmol/l	50 h	21 kb,	6	796
Tissue plasminogen activator	68 000	0.005	70 pmol/l	5 min	>20 kb,	8	530
Urokinase	54 000	0.008	150 pmol/l	6 min	6.4 kb,	10	411
tPA inhibitor type 1	52 000	0.05	1 nmol/l	?	15 kb	7	379
tPA inhibitor type 2	70 000	0.005	100 pmol/l	?	—	—	—
Alpha$_2$antiplasmin	70 000	70	1 μmol/l	75 h	—	—	452
Histidine-rich glycoprotein	75 000	100	1.3 μmol/l	?	—	—	507
Alpha$_2$macroglobulin	725 000	2500	3 μmol/l	?	—	12	1451

* C = chromosome.
AAs = amino acids.

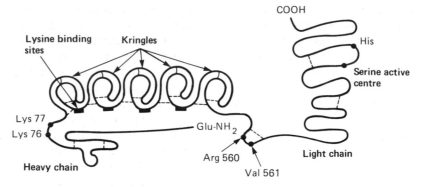

Fig. 21.15. *Diagrammatic representation of a plasminogen molecule.*

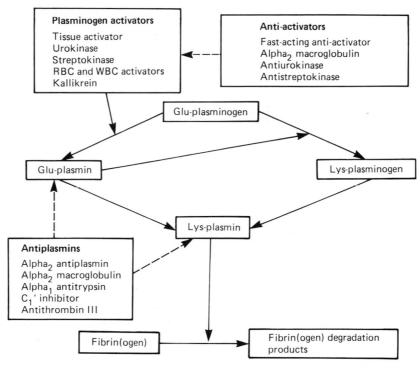

Fig. 21.16. *The fibrinolytic pathway.*

Conversion of plasminogen to plasmin can proceed via two routes (Fig. 21.16). Most plasminogen activators (see below) cleave the arg_{560}–val_{561} bond to form glu-plasmin, which has two chains joined by a single disulphide bridge. The heavy chain is derived from the N-terminal and bears the lysine-binding sites, while the C-terminal light chain contains the serine active centre. Glu-plasmin, despite being a serine protease, is functionally ineffective since its lysine-binding sites remain masked. It is converted to lys-plasmin autocatalytically by cleavage, chiefly between lys_{76} and lys_{77}, which exposes the lysine-binding sites and thus markedly enhances its interaction with fibrin. Both glu-plasmin and lys-plasmin attack the lys_{76}–lys_{77} bond in glu-plasminogen to form lys-plasminogen. This binds to fibrin before it develops protease activity and is thus brought into close proximity with the physiological plasminogen activators (which may themselves bind to fibrin) that convert it to lys-plasmin. These events serve to localize the fibrinolytic response to the fibrin clot where plasmin is to some extent protected from the effects of circulating antiplasmins which, as indicated below, would otherwise neutralize plasmin extremely rapidly (< 50 milliseconds). The fact that lys-plasminogen is potentially a much more effective fibrinolysin than glu-plasminogen is reflected in its half-life, which is around 20 hours, compared to 50 hours for the latter.

Plasminogen Activators

These can be broadly divided into three categories according to their origin.

Intrinsic (Blood) Activators

Intrinsic (blood) activators are those derived from the plasma and the blood cells. As has been previously discussed, fibrinolytic activity is generated during the contact activation stage of blood coagulation, and is generally attributed to kallikrein. Although deficiencies of any of the contact factors result in an impairment of surface-enhanced fibrinolysis in vitro, there appear to be few, if any, clinically important sequelae of this. Erythrocytes and granulocytes also synthesize plasminogen activators which may be released in certain pathological states, although their physiological importance is uncertain.

Tissue-type Plasminogen Activators

These are synthesized in virtually every organ of the body, except the liver, and are found in low concentration in many body fluids including plasma, saliva, milk, bile, cerebrospinal fluid and urine. The two best-characterized tissue activators are vascular activator (commonly called tissue plasminogen activator, or simply t-PA) and urokinase. There is great current interest in the former since, as mentioned earlier, genetically engineered t-PA is now becoming available for clinical use (see also Chapter 25).

Human t-PA is a single-chain glycoprotein with molecular weight of around 65 000, which is synthesized by endothelial cells where, under resting conditions, it mainly remains stored. Any which does leak into the plasma is quickly cleared by the liver or inactivated by the fast-acting t-PA inhibitor (see below), the half-life of t-PA being approximately 2 minutes. The resting level of t-PA in plasma is around 5 ng/ml, most of which is in an inactive complex with t-PA inhibitors (see below).

A number of physical and biochemical stimuli, including venous occlusion, strenuous exercise, thrombin, adrenaline and vasopressin or its analogues such as DDAVP (see Chapter 23), markedly increase the rate of t-PA release, although its biological activity remains negligible until it becomes bound to fibrin, whereupon its affinity for and action upon plasminogen are greatly potentiated. The effect of t-PA is further enhanced by plasmin itself which cleaves t-PA into a two-chain molecule whose binding sites are exposed, thus enabling it to form a complex with plasminogen and fibrinogen more readily. The ability of venous occlusion to stimulate t-PA release from endothelial cells forms the basis of a test of fibrinolytic activity known as the cuff test (see Appendix, p. 597).

Urokinase

Urokinase is a serine protease, the native form of which is pro-urokinase, a single-chain polypeptide with molecular weight of 54 000. The principal site of production of pro-urokinase is the kidney (hence its name) but it is also synthesized in small amounts in many other organs and by endothelial cells. It is, however, immunologically distinct from t-PA. Pro-urokinase is cleaved by plasmin or thrombin to two-chain urokinase, which attacks the arg_{560}–val_{561} bond in plasminogen, as described above. The protease activity of urokinase is associated with the heavy chain (mol. wt 33 000) which may dissociate from the light chain which carries the plasminogen-binding site. The isolated heavy chains, which are also known as low molecular weight urokinase, therefore have weaker plasminogen-activating activity than the two-chain form.

Exogenous Plasminogen Activators

Exogenous plasminogen activators are those derived from non-human sources, including animals (e.g. the saliva of the vampire bat and the venom of some snakes) and certain plants and micro-organisms. The best known of these is streptokinase, which is derived from some strains of beta-haemolytic streptococci and which has for many years been used, with moderate success, for the treatment of life-threatening thrombotic states (see Chapter 25). Streptokinase is a non-enzymatic polypeptide, molecular weight 47 000, which forms a stable, 1:1 stoichiometric complex with plasminogen, as a result of which the latter undergoes a conformational change, unmasking its serine active centre. The plasmin which is formed remains associated with the streptokinase but can convert free plasminogen to plasmin.

The main problem with streptokinase in clinical use is that the streptokinase–plasmin(ogen) complexes are rapidly removed from the circulation so that continuous or repeated administration of large doses of streptokinase is required. This creates difficulties in controlling therapy and frequently results in systemic fibrinolysis, and marked hypofibrinogenaemia with the attendant high risk of bleeding. The problem is compounded by the antigenicity of streptokinase and the fact that most people have fluctuating levels of anti-streptokinase antibodies consequent upon previous streptococcal infections.

Inhibitors of Fibrinolysis

The plasmin-generating potential of plasma is sufficient to degrade all of the fibrinogen in the body completely in a very short period of time. It is prevented from doing so by a number of circulating inhibitors of plasmin itself and/or the plasminogen activators.

Inhibitors of Plasminogen Activators

The most important of these appears to be the recently described specific, fast-acting t-PA inhibitor (PAI-1), a 52 000 molecular weight glycoprotein which is synthesized by endothelial cells. Its plasma concentration is low and, in the presence of activated protein C, is decreased still further, thus effectively promoting fibrinolysis. The precise mechanisms involved in these reactions have not yet been defined. A second t-PA inhibitor (PAI-2) is produced by the placenta and this may contribute

to the inhibition of fibrinolysis which occurs during pregnancy.

Other protease inhibitors, such as $alpha_1$ antitrypsin, C_1 esterase inhibitor, $alpha_2$ antiplasmin and $alpha_2$ macroglobulin, also neutralize t-PA, but at a rate which is too slow to be of physiological significance. $Alpha_2$ macroglobulin is, however, thought to be the major inhibitor of the streptokinase–plasminogen complex.

Inhibitors of Plasmin

As with thrombin, a number of the broad spectrum inhibitors contribute to plasmin neutralization (see Fig. 21.16). By far the most potent of these is $alpha_2$ antiplasmin, a single-chain glycoprotein with a molecular weight of 70 000 which shows considerable sequence homology with antithrombin III and $alpha_1$ antitrypsin. Its physiological importance is supported by the fact that a congenital deficiency is associated with a clinically significant bleeding disorder due to uncontrolled fibrinolytic activity and that levels are reduced in DIC and during thrombolytic therapy. It is synthesized in the liver, has a half-life of about 60 hours and a plasma concentration of around 80 μg/ml (approximately 1 μmol/l).

$Alpha_2$ antiplasmin forms a stable, 1:1 stoichiometric complex with plasmin in which the plasmin is completely inactivated. The reaction appears to involve the cleavage by plasmin of a specific leucine–methionine bond in the inhibitor, whose lysine-binding sites are thereby exposed. It then interacts with, and neutralizes, plasmin by the formation of a bond between the newly exposed leucine group and the serine active centre on the light chain of plasmin. Plasmin-modified $alpha_2$ antiplasmin can also bind to plasminogen and to fibrin, the latter reaction being reinforced by factor XIIIa-mediated cross-linking. Thus, in addition to inactivating plasmin, $alpha_2$ antiplasmin retards fibrinolysis by masking the lysine-binding sites through which plasminogen interacts with fibrin.

The plasma concentration of plasminogen (*c.* 2 μmol/l) exceeds that of $alpha_2$ antiplasmin (*c.* 1 μmol/l) so that, in certain pathological conditions where extreme activation of fibrinolysis occurs, the latter may be swamped. Under these circumstances, other inhibitors, in particular $alpha_2$ macroglobulin and histidine-rich glycoprotein, may become clinically important. The action of alpha$_2$ macroglobulin on plasmin is similar to its effect on thrombin. Following the plasmin-induced cleavage of a specific arginine–leucine bond in the inhibitor, the latter forms a 1:1 molecular complex with the light chain of plasmin. The serine active centre of plasmin is not involved and the complex retains weak biological activity, albeit only briefly until it is removed by the liver.

Histidine-rich glycoprotein has a molecular weight of around 75 000, a half-life of 70 hours and a plasma concentration of approximately 100 μg/ml (1.5 μmol/l). It inhibits fibrinolysis by blocking the lysine-binding sites of plasminogen, thus preventing its interaction with fibrinogen.

Action of Plasmin on Fibrin(ogen)

Plasmin hydrolyses arginine and lysine bonds in a variety of substrates including factors V and VIII, casein, gelatin and some arginine or lysine esters. Its major physiological effect, however, is on fibrin and fibrinogen, which are split progressively into a heterogeneous mixture of small peptides (plasmin attacks at least 50 cleavage sites in fibrinogen)

known collectively as fibrin(ogen) degradation products (FDP). A simplified scheme of these reactions is shown in Figure 21.17. The first stage in the proteolysis of fibrinogen involves the removal of several small peptides (fragments A, B and C) from the C-terminal of the Aα chains, each involving cleavage of a lysine bond. This is rapidly followed by removal of the first 42 amino acids from the N-terminal end of the Bβ chain. The large residual portion, which is known as fragment X and still contains fibrinopeptide A, remains thrombin clottable and will agglutinate some species of *Staphylococcus*. Assay of the Bβ 1–42 fragment released from fibrinogen by plasmin gives a sensitive index of fibrinogenolytic activity.

Asymmetrical digestion of all three chains then occurs, with the release of the D-fragment in which the chains remained linked by disulphide bonds. The residue, known as fragment Y, is again attacked by plasmin, cleaving a second fragment D and leaving the disulphide-linked N-terminal ends of all six chains, which are referred to as fragment E. Fragments Y, D and E are not thrombin clottable and do not agglutinate staphylococci. Their presence can be detected immunologically using a latex

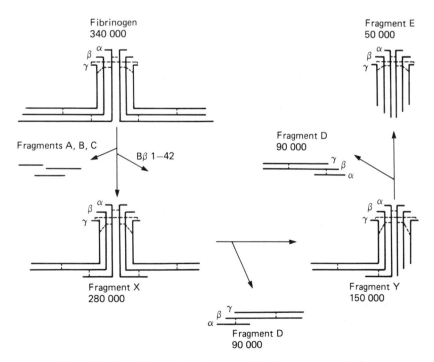

Fig. 21.17. *Schematic diagram of fibrinogen degradation.*

agglutination assay, which provides a simple test for most FDPs.

Degradation of non-cross-linked fibrin produces virtually identical products, but inter- or intramolecular transamidation of the γ or α chains by factor XIIIa yields characteristic D-dimer and D-dimer-E fragments and oligomers of fragments X and Y, in addition to X, Y, D and E. Furthermore, cleavage of the N-terminal of the β chain of fibrin produces a 15–42 fragment, the 1–14 fragment (fibrinopeptide B) having been previously removed by thrombin. Assays for cross-linked FDPs and for fragments $B\beta$ 1–42 and β 15–42 are available and these may prove to be clinically useful by providing information about whether fibrinogen or fibrin has been degraded, hence suggesting whether any fibrinolytic process is primary or secondary.

HAEMOSTATIC CHANGES DURING PREGNANCY AND IN THE NEONATE

Considerable fluctuation in the levels of individual haemostatic factors can occur in normal healthy subjects, due either to physiological variability, e.g. age, sex, racial origin, blood group or hormonal influence, or secondary to some environmental factor, such as diet, smoking habits, ambient temperature or even noise. This must be taken into account when interpreting the results obtained in patients being investigated for bleeding or thrombotic disorders.

Detailed consideration of such factors is beyond the scope of this chapter and, for a comprehensive review, the reader should refer to the excellent monograph by Ogston (see references).

Table 21.8
Haemostasis during pregnancy

Platelet count	No consistent change
Platelet volume	Slight progressive increase
Platelet aggregation	Progressive enhancement; functional defects may show clinical improvement
Fibrinogen	Marked progressive rise (up to 4 × basal)
Factor II	No consistent change
Factor V	No consistent change
Factor VII	Progressive rise (up to 3 × basal)
Factor VIII	Marked progressive rise (up to 5 × basal)
von Willebrand factor	Marked progressive rise (up to 10 × basal)
Factor IX	Variable but no consistent change
Factor X	No consistent change
Factor XI	Progressive fall (to around half basal)
Factor XII	No consistent change
Factor XIII	Progressive fall (to around half basal)
AT III	No consistent change
HC II	No consistent change
α_1 antitrypsin	Progressive rise (up to 3 × basal)
α_1 macroglobulin	No consistent change
Protein C	No consistent change
Protein S	Progressive fall (to around half basal)
C4b-binding protein	No consistent change
Plasminogen	Progressive rise (up to 3 × basal)
t-PA	No consistent change
α_2 antiplasmin	Progressive rise (up to 3 × basal)
t-PA inhibitor	Marked progressive rise (up to 5 × basal)
FDP	Slight increase
Fibrinopeptide A	Progressive rise (up to 3 × basal)
Euglobulin lysis time	Progressive prolongation (up to 6 × basal)

Haemostasis during Pregnancy

There is considerable individual fluctuation, and many of the changes observed are related to the stage of gestation, becoming more pronounced as pregnancy progresses. Some of the haemostatic changes associated with normal pregnancy are presented in Table 21.8. Platelet responsiveness and the levels of some coagulation factors increase, whereas fibrinolysis is somewhat impaired and some coagulation inhibitors are reduced. Overall, this leads to a mild hypercoagulable state which may contribute to the increased incidence of venous thrombosis during pregnancy.

Haemostasis in Neonates

In general, haemostasis is slightly impaired in the newborn, largely due to the immaturity of the liver. The vitamin-K-dependent factors are particularly susceptible, and prophylactic administration of vitamin K (1 mg, intramuscularly) to all neonates is advocated by many clinicians. Although adult

Table 21.9

Haemostasis in the neonate

Platelet count	Similar to adult
Platelet volume	Similar to adult
Platelet aggregation	Unresponsive to adrenaline; variable but often reduced with ADP, collagen, arachidonate; normal or enhanced with ristocetin
Fibrinogen	Similar to adult; fetal fibrinogen present
Factor II	30–50% of adult level; normal by 1–3 months
Factor V	Similar to adult
Factor VII	30–50% of adult level; normal by 1 month
Factor VIII	Variable; 50–200% of adult level
von Willebrand factor	Usually raised (up to 3 × adult level)
Factor IX	20–50% of adult level; normal by 1 month
Factor X	30–50% of adult level; normal by 1 month
Factor XI	20–50% of adult level; normal by 1 year
Factor XII	20–50% of adult level; normal by 3 months
Factor XIII	50–100% of adult level; normal by 1 month
Prekallikrein	20–50% of adult level; normal by 3 months
High molecular weight kininogen	50–100% of adult level; normal by 3 months
AT III	50–80% of adult level; normal by 6–12 months
HC II	30–50% of adult level; normal by 6 months
C_1E inhibitor	50–100% of adult level; normal by 1 week
α_1 antitrypsin	Up to 2 × adult level; normal by 12 months
α_2 macroglobulin	Up to 2 × adult level; normal by puberty
Protein C	30–50% of adult level; normal by 3 months
Protein S	30–50% of adult level; normal by 3 months
C4b-binding protein	5–30% of adult level; normal by 6 months
Plasminogen	30–80% of adult level; normal by 2 weeks
t-PA	Normal or slightly raised
α_2 antiplasmin	Up to twice adult level; normal by 3 months
t-PA inhibitor	?
FDP	Up to 20 μg/ml; normal by 1 week
Euglobulin lysis time	Usually shortened

levels of some factors are not achieved for many months (Table 21.9), most healthy, non-premature infants are haemostatically competent within a week or two of birth.

SELECTED BIBLIOGRAPHY

Berridge M. J. (1984). Inositol triphosphate and diacyl-glycerol as second messengers. *Biochemical Journal*, **220**, 345–360.

Bloom A. L., Thomas D. P. (Eds.) (1987). *Thrombosis and haemostasis*, 2nd edn. Edinburgh: Churchill-Living-stone.

Colman R. W., Hirsh J., Marder V. J., Salzman E. W. (Eds.) (1987). *Haemostasis and thrombosis*, 2nd edn. Philadelphia: Lippincott.

Furie B., Furie B. C. (1988). The molecular basis of blood coagulation. *Cell*, **53**, 505–518.

Holmsen H. (1985). Platelet metabolism and activation. *Seminars in Hematology*, **22**, 219–240.

Hutton R. A. (1987). Chromogenic substrates in haemo-stasis. *Blood Reviews*, **1**, 201–206.

Mullertz S. (1987). Fibrinolysis. General aspects, charac-teristic features and perspectives. *Fibrinolysis*, **1**, 3–12.

Ogston D. (1983). *The physiology of haemostasis*. London: Croom Helm.

Triplett D. A. (1985). *Haemostasis: A case-oriented ap-proach*. New York: Igaku-Shoin.

Verstraete M., Vermylen J., Lijnen R., Arnout J. (1987). *Thrombosis and haemostasis 1987*. Leuven: Leuven University Press.

Appendix

Some tests of haemostatic function

Test	Abbreviations	Factors involved	Comments
Activated partial thromboplastin time (kaolin-cephalin clotting time)	APTT, PTTK KCCT	I, II, V, VIII, IX, X, XI, XII, prekallikrein. high molecular weight kininogen	Measures intrinsic system and common pathway factors. Forms the basis of one-stage clotting factor assays
Kaolin clotting time	KCT	As above	Using platelet-rich plasma, the KCT also measures PF3a
Recalcification time	RCT	As above	Wide normal range due to variable activation of contact factors
Whole blood clotting time	WBCT	As above + platelets	Wide normal range due to variable activation of platelets and contact factors
Thromboplastin generation test	TGT	V, VIII, IX, X, XI, XII	Largely replaced by APTT. Forms the basis of the two-stage assay of factors VIII and IX and the anti-VIII inhibitor assay
Prothrombin consumption index	PCI	V, VII, VIII, IX, X, XI, XII	Measures residual prothrombin in serum at a fixed interval after coagulation of whole blood. Rather insensitive (see WBCT)
Prothrombin time (Quick's method)	PT(Q)	I, II, V, VII, X	Measures extrinsic and common pathway factors
Prothrombin time (Owren's method)	P & P*	II, VII, X	Prothrombin and proconvertin (factor VII). Designed for oral anticoagulant control

Appendix (continued)
Some tests of haemostatic function

Test	Abbreviations	Factors involved	Comments
Thrombotest	—	II, VII, X, ?IX	Designed for oral anticoagulant control. Venous or capillary whole blood used in test. Sensitive to PIVKA (see text)
Thrombin time	TT	I	Also sensitive to FDPs, fibrin monomers, abnormal fibrinogens and heparin; basis of Clauss fibrinogen assay
Reptilase time	—	I	As TT but unaffected by heparin. Uses venom of *Bothrops atrox*
Arvin time	—	I	As TT but unaffected by heparin. Uses venom of *Agkistrodon rhodostoma*
Stypven time	SVT	I, II, V, X	Measures common pathway factors. Can be modified to measure PF3a. Uses venom of Russell's viper (*Vipera russelli*)
Clot solubility test	—	XIII	Measures solubility of clot in 5 mol/l urea or 1% monochloracetic acid
Ethanol gelation test	—	Soluble fibrin monomer complexes	May also measure fibrinogen–fibrin degradation product complexes
Protamine sulphate test	—	Soluble fibrin monomer complexes	Also measures fibrinogen–fibrin degradation product complexes
Staphylococcal clumping test	—	Large fibrinogen/fibrin degradation products fibrinogen	Measures fragments X and Y but not D and E. Uses serum

Appendix (continued)

Some tests of haemostatic function

Test	Abbreviations	Factors involved	Comments
FDP tests (e.g. Thrombowellcotest, Diagen FDP test)	FDP	Fibrinogen/fibrin degradation products, fibrinogen	Measures most FDP/fdps. Immunological method. Uses serum
Dimertest	XDP	Cross-linked fibrin degradation products	Uses citrated plasma
Euglobulin lysis time	ELT	Plasmin, plasminogen activators	Largely unaffected by antiplasmins but fibrinogen and plasminogen as substrates are required
Venous occlusion test (cuff test)	—	Vascular plasminogen activators	Tissue ischaemia due to occlusion may cause severe pain
Bleeding time (Duke, Ivy, Template)	BT	Platelet count. Platelet function. Vascular integrity. vWF	Widely used screening test of platelet numbers and function
Platelet aggregometry	—	Platelet function, vWF	Reagents used include ADP, adrenaline, collagen, ristocetin and arachidonic acid
Platelet–glass bead adhesion test	—	Platelet adhesiveness and aggregability + vWF	Non-specific test of platelet function and of von Willebrand factor
Platelet factor 3 availability assay	PF3a	Platelet adhesion, aggregation and coagulant activity	Non-specific test of platelet function (*see* KCT and SVT)
Clot retraction	CR	Platelet aggregability and coagulant activity	Non-specific and insensitive test of platelet numbers and function

*P & P = prothrombin and proconvertin.

Chapter 22

PLATELET DISORDERS

R. M. HARDISTY

An adequate number of normally functioning platelets is essential not only for the arrest of haemorrhage after obvious vascular injury, but also to prevent the leakage of red cells from apparently uninjured vessels. Failure of these two aspects of haemostasis is expressed respectively by a prolonged bleeding time and the spontaneous appearance of purpuric lesions—both hallmarks of platelet disorders. It is conventional and convenient to consider these under the general headings of thrombocytopenia, thrombocytosis, and abnormalities of function. In adopting this practice here, it must be pointed out that such a classification is not mutually exclusive: in many disorders involving platelet number, both hereditary and acquired, the platelets are also functionally defective. In chronic renal disease, for example, as well as in thrombocythaemia, haemorrhage may be attributable to both types of abnormality.

The commonest symptoms and signs of haemorrhage in the platelet disorders are of purpuric type: spontaneous skin purpura and ecchymoses, bleeding from mucous membranes, particularly the nose, multiple small subcutaneous bruises and menorrhagia. Purpura is most often seen on the legs, at flexures and pressure points and in relation to scratch marks. Large spreading haematomata are rare, and haemarthroses hardly ever occur. Conjunctival and retinal haemorrhages are common in severe cases, and vitreous haemorrhages may also occur. The most serious complication, and the most important cause of death, is intracranial haemorrhage, and massive gastrointestinal bleeding may also threaten life. Bleeding from superficial cuts and grazes tends to be prolonged—as expressed in a semiquantitative manner by the bleed-ing time—and in severe cases bleeding is apt to occur from venepuncture and injection sites.

THROMBOCYTOPENIA

Pathogenesis

Thrombocytopenia occurs when platelets are lost from the circulation faster than they can be replaced by the bone marrow. It may therefore result from a failure of platelet production, an increased rate of removal from the circulation, or a combination of both mechanisms. A pathogenetic classification of the thrombocytopenias is presented in Table 22.1, but this must be recognized as an oversimplification in that more than one mechanism often operates. In viral infections, for instance, aggregation and destruction of circulating platelets by the virus itself, or by antigen–antibody complexes, may combine with failure of platelet production, as a result of infection of the megakaryocytes, to produce acute transient thrombocytopenia; in chronic lymphocytic leukaemia, defective platelet production may be associated with the presence of autoantibodies against the circulating platelets, and also with excessive platelet pooling in an enlarged spleen; again, the diminished survival of platelets in some of the hereditary thrombocytopenias is a direct consequence of their structural abnormality, and thus of the underlying defect of production. Nevertheless, a classification of this sort is useful as an aide-mémoire, and has the practical advantage of being related to the bone marrow findings: in thrombocytopenia due chiefly to defective platelet production, the megakaryocytes tend to be reduced in number, while in the other categories their numbers are usually normal or increased. Besides helping to appraise the mechanism of the thrombocytopenia in this way, examination of the marrow may, of course, establish its cause by identifying the underlying disease. Unless the cause is obvious, bone marrow aspiration forms an essential part of the investigation of thrombocytopenia.

Table 22.1
Thrombocytopenia: pathogenetic classification

Defective platelet production
Bone marrow aplasia
  Hereditary, acquired
Metabolic disorders
  Megaloblastic anaemias
  Uraemia
  Alcoholism
  Drugs
Megakaryocyte abnormalities
  TAR syndrome
  Hereditary thrombocytopenias
  Dyshaemopoiesis (preleukaemia)
  Virus infections
Bone marrow infiltration
  Leukaemias, lymphomas
  Myeloma
  Carcinomatosis
  Myelofibrosis
  Osteopetrosis

Diminished platelet survival
Immune mediated
  Platelet alloantibodies
    Neonatal
    Post-transfusion purpura
    Antilymphocyte globulin
  Platelet autoantibodies
    Idiopathic thrombocytopenic purpura
    Evans' syndrome
    Following bone marrow transplantation
  Other mechanisms
    Systemic lupus erythematosus, other
      autoimmune disorders
    Malaria
    AIDS-related thrombocytopenia
    Infectious mononucleosis
    Other virus infections
    Lymphoproliferative disorders
    Drug induced

Excessive platelet consumption
  Disseminated intravascular coagulation
  Giant haemangioma
  Microangiopathic processes
    Haemolytic–uraemic syndrome
    Thrombotic thrombocytopenic purpura
    Prosthetic heart valves, etc.
  Extracorporeal circulations

Structural platelet defects
  Hereditary thrombocytopenias

Loss of platelets from the systemic circulation
Massive or exchange transfusion
Splenomegaly

Thrombocytopenia seldom results in abnormal bleeding until the platelet count falls below about $80–100 \times 10^9/l$. With lower counts, there is no very close relationship between the number of platelets and the severity of symptoms, but spontaneous haemorrhage is to be increasingly expected as the count falls below about $50 \times 10^9/l$, and is usual in the $10–20 \times 10^9/l$ range. This variability of effect is presumably due partly to differences in various aspects of platelet function, some of which may be related to platelet age and therefore turnover rate, and partly to variation in the integrity of vessel walls and their supporting tissues. The bleeding time, particularly if measured by a well-standardized technique such as the template method, correlates rather more closely with the platelet count, and is usually progressively prolonged as this falls below $100 \times 10^9/l$ as a result of a defect of platelet production. In the immune thrombocytopenias, when there is a rapid platelet turnover with many young forms in the circulation, the bleeding time is relatively less affected. A persistently long bleeding time in the presence of a relatively normal platelet count calls for an investigation of platelet function (see below).

From the point of view of clinical awareness and diagnosis, it is appropriate to consider the many causes of thrombocytopenia in three separate age groups—the newborn infant, the child and the adult—since the chief causes differ widely between them.

Neonatal Thrombocytopenia

The normal range of platelet counts in newborn infants, whether full-term or premature, is slightly lower than in older children and adults, being between $100 \times 10^9/l$ and $300 \times 10^9/l$. Lower counts than this may lead to purpuric lesions, but it must also be remembered that localized crops of petechiae are very common in normal infants at birth, particularly over the presenting part, as a result of mechanical compression of veins during delivery. A platelet count should always form part of the investigation of more generalized purpura or when other haemorrhagic signs are present.

The chief causes of neonatal thrombocytopenia are listed in Table 22.2, and some of them are further discussed below. It will be seen that many of them, whether hereditary or due to intrauterine influences or complications of delivery, produce well-recognized syndromes of which the thrombocytopenia is only a part.

Table 22.2
Neonatal thrombocytopenia

Intrauterine infections
    Rubella, cytomegalovirus, herpes simplex
    Toxoplasmosis
    Syphilis
Platelet antibodies
    Autoimmune: maternal ITP and SLE
    Alloimmune: fetomaternal incompatibility
    Drug induced
Disseminated intravascular coagulation
    Maternal pre-eclampsia
    Hypothermia, asphyxia, shock, sepsis
    Rh isoimmunization
    Necrotizing enterocolitis
Congenital megakaryocytic hypoplasia
    TAR syndrome
    Maternal drug ingestion
Hereditary thrombocytopenias
    Wiskott–Aldrich syndrome
    May–Hegglin anomaly
    Others
Giant haemangioma
Congenital and neonatal leukaemia and histiocytosis
Metabolic disorders: hyperglycinaemia, methyl-
    malonic acidaemia, etc.
Post-exchange transfusion

Intrauterine Infections

Thrombocytopenia occurs as part of the congenital rubella syndrome in 40–80% of cases, its incidence varying between epidemics. It is usually associated with one or more of the other features, which include low birth weight, congenital heart disease, hepatosplenomegaly, cataracts, deafness and hepatitis. Purpura is maximal on the first day of life and disappears during the first weeks, requiring no specific treatment. Thrombocytopenic purpura of similar duration is seen in about 50% of cases of congenital cytomegalovirus (CMV) infection, and occasionally in congenital toxoplasmosis and syphilis. In all these conditions, and also in generalized herpes simplex of the newborn, thrombocytopenia may result at least partly from disseminated intravascular coagulation (DIC), sometimes being associated with deficiency of factors V and VIII and fibrinogen. Hypoplasia of the megakaryocytes has also been reported in the congenital rubella syndrome.

Immune Thrombocytopenias in the Newborn

Infants born to mothers with idiopathic thrombocytopenic purpura (ITP; see p. 606) are likely to be thrombocytopenic at birth, even when the mother is in remission following splenectomy. The condition in the infant is due to the passive transfer across the placenta of IgG platelet autoantibodies which are not group specific. Infants of mothers with systemic lupus erythematosus (SLE) may be similarly affected. Alloimmune thrombocytopenia may occur in infants of healthy mothers, due to group-specific immunization of the mother against fetal platelet antigens, in a manner analogous to the red-cell antibody production responsible for haemolytic disease of the newborn. The platelet antigen Pl^{A1} is implicated in about half the cases, antibodies being formed by mothers who belong to the 2% of the population who are Pl^{A1} negative against the platelets of their Pl^{A1}-positive infants. Other platelet-specific and histocompatibility (HLA) antigen systems have also been involved; in the latter case, the resulting thrombocytopenia is usually less severe.

Infants suffering from immune thrombocytopenia are otherwise healthy, though they are obviously at risk of serious internal haemorrhage from birth injury. Generalized purpura or ecchymoses appear within a few hours of birth, and gastrointestinal or umbilical haemorrhage may also occur. In the absence of serious haemorrhage, the condition is self-limiting, the platelet count eventually rising when the titre of maternal antibodies in the infant's plasma falls; this usually takes 3–4 weeks, but the thrombocytopenia may last as long as 3 months. In the occasional case of alloimmune thrombocytopenia severe enough to require treatment, platelet concentrates may be prepared from the mother and transfused to the infant; the use of maternal whole blood or platelet-rich plasma should be avoided in order not to increase the titre of antiplatelet antibodies in the infant's circulation. Transfusion of maternal platelets will, of course, not be applicable to infants of women with ITP or SLE, but here exchange transfusion may have a place, with the aim of removing antibodies rather than raising the platelet count directly. Corticosteroids have often been used empirically for the first few days of life; though they clearly cannot be expected to influence the underlying cause, they may inhibit the removal of antibody-coated platelets from the circulation. Good results have also been claimed for intravenous immunoglobulin therapy. In the case of maternal ITP, treatment of the mother with prednisone (10–20 mg/day for 1–2 weeks before and during delivery), or with intravenous immunoglobulin, has been found to be effective in protecting the infant from serious thrombocytopenia. Particular care should obviously be taken during delivery when the mother is known to have ITP or to have borne a thrombocytopenic infant previously, and caesarean section is probably advisable.

Drug-induced immune thrombocytopenia (see below) may also be transmitted from mother to infant when both drug and antibody cross the placenta: quinidine and tolbutamide have been implicated in this way.

Disseminated Intravascular Coagulation in the Newborn

This condition, in which thrombocytopenia plays an essential part, is considered in more detail in Chapter 24. It must be mentioned here in order to contrast its clinical presentation with that of other causes of neonatal thrombocytopenia. It occurs in seriously ill infants in association with hypoxia, birth asphyxia, hypothermia and shock. Prematurity, sepsis, Rh isoimmunization, preeclampsia and premature separation of the placenta are other predisposing factors, and DIC may also complicate necrotizing enterocolitis. Unlike infants with immune thrombocytopenia, therefore, these infants present as acute emergencies in which the bleeding disorder is often not the most urgent problem. Besides the low platelet count, there is prolongation of the prothrombin and thrombin times, low plasma fibrinogen and raised fibrinogen degradation products. Red-cell fragmentation will usually be seen on the blood film. Replacement therapy, and possibly heparin, may be indicated, but prompt attention to resuscitation and the treatment of the underlying disease are the overriding considerations.

Thrombocytopenia with Absent Radii (TAR Syndrome)

The striking combination of neonatal purpura with bilateral absence of the radii characterizes a syndrome in which thrombocytopenia is due to profound hypoplasia or aplasia of the megakaryocytes, but red-cell and white-cell production are not depressed. Indeed many of these infants have a leukaemoid blood picture, with high leucocyte counts. Various other skeletal abnormalities may also be present, and congenital heart defects are found in about one-third of cases.

Purpuric bleeding is typically first observed in the neonatal period, and nearly half of these infants die within the first few months of life, often of cerebral haemorrhage. For those who survive the first year, however, the prognosis is surprisingly good, the platelet count tending to rise as the child becomes older, with a corresponding decrease in the severity of symptoms. Platelet transfusions may be useful in the management of serious bleeding episodes, but no form of treatment has been found to influence platelet production. The aetiology is obscure: there is no convincing evidence for a genetic origin, and intrauterine environmental influences may be responsible. In contrast to Fanconi's anaemia, cytogenetic abnormalities have not been found.

Wiskott–Aldrich Syndrome

This is an X-borne recessive trait characterized by thrombocytopenia, eczema and an immunological disorder affecting both cellular and humoral immune mechanisms and resulting in recurrent infections. All the clinical features usually occur during the first year of life, and purpura and rectal haemorrhage are commonly seen in the neonatal period. The thrombocytopenia is due to impaired production of small, functionally defective platelets, which have a short lifespan. The bone marrow usually contains normal numbers of megakaryocytes, and does not distinguish the condition clearly from others in which thrombocytopenia is due chiefly to diminished platelet survival. The diagnosis can seldom be made in the newborn unless the male infant has an affected elder brother; later on, it rests on the appearance of the other components of the syndrome. The untreated condition is commonly fatal within the first few years of life, usually from infection but occasionally from haemorrhage.

Bone marrow transplantation is the treatment of choice if a histocompatible sibling donor is available; in contrast to severe combined immunodeficiency, cell-mediated immunity is not completely deficient, so that immunosuppressive priming of the recipient is necessary. In boys without a sibling donor, a few successful transplants of haploidentical parental marrow have been recorded, but the early claims of improvement on treatment with transfer factor have not been substantiated. Splenectomy has been found to result in a significant improvement in platelet number, survival and function in most patients, and the increased susceptibility to infection can be effectively overcome by the use of prophylactic antibiotics on a long-term basis. Corticosteroids have no place in the management of the thrombocytopenia.

Other hereditary forms of thrombocytopenia more commonly present in infancy or childhood than in the newborn period and are considered below.

Giant Haemangioma (Kasabach–Merritt Syndrome)

Massive, often rapidly enlarging, haemangiomata lead to thrombocytopenia as a result of excessive platelet consumption in the course of thrombus formation within the tumour. Fibrinogen and factors V and VIII are also often depleted, so that the condition represents a subacute or chronic form of DIC. The syndrome may be apparent at birth, or develop as the tumour enlarges in early infancy. The haemangioma is usually obvious, involving a large area of the body surface, but may be confined to deeper structures (e.g. spleen, liver). The haemostatic defects can be temporarily corrected by heparin therapy, but permanent correction depends on regression of the tumour, whether spontaneous or in response to prednisone, radiotherapy or surgical removal. Management of the individual case depends primarily on the anatomical site and behaviour of the tumour: eventual spontaneous regression can be expected in most instances.

Thrombocytopenia in Childhood

The causes of thrombocytopenia in childhood (Table 22.3) include some of those (Wiskott–Aldrich syndrome, giant haemangioma) which may present at or soon after birth, and have therefore been considered above, and others (leukaemia, splenomegaly, drugs) which are seen at all ages. The

Table 22.3
Thrombocytopenia in childhood

Idiopathic thrombocytopenic purpura
  Acute
  Chronic
Acute leukaemias
Bone marrow aplasia
  Hereditary (Fanconi's anaemia)
  Acquired
Hereditary thrombocytopenias
  Wiskott–Aldrich syndrome
  Bernard–Soulier syndrome
  May–Hegglin anomaly
  Others
Haemolytic–uraemic syndrome
Acute viral and rickettsial infections
Septicaemia, purpura fulminans
Giant haemangioma
Splenomegaly
Cyanotic congenital heart disease
Chronic relapsing thrombocytopenia
Osteopetrosis

commonest is acute idiopathic thrombocytopenic purpura (ITP), and the most important diagnostic distinction is between this and the more serious causes—leukaemia and aplastic anaemia in particular.

Idiopathic (Immune) Thrombocytopenic Purpura in Childhood

Originally, ITP was a diagnosis by exclusion: thrombocytopenic purpura in the absence of evidence of underlying disease, genetic origin or drug toxicity, and with normal or increased numbers of megakaryocytes in the bone marrow. After many years of argument, aggravated by the technical difficulties inherent in platelet antibody testing, it is now generally agreed to be an immune disorder characterized by the presence of platelet-bound antibody (see p. 607). This definition of ITP encompasses at least two separate clinical conditions: acute ITP, usually self-limiting, which is the commonest form in children, to whom it is largely confined; and chronic ITP, which is predominantly a disease of young adults, particularly women. The main contrasting features of the two conditions are set out in Table 22.4. The acute form will be discussed here, and the chronic form in the next section (p. 606).

Acute ITP in children usually starts abruptly within about 2–3 weeks after an acute viral infection, or occasionally after vaccination against a viral disease. Rubella is a common precipitating cause, but measles, chicken-pox and other specific fevers may be responsible, as well as various unidentified upper respiratory infections. The peak age incidence is at about 3 years, and there tends to be a seasonal fluctuation, with a maximal incidence in the spring. The platelet count is usually less than $20 \times 10^9/l$, and there may be extensive skin purpura, superficial bruising and epistaxis. The child is usually in good general health, however; blood loss is seldom sufficient to cause significant anaemia, and serious internal haemorrhage very rarely occurs. The white cell count is usually normal or slightly raised, and mild eosinophilia is sometimes seen. The few platelets on the blood film usually include giant forms. The tip of the spleen may be palpable, but greater splenic enlargement strongly suggests an alternative diagnosis. The bone marrow megakaryocytes are usually increased in number and show an increase in immature forms, and eosinophil precursors are often prominent. Leukaemia and aplastic anaemia, which usually have a rather more insidious onset and tend to produce more widespread systemic effects, will be finally excluded by the bone marrow examination.

Very high levels of platelet-bound immunoglobulin are usually found in acute ITP of childhood: IgG and IgM are nearly always raised together, the mean values of each being four to five times as high as those seen in the chronic form of the disease; C3d is also raised, though perhaps to a rather lesser extent. While there is much evidence that the platelet-bound immunoglobulin of chronic ITP represents platelet-specific antibody, it seems likely that acute ITP is caused by immune complexes bound to the platelets through their Fc receptors. Such viral antigen–antibody complexes can cause platelet aggregation, with removal of aggregates by the reticuloendothelial system, and may also cause

Table 22.4

Idiopathic thrombocytopenic purpura in childhood and adult life

	Childhood	*Adult*
Peak age incidence (years)	2–6	20–30
Sex incidence (M:F)	1:1	1:3
Onset	Acute	Insidious
Preceding infection	Common	Unusual
Platelet count ($\times 10^9/l$)	Often <20	Usually >20
Spontaneous remission rate (%)	>80	<20
Usual duration	2–4 weeks	Months or years

widespread damage to vascular endothelium, leading to increased utilization of platelets as a result of their adhesion to the damaged vessel walls. This dual mechanism of platelet depletion might at least temporarily outstrip the proliferative capacity of the megakaryocytes.

Treatment

About 80% of children with acute ITP will remit spontaneously and permanently, and no treatment is indicated other than avoidance of injury. The risk of serious (e.g. intracranial) haemorrhage is very small (about 1%) and admission to hospital is seldom necessary. Corticosteroids are of doubtful benefit, though they have been claimed to accelerate the return of the platelet count to normal levels; a similar claim has been made for intravenous immunoglobulin.

Occasional patients will take up to 6 months to remit, and a few will develop chronic or recurrent ITP. The latter course is more usual in those without a clear history of antecedent infection, and with a more insidious onset: these cases resemble the adult type of ITP (see p. 606), and presumably have a similar aetiology. Even chronic ITP is essentially a benign disease in childhood, however, with eventual recovery, though sometimes not for a few years, and symptoms are usually confined to easy bruising, even in the presence of a platelet count persistently in the $10–20 \times 10^9$/l range. The temptation to treat the platelet count rather than the patient should therefore be resisted; only if distressing symptoms (e.g. repeated epistaxes) occur should active measures be taken. The side-effects of long-term steroid therapy outweigh any possible usefulness, and splenectomy should certainly be avoided, at least until the age of 5–6 years, because of the postoperative risk of infections. In those patients who do require treatment, intravenous immunoglobulin is probably now the treatment of choice: some patients will have a lasting remission after a single 5-day course (400 mg/kg per day), while the majority will have only a transient response, and may need further doses from time to time. Short courses may be used in such patients to cover traumatic episodes such as tooth extractions or accidental injuries. The possible mode of action

of intravenous immunoglobulin in thrombocytopenic states, and further indications for its use, are considered below (p. 608).

Hereditary Thrombocytopenias

The Wiskott–Aldrich syndrome has been considered amongst the neonatal purpuras (p. 602), and the Bernard–Soulier and grey platelet syndromes will be described under the heading of disorders of platelet function (p. 614). In addition to these well-defined syndromes, a number of instances have been reported of thrombocytopenic purpura occurring as a familial disorder, unassociated with immunodeficiency or other developmental abnormalities. Although the genetic evidence has not always been convincing, it seems probable that autosomal dominant and recessive and X-linked patterns of inheritance may all occur. Most cases have presented in infancy or childhood, and the clinical severity has ranged from mild to fatal. Platelet size may be abnormal in either direction and autologous platelet survival has been found to be reduced in some families. The bone marrow contains normal or increased numbers of megakaryocytes, and the important distinction from chronic ITP rests on the family history, the early onset, the absence of platelet antibodies in the serum and the presence of normal levels of platelet-associated IgG. The survival of labelled donor platelets will be found to be normal, so that platelet transfusion is appropriate for the treatment of serious bleeding episodes. Corticosteroids and intravenous immunoglobulin have no place in the management of hereditary thrombocytopenias, but splenectomy may result in some improvement of the platelet count.

Thrombocytopenia has been observed in about one-third of patients with the May–Hegglin anomaly, an autosomal dominant trait characterized by giant platelets and the presence of inclusions resembling Döhle bodies in the granulocytes; the resulting bleeding tendency is usually mild. Other hereditary disorders of which thrombocytopenia may form part are the Chediak–Higashi syndrome (pp. 313, 617) and Epstein's syndrome, in which the thrombocytopenia is associated with the presence of giant platelets, congenital nephritis and nerve deafness.

Haemolytic–Uraemic Syndrome (see also pp. 196, 667)

Haemolytic–uraemic syndrome (HUS) comprises a heterogeneous group of disorders, which are amongst the commonest causes of acute renal failure in childhood, but relatively less common in adults. The hallmarks of the syndrome are the triad of acute renal failure, microangiopathic haemolytic anaemia and thrombocytopenia. In childhood, two major subgroups of the disorder are recognized— the epidemic and sporadic forms.

Typical (epidemic) HUS of childhood occurs in small outbreaks in the summer months, and usually affects children between 6 months and 6 years of age. A diarrhoeal prodrome is followed after 3–10 days by the acute onset of microangiopathic haemolytic anaemia, thrombocytopenia and renal failure; involvement of other organs, especially the CNS, may occur. Despite the severity of the initial illness, the prognosis is good, and most affected children recover completely.

Atypical (sporadic) HUS develops insidiously without prodromal diarrhoea or follows an upper respiratory illness. It may occur in the first year of life, but usually affects older children than the epidemic form. Renal failure develops gradually, and the haematological manifestations may be the presenting feature. This form of HUS is often familial, and both autosomal dominant and recessive inheritance have been reported. The prognosis is poor, with relapses and progressive deterioration of renal function. CNS involvement also occurs, and the disorder is probably indistinguishable from adult thrombotic thrombocytopenic purpura (TTP).

The red cell fragmentation and haemolysis are probably due to microvascular damage. The earlier suggestion of a pathogenetic role for fibrin deposition in small vessels has not been supported by evidence of increased fibrinogen turnover, and it is more likely that endothelial swelling and disruption, resulting in platelet deposition on the vessel wall, are the underlying mechanisms.

The epidemic occurrence and prodromal diarrhoea suggest an infective or toxic aetiology for typical childhood HUS, and a number of organisms have been implicated, including *Shigella* in India and toxin-producing *Escherichia coli* in developed countries. Other cases have been associated with *Campylobacter*, *Yersinia* and a number of viral infections, but usually no organism is identified. In some non-diarrhoeal cases, neuraminidase-producing pneumococci have been shown to induce HUS by exposing the Thomsen–Friedenreich antigen as a result of sialic acid degradation, and inducing polyagglutination.

In the atypical (sporadic) form of the disease, an inherited defect in vascular haemostasis seems likely. Defective prostacyclin production by endothelial cells incubated with the patient's plasma has been observed in many cases, while the plasma of others has been found to aggregate normal platelets directly. Abnormal production of high-molecular-weight multimers of von Willebrand factor has been implicated in some cases.

Endothelial cell swelling and separation from the basement membrane are the major histological features of the epidemic form, while proliferation of subendothelial smooth muscle and connective tissue in arteries and arterioles is commonly seen in the sporadic form. These vascular changes may occur in many organs in addition to the kidney, especially the gastrointestinal tract and the CNS. Despite a marked shortening of RBC and platelet survival, DIC is not a usual feature: FDPs may be moderately raised, but fibrinogen and factor V and VIII are usually normal or increased. Platelet survival is shortened.

In the typical form of HUS, treatment is purely supportive. Early dialysis to prevent electrolyte imbalance and fluid overload, and blood transfusion to maintain haemoglobin, have reduced the mortality to below 10% in most centres. Control of hypertension and maintenance of nutrition are other important measures. No benefit from anticoagulant or fibrinolytic therapy has been demonstrated in a number of controlled trials, and only uncontrolled trials of antiplatelet agents have been performed.

In the atypical, familial and relapsing forms of HUS, the prognosis with dialysis and transfusion alone is poor, and more aggressive specific treatments are indicated. Some patients respond to fresh plasma infusions, but others require plasma-pheresis, often repeated with successive relapses, to induce remission. Control of hypertension is an important aspect of the management of these patients.

Thrombocytopenia in Infections

Apart from their role in precipitating acute post-infective ITP in children, a variety of acute viral and rickettsial infections may cause thrombocytopenia during the acute febrile phase of the disease. These include influenza, chicken-pox, infectious mono-nucleosis, rubella and measles, as well as typhus and the various epidemic haemorrhagic fevers. Thrombocytopenia in acute bacterial infections, particularly gram-negative septicaemias, is usually the result of DIC (Chapter 24).

Splenomegaly

About one-third of the body's platelets are normally contained in the splenic pool, and in splenomegaly from any cause this proportion may increase, even to 80–90%, so that the compensatory increase in production is insufficient to maintain a normal platelet count. Amongst the main causes in childhood of splenomegaly leading to excessive splenic sequestration of platelets are portal hypertension, thalassaemia, Gaucher's disease and other storage diseases, chronic malaria and infantile kala-azar. The thrombocytopenia is seldom of profound degree, and does not constitute an indication for splenectomy in its own right.

Other Causes of Thrombocytopenia in Childhood

Two of the most important causes of thrombocytopenia in childhood, acute leukaemia and bone marrow aplasia, are discussed in detail in Chapters 14 and 4 respectively. The great majority of patients with acute myeloid leukaemia, and about 80% of children with acute lymphoblastic leukaemia, have some degree of thrombocytopenia at diagnosis. Purpuric symptoms due to thrombocytopenia are a frequent presenting feature of aplastic anaemias, whether hereditary or acquired, and megakaryo-cytic hypoplasia may antedate involvement of the other cell series by weeks or months; it is obviously particularly important to distinguish such cases from chronic ITP. In cyanotic congenital heart disease, the platelet count tends to be somewhat lower than normal, and to fall in proportion to the degree of hypoxia and of polycythaemia. A cyclical variation in platelet count has been observed in some such patients.

A very rare cause of thrombocytopenia in childhood is a congenital form of chronic relapsing thrombocytopenic purpura which responds to the infusion of plasma or plasma fractions. One such patient, who has been successfully maintained on plasma infusions every few weeks for over 20 years, was originally postulated to have a deficiency of thrombopoietin production, but subsequent investigations have shown similarities to the chronic relapsing form of thrombotic thrombocytopenic purpura, though without the neurological and renal manifestations. A similar patient of the author's responds regularly to infusions of cryoprecipitate or factor-VIII concentrate, the platelet count rising over the next week or so and then falling steadily until the next infusion.

In osteopetrosis (Albers–Schönberg disease), thrombocytopenia results partly from encroach-ment of bone on the marrow cavity, leading to generalized marrow failure. Splenic sequestration must also play a part, however, since several children have been reported in whom the thrombo-cytopenia was relieved by splenectomy. Early bone marrow transplantation, by providing normal osteoclast precursors, can restore cancellous bone formation and effectively cure the disease.

Thrombocytopenia in Adults

The main causes of thrombocytopenia in adult life are listed in Table 22.5. Although many of them also operate in childhood, the spectrum of diseases with which they are associated is for the most part very different.

Idiopathic Thrombocytopenic Purpura in Adults

The childhood and adult forms of ITP are con-trasted in Table 22.4 (p. 603). The adult disease predominantly affects young women, has an insidious onset without obvious precipitating cause, and usually runs a chronic course over months or years.

Table 22.5
Thrombocytopenia in adults

Idiopathic (autoimmune) thrombocytopenic purpura
Other immune thrombocytopenias
   Evans' syndrome
   Antilymphocyte globulin
   After bone marrow transplantation
   Malaria
   AIDS associated
   Other virus diseases
   Lymphoproliferative disorders
   Systemic lupus erythematosus
   Other autoimmune disorders
   Post-transfusion purpura
Drug induced (see Table 22.6)
Thrombotic thrombocytopenic purpura
Bone marrow aplasia
Disseminated intravascular coagulation
   Obstetric complications
   Malignancy
   Infections, etc.
Acute leukaemias
Myelofibrosis, myelomatosis, carcinomatosis
Megaloblastic anaemia
Splenomegaly

Pathogenesis

Platelet survival is very short, being measured in hours rather than days in severe cases. The survival of labelled isologous platelets has been found to be reduced in proportion to the patient's platelet count. It has been known since the classical experiment of Harrington in 1951, who infused plasma from a patient with ITP into himself and rapidly developed thrombocytopenia, that the rapid platelet destruction was due to a humoral factor, and this is clearly also borne out by the transmission of the disease from mother to newborn infant (see p. 600). For many years, however, the variable and conflicting results of tests for platelet antibodies in patients' sera, using various conventional immunological techniques, delayed the general acceptance of ITP as an autoimmune disease. This era of doubt was effectively ended by Rosse and his coworkers in 1975, when they developed a quantitative test for platelet-bound IgG based on red-cell lysis inhibition, and showed much higher values in

patients with ITP than in normal controls. This work has been abundantly confirmed by many other groups using a variety of different techniques for the quantitation of the platelet-bound antibody. Although reported normal ranges vary quite widely, there is general agreement that the great majority of patients with ITP have five to ten times as much IgG per platelet as normal individuals. The quantity per platelet correlates well with the severity of the disease and is inversely proportional to the platelet count and platelet survival. The bound IgG is not restricted to any one subclass, and IgM may also be present. Platelet-bound complement (C3) is usually also found.

Although in other conditions — notably systemic lupus erythematosus and AIDS-related thrombocytopenia (p. 609) — raised platelet-bound IgG appears to represent the binding of immune complexes to the platelet Fc receptor, the weight of evidence suggests that in chronic ITP it is specific antiplatelet immunoglobulin which is bound. It has recently been shown that in many cases of ITP the antibody is directed against antigen sites on the glycoprotein IIb–IIIa complex, which also carries the fibrinogen-binding site necessary for aggregation, and is missing from thrombasthenic platelets (see p. 615).

Chronic ITP can therefore be regarded as an autoimmune disorder, and indeed there are those who would replace the word 'idiopathic' by 'autoimmune' in its title. The reason for the production of the autoantibody remains unknown, however. The spleen has been shown to synthesize specific antiplatelet IgG; it is probably the main, if not the only, source of the antibody in most cases, and is also the chief site of removal of antibody-coated platelets from the circulation. There is evidence, on the other hand, that heavily coated platelets are removed mainly in the liver, and that patients with very high levels of platelet-bound antibody are unlikely to benefit from splenectomy.

The short platelet survival leads to positive-feedback stimulation of thrombopoiesis, and the bone marrow characteristically shows an increased number of megakaryocytes with a preponderance of early (low ploidy) forms. Kinetic studies have shown that both total megakaryocyte mass and platelet turnover are increased in parallel up to about five times normal.

Clinical and Haematological Features

The onset is usually insidious, without any antecedent illness. Skin purpura, multiple superficial bruises, epistaxis and menorrhagia are the commonest symptoms. The course is often fluctuating, and may even be cyclical, with periods in which the platelet count returns to normal. Indeed, some patients may have well-compensated subclinical thrombocytopenia, which reveals itself only when platelet production or survival is adversely affected by an acute infection or drug toxicity. The platelets are often irregular in size and shape, with a high proportion of giant forms, representative of the accelerated thrombocytopoiesis. The fact that the bleeding time and clinical severity are often less than might be expected from the platelet count suggests that these 'megathrombocytes' are functionally very efficient. Raised platelet-bound IgG will be present in the great majority of cases, but is not diagnostic of ITP since it is found in various other immune thrombocytopenias. The haemoglobin and leucocyte count may be affected by acute blood loss, but are otherwise normal. The bone marrow appearances are essentially normal apart from the megakaryocyte changes described above, and perhaps also normoblastic and granulopoietic hyperplasia in response to haemorrhage. Bone marrow examination is invaluable in excluding other causes of thrombocytopenia, and tests for systemic lupus erythematosus and thyroid dysfunction, both of which are often associated with immune thrombocytopenia, should be performed.

Treatment

In contrast to the childhood disease, ITP in adult life does not usually remit spontaneously, nor can it be regarded as such a relatively harmless condition in the chronic state, especially in young women, for whom severe menorrhagia is a particular hazard. Mild cases, however, with platelet counts above about $50 \times 10^9/l$, can often be managed conservatively. The main forms of treatment available are corticosteroids, intravenous immunoglobulin and splenectomy with immunosuppressive drugs and vincristine to fall back on for resistant cases. Opinions differ with regard to the exact indications, but the usual approach is to use corticosteroids in full dosage (e.g. prednisolone, 60 mg daily) initially.

If a response is achieved—usually within a week or so—the drug should be gradually withdrawn, either completely or to the smallest dose compatible with acceptable clinical effect; if no response occurs within 3 weeks, nothing is to be gained by continuing steroid therapy for longer. Even low doses of corticosteroids should not be continued indefinitely: recurrence of unacceptable haemorrhagic symptoms on withdrawing them completely constitutes an indication for alternative therapy.

Although 70–80% of patients with chronic ITP show some degree of response to steroid therapy, and about half this number achieve a platelet count above $100 \times 10^9/l$, most of them relapse again on stopping treatment, and permanent complete remissions occur in less than 20% of cases. In general, older patients respond less to steroids (and other forms of treatment) than younger patients. For those who continue to have troublesome symptoms or whose platelet count falls to dangerous levels, splenectomy is probably still the treatment of choice. Although most patients with chronic ITP will respond to a 5-day course of intravenous immunoglobulin, the platelet count nearly always falls again within about 3 weeks, so that this form of treatment lends itself to the control of acute bleeding episodes or the preparation of the patient for surgery rather than to maintenance. It has also been successfully used in the management of ITP in late pregnancy, to the benefit of both mother and infant. The mode of action of intravenous immunoglobulin in immune thrombocytopenia is still not completely understood. The main mechanism of the short-term effect seems to be Fc receptor blockade of the reticuloendothelial system, and inhibition of platelet antibody synthesis and its binding to platelets have also been suggested to account for the more lasting responses, though without objective supporting evidence. In those forms of thrombocytopenia due to the binding of immune complexes to the platelets, the elimination of such complexes or of free viral antigens is likely to be of prime importance.

Splenectomy is indicated, after 6 months or so of observation, in patients who have not maintained a remission, whether spontaneous or in response to steroids or intravenous immunoglobulin, and whose symptoms are severe enough to require treatment. Splenectomy should not as a rule be performed in the early phase of the disease, in children under the age of 5–6 years or in pregnancy. Neither the response to steroids nor the site of sequestration of labelled platelets is a useful guide to the probable effect of splenectomy. Most patients with chronic ITP respond at least temporarily with a rise of platelet count, and complete and lasting remissions occur in about 80% of cases. Some of the remainder will be clinically improved, despite a degree of continuing thrombocytopenia, and others may be controlled more readily on small doses of steroids, or achieve a more lasting response to intravenous immunoglobulin, than before operation. In those with continuing severe thrombocytopenia, immunosuppressive drugs such as azathioprine or cyclophosphamide are occasionally effective, the latter being perhaps more likely to succeed, though potentially more toxic. Neither can be expected to achieve an effect in under 2–3 months. The vinca alkaloids, which stimulate thrombocytopoiesis as well as being immunosuppressive, have also been used with success in some such cases—both by direct intravenous injection and after incubation in vitro with the patient's platelets. The rationale of this latter approach is to deliver the vinblastine-loaded platelets directly to the patient's reticuloendothelial system with the aim of impairing its function and so allowing the antibody-coated platelets to continue to circulate. Not enough patients have been treated in this way to allow a proper appraisal of its efficacy.

Other Immune Thrombocytopenias

Raised levels of platelet-associated IgG (PAIgG) are found in many conditions besides ITP, and are not in themselves diagnostic of any single disorder. They may be due to specific binding of autoantibody or alloantibody to a platelet antigen, or of an antibody to a non-platelet antigen adsorbed to the platelet surface, or to immune complexes bound to the platelet membrane through IgG Fc receptors. Any of these processes can lead to complement-mediated lysis of platelets, or to their removal by the reticuloendothelial system. Apart from ITP, there is good evidence for specific binding to platelet antibodies in Evans' syndrome of autoimmune thrombocytopenia and haemolytic anaemia, and in the transient thrombocytopenia caused by anti-lymphocyte or antithrombocyte globulin, which is due to antibodies against HLA antigens on the platelet surface. The platelet antibodies which have been demonstrated in a high proportion of patients after both autologous and allogeneic bone marrow transplantation appear to be true autoantibodies, of donor origin; the mechanism of their production remains to be explained. They may lead to severe and persistent thrombocytopenia but may also be detected in the presence of a relatively normal platelet count.

It seems likely that the thrombocytopenia associated with many viral and protozoal infections is immune mediated, and in malaria it has been shown that the IgG antibodies are directed against malarial antigen bound to the platelet membrane. The raised PAIgG in viral infections, including infectious mononucleosis, probably represents bound immune complexes, and this seems to be the mechanism underlying the AIDS-associated thrombocytopenia seen in homosexual men and some haemophiliacs. Raised levels of PAIgG are also seen in association with thrombocytopenia in lymphoproliferative disorders, especially chronic lymphocytic leukaemia and Hodgkin's disease, and in systemic lupus erythematosus (SLE). Some degree of thrombocytopenia—usually mild—occurs in 20–30% of cases of SLE, and occasionally in other autoimmune disorders including rheumatoid arthritis and thyroid diseases, but raised PAIgG is often found in association with a normal platelet count: there is evidence that it represents bound immune complexes rather than platelet-specific antibody.

Immune mechanisms are also involved in some drug-induced thrombocytopenias and in post-transfusion purpura. These are considered separately below.

Thrombocytopenia Due to Drugs

Drugs may produce thrombocytopenia as a result of suppression of megakaryocytes, through immune mechanisms or by direct aggregation of the platelets in vivo. The drugs which have been most clearly implicated are listed in Table 22.6, but many others have been suspected of causing thrombocytopenia on rare occasions, as well as some foods, including citrus fruits and beans. In most such instances, the

Table 22.6
Thrombocytopenia due to drugs

Bone marrow suppression
Predictable (dose related)
  Ionizing radiation, cytotoxic drugs, ethanol
Occasional
  Chloramphenicol, co-trimoxazole, idoxuridine, phenylbutazone, penicill-
    amine, organic arsenicals, etc.
Immune mechanisms (proven or probable)
Analgesics, anti-inflammatory drugs
  Aspirin, paracetamol, phenacetin, gold salts, rifampicin
Antimicrobials
  Penicillins, sulphonamides, trimethoprim, para-aminosalicylate
Sedatives, anticonvulsants
  Apronal (Sedormid), diazepam, sodium valproate
Diuretics
  Acetzaolamide, chlorothiazides, frusemide
Antidiabetics
  Chlorpropamide, tolbutamide
Others
  Digitoxin, heparin, methyldopa, oxprenolol, quinine, quinidine
Platelet aggregation
Ristocetin, heparin

---

mechanism has not been clearly identified, though an immunological one seems likely. Bone marrow aplasia due to drugs is discussed in Chapter 4, and the rest of this section is confined to the drug-induced immune thrombocytopenias. Although these affect only a very small proportion of people receiving the drugs in question, the overall incidence of drug-induced thrombocytopenia is substantial. Heparin, quinine and quinidine, gold salts and chlorothiazides are the most frequent offenders.

The condition usually develops suddenly within about 12 hours of taking a single dose of a drug to which the patient has been previously exposed, or in the course of a period of continuous treatment which may even have lasted for months or years before the development of hypersensitivity. The purpuric symptoms may be accompanied by other signs of allergy, such as fever, joint pains and skin rashes, and sometimes by neutropenia or haemolytic anaemia. Amongst methods used for the detection of antibodies leading to platelet destruction in the presence of the offending drug are complement fixation, antiglobulin consumption, lymphocyte transformation and measurement of the release of ^{51}Cr or platelet factor 3 from the platelets. Such

tests have given positive results in thrombocytopenia induced by quinine, quinidine, gold and sedormid, but results are often negative in the presence of other offending drugs, perhaps because it is a metabolite, rather than the drug itself, which provides the antigenic stimulus: evidence for such a mechanism has been adduced in the case of paracetamol and p-aminosalicylate. The platelets may be involved either through Fc receptor binding of immune complexes formed between the drug or its metabolite and IgG (or, more rarely, IgM) antibody, or by the reaction of antibody with drug already bound to the platelet membrane; the platelet destruction results in either case from binding of complement. These two mechanisms are typified by quinine and penicillin-induced thrombocytopenia respectively. Heparin appears to cause thrombocytopenia by direct platelet aggregation as well as through an immune mechanism (see also p. 621), and this effect of ristocetin has led to its withdrawal from use as an antibiotic.

The bone marrow contains abundant megakaryocytes, but the thrombocytopenia continues as long as the drug is taken, recovering spontaneously within a week or two of withdrawing the drug: the speed of recovery depends on its rate of metabolism or excretion. No other treatment is usually necessary, but platelet transfusion can be used if serious haemorrhage occurs. Further use of the offending drug is strictly contraindicated.

Post-transfusion Thrombocytopenia

Due to Dilution

The rapid replacement of large volumes of blood lost by transfusion may lead to thrombocytopenia as a result of dilution, such platelets as may remain in stored blood being non-viable. The thrombocytopenia caused in this way is not likely to reach dangerous levels unless the patient receives a transfusion equivalent to more than his own blood volume within a few hours. Since such a situation arises most commonly in association with continuing uncontrolled bleeding and shock, however, dilution of platelets may be only one of several factors contributing to a vicious circle of haemostatic failure: dilution of labile plasma clotting factors, particularly factor VIII, and DIC are also likely to occur. Dilutional thrombocytopenia may also result from exchange transfusions or from the use of extracorporeal circulations; in the latter case, activation of the platelets also plays a part, as well as disturbances of coagulation and fibrinolysis. In all these circumstances, the thrombocytopenia can be prevented, or reduced to insignificant degree, by the use of platelet concentrates in addition to whole blood.

Another cause of transient thrombocytopenia in some patients undergoing cardiac surgery is hypothermia. At temperatures of 25°C or below, the platelets swell and undergo reversible aggregation, and this may lead to their sequestration in the spleen and contribute to postoperative bleeding.

Due to Alloantibodies

A few cases have been reported of severe thrombocytopenia developing, usually in a multiparous woman, within about a week after a blood transfusion. In nearly every case, the patient's serum has been found to contain alloantibody specific for the Pl^{A1} (Zw^a) platelet antigen, her own platelets being Pl^{A1} negative. The patient has presumably been sensitized to the Pl^{A1} antigen by a previous preg-

nancy or transfusion, but the destruction of her own Pl^{A1}-negative platelets by the alloantibody is difficult to explain. It has been suggested that the Pl^{A1} antigen released from donor platelets by the antibody binds to the recipient's platelets and renders them susceptible to antibody-mediated destruction. Alternatively, complement-mediated lysis may result from the binding of Pl^{A1} antigen–antibody complexes to the recipient's platelets. The most appropriate treatment is exchange transfusion or plasmapheresis with transfusion of Pl^{A1}-negative platelets. Corticosteroids have not usually influenced the speed of recovery, which can be expected to occur spontaneously within a few weeks, but one patient remitted in 5 days on intravenous methylprednisolone.

Alcoholism

This is mentioned separately from the other causes of drug-induced thrombocytopenia since its very frequency often causes it to be overlooked. The thrombocytopenia of chronic alcoholism occurs independently of folate deficiency and cirrhosis, which are likely to be additional contributory factors, and seems to result both from bone marrow depression and from shortening of platelet lifespan; the platelets may also be functionally abnormal (see p. 621). Withdrawal of alcohol results in a rapid rise of platelet count to normal levels within a few days, and often leads to a transitory rebound thrombocytosis.

Thrombotic Thrombocytopenic Purpura

This is a rare but serious disorder, usually seen in young adults, and characterized by fever, microangiopathic haemolytic anaemia, thrombocytopenia, fluctuating neurological signs and renal disease. It sometimes appears to be triggered by pregnancy, oral contraceptives or the use of drugs, including cyclosporin A and mitomycin, and there is occasionally a familial predisposition. The clinical effects are due to widespread arteriolar lesions and resulting thrombotic occlusions, but the pathogenesis is imperfectly understood. The condition appears to be essentially the same as the sporadic type of haemolytic–uraemic syndrome (see p. 605), but central nervous system involvement is often a more prominent feature in adults. The pathological basis of the disease is widespread arteriolar microthrombi, but debate continues as to whether these lesions are primarily due to vessel wall damage, probably immune mediated, or platelet hyperaggregability. On the one hand, diminished production of prostaglandin I_2 (prostacyclin) by the vessel wall has been demonstrated and attributed both to the lack of a plasma factor and to the presence of an inhibitor of PGI_2 production; on the other hand, the plasma of many patients with thrombotic thrombocytopenic purpura (TTP) agglutinates normal platelets in vitro, and there is evidence that a platelet-agglutinating factor interacts with large multimers of von Willebrand factor—also shown to be present in increased amounts in these patients—to cause platelet agglutination in vivo. The agglutinating factor has been shown to be inhibited by IgG from normal plasma, but not from TTP plasma.

Whatever the mechanism, the response of 60–80% of these patients to plasma infusion or exchange makes it clear that it must be mediated by some plasma factor. Such treatment, repeated on several successive days, will produce lasting remissions in many patients, while others may relapse and require repeated courses or even maintenance infusions. For the minority who fail to respond, intravenous prostacyclin infusions and oral antiplatelet agents have occasionally proved helpful.

Splenomegaly

The causes of hypersplenism in adult life include portal hypertension, Felty's syndrome, Hodgkin's disease and other lymphomas, chronic malaria and kala-azar (see p. 19). The thrombocytopenia associated with splenomegaly is chiefly due to sequestration within the organ: when there is massive enlargement, the splenic platelet pool may increase from the normal one-third of the total platelet mass to as much as 90%. Unless bone marrow function is defective, as for example in chronic lymphocytic leukaemia or lymphomas, a compensatory increase in megakaryocytopoiesis will result, and the degree of thrombocytopenia is seldom severe enough to be more than a minor contributory reason for splenectomy. If the spleen is removed, the platelet count usually returns to normal.

THROMBOCYTOSIS

The main causes of an increase in platelet count are listed in Table 22.7. Vigorous exercise and adrenaline appear to act by mobilizing platelets from outside the circulating pool, especially from the spleen; they produce their effect within minutes, but the other causes of reactive thrombocytosis, which are mediated by increased output of platelets from the megakaryocytes, lead to a rise and fall of platelet count over several days.

Thrombocythaemia

Autonomous hyperplasia of the megakaryocytes, leading to a raised platelet count, may occur as part of any of the myeloproliferative disorders. The least common of these clonal proliferations of haemopoietic stem cells is essential thrombocythaemia, in which the megakaryocytes are the predominant progeny, and the chief symptoms are related to the high platelet count. This is a disorder of middle age and after, which usually runs a chronic or fluctuat-

Table 22.7
Causes of a raised platelet count

Reactive thrombocytosis
  Exercise, adrenaline
  Post-partum
  Post-haemorrhagic
  Rebound: recovery from thrombocytopenia
  Postoperative
Myeloproliferative disorders
  Essential thrombocythaemia
  Chronic granulocytic leukaemia
  Polycythaemia vera
  Myelofibrosis
Asplenic states
  After splenectomy
  Splenic agenesis or atrophy
Drugs
  Vinca alkaloids, corticosteroids
Miscellaneous
  Malignant disease: carcinoma, lymphoma
  Chronic inflammatory disorders
    Rheumatoid arthritis
    Ulcerative colitis
    Crohn's disease
    Polyarteritis nodosa

---

ing course over many years, characterized both by episodes of haemorrhage, which may include spontaneous painful superficial bruises, spreading ecchymoses and bleeding from the gastrointestinal tract, and by venous and arterial thromboses. The latter usually involve the smaller arteries, and may result in peripheral gangrene or in transient cerebral ischaemic attacks. Most patients have some degree of splenomegaly, but splenic infarcts and atrophy may also occur. Patients may have long asymptomatic periods and the diagnosis is not infrequently made incidentally on routine blood examination. The thrombotic lesions may cause considerable morbidity or even prove fatal, but the prognosis for the treated patient is reasonably good. Transition to myelofibrosis may occur, but acute leukaemic transformation, as in chronic myeloid leukaemia, is very seldom seen.

The platelet count is always above $500 \times 10^9/l$, and usually over $10^{12}/l$; giant and irregular forms are common. The total leucocyte count is usually raised, often to levels of $15–30 \times 10^9/l$, with a shift to the left in the granulocytes, and there may be a mild degree of polycythaemia, though anaemia may also occur as a result of chronic blood loss. The neutrophil alkaline phosphatase score is typically normal or raised. The bone marrow is hyperplastic, particularly the megakaryocytes, which are larger than normal and may show structural abnormalities. Bone marrow culture yields an excess of megakaryocyte colony-forming units (CFU–Mk), both in the presence and absence of conditioned medium. Histology of the marrow usually shows an increase in reticulin as well as providing the most effective way of demonstrating the megakaryocytic hyperplasia. There is no characteristic chromosomal abnormality: the Ph^1 chromosome is not found. Despite the high platelet count, the bleeding time is often prolonged, and various abnormalities of platelet function have been observed; these are further discussed on p. 619. Reducation of the platelet count is usually accompanied by reversion of platelet function towards normal, as well as by relief of haemorrhagic and thrombotic symptoms. Busulphan is probably the drug of choice, though hydroxyurea, melphalan and ^{32}P have also been used effectively. Splenectomy is contraindicated, since it is often followed by a further sustained rise in platelet count, and may lead to fatal thrombotic

or haemorrhagic complications. Aspirin may produce striking symptomatic relief when peripheral vascular ischaemia is present, but is probably better not used prophylactically because of the increased risk of bleeding.

Other Causes of Thrombocytosis

Essential thrombocythaemia is the only condition in which the platelet count remains in excess of $10^{12}/l$ for long periods of time, and the only one in which the primary aim of treatment is reduction of the platelet count to normal levels (see Chapter 20). In the other myeloproliferative disorders, lesser degrees of thrombocytosis may persist for months at a time, and abnormalities of platelet function may be observed, but thrombocytosis due to other causes is usually of a transient nature, seldom exceeds $10^{12}/l$, and is not associated with functional defects. Indeed, an increased turnover of normal platelets is likely to lead to an enhancement of platelet function, since young platelets are haemostatically more effective than old ones. It may therefore occasionally be felt prudent to administer an inhibitor of platelet function to cover a period of extreme thrombocytosis, particularly when other thrombogenic factors may operate (e.g. during the first 10–14 days after splenectomy), but no active measures to reduce the platelet count are necessary.

Post-splenectomy thrombocytosis is largely attributable to the combination of postoperative reactive thrombocytosis with removal of the splenic pool. The peak is usually reached within 2–3 weeks, to be followed by a gradual decline to near-normal levels. Continuing postoperative anaemia, however, often results in persistence of the thrombocytosis, with the risk of thromboembolic complications, particularly when erythropoiesis is active, as in an uncorrected haemolytic anaemia.

The pathogenesis of the thrombocytosis seen in malignant disease is not understood, except when it follows acute haemorrhage. Hodgkin's disease and carcinoma of the breast and lung are the tumours with which high platelet counts have been most frequently associated. Occult malignancy must always be considered as a possible cause of unexplained thrombocytosis. Chronic inflammatory disorders of the bowel—particularly Crohn's disease and ulcerative colitis—and also rheumatoid arthritis, chronic tuberculosis and sarcoidosis, may also be associated with high platelet counts, as may haemolytic or iron-deficiency anaemia. The vinca alkaloids and corticosteroids, alone or in combination, may raise the platelet count above normal levels, whether it was previously low or normal.

DISORDERS OF PLATELET FUNCTION

The haemostatic properties of platelets are described in Chapter 21. Following injury to a blood vessel, platelets adhere to structures within the vessel wall, particularly to the subendothelium and to collagen in the deeper layers. This adhesion is rapidly followed by activation of the platelets, leading to the secretion of adenine nucleotides and 5-hydroxytryptamine from the dense bodies, and of many proteins, including thrombospondin, fibrinogen and von Willebrand factor, from the α-granules. Together with the prostaglandin endoperoxides and thromboxane A_2 formed from arachidonic acid released from platelet membrane phospholipids, these various active principles lead to platelet aggregation and so to the formation and propagation of a platelet plug, in turn to be reinforced by local fibrin formation. Haemorrhagic disorders may result not only from thrombocytopenia but from abnormalities of platelet function affecting any of the steps leading to platelet plug formation—adhesion, thromboxane synthesis, secretion, aggregation or blood coagulation. Such disorders may be hereditary or acquired: although acquired disorders are met more commonly in practice, the hereditary abnormalities are better understood in terms of the pathophysiological mechanisms involved, and they will be considered first.

Hereditary Disorders of Platelet Function

Defective platelet function may result from hereditary abnormalities of the connective tissue with which the platelets normally react (e.g. Ehlers–Danlos syndrome), or of plasma proteins necessary for their interaction, as in von Willebrand's disease or afibrinogenaemia, as well as from defects of the platelets themselves. The plasma protein disorders are dealt with in Chapter 23, and disorders of connective tissue on p. 625; this section

Table 22.8
Hereditary disorders of platelet function

Defects of the plasma membrane
  Bernard–Soulier syndrome
  Platelet-type von Willebrand's disease
  Glanzmann's thrombasthenia
  Defect of response to collagen
  Primary platelet coagulant defect
Deficiency of storage organelles
  Dense body deficiency (δ-SPD)
    Idiopathic (storage pool disease)
    Hermansky–Pudlak syndrome
    Wiskott–Aldrich syndrome
    Chediak–Higashi syndrome
    Thrombocytopenia with absent radii
  α-granule deficiency (α-SDP)
    Grey platelet syndrome
Deficiency of dense bodies and α-granules
  ($\alpha\delta$-SPD)
Defects of thromboxane synthesis
  Cyclo-oxygenase deficiency
  Thromboxane synthetase deficiency
Defects of response to thromboxane A_2 and ionophores
Miscellaneous
  Montreal platelet syndrome
  Defects of response to adrenaline
  Epstein's syndrome

will be concerned mainly with primary platelet abnormalities. The classification set out in Table 22.8 is based as far as possible on ultrastructural and functional evidence relating to the various defects.

Bernard–Soulier Syndrome

This is an autosomal recessive trait characterized by a long bleeding time, variable and inconstant thrombocytopenia, defective prothrombin consumption and giant platelets which usually show wide variation in size and morphology. The clinical severity varies from one patient to another, but is characteristically disproportionate to the degree of thrombocytopenia. Multiple superficial bruises and other lesions of purpuric type are usually seen from an early age, and several reported patients have died in childhood from haemorrhagic complications.

The patient's platelets adhere normally to collagen in vitro and aggregate normally in response to ADP, adrenaline or collagen; they fail to agglutinate, however, in the presence of bovine factor VIII or ristocetin. The highly artificial system of ristocetin agglutination acts as an indicator of the ability of platelets to adhere to exposed vascular subendothelium, a reaction involving the binding of von Willebrand factor (VWF) both to the subendothelium and to the platelet surface membrane. While the plasma factor is deficient or defective in von Willebrand's disease, the defect in the Bernard–Soulier syndrome is in the sialic acid-rich glycoprotein (GP) Ib of the platelet membrane, which carries specific receptors for factor VIII. The deficiency of the GP Ib complex (including also GP V and GP IX) is also probably responsible for the defective coagulant activity of Bernard–Soulier platelets, and for their short survival, which in turn probably contributes to the thrombocytopenia. The GP Ib complex also carries receptors for quinine- and quinidine-dependent antibodies.

No specific therapy is available for the Bernard–Soulier syndrome. Local measures are of paramount importance in the control of bleeding, and are usually effective when the bleeding point is accessible, as in the case of tooth extractions. Platelet transfusions may be required in the management of more serious bleeding episodes: donor platelets can be expected to survive normally, but one patient who had received multiple transfusions developed an antibody to GP Ib which agglutinated all donor platelets. Splenectomy is potentially hazardous, and should not be undertaken lightly, or in the hope of dramatic success. Some patients have, however, experienced a modest diminution in bleeding symptoms after splenectomy, perhaps because of improved platelet survival, and the operation should not be regarded as wholly contraindicated. Corticosteroids have no place, but menorrhagia may call for the use of anti-ovulatory agents.

Platelet-type von Willebrand's Disease

This name has been applied to an autosomal dominant bleeding disorder, also described as pseudo-von Willebrand's disease, in which mild thrombocytopenia is associated with increased ristocetin-induced platelet agglutination and a deficiency of the higher multimers of vWF in the plasma. The abnormality appears to consist of an abnormally high avidity of the platelet membrane for these higher multimers, which are thus preferentially removed from the plasma. No increase of glycoprotein Ib or other glycoprotein abnormality of the platelets has been observed.

Thrombasthenia (Glanzmann's Disease)

This is an autosomal recessive disorder resulting in a moderately severe lifelong haemorrhagic tendency, with multiple superficial bruises from childhood onwards, epistaxis and menorrhagia. The clinical severity tends to lessen with age, and varies between one affected individual and another, but this cannot be explained in terms of the defect of aggregation, which is characteristically absolute.

The platelet count, size and morphology are normal, but the bleeding time is greatly prolonged and clot retraction defective. The platelets completely fail to aggregate in response to any concentration of ADP, adrenaline, collagen, arachidonate or thrombin, but agglutinate normally with bovine factor VIII and with ristocetin. They also adhere normally to collagen fibres in vitro, and secrete their granule contents normally in response to thrombin, but no aggregation results.

This failure to aggregate is due to a profound deficiency of two closely associated membrane glycoproteins—GP IIb and IIIa. These form a dissociable calcium-dependent complex in normal platelet membranes, on which receptors for fibrinogen (and also for von Willebrand factor and fibronectin) are exposed in response to stimulation by ADP and other aggregating agents. Although thrombasthenic platelets bind such agonists normally, and undergo the normal initial shape change from discs to spheres in response to them, they fail to bind fibrinogen and hence to aggregate. They also fail to adhere to glass and other inorganic surfaces or to make their membrane phospholipid available for blood coagulation on stimulation by kaolin or ADP. Although, in contrast to Bernard–Soulier platelets, they adhere normally to vascular subendothelium at low shear rates, a defect can be demonstrated at very high shear rates such as those which obtain in small arterioles—perhaps as a result of the defect of binding of von Willebrand factor.

Although the platelets of most patients with thrombasthenia are profoundly deficient in GP IIb–IIIa, the patients can be divided on the basis of clinical severity into types I and II: the former group, consisting of more severely affected patients, is characterized by a lower platelet fibrinogen and a more profound deficiency of GPIIb–IIIa than the latter. More recently, variants of thrombasthenia have been described in which the failure of fibrinogen binding and aggregation is due to a molecular abnormality of GP IIb–IIIa rather than an absolute deficiency of the complex. The platelet specific alloantigens Zw^a (Pl^{A1}) and Lek^a are located on the GP IIb–IIIa complex, and are therefore not expressed on thrombasthenic platelets, though they are distinct from the fibrinogen-binding site.

No specific treatment is available for thrombasthenia. As in the case of Bernard–Soulier syndrome, local measures and platelet transfusions are the main methods of controlling haemorrhage, but antibodies directed against the missing glycoprotein complex have developed in one case. Hormonal suppression of menstruation may be necessary for the prevention of menorrhagia. There is no place for splenectomy. Heterozygotes are clinically unaffected, but have only about half the normal number of GP IIb–IIIa complexes on their platelet membranes: this provides a method for carrier detection.

Other Platelet Membrane Defects

A single case has been reported of a mild bleeding disorder characterized by a specific failure of platelets to respond to collagen—by adhesion, aggregation, secretion or thromboxane synthesis—and by a deficiency of glycoprotein Ia, suggesting that this may be the site of a collagen receptor. Another patient has been shown to have a defect of platelet procoagulant activity due to a deficiency of factor-V-binding sites on the membrane, though no abnormality of membrane proteins or phospholipids could be demonstrated. In the absence of a family history in either of these cases, the genetic nature of the defects must remain in doubt.

Intracellular Abnormalities

This group of disorders can be divided into those due to deficiency of storage organelles and those in which these are normally present but the mechanisms leading to the secretion of their contents are in some way impaired. All result in relatively mild haemorrhagic states, less severe, for example, than either thrombasthenia or the Bernard–Soulier syndrome, and special therapeutic measures are seldom required except in the case of serious accidental or surgical trauma, when platelet transfusion is the logical form of replacement therapy. Somewhat surprisingly, however, cryoprecipitate, DDAVP and prednisone have all been claimed to shorten the bleeding time and achieve adequate surgical haemostasis in this group of disorders, although the underlying platelet abnormalities were not corrected.

Storage Pool Deficiency (SPD)

This is the term first applied to a deficiency of the dense osmiophilic granules within which the secretable pool of adenine nucleotides and 5-hydroxytryptamine is normally stored. More recently, the term has been extended to include deficiency of the α-granules—the site of storage of many platelet-specific and other proteins (see Chapter 21); thus pure deficiency of dense bodies is conveniently referred to as δ-SPD, deficiency of α-granules (the 'grey platelet syndrome') as α-SPD, and the combined deficiency as αδ-SPD.

δ-SPD may occur as part of a number of distinct syndromes (Table 22.8), or as an isolated hereditary abnormality; several of the latter group have shown autosomal dominant inheritance. The bleeding time is often somewhat prolonged, and the characteristic laboratory features are defective aggregation and secretion of dense body contents in response to collagen, failure of second-phase aggregation in response to ADP or adrenaline, defective uptake of 5HT and reduced platelet content of 5HT and adenine nucleotides, particularly ADP. The lack of dense bodies can also be demonstrated by electron or fluorescence microscopy.

In the Hermansky–Pudlak syndrome, δ-SPD is associated with oculocutaneous albinism of the tyrosinase-positive type and the presence of ceroid-like pigment in macrophages in the bone marrow and throughout the reticuloendothelial system. The storage disorder may lead to pulmonary fibrosis and inflammatory bowel disease. The platelet count is normal but the bleeding time prolonged. Easy bruising, ecchymoses, epistaxis and menorrhagia are the commonest symptoms, and inheritance is autosomal recessive, heterozygotes being unaffected.

δ-SPD is seen in the Chediak–Higashi syndrome in both humans and animals, and is also combined with hereditary lysosomal and pigmentation defects in various inbred strains of mice. Children with the Wiskott–Aldrich syndrome and with thrombocytopenia with absent radii (the TAR syndrome) have also been shown to lack platelet dense bodies, but the bleeding tendency in these conditions is of course chiefly attributable to the thrombocytopenia.

α-SPD (*Grey Platelet Syndrome*)

This rare autosomal dominant disorder takes its name from the appearance of the platelets on a stained blood film. They are larger than normal and often somewhat reduced in number, and their homogeneous grey appearance is due to a virtually complete absence of α-granules, all other platelet organelles being normally present. The platelets are profoundly deficient in all those proteins which are normally stored in the α-granules, including platelet factor 4, β-thromboglobulin, thrombospondin, fibrinogen, von Willebrand factor, fibronectin and the platelet-derived growth factor. Defects of aggregation and secretion have been described, though the relation of these to the α-granule deficiency is not clear. The bleeding tendency is surprisingly mild considering the profound platelet abnormality. Some patients have been found to have a degree of myelofibrosis, presumably due to the leakage of platelet-derived growth factor into the extracellular space from megakaryocytes lacking the α-granules in which it is normally stored.

$\alpha\delta$-SPD

The platelets of some patients with SPD, particularly those unassociated with other clinical features, are deficient in α-granules as well as in dense bodies. Those with the combined defect do not seem to have more serious bleeding problems than those

with pure δ-SPD, and the distinction is clinically unimportant.

Defects of the Secretory Mechanism

The commonest cause of failure of dense body secretion in the presence of a normal storage pool is ingestion of aspirin, which inhibits cyclo-oxygenase and so prevents the formation of prostaglandin endoperoxides and thromboxane A_2. A few patients have been described, however, in which a similar defect was evidently due to congenital deficiency of either cyclo-oxygenase or thromboxane synthetase. Two kindreds with the latter deficiency suggest autosomal dominant inheritance. Other patients with lifelong mild bleeding disorders have been shown to synthesize thromboxane normally but to fail to respond to it by aggregation and secretion. This group is probably heterogeneous, including various defects of intracellular calcium transport or utilization; patients with the hereditary attention deficit disorder, who suffer from easy bruising, seem to have a similar type of platelet disorder.

Miscellaneous Hereditary Disorders

A variety of platelet abnormalities have been described in patients with lifelong bleeding tendencies which do not fit into any of the categories described above. These include the Montreal platelet syndrome, an autosomal dominant trait with thrombocytopenia and giant platelets, defective response to thrombin but normal ristocetin-induced agglutination; patients with a defective response of their platelets to adrenaline, which has been described in normal individuals as well as some with bleeding symptoms; and Epstein's syndrome, in which mild thrombocytopenia and giant platelets are associated with nephritis and nerve deafness as an autosomal dominant trait.

Diagnosis of Hereditary Disorders of Platelet Function

This group of disorders cannot be clearly distinguished from one another, or from von Willebrand's disease, by the nature of their bleeding symptoms or signs, but genetic considerations and associated abnormalities, together with appropriate

Table 22.9

Hereditary disorders of platelet function: diagnosis

	Platelet count	Platelet size	Platelet aggregation				Hereditary pattern	Associated abnormalities
			ADP	Collagen	Arachidonic acid	Ristocetin		
Thrombasthenia	N	N	O	O	O	(1)	Autosomal recessive	
Bernard–Soulier syndrome	↓(or N)	↑	N	N	N	O	Autosomal recessive	
Hermansky–Pudlak syndrome	N	N	(1)	↓	N	(1)	Autosomal recessive	Albinism; pigmented macrophages in bone marrow
Isolated storage pool deficiency	N	N or ↓	(1)	↓	N	(1)	Autosomal dominant	
Wiskott–Aldrich syndrome	↓	↓	↓	↓			X-borne recessive	Eczema; recurrent infections
Chediak–Higashi syndrome	N or ↓	N	(1)	↓			Autosomal recessive	Partial albinism; recurrent infections; lysosomal abnormality of granulocytes
Cyclo-oxygenase deficiency	N	N	(1)	↓			?	
Thromboxane synthetase deficiency					→			
Grey platelet syndrome	↓	↑	N or ↓	N or ↓	N	N	Autosomal dominant	Myelofibrosis

(1) = first phase aggregation only.
N = Normal.

laboratory investigations, will usually enable an accurate diagnosis to be made.

The first steps in laboratory diagnosis include a bleeding time, platelet count and size distribution, examination of a stained blood film and platelet aggregation in response to ADP, collagen, arachidonate and ristocetin; characteristic patterns of results of these tests are shown in Table 22.9. It is important to distinguish hereditary from acquired disorders of aggregation, and especially from the effects of aspirin and other drugs (see below); particular care should be taken to ensure that the patient has taken no such drugs for at least 10 days before platelet function is tested. Further tests which may be used for confirmation of the diagnosis include the measurement of uptake and secretion of 5HT, secretion of adenine nucleotides and granule constituents, and thromboxane B_2 production; all these will help to distinguish the various intracellular abnormalities from each other. In the investigation of the membrane defects, specific monoclonal antibodies against the various glycoproteins have proved very useful, and can be used for diagnosis when only small amounts of blood are available, as for example in fetal or neonatal samples.

Acquired Disorders of Platelet Function

Platelet function is disturbed in a wide variety of conditions, and the most important of these are listed in Table 22.10. The nature of the platelet abnormality is less clearly identified in most of these conditions than in the hereditary platelet disorders, so that they do not easily lend themselves to a pathogenetic classification. In many of them, other aspects of the haemostatic mechanism are affected as well as platelet function.

Myeloproliferative Disorders

Essential thrombocythaemia is described above (p. 612) and in Chapter 20, and the other myeloproliferative disorders in Chapters 15, 16 and 20. It is well recognized that patients with this group of disorders may suffer from a moderate to severe bleeding tendency, in the presence of a normal or even greatly raised platelet count. Purpura, large spreading ecchymoses, epistaxes and gastrointesti-

Table 22.10
Causes of acquired platelet dysfunction

Myeloproliferative disorders
  Thrombocythaemia
  Chronic myeloid leukaemia
  Polycythaemia vera
  Myelofibrosis
Acute leukaemias, preleukaemic states
Renal disease
Dysproteinaemias
Acquired storage pool deficiency
  Autoimmune diseases
  Disseminated intravascular coagulation
  Haemolytic–uraemic syndrome
  Thrombotic thrombocytopenic purpura
  Renal transplant rejection
  Severe burns
  Valvular heart disease
  Cardiopulmonary bypass
Chronic hypoglycaemia
  Glycogen storage disease type I
  Fructose-1,6-diphosphatase deficiency
Bartter's syndrome
Drugs
  See Table 22.11

nal haemorrhage are the commonest symptoms, and may be associated with evidence of peripheral arterial thrombosis, particularly in thrombocythaemic patients. Many different defects of platelet function have been described, as well as morphological abnormalities, but in general the results of laboratory tests of platelet function correlate poorly with the incidence of either bleeding or thrombotic manifestations. Nor is any particular type of platelet abnormality associated with any one of the myeloproliferative disorders. The most commonly recorded defect of aggregation is a failure of response to adrenaline, probably due to a deficiency of α_2-adrenergic receptors, but dense-body deficiency and defects of arachidonate metabolism have also been described, as have various disturbances of membrane glycoproteins and of platelet coagulant activity. Some patients with thrombotic episodes have been found to have hyperaggregable platelets; this hyperaggregability may be due to the lack of specific receptors for the aggregation inhibitor prostaglandin D_2 on the platelet membrane.

In thrombocythaemia, both thrombotic and haemorrhagic complications can usually be controlled by lowering the platelet count, and in polycythaemia the risk of thrombosis can be reduced by lowering the haematocrit. Aspirin has a place in the management of arterial occlusive disease in this group of disorders, but the prophylactic use of antiplatelet drugs may be hazardous when bleeding and thrombotic tendencies coexist.

Acute Leukaemias, Preleukaemic States

Various defects of platelet function have been described in this group of disorders, but the primary cause of haemostatic failure is thrombocytopenia.

Renal Disease

Although the bleeding tendency associated with uraemia often has a complex aetiology, including some degree of thrombocytopenia and of coagulation defects, disordered platelet function is probably the most important contributory cause. The bleeding time is usually prolonged, and amongst the other abnormalities that have been demonstrated are reduced in-vivo platelet adhesiveness and retention in glass-bead columns, and defective aggregation, platelet factor-3 availability and clot retraction. The bleeding tendency, as well as the laboratory abnormalities, can be corrected by haemodialysis or peritoneal dialysis, suggesting that the observed defects are due to inhibition of platelet function by retained metabolites. Amongst the substances which have been held responsible for the inhibition are urea, guanidinosuccinic acid and various phenolic compounds. More recently, it has been suggested that the aggregation defect in uraemia is due to an abnormality of arachidonate metabolism, leading to a reduced rate of synthesis of thromboxanes. The raised levels of parathyroid hormone found in uraemic plasma have also been found to inhibit platelet aggregation and 5HT secretion.

Although the long bleeding time of uraemic patients is usually associated with raised plasma levels of factor VIII and von Willebrand factor, both cryoprecipitate and DDAVP have been claimed to shorten the bleeding time and correct the bleeding tendency, without affecting the results of platelet function tests. Correction of the anaemia will also lessen the bleeding tendency: the bleeding time is inversely related to the PCV of uraemic patients.

In the nephrotic syndrome, a thrombotic tendency is often associated with hyperaggregability of the platelets. This is partly attributable to the low plasma albumin, which results in increased availability of arachidonic acid, but there is evidence that partial neutralization of the negative surface charge of the platelets by a cationic macromolecule may also play an important part.

Dysproteinaemias

Although disorders of coagulation and fibrinolysis are also seen in this group of disorders, defects of platelet function and hyperviscosity seem to be more closely correlated with the bleeding tendency. Platelet adhesion and aggregation have both been found to be defective, probably because of binding of the paraprotein to the platelet membrane.

Acquired Storage Pool Deficiency

Damage to circulating platelets, whether mechanical or immune mediated, stimulates the release of their dense body and α-granule contents, and the continued circulation of such depleted platelets may lead to haemostatic failure. This mechanism operates in a wide variety of conditions, in many of which thrombocytopenia may subsequently develop as the damaged platelets are removed from the circulation. Thus, acquired SPD has been described in various types of autoimmune disease, including systemic lupus erythematosus and ITP, and also in conditions associated with increased platelet consumption—the most important of these are listed in Table 22.10. Storage of platelets for transfusion may also result in depletion of their granule contents.

Chronic Hypoglycaemia

The syndrome resulting from glycogen storage disease type I (glucose-6-phosphatase deficiency) includes a mild bleeding tendency characterized by easy bruising, epistaxis and prolonged haemorrhage after injury, and a long bleeding time. This is due to a disorder of platelet function, involving deficiency of adenine nucleotides in both the storage and metabolic pools and a defect of ADP secretion, which appears to be secondary to the chronic hypoglycaemia resulting from the hereditary metabolic defect, and can be temporarily corrected by intravenous administration of glucose. A similar platelet abnormality has been observed in fructose-1,6-diphosphatase deficiency.

Bartter's Syndrome

This uncommon metabolic disorder involves hyperplasia of the juxtaglomerular apparatus, with hypokalaemic acidosis, hyperreninaemia, aldosteronism and increased urinary excretion of prostaglandins. Although it is not associated with a bleeding tendency, defective platelet aggregation has been reported, and probably results from overproduction of inhibitory prostaglandins. It has been shown to be corrected by a high sodium intake.

Drugs

Many different classes of drugs interfere with platelet function, and several of them have been used, or at least considered, as potential antithrombotic agents (see Chapter 25). This section relates only to those drugs which may provoke bleeding as a side-effect of their use for other purposes (Table 22.11).

Aspirin has long been known to cause bleeding in some patients, and to prolong the bleeding time.

Table 22.11
Drugs which interfere with platelet function

Non-steroidal anti-inflammatory drugs
  Acetylsalicylic acid
  Indomethacin
  Sulphinpyrazone
  Phenylbutazone
Antimicrobials
  Penicillins
  Cephalosporins
Heparin
Dextrans
Ethanol
Radiographic contrast agents

These effects are due to its inhibition of cyclo-oxygenase, resulting in a failure of the platelets to synthesize prostaglandin endoperoxides and thromboxane A_2. Aspirin acetylates platelet cyclo-oxygenase irreversibly, so that the effect of a single pharmacological dose of aspirin may last up to 10 days. It must therefore be withheld for at least this period before blood is taken for platelet function tests. The other non-steroidal anti-inflammatory agents have a similar but shorter lived effect, and some of them have been claimed to inhibit platelet adhesion to subendothelium. Aspirin also inhibits the cyclo-oxygenase of vascular endothelial cells, and so blocks the synthesis of prostaglandin I_2, but the endothelial enzyme recovers much more rapidly than the platelet enzyme, so that the effect is short lived. It is because of this differential effect that low-dose aspirin is likely to diminish platelet aggregability in vivo.

Various penicillins and cephalosporins, when given in high dosage, interfere with ADP-induced platelet aggregation and secretion, and may also impair adhesion to collagen. These effects are thought to be due to coating of the cell membrane by the drugs or their metabolites, with consequent blocking of receptor sites. Purpuric symptoms and a long bleeding time may result. Patients in renal failure are particularly at risk of this side-effect, since their platelet function may already be impaired (see above), and unusually high concentrations of the drugs or their metabolites may result from defective clearance. The effect may persist for several days after withdrawal of the drug, suggesting an irreversible effect on circulating platelets.

Heparin in high concentrations has been found to inhibit platelet aggregation and secretion, and this effect might sometimes contribute to the bleeding tendency resulting from overdosage. Dextrans have a similar effect, and can prolong the bleeding time at clinical dosage. The inhibitory activity of both these drugs seems to be due to the induction of a refractory state following transient activation of the platelets; in each case the effect is more pronounced with high molecular weight forms.

Acute ethanol ingestion may cause both thrombocytopenia and disorders of platelet function including defects of aggregation, secretion and thromboxane synthesis. It potentiates the prolongation of the bleeding time by aspirin, and inhibits the pro-aggregatory effect of saturated fats. Withdrawal of ethanol from acute alcoholics not only corrects the defects but may result in an overswing to a transitory thrombotic tendency during the next 2–3 weeks.

Long bleeding times and defective platelet aggregation and secretion have been found to follow the use of various intravenous radiographic contrast agents for angiography, and to persist for hours or days.

Amongst foods which have been observed to interfere with platelet function are onions, garlic, ginger and Chinese black tree fungus. Although none of these causes a bleeding tendency, they may cause confusion by upsetting the results of laboratory tests.

PLATELET TRANSFUSION

Platelet transfusion may be required in the conditions listed in Table 22.12; the specific indications are discussed below, and the immunological and technical aspects are considered in Chapters 8–10. Platelet concentrations are the preparation of choice in every case, though in the case of massive blood transfusion, thrombocytopenia can usually be prevented or controlled by giving fresh whole blood in a proportion of 1 unit for every 5 units of stored blood. There is no place for platelet transfusion (except in extreme emergency) in most of the immune thrombocytopenias, or when shortened platelet survival is due to vascular lesions, since the donor platelets are likely to be removed from the circulation as rapidly as the patient's own.

Platelet transfusion is seldom required in thrombocytopenia from any cause unless the platelet count falls below 20×10^9/l, and only then when serious haemorrhage is present, or is likely to occur—as, for example, during intensive chemotherapy of leukaemia. Severe epistaxis or gastro-intestinal haemorrhage, and bleeding into the CNS, are immediate indications for platelet transfusion if the platelet count is below 50×10^9/l; the presence of fever, especially with known infection, makes haemorrhage more likely and may call for prophylactic platelet transfusion in the attempt to forestall bleeding. Surgery is another indication: 100×10^9/l is a reasonable goal during the operative procedure. For most other purposes the aim of a single platelet transfusion should be to raise the platelet count to $40–60 \times 10^9$/l immediately after transfusion. This requires something of the order of 4–6 units/m^2 of fresh platelets, and this figure should be doubled if the patient has fever or splenomegaly. Higher doses are also needed if stored or frozen platelets are used (see Chapter 10). Although haemostasis may be temporarily achieved in the absence of an increase of circulating platelets, it is much more likely to result when a significant increment is observed.

The most frequent and important indications for platelet transfusion are in the leukaemias and aplastic anaemias. Adequate replacement therapy with platelets is an essential component of aggressive antileukaemic chemotherapy and of bone marrow transplantation regimes. Such patients may require platelet support for days or weeks, pending bone marrow recovery or engraftment. In aplastic anaemia, however, profound thrombocytopenia may persist for months, and if such patients are regularly transfused, antiplatelet antibodies, with consequent refractoriness to platelet transfusion, are particularly likely to develop. The use of HLA-matched platelets will greatly lessen this risk, but nevertheless platelet transfusion should be used only for serious bleeding episodes, and should be from unrelated donors in order to avoid sensitization against antigens present in family members who might become bone marrow donors.

In alloimmune neonatal thrombocytopenia, the infant may be transfused with platelets lacking the

Table 22.12
Conditions in which platelet transfusion may be needed

Failure of platelet production
  Acute leukaemias
  Bone marrow aplasia
Acute loss of platelets
  Massive blood transfusion
  Extracorporeal circulation
Alloimmune neonatal thrombocytopenia
Disseminated intravascular coagulation
Hereditary thrombocytopenias
Disorders of platelet function

---

offending antigen (usually Pl^{A1}); the mother's platelets may be used but must be washed to remove antibody. This is the only form of immune thrombocytopenia in which platelet transfusion has a place; in autoimmune or immune complex-mediated thrombocytopenia, the transfused platelets are likely to be removed from the circulation so rapidly as to be of little therapeutic value, and in the former case may also stimulate further antibody production. Similarly, platelet transfusions will be ineffective in drug-induced thrombocytopenia until the offending drug has been eliminated from the circulation, when there is seldom any further need for treatment. Platelet transfusion may have a place in supportive care of some cases of acute DIC, but must be combined with treatment of the underlying condition and with measures to prevent further intravascular coagulation.

Platelet transfusions may be required in the hereditary thrombocytopenias or in disorders of platelet function, chiefly to control accidental haemorrhage or as cover for necessary surgical procedures. Since such patients may require platelet transfusions from time to time throughout their life, they are at risk of developing platelet antibodies, and HLA-compatible platelets should be used if possible.

DISORDERS OF BLOOD VESSELS: THE NON-THROMBOCYTOPENIC PURPURAS

Focal or generalized vascular abnormalities may be a cause of haemorrhagic symptoms, either on their own account or in association with defects of the platelets or coagulation mechanism. The conditions in which abnormal bleeding is mainly due to disorders affecting the blood vessels or their supporting structures are listed in Table 22.13, and some of them are discussed further below. Since there are no reliable tests of vascular function, the diagnosis of these disorders is chiefly a clinical one, supported by the exclusion of other haemostatic defects.

Mechanical Purpuras

Purpura in a restricted area of the body may result from local venous compression, as for example over

Table 22.13

Bleeding disorders due to vascular and connective tissue disorders

---

Mechanical
  Venous compression
  Orthostatic purpura
  Pigmented dermatoses
Allergic
  Henoch–Schönlein syndrome
  Drugs, foods
Atrophic
  Senile purpura
  Steroid purpura, Cushing's syndrome
  Penicillamine
  Scurvy
Infections
  Bacterial, viral, rickettsial
Hereditary
  Hereditary haemorrhagic telangiectasia
  Ehlers–Danlos syndrome
  Pseudoxanthoma elasticum
  Marfan's syndrome
  Osteogenesis imperfecta
  Fabry's disease
Paraproteinaemias, amyloidosis (see Chapter 18)
Miscellaneous
  Purpura simplex
  Factitious purpura
  Autoerythrocyte sensitization, DNA sensitivity
  Fat embolism

---

the presenting part in newborn infants, or on the face and neck after prolonged bouts of coughing or vomiting. In the elderly, orthostatic purpura results from poor venous return combined with atrophy of supporting connective tissues, and leads to permanent discoloration from the deposition of haemosiderin. The pigmented dermatoses (Majocchi; Schamberg; Gougerot and Blum) have a similar end result.

Allergic Purpuras

These constitute a group of non-thrombocytopenic purpuras characterized by aseptic vasculitis of the skin and other tissues, together with other allergic features such as oedema and urticaria. The syndrome may occur acutely as a transient allergic response to foods or drugs, including penicillins, sulphonamides, salicylates, iodides and many others; it is also seen as a more chronic disorder, often without obvious precipitating cause. When the skin lesions are associated with gastrointestinal symptoms and/or joint pains, the condition is known as the Henoch–Schönlein syndrome.

Henoch–Schönlein Syndrome

The syndrome is seen mainly in children, with a peak incidence between 3 and 6 years of age. The characteristic rash usually appears 1–3 weeks after an acute infection or occasionally vaccination, and may be accompanied by painful periarticular swellings, abdominal colic and melaena, subcutaneous oedema and/or haematuria. The rash itself is seen mainly on the buttocks and extensor surfaces of the limbs, and has urticarial and maculopapular as well as petechial components; it tends to occur in crops over a period of weeks. Oedema usually affects the dorsum of the hands and feet, and may also involve the face and scalp, particularly in younger children. The condition eventually resolves spontaneously in the great majority of cases, but early renal involvement may progress to chronic renal failure in a small minority—perhaps 2–3%. In about half of all cases, one or more symptoms may recur from time to time, but seldom for more than a few months, and the ultimate prognosis remains good so long as renal function remains unimpaired.

The aseptic vasculitis seems to be attributable to the deposition of circulating immune complexes on vessel walls in skin, glomeruli and elsewhere, with resulting complement activation. Most patients can be shown to have raised levels of IgA immune complexes in their serum, but there is evidence that the renal damage may be mediated by IgG complexes, which are seen only in those children who develop nephritis. Laboratory tests do not contribute to the diagnosis, which is essentially clinical; the platelet count and bleeding time are normal.

Treatment does not significantly modify the course of the disease. Corticosteroids may give relief from joint and abdominal symptoms but do not seem to influence the skin or renal lesions. Dapsone is said to control cutaneous recurrences in about 50% of cases. If precipitating factors such as foods or drugs can be identified, they should obviously be eliminated.

Atrophic Disorders of Connective Tissues

Senile Purpura

This occurs with increasing frequency in both sexes from the seventh decade of life onwards, and consists of large irregular superficial ecchymotic lesions on the extensor surface of the forearms and hands, and sometimes the back of the neck. These are dark purple, fading to brown, and the surrounding skin is thin, inelastic and pigmented. Fresh lesions can be produced in the same areas by blunt pressure, the vessel walls being unduly friable as a result of the atrophy of the surrounding subcutaneous tissues. The platelets are normal and treatment is neither effective nor necessary.

Steroid Purpura

Long continued steroid therapy, whether systemic or topical, may cause atrophy of the dermis and so lead to a form of purpura closely similar to senile purpura, but often on the lower legs as well as the forearms and hands. The same type of purpura may occur in Cushing's syndrome, and is sometimes seen in long-standing rheumatoid disease, even in the absence of steroid therapy. The purpura which may develop in patients on high doses of penicillamine probably has a similar pathogenesis.

Scurvy

Haemorrhage is usually a presenting feature in scurvy: acute periosteal haemorrhage in infants, and a more insidious onset of skin and gum bleeding in the elderly, sometimes accompanied by deep haematomata. The perifollicular distribution of the ecchymotic lesions is characteristic. The bleeding results from defective collagen synthesis in and around the vessel wall; defects of platelet function have also been described but are of doubtful significance. The condition responds rapidly to oral ascorbic acid.

Purpura Associated with Infections

Apart from the thrombocytopenic purpura which may follow acute infections (pp. 603, 606), and disseminated intravascular coagulation due to septicaemias (see Chapter 24), many bacterial, viral and rickettsial infections may cause purpura as a result of vascular damage, either by the organism itself or as a result of immune complex formation. Examples are measles, meningococcal septicaemia and Dengue fever.

Hereditary Disorders

Hereditary Haemorrhagic Telangiectasia (Rendu–Osler–Weber Disease)

This autosomal dominant trait results in the development of small thin-walled venous angiomatous malformations in skin, mucous membranes and many internal organs. The bleeding is confined to these lesions, which do not usually cause symptoms until the second or third decade. Recurrent epistaxis is the commonest symptom, but gastrointestinal haemorrhage or haematuria may occur. Tests of the haemostatic mechanism give normal results, and the diagnosis depends on the recognition of telangiectases in the skin, buccal mucosa, or elsewhere. The severity tends to increase with age as more lesions develop and enlarge, and severe iron-deficiency anaemia commonly results. Pulmonary arteriovenous fistulae are common, particularly in older patients.

Accessible bleeding points can be controlled by local measures, but surgery may be required for gastrointestinal or pulmonary lesions; surgical wounds do not bleed excessively provided telangiectases are not injured. Cautery may provide temporary relief from epistaxis, and systemic oestrogen therapy has been advocated for its long-term control, but its side-effects probably outweigh its effectiveness. Most patients require regular iron replacement therapy.

Connective Tissue Disorders

Several of the hereditary disorders of connective tissues result in a bleeding tendency, as a result either of lack of support to the vessels by the surrounding connective tissue, or of defective interaction of the abnormal vascular collagen with the platelets.

Ehlers–Danlos syndrome comprises a heterogeneous group of hereditary collagen abnormalities characterized by hyperextensibility of joints and hyperelastic, friable skin. Of the eight subtypes

currently recognized, the bleeding tendency is most severe in type IV, in which type III collagen is defective.

Pseudoxanthoma elasticum is a rare autosomal recessive disorder of elastic tissue, of which arterial haemorrhage and thrombosis are the chief results. Haemorrhage may involve the central nervous system, gastrointestinal tract and many other organs, and is the commonest cause of death. Milder cases may result in only superficial bruising following minor trauma. The diagnosis can be confirmed by skin biopsy.

Easy bruising and epistaxis may also occur in Marfan's syndrome and osteogenesis imperfecta, but these conditions seldom result in serious bleeding. In Fabry's disease (angiokeratoma corporis diffusum universale), an X-linked disorder of glycolipid metabolism, the telangiectatic spots require to be distinguished from other purpuric lesions and from those of hereditary haemorrhagic telangiectasia.

Other Non-Thrombocytopenic Purpuras

Purpura Simplex (Simple Easy Bruising)

Apparently spontaneous bruising of the legs is a fairly common complaint of adolescent girls and young women, chiefly on cosmetic grounds and unassociated with other symptoms except anxiety. Some such cases may prove to be due to minor defects of platelet function, but laboratory tests usually give entirely normal results, and reassurance based on such findings is the only treatment necessary. It is important to distinguish the condition from factitious purpura, in which an unusual distribution of lesions is likely to be associated with other evidence of psychological disturbance.

Autoerythrocyte Sensitization

This curious condition of adult women consists of painful ecchymoses with surrounding oedema, mainly on the limbs, usually developing after injury or operations, though not necessarily at the same site. The lesions last for a week or two, tend to recur at intervals, and may be accompanied by headaches, vomiting, abdominal pain and even melaena and haematuria, so coming to resemble the Henoch–Schönlein syndrome. The patient is often profoundly emotionally disturbed, and the condition seems to be psychosomatic in origin. Tests of the haemostatic mechanism give normal results but the intradermal injection of 0.1 ml of the patient's own blood or red cells induces, during the succeeding 24 hours, a painful ecchymosis similar to the naturally occurring lesion. No form of therapy has been consistently successful, and psychotherapy may be the treatment of choice.

DNA sensitivity is a similar condition, also of women, in which the lesions can be induced by the intradermal injection of autologous leucocytes or of DNA, but not by red cells. The lesions usually occur only on the limbs, the skin of the trunk being insensitive to provocation. Treatment with chloroquine has proved effective.

Fat Embolism

A petechial rash is a characteristic feature of fat embolism following major trauma, although thrombocytopenia occurs in only a minority of cases. Damage to skin capillaries by the fat droplets seems the most likely mechanism.

SELECTED BIBLIOGRAPHY

Barratt T. M., Drummond K. N. (1981). The vasculitis syndromes: Henoch–Schönlein syndrome or anaphylactoid purpura. In *Practice of pediatrics* (Ed. Wedgwood R. V.). Hagerstown: Harper and Row.

Bussel J. B., Hilgartner M. W. (1984). The use and mechanism of action of intravenous immunoglobulin in the treatment of immune haematologic disease. *British Journal of Haematology*, **56**, 1–7.

Burstein S. A., McMillan R. M., Harker L. A. (1987). In *Haemostasis and thrombosis*, 2nd edn. (Eds. A. L. Bloom and D. P. Thomas) pp. 333–364. Edinburgh: Churchill Livingstone.

Hardisty R. M., Caen J. P. (1987). Disorders of platelet function. In *Haemostasis and thrombosis*, 2nd edn (Eds. A. L. Bloom, D. P. Thomas) pp. 365–392. Edinburgh: Churchill Livingstone.

Harker L. A., Zimmerman T. S. (Eds.) (1983). Platelet disorders. *Clinics in Haematology*, **12**, 1–360.

Harker L. A., Zimmerman T. S. (Eds.) (1983). *Measurement of platelet function*. Edinburgh: Churchill-Livingstone.

Kelton J. G. (1983). The measurement of platelet-bound immunoglobulins: an overview of the methods and the biological relevance of platelet-associated IgG. *Progress in Hematology*, **13**, 163–199.

Machin S. J. (1984). Thrombotic thrombocytopenic purpura. *British Journal of Haematology*, **56**, 191–197.

Pope F. M., Nicholls A. C., Dorling J., Webb J. (1983). Molecular abnormalities of collagen: a review. *Journal of the Royal Society of Medicine*, **76**, 1050–1062.

Walker R. W., Walker W. (1984). Idiopathic thrombocytopenia, initial illness and long term follow up. *Archives of Disease in Childhood*, **59**, 316–322.

Walsh C. M., Nardi M. A., Karpatkin S. (1984). On the mechanisms of thrombocytopenic purpura in sexually active homosexual men. *New England Journal of Medicine*, **311**, 635–639.

Waters A. H., Webster A. D. B. (Eds.) (1985). Intravenous immunoglobulins in immunodeficiency syndromes and idiopathic thrombocytopenic purpura. *RSM International Congress and Symposium Series*, **84**, 63–112.

Chapter 23

INHERITED BLEEDING DISORDERS

E. G. D. TUDDENHAM

The existence of lifelong bleeding disorders and their familial occurrence was noted very early in the medical literature by Alsaharavius in 1519. No doubt this was because the clinical syndrome of haemophilia is highly distinctive. The medical practitioner's helplessness in the face of exsanguinating haemophilic blood loss profoundly impressed the early writers. A full understanding of the pathophysiology and genetics of these disorders was long delayed by the complexities of the clotting mechanism. Recent advances in protein chemistry and recombinant DNA technology have produced a comprehensive account both of normal coagulation and of the molecular genetics of some types of haemophilia. The coagulation mechanism is outlined in Chapter 21. In this chapter, the clinical features of inherited bleeding disorders will be described together with what is known of the underlying genetics. Advances in therapy that will arise from this new knowledge have not yet reached the clinic, but since these developments are imminent, an attempt will be made to predict their likely effect on current practice.

Restriction fragment length polymorphisms are now routinely used to determine the carrier state for the two X-linked haemophilias and it is therefore appropriate to discuss this methodology in some detail.

Table 23.1 lists the hereditary bleeding disorders in approximately their order of incidence, which is the order followed in this account.

HAEMOPHILIA A

Clinical Features

Almost but not quite all patients are male (see 'Female haemophiliacs' below). The severity and frequency of bleeding in X-linked factor VIII deficiency are inversely correlated with the residual factor VIII level. Table 23.2 summarizes this relationship and gives the relative frequency of categories based on UK national data. The joints most affected are the main load- or strain-bearing articulations—ankles, knees, hips and elbows — but any joint can be the site of bleeding. Untreated, this intracapsular bleeding causes severe swelling, pain, stiffness and inflammation which gradually resolves over days or weeks. A vivid account of a classical case is given in *Journey* by Robert and Anne Massey (1973). Blood is highly irritant to the synovium and causes synovial overgrowth with a tendency to rebleed from friable vascular tissue, setting up a vicious circle. Probably through accumulation of iron in chondrocytes, a rapid degenerative arthritis occurs leading to irregularity of articular contour, then thinning of the cartilage, bony overgrowth and subchondral cysts, and finally, ankylosis (Fig. 23.1). A particular joint or joints tend to be the target for this destructive process in a given patient, whilst other joints may be relatively spared.

Muscle bleeding can be seen in any anatomical site but most often presents in the large load-bearing groups of the thigh, calf, posterior abdominal wall and buttocks. Local pressure effects often cause entrapment neuropathy, particularly of the femoral nerve, with iliopsoas bleeding. The latter causes a common symptom triad of groin pain, hip flexure and cutaneous sensory loss over the femoral nerve distribution. Bleeding into the calf, forearm or peroneal muscles can lead to ischaemic necrosis and contracture.

Haematuria is less common than joint or muscle bleeding in haemophiliacs but most severely affected cases have one or two episodes per decade.

Table 23.1

Inherited bleeding disorders

Disorder (synonyms)	Pathophysiology	Mode of Inheritance*	Molecular genetics	Approximate incidence per 10^6 population‡
Common group				
Haemophilia A (classical haemophilia)	Factor VIII deficient or defective	XL	Deletions, missense, nonsense, insertions	100
von Willebrand's disease	von Willebrand factor deficient or defective	AD or AR	Deletions	AD-100 or more† AR-1
Haemophilia B (Christmas disease)	Factor IX deficient or defective	XL	Deletions, missense nonsense, splicing errors	20
Haemophilia C (PTA deficiency)	Factor XI deficiency	AD	?	5% in Ashkenazi Jews, others rare
Rare group				
Factor X deficiency		AR	Deletions	1
Factor V deficiency		AR	?	1
Factor VII deficiency		AR	?	1
Factor II (prothrombin) deficiency		AR	?	1
Afibrinogenaemia		AR	?	1
Dysfibrinogenaemia		AD	Missense	1
Factor XIII deficiency		AR	?	1
Factor V plus VIII deficiency		AR	?	1
Hyperplasminaemia: α_2 antiplasmin deficiency		AR	?	Very rare

* XL, X-linked recessive. AD, Autosomal dominant. AR, Autosomal recessive.

† Recent population surveys indicate much higher incidence of mild von Willebrand's disease.

‡ Figures applicable to developed countries. Incidence is lower in developing countries due to very high early mortality and low reproductive fitness of sufferers.

Table 23.2
Haemophilia A: clinical severity*

Factor VIII (units/dl)	Bleeding tendency	Relative incidence (% of cases)
<2	Severe; frequent spontaneous[+] bleeding into joints, muscles and internal organs	50
2–10	Moderately severe; some 'spontaneous bleeds', bleeding after minor trauma	30
>10–30	Mild; bleeding only after significant trauma, surgery	20

* This table is also applicable to factor IX, X, VII and II deficiencies but not to factor XI, V, XIII or von Willebrand factor deficiencies (see text).
[+] 'Spontaneous' bleeding refers to those episodes where no obvious precipitating event preceded the bleed. No doubt minor tissue damage consequent on everyday activities actually initiates bleeding.

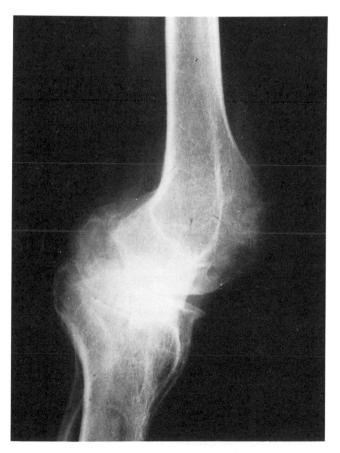

Fig. 23.1 *X-ray of knee joint showing advanced haemophilic arthropathy. Note loss of cartilage, bony overgrowth, deformity subluxation, osteophytes, sub-chondral cysts and irregularity of joint contours.*

These may be painless and resolve spontaneously, but if bleeding is heavy, it can produce clot colic. No anatomical abnormality is usually found to account for the haematuria on radiological investigation.

Central nervous system bleeding is uncommon but can occur after slight head injury and was formerly the commonest cause of death in haemophilia A. Intestinal tract bleeding usually presents as obstruction due to intramural haemorrhage, but haematemesis and melaena also occasionally occur and should be routinely investigated since they may be due to peptic ulcer or malignancy.

Oropharyngeal bleeding, although uncommon, is clinically dangerous since extension through the soft tissues of the floor of the mouth can lead to respiratory obstruction. Bleeding from the tongue can be very persistent and troublesome after laceration due to fibrinolytic substances in saliva and the impossibility of immobilizing the part.

Surgery and open trauma invariably lead to dangerous haemorrhage in the untreated haemophiliac. The most impressive feature is not the rate of haemorrhage but its persistence, often after an initial short-lived period of haemostasis. Clots, if formed, are bulky and friable and break off, with renewed haemorrhage occurring intermittently over days and weeks. This is only seen today in patients who are resistant to conventional replacement therapy due to the presence of inhibitors (see below).

Bruising is a feature of haemophilia A, but usually only of cosmetic significance since it remains superficial and self-limiting. Large extending echymoses may occasionally require treatment.

Presentation

Where a woman is known to be a carrier or at high risk, the cord blood factor VIII level will establish the diagnosis in her infant. One-third of cases are sporadic, however, and in these the haemophilic condition may come to light in the neonatal period with cephalohaematoma or prolonged bleeding from the cord. In cultures where early circumcision is the rule this will cause prolonged haemorrhage, as was noted in the Babylonian Talmud almost 2000 years ago. Quite often the diagnosis is delayed until it is noticed that the infant has many large bruises from hand pressure where picked up or from minor

knocks on the cot. These sometimes cause diagnostic confusion and the erroneous label of 'battered baby syndrome', with needless psychological trauma to the parents. As soon as the infant starts to crawl actively, joint bleeding will begin to appear. Excessive bleeding from eruption of primary dentition or from lacerations leads to performance of diagnostic tests in other children. Mild cases may only present in later life when severe trauma or surgery provokes unusual bleeding.

Pathophysiology

All the clinical features of haemophilia A are due directly or indirectly to lack of the clotting factor VIII. The gene for this protein cofactor is located near the tip of the long arm of the X chromosome (Xq 2.8/Ter) which accounts for the sex-linked pattern of inheritance. Sufferers are unable to produce factor VIII due to various mutations (see below) at the factor VIII locus. Lack of the cofactor drastically slows the rate of generation of factor Xa, despite the presence of all other coagulation factors and platelets in normal amounts. Conversely, replacement by intravenous infusion of factor VIII can normalize the haemophiliac's haemostatic mechanism for the duration that the infused factor resides in his circulation at physiological concentration

Laboratory Diagnosis

Screening tests show a long PTTK, normal prothrombin time (PT), thrombin clotting time (TCT) and bleeding time and normal platelet count (Table 23.3). Specific assays show factor VIII clotting activity below 35 u/dl with all other factors normal and normal von Willebrand factor antigen and ristocetin cofactor. The bleeding time as performed by the standardized template method is normal (c. f. von Willebrand's disease). A test for antibodies to factor VIII should also be performed.

Treatment

The mainstay for treatment is replacement therapy by means of intravenous infusion with factor VIII. Up to now, all factor VIII used has been blood derived (Table 23.4). Ideally, all severely affected

Table 23.3

Laboratory diagnosis of inherited bleeding disorders

Disorder	Screening tests*				Specific assays†(units/dl)
	PT	PTTK	TCT	BT	
Haemophilia A	N	↑	N	N	Factor VIII < 50 vWF:Ag N Ricof. N
von Willebrand's disease	N	↑ or N	N	↑ or N	Factor VIII < 50 vWF:Ag < 50 or N Ricof. < 50 or N
Haemophilia B	N	↑	N	N	Factor IX < 50
Factor XI deficiency	N	↑	N	N	Factor XI < 35
Factor X deficiency	↑	↑	N	N	Factor X < 50
Factor V deficiency	↑	↑	N	N or ↑	Factor V < 50
Factor VII	↑	N	N	N	Factor VII < 50
Factor II	↑	↑	N	N	Factor II < 50
Afibrinogenaemia	↑	↑	↑	↑	Fibrinogen undetectable
Dysfibrinogenaemia	↑	↑	↑	N	Fibrinogen N or ↓
Factor XIII deficiency	N	N	N	N	Fibrin solubility ↑ Factor XIII < 1
Factor V plus VIII deficiency	↑	↑	N	N	Factor V < 50 Factor VIII < 50
Hyperplasminaemia	N	N	N	N	Euglobulin clot lysis time short, α_2 antiplasmin absent

* PT, prothrombin time. PTTK, activated partial thromboplastin time. TCT, thrombin clotting time. BT, bleeding time.
† Factor VIII (formerly VIII:c). vWF:Ag, von Willebrand factor antigen (formerly VIIIR:Ag). Ricof., Ristocetin cofactor.
↑ = Increased, ↓ = decreased, N = normal.

patients would be maintained on long-term prophylaxis with daily or alternate-day infusions to keep spontaneous haemorrhages to a minimum. This is impossible due to the limitations of supply and finance. The half-life of factor VIII of 8–10 hours means that twice-daily infusions are needed to maintain a normal level at all times; however, for prophylactic purposes a fairly wide fluctuation is still very effective. In practice, most patients are treated on demand. That is, they receive (or give themselves) an infusion of factor at the earliest symptom of bleeding. Patients become skilled at recognizing very early joint bleeding, and provided that an infusion of factor VIII is given within a few minutes to 1 hour of onset, the bleeding will be halted before a significant amount of blood has leaked into the joint. Normal activities can then be resumed almost immediately.

It was realized in the 1960s that such prompt treatment could only be achieved if the patient or his relatives gave the injection and so home therapy programmes were instituted. The results of these programmes were a dramatic fall in time lost from work or school and a marked reduction in the onset of new and the progression of old joint damage. Severely affected patients who have grown up under this regime are now reaching their twenties with little or no arthritis, in marked contrast to the older patients or patients from developing countries who nearly all have severe damage in several joints, increasing relentlessly with age and number of bleeds.

Dosage of factor VIII is adjusted approximately to obtain a desired level in the circulation (Table 23.5). Formulae based on plasma volume and expected recovery give a rough guide to dosage,

Table 23.4

Therapeutic materials for treatment of haemophilia A and von Willebrand's disease

Material	Factor VIII (u/ml)	vWF (u/ml)	Donors per unit‡	Advantages	Disadvantages
Fresh frozen plasma (FFP)	1	1	1	Low infection hazard	Storage at −20°C / High volume/low potency / Allergic reactions
Cryoprecipitate	5–10	5–10	1	Low infection hazard (unless many units used)	Storage at −20°C / Allergic reactions / Not heat treated in UK / Potency not assayed
Heat-treated factor VIII concentrate	20–50	Low*	3000–15000	Assayed high potency, low or absent HIV and hepatitis B infectivity. Store at 4°C. Few allergic reactions	Infective for non-A–non-B, cost 15p/unit. Heavy load of non-F VIII proteins including iso-anti A, anti B, β_2 microglobulin, fibrinogen etc.
DDAVP	—	—	0	No infection risk, totally synthetic	Only effective in mild cases
Porcine factor VIII† (Hyate C)	20–50	Low	—	No infection risk, high purity	Animal protein, allergic reactions / Alloantibody to porcine factor VIII
Recombinant factor VIII	5000 u/mg	0	0	No infection risk, totally pure	Cost at least 15p/unit / Not yet available
Recombinant von Willebrand factor	0	100 u/mg	0	No infection risk, totally pure	Not yet available

* Although high concentrations of vWF antigen are present, the size distribution is altered with loss of highly polymerized forms and consequently little effect on the bleeding time in von Willebrand's disease.
† Generally reserved for treatment of inhibitor cases.
‡ Number of individuals whose blood donation contributes to a single unit of treatment, i.e. pack of plasma or bottle of concentrate.

Table 23.5

Plasma levels of factor VIII required for haemostasis

Clinical indication	Plasma factor VIII (units/dl)	Dosage (units/kg)
Early haemarthrosis or muscle bleed	15–20	8–10
More severe bleeding, minor trauma	30–50	15–25
Surgery, major trauma, head injury	80–120	40–60

but where the level is critical, as for surgery or in case of serious bleeding, it should always be checked by assay after infusion. On average, factor VIII infusion produces a plasma increment of 2 units/dl per unit infused per kilogram body weight. From this a simple formula can be derived, as follows:

dose to be infused (units)

$$= \frac{\text{weight (kg)} \times \text{increment needed (u/dl)}}{2.0}.$$

Assessing the period of treatment required is a matter of clinical judgement of the individual episode or lesion. An early joint bleed will often resolve with a single infusion. Cover for surgery other than very minor procedures will need to be continued at full twice-daily dosage, adjusted according to pre- and post-treatment assays, for a week or more, followed by a period at reduced dosage during convalescence.

Detailed discussion of the orthopaedic management of haemophilic arthropathy is beyond the scope of this chapter, and the reader is referred to the texts on comprehensive care listed in the bibliography at the end of the chapter. Suffice to say that large numbers of patients have had total hip or knee joint replacements with good results and that arthrodesis of the knee or ankle can provide pain relief and improved locomotor function where arthroplasty is impractical.

Physiotherapy plays a very important role in maintaining and improving the function of joints and muscles damaged or weakened by bleeding and enforced periods of immobilization.

Factor VIII concentrate, with its advantages of storage, convenience and assayed potency, is the material of choice in severe haemophilia and treatment of major bleeding where it is essential to maintain high levels. The realization of its infective hazard (see below, 'Complications') has given prominence to the use of a non-blood-derived alternative—DDAVP (desamino D-arginyl vasopressin). This synthetic analogue of vasopressin was noted to cause a rise in factor VIII and von Willebrand factor levels without pressor effects. DDAVP retains the antidiuretic action of the natural hormone and also stimulates the release of vascular plasminogen activator. In practice, these effects can be used to elevate the plasma factor VIII level two- to four-fold above baseline, presumably by release from storage site(s).

Given together with a fibrinolytic inhibitor such as tranexamic acid (to neutralize the fibrinolytic stimulus), DDAVP can correct the haemostatic defect in mild haemophilia A or von Willebrand's disease enough to cover minor surgery or treat a minor bleeding episode. A typical regimen would be to give 4 μg/kg body weight by slow intravenous infusion over 20 minutes together with 1 g tranexamic acid. The effect reaches a maximum at 1 hour, when the factor VIII level may have risen, for example in a mild haemophiliac, from 10 u/dl to 40 u/dl. The half-life of the endogenously released factor VIII is about 8 hours, and repeat doses can be given, but with progressively diminishing response. The maximum useful number of doses is three in 24 hours, after which a rest period is needed to allow stores to reaccumulate. Fibrinolytic inhibition is also useful for the management of oral and intestinal tract bleeding. It must be strictly avoided where there is upper urinary tract bleeding since it can cause obstructive nephropathy and acute renal failure due to mechanical outflow occlusion by blood clot.

Complications of Therapy

Inhibitors

Development of antibodies to factor VIII (often termed inhibitors) occurs in about 5% of all patients with haemophilia A, but in 10–15% of severely affected individuals after exposure to factor VIII. The time of appearance of such antibodies is unpredictable and can occur after the first exposure or many years later after thousands of treatments. Routine testing for factor VIII antibodies is therefore always performed prior to elective surgery and regularly at follow-up of severe cases. Laboratory tests for antibody rely on neutralization of clotting activity in mixtures of normal and patient plasma. Since the plasma concentration of factor VIII is very low (200 ng/ml or 0.5 nmol/l), it is necessary to prolong the incubation of the mixture to 1–4 hours to attain equilibrium binding of antibody to antigen. Several tests have been devised with different periods of incubation and different units that are not strictly interconvertible. This is important when one considers therapeutic alternatives (below). Thus, old Oxford units are based on 1 hour incubation, Bethesda units on 2 hour incubation and New Oxford units on 4 hour incubation. The most widely used at present are Bethesda units. Lack of interconvertability is due to differing kinetics of inactivation of different antibodies. This is a vexed subject which fortunately in practice can be resolved by a pragmatic approach, the important issue being whether a patient's antibody can be neutralized in the short term and by what dose of factor VIII.

Three aspects of the individual patient's antibody are of clinical importance: level in units at time of treatment, type of immune response to infusion of factor VIII (low or high), and cross-reaction with porcine factor VIII. When the antibody is low (Table 23.6), an increased dose to neutralize circulating inhibitor, plus additional factor to attain a haemostatic level, will be effective. In some patients the level of antibody remains low to moderate (low responders) but in others treatment with factor VIII elicits a sharp anamnestic response (high responders). The low responders can be treated repeatedly but high responders become refractory so that alternative therapies have been developed. Most often the antibody is species specific to human factor VIII, having little or no cross-reactivity with porcine factor VIII. A new concentrate from pig plasma (Hyate C, see Table 23.4) is available which has greatly improved clinical characteristics compared to earlier animal factor VIII. This material is effective on many occasions when the titre against human factor VIII is too high to be neutralized.

Table 23.6
Guidelines for treatment of patients with factor VIII inhibitors*

Inhibitor level (B. U./ml)[†] Antihuman	Antiporcine	Type of responder	Therapeutic strategies
1–5	1–5	Low High	Human factor VIII at increased dosage a) give factor IX for minor bleeds, or b) institute immune tolerance-inducing regimen
5–13	1–5	Low High developing anti-porcine antibodies	Hyate C for all bleeds (could use plasmapheresis and human VIII) a) Factor IX for minor bleeds, reserve Hyate C for major bleeds, or b) attempt to induce tolerance
> 13	> 13	High	a) Treat acute bleeds with activated factor complex, or b) institute immune tolerance-inducing regimen

*These suggestions are the author's own practice; other clinicians may advocate alternatives.
†B.U. = 1 Bethesda unit inhibits 0.5 units factor VIII activity after 2 hours incubation at 37°C.

About half of the patients treated with Hyate C have become resistant due to development of an alloantibody, but the remainder can be treated repeatedly with good response. When the factor VIII inhibitor titre rises strongly to hundreds or even thousands of units per millilitre, factor VIII therapy is ineffective. In this situation an alternative strategy is to attempt to bypass factor VIII with partly activated mixtures of the vitamin-K-dependent factors. Conventional factor IX concentrate contains activated species (and is, in fact, liable to produce thrombosis, particularly in patients with liver damage). Controlled trials have shown it to be more effective than albumin solution in hastening recovery from a haemarthrosis. Somewhat more effective (but much more expensive) are the deliberately activated coagulation factor mixtures FEIBA and Autoplex. It is not entirely clear what the active principle in these products consists of, nor how to monitor the response by blood tests. Empirical dosage regimens have been established (see manufacturer's product literature) and the fact remains that these products have been strikingly effective on some occasions, but fail to control bleeding on others. Few clinicians would recommend undertaking elective surgical procedures under cover of these products.

Induction of immune tolerance has been attempted on many occasions. Immunosuppressives such as glucocorticoids and alkylating agents are of no benefit (although probably valuable for treatment of spontaneous acquired autoantibodies to factor VIII). It has been demonstrated that a megadose regimen continued over many months of factor VIII infusion is effective in abolishing inhibitory antibodies in over 90% of cases. The cost of this is prohibitive in most economies. A medium dose intermittent regimen is also fairly effective in the long term in blunting or abolishing immune response to factor VIII. Various schemes have been proposed for inducing specific immune tolerance, but to date no consistently successful protocol has been reported. Infusion of intravenous gammaglobulin has been successful in temporarily lowering inhibitor titres, presumably through the action of anti-idiotype antibodies. New combinations of these modalities offer hope.

The multiplicity of therapies proposed and the space devoted to this topic reflect the present lack of any one universally successful regimen, and the disproportionate amount of time, expense and effort which managing these unfortunate patients demands.

Blood-transmitted Infections

Multiple donor concentrates were introduced in the late 1960s. Very soon it was noted that a high incidence of hepatitis occurred and the newly discovered Australia antigen was present in most attacks. At the present time, most older patients test positive for hepatitis B antibody or are chronically antigen positive. During the 1970s, despite screening of blood for hepatitis B antigen, hepatitis, both acute and chronic, continued to appear in haemophiliacs and it was realized that this was mainly due to another virus or transmissible agent, non-A–non-B. This agent is relatively heat resistant and continues to contaminate all multiple donor concentrates, with an 80–100% attack rate after a single dose. No screening test is available that directly detects the virus or viruses, but some advocate rejection of blood with elevated liver enzymes. Up to half of haemophiliacs have chronically or intermittently elevated liver enzymes following a first attack of non-A–non-B hepatitis, which may cause a very severe acute episode before converting to chronicity. Liver biopsies show characteristic histological features and chronic active or chronic persistent hepatitis in a high proportion of cases. The long-term effect of this process can only be guessed at, but already a few patients have entered end-stage liver failure mainly or partly due to this pathogen. Prevention of hepatitis B is now assured by vaccinating all non-immune patients. The management of chronic hepatitis B antigenaemia, especially with coexistent delta agent, may include interferon, since there is a very real risk of later developing hepatocellular carcinoma if infection remains chronic.

The first haemophilic patient to develop AIDS was reported from the USA in 1983. Retrospective survey of stored blood serum of haemophiliacs in the UK and USA. shows that seroconversion to HIV antibody positivity began to occur from 1978 onwards. In the UK this was nearly always associated with the use of imported commercial factor VIII concentrate. However, a few well-documented instances of contamination of UK blood-derived factor VIII by HIV have occurred. Currently, all factor concentrates are from HIV-antibody-negative plasma and are heat treated. HIV is quite heat sensitive so that reasonable recovery of factor VIII is obtained, if conditions for inactivation are carefully adjusted. Hepatitis B is also inactivated but not the agent causing non-A–non-B hepatitis. Tragically, 30% of the UK haemophiliacs were infected by HIV (up to 90% of severely affected patients) before the cause and means of avoiding AIDS were discovered. The attack rate for conversion of HIV antibody positive to clinical AIDS is apparently somewhat lower for haemophiliacs (at 10%) than for other high-risk groups: homosexuals, intravenous drug abusers and Africans have an attack rate up to 70% which may cumulatively reach 100%.

Nevertheless, AIDS has now become the commonest cause of death in haemophilia, with 80 cases reported in the UK up to February 1988 and 58 deaths. The only clinical point of difference between AIDS in haemophiliacs and the syndrome seen in homosexuals is that Kaposi's sarcoma is very uncommon in the former. Surveys of the families of HIV-antibody-positive haemophiliacs show up to 5% positive tests in wives and sexual partners but no positives in other household contacts. Several wives of haemophiliacs have died of AIDS. This devastating situation has thrown a great strain on patients, their families and carers. Intensive counselling and palliative treatment of the condition once it develops are all that can be offered at present. Patients have been strongly advised if they test positive to use barrier contraception and delay starting a family whether their wives test positive or not.

Molecular Genetics of Haemophilia A

Haemophilia A demonstrates typical X-linked recessive inheritance (Fig. 23.2), of which it is the classic example. Population genetic considerations lead to the conclusion that new mutations must account for the observed incidence of sex-linked haemophilia. Haldane, in a famous paper (Haldane,

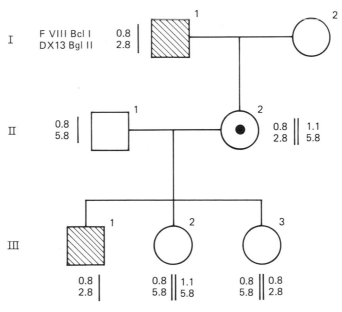

Fig. 23.2. *Family segregating haemophilia A.* ▨ *affected male,* ⊙ *obligate carrier female,* ☐ *normal male,* ○ *normal female or possible carrier. F VIII Bc1 I, RFLP size of allele in kb. DX13 Bg1 II, RFLP size of allele in kb. II_2 and III_3 have a 50% chance of carriership on pedigree analysis. Status determined by linkage analysis (see text).*

1935), argued as follows. In any generation, one-third of affected X chromosomes are in males and two-thirds in females. Due to the near lethality and at best low reproductive fitness associated with the disease, almost a third of the mutant alleles will be lost per generation. Therefore, to maintain a constant frequency in the population, new mutations are required and about one-third of cases will be due to recent mutation events. Conversely, if this were not so, a *reductio ad absurdum* argument shows that at the time of the Norman Conquest every male would have to have been a haemophiliac to provide the present proportion of cases in the British population. Haldane also demonstrated linkage between colour blindness and haemophilia. Later work — after the crucial recognition that sex-linked haemophilia includes both factor VIII deficiency (haemophilia A) and the clinically identical factor IX deficiency (haemophilia B) — showed that haemophilia A is also linked to the glucose-6-phosphate

dehydrogenase locus (Fig. 23.3). There the matter rested until the advent of the new genetics. The factor VIII gene was cloned using sequence information from purified protein to design an oligonucleotide probe.

The factor VIII gene (Fig. 23.4) spans 190-kilobase pairs of the X chromosome. The protein-coding regions (exons) are separated by 25 introns, some of very large size (e. g. intron 22 is over 35 kb). The processed messenger RNA specifies a protein of 2351 amino acids which is synthesized in the liver, spleen and lymph nodes, and from which a 19 amino acid N-terminal leader sequence is cleaved upon secretion. The mature plasma protein initially consists of a single chain of 2332 amino acids, but partially proteolysed derivatives are present in plasma as well. The sequence contains a triplicated region (A1, A2 and A3 in Fig. 23.4) whose elements are more than 30% homologous to each other and to similar regions of caeruloplasmin (the copper transport enzyme). This is presumed to indicate only common ancestry, since function has diverged markedly for these two plasma proteins. A second duplicated homology region (C1, C2) bears resemblance to a lectin from slime mould. The third type of sequence in the protein is the heavily glycosylated B domain which is coded entirely within exon 14, connects A2 to A3 and is removed upon thrombin activation of factor VIII. After thrombin activation the cofactor consists of an N-terminal heavy chain corresponding to region A1, A2 (with a single nick at residue 372) which is held by a divalent cation-dependent linkage to the C-terminal light chain corresponding to part of A3 plus C1 and C2 (Fig. 23.5).

Protein C makes a single nick at residue 336, totally inactivating the cofactor. It seems that binding to von Willebrand factor is partly via the light chain, but other structure–function relationships such as the factor IXa, factor X and phospholipid-binding sites have not yet been resolved. However, quite small regions of this large protein are critical for function since it can be totally inactivated by certain monoclonal antibodies whose binding epitopes are significantly restricted in size. Antibodies to the B domain have no effect on function. Attempts to locate specific mutations in haemophilic DNA are hampered by the lack of any general method, short of sequencing, that can detect all

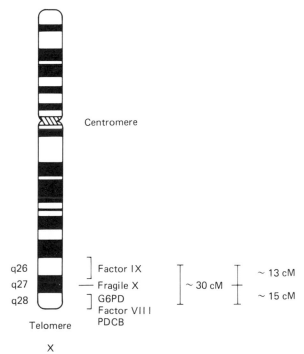

Fig. 23.3. *X chromosome showing map locations of loci for factor IX haemophilia B, fragile X/mental retardation, G6PD/haemolytic anaemia, factor VIII/haemophilia A. (PDCB = protan–deutan colour blindness.) Approximate distances in centimorgans (cM). (Reproduced from Antonarakis S. E. (1988), with permission.)*

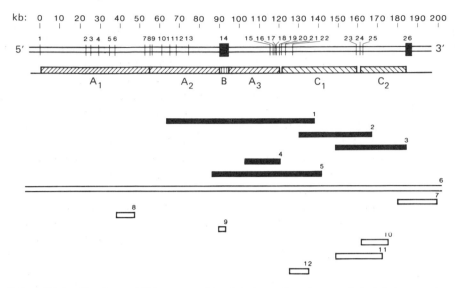

Fig. 23.4. *The factor VIII gene and its deletions. Top line: scale in kilobase pairs of DNA. Second line: map of exons (shaded bars) and introns (unshaded bars). Third line: corresponding regions of secreted protein. $A_1 A_2 A_3$, ceruloplasmin homology. B, activation peptide. $C_1 C_2$ lectin homology. Solid bars 1–5: deletions associated with inhibitor phenotype. Open bars 6–12: deletions not associated with inhibitors of factor VIII.*

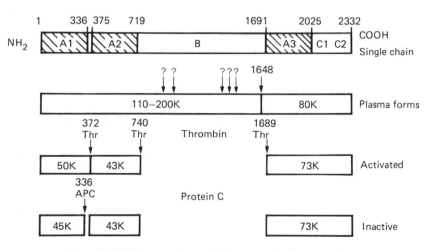

Fig. 23.5. *Human factor VIII, proteolytic processing.*

sequence variation. Clearly it is impractical to sequence 190 kb of DNA for each family. Therefore researchers have screened haemophilic DNA with labelled wild-type cDNA as probe, by means of Southern blotting. With this approach, a series of bands can be resolved corresponding to genomic restriction fragments containing exons. A missing band, or additional band, will indicate a deletion larger than 1 kb, or the loss of a restriction enzyme site or introduction of a new restriction site. Only about 5% of random mutations can be expected to be picked up by this means, and indeed 95% of patient DNA when so analysed has shown no aberrant banding—indicating only that there is a small deletion or point mutation not affecting a restriction site.

All the deletions reported to date are summarized in Fig. 23.4. These deletions range in size from about 5 kb (number 9) to over 200 kb (number 6), the latter spanning the whole factor VIII gene. Each deletion was found in a different family and they are entirely diverse in size and location. Nor is there any clear relation between type of deletion and presence (filled-in bars) or absence (open bars) of antibodies to factor VIII. This is in contrast to the situation in haemophilia B (see below). Shown in Figure 23.6 are the point mutations that have been detected, in each case by Southern blotting after digesting DNA with the enzyme Taq 1. Mutants 1,3,4 and 5 are due to substitution of T for C, destroying the Taq 1 recognition sequence (TCGA) and introducing a premature stop codon. Each of these patients has severe haemophilia A, and patients 3 and 5 also have antibodies to factor VIII. Patient number 2 has what appears to be a different type of mutation with G to A transition, however this is equivalent to a C to T transition on the opposite strand. The effect is to produce substitution of glutamine for arginine and the patient has mild haemophilia A (factor VIII activity 5%). The relatively frequent occurrence of C-to-T mutations of this type is due to the fact that vertebrate DNA is methylated at the cytosine of CpG dimers. Methyl cytosine can undergo spontaneous deamination to thymidine, which is not recognized by DNA repair mechanisms. If correctly in frame, the transition will cause premature chain termination or other substitution as shown here. The specific mutation can be used to identify carriers and for antenatal diagnosis. As predicted, about a third of these mutations were of demonstrably recent origin. For the majority of families, the mutation remains obscure, so that carrier detection must rely on phenotype analysis (Fig. 23.7) and linkage to DNA markers (Fig. 23.8).

Carriers of haemophilia A have on average 50% of the normal mean level of the clotting factor (or its antigen VIII:Ag). However, owing to the wide scatter of normal values (50–150%), an individual will often be within the normal range. By measuring the level of von Willebrand factor antigen (vWF:Ag), the autosomally coded carrier protein for factor VIII, it is possible to improve discrimination since carriers will tend to have lower levels of VIII than of vWF. Even so, there is still some overlap (about 15%) where carriers fall into the normal ratio (see Fig. 23.7). This is due to the 'lyonization' effect whereby random X inactivation can cause predominantly the X chromosome bearing the mutant allele to be inactivated. In brief, one can obtain very strong evidence for carriership by this method but never definitively rule it out.

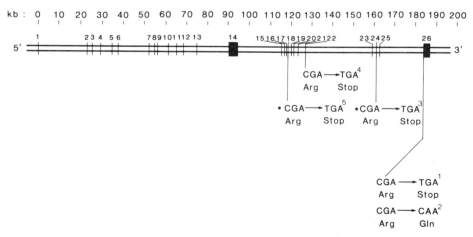

Fig. 23.6. *Point mutations in the factor VIII gene. Top two lines as Fig. 23.4. CGA/Arg: wild type sequence is indicated, where mutation has produced nonsense or missense error in one or more unrelated families. *Indicates presence of inhibitors in some affected individuals.*

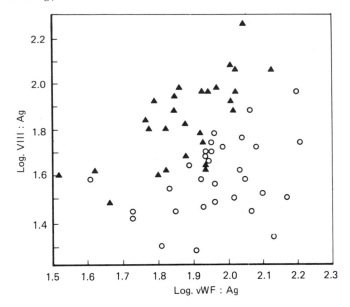

Fig. 23.7. *Phenotype assays used for carrier detection.* ▲, *normal females;* ○, *obligate carriers; VIII:Ag, factor VIII antigen, measured with human antibody; vWF:Ag, von Willebrand factor antigen, heteroantibody assay.*

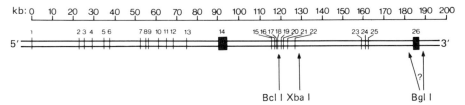

Fig. 23.8. *Polymorphic restriction sites in the factor VIII gene. Bc1 I, site present in intron 18; Bgl I, site adjacent to exon 26; Xba I site present in intron 22.*

The principle of linkage using DNA markers is now widely applied to genetic disease. Polymorphic variation in DNA affecting restriction enzyme recognition sequences is detected by Southern blotting using DNA probes within or adjacent to the genetic locus of the disease in question. Presence or absence of that restriction site will produce variation in the fragment size produced, referred to as restriction fragment length polymorphism (RFLP). Figure 23.8 indicates the site of three RFLPs within the factor VIII gene. Although RFLPs are quite unrelated to specific mutations, they can be used to track the mutant X chromosome in a given family. For example, in the family shown in Figure 23.2, II_2 is an obligate carrier (being the daughter of a haemophiliac). Since she is heterozygous for the

factor VIII–BcII RFLP, one can track linkage between haemophilia A and the smaller allele (0.8 kb) to her daughters, III_2 and III_3. On pedigree alone they each have a 50% chance of carriership. By linkage, II_2 is not a carrier since she must have inherited the 1.1 non-haemophilic allele from her mother, whereas the other sister is a carrier. III_3 is herself homozygous for this RFLP so cannot have antenatal diagnosis based on that marker. Also shown on the figure are RFLP alleles for the linked marker DX13–BgIII. This marker is located about 4.5 centimorgans* distant from factor VIII, tight

* 1 centimorgan is defined as the distance between genetic loci such that crossover occurs at 1% of meioses on average. It corresponds to about 10^6 base pairs.

linkage but with 4.5% chance of crossover per meiosis. III_3 is heterozygous for DX13, haemophilia being associated with the smaller allele, 2.8 kb. Note that no identifiable crossover has occurred between factor VIII BcII and DX13 from II_2 to her three offspring, but crossover can occur for each gamete that III_3 produces. Therefore antenatal diagnosis based on DX13 linkage would need to be checked by fetoscopy at 18 weeks.

Figure 23.9 shows the results by Gitschier *et al.* (1985) of the first successful antenatal diagnosis for haemophilia A by analysis of DNA extracted from a chorion biopsy at 8 weeks gestation. The finding of the large allele in III_1 (a male fetus) excluded haemophilia since that X chromosome must have come from his normal grandfather, I_2.

Figure 23.10 shows the additional discrimination available when two intragenic markers are used. In the absence of I_1 and I_2, the phase of the alleles in II_2 is not obvious. However, by examining her husband and daughter, III_3 (the individual requesting diagnosis and pregnant with IV?), it is clear what her haplotype must be. This haplotype is incompatible with the haemophilic haplotype in this kindred. Therefore II_2 cannot be a carrier, which of course also excludes III_2, III_3 and IV_2. The pregnancy was allowed to continue undisturbed by any direct investigation.

With present intragenic RFLPs, about 70% of European females are informative (frequencies differ markedly in different populations). For the other 30%, linked markers (DXI3 or ST14, a highly polymorphic marker) give linkage information in 95% of women. A 4% risk of crossover is found for both markers, which unfortunately are on the same side (centromeric) of the factor VIII gene. There is a need to locate more intragenic and telomeric markers.

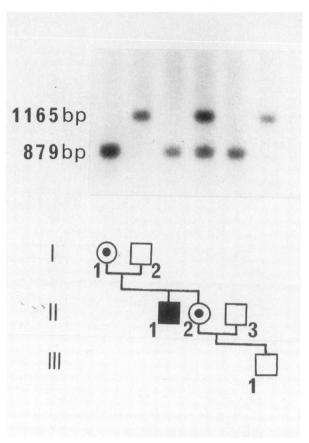

Fig. 23.9. *The first use of intragenic RFLP linkage for antenatal diagnosis of haemophilia A. Top panel: Southern blot showing Bcl I restriction fragments probed with factor VIII exon 17, 18, aligned vertically with family members in lower panel. (Symbols as Fig. 23.1.) Obligate carrier status of I_1 was evident from pedigree (as she had a haemophilic brother). II_2 was predicted to be a carrier by linkage analysis using DX13 probe. III_1, a male fetus, has the alternative allele to his haemophilic uncle (II_1) and therefore cannot be affected, as proved to be the case 7 months later.*

Haemophilia A in Females

True homozygous haemophilia A is rare but well described, being due to marriage of a carrier to an affected male, usually a cousin. Severe menstrual haemorrhage occurs but responds to factor VIII infusion. About 5% of carriers have a low enough factor VIII level to be classified as mild haemophiliacs, requiring precautions to cover surgery and occasionally experiencing traumatic bleeding. Due to sperm mutation in the father, such a carrier can present de novo with no haemophilic relative. Acquired autoantibodies to factor VIII arise in previously normal people, sometimes in association with rheumatoid arthritis or in the puerperium. This is called acquired haemophilia but has no genetic basis. Treatment resembles that described above under inhibitors. Haemophilia A has been described in a female with Turner's syndrome. One family with apparently clear-cut dominant factor

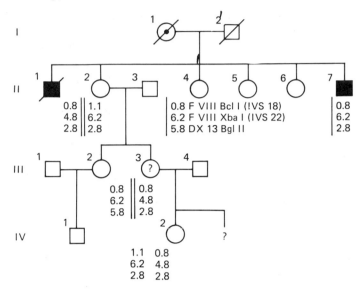

Fig. 23.10. *Haemophilia A, linkage analysis using two intragenic and one linked probe. Haplotypes inferred from II_3 and III_3 show that II_2 cannot be a carrier, hence also excluding III_2, III_3, IV_2 and the fetus IV?. ($\odot$, obligate carrier: $\blacksquare$, affected male; ϕ, deceased.)*

VIII deficiency affecting females has been described. The genetic basis for this last disorder awaits clarification. The most usual reason for finding a low factor VIII in a female if the above have been excluded is von Willebrand's disease. This should usually be evident from assays of von Willebrand factor and a prolonged bleeding time. Of course, von Willebrand's disease and haemophilia A can coexist in the same family, which makes carrier detection difficult.

Biosynthetic Factor VIII and the Future of Haemophilia

The economics of factor VIII production (summarized in Table 23.7) were the stimulus for intense efforts to achieve synthesis by recombinant DNA technology. Success was announced by Genentech Inc. in April 1984, followed fairly closely by other companies. As with all new drugs, the interval from synthesis to clinical introduction is to be measured in years, but with added pressure from fears of AIDS and other infections, full-scale clinical trials were planned to begin as early as 1988. There seems little doubt that some form of recombinant factor VIII will take over from the plasma-derived product in the 1990s. Will haemophilia A then be solved? In many respects the answer must be yes. Patients would prefer, of course, an easier route of administration, and possibly an orally absorbable form will be devised. Presumably megadoses of synthetic factor VIII will be used to induce toler-

Table 23.7
Economics of factor VIII

Specific activity	5000 units* per kg
Average dose	100 μg = 1000 units
Cost per dose at 15 pence per unit	£150
World usage per year	1 kg
World market per year	£750 million

* 1 unit is the amount present in 1 ml of plasma.

ance in patients with inhibitors. In the never-ending search for better therapy, attention will inevitably turn to prospects of gene therapy. Haemophilia is a reasonable candidate for this since close control of plasma levels is not required and even an increase from 0% to 5% would markedly improve the clinical status. Many problems remain to be solved in the tissue-specific localization and safe, functional integration of foreign genes before the final solution to haemophilia A is with us.

VON WILLEBRAND's DISEASE

Although first described in 1926, our understanding of this complex and variable bleeding disorder continues to grow. The basic defect common to all variants is abnormal production of von Willebrand factor (vWF). The abnormality may be quantitative and/or qualitative. Von Willebrand factor is coded by a gene, on chromosome 12, which was recently cloned by several groups. The primary gene product is an extremely long protein monomer of some 2791 amino acids. This is produced predominantly in vascular endothelial cells, but also in megakaryocytes, and undergoes a series of post-translational modifications. Dimers are formed and a very large propeptide is excised. The propeptide is detectable in plasma as von Willebrand antigen II, but its function other than to aid protomer assembly is unknown. Dimers of the main protein chain are assembled into tetramers which then further polymerize to form a series of multimers with molecular weights ranging from 1×10^6 to 20×10^6 daltons. These are stored prior to release in the Weibel–Palade bodies of endothelial cells and the α-

granules of platelets. Von Willebrand factor is released into plasma at a steady rate from the endothelial cells where it is detectable immunologically using heteroantibodies as von Willebrand factor antigen (vWF:Ag). (This was formerly called factor VIII-related antigen due to confusion about the composition of the factor VIII complex.) The key to understanding the relationship between von Willebrand's disease (vWD) and haemophilia A is to realize that factor VIII and vWF are entirely distinct entities with separate functions (Fig. 23.11). However, vWF acts as a protective carrier for factor VIII in the circulation, as well as being involved in platelet adhesion to subendothelium at high shear rates. Therefore deficiency of von Willebrand factor gives rise to a dual haemostatic defect, reduced plasma levels of factor VIII (which though synthesized normally has a shorter half-life in the absence of its carrier) and prolonged bleeding time due to failure of platelets to adhere to the cut edges of small blood vessels. Platelet adhesion is mediated by the higher molecular weight multimers of vWF and is thought to involve physical cross-linking from the platelet membrane glycoprotein I, via vWF to collagen. It should be evident that in the multistep synthesis, assembly and secretion of vWF, and with its multifunctional involvement in haemostasis, there are many ways in which mutations of the von Willebrand factor gene could be expressed as varying types of disease. Rapid release of vWF from storage sites can be induced by infusion of DDAVP, acute exercise or adrenaline. The physiological mediator(s) of this response are not fully understood. Chronic elevation of vWF due to increased synthesis occurs as part of the 'acute phase' response to injury, inflammation, infection and

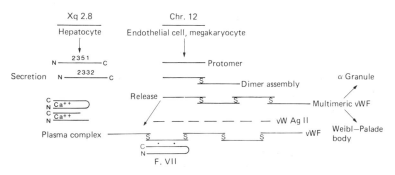

Fig. 23.11. *Assembly of the factor VIII–von Willebrand factor complex.*

neoplasia, and in pregnancy and hyperthyroidism. These responses are presumed to be physiological in promoting enhanced haemostasis but could reach pathological expression in being associated with increased risk of thrombosis. These effects need to be taken into account when measuring vWF levels in attempting to diagnose vWD.

Clinical Features of von Willebrand's Disease

The classical picture is of an autosomal dominant, mild to moderately severe bleeding tendency. Patients suffer from bruising, epistaxes, prolonged bleeding from minor cuts, menorrhagia and excessive but not often life-threatening bleeding after trauma or surgery. Patients often present for investigation in the second or third decade after prolonged bleeding from dental extraction has aroused clinical suspicion. Menorrhagia inexplicable by local or hormonal factors can also be the presenting symptom. Haemarthroses do not occur in typical mild dominant von Willebrand's disease. Much less common is autosomal recessive vWD, where vWF is undetectable and VIII:C levels are usually around 1 or 2 u/dl. These patients have a bleeding tendency that clinically resembles severe haemophilia A, with haemarthroses, muscle bleeds and life-threatening haemorrhage after trauma, as well as the proneness to small vessel bleeding that is not a feature of haemophilia A. The distribution of bleeding in vWD can be explained on the basis that vWF is required for platelet adhesion at high shear rate—the condition of flow found in the smallest blood vessels exposed to trauma in skin and mucous membranes.

Laboratory Diagnosis

The following tests are necessary to make the diagnosis: factor VIII, von Willebrand factor antigen, ristocetin cofactor activity (ricof), platelet count, and template bleeding time. When factor VIII, vWF:Ag and ricof are all below 40 u/dl, the platelet count is normal and the bleeding time is longer than 10 minutes, the diagnosis is easily made. Unfortunately, due to the variability of the disease and varying levels of vWF release or synthesis in individuals over time, all of these tests can give normal results on some occasions but clearly abnormal results on others. This is especially true of the milder cases of type I vWD (see below). It is necessary to perform carefully standardized sets of assays and a bleeding time on three occasions in some cases to be sure of the diagnosis. Additional tests are necessary to establish the subtype, principally vWF multimer size analysis at low and high resolution. This will demonstrate the distribution of von Willebrand factor polymers and the pattern of flanking bands (Fig. 23.12) adjacent to the main multimer bands. Table 23.8 lists the main variants and their characteristics. In type IIB there is excessive response to ristocetin at low concentration (0.5 mg/ml) in stirred patient's platelet-rich plasma. If normal washed platelets are resuspended in patient's plasma, the phenomenon is reproduced, demonstrating that the abnormality is in the plasma. Studies with purified type IIB vWF show that it binds directly to unactivated platelets (unlike normal vWF). This evidently results in loss of high molecular weight multimers and platelets due to in - vivo formation of platelet aggregates in the circulation. Routine platelet aggregation studies with a range of ristocetin dosages should be performed as part of the diagnostic work up, since it is important to detect this variant (see below), which does not always show up in the other tests.

The majority of cases are found to be types IA or IB, accounting for 80% of kindreds. Types IIA and IIB are fairly common, together amounting to about 15% of kindreds. The remainder of subtypes are rare. All the subtypes are inherited dominantly, except for type III recessive and type IIc double heterozygote. Type III cases are commoner in cultures where intermarriage is usual, such as the Middle East. Type IIc cases are always double heterozygotes, inheriting a type I gene from one parent and the IIc gene affecting polymerization from the other. Heterozygotes of all subtypes sometimes have quite low levels (15–25%) of vWF:Ag when presumably they have one normally functioning allele. No doubt the presence of an abnormal protomer can interfere with the polymerization and secretion of the normal gene product. Recent studies have shown differential sensitivity of variant vWF to proteases affecting the apparent distribution of multimers in plasma.

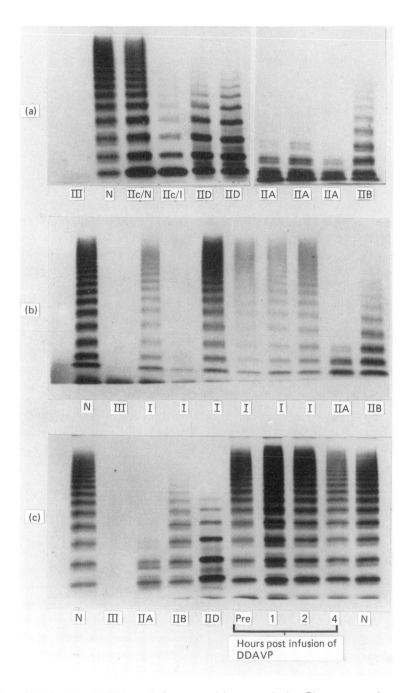

Fig. 23.12. *Von Willebrand factor multimer analysis. Plasma samples were boiled in SDS buffer and electrophoresed in 1.6% agarose. vWF was detected after fixation in situ with rabbit antibodies labelled with ^{125}I and autoradiographed. (N, normal plasma; III, homozygous severe vWD; IIA etc., subtypes as indicated.) (These multimer analyses were carried out by K. Matthews, Haemophilia Centre, The Royal Free Hospital, London.)*

Table 23.8

Variants of von Willebrand's disease

Subtype	Factor VIII	vWF:Ag	Ristocetin cofactor	Bleeding time	Platelet count	Multimer bands			
						Higher	Middle	Lower	Flanking
I A	↓ or N	↓ or N	↓ or N	↑ or N	N	↓	↓	↓	Normal
B	↓	↓	↓	↑	N	↓↓	↓	↓	Normal
C	↓ or N	↓	↓	↑	N	↓	↓	↓	Absent
II A	↓	↓	↓↓	↑	N	Absent	↑	↑	Upper band decreased, middle and lower bands equal
B	↓ or N	↓ or N	N or ↓*	↑	↓ or N	Absent	N	N	Enhanced
C	↓	↓	Absent	↑	N	Absent	Absent	↑	Absent
D	↓ or N	↓ or N	↓	↑	N	Absent	↓	↑	Additional abnormal bands
E	↓	↓	↓	↑	N	Absent	↓	N	Absent
F	↓	↓	↓	↑	N	Absent	N	↑	Absent†
III	<5%	Absent	Absent	↑	N	Absent	Absent	Absent	Absent

* Enhanced response of patients' PRP to low concentration of ristocetin but normal or reduced level in standard cofactor test systems.
† The cardinal feature distinguishing this variant from IIE is that platelet vWF is normal.
↓ Decreased. ↓↓ Strongly decreased. N, Normal amount. ↑ Increased.

Treatment

Patients with mild or moderate von Willebrand's disease (clinical severity correlates roughly inversely with ristocetin cofactor activity) attend infrequently for treatment. The first-line treatment for minor bleeding after local measures have failed in type I vWD is DDAVP. This will produce a brisk rise in vWF and factor VIII levels and a shortening of the bleeding time (see discussion under mild haemophilia A for details of therapy). DDAVP is much less effective in types IIA and IIC vWD, presumably because the patient's released vWF is highly abnormal and still unable to promote platelet adhesion. DDAVP is contraindicated in IIB vWD since the released abnormal vWF will cause circulatory platelet aggregates to form, with a further fall in the platelet count.

It is still worth a therapeutic trial in type IIA since some families do respond well. DDAVP is effective in types IID and IC.

In cases where DDAVP is ineffective or contraindicated, the next line of treatment is cryoprecipitate. This low-purity product is rich in von Willebrand factor and normalizes the bleeding time whilst also elevating factor VIII. The correction of bleeding time usually lasts only a few hours, but the factor VIII levels do not fall off and may rise to a post-infusion peak at 12–24 hours. The explanation for this de novo synthesis, which excited much interest and speculation when it was first observed in the early 1960s, is that the infused von Willebrand factor acts as a carrier for endogenously synthesized factor VIII. This bonus means that postoperative cover can be continued on a daily dosage basis. Because of the variable content of individual donor packs of cryoprecipitate, it is usual to give a minimum dose of 5 units. The initial dose can be calculated based on 100 units VIII per bag, using the same formula as given for haemophilia A to produce a desired rise. The response should be checked by assay.

Factor VIII concentrates are contraindicated (except in severe type III von Willebrand's disease) since they contain little functional von Willebrand factor and pose a high risk of transmitting non-A–non-B hepatitis to infrequently treated patients. Type III patients who bleed very frequently may require concentrate, but some bleed less often and can be managed with cryoprecipitate. There is a need for a highly purified, safe von Willebrand factor concentrate and this may be supplied in future by recombinant DNA methods.

Clinical Course and Complications

Type I and II von Willebrand's disease patients lead relatively normal lives with normal expectancy. Menstruation is seldom a cause of severe blood loss though menorrhagia is common. This can usually be managed satisfactorily with antifibrinolytics or by oral contraceptive oestrogen/progesterone combinations. In later years some patients require hysterectomy. During pregnancy the vWF levels rise spontaneously to the normal or low-normal range in all but the severely affected cases.

Type III severe cases have a clinical course resembling severe or moderately severe haemophilia A. Some of these patients develop antibodies to vWF which inhibit its platelet adhesion-promoting property and cause rapid removal from the circulation of infused material.

Molecular Genetics

The cloning of von Willebrand factor cDNA and its gene should lead to progress in identifying the underlying mutations responsible for the various phenotypes. As with the factor VIII gene, the large size of the DNA region involved presents problems of localization. It is to be expected that the mutations will be highly diverse to account for the variable phenotypes both between and within subtypes. So far it has been reported by Shelton-Inloes, *et al.* (1987) that the rare patients who develop antibodies to vWF have large deletions of their vWF gene. It has been demonstrated that functional vWF can be produced in tissue culture by cells transfected with a recombinant expression vector containing human vWF cDNA. Despite the fact that the cells transfected (fibroblasts) do not normally produce vWF, the recombinant protein was correctly modified and polymerized. Material for clinical use derived from this source will need to be given together with recombinant factor VIII, at least in the first dose of a treatment course.

Pseudo von Willebrand's Disease (Platelet-type vWD)

Several families have been described with a disorder closely resembling type IIB vWD but in whom mixing experiments show the defect to be in their platelets rather than their plasma. Patients with pseudo vWD have moderately reduced levels of vWF:Ag and platelets, with enhanced response of their platelet-rich plasma to low levels of ristocetin (0.5 mg/ml). Addition of normal cryoprecipitate to their washed platelets causes spontaneous aggregation, whereas the reverse experiment is without effect (c.f. type IIB vWD). An abnormality of platelet membrane GP I such that it spontaneously binds higher multimers of vWF is postulated as the underlying cause of this autosomal dominant mild bleeding syndrome. Treatment has not been extensively evaluated but should probably be with normal platelet concentrates, not DDAVP or cryoprecipitate.

HAEMOPHILIA B (FACTOR IX DEFICIENCY)

Clinically, haemophilia B resembles haemophilia A to the extent that they cannot be distinguished (and historically were not) until specific factor assays are performed. Both disorders are X linked (see Fig. 23.3), their genes being within 30 cM at the tip of the long arm of the X chromosome. The phenotype resemblance is to be expected as factor VIII is the cofactor for factor IXa's attack on factor X and is reminiscent of the clinical resemblance of folate to B_{12} deficiency. Factor IX, unlike factor VIII, is vitamin K dependent, with 12 γ-carboxy glutamate residues near the N-terminus which are involved in binding to phospholipid. The plasma level of factor IX activity falls in vitamin K deficiency and liver disease but this should not give rise to diagnostic confusion when the clinical picture and additional factor assays are taken into consideration. Isolated factor IX deficiency is always hereditary, and the clinical severity of haemophilia B shows the same relationship with residual factor level as for factor VIII in haemophilia A (see Table 23.2).

Treatment

The mainstay of treatment is factor IX concentrate, which has been available from the Blood Products Laboratory in the UK and is sufficient to meet all national needs since the early 1970s. The product contains all the vitamin-K-dependent factor proteins (factors X, VII, II, protein C) as well as factor IX, since the method of fractionation (ion-exchange chromatography) does not separate these very homologous proteins efficiently. Recent National Health Service factor IX concentrates are relatively poor in factor VII, which is fractionated into a separate concentrate. All prothrombin complex preparations have a greater or lesser tendency to promote thrombosis due to the presence of activated clotting enzymes. This can be used to advantage in the treatment of factor VIII antibodies but is a distinct hazard to haemophilia B patients, especially when full dosage has to be given to cover surgery. It has long been the rule to give heparin together with factor IX concentrate in the US. The author's preference is to give low-dose subcutaneous heparin, 5000 units t.d.s., before and for 1 week after major surgery (or as long as full-dose factor IX has to be given).

Dosage calculation in the treatment of haemophilia B follows the same principles as set out for factor VIII deficiency except that a higher initial dosage is required due to an apparently lower recovery. Thus:

dose to be infused (units)

$$= \frac{\text{weight (kg)} \times \text{increment needed (u/dl)}}{0.9}.$$

Also, the longer half-life (at 18 hours) means that daily infusions often suffice to maintain good levels after surgery. Severely affected patients are usually maintained on once- or twice-weekly prophylaxis to prevent spontaneous bleeds. This is practicable because of the better supply and longer half-life of the factor. All presently used factor IX is heat treated and probably HIV inactivated, but still capable of transmitting non-A–non-B hepatitis.

Clinical Course and Complications

Factor-IX-deficient patients who grew up before the concentrate was easily available have similar joint problems to haemophilia A patients. Liver disease is common due to the same viruses that have infected other recipients of multiple donor concentrates. In the UK at least, the incidence of HIV antibody positivity is much lower, at 5%, in haemophilia B than A. This is due to the concentrate having all been from UK source plasma. In Germany, where imported concentrates were used, the HIV-antibody-positive rate is equal in haemophilia A and B.

Antibodies to factor IX are rare in haemophilia B, affecting about 1% of cases, and most often associated with gene deletion (see below). Treatments used have included activated prothrombin complex, absorption of antibody onto immobilized factor IX in an extracorporeal circuit, and immunosuppression. The last-mentioned holds out great promise.

Molecular Genetics

The factor IX gene was cloned in 1982 by three independent groups and considerable progress has been made on the analysis of molecular defects associated with haemophilia B. Figure 23.13 is a diagram of the factor IX gene which spans 35 kb of Xq 2.6. The protein-coding domains are labelled a to h, separated by seven introns. It is interesting to note that the ratio of haemophilia B to haemophilia A (1:6) is the same as the ratio of the sizes of the respective genes, suggesting a random hit basis of mutation. Eleven deletions (extent shown as shaded bar) have been found in different haemophilia B kindreds, ranging from over 70 kb to 8 kb. In all but one of these families the affected individuals have made antibodies to factor IX. There is therefore a strong association between deletion genotype and inhibitor phenotype. However, only about half of all patients with factor IX antibodies have a detectable deletion. A number of point mutations associated with haemophilia B have been discovered and these are summarized on Figure 23.14. They constitute a heterogeneous group with two splice donor site mutants (introns 3 and 6) and three point mutations (variant inactive protein is present in the plasma of these cases). Two are of the methyl cytosine to thymidine transition type, therefore resembling the six factor VIII point mutations shown in Figure 23.6.

Carrier detection of females heterozygous for these mutants is straightforward but they are in the minority. Therefore linkage to comon RFLPs must be used for most families to track haemophilia-associated alleles. Five RFLPs have been discovered in the factor IX gene (Fig. 23.15) but, due to linkage disequilibrium, these are informative for only about 65% of females. One DNA variation produces a protein polymorphism located within the activation peptide. This can be detected by a

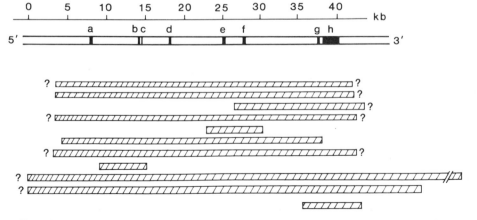

Fig. 23.13. *The factor IX gene and its deletions. Top line: scale in kilobase pairs. Second line: map of exons (solid bars) and introns (open bars). Hatched bars: deleted regions in different families. All except one have inhibitors to factor IX. (Reproduced from Antonarakis S. E. (1988), with permission.)*

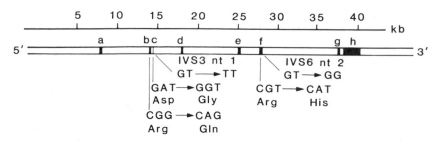

Fig. 23.14. *Point mutations in the factor IX gene. Wild-type sequence to left of arrows, mutated sequence to right. (IVS, intron; nt, nucleotide number after splice junction.)*

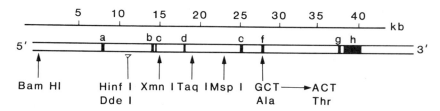

Fig. 23.15. *Polymorphic restriction sites in the factor IX gene and one amino acid polymorphism.*

(Figs. 23.14 and 23.15 are reproduced from Antonarakis S. E. (1988), with permission.)

monoclonal antibody that binds only one alternative sequence. Reduced amounts of normal or variant factor IX antigen can be detected in 30% of cases of haemophilia B.

Biosynthetic factor IX has been produced in various cell lines transfected with vectors containing human factor IX cDNA. The recombinant protein is correctly glycosylated and carboxylated and fully functional. It is to be expected that recombinant factor IX will be introduced and take over from plasma-derived concentrate during the next decade.

FACTOR XI DEFICIENCY (PTA DEFICIENCY)

The inheritance of this mild bleeding disorder is unusual, being almost confined to Ashkenazi (Eastern diaspora) Jews and common in that racial group. Seligsohn (1978) found 8% of healthy Jews to have a low factor XI level, which may be the heterozygote gene frequency. Homozygous patients have factor XI levels of less than 4 u/dl. Clinically, bleeding is infrequent and only occurs after trauma

or surgery. Haemarthroses and muscle bleeds occur as in mild haemophilia A. Heterozygotes have factor XI levels ranging from 15 to 65 u/dl. The relationship between residual factor level and bleeding tendency is not clear cut, since some patients with levels in the 20–40 u/dl range bleed excessively after trauma but others do not.

Diagnosis

Any Jewish patient with a history of bleeding should be investigated with PTA deficiency in mind. A long PTT and normal PT point to the diagnosis, and a reduced factor XI, with normal factor VIII and factor IX assays, establishes the diagnosis. Prolonged bleeding after circumcision, ritually performed at 8 days, can be the presenting problem.

Treatment

Factor XI concentrate only recently became available from the Blood Products Laboratory. Since it is heat treated, it is probably the treatment of choice. Formerly, fresh frozen plasma was used exclusively with good results. The long half-life, at

60 hours, and the relatively low level necessary to achieve haemostasis mean that infusions of plasma in adults are sufficient to control or prevent bleeding. These can be given at 1–3-day intervals to sustain an acceptable plasma level of 40 u/dl.

FACTOR VII DEFICIENCY

This rare autosomal recessive disorder causes bleeding similar to that seen in haemophilia A or B. Variants with non-functional protein present in the plasma have been described, but since the gene was only cloned in 1986 no information on the genotype of deficient patients is available as yet. Investigation shows a long PT and a normal PTT. The factor assay is confirmatory. Treatment with specific factor VII concentrate is similar to that for factor IX deficiency but with the real added difficulty that the half-life of factor VII is only 3 hours. This means that infusions to cover surgery have to be very frequent.

FACTOR V DEFICIENCY

This is another rare autosomal recessive bleeding disorder, with a curious feature in that the plasma factor levels do not correlate at all closely with the bleeding tendency. However, it has been shown that the platelet content or surface-associated factor V level is the critical determinant of bleeding tendency. Thus patients may have no detectable plasma factor V but little bleeding. These cases have normal or slightly reduced platelet factor V. Other cases have no platelet or plasma factor V and these patients bleed readily, especially after trauma or surgery. Many such cases have a prolonged bleeding time, emphasizing the close relationship between factor V and platelet function. Treatment with plasma is effective, and the haemostatic level may be sufficient at 20 u/dl. Some cases are reported to have non-functional factor V antigen in their plasma, but there is no further information on the underlying genotype.

FACTOR X DEFICIENCY

The parents of patients with this rare disorder are nearly always related. Bleeding is typically haemophilia like. A number of variant factor X proteins have been described based on antigen assays and response to different animal tissue thromboplastins. Bleeding tendency correlates with residual factor level. The most severely affected cases have no effective intrinsic or extrinsic clotting pathway and bleed even more severely than patients with haemophilia A or B. There is a very high risk of spontaneous intracerebral haemorrhage in such patients, whose lives can only be maintained by daily infusion of factor X concentrate (the standard factor IX concentrate is suitable as it contains approximately equal amounts of the two factors). Several factor-X-deficient patients have now been found to have large deletions of their factor X gene.

PROTHROMBIN DEFICIENCY

This extremely rare bleeding disorder has only been reported in about 50 cases but these appear highly diverse. True hypoprothrombinaemia encompasses those cases with reduced factor II activity and antigen. The disorder is autosomal recessive and associated with a bleeding tendency inversely proportional to the residual factor. The lowest level noted was 2% and no cases with undetectable prothrombin have been found. Dysprothrombinaemia refers to patients in whom the factor II activity is about half the antigen level. Many of these cases have a demonstrably abnormal proteolytic fragmentation pattern of half their circulating factor II. The disorder is autosomal dominant in most families and associated with mild bleeding after trauma or surgery.

The diagnosis may be suspected where the prothrombin time is slightly to moderately prolonged (16–23 seconds) and factor II assay is reduced whilst other vitamin-K-dependent factors are normal.

Treatment with prothrombin complex or plasma is straightforward, a haemostatic level of factor II being 50 u/dl and the half-life of 2–3 days requiring only infrequent infusions for maintenance.

Presumably the dysprothrombinaemias are due to point mutations affecting the primary amino acid sequence adjacent to activation cleavage sites, or introducing new sites, but detailed studies on this have not yet been reported.

INHERITED DISORDERS OF FIBRINOGEN

These are slightly more frequent than the preceding four deficiencies. As with prothrombin deficiency, the cases fall into two groups: hypo- and afibrinogenaemias being the quantitative defects and dysfibrogenaemias the qualitative defects of factor I.

Quantitative Deficiency

Afibrinogenaemia has been reported in about 150 cases worldwide and is associated with a moderate to very severe bleeding tendency. Bruising and bleeding after minimal trauma occur, and all the internal organs are susceptible to bleeding. Some patients have haemarthroses but others are free of this type of bleed. Investigation shows prolongation of all the screening tests with no clot formation. Fibrinogen is generally unmeasurable except with sensitive immunoassays. The bleeding time is usually prolonged and platelet aggregation studies show defective aggregation with all agonists (due to the involvement of fibrinogen in platelet–platelet interaction).

Hypofibrinogenaemia is a less well-defined disorder in which, whilst fibrinogen levels are reduced, there may be no bleeding or only a mild bleeding tendency. Both disorders are autosomal recessive, with consanguinity in about half the parents of affected individuals. Fibrinogen concentrate is not suitable for treatment as it causes thrombosis and hepatitis. Treatment with plasma or cryoprecipitate is very effective but some patients with afibrinogenaemia have developed antibodies to fibrinogen and severe reactions to infusion. A plasma level of 1 g/l is haemostatically sufficient and can be maintained by weekly infusion.

Qualitative Abnormality

The dysfibrinogenaemias constitute a diverse group which can be broadly classified according to functional abnormality. In group I, typified by fibrinogen Zurich, there is defective fibrin monomer aggregation. In group II the fibrinopeptide release is delayed or absent, e.g. fibrinogen Bethesda I. Many cases of group I aggregation defect are asymptomatic and only detected on routine screening. Most cases of group II fibrinopeptide release defect have either bleeding or, paradoxically, a thrombotic tendency.

Laboratory investigation shows prolonged PT, TCT or reptilase time. Fibrinogen level is variable, with normal results by immunologic and gravimetric methods, but reduced values according to the Clauss thrombin clotting time procedure. Since the disorder is autosomal dominant, detailed studies reveal two populations of fibrinogen, the normal and the dysfibrinogen in patient's plasma. One fibrinogen—Oslo—has shortened clotting times and this is associated with a thrombotic tendency.

Recent biochemical studies have now located the defect in many of these abnormal fibrinogens and, as might be predicted, a variety of point substitutions in critical regions of the fibrinogen chains have been found which affect peptide release or interchain interaction.

Treatment for bleeding has occasionally been necessary and various infusions have been given including fresh blood, plasma and cryoprecipitate. Commercial fibrinogen concentrate is definitely contraindicated as it transmits hepatitis and cannot be pasteurized. Patients with a thrombotic tendency have been successfully managed by oral anticoagulation therapy.

FACTOR XIII DEFICIENCY

This rare autosomal recessive disorder is characterized by a severe haemorrhagic tendency and poor wound healing. Nearly all cases present in early life with prolonged bleeding from the umbilical cord. There is a high incidence of intracerebral haemorrhage, bruising, haematomas and, in women, recurrent spontaneous abortion. Coagulation screening tests are normal, but plasma clots are soluble in 5 mol/l urea due to a lack of cross-linking. Quantitative assay shows fibrinoligase (factor XIII) activity below 1%. Bleeding time and platelet function studies are normal. The basis of the disorder is absence of factor XIIIa chain from plasma and platelets. Factor XIIIb chain is present in normal amounts, but this is the catalytically inactive carrier molecule for the a chain which alone possesses transamidase activity.

Treatment with cryoprecipitate or specific factor XIII concentrate is highly effective and can be given weekly, as a low level (above 5%) is haemostatically effective and the half-life is about 7 days in the circulation.

COMBINED FACTOR V AND FACTOR VIII DEFICIENCY

About 50 families with this surprising combined defect, inherited as an autosomal recessive, have been described worldwide. Bleeding is mild and no more than would be expected for moderate deficiency of V or VIII alone. No good genetic or physiological explanation for this combination has been advanced, although it was thought that excessive protein C activity due to deficiency of its inhibitor might be the unifying defect. Further studies showed that the protein C inhibitor (which is labile) is normal in the plasma of the combined deficiency cases.

Laboratory tests show prolonged PT and PTT, with factor V and factor VIII both in the range of 15–35 u/dl. The corresponding antigens are depressed to a similar extent and no abnormal inhibitor is present. Treatment with fresh frozen plasma is effective.

FACTOR XII, HIGH MOLECULAR WEIGHT KININOGEN (FITZGERALD FACTOR) AND PREKALLIKREIN (FLETCHER FACTOR) DEFICIENCIES

These traits, inherited in an autosomal recessive manner, produce prolonged partial thromboplastin times due to defective surface activation of the intrinsic pathway, but *no* bleeding tendency. Their only clinical importance is that they are occasionally picked up by routine coagulation screening and need to be identified by specific factor assays so that reassurance can be given to surgical colleagues.

GENERAL ORGANIZATION OF HAEMOPHILIA CARE

As these are relatively uncommon disorders, with many and varied effects on the patient and his family at all stages of life, requiring care and support services across the whole field of medicine and social services, it is now accepted that this care can best be delivered comprehensively by referral centres. The staff of a major comprehensive care centre will include physicians, nurses, social workers, laboratory scientists and physiotherapists, devoting all or a substantial part of their time to haemophilia care. An orthopaedic surgeon prepared to see haemophilic patients regularly in a clinic set aside for their problems is a vital addition to this team. The haemophilia centre network in the United Kingdom was set up in the late 1960s and early 1970s. It is recognized that not every centre can provide every facility and that there should be a fairly wide distribution according to population density which determines numbers of patients. As defined by health service circulars, the functions of a centre are to provide 24-hour emergency treatment for haemophiliacs and a full range of diagnostic tests for identifying new cases and monitoring treatment. Full records should be kept of all treatments whether given in hospital or as home therapy. The patients' progress should be monitored through regular follow-up: paediatric, dental and orthopaedic referrals being organized by the centre as necessary. (Many centres are, in fact, in paediatric departments or run by paediatricians.) Genetic counselling must be available for families of haemophilic patients including carrier detection and antenatal diagnosis. In order to maintain interest and expertise, at least 10 patients with severe haemophilia should be registered at the centre to merit the designation. A part- or whole-time social worker who can review the wider problems of living affecting the haemophiliac at school, home and work should be part of the team. Many centres now have AIDS counsellors and of course are closely monitoring all their patients by clinical and laboratory indices for signs of HIV-related disease. All patients upon diagnosis are issued with a special medical card indicating laboratory test results, inhibitor status, main centre and local centre for treatment.

Caring for haemophiliacs is demanding but rewarding. Until the recent setbacks, the trend has been towards an ever-improving life expectancy and social participation for haemophiliacs based on continuing medical progress and the skill and devotion of many professionals. It is both tragic and ironic that the main foundation upon which this progress rested— factor concentrate—has also been the route by which life-threatening infections have been introduced, to a high proportion of the most severely affected patients. During the period of fear and uncertainty which we have entered, the haemophiliac and his family will need even more of our professional help to endure and if possible overcome the handicap dealt him by the genetic lottery.

SELECTED BIBLIOGRAPHY

Abildgaard C. F., Suzuki Z., Harrison J., Jefcoat K., Zimmerman T. S. (1980). Serial studies in Von Willebrands disease. Variability versus variants. *Blood* **56**, 712–716.

Aledort L. M., Levine P. H., Hilgartner M. *et al.* (1985). A study of liver biopsies and liver disease among haemophiliacs. *Blood*, **66**, 367–372.

Antonarakis S. E. (1988). The molecular genetics of hemophilia A and B in man. In *Advances in human genetics*, Vol. 17. (Eds. H. Harris and K. Wirschhorn). New York: Plenum Press.

Antonarakis S. E., Waber P. G., Kittur S. D. *et al.* (1985). Haemophilia A: Molecular defects and carrier detection by DNA analysis. *New England Journal of Medicine*, **313**, 842–848.

Antonarakis S. E., Youssoufian H., Kazazian H. K. (1987). Molecular genetics of hemophilia A in man. *Molecular Biology and Medicine*, **4**, 81–94.

Biggs R. (1978). *The treatment of haemophilia A and B and Von Willebrand's disease.* Oxford: Blackwell Scientific.

Biggs R., Rizza C. R. (1984). *Human blood coagulation, haemostasis and thrombosis* Oxford: Blackwell Scientific.

Boone D. C. (1976). *Comprehensive management of haemophilia.* Philadelphia: F. A. Davis.

Brackman H. H. (1982). The treatment of inhibitor against factor VIII by continuous treatment with factor VIII and activated prothrombin complex concentrate. In *Activated prothrombin complex concentrates* (Eds. G. Mariani, M. A. Russo and F. Mandelli) New York: Praeger.

Brownlee G. G. (1988). Haemophilia B: a review of patient defects, diagnosis with gene probes and prospects for gene therapy. In *Recent advances in haematology*, Vol. 5. (Ed. A. V. Hoffbrand). Edinburgh: Churchill Livingstone.

Eaton D., Rodriguez H., Vehar G. A. (1986). Proteolytic processing of Human factor VIII. Correlation of specific cleavages by thrombin, Factor Xa and activated protein C with activation and inactivation of factor VIII coagulation activity. *Biochemistry*, **25**, 505–512.

Eyster M. E., Whitehurst D. A., Catalano P. M. *et al.* (1985). Long term follow-up of hemophiliacs with lymphocytopenia or thrombocytopenia. *Blood*, **66**, 1317–1320.

Gitschier J., Lawn R. M., Rotblat F., Goldman E., Tuddenham E. G. D. (1985). Antenatal diagnosis and carrier detection of haemophilia A using a factor VIII gene probe. *Lancet*, i, 1093–1094.

Gitschier J., Wood W. I., Tuddenham E. G. D., Shuman M. A., Goralka T. M., Chen E. Y., Lawn R. M. (1985). Detection and sequence of mutations in the factor VIII gene of haemophiliacs. *Nature*, **315**, 427–430.

Haldane J. B. S. (1935). The rate of spontaneous mutation of a human gene. *Journal of Genetics*, **31**, 317–326.

Lynch D. C., Zimmerman T. S., Ruggeri Z. M. (1986). von Willebrand Factor now cloned. Annotation. *British Journal of Haematology*, **64**, 15–20.

Massey R., Massey S. (1973). *Journey.* New York: Alfred A. Knopf.

Nillson I. M., Berntorp E., Zettervall O. (1986). Induction of split tolerance and clinical cure in high responding hemophiliacs with factor IX antibodies. *Proceedings of the National Academy of Sciences, USA*, **83**, 9169–9173.

Rizza C. R., Matthews J. M. (1982). Effect of frequent factor VIII replacement on the level of factor VIII antibodies in haemophiliacs. *British Journal of Haematology*, **52**, 13–24.

Rizza C. R., Spooner R. J. D. (1983). Treatment of haemophilia and related disorders in Britain and Northern Ireland during 1976–80: report on behalf of the directors of haemophilia centres in the United Kingdom. *British Medical Journal*, **286**, 929–933.

Rotblat F., Goodal A. H., O'Brien D. P., Rawlings E., Middleton S., Tuddenham E. G. D. (1983). Monoclonal antibodies to human procoagulant factor VIII. *Journal of Laboratory and Clinical Medicine*, **101**, 736–746.

Ruggeri Z. M. (Ed.) (1985). *Coagulation disorders. Clinics in Haematology*, Vol. 14, No. 2. London: W. B. Saunders.

Ruggeri Z. M., Zimmerman T. S. (1987). von Willebrand's factor and von Willebrand's disease. *Blood*, **70**, 895–904.

Shelton-Inloes B., Chehab F. F., Mannucci P. M., Federici A. B., Sadler J. E. (1987). Gene deletions correlate with development of allo antibodies in von Willebrand disease. *Journal of Clinical Investigation*, **79**, 1459–1465.

Seligsohn U. (1978). High gene frequency of factor XI (PTA) deficiency in Ashkenazi Jews. *Blood*, **51**, 1223–1228.

Tuddenham E. G. D. (1984). The varieties of von Willebrand's disease. *Clinical and Laboratory Haematology*, **6**, 307–323.

Vehar G. A., Keyt B., Eaton D. *et al.* (1984). Structure of human factor VIII. *Nature*, **312**, 337–342.

Wood W. I., Capon D. J., Simonsen C. C. *et al.* (1984). Expression of active factor VIII from recombinant DNA clones. *Nature*, **312**, 330–337.

Chapter 24

ACQUIRED DISORDERS OF HAEMOSTASIS

S. J. MACHIN

The normal haemostatic process is carefully balanced so that haemorrhage is promptly arrested and inappropriate thrombosis does not occur. There are numerous causes of acquired defects of haemostatic failure and these are often associated with multisystem disease, drug therapy or particular physiological events such as pregnancy, in the newborn infant or in old age. The initial problem is to recognize a bleeding tendency clinically and then to define the defect by specific laboratory tests before the appropriate prophylactic or therapeutic measures can be instigated.

A careful clinical history and physical examination should be undertaken and the initial difficulty is often to determine whether bleeding is due to a local factor, such as a peptic ulcer, or to an underlying haemostatic defect. In particular, continual oozing from venepuncture and drip sites, extensive petechiae and bruising at pressure areas or the site of recent intramuscular injections, and steady blood loss from postoperative drainage tubes are often signs of impending haemostatic failure. Paradoxically, patchy skin cyanosis with the later development of superficial gangrene of the limbs or face may signify a consumptive coagulopathy before excessive clinical bleeding is apparent.

Initially a series of simple laboratory screening tests which are easy to perform and give reliable results quickly should be undertaken. A suggested widely available screening procedure is given in Table 24.1. The normal range for each test performed in the particular laboratory involved should be known before any results can be interpreted. If the screening tests suggest an abnormality, further specialized investigations such as specific coagulant factor assays and immunological studies should be carried out to define precisely the defect and its severity. The technical details of these various tests will not be discussed as these are available in numerous practical manuals. Specific acquired disorders of platelets have been covered in Chapter 22 and will only be briefly mentioned in this section when they are involved in the various causes of generalized haemostatic failure.

HAEMOSTASIS IN THE NEWBORN

Haemorrhage and thrombosis occur relatively frequently in the sick neonate, particularly if the infant is premature. Coagulation testing is technically difficult and very often only 1 ml of plasma is available for analysis, although umbilical vein samples are suitable. Micromethods have to be developed for routine screening and specific factor assays. Due to liver immaturity, which is more marked in the premature infant, deficiencies of the vitamin-K dependent clotting factors (II, VII, IX, X, proteins C and S), the contact factors, plasminogen and antithrombin III regularly occur. However, even in the extremely premature infant, coagulant levels of the factor VIII complex, factor V, fibrinogen and platelets are within the normal adult range. Approximate ranges for the haemostasis screening tests and specific factor assays of premature and full-term infants are shown in Table 24.2.

Of particular concern is the development of vitamin K deficiency or disseminated intravascular coagulation (DIC), and because premature infants have less reserve to compensate for decreased procoagulant levels they can very easily develop clini-

Table 24.1

Laboratory screening tests for haemostatic defects

Platelet count
Bleeding time

Prothrombin time
Thrombin time
Activated partial thromboplastin time

Assessment of fibrinogen (titre or Clauss)*
Euglobin lysis time

*see p. 596.

cal bleeding, often associated with other pathological conditions.

VITAMIN K DEFICIENCY

The K vitamins bring about the γ-carboxylation of the glutamic acid residues at the amino-terminal domain of the vitamin-K dependent clotting factors. Factors II, VII, IX and X are thereby able to bind calcium ions and thus become biologically active in the coagulation mechanism. The carboxylation process is a post-translational process of the rough endoplasmic reticulum of the normal hepatocyte. Vitamin K_1, known as phylloquinone, is only produced by plants whereas the components of vitamin K_2, the menaquinones, are only synthesized by micro-organisms. Vitamin K is fat soluble and is absorbed in the upper part of the small intestine in the presence of bile. Most of the absorbed vitamin K passes to the hepatic cell but liver stores are always relatively low with a short half-life of only a few days. It is now possible to quantitate serum vitamin K levels by high-pressure liquid chromatography (HPLC) techniques, and normal levels in fasting healthy adults range between approximately 150 pg/ml and 800 pg/ml. Patients with vitamin K deficiency or who are receiving vitamin K antagonists such as the oral 4-hydroxycoumarin anticoagulants (i.e. warfarin) are unable to γ-carboxylase the K-dependent coagulation proteins fully. Inactive precursors with reduced carboxylation of the glutamic acid residues of these factors are then released into the circulation. These have been termed PIVKAs (protein induced by vitamin K absence or antagonism).

Laboratory diagnosis of vitamin K deficiency or antagonism is usually determined by prolongation of the prothrombin time with a normal thrombin time but with decreased coagulant factor assays of factors II, VII, IX and X. However, the prothrombin time is relatively insensitive to the early stages of vitamin K deficiency and the appearance of abnormal non- or under-γ-carboxylated PIVKAs such as descarboxyprothrombin (PIVKA II) can now be detected by sensitive immunoassays utilizing specific antibodies to abnormal undercarboxylated prothrombin molecules. Decarboxyprothrombin and other PIVKAs are not found in plasma samples from normal persons with normal vitamin K stores.

Proteins C and S are also γ-carboxylated by vitamin K in the liver cell and act as natural

Table 24.2

Haemostasis screening tests and factor assays in premature infants and term infants compared to the normal adult range

	Premature infant (28–34 weeks)	Term infant (38–41 weeks)	Normal adults
PT (seconds)	16–20	14–17	12–14
TT (seconds)	15–24	14–18	12–14
APTT (seconds)	50–65	40–50	30–40
Factor IX (%)	15–20	20–40	50–200
Factor VII (%)	20–60	35–70	50–200
AT III (%)	25–35	45–75	80–120

PT, prothrombin time; TT, thrombin time; APTT, activated partial thromboplastin time; AT III, antithrombin III.

anticoagulants by inhibiting the active forms of factors V and VIII:C. Protein C has a short half-life of 8–12 hours, so that when vitamin K deficiency or antagonism first develops, for example 2–6 days after the initiation of warfarin therapy, active protein C may be significantly reduced and induce a hypercoagulable prothrombotic state before the coagulant level of the other vitamin-K-dependent factors are significantly decreased. Clinically this may present with extensive skin necrosis due to dermal capillary thrombosis.

Haemorrhagic Disease of the Newborn

Neonatal bleeding occurring shortly after birth may be due to a deficiency of the vitamin-K dependent coagulation factors. To prevent this the prophylactic administration of 1 mg vitamin K_1 intramuscularly within 24 hours of birth should now be standard practice. Approximately 20–30% of cord blood samples from healthy full-term infants have detectable levels of descarboxyprothrombin (PIVKA II), which is indicative of vitamin K deficiency. Among full-term infants not given vitamin K_1 at birth, 50–60% become PIVKA II positive at 3–5 days of age, with raised levels compared to birth and significant lengthening of the prothrombin time. In contrast, following vitamin K_1 administration only 10% are PIVKA II positive when 3–5 days old. This latent deficiency of the vitamin-K-dependent clotting factors is caused by insufficient dietary intake of vitamin K and the very low liver stores of vitamin K at birth. Neonatal bleeding can also result from impaired production of the core protein of the vitamin-K dependent and other coagulation factors by the hepatocyte due to liver immaturity. This is more marked in premature infants, particularly when associated with generalized sepsis. These infants have a prolonged prothrombin time with reduced coagulation factor levels which do not respond to vitamin K_1 administration and do not have raised PIVKA II levels.

A baby's vitamin K supply depends on the vitamin K content of the milk and the amount of milk given. Maternal breast milk contains a considerably lower amount of vitamin K than formula or cow's milk. This may be responsible for severe haemorrhagic events, particularly spontaneous ventricular haemorrhages, which may occur in breast-fed infants aged 2–6 weeks due to latent vitamin K deficiency occurring beyond the perinatal period

Vitamin K Deficiency in Gastrointestinal Disorders

The minimal daily requirement of vitamin K in humans is in the order of 0.1–0.5 $\mu g/kg$. Patients with obstructive jaundice invariably develop a prolonged prothrombin time due to decreased synthesis of the γ-carboxylated vitamin-K dependent clotting factors. Absence of bile salts in the small intestine virtually abolishes the absorption of vitamin K. Other malabsorption states will also cause various degrees of vitamin K deficiency. This is particularly likely to occur in coeliac disease and after major surgical resection of the small intestine. Minor degrees of subclinical vitamin K deficiency, very often with a normal prothrombin time but reduced serum vitamin K levels and the presence of abnormal PIVKAs in the circulation, may be found in many chronic gastrointestinal disease states. For example, patients with inflammatory bowel disease, ulcerative colitis, tropical sprue, cystic fibrosis and intestinal fistulae may all develop vitamin K deficiency. This is often associated with an inadequate dietary intake. As well as being at risk from vitamin K deficiency, patients with poor nutrition are also liable to develop multiple vitamin deficiencies, particularly of vitamin C and folic acid which will also predispose towards a haemorrhagic tendency.

Patients receiving total parenteral nutrition will require weekly vitamin K supplements although a fat-soluble vitamin mixture such as Vitlipid once a week, which contains 0.15 mg of vitamin K, is usually adequate. However, antibiotic therapy may increase the vitamin K requirements of these patients to 10 mg per week to maintain a normal prothrombin time.

Broad-spectrum antibiotics, particularly the oral non-absorbable ones, have all been widely reported to cause vitamin K deficiency. However, the mechanism by which this occurs is unclear. It is widely quoted that these antibiotics inhibit the production of vitamin K_2 by the gut bacterial flora by suppressing bacterial growth in the bowel. Whilst the intestinal bacteria, mainly *Escherichia coli* and *Bacteroides* species, do produce menaquinones, this occurs mainly in the large intestine and there is no convincing evidence that these compounds are absorbed in the large intestine by humans. Only vitamin K_2 (menaquinones) present in dietary sources have been shown to be significantly absorbed.

All these gastrointestinal causes of vitamin K deficiency can be prevented by an intravenous injection of 10 mg of vitamin K_1 once per week.

Vitamin K Antagonists

The oral anticoagulants (coumarin and phenindione derivatives) are competitive inhibitors of the vitamin K–epoxide reductase enzyme complex. Their mode of therapeutic action is to decrease the availability of reduced vitamin K in the hepatocyte and thus inhibit the γ-carboxylation of the K-dependent clotting factors. The clinical indications and control of oral anticoagulant therapy are discussed in Chapter 25. A major complication of oral anticoagulation is haemorrhage due to overdosage. The usual therapeutic range for oral anticoagulant control using the prothrombin time test is an international normalized ratio (INR) of between 2.0 and 4.0. However, control is often erratic and there are numerous drugs which can increase or decrease the biological effect of oral anticoagulants. Table 24.3 summarizes most of the common drugs which interfere with oral anticoagulant control. When a patient has an increased INR of >4.0 without any clinical bleeding event, it is usually sufficient to stop anticoagulant therapy for one or two days and then to restart with a lower regular dosage. If the INR is increased to between 4.0 and 7.0 and is associated with minor haemorrhagic episodes such as mild haematuria or skin ecchymoses, a small dose of between 0.5 mg and 2.0 mg of vitamin K_1 should be given intravenously as well. Following an intravenous dose of vitamin K_1, effective liver cell synthesis of γ-carboxylated clotting factors does not begin for 6 hours and is not maximal until 24–36 hours later. If a larger dose of vitamin K_1 such as 10 mg is administered, it excludes the reintroduction of effective oral anticoagulation for approximately the next 2 weeks. If the INR is increased above 7.0 or there is a major clinical haemorrhagic episode, it is essential to shorten the prothrombin time immediately by an infusion of fresh frozen plasma

Table 24.3

Commonly used drugs which interfere with oral anticoagulant control (see also Table 25.5, p. 687)

*Drugs which **increase** the effect of coumarins*
Reduced coumarin binding to serum albumin
  phenylbutazone
  sulphonamides

Decreased rate of coumarin breakdown
  cimetidine
  allopurinol
  tricyclic antidepressants
  metronidazole
  sulphonamides

Alteration of hepatic receptor site for drug
  thyroxine
  quinidine

Decreased synthesis of vitamin-K factors
  high doses of salicylates
  cephalosporins with NMTT side-chains

Antiplatelet agents
  non-steroidal anti-inflammatory drugs
  dipyridamole
  aspirin

*Drugs which **depress** the action of coumarins*
Accelerate coumarin metabolism by inducing hepatic
    microsomal enzyme activity
  barbiturates
  rifampicin
  glutethimide

Enhanced synthesis of clotting factors
  oral contraceptives
  stanozolol

or factor IX (prothrombin complex) concentrate as well as giving vitamin K_1.

Recently, certain cephalosporin antibiotics containing an N-methyltetrazole side-chain (such as latamoxef and cephamandole) have been shown occasionally to cause a prolonged prothrombin time. These antibiotics inhibit liver cell vitamin K–epoxide reductase activity and thus act like mild oral anticoagulants. Especially in situations with marginal vitamin K stores and intake, clinical bleeding episodes may occur. These can be readily corrected by vitamin K_1 administration.

DISSEMINATED INTRAVASCULAR COAGULATION

Disseminated intravascular coagulation (DIC) occurs due to inappropriate and excessive activation of the haemostatic process. This is initially present in a compensated state when the process produces no clinical symptoms and can only be demonstrated by laboratory tests. In the subacute or chronic form there is a slow activation of the haemostatic system with spontaneous bruising rather than major clinical bleeding episodes. If the triggering factor is severe enough, the clinical syndrome of uncompensated acute DIC will result with a generalized haemorrhagic state and/or end-organ failure following blockade of the microvasculature by thrombus formation.

The major clinical problem and presenting feature of acute DIC is bleeding. This may manifest itself as generalized bruising, especially over dependent areas and pressure sites, or there may be generalized oozing or even more profuse bleeding. In surgical practice this may occur during the operative periods, especially in situations involving extracorporeal circulations, massive blood transfusions and complicated prolonged procedures. Usually, however, it presents in the immediate 24-hour postoperative phase, often whilst the patient is in an intensive care unit. The bleeding occurs from venepuncture sites, around intravenous lines, from the surgical incision and in-dwelling drainage tubes and may also be generalized throughout the gastrointestinal tract, from the oronasopharynx with pulmonary haemorrhage and from the urogenital tract. In obstetric units, postpartum bleeding from the vagina may be particularly severe. In approximately 5–10% of cases microthrombotic lesions are present initially as clinical features. These usually present with gangrene of the fingers or toes. Fibrin thrombi are most commonly observed in the microarterioles of the renal glomeruli and may cause acute renal failure. A variety of thrombotic skin lesions, including purpura fulminans, gangrene, acrocyanosis and haemorrhagic bullae, may result from dermal capillary thrombosis. The involved vessels and surrounding tissue show necrosis and haemorrhage. Platelet–fibrin thrombi in the pulmonary vasculature may cause the acute respiratory distress syndrome or shock lung. Transient central nervous system disturbances are also common due to focal ischaemia.

Pathogenesis

The potential underlying triggering mechanisms are numerous, but DIC may be initiated in three basic ways.

1. Stimulation of the coagulation cascade by the entry of tissue thromboplastins containing a high phospholipid concentration into the bloodstream. This occurs following extensive tissue trauma during surgery, by dissemination of malignant tissue and during an acute intravascular haemolytic episode (i.e. following an incompatible blood transfusion).

2. Severe endothelial injury of the vessel wall will cause platelet activation and activation of the coagulation cascade, mainly by the intrinsic pathway. This occurs in patients with Gram-negative septicaemia due to released endotoxins, with virus diseases, following extensive burns, and may be exacerbated by prolonged hypotension, hypoxia or acidosis.

3. Direct induction of platelet activation. This can occur primarily in septicaemic and viraemic states and by antigen–antibody complexes. Platelet activation will also result secondarily from vessel wall endothelial damage and following thrombin generation by the coagulation cascade.

The final consequence following activation of the coagulation cascade is fibrin formation. Fibrinogen is a glycoprotein with a molecular weight of 340 000. It consists of a dimer with two identical subunits. Each subunit has three polypeptide chains termed Aα (mol. wt 66 500), Bβ (mol. wt 52 000) and γ (mol. wt 46 500). Thrombin cleaves sequentially fibrinopeptides A and B from the Aα and Bβ chains forming fibrin monomers. These monomers spontaneously polymerize to form the fibrin clot. Factor XIIIa then catalyses the formation of new peptide bonds between the chains of adjacent fibrin molecules, followed by cross-linking of the chains. This stabilizes and increases the tensile strength of the fibrin clot. Circulating plasminogen is incorporated into the fibrin clot. Excessive fibrin strands and aggregates of activated platelets will cause partial blockage initially of the arterial microcirculation.

Fibrin–platelet plugs act rather like a fine-mesh sieve and passing red cells are traumatized, leading to distorted fragmented microcytic red cells and a resultant intravascular haemolytic process.

Following intravascular thrombosis there is a localized secondary activation of the fibrinolytic pathway in an attempt to limit thrombus formation and to begin the repair process by lysing the formed platelet–fibrin plug. Tissue-type plasminogen activator (tPA) is released locally from the vascular endothelium at sites of fibrin deposition and binds readily with plasminogen incorporated into the fibrin–platelet clot. Plasmin generated in the fibrin clot is protected from the inhibitory action of α_2-antiplasmin. If an excessive generalized release of tPA occurs, plasmin generation is initially rapidly neutralized by plasmin–α_2-antiplasmin complexes. Following the decrease in non-complexed α_2-antiplasmin, generalized free plasmin generation occurs leading to lysis and breakdown of circulating fibrinogen as well as that of preformed cross-linked fibrin. Progressive degradation of fibrinogen leads to the formation of the core fragments D and E via the intermediate fragments X and Y. These reactions are simplistically shown in Figure 24.1. The lysis of fibrin also leads to the formation of a variety of cross-linked complexes including D–D dimers which differ antigenically from fibrinogen breakdown products. Raised levels of circulating fibrin complexes and fibrin/fibrinogen degradation products (FDPs) inhibit the action of thrombin and inhibit platelet function by binding to the platelet membrane. Free plasmin also non-specifically cleaves a variety of peptides with arginyl–lysine

bonds, including factors V and VIII and the first component of complement.

Due to continual excessive fibrin formation, liver cell synthesis of the coagulation factor proteins is unable to compensate fully for their consumption. This causes decreased circulating levels of all the coagulation factors but particularly of factors V, VIII, XIII and fibrinogen. Similarly, bone marrow megakaryocyte production of platelets is unable to maintain a normal platelet count and thrombocytopenia results. A combination of coagulation factor deficiency, thrombocytopenia and the inhibitory actions of raised FDPs causes the generalized and continuing bleeding tendency. These pathogenetic mechanisms are summarized in Figure 24.2

Associated Diseases

The main causes of DIC encountered in clinical practice in the UK are shown in Table 24.4. Approximately 60% of clinical cases of DIC are associated with a septicaemic infection, with Gram-negative bacteria being the most frequent organisms. Severe haemorrhage and hypovolaemic shock may occur acutely in pregnancy, usually related to labour. During the latter months of pregnancy there already exists an hypercoagulable state with increased activity of all the coagulation factors, particularly factor VII, a slight lowering of antithrombin III activity and decreased overall fibrinolytic activity. These changes are consistent with local placental activation of the coagulation system, with fibrin deposition occurring to some

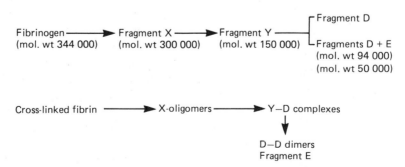

Fig. 24.1. *Schematic representation of the progressive degradation products of fibrinogen and cross-linked fibrin.*

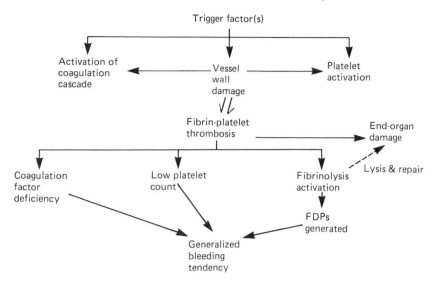

Fig. 24.2 *Pathogenesis of acute DIC.*

extent in normal pregnancy. Abruptio placentae, amniotic fluid embolus, intra-uterine fetal death and sepsis associated with abortion or premature rupture of the membranes are the most frequent obstetric emergencies to be complicated by acute life-threatening DIC. In patients with abruptio placentae, entrance of cellular elements of decidua and placenta with thromboplastin-like activity into the maternal circulation from the retroplacental area causes generalized coagulation and platelet activation. Similarly, in amniotic fluid embolism, the entrance of meconium and fetal squamous cells from the amniotic fluid into the maternal circulation activates the haemostatic system.

Malignancies of various types can lead to serious DIC. This is usually associated with metastatic disease, particularly with carcinoma of the pancreas, lungs and stomach. DIC can also occur in all the various forms of leukaemia but has a high incidence in association with the hypergranular form of acute promyelocytic leukaemia. It is triggered by the breakdown of the abnormal promyelocytic blast cells and the entrance of the thromboplastic granular material into the circulation following the initiation of cytotoxic chemotherapy during remission induction. Following surgery for carcinoma of the prostate there is an increased risk of local urogenital and generalized bleeding. This is predominantly due to the release

from prostatic tissue or metastatic lesions of material with plasminogen activator activity. Initially this causes local then systemic primary fibrinolysis but secondary DIC may also be present.

Laboratory Diagnosis of Acute DIC

In the acute state of DIC it is essential to demonstrate the abnormal laboratory parameters accurately and quickly so that the appropriate therapy can be instigated. Ideally the results of the screening tests should be available within 30 minutes after the laboratory receives the sample. To demonstrate depletion or consumption of clotting factors and platelets, the presence of intravascular haemolysis and the degree of the process, the following simple tests should be performed: haemoglobin, platelet count, thrombin time, prothrombin time and an assessment of clottable fibrinogen. The main abnormalities are reflected by a prolonged thrombin time, hypofibrinogenaemia and thrombocytopenia. A fibrinogen level below 1.0 g/l (normal range 1.5–4.0 g/l) and a platelet count below $100 \times 10^9/l$ are regarded as virtually diagnostic, especially if associated with a generalized bleeding state. Although patients will also have decreased levels of other coagulation factors, particularly factors II, V and VIII, specific factor assays, apart from that of fibrinogen, are of limited immediate value.

Table 24.4
Main causes of DIC encountered in clinical practice

Infections	Septicaemia
	Viraemia
	Protozoal (malaria)
Malignancy	Especially when disseminated, metastatic carcinomas
	Leukaemia, especially acute promyelocytic
Obstetric disorders	Septic abortion
	Abruptio placentae
	Eclampsia
	Amniotic fluid embolism
	Placenta praevia
Shock	Extensive surgical trauma
	Burns
	Heat stroke
Liver disease	Cirrhosis
	Acute hepatic necrosis
Transplantation	Tissue rejection
Extracorporeal circulations	Cardiac bypass surgery
Severe blood transfusion reaction	ABO-incompatible transfusion
Certain snake bites	
Vascular malformations	
Extensive intravascular haemolysis	

The thrombin time is prolonged by a deficiency of clottable fibrinogen, elevated FDP levels which inhibit thrombin activity or the presence of circulating heparin. The thrombin time acts as the best practical guide to the clinical significance of raised FDPs and a low fibrinogen level. A prolonged thrombin time more than double the control time is usually indicative of impending overt clinical bleeding and support therapy should be instigated.

Secondary fibrinolytic activity causes raised levels of circulating fibrin complexes and fibrin degradation products (FDPs). Plasma containing the earlier formed high molecular weight FDPs (fragments X and Y) and fibrin complexes can be detected by the so-called paracoagulation tests which rely on gel formation after exposure to ethanol or protamine. These tests, although simple, are unreliable as non-specific positive reactions frequently occur. Commercial kits to detect FDPs are now readily available and are more reliable as rapid screening tests. Levels above 100 μg/ml are usually found in acute DIC (normal values less than 10 μg/ml). However, some patients with severe DIC have no elevation of FDPs due to a general inhibition of their fibrinolytic response. These patients have a particularly poor prognosis due to irreversible organ failure. More sophisticated radio-immunoassays of specific FDP fragments (i.e. fragment X and D–D dimers) have recently become available and may be useful in the diagnosis of the chronic compensated form of DIC without overt clinical symptoms.

The basic haemostatic abnormalities encountered in acute DIC have been outlined above. More sophisticated and time-consuming tests, often only available in the specialist haemostasis unit, may be useful in the diagnosis of the early stages of compensated subacute DIC before excessive haemorrhage occurs. Platelet activation can be detected by raised plasma levels of the platelet secretory products such as platelet factor 4, β thromboglobulin and thromboxane A_2. Increased coagulation factor activation and thrombin generation are indicated by raised levels of fibrinopeptide A (the small peptide released from the N-terminal end of the Aα chains of fibrinogen initially by thrombin) and decreased levels of the two main inhibitory proteins antithrombin III and protein C.

Secondary activation of the fibrinolytic system is detected by depletion of plasminogen and α_2-antiplasmin levels and raised levels of the peptide Bβ 15–42 (released by plasmin-induced lysis of fibrin) and plasmin–antiplasmin complexes. Recently an acquired type II von Willebrand's disease defect has been described in patients with acute DIC with absence of the high molecular weight vWF multimers. This is possibly caused by cleavage of the vWF multimers into smaller forms by excessive proteolytic enzyme activity with plasmin- or calcium-activated proteases.

Reduced levels of plasma fibronectin also occur in acute DIC, and fibronectin levels have been reported to correlate with elevated fibrin degradation products and reduced antithrombin III levels. It is probable that fibronectin is deposited in the intravascular thrombi, through cross-linkage mediated by factor XIIIa with fibrin, and also has an increased consumption as a non-specific opsonin, especially in septicaemic states. Decreased fibronectin levels further impair the clearance of infective organisms and other foreign material by the reticuloendothelial system and may impede correction of the pathogenetic triggering factors.

Management of Acute DIC

Certain aspects of the management of acute DIC are extremely controversial and several widely different approaches are advocated. The first essential, if at all possible, is to eliminate the precipitating trigger factors. Wide-spectrum antibiotics (usually an aminoglycoside and a β-lactam penicillin) must be given intravenously and shock should be vigorously treated to maintain the blood volume and to avoid excess vascular stasis, hypoxia or acidosis. In obstetric situations rapid complete evacuation of the uterus may be life saving. However, in the presence of widespread uncontrollable bleeding, specific replacement therapy should be immediately instigated.

Fresh frozen plasma (FFP) contains all the coagulation factors and the main inhibitors, antithrombin III and protein C, in near normal quantities, and 4–5 units (approximately 200 ml/unit) should be rapidly infused. The FFP will also act as a valuable plasma expander. Cryoprecipitate, which contains all components of the factor VIII complex as well as fibrinogen, factor XIII and fibronectin in concentrated form, is a useful additional component, and 5–10 units should be infused initially along with the fresh frozen plasma. Platelet concentrates are the third essential blood component, and 5–10 units should also be infused as soon as they are available. As soon as this initial replacement therapy with FFP, cryoprecipitate and platelet concentrates has been given, a further blood sample should be taken to reassess their effect on the haemostatic process by repeating the simple screening tests. During this initial period, packed red cells should be transfused to maintain the haematocrit above 0.30 and the blood volume should be maintained with human plasma protein fraction or crystalloid solution. These products do not contain any viable coagulation factors or platelets. The various factor IX (prothrombin complex) concentrates and specific fibrinogen preparations should not be used as they may potentiate the microvascular thrombotic tendency. In particular, the various factor IX concentrates have been shown to contain variable amounts of activated coagulation factors including factors Xa and IXa which may enhance local fibrin deposition.

Following repetition of the haemostatic screening tests, further replacement therapy should be judged by the response of the thrombin time, fibrinogen level, platelet count and degree of clinical bleeding. The use of heparin therapy in DIC remains controversial. Reports of both benefit and marked deterioration are present in the literature. As a general guideline, heparin should only be used after initial adequate replacement therapy has failed to control excessive bleeding. If used, a low-dose continuous intravenous regimen using an automatic pump should be started of between 500 and 1000 units per hour with continuing replacement therapy. However, in certain specific situations, clinical trials have shown early low-dose continuous heparin therapy to be clearly beneficial. These include before and during induction therapy for acute promyelocytic leukaemia, the early stages of amniotic fluid embolism and immediately a severe incompatible blood transfusion (i.e. an ABO mismatch) has been recognized to have occurred.

The use of fibrinolytic inhibitors, such as EACA or tranexamic acid, should not be considered as this may result in the failure to remove fibrin thrombi from important organs such as the kidney.

During acute DIC there is also a rapid consumption of antithrombin III and protein C. These are the two main physiological inhibitors of inappropriate activation of the coagulation cascade. Antithrombin III inhibits mainly activated factor X and thrombin, whereas heparin considerably augments this activity. Recent reports of specific replacement therapy with antithrombin III concentrates have been encouraging and should now be considered in severe cases if available. In certain circumstances where platelet activation is the main pathogenetic factor, specific inhibition of platelet activation with an intravenous infusion of prostacyclin may be useful, particularly to maintain pulmonary and renal function.

LIVER DISEASE

All the coagulation factors and their main inhibitors are produced by the hepatocyte, whereas the synthesis of factor VIII:C probably occurs in different cells of the liver as well as in other organs. In addition, the liver synthesizes plasminogen and α_2-antiplasmin and is responsible for the clearance of activated coagulation factors through the activity of the reticuloendothelial system.

Bleeding is a major complication of acute and chronic liver disease and cirrhosis. This is usually multifactorial and the overall severity of the problem can be readily assessed by the simple screening tests for haemostasis. In hepatic cell failure there is defective synthesis of all the coagulation factors, apart from factor VIII:C, levels of which are usually increased. To distinguish pure hepatocellular damage from vitamin K deficiency the level of factor V activity is a good indicator. A prolonged thrombin time is frequently encountered in chronic liver failure and may be caused by hypofibrinogenaemia, dysfibrinogenaemia or raised levels of fibrin degradation products. Hypofibrinogenaemia is due to reduced hepatic synthesis and usually is a relatively late complication of cirrhosis. Dysfibrinogenaemia is the synthesis of an abnormal fibrinogen molecule with an increased sialic acid content. The removal of fibrinopeptides A and B appears normal but fibrin polymerization is delayed. Primary hepatocellular carcinoma is associated with the synthesis of aberrant proteins, including α-fetoprotein. Dysfibrinogens and descarboxyprothrombin (PIVKA II) due to defective γ-carboxylation of prothrombin not due to vitamin K deficiency may also occur in hepatoma patients. To confirm that a prolonged thrombin time is caused by a dysfibrinogenaemia, a clotting time using the snake venom Reptilase or Arvin instead of thrombin to activate fibrinogen should be performed. These enzymes only remove fibrinopeptide A and this exaggerates the polymerization defect and also corrects for any heparin which may inadvertently be present in the plasma sample. It has been claimed that assays of factors XIII, V and plasminogen are of prognostic value in patients with chronic liver disease but these are probably no more reliable than the simple screening tests.

In acute fulminant hepatitis of infectious or toxic aetiology, similar defects of the coagulation factors are found. Because of the short half-life of factor VII activity (3–6 hours), this shows an early decrease in acute liver failure and levels below 10% have been shown to be associated with a very poor prognosis. Conversely, subsequent increases in factor VII activity can be considered as an early sign of recovery.

Disseminated intravascular coagulation may occur in both acute and chronic liver failure. This is related to the increased activation of clotting factors due to the release of thromboplastic material from the damaged liver and reduced concentrations of the main inhibitory proteins antithrombin III, protein C and α_2-antiplasmin. In addition there is impaired removal of activated clotting factors and increased fibrinolytic activity. The diagnosis and therapy of DIC have been outlined previously in this chapter. Thrombocytopenia and platelet dysfunction will occur in DIC but may also occur in liver failure alone. This may be exacerbated by hypersplenism or other aetiological factors such as alcoholism of folate deficiency. Patients with cirrhosis or certain metastatic malignancies (i.e. of the breast or ovary) may develop large disabling amounts of ascitic fluid in the peritoneal cavity. Shunting procedures such as a Levene shunt to divert the ascitic fluid back into the vascular circulation are often associated with a chronic DIC state. This is related to the thromboplastic nature of the mesothelial cells and macrophages in the ascitic fluid.

The therapy for bleeding problems encountered in liver disease should be correlated with any abnormalities found in the haemostatic screening tests. Very often major haemorrhagic events, such as bleeding oesophageal varices, are encountered in the presence of virtually normal laboratory tests. These patients do not respond to haemostatic replacement therapy. Obviously vitamin K_1 should be given if there is any evidence of vitamin K deficiency, but if there is no response after 2 days' therapy with 10 mg daily, this should be discontinued. Fresh frozen plasma supplies all the missing clotting factors but will never completely correct the prolonged prothrombin and thrombin times in hepatocellular failure and problems with fluid overload may arise. The use of prothrombin complex concentrates may be helpful but it is important to use one containing factor VII activity if this is available on account of the short half-life of factor VII activity. Platelet concentrates should be given to correct thrombocytopenia and platelet dysfunction disorders. Fibrinolytic inhibitors should not generally be used as they may predispose to intravascular coagulation. The use of heparin in DIC-like states has not been shown to be helpful in liver disease. The development of extracorporeal columns for the treatment of acute liver failure

potentially causes further haemostatic defects. This leads to further thrombocytopenia, platelet function defects and haemodynamic problems related to vasoactive amine release from the activated platelets. Prostacyclin infusion during charcoal perfusion reduces the incidence and severity of these problems. Before a liver biopsy can be performed a prothrombin time test is mandatory. Only if the prothrombin time is within 4 seconds of the control value can this procedure be performed without an increased risk of haemorrhagic complications occurring.

HAEMOSTATIC DEFECTS ASSOCIATED WITH MASSIVE TRANSFUSIONS

When the patient's blood volume is replaced by the administration of large quantities of stored banked blood in a short period of time, haemorrhagic manifestations are liable to follow. In previously healthy individuals, clotting factor deficiency is unlikely to occur until 80% of their original blood volume has been replaced. Stored whole blood contains approximately 10% functional factor V and VIII, 20% factor XI, variable reduced levels of the other coagulation factors and no viable platelets. If plasma-reduced red cells or red cells collected into an optional additive solution are transfused, further dilution of coagulation factors will occur. Obviously additional infusion of crystalloids or human albumin preparations such as PPF or one of the artificial colloid substitutes will also cause further dilution of coagulation factors and platelets. These dilutional effects should be anticipated and, in adults, 2 units of fresh frozen plasma and 5 units of platelet concentrates should be administered with every 8–10 units of stored blood or equivalent infused fluid. The various available red cell preparations may also precipitate disseminated intravascular coagulation owing to a combination of partial activation of clotting factors and breakdown of platelets, leucocytes and red cells releasing thromboplastin-like material during storage. There is also evidence that platelet function may be impaired in the massively transfused patient.

To maintain blood volume during the acute stages of hypovolaemic shock, large volumes of synthetic colloids such as dextrans, gelatin solutions or hydroxyethyl starch or human albumin solutions are frequently infused. In addition to their simple dilutional effect on all the coagulation factors and platelet count, they may further interfere with and inhibit haemostasis to variable degrees. Dextran has been shown to accelerate the action of thrombin on fibrinogen (thus shortening the thrombin time), to reduce the plasma levels of vWF:Ag and vWF and induce an acquired von Willebrand's disease and, due to absorption onto the platelet surface, cause decreased platelet adhesiveness and aggregation by steric blockage of the surface membrane receptors. These defects are additive and dose dependent and may significantly prolong the bleeding time and activated partial thromboplastin time and predispose to clinical bleeding episodes. Similarly, hydroxyethyl starch, due to its macromolecular properties, will induce a slight shortening of the thrombin time and similar factor VIII defects in vitro, but these effects are of negligible clinical significance with infused volumes of up to 1500 ml. Human albumin solutions infused in large volumes have also been shown to inhibit haemostasis further, possibly by decreasing hepatic protein synthesis or due to the presence of prekallikrein activator in the infused solution stimulating fibrinolysis. The modified gelatins, although adsorbed onto the platelet surface, do not induce any inhibitory haemostatic defect. However, gelatin solutions have been shown to decrease plasma fibronectin levels significantly and to inhibit fibronectin function by gelatin–fibronectin interactions. This may potentially decrease the opsonization of noxious material and subsequent phagocytosis by the reticuloendothelial system and delay early wound healing and cross-linkage of fibrin by factor XIIIa.

EXTRACORPOREAL CIRCULATIONS

Cardiopulmonary bypass surgery is frequently associated with laboratory abnormalities but only rarely now is their associated excessive peri- or postoperative bleeding related to specific haemostatic defects. The causes of postoperative bleeding include thrombocytopenia, functional platelet defects, coagulation factor deficiencies, inadequate heparin neutralization, and disseminated intravascular coagulation. Most clinical problems arise in patients with preoperative liver dysfunction due to venous congestion, a raised haematocrit over 0.55 or following repeat coronary artery grafting. Heparinization is achieved by a loading dose of 200–300 units of heparin per kilogram followed by additional boluses as required. Control of heparin dosage is usually performed in theatre by means of an activated clotting time (ACT) using the Hemocron. An ACT of between 400 and 600 seconds maintains adequate anticoagulation. At the end of the bypass procedure the heparin effect is reversed by a slow infusion of protamine sulphate. Approximately 1 mg of protamine neutralizes 100 units of heparin. Excess protamine can itself predispose to clinical bleeding by producing a consumptive coagulopathy. Following initial adequate heparin neutralization, the reappearance of active heparin in the bloodstream may occur 2–6 hours later. This rebound effect is caused by the delayed return of sequestered extravascular heparin, which occurs when peripheral perfusion improves, and possibly also the release of some free heparin from bound heparin–protamine complexes. Thrombocytopenia to some degree occurs in all patients undergoing bypass surgery due to platelet damage in the pump and oxygenator system. However, with the continual improvement in the use of non-thrombogenic material in the bypass equipment, this is now rarely severe. Partial platelet activation with release of α-granule contents with associated platelet aggregation defects and a prolonged bleeding time also occurs to some extent during all bypass procedures. These functional defects correct themselves within 1 hour after termination of bypass. Severe postbypass thrombocytopenia of $< 50 \times 10^9/l$ and more persistent functional defects occur in patients having prolonged complicated operations and bleeding can be controlled by the infusion of platelet concentrates. It has recently been shown that the infusion of DDAVP or aprotinin may preserve platelet function and reduce postoperative bleeding in high-risk cases. Haemodilution of clotting factor levels by the priming fluid and the use of stored bank blood and consumption in the pump system occur to a variable degree, and fresh frozen plasma may be required postoperatively.

RENAL DISEASE

In acute and chronic renal disease there is often a bleeding tendency associated with several haemostatic disorders. These are most frequently related to a prolonged bleeding time caused by thrombocytopenia, an acquired platelet function abnormality or severe anaemia. These disorders are reviewed in Chapter 22. However, variable coagulation factor abnormalities do occur and are detected by moderate prolongation of the coagulation screening tests. Deficiency of the vitamin-K-dependent factors occurs due to vitamin K deficiency related to malnutrition, antibiotic therapy or uraemic enteritis or results from associated liver impairment with factor V deficiency in addition.

Isolated deficiencies of factors IX and XII have been reported in the nephrotic syndrome and are related to an excessive urinary loss of these proteins. Conversely, thromboembolic complications frequently occur in nephrotic patients and are related to antithrombin III and plasminogen deficiency secondary to excess urinary excretion.

There is generally an increased incidence of low-grade compensated DIC in renal disease, often related to intraglomerular fibrin deposits. Fibrinolytic activity is variable, with reports of both an overall decreased response and increased local glomeruli activity. Patients receiving regular haemodialysis with heparin anticoagulation may develop subnormal antithrombin III levels related to prolonged heparin therapy. This further predisposes to low-grade DIC.

Levels of fibrinogen and the factor VIII complex are frequently raised in chronic renal disease. There is often a disproportionate rise in vWF and vWF:Ag activity in comparison with factor VIII:C levels. This may be related to episodes of acute vascular injury and may become a useful marker to detect allograft rejection or cyclosporin toxicity following renal transplantation.

Defects in the factor VIII complex have also been associated by some reports with the bleeding tendency in uraemia. Selective deficiency of larger factor VIII:vWF multimers results in impaired platelet adhesiveness and a prolonged bleeding time despite the generally raised levels of vWF:Ag usually encountered. This may explain the successful treatment of uraemic bleeding in some instances by cryoprecipitate or DDAVP infusions.

MICROANGIOPATHIC HAEMOLYTIC ANAEMIA AND THROMBOTIC THROMBOCYTOPENIC PURPURA
(see also pp. 196, 198, 605)

Thrombotic thrombocytopenic purpura (TTP) is a multisystem disease characterized by fever, fluctuating central neurological abnormalities, progressive renal failure, microangiopathic haemolytic anaemia and thrombocytopenia. A microangiopathic haemolytic anaemia is present in virtually all cases with numerous bizarre fragmented red cells on the peripheral blood film. Peripheral thrombocytopenia is accompanied by marked marrow megakaryocytic hyperplasia and a shortened platelet survival. A coagulation screen and fibrinogen level usually show only minimal changes and so distinguish these cases from disseminated intravascular coagulation (DIC). However, some cases of severe TTP with extensive haemolysis or septicaemia may be further complicated by the added features of DIC. Several biochemical changes reflect intravascular haemolysis with elevated bilirubin and lactate dehydrogenase (LDH) values. Repeated monitoring of LDH levels is a useful assessment of changes of the degree of haemolysis and disease progression. TTP is not a single disease entity but a clinical syndrome which has been associated with systemic lupus erythematosus, other connective tissue disorders, pregnancy, oral contraceptives and related to drug therapy with several compounds including cyclosporin and mitomycin. In addition, in certain rare instances there seems to be a familial association and recurrent episodes or relapses have also been reported. However, in the majority of cases there is no known causal event or associated disease process. It is found in both sexes at all ages with a slight predominance in females and a peak incidence between 30 and 40 years of age.

Pathologically there are intravascular thrombi consisting of platelet aggregates and fibrin in capillaries and precapillary arterioles, predominantly involving the pancreas, adrenals, brain, heart, and kidney. The haemolytic uraemic syndrome (HUS) overlaps considerably with the clinical and pathological features of TTP but is often preceded by an acute infective illness which may be epidemic in nature and the intravascular thrombi are usually confined to the kidneys. HUS is seen most frequently in children, varies considerably in its severity and has a much lower mortality rate than adult TTP. However, it is believed that the pathogenesis of both conditions is similar, only differing in the distribution of the thrombotic lesions. The pathogenesis of the diffuse microvascular thrombosis remains unknown. Presumably the initiating event is inappropriate platelet adhesion, aggregation and release on the microarterial endothelial surfaces.

Several workers have shown that plasma from patients with TTP and HUS lacks a prostacyclin stimulatory factor and thus postulate that deficiency of such a factor was primarily responsible for reduced vascular PGI_2 synthesis and release and the initiation of platelet thrombi. Subsequently, in support of this hypothesis, it has been reported that cultured endothelial cells have decreased PGI_2 production in the presence of TTP plasma compared to normal plasma. PGI_2 is an unstable compound with a half-life in vitro of 2–4 minutes at a pH of 7.4, but when incubated in human plasma the half-life has been reported to be stabilized for up to 2 hours. It has been suggested that plasma contains an active compound, other than albumin, which prolongs the activity of PGI_2 and that deficiency of this stabilizing factor will lead to reduced PGI_2 levels and thus favour platelet deposition and microvascular thrombosis.

It has also been demonstrated that the plasma from some patients with TTP induces aggregation of both normal and TTP platelets. Normal plasma contains an IgG which inhibits the platelet-aggregating factor of TTP plasma, whereas IgG purified from TTP plasma fails to inhibit this platelet-aggregating activity. It is therefore proposed that deficiency of an IgG which inhibits a platelet-aggregating factor present in normal plasma is responsible for inappropriate and excessive platelet activation in some cases of TTP. Another related finding is the report of unusually large VIII:vWF multimers in plasma from patients with acute HUS and TTP. It is postulated that vascular damage causes release of factor VIII:vWF with an abnormal multimer pattern and that these abnormal multimers cause secondary platelet agglutination to the exposed subendothelium.

Therapy of TTP and HUS in the past has largely been empirical, but with some basic understanding of the pathogenesis of this condition having recently emerged, a more reasoned approach can now be adopted. Because both are uncommon disorders and the use of multiple agents in severe cases of the disease is frequently employed, assessment of therapy is difficult to define accurately. Supportive therapy for acute renal failure and antibiotic prophylaxis should be instigated when appropriate.

Infusion of fresh frozen plasma should be started immediately after the diagnosis is confirmed. The initial limitations to continual plasma infusions are the hazards of volume overload and the length of time required to infuse a large volume. It has been proposed that a plasma infusion would provide the so-called important plasma factor which is presumably deficient. There is also evidence that cryoprecipitate infusions may be helpful in selected cases with factor VIII complex abnormalities. Approximately 60–70% of patients respond to plasma infusions, showing initially an improvement in neurological status followed by a spontaneous increase in the platelet count and a progressive decrease in the serum LDH levels. There seems to be very little correlation between disease severity and response rate. Those patients responding to plasma infusions exhibit a wide range in the volume infused and the duration the infusions should continue for.

Plasmapheresis on a cell separator and replacement with fresh frozen plasma should be instituted for all patients not responding to plasma infusions alone after 48 hours, or earlier if the facilities are readily available or if the disease is becoming rapidly progressive. This allows 2–3 litres of plasma to be replaced daily with each exchange. Reported response rates are slightly improved, ranging from 60% to 80% using an intensive plasma exchange and replacement regime. It is possible that the removal of a platelet-aggregating factor provides an additional benefit of exchange over simple plasma infusions. When replacement solutions other than plasma have been used, such as artificial volume expanders or human albumin fractions, the results have been very disappointing.

Although a significant number of patients will be severely thrombopenic with spontaneous bleeding and purpura, the use of platelet concentrate infusions should be avoided. There are reports that platelet infusions may accelerate the disease process and these are consistent with the view that intravascular platelet aggregation is probably the initiating event.

The management of the small number of patients who do not respond to plasmapheresis and plasma replacement is extremely difficult. As local prostacyclin deficiency may be the primary defect at the vascular sites of platelet thrombi formation, an intravenous infusion of prostacyclin may be helpful in refractory cases. There have also been reports of the successful use of low-dose vincristine infusions in such circumstances.

The role of oral antiplatelet agents is difficult to assess. Used alone they probably do not affect the underlying mechanisms causing the disorder. However, they do appear to supplement plasma exchange in some reports and may be a useful form of maintenance therapy to prevent relapse. The ideal oral antiplatelet regimen is also undetermined, but low-dose aspirin or dipyridamole, 400–600 mg daily in divided doses, is the most widely used.

ACQUIRED INHIBITORS

Acquired inhibitors or circulating naturally occurring anticoagulants can be classified into two pathological groups. The first group comprises autoantibodies to specific coagulation factors and may develop in patients with congenital defects of coagulation or may arise de novo in people who were previously haemostatically normal. The second group comprises anticoagulants which act against certain activation complexes in the coagulation cascade and usually inhibit interactions which occur on phospholipid surfaces. The initial laboratory diagnosis of these conditions is usually suspected by the finding of a prolonged prothrombin time, activated partial thromboplastin time or thrombin time. The prolonged clotting time is not appreciably corrected by the addition of various proportions of normal plasma. Usually antibodies

against specific coagulation factors produce a progressive inhibitory effect on prolonged incubation whereas the anticoagulant type of inhibitors produce a maximal immediate effect.

Specific Coagulation Factor Inhibitors

Specific antibodies have been reported against factors VIII:C, VIII:vWF, V, IX, XII, XIII and fibrinogen. Approximately 5–10% of patients with haemophilia A develop an IgG antibody against factor VIII:C. This is more likely to occur in severe haemophiliacs but does occasionally develop in patients with mild forms of haemophilia but only following exposure to human blood products. An antibody with similar properties occurs rarely in non-haemophiliac patients associated with rheumatoid arthritis, other collagen disorders and skin conditions, syphilis, drug sensitivity reactions (particularly penicillin), postpartum, or sometimes in elderly persons for no apparent reason. The clinical and laboratory features of haemophiliacs with inhibitors are discussed in Chapter 23. Non-haemophiliac patients present with severe and persistent bleeding lesions, usually from the gastrointestinal or genitourinary tract, skin bruises or postoperative incisions with wound haematomas. Many antibodies which develop in non-haemophiliac patients show complex reaction kinetics with initial rapid inactivation of factor VIII:C activity which then slows down but does not plateau. This suggests dissociation of the immune complex or that the immune complex retains some biological VIII:C activity. This renders conventional Bethesda-type inhibitor assays unreliable indicators of disease state or treatment response. The treatment of bleeding episodes involves replacement therapy with high doses of factor VIII concentrates, often in association with regular plasma exchange on a cell separator. If this fails to control the bleeding episodes, regular 6–8-hourly infusions of an activated prothrombin complex concentrate (i.e. FEIBA or Autoplex) or polyelectrolyte porcine factor VIII concentrate may help. Generally steroid therapy or immunosuppressive drugs are not helpful in the acute situation but may be beneficial for the long-term management of patients with chronic haemorrhagic events.

Autoantibodies to factor VIII:vWF occur even less frequently, either in patients with congenital von Willebrand's disease or as acquired events related to other immunological or lymphoproliferative disorders. These antibodies are usually precipitating and act specifically against vWF:Ag, inhibiting the formation of the high molecular weight oligomers and ristocetin cofactor activity. Factor VIII:C activity is reduced to a variable extent. However, in many cases of acquired von Willebrand's disease, specific immunoglobulin inhibitors cannot be detected. Treatment of bleeding events is similar to that employed with factor VIII:C inhibitors although cryoprecipitate infusions should also be used as a source of the high molecular weight multimers of factor VIII:vWF which are absent from most factor VIII concentrate preparations. Some patients will also respond to an infusion of the desmopressin DDAVP (desamino D-arginyl vasopressin).

Inhibitors to the other coagulation factors occur exceedingly rarely. They may be associated with lymphoproliferative disorders, specific drug therapy (i.e. streptomycin and factor V inhibitors, isoniazid and factor XIII inhibitors) or following recent blood transfusion. In view of the rarity of these cases, the effects of specific therapy are difficult to assess, although regular high doses of replacement therapy for the factor inhibited using cryoprecipitate, fresh frozen plasma or a prothrombin complex concentrate in conjunction with plasma exchange should control any bleeding episodes.

Lupus-Type Anticoagulant

The lupus-type anticoagulant non-specifically prolongs the activated partial thromboplastin time. This type of anticoagulant occurs relatively frequently in patients with systemic lupus erythematosus but also has been reported in association with other collagen disorders. More detailed studies have shown immune complexes that inhibit reactions occurring on phospholipid surfaces (i.e. the platelet membrane), such as factor X activation, to be responsible. The exact frequency of this type of anticoagulant has probably been underestimated in the past, but heightened awareness has resulted from the use of more sensitive tests such as the dilute Russell's viper venom test, kaolin clotting time and anticardiolipin assay. Paradoxically this laboratory finding is associated with a thrombotic tendency rather than a haemorrhagic diathesis (see Chapter 25). Occasional cases have been reported with bleeding episodes but these are usually associated with thrombocytopenia related to immune-mediated platelet destruction or specific inhibitory activity against prothrombin. In the absence of thrombocytopenia, surgical operations and invasive procedures can be performed safely without any special precautions in patients with a lupus-type anticoagulant.

VASCULAR DISORDERS

A diagnosis of a vascular defect is usually suspected when bleeding is confined to the skin and mucous membranes and the standard laboratory screening tests show no abnormality. The tourniquet (Hess) test may be positive and occasionally the bleeding time will be prolonged. Bleeding is usually minor with an easy bruising tendency and spontaneous bleeding from small vessels, and is commonly seen in elderly people. The underlying defect is in the vessel wall which may be structurally weak or suffer damage due to inflammatory or immune processes, or in the supporting connective tissue.

Senile purpura is the commonest cause of an easy bruising and bleeding tendency in elderly people, being present to some extent in approximately 30–40% of patients over 70 years of age when admitted to hospital. This is a benign condition in which purpuric spots appear spontaneously on the extensor surfaces of the forearms and hands and also on the face and neck. These spots tend to coalesce, giving the skin a reddish purple colour which may remain for several weeks, often leaving a brown stain when they eventually disappear. The lesions develop because the small skin capillary vessels lack the support of subendothelial collagen fibres which atrophy as part of the ageing process. This is associated with loss of supporting subcutaneous fat and elastic fibres which renders the vessels very fragile and liable to leakage of blood following the slightest touch or shearing stress. A similar form of purpura is seen in Cushing's syndrome and following excessive steroid administration. Steroids also cause atrophy of dermal connective tissue. If the purpuric bruising is widespread, it is important to exclude any other defect in the haemostatic system and avoid any form of steroid administration which will only exacerbate the bruising tendency. There is no specific therapy apart from avoiding excessive trauma and ensuring the patient is well nourished.

The severely malnourished or alcoholic patient may present with gingival bleeding, perifollicular skin haemorrhages and widespread purpura caused by vitamin C deficiency. This will cause defective collagen formation, making the skin capillary vessels more fragile, and abnormal platelet function predisposing to a bleeding tendency. This is easily corrected by regular vitamin C replacement therapy.

Damage of the vascular endothelium can be associated with infections, drug reactions and anaphylactoid purpura (Henoch–Schönlein syndrome). A variety of infective agents during the septicaemic or viraemic stage cause purpura by direct endothelial injury, an autoimmune process or toxin-mediated damage. Organisms most frequently responsible are meningococci, streptococci and salmonella. A wide variety of drugs have been reported to cause a vasculitis by a type III hypersensitivity mechanism (i.e. penicillins, sulphonamides, thiazides), and purpura develops due to changes in vessel permeability. A specific drug can be proved responsible by a positive patch test result. Henoch–Schönlein purpura presents with purpura on the extensor aspects of the limbs often associated with abdominal pain and arthralgia. Renal impairment with microscopic haematuria and albuminuria occurs in approximately 50% of cases. It usually affects young children but may occur at any age. The process is mediated by IgA complexes which become fixed on the vessel wall. There is often a preceding upper respiratory tract infection or certain triggering factors such as insect bites or food allergy. Steroid therapy may give symptomatic relief and dapsone may control the cutaneous lesions. The dysproteinaemias including macroglobulinaemia, cryoglobulinaemia, multiple myeloma and amyloid may all present with vascular purpura. This results from infiltration of the abnormal protein into the endothelium and perivascular tissues causing vascular weakness.

Occasionally patients present with excessive bruising for which no apparent cause can be found. In these circumstances one should always be aware of the possibility of the psychiatrically disturbed person inflicting self-injury or of relatives or other people in close attendance repeatedly mistreating them. Self-administration of oral anticoagulants, usually in paramedical personnel, with a variable effect on the prothrombin time may also cause a bizarre bleeding disorder which may be difficult to diagnose.

SELECTED BIBLIOGRAPHY

Bowie E. J. W., Sharp A. A. (1985). *Haemostasis and thrombosis.* London: Butterworths.

Bull H. A., Machin S. J. (1987). The haemostatic function of the vascular endothelial cell. *Blut*, **55**, 71–80.

Chesterman C. N. (Ed.) (1986). Thrombosis and the vessel wall. *Clinics in haematology*, Vol. 15 (2). London: W. B. Saunders.

Machin S. J. (1984). Clinical annotation—Thrombotic thrombocytopenic purpura. *British Journal of Haematology*, **56**, 191–197.

Machin S. J., Schey S. (1986). Disseminated intravascular coagulation. *Surgery*, **1** (33), 781–784.

Mishler J. M. (1984). Synthetic plasma volume expanders—their pharmacology, safety and clinical efficacy. *Clinics in Haematology*, **13**, 75–92.

Moia M., Mannucci P. M., Vizzotto L., *et al.* (1987). Improvement in the haemostatic defect of uraemia after treatment with recombinant human erythropoietin. *Lancet*, **ii**, 1227–1229.

Ruggeri Z. M. (Ed.) (1985). Coagulation disorders. *Clinics in haematology*, Vol. 14 (2). London: W. B. Saunders.

Shepard K. V., Bukowski R. M. (1987). The treatment of thrombotic thrombocytopenic purpura with exchange transfusions, plasma infusion, and plasma exchange. *Seminars in Hematology*, **24**, 178–193.

Verstraete M., Vermylen J., Lijnen R., Arnout J. (1987). *Thrombosis and haemostasis.* Belgium: Leuven University Press.

Chapter 25

THROMBOSIS AND ANTITHROMBOTIC THERAPY

P. B. A. KERNOFF

Despite recent developments in our understanding of the mechanisms, diagnosis, prophylaxis and treatment of venous and arterial thrombosis, these diseases remain major medical problems, particularly in countries with advanced economies.

The effects of a thrombus depend upon its extent, its location and the events which follow its formation. Venous thrombosis occurs particularly in the calf veins and the main venous channels of the lower limbs. Many venous thrombi remain symptomless, are confined to the calf and undergo lysis, organization or recanalization, while others propagate in the main veins and produce symptoms due to venous obstruction or pulmonary embolism. An important late effect of venous thrombosis is venous insufficiency due either to permanent obstruction of veins or to incompetence of valves, producing the post-thrombotic syndrome. Arterial thrombosis produces its effects mainly by obstructing arterial blood flow and causing infarction of tissue, but non-occlusive thrombi in large arteries may embolize to cause distal obstruction. Thrombi occurring on prosthetic heart valves or in the chambers of the heart also produce their effects mainly by embolization. Multiple thrombi in the microcirculation give rise to the clinical and laboratory features of disseminated intravascular coagulation.

PATHOGENESIS OF THROMBOSIS

Probably, mechanisms of thrombosis differ according to the part of the vascular system that is involved. Increasing understanding of these pathogenetic mechanisms is having a growing impact on therapy. Venous thrombosis in the deep veins of the leg (DVT) probably originates in most cases in the venous saccules in the calf or in valve pockets in the femoral vein, areas where stasis of blood or eddy currents occur. For reasons which are largely not understood, excessive local production of thrombin results in fibrin deposition and platelet aggregation, forming the nidus of a thrombus. There may be a background hypercoagulability, detectable by tests carried out on blood obtained from sites remote from thrombus formation. Probably local vessel wall damage does not contribute significantly to most cases of DVT.

Whether or not a venous thrombus propagates from its site of origin depends upon a balance of enhancing and inhibitory factors (Table 25.1). A rapid blood flow through the vessels may, by a mechanical scouring action, wash away the platelet–fibrin nidus and prevent growth of the thrombus. Furthermore, a flowing stream of blood will disperse thrombin and other activated intermediates of coagulation, and may allow the more effective neutralization of these activated factors by physiological inhibitors such as antithrombin III and protein C. Another protective mechanism is the natural fibrinolytic activity of the blood and vessel wall, which may cause fibrin to be digested as fast as it is deposited. Increased blood viscosity due either to a raised haematocrit or increased plasma concentrations of fibrinogen or globulins will result in slowing of blood flow and enhance the growth of a thrombus.

Arterial thrombosis is usually the result of atheroma causing vascular endothelial damage and exposure of components of the blood to subendothelial tissue. The sequence of events which follow is similar to that which produces haemostatic plug

Table 25.1

Factors involved in the propagation of venous thrombi

Enhancing factors
    Stasis of blood
    Increased blood viscosity
    Hypercoagulability

Inhibitory factors
    Rapid blood flow
    Activity of the calf muscle pump
    Adequate hydration
    Normal coagulation and fibrinolytic mechanisms

---

formation. Platelets fall out of the coaxial stream of blood and adhere to the vessel wall at the site of endothelial damage. Collagen activates platelet phospholipase with the production of cyclic (prostaglandin) endoperoxides, which are the precursors of thromboxane A_2, a potent platelet-aggregating substance. Prostacyclin, an inhibitor of platelet aggregation, is also produced from cyclic endoperoxides by vascular endothelium, and the balance of the interaction between the effects of thromboxane A_2 and prostacyclin may be critical in determining whether a mass of aggregated platelets continues to develop and propagate. Platelet aggregation is enhanced by the liberation of adenosine diphosphate (ADP) from damaged platelets, from the vessel walls and possibly from damaged red cells. The platelet aggregate becomes bound on its external surface with fibrin derived from plasma fibrinogen through the action of thrombin generated by local activation of the blood coagulation mechanism. Such activation may be triggered by exposure of blood to collagen, by release of thromboplastin from the vessel wall or by release of the coagulant activity of platelets.

Thrombin production also causes irreversible aggregation of platelets so that a firm platelet–fibrin mass develops. This is the nidus of the arterial thrombus. Increased platelet numbers and hyper-reactive platelets would be expected to enhance the formation of arterial thrombi, while antithrombin III, protein C, and vessel-wall fibrinolysis would act in the opposite manner.

Thrombosis occurring throughout the microcirculation may be due either to vascular endothelial damage or to blood hypercoagulability. In viraemia and bacterial sepsis, vessel wall damage is the likely mechanism, whereas in intravascular coagulation due to snake bite or disseminated carcinoma, thromboplastic material in the circulation activates blood coagulation.

DIAGNOSIS OF THROMBOSIS

Venous Thrombosis

Appropriate management of venous thrombosis depends upon correct diagnosis. Most methods of treatment carry major risks, particularly of bleeding, and it is clearly inappropriate to expose a patient to these risks if thrombosis is not present. A further problem resulting from an incorrect positive diagnosis is that of 'labelling', which may carry lifelong consequences for the patient. For example, a young woman incorrectly diagnosed as having DVT may be advised to avoid taking oral contraceptives for ever, and may be inappropriately treated with anticoagulant prophylaxis during pregnancy.

It is now well established that the diagnosis of venous thrombosis by clinical criteria alone is commonly fallacious. Probably, up to two-thirds of venous thrombi are not detected clinically, and thrombi are present only half the time when signs and symptoms suggest their presence. The classical features of clinical calf-vein thrombosis are pain and stiffness in the back of the calf with swelling of the calf and oedema around the ankle. The calf is warm and tender to pressure over the course of the posterior tibial vessels, often with a localized area of increased tenderness at the junction of the upper one-third and lower two-thirds of the calf. Homan's sign may be positive. Identical signs may be produced by excessive muscular activity or by rupture of a popliteal cyst into the calf. In the painful vein syndrome, which is more common in women, recurrent episodes of pain and tenderness in the calf occur without confirmatory evidence of thrombosis when venography is performed. In occlusive ilio-femoral thrombosis, the whole thigh and the leg become swollen and painful. Examination reveals that the affected limb is warmer to the touch and there is skin hyperaemia due to the opening up of collateral vessels. Even these signs are not diagnostic of thrombus as similar findings may be produced by external compression of the iliac veins within the pelvis.

Major pulmonary emboli usually originate from the large veins of the thigh and pelvis. However, the presence of DVT may be indicated for the first time only when the patient suffers a massive embolism. Smaller thrombi may produce transient spikes in temperature, transient cardiac arrhythmias or nonspecific shadowing in the chest radiograph with or without chest pain. Such findings in the postoperative patient or the seriously ill medical patient should alert the clinician to the possibility of venous thrombosis and pulmonary embolism despite the absence of signs and symptoms referable to the lower limbs.

The 'gold standard' for diagnosis of deep vein thrombosis is radiographic venography. However, the costs and logistic difficulties of this procedure preclude its application in many patients. Also, it is associated with a not insignificant morbidity—local pain, allergic reactions to contrast material and thrombosis induced by the procedure itself. Radioisotopic scanning, using labelled fibrinogen or other isotopes, is generally unhelpful for the detection of thrombi above the mid-thigh level, and more applicable to prospective screening rather than immediate diagnosis. Methods which detect venous obstruction, including ultrasound and impedance plethysmography (IPG), are non-invasive and of particular value in the detection of occlusive proximal thrombi. IPG in particular has been subjected to extensive formalized studies and has been shown, when used in combination with radiofibrinogen scanning, to have a sensitivity and specificity in excess of 90% in symptomatic patients. Whether its routine application in clinical practice can be expected to yield similarly impressive results is somewhat doubtful. Thermography is a non-invasive alternative to isotopic scanning and IPG. It appears to have equivalent sensitivity, but rather inferior specificity.

In short, there is no ideal method for the routine objective diagnosis of DVT. However, it is important to remember the inadequacies of clinical diagnosis, and to attempt to prove the diagnosis whenever possible by whatever investigative methods are most easily available.

Arterial Thrombosis

A full discussion of methods of diagnosis and investigation of arterial thrombotic disease is beyond the scope of this chapter. However, one fundamental point will be mentioned. This is that evidence of a dominant *thrombotic* component of many occlusive arterial diseases or events is often lacking. Clearly, drugs which modify haemostatic function cannot be expected to be therapeutically useful if haemostatic mechanisms in general, and thrombus formation in particular, are not relevant to the pathogenesis of the disease under consideration. In myocardial infarction, for example, there has been cycling opinion for many years on the question of whether thrombus formation is a primary pathogenetic event. At present, it is regarded as being so, and therapy with fibrinolytic agents therefore has got a rational basis. If, however, the dominant cause of myocardial infarction were vascular spasm, then fibrinolytic therapy would be unlikely to be of benefit, not because it did not affect the haemostatic mechanism, but because the target was wrong. As will be discussed later, lytic therapy *does* seem to be of benefit in acute myocardial infarction, which provides evidence in support of the concept that thrombosis *is* important in pathogenesis.

IDENTIFICATION OF PATIENTS AT RISK FROM THROMBOSIS

Clinical Risk Factors for Venous Thrombosis

A number of clinical risk factors for the development of venous thrombosis can readily be identified (Table 25.2). Postoperative venous thrombosis is the major clinical problem and this is more likely to occur in the aged, the obese, patients with a previous history of venous thrombosis, patients with cancer and patients in whom major abdominal and hip operations are performed. Calculated indices using simple clinical and laboratory criteria can be used to predict, with considerable accuracy, patients likely to develop postoperative DVT. Such predictive indices can be used to select patients for prophylactic antithrombotic therapy. The incidence of postoperative DVT is increased fourfold in women taking full dosage oestrogen-containing

Table 25.2
Clinical risk factors for venous thrombosis

Increasing age
Obesity
Immobility
Previous history of deep vein thrombosis
Varicose veins
Cancer
Major abdominal and hip operations
Trauma to lower limb, especially fractured neck of femur
Oestrogen therapy or contraceptive medication
Pregnancy and puerperium
Polycythaemia, haemoconcentration, increased blood viscosity
Family history of venous thrombosis

oral contraceptives, but the risk is probably much less with low dosage preparations. There is no evidence that progestogen-only oral contraceptives are hazardous in this respect. Patients with congestive cardiac failure, acute myocardial infarction and those with paralysis of one or both lower limbs are also at high risk from venous thrombosis because of venous stasis and immobility.

The incidence of deep vein thrombosis is increased during corticosteroid therapy, in paroxysmal nocturnal haemoglobinuria, sickle cell disease, autoimmune haemolytic anaemia, Behçet's syndrome, homocystinaemia and in both polycythaemia vera and secondary polycythaemia. Patients who have undergone splenectomy for blood diseases and who remain anaemic after operation are likely to develop thrombocytosis and an increased risk of thromboembolism. An unexplained observation is that postoperative venous thrombosis is more frequent in cold climates than in the Tropics. Curiously, cigarette smoking has been found in several studies to be a *negative* risk factor for venous thrombosis. Why this should be so is uncertain.

Clinical Risk Factors for Arterial Thrombosis

Risk factors for arterial thrombosis are essentially those related to the development of atherosclerosis. Hypertension, hyperlipidaemia, diabetes mellitus, gout, polycythaemia, cigarette smoking and genetic influences are all predisposing factors. Identification of the patient at risk is based on clinical assessment. Coronary risk profiles, derived from Framingham and other epidemiological studies, have been constructed for groups of persons based on sex, age, cigarette smoking habit, elevated blood pressure, high levels of serum cholesterol, glucose intolerance and electrocardiograph abnormalities. In general, the more risk factors present, and the greater the degree of abnormality of any factor, the greater the risk of coronary heart disease. These profiles allow presymptomatic assessment of apparently fit subjects and should be valuable in the counselling of individuals at risk.

HYPERCOAGULABILITY

The terms hypercoagulable state, prethrombotic state, and prothrombotic state are usually considered synonymous. They imply changes in the blood which may be conducive to thrombosis formation if additional trigger factors, such as stasis, are present. Indications of hypercoagulability may include changes in coagulation factors, platelets, the fibrinolytic system or physiological inhibitors of haemostasis which have either been proved, or are considered likely on theoretical grounds, to be pathogenetically important in thrombosis formation. A source of confusion in the literature is that some authors have broadened the concept of hypercoagulability to include any changes indicative of activation of blood coagulation in vivo, or changes which may be useful as diagnostic markers of thrombus formation.

Although it is widely accepted that changes in haemostatic factors in the blood can contribute to the pathogenesis of thrombotic disease, this concept has been difficult to prove in patients. One fundamental problem is that test abnormalities detected in *association* with thrombosis may be a result, rather than a cause, of the disease. Although such abnormalities may be useful as diagnostic markers, they do not necessarily provide information about pathogenesis or risk. To prove a causal relationship, changes in the blood need to be present *before* a thrombotic episode occurs. A widely used clinical model has been to study patients before major surgery, and then to examine the relationships between the results of preoperative blood tests and postoperative thrombosis. A second major problem in the interpretation of blood test abnormalities in thrombotic disease is that although thrombosis may occur against the background of systemic hypercoagulability, it is usually a localized disease. Therefore, tests carried out on blood samples obtained from a remote site—usually a peripheral arm vein—may well be irrelevant to the pathological processes occurring in a deep leg vein. Certainly, background 'noise' will confuse interpretation. Probably mainly for this reason, blood tests for hypercoagulability have been found to be of little use in the diagnosis of thrombotic disease. They are of much more potential value to investigate the related matters of causation and risk.

Tests for Hypercoagulability

Because activation of coagulation leading to thrombin generation and fibrin formation is considered to be of dominant importance in the initiation and propagation of *venous* thrombi, tests for hypercoagulability in this situation are largely focused upon abnormalities of coagulation and fibrinolysis. For the same reason, therapy for venous thrombotic disease is usually designed to suppress coagulation or enhance fibrinolysis. In *arterial* disease,where platelets are thought to have a more dominant pathogenetic role, tests of platelet function may be more relevant, and platelet suppressive therapy is increasingly being used instead of anticoagulants.

Tests for Activated Coagulation

There is little evidence that increased levels of unactivated clotting factors lead to an increased rate of fibrin formation, or can be used to diagnose hypercoagulability, although it is interesting to note that raised levels of factor VII and fibrinogen are predictive of an increased risk of ischaemic heart disease. However, evidence from experimental animals suggests that the presence of activated clotting factors may help to trigger thrombosis formation. In the absence of direct tests for such activated factors in the circulation—a situation which may change in the near future—a large number of indirect approaches have been taken in attempts to detect the effects of increased thrombin generation. At the most simple level, shortening of the partial thromboplastin time (PTT) is often seen in thrombotic states, and soluble polymers of fibrinogen-derived fragments can be detected using the protamine sulphate and ethanol gelation tests. Gel exclusion chromatography is a more sensitive method of detecting similar fragments, but not applicable outside the research area. The primary action of thrombin is the conversion of fibrinogen to fibrin monomer, brought about by splitting off fibrinopeptides A and B (FPA, FPB). High levels of FPA, measured by radioimmunoassay, can be detected in patients with thrombosis, or other evidence of activation of coagulation. Levels of fibrin/fibrinogen degradation products (FDPs), measured by various immunological techniques, have been known for many years to be raised in some patients with venous thromboembolism; increased concentrations indicate activation of fibrinolysis which is probably secondary to the deposition of fibrin. More recently, specific immunological tests using monoclonal antibodies have been introduced for the assay of cross-linked fibrin derivatives (D dimer, XDP). Thrombin also causes degranulation of platelets with release of intracellular constituents into the plasma. Radioimmunoassays for two of these, platelet factor 4 (PF4) and beta-thromboglobulin (BTG), are available. Levels of both can be raised in thrombotic disease. PF4 has antiheparin activity and raised levels in the circulation, a consequence, for example, of the disruption of platelets incorporated into propagating thrombi, are reflected in shortening of the heparin–thrombin clotting time.

With the possible exception of tests for XDP, which have not yet been fully evaluated, all these tests, whatever their degree of sophistication, suffer the disadvantage of a lack of specificity for thrombosis. They are therefore of limited practical value in individual patients, either as diagnostic markers or as indicators of risk.

Tests of Fibrinolysis

There is good evidence that diminished fibrinolysis can constitute a risk factor for venous thrombosis, and tests of lytic function and components can usefully form part of the laboratory investigation of the hypercoagulable state. The value of simple non-specific tests such as the euglobulin lysis time (ELT) can be enhanced by assessing the response to venous tourniquet occlusion, which provides a measure of fibrinolytic potential. Specific assays for antiplasmin, tissue plasminogen activator (TPA), and TPA inhibitor are becoming increasingly available. Rarely, congenital plasminogen deficiency or dysplasminogenaemia may present with thrombosis, and may be identified by functional, chromogenic and immunoassays. Simple screening using the thrombin and Reptilase time tests can exclude the presence of several congenital dysfibrinogenaemias which are now recognized to be causally associated with a thrombotic tendency.

Tests for Physiological Inhibitors of Coagulation

Physiological inhibitors of activated clotting factors include α_2-macroglobulin, α_1-antitrypsin, C_1 esterase inhibitor, antithrombin III (AT III), and proteins C and S. Congenital deficiencies of AT III and proteins C and S are characterized by an hereditary predisposition to thrombotic disease, which provides strong evidence in support of the concept that hypercoagulability is of pathogenetic importance in thrombosis.

Antithrombin III (see also Chapter 21, p. 582)

Antithrombin III (AT III) accounts for approximately 70% of the antithrombin activity of plasma. It is an inhibitor of serine proteases, which include factors XIIa, XIa, IXa, Xa, thrombin and plasmin, and its activity is increased markedly in the presence of heparin. Concentrations of antithrombin III may be measured by functional and immunological assays.

Congenital deficiency of AT III is inherited as an autosomal dominant trait, individuals having less than about 70% of average normal values having an increased tendency to venous thrombotic disease. The deficiency probably accounts for 2–4% of unexplained thrombosis occurring at a young age. Acquired deficiencies of AT III are not uncommon. Low values have been reported in liver disease, disseminated intravascular coagulation (DIC), nephrotic syndrome, and in association with heparin therapy. Results are variable in patients at risk from thrombosis. Some authors have reported values 10–20% lower than normal in women taking oral contraceptives while others have observed no change. Some have reported significant falls in AT III concentrations postoperatively while others have not. No consistent changes have been observed in venous thrombosis or in myocardial infarction.

Functional antithrombin activity may be measured by the ability of plasma to neutralize added thrombin or factor Xa. The activity of antithrombin is increased greatly in the presence of heparin and functional assays may be performed with and without the addition of heparin to the test system. Such functional assays are probably more relevant to the detection of hypercoagulability than are immunoassays, since patients with recurrent venous thrombosis have been described in whom immunoassay for antithrombin III was normal but functional assays were reduced. In patients with AT III deficiency, either congenital or acquired, a tendency to thrombosis can be controlled by anticoagulant therapy. AT III concentrates are available, but indications for their use are uncertain. Most commonly, they have been used in severe DIC, or for prophylaxis in AT III-deficient patients going through high risk events such as surgery or pregnancy.

Proteins C and S (see also Chapter 21, p. 585)

Proteins C and S are physiological anticoagulants which, like the procoagulant factors II, VII, IX, and X, require vitamin K for synthesis of their complete γ-carboxylated forms. Coumarin derivatives such as warfarin prevent the vitamin-K-dependent modification of these proteins, which in their unmodified forms do not function in haemostasis.

For protein C to function as an anticoagulant, it needs to be activated to protein Ca. This conversion is brought about by the combined activities of thrombin and thrombomodulin, a protein located on endothelial cells. The anticoagulant effect of protein C is due to inactivation of factors V and VIII, especially in their activated forms Va and VIIIa. The reaction is phospholipid and calcium dependent, and requires protein S as a cofactor. Protein Ca inactivates both platelet-bound and free Va and VIIIa, and may also neutralize TPA inhibitor, thereby potentially enhancing fibrinolytic activity. Protein Ca is itself neutralized by a plasma inhibitor.

Congenital protein C deficiency is usually inherited as an autosomal dominant trait, with variable penetrance. Complete deficiency of protein C may not be compatible with survival. The usual clinical picture is one of purpura fulminans, presenting within hours of birth, or massive venous thromboembolism. Protein C replacement using either fresh frozen plasma or prothrombin complex concentrates (PCCs, 'factor IX' concentrates), which contain protein C, has been reported to allow survival. Lesser degrees of protein C deficiency (e.g. levels less than about 60 u/dl) are clearly associated with an increased risk of deep vein thrombosis and pulmonary embolism, but presentation with thrombotic problems is not common until additional risk factors, such as surgery, are encountered. The deficiency probably accounts for 5–8% of unexplained venous thrombosis in patients aged less than 40–45 years. Treatment is normally with long-term oral anticoagulants, but because there appears to be an increased risk of thromboembolic problems and skin necrosis reactions when warfarin therapy is started, heparin should be begun before warfarin, and given for 4 or 5 days concurrently. Acquired deficiencies of protein C can occur in disseminated intravascular coagulation (DIC) and liver disease and, of course, with oral anticoagulant therapy.

Protein S occurs in plasma both free and bound to C4b-binding protein, an inhibitory protein of the complement system. Bound protein S is not functionally active. Partial deficiency of protein S, probably inherited as an autosomal dominant trait, is associated with a thrombotic tendency.

Immunoassays are available for both protein C and protein S, but because functional defects of protein C with normal antigenic levels have been recognized, and because immunoassays measure total rather than free protein S, application of both functional and immunoassays is required to detect deficiencies. A common problem in diagnosis is that patients referred for investigation may be taking warfarin. Comparison of levels of proteins C and S with those of other vitamin-K-dependent factors may help to elucidate whether apparent deficiencies are likely to be wholly due to warfarin therapy. Alternatively, heparin may be substituted for a short period to allow the protein C- and S-suppressing effects of warfarin to wear off.

Tests for Platelet Hyperactivity

Although platelets are undoubtedly of importance in the pathogenesis of thrombosis, there is only scanty evidence that 'hyperactive' platelets predispose to thrombosis, or that tests of platelet function can predict risk. While investigating patients with thrombosis, therefore, there is less indication to carry out tests on platelets than there is to carry out tests of coagulation or fibrinolysis. Where investigation of platelet function is considered necessary, it is usually in the context of arterial rather than venous disease.

Although there is no definite evidence that thrombocytosis per se predisposes to thrombosis, high platelet counts in patients with myeloproliferative disorders, and in some patient groups after splenectomy, have been reported to be associated with thrombosis. Therefore, a full blood count forms part of a normal workup. The most commonly used method of assessment of platelet function is aggregometry, and heightened responses to various agents have been observed in many conditions associated with increased risk of arterial thrombosis. Similarly, there are many reports of abnormalities of in-vitro adhesiveness (glass bead retention) in these conditions. Probably, the best evidence of a pathogenetic relationship between an in-vitro test and in-vivo thrombosis is the observation of spontaneous aggregation in vitro in citrated platelet-rich plasma obtained from some patients with thrombocytosis and small vessel occlusion. Both the in-vitro abnormality and the clinical ischaemia can resolve on treatment with aspirin. Tests of platelet coagulant activities have been claimed to show an association with thrombotic disease, but the relationship is weak and the tests are technically difficult. A similar situation exists with platelet turnover and survival studies, which are rarely applicable in routine clinical practice. A simple method of detecting 'in-vivo' aggregates is available, in which blood is taken directly into formalin to 'fix' any circulating aggregates. Abnormalities can be detected in many patients with occlusive arterial disease, and may sometimes be reversed by therapy with aspirin or other platelet-suppressing agents.

A problem common to all these tests is that a drug-induced reversal of test abnormality in vitro only very rarely provides evidence of likely therapeutic efficacy in vivo. This problem is fundamental to the search for new antithrombotic agents which might be beneficial in arterial disease.

Haematological Investigation of Patients with Thrombosis

Increasingly, haematologists are asked to investigate patients with thrombosis. Before embarking on what is likely to be a very costly and time-consuming exercise, it is important to establish clearly both the reasons for investigation and the questions that are hoped to be answered. The most common reasons for investigation are: (a) recurrent deep venous thrombosis or pulmonary embolism, especially while taking warfarin; (b) thrombosis at an unexpectedly young age; and (c) an apparent familial tendency to thrombosis. The most common questions are: (a) is there a haematological cause for thrombosis? (b) is the patient at risk of (further) thrombosis? and (c) is any particular treatment indicated?

Although the number of positive haematological diagnoses resulting from investigation of patients with thrombotic disorders is undoubtedly increasing, these 'pickups' still represent only a small proportion of the total patients investigated. Usually, even full investigation yields no abnormalities, and treatment in most cases remains empirical. In assessing patients prior to investigation, it is crucial to obtain a full clinical history, and to make an assessment of the security of the diagnosis of thrombosis, particularly if it is claimed to be 'recurrent'. As noted previously, diagnoses based on clinical criteria alone are notoriously unreliable. In focusing on haematological diagnostic possibilities, non-haematological factors are sometimes forgotten. Clearly, it will be very relevant to management to recognize obesity as a risk factor, or the possibilities of occult malignancy or an 'autoimmune' disorder. A positive family history, particularly if parental consanguinity is present, will increase the likelihood of a congential disorder, especially protein C deficiency. However, most cases of thrombosis are probably due to acquired defects, and a search for the presence of a 'lupus' coagulation inhibitor (Chapter 24) must always be included in laboratory workup. In the search for a diagnosis, advice on treatment tends to be neglected. It should not be, since investigation is only a small part of total management. In patients who have recurrent episodes of thrombosis while taking warfarin, for example, the answer to the patient's problem does not usually lie in the results of extensive tests. Much more often, the level of anticoagulation is inadequate, and increasing dosage with effective control is a quicker and simpler route to both patient and physician satisfaction!

A suggested profile of tests which might be used in the haematological investigation of causation and risk in a patient with a significant thrombotic problem is shown in Table 25.3.

GENERAL APPROACHES TO THE PREVENTION OF THROMBOSIS

The availability of pharmacological methods for the prevention of thrombotic disease does not obviate the need, in planning patient management, to attempt to minimize risk by other methods. Most importantly, *recognition* of increased risk by detailed history taking and consideration of clinical circumstances can go a long way towards risk reduction in individual patients provided, of course, that appropriate action is taken when increased risk has been identified. This is perhaps easier said than done, for example, on a busy surgical ward, where there may be a temptation to rely on subcutaneous

Table 25.3

Haematological tests which may usefully be applied to the investigation of causation of thrombotic disease

---

General tests and tests of coagulation
Full blood count and film, haematocrit and platelet count
Erythrocyte sedimentation rate (ESR)
Prothrombin time (PT)
Partial thromboplastin time (PTT)
Thrombin time (TT)
Reptilase time (RT)
Tests for 'lupus' inhibitor
Antithrombin III, functional and immunoassays
Protein C, functional and immunoassays
Protein S, functional and immunoassays
Heparin cofactor II

Tests of fibrinolysis
Euglobulin lysis time (ELT), with and without occlusion, or fibrin plate assays
Plasminogen, functional and immunoassays
Screening test for fibrinolytic inhibitors (e.g. urokinase sensitivity test)
Antiplasmin
Tissue plasminogen activator (TPA)
Inhibitor to TPA

Tests for platelet hyperactivity
Aggregation to low concentrates of agonists
In-vitro spontaneous aggregation
In-vivo aggregates

---

heparin prophylaxis, rather than spend time and trouble on full preoperative assessment. Such short-cut approaches to management can lead to major problems.

Any attempt to reduce the incidence of arterial thrombosis must be directed primarily at the elimination of the preventable or treatable risk factors described previously. Platelet suppressive therapy is a poor second best. For venous disease, prevention is generally more easily attainable, mainly because venous thrombosis is particularly associated with high risk events such as surgery and pregnancy, which are of limited duration and have a known starting point. Studies with the ^{125}I-labelled fibrinogen test indicate that postoperative deep vein thrombosis usually starts in the calf veins during or shortly after operation. In some cases, however, and especially when the patient has been immobile or confined to bed, DVT may be present before surgery. Immobility of the legs during operation favours stasis of blood in the venous saccules of the soleus plexus, and stasis may be accentuated by the use of muscle relaxants during anaesthesia. Poor respiratory movements in the obese and the elderly also impair venous return from the lower limbs, while prolonged venous stasis is more likely during lengthy major abdominal operations. Prophylaxis of postoperative venous thrombosis commences in the preoperative period by correcting dehydration, if present, and keeping the patient as mobile as possible. If practical, obese patients should lose weight before major elective surgery and conditions such as congestive cardiac failure should be controlled. It is probably unnecessary to suspend oral contraceptive therapy. A number of procedures have been employed during the operative procedure to reduce venous stasis. These include elevation of the legs, the wearing of elastic stockings, intermittent compression of the calf with a pneumatic cuff, and electrical stimulation of the calf muscles to cause intermittent contraction. Active leg exercises should be started as soon as the patient is able to co-operate and early ambulation encouraged. In some centres, haemodilution by phlebotomy and postoperative autotransfusion has been used as a method of reducing blood viscosity during the high risk period.

ANTICOAGULANT THERAPY

The rationale of the use of anticoagulant drugs to prevent and treat thrombotic disease is based on the assumption that blood coagulation, thrombin generation, and fibrin formation are important in the pathogenesis of thrombosis, and that inhibition of these processes will prevent initiation of thrombus formation, or growth of formed thrombi. Hence, in disorders where accelerated blood coagulation may not be a dominant pathogenetic mechanism, anticoagulants would not be expected to be of benefit. This is one main reason for the increasing tendency to use platelet-suppressive agents instead of anticoagulant drugs in some types of arterial thrombotic disease. Anticoagulant therapy can be regarded as a rather passive means of treating existing thrombotic disease because it is clearly unlikely to result in lysis or clearance of formed thrombi. Reliance is being placed on physiological fibrinolytic mechanisms to accomplish this process, which may take many weeks or months, or not occur at all.

Use of agents which either inhibit coagulation or enhance fibrinolysis is inevitably accompanied by an increased risk of bleeding and it is this risk which constrains the intensity of treatment. The ideal objective of control of anticoagulant therapy would be to achieve a level of anticoagulation at which there was a complete antithrombotic effect, but no increased risk of bleeding. This ideal is not achievable using current drugs, and recommendations for control are therefore based on a compromise between efficacy and risk. Although the risk of bleeding is clearly related to the intensity of anticoagulation, it is important to remember that serious bleeding can occur even in 'perfectly' controlled patients, particularly if other risk factors are present. In any patient being considered for anticoagulant therapy, therefore, it is essential to make a complete evaluation of risk for bleeding before starting treatment, and to avoid provoking problems by injudicious invasive procedures or the prescription of high risk medications. *Absolute* contraindications to anticoagulant therapy are few, if any. However, the list of risk factors is long, and includes pre-existing bleeding states or test abnormalities, renal and hepatic disease, surgical wounds, intramuscular injections, peptic ulceration, recent stroke, severe hypertension and advanced age. Of the many drugs which can provoke bleeding problems in patients taking anticoagulants, aspirin-containing preparations are prime offenders, and should normally be avoided.

Heparin

Heparin is a naturally occurring sulphated glycosaminoglycan with powerful anticoagulant properties, which is prepared commercially from either bovine lung or porcine intestinal mucosa. Originally, it was purified from the liver, hence its name. Heparin available for normal clinical use is not a homogeneous substance, but a mixture of polysaccharide molecules which vary in molecular weight from about 2000 to 40 000, averaging 15 000–18 000. Recently, there has been particular interest in the clinical use of small molecular weight varieties (see below). Heparin is normally available as either the sodium or calcium salt. Its anticoagulant activity reflects its ability to potentiate the inhibitory effect of antithrombin III (heparin cofactor) on the activated forms of factors XII, XI, IX, X and thrombin (factor IIa), which is achieved by accelerating the formation of molecular complexes between AT III and the activated clotting factors. Additionally, heparin probably has a direct anticoagulant effect independent of AT III. The principal clinical uses of heparin are to prevent venous thromboembolism in high risk patients, when it is usually given subcutaneously in low dosage, and to treat venous thromboembolism, when it is usually given intravenously in full dosage. The rationale of this difference in dosage is based on evidence which suggests that less heparin is needed to *prevent* thrombin generation than is needed to *neutralize* formed thrombin. The anti-Xa activity of AT III/-heparin, as opposed to its antithrombin activity, has been held to be of greater relevance to its antithrombotic effects. Whether this is in fact the case is becoming increasingly doubtful.

Low-dose Heparin Prophylaxis

Following the subcutaneous injection of 5000 units of heparin, sensitive assay techniques can demonstrate the presence of small concentrations of heparin in the plasma which peak about 4 hours after the injection and have mostly disappeared at 8 hours. There is considerable variation in peak concentrations between subjects. The peak concentration is influenced by the type of heparin, higher values being achieved with the sodium than the calcium salt.

The usual prophylactic procedure in surgical patients is to inject 5000 units of heparin subcutaneously 2 hours preoperatively and then 8–12 hourly after operation. Control by laboratory tests is not usually needed. This procedure has now become routine for major abdominal and gynaecological surgery in many parts of the world, especially for patients over the age of 45 years and those considered to be at particular risk. Many clinical trials have shown significant reductions in the incidence of postoperative venous thrombosis. Less well proven, but still very probable, are reductions in the incidence of fatal pulmonary embolism and the post-thrombotic syndrome. Low-dose heparin prophylaxis has also been shown to be effective in reducing the incidence of venous thrombosis following acute myocardial infarction and such therapy also may be indicated in other high risk medical illnesses and in patients confined to bed for long periods.

Conventional heparin prophylaxis is less effective in reducing the incidence of venous thromboembolism in patients with fractured necks of femur or those undergoing total hip replacement. In these situations, alternative possibilities are to use larger, titrated doses of heparin, controlling dosage by heparin assay based on anti-Xa inactivation or the PTT; or carefully adjusted low-dose warfarin; or a combination of fixed dosage heparin and dihydro-ergotamine, which appears to be superior to heparin alone. Of course, any of these methods should be combined with the general methods of risk reduction described previously.

Adverse effects associated with low-dose heparin

prophylaxis are uncommon, and rarely severe. In some studies, mildly increased blood loss has been noted, but this has usually only been evident on group rather than individual patient analysis. However, even this small risk is usually unacceptable in certain patients, such as those having cerebral and eye surgery, where even minimal bleeding may have serious consequences. Probably, bleeding problems are more common using 8-hourly rather than 12-hourly dosing schedules. Subcutaneous haematomas at injection sites can occur, but can be minimized by good technique. Very rarely, skin necrosis reactions can occur.

Thrombocytopenia is a well-recognized complication, which may be detected more frequently if serial platelet counts are performed during treatment. Immune-mediated and direct mechanisms have been described. Possibly, an element of heparin-associated bleeding is attributable to platelet dysfunction rather than inhibition of coagulation. Although rarely clinically significant, osteoporosis is well described and dose related. It is only likely to be encountered when therapy is continued for at least many months, for example in recurrent DVT or pregnancy.

Full-dosage Heparin Treatment

Used intravenously, heparin has an immediate anticoagulant effect, and is therefore the most usually preferred agent for the initial treatment of acute DVT and pulmonary embolism (PE). After intravenous injection, it has a very short half-life of 30–120 min. Heparin should never be administered intramuscularly because of the risk of haematoma formation. For the same reason, intramuscular injections of any sort are forbidden in a patient receiving therapeutic heparin. Heparin therapy is best given by constant infusion pump as relatively constant plasma levels can be obtained by this method. It is practical to mix the total 24–hour dose diluted with physiological saline in a 50-ml syringe and infuse at a constant rate of 2 ml per hour. A less satisfactory method is to mix the dose of heparin with 500 ml saline and infuse with a paediatric drip set. Intermittent injections through an indwelling needle are not advised as the incidence of haemorrhagic complications is significantly increased.

In the management of acute DVT/PE in an adult,

the usual practice is to inject a loading dose of about 5000 units of heparin followed by a constant infusion for 5–10 days. The initial daily dose is usually 24 000–48 000 units, depending on the patient's size and age, and the severity of the clinical problem, and dosage is adjusted up or down according to the results of laboratory tests. Usually, heparin requirements are greatest in the first few days of therapy. On about the seventh day, oral anticoagulant therapy is started to allow a 3-day overlap. The patient may be got out of bed safely by the seventh day as organization of the thrombus and fixation to the vessel wall should be well established. During mobilization, it may be necessary to provide the patient with an elastic support stocking if there is much oedema. A diuretic may help as well. The common practice of bandaging the legs serves no useful purpose. Heparin therapy does not influence the probability of post-thrombotic symptoms if the perforator veins have been rendered incompetent or if valves in the femoral vein have been involved in the thrombus.

The most widely used test for the control of intravenous heparin therapy is the partial thromboplastin time (PTT), or a variant of it, and the usual objective for therapeutic heparinization is to keep the PTT about 1.5–2.0 times the clotting time of the control plasma. Different reagents used in the PTT show marked differences in their sensitivities, and can produce a range of results on the same plasma sample. However, standardization of reagents and methodology, or the use of any of the large number of alternative tests, offers no proven advantages in controlling full-dose heparin therapy. The main problems of heparin control are not so much deficiencies in test systems, but the difficulties of ensuring a smooth delivery of the prescribed dose of drug. Without using a constant infusion pump, which has its own problems, meaningful control is difficult to achieve. This is probably one reason why heparin is a dominant cause of drug-induced morbidity in hospitalized patients.

Because of its short half-life after intravenous administration, cessation of therapy is usually all that is needed if over-anticoagulation is recognized, or bleeding problems are encountered. Neutralization by protamine sulphate is not often required and, because protamine itself has anticoagulant activity, it may carry risks if large doses are used.

Low Molecular Weight Heparin

The anticoagulant activity of heparin is a function of its molecular size. Compared with standard heparin, low molecular weight heparin of about 5000 daltons has a relatively greater capacity to potentiate the inhibition of factor Xa than it does to potentiate the inhibition of thrombin or overall clotting (as measured by PTT). Also, low molecular weight heparin tends to interact less with platelets. For both these reasons, it has been suggested that low molecular weight heparin might have advantages in therapeutic anticoagulation, in perhaps having a similar antithrombotic activity to standard heparin, but a lesser tendency to cause bleeding.

Low molecular weight heparin can be produced either by fractionation from standard heparin, or (more economically) by chemical hydrolysis. In animal studies and limited clinical trials it clearly has the capability to inhibit thrombosis formation, and it has the advantage of having a half-life after subcutaneous injection about twice that of standard heparin. Once-daily administration would clearly be advantageous. However, there is no clear evidence yet that low molecular weight heparin is associated with a lesser risk of bleeding in clinical studies, and this would be the main reason for preferring it to conventional heparin.

Oral Anticoagulant Therapy

Mechanism of Action

The oral anticoagulants consist of two classes of compounds, the coumarins and the indanediones. Only coumarin drugs are now recommended because of the more frequent side-effects of indanediones. Warfarin sodium, the most widely used agent, is the water-soluble form of the insoluble rat poison warfarin, and was named from the initials of the Wisconsin Alumni Research Foundation, where it was first synthesized.

Oral anticoagulants act by interfering with the action of vitamin K in the hepatic synthesis of factors II, VII, IX and X, which require vitamin-K-dependent gamma carboxylation of their terminal glutamic acid residues to be able to bind phospholipid and calcium ions, a reaction necessary for their conversion from inactive zymogens to active serine proteases. During oral anticoagulant therapy or in states of vitamin K depletion, inactive molecular forms of these clotting factors appear in the blood, where they may be detected by immunological methods. These abnormal proteins (PIVKA: protein induced by vitamin K absence or antagonism) have some anticoagulant effect themselves, to which not all thromboplastins are sensitive. It is unlikely, however, that sensitivity of test reagents to PIVKA is necessary for good anticoagulant control.

After warfarin ingestion, the rates at which plasma levels of the vitamin-K-dependent clotting factors fall depend on their respective biological half-lives. Factor VII activity falls first, together with protein C, which has a similar half-life (6 hours); then factor IX (24 hours), factor X (40 hours) and factor II (60 hours). Reduction in factor VII activity is the main cause of the coagulation defect in the first two days. Thereafter, a steady state reduction of all the factors is achieved. Parenteral administration of vitamin K is followed within a few hours by a rapid synthesis of active clotting factors despite the presence of the anticoagulant drug in the plasma.

Oral anticoagulant therapy is monitored by the one-stage prothrombin time (PT), or a variant of it. The optimal therapeutic range for laboratory control under different clinical circumstances has been debated for over 40 years, because it has rarely been assessed in properly designed studies. A fundamental problem until recently has been the varying sensitivities of different thromboplastins used in the PT, and the resulting non-comparability of levels of control used in different studies. Thromboplastins are usually made from rabbit, human or bovine brain. Most rabbit brain thromboplastins are less sensitive than human and bovine preparations to reductions in levels of vitamin-K-dependent clotting factors. Hence, the usually advised optimal therapeutic range for the PT in North America (2–2.5 times the control value), where rabbit brain thromboplastins are generally preferred, represents a much higher level of anticoagulation than numerically similar ranges obtained using human or bovine reagents, which have been more widely used in Europe. Until recently, a human brain thromboplastin (the Manchester Comparative Reagent, MCR) was most commonly used in the UK. Because of concerns about risks of viral contamin-

ation, however, production of this reagent has now been stopped, and most UK laboratories have adopted one of several available rabbit brain preparations. The most widely used bovine brain reagent (Thrombotest) remains popular in many laboratories.

In an attempt to overcome the problem of differing reagent sensitivities, and therefore differing therapeutic ranges for anticoagulation, thromboplastins are now assigned an International Sensitivity Index (ISI), which is assessed by comparison with a WHO international reference thromboplastin or a secondary standard derived from it. By definition, the primary reference preparation has an ISI of 1.0. Using the ISI for any particular reagent, an International Normalized Ratio (INR) can be derived from the prothrombin time ratio (PTR)— i.e. the ratio between the patient's PT and the control—using the relationship:

$$INR = PTR^{ISI}$$
or $INR = $ antilog (ISI $\times$ log PTR).

The ISI for a thromboplastin is now supplied by the manufacturer, who will normally also supply a conversion table which obviates the need to calculate INRs from PTRs. Use of the INR, rather than PTR, is now internationally recommended for expression of the degree of anticoagulation induced by oral anticoagulant drugs.

Indications

Oral anticoagulants may be used either for the prevention or treatment of thrombotic disease, and varying therapeutic ranges for the INR are recommended in different circumstances (Table 25.4). In general, evidence of efficacy is stronger for venous than for arterial disease.

Patients with deep vein thrombosis or pulmonary embolism are usually treated with warfarin for 3–6 months, the risk of recurrence being greatest in the first few weeks following the start of therapy. *Recurrent* DVT or PE, seen particularly in elderly patients with continuing ill health, immobility or obesity, is normally an indication for life-long treatment. As mentioned earlier, recurrent thrombosis which occurs *during* anticoagulant therapy usually responds to an increase in dosage, and a higher level of anticoagulation. In resistant cases, the addition

Table 25.4

Recommended therapeutic ranges for oral anticoagulant therapy (British Society for Haematology, 1984)

INR	Clinical state
2.0–2.5	Prophylaxis of deep vein thrombosis including high risk surgery (2.0–3.0 for hip surgery and fractured femur operations)
2.0–3.0	Treatment of deep vein thrombosis Pulmonary embolism Transient ischaemic attacks
3.0–4.5	Recurrent deep vein thrombosis and pulmonary embolism Arterial disease including myocardial infarction Arterial grafts Cardiac prosthetic valves and grafts

INR, International Normalized Ratio.

of antiplatelet agents such as aspirin or dipyridamole may help but use of the former agent, in particular, is accompanied by an increased risk of bleeding, and should not be considered unless the need is compelling. There is strong evidence that oral anticoagulant therapy is effective in the prevention of venous thromboembolism, especially in high risk patients undergoing surgical operations. Although formal clinical studies have shown that the risk of bleeding is very low—provided, of course, that the INR is maintained within an appropriate range (Table 25.4)—surgeons have generally been reluctant to use warfarin for routine prophylaxis, even in high risk patients.

Routine long-term anticoagulation after myocardial infarction is not now generally recommended. Although several studies have shown reduced mortality in treated patients, the difficulties of long-term dosage supervision, and the increased risks of bleeding, usually outweigh the benefits of therapy. In unstable angina, anticoagulant therapy has not been found to be beneficial. In the past, warfarin was widely used to treat transient cerebral ischaemic attacks (TIA), but there is no good evidence that such treatment reduces either the risk of recurrence or the incidence of subsequent stroke. Treatment with low-dose aspirin is now generally preferred. Although there is a lack of evidence from controlled trials, oral anticoagulant therapy probably reduces the incidence of embolism in patients

with atrial fibrillation (AF) due to mitral stenosis, thyrotoxicosis, congestive cardiomyopathy and chronic sinoatrial disease. However, it is not usually indicated in patients with AF associated with mitral valve prolapse, and is of debatable value in those with mitral stenosis who remain in sinus rhythm. The original artificial aortic and mitral valves were associated with a high incidence of thromboembolism and, even with improvements in valve design, long-term anticoagulation is usually regarded as mandatory. Tissue valve replacements, particularly of the aortic valve, are less likely to be associated with problems in this respect, and anticoagulant therapy is not normally required. Warfarin is commonly used after coronary bypass surgery, but the optimal duration of therapy, and the intensity of anticoagulation, remain to be firmly established. Usually, therapy is given for at least several months, and an antiplatelet agent then substituted. However, long-term anticoagulation, with or without antiplatelet therapy, has also been claimed to be advantageous.

Practical Aspects of Oral Anticoagulant Therapy

Whenever possible, a baseline prothrombin time and INR should be determined before the initial dose is given. Although in the past it was common practice to initiate therapy with a large loading dose, this is no longer recommended, particularly because of the risk of 'over-shooting' the therapeutic range, and consequent bleeding problems. Most usually, warfarin is started in a dosage of 10 mg daily for 3 days, but this should be reduced if the baseline PT is prolonged, if liver function tests are abnormal, or if the patient is in cardiac failure, is on parenteral feeding, is less than average weight, is particularly elderly, or is taking concomitant medication which is known to heighten the anticoagulant effect of warfarin (see below). The daily dose is best given at a fixed time in the evening and the INR determined in the morning, initially on the second and third days of treatment, then on alternate days with longer intervals once stability of dosage has been achieved. The usual maintenance dose of warfarin is 3–9 mg daily, but individual patient responses vary greatly. Occasionally patients require excessively large doses of warfarin to maintain an anticoagulant effect. Although genetic resistance to warfarin has been described, much more common reasons for apparent resistance are patient variability and non-compliance. The latter possibility, in particular, may be investigated by biochemical estimation of the plasma warfarin level. In patients receiving concurrent heparin and warfarin, the INR will usually reflect the effect of warfarin, provided that the PTT is less than about 2.5 times the control value.

When the patient's warfarin dosage is stabilized, testing intervals can be gradually extended, usually to a maximum of 8 weeks. If there is a change in the patient's clinical state or drug therapy, especially involving a drug known to interact with warfarin, the INR should be checked more frequently. In most hospitals, out-patient control of warfarin therapy is carried out in formalized anticoagulant clinics. When patients are discharged from hospital, it is important for the clinicians arranging treatment— often with several different drugs—to make sure that the patient understands the problems relating to control of anticoagulant therapy, and the risks of drug interactions and mistakes in taking the correct dosage. All too frequently, doctors prescribe for an unrelated condition which has become apparent after discharge from hospital, without recognizing that the new drug will potentiate or inhibit the level of anticoagulation. Such careless prescribing, poor laboratory control, and incorrect dosage or wrong information transmitted by telephone can lead to imperfect control, with its attendant risks of re-thrombosis or bleeding. After completion of the prescribed course of therapy, warfarin may be stopped abruptly. There is little convincing clinical or laboratory evidence of rebound hypercoagulability, and tailing off dosage over several weeks has neither a well-found theoretical nor practical basis. With patients who are aware of this time-honoured practice, however, and particularly when a request is made for its implementation, it may be prudent to acquiesce without argument!

Bleeding is the most important complication of oral anticoagulant therapy, and usually requires active intervention. It should be appreciated, however, as in patients with congenital coagulation disorders, that bleeding may not always be due to the coagulation defect alone, but may possibly be an early presenting feature of local pathology. Hence, appropriate investigation needs to be carefully considered, even if an excessive degree of anticoagulation is identified as a main causative factor. Recommendations on reversal of oral anticoagulant therapy are necessarily influenced by the degree of the laboratory abnormality, the severity of clinical bleeding, and the risks associated with vitamin K, plasma and plasma product therapy. Vitamin K, given intravenously, can completely reverse the effect of warfarin within 12–24 hours, but may render patients refractory to warfarin therapy for unpredictable lengths of time, varying from several days to several weeks. Small doses (e. g. 2.5 mg) are therefore advised. Fresh frozen plasma (FFP) will induce a more rapid and easily controllable correction of the warfarin-induced defect, but carries the attendant risk of all blood products, including those of virus transmission. Also, the large volume of FFP may be a problem in patients with cardiac impairment. The risk of disease transmission is a particular problem with prothrombin complex concentrates (PCCs, 'factor IX' concentrates), which are prepared from plasma obtained from many thousands of donors. At present, in the absence of products of proven safety in this respect, concentrates are probably best avoided for the reversal of anticoagulant therapy unless a life-threatening event is encountered.

The following recommendations are adapted from those suggested by the British Society for Haematology (1984).

INR > 4.5 without bleeding: withhold warfarin for one or more days, according to INR.

Minor bleeding: withhold warfarin and consider giving vitamin K, 2.5 mg i.v.

Major bleeding: withhold warfarin and give vitamin K, 2.5–10 mg i.v. and FFP/PCC.

Therapeutic regimens for patients taking anticoagulants who require surgery or invasive diagnostic procedures should be planned well in advance, and should not include reversal of the anticoagulant effect using either vitamin K or blood products. A preoperative check of the INR is mandatory. The 'safe' range depends on the procedure. For most operations, including dental surgery, an INR of less than 2.5 is generally recommended

Drug Interactions and Warfarin Therapy

Warfarin is almost completely absorbed after oral administration, peak plasma levels being achieved in 2–12 hours. The drug has a mean half-life of about 40 hours. At least 97% of the absorbed drug is protein bound, mainly to albumin, and it is the unbound fraction which is pharmacologically active, being metabolized through hydroxylation by hepatic microsomal enzymes. The ingestion of drugs which compete with warfarin for plasma protein binding sites will result in less of the absorbed warfarin being bound and more remaining free and pharmacologically active, thereby increasing the anticoagulant effect of the dose. Drugs which increase the activity of hepatic microsomal enzymes will result in more rapid degradation of free warfarin in the plasma, with a lessening of the anticoagulant effect, whereas drugs or agents which suppress hepatic microsomal enzyme activity will increase the anticoagulant effect. A further complication is introduced by variable intake of vitamin K, since there is competition between the oral anticoagulants and vitamin K at the liver cell site. A variable intake may be due to alterations in the diet, to the use of broad-spectrum antibiotics which have

Table 25.5
Drugs which affect the anticoagulant effect of warfarin

Drugs which increase the anticoagulant effect of warfarin
Alcohol
Antibiotics (cephalosporins, penicillin, sulphonamides, tetracyclines)
Anti-inflammatory analgesics (aspirin, indomethacin, phenylbutazone)
Oral hypoglycaemic agents (tolbutamide, chlorpropamide, phenformin)
Anti-hyperlipidaemic agents (clofibrate, cholestyramine)
Antidepressants (tricyclic antidepressants, phenothiazines)
Anabolic steroids
Allopurinol
Laxatives
Glucagon
Quinine
Thyroxine

Drugs which decrease the anticoagulant effect of warfarin
Barbiturates
Phenytoin
Glutethimide
Spironolactone
Rifampicin
Griseofulvin
Haloperidol
Oral contraceptives
(See also Table 24.3, p. 658)

an effect on gut flora, or to the use of laxatives which increase gut motility with reduced absorption of vitamin K.

These potential interactions offer a challenge to smooth anticoagulant control and indicate that careful attention must be given to the patient's dietary habits and other drug therapy. Unreliability in following instructions or inability to attend for regular blood tests is a contraindication to oral anticoagulant therapy. It is advisable to issue each patient with a booklet describing the rationale of anticoagulant therapy in simple terms and giving practical advice concerning diet, alcohol and other medications and what to do in the event of bleeding or during intercurrent infection. The booklet also serves to warn dentists or other medical practitioners who may attend the patient that he is receiving an anticoagulant drug. A patient on anticoagulants may have other medication prescribed by the hospital doctor or by his general practitioner or he may take self-medication unknown to either; furthermore, there may be a lack of communication between the anticoagulant clinic and the general practitioner. In one survey conducted by an anticoagulant clinic in a large teaching hospital, patients were taking on average three drugs prescribed by general practitioners as well as the drugs listed in the patients' records. In addition, drugs were being taken as self-medication by 35% of the men and 43% of the women. A potential drug interaction with warfarin was noted in 33% of patients with drugs supplied by prescription and in 30% of patients with drugs taken as self-medication.

A list of drugs which, when taken concurrently, may affect the anticoagulant effect of warfarin is shown in Table 25.5. The most important members of this list are alcohol, anti-inflammatory compounds and barbiturates. Alcohol ingestion prolongs the plasma clearance rate of warfarin and alcoholic indiscretions may explain the poor control achieved in a number of patients and may be the most common cause of bleeding. Aspirin, indomethacin and phenylbutazone displace warfarin from its binding to plasma protein and these agents also cause impairment of platelet function. Barbiturates are an important group of enzyme inducers which increase the rate of clearance of warfarin from the blood. On the other hand, nitrazepam and diazepam do not appear to affect warfarin requirements.

ANTITHROMBOTIC THERAPY AND PREGNANCY

Venous thrombosis is the commonest vascular complication which can arise in pregnancy or the puerperium, and pulmonary embolism is now the major single cause of maternal death associated with pregnancy. The management of thrombotic disease occurring during pregnancy, and patients receiving long-term anticoagulant therapy who become pregnant, present particular problems.

Oral anticoagulants cross the placenta and can have adverse effects on the fetus throughout the antenatal period, reducing the overall chance of a normal outcome by as much as a third in some estimates. This is as a result of spontaneous abortion, bleeding problems—the fetus is likely to be considerably overdosed at 'therapeutic' levels of maternal anticoagulation because of the immaturity of fetal hepatic enzyme systems—and warfarin embryopathy. The last is particularly associated with use of warfarin in the first trimester, features of the syndrome including saddle nose, nasal hypoplasia, low birth weight, short stature and stippled epiphyses (the Conradi–Hunerman syndrome). However, maternal exposure to warfarin in the second and third trimesters may also result in fetal abnormalities, particularly blindness, mental retardation, and other defects of the central nervous system. Some of these problems may be related to cerebral haemorrhage due to birth trauma. While it is likely that the reported incidence of complications due to warfarin therapy represent an overestimate of that which might be expected in clinical practice, oral anticoagulants are now generally avoided in pregnancy, especially in the first trimester, unless there are compelling reasons for their use. To a large extent, heparin is preferred for treatment and prophylaxis, both because it does not cross into the fetal circulation, and because its effect is short lived and can be rapidly neutralized if a bleeding complication should arise. However, administration of heparin, either intravenously or subcutaneously, is unpleasant for the patient, and there are some concerns about the risk of bone demineralization (referred to earlier), which appears to increase when larger doses are given for long periods, as may sometimes be the case in pregnancy. The need for treatment and the choice of therapy for any individual patient therefore depend upon a careful evaluation of the balance of risks. Thrombosis which is shown to be confined to the calf veins and not extending above the knee is probably *not* an indication for anticoagulant drugs.

Treatment of venous thromboembolism arising in pregnancy is initially with intravenous heparin, which usually needs to be given in higher dosage than is normally required in non-pregnant patients. A reasonable starting level is 40 000 units daily, with subsequent dosage adjustment according to the PTT. After about a week of therapy, the regimen can be changed to subcutaneous heparin 10 000 units twice daily, which may be adjusted to maintain a heparin level, measured by weekly or bi-weekly anti-Xa assay, of less than 0.3 units/ml. The patient may be taught to administer the subcutaneous injections herself. Heparin is continued through labour, and the dose reduced to about 7500 units twice daily after delivery. After about 10 days, when the risk of secondary postpartum bleeding is much reduced, most patients prefer to change to warfarin, which should be continued for about 6 weeks. Contrary to widespread belief, warfarin is not secreted in breast-milk in significant quantities and mothers receiving warfarin may safely breast-feed their babies. However, this is not the case with phenindione, which is secreted in breast-milk and should not be used in pregnancy. Treatment with any anticoagulant drug at the time of delivery precludes the use of epidural anaesthesia, which is a major disadvantage for some patients.

The use of prophylactic anticoagulants in pregnant women who have previously had venous thromboembolism is controversial, since the overall risks of a recurrence are relatively low—perhaps about 12%. One possibility is to start subcutaneous heparin only after 34 weeks gestation, which may help to reduce the risks of bone demineralization which, as mentioned earlier, are dose dependent. Alternatively, anticoagulant drugs can be used in the postpartum period only. Whether or not to embark on a course of prophylaxis depends on a careful evaluation of risks in the individual patient. In women whose past history is confined, for ex-

ample, to a single episode of calf vein DVT, and who appear to have no other risk factors, prophylactic anticoagulants throughout pregnancy are probably not justified. On the other hand, the balance of risks may be quite different in a patient who has had a major proximal vessel thrombosis in a previous pregnancy, and is overweight. Patients with 'lupus' inhibitors are at particular risk in pregnancy, both from maternal thromboembolism and from spontaneous abortion. Suppression of the inhibitor with prednisolone and antithrombotic therapy with low-dose aspirin have been claimed to reduce the fetal loss rate, though clearly steroid therapy, in particular, is not without its problems. The one situation in which warfarin is still widely advocated during pregnancy is for patients with prosthetic heart valves, or others with cardiac disease who are receiving long-term anticoagulant therapy. If a decision is made to continue warfarin, the balance of risks should be carefully explained to the patient, ideally before she becomes pregnant. One compromise is to use heparin in the first trimester, then warfarin thereafter.

THROMBOLYTIC (FIBRINOLYTIC) THERAPY

Thrombolytic therapy has potential advantages over anticoagulation in the treatment of patients with thrombosis, since it is capable of inducing dissolution of formed thrombi rather than merely preventing propagation. The more rapid removal of thrombus should not only result in a more rapid reversal of the acute effects of thrombotic disease, such as shock in severe pulmonary embolism, but also in improved prevention of longer term sequelae, such as the post-thrombotic syndrome. However, the disadvantage of thrombolytic therapy is equally apparent: thrombolytic agents are fibrinolysins, and their target is not only the fibrin contained in thrombi, but also fibrin deposited elsewhere. Maintenance of physiological haemostatic integrity is probably dependent upon a continuous process of fibrin deposition on small breaks in vessels. In some circumstances, such as after surgery, fibrin is clearly essential for wound healing and tissue repair. Use of thrombolytic drugs without due regard for risk factors for bleeding is accompanied by a serious risk of major haemorrhagic complications, and it is the perception of this risk, above all, which has constrained the wider clinical use of these agents in clinical practice.

Although proteolytic enzymes such as porcine plasmin and Brinase (obtained from *Aspergillus oryzae*) have been claimed to be effective in lysing intravascular thrombi, the most widely used agents are plasminogen activators which, by various mechanisms, convert plasminogen to the active enzyme plasmin. Both plasminogen and, to variable extents, plasminogen activators have an affinity for formed fibrin, and for effective thrombolysis to occur the conversion of plasminogen to plasmin needs to take place on the fibrin surface, where generated plasmin is protected from the inhibitory effects of circulating antiplasmin. Where therapeutic agents are relatively 'non-selective' for fibrin, because of their low ratio of activity for fibrin-bound plasminogen as compared with plasma plasminogen, conversion of circulating plasminogen to plasmin may occur to an extent at which inhibitory mechanisms are overwhelmed, and free plasmin appears in the circulation. The proteolytic specificity of plasmin is not restricted to fibrin, and degradation of fibrinogen, clotting factors V and VIII, and other plasma proteins may occur. It is held that such systemic generation of plasmin contributes to the haemorrhagic complications of thrombolytic therapy, and that agents which are more 'fibrin selective' might carry a reduced risk of bleeding. This potential benefit has yet to be proved convincingly in clinical trials. The lytic effects of the various available agents depend not only on their relative selectivities for fibrin, but also their plasma half-lives, which differ substantially.

Streptokinase

Streptokinase, the most widely used thrombolytic agent, is produced from the filtrate obtained from cultures of β-haemolytic streptococci, and invokes intense fibrinolytic activity in the blood when injected intravenously. There is a severe derangement of haemostasis manifested by a profound fall in the concentration of plasminogen, variable reductions in the levels of fibrinogen and other clotting factors, and a large increase in fibrin/fibrinogen degradation products (FDPs). Streptokinase is relatively cheap compared with other available agents, but suffers from three main disadvantages: it shares with other streptococcal proteins the ability to act as immunogen in humans; its administration may cause febrile reactions; and it is not very selective in causing activation of fibrin-bound plasminogen in preference to circulating plasminogen. Although the systemic hypocoaguable state invoked by streptokinase therapy has usually been perceived as a drawback, it may possibly be advantageous in reducing the likelihood of rethrombosis, especially in vessels with a tight residual stenosis.

Urokinase

Urokinase is either extracted from human urine or produced by the culture of fetal kidney cells. It is non-antigenic, does not cause allergic reactions, and has a greater affinity for fibrin-bound rather than soluble phase plasma plasminogen. In theory at any rate, therefore, infusion of urokinase should cause less systemic activation of plasminogen than streptokinase, and have a lesser propensity to cause haemorrhagic complications. A main disadvantage of urokinase, and the factor which has prevented its substitution for streptokinase on a wide scale, is its high cost. Its plasma half-life (16 min) is only slightly shorter than that of streptokinase (23 min).

Newer Fibrinolytic Agents

More recently developed fibrinolytic agents include tissue plasminogen activator (t-PA), single chain urokinase (scu-PA), and acylated plasminogen streptokinase activated complex (APSAC). t-PA is produced on an industrial scale by recombinant DNA (r-DNA) technology, and has a low affinity for circulating plasminogen. In the presence of fibrin, its affinity for plasminogen increases considerably, thereby conferring relative selectively. However, large doses can cause some activation of circulating plasminogen and a mild hypocoagulable state, which resolves rapidly after cessation of infusion of the drug. Possibly, this is a disadvantage compared with streptokinase. scu-PA, also manufactured by r-DNA technology, has, in contrast to t-PA, a high affinity for plasminogen but a low affinity for fibrin. The activation of plasminogen by scu-PA is inhibited by plasma, and this inhibitory effect is reversed by addition of soluble fibrin. Because of their different modes of action, t-PA and scu-PA might act synergistically. Their plasma half-lives are short, of the order of 5–8 min. APSAC has a more sustained duration of action than either streptokinase or t-PA, (half-life 90 min), and has the advantage of being administered by bolus injection. The active site on the plasminogen molecule is protected by acyl groups, but the fibrin-binding sites are unaffected. After injection, therefore, APSAC can bind immediately to fibrin. Deacylation by hydrolysis in plasma proceeds more slowly, resulting in a controlled thrombolytic effect which may be enhanced by greater fibrin binding and retention.

Clinical Use of Thrombolytic Agents

Thrombolytic drugs have been used in numerous clinical situations and there is good evidence, from radiographic studies, that they are capable of promoting a more rapid and complete dissolution of thrombus than is achievable by anticoagulant therapy. However, many uncertainties still remain about optimum dosage, duration of treatment, and precise indications. One point seems clear: lytic therapy is much more likely to be successful when started soon after the onset of symptoms. Because of their hazards, lytic agents are usually reserved for more serious clinical problems, and it is normally essential to have radiographic evidence of the thrombotic 'target' before starting treatment. However, in some circumstances, such as myocardial infarction, the logistic difficulties of obtaining such evidence may make this ideal impossible to achieve.

Lytic therapy for *deep vein thrombosis* is usually reserved for patients with major occlusive thrombi of proximal veins. There is little to suggest that an increased risk of pulmonary embolism may result from such treatment; however, the risk of embolism is not reduced below that achieved by conventional anticoagulation. In some studies, a good initial result has been followed by proven long-lasting benefit in terms of venous function and valve preservation. In *pulmonary embolism*, thrombolytic therapy is usually only considered when the degree of vascular occlusion is sufficiently major to have caused shock or impending shock. In such patients, treatment with urokinase/streptokinase for 12/24 hours has been shown to be superior to heparin in lowering the pulmonary artery pressure and improving angiographic findings. However, large-scale studies have not been able to demonstrate a difference in ultimate mortality. In both DVT and PE, cessation of thrombolytic therapy should be followed by a course of conventional anticoagulation.

Lytic therapy has been used either systemically or locally in a wide variety of other disorders, including peripheral arterial occlusion, retinal vein thrombosis, arteriovenous cannula occlusion, and priapism. Based on the belief that many cases of *acute myocardial infarction* are due to thrombosis in a coronary vessel, and that secondary thrombosis may be instrumental in causing extension of infarcted cardiac muscle, there has been fluctuating interest for many years in the possibility of using thrombolytic agents to limit heart muscle damage in myocardial infarction. The recent widespread development and availability of coronary angiography have rekindled interest in this area, because of the technical feasibility of infusing lytic agents directly into the coronary circulation, and objectively assessing the degree of thrombus dissolution. On a mass scale, however, such an approach to therapy would clearly be impracticable—more than 160 000 people die each year of myocardial infarction in Britain alone—and attention has therefore focused on mounting large-scale clinical trials of both old and new lytic agents which are administered into peripheral veins. In contrast to the somewhat equivocal data on the long-term clinical benefits of thrombolytic therapy in DVT, PE and peripheral arterial disease, results of recent studies have provided strong evidence that such treatment produces functional improvement and reduction in mortality in patients with myocardial infarction, especially when treatment is started within a few hours of the onset of pain. As a result of this evidence, use of lytic agents has become established as routine in this stiuation, and seems not unlikely to be adopted in the near future by general practitioners and ambulance crew. Current evidence on reduction of mortality relates mainly to the use of streptokinase, given intravenously in a dosage of 1.5 million units over 60 min. Other studies, now in progress, will doubtless provide data on the comparative efficacy and safety of the newer agents, ancilliary therapy, optimum dosage, and cost.

As stressed earlier, the main problem with thrombolytic therapy is not so much the question of its efficacy, but the risk of bleeding complications. As with anticoagulant therapy, the bleeding hazard is primarily related to clinical risk factors, which must be positively excluded before a decision is made to embark on treatment. Contraindications to systemic lytic therapy, some of which may be outweighed in patients with major thrombotic disease, include: a surgical procedure within the previous 10 days, including invasive biopsy, thoracentesis or paracentesis; active gastrointestinal bleeding or a condition with a high potential for bleeding; defective haemostasis indicated by laboratory tests; a recent stroke (within 2 months) or a condition such as mitral valve disease which is associated with a significant risk of central nervous system embolism; recent trauma with possible internal injuries or external cardiac massage; intracranial neoplasia; severe hypertension; hepatic or renal disease; and pregnancy. Unfortunately, several of these contraindications are also associated with an increased risk of thrombosis, and are therefore precisely those situations in which, were it not for the risk of bleeding, thrombolytic therapy might be considered appropriate.

For patients receiving treatment with lytic drugs, close clinical monitoring is essential and all invasive procedures should be avoided except carefully performed venepunctures using small needles. If arterial samples are needed, the radial or brachial arteries should be used rather than the femoral artery, and a pressure dressing applied. Control of therapy by laboratory tests is generally unrewarding, either for predicting the degree of thrombolysis or for predicting bleeding, and is unnecessary where treatment is of only short duration, such as after myocardial infarction. For longer courses of therapy, however, monitoring with the thrombin time is usually recommended, and this should be maintained at a value of between two and five times the control plasma. A value of more than five times the control suggests a need to stop therapy, which can be reintroduced at a lower dosage when the thrombin time has fallen into the 'therapeutic range'. When the course of thrombolytic therapy has finished, heparin should be started when the thrombin time has fallen to less than twice the control value, which usually takes 2–4 hours. Whatever the thrombin time, significant bleeding while receiving a lytic agent requires cessation of therapy. If bleeding is uncontrollable, antifibrinolytic treatment with tranexamic acid is indicated.

Although thrombolytic therapy can be more effective than conventional anticoagulation, it should only be administered after a very thorough consideration of its risks and benefits in the individual patient, since its indiscriminate and improper use may clearly have serious consequences.

THERAPEUTIC DEFIBRINATION

The use of snake venoms to prevent and treat thrombotic disease was suggested by clinical observations that victims of bites from the Malayan pit viper (*Agkistrodon rhodostoma*) developed severe hypofibrinogenaemia without haemorrhagic symptoms. Fractionation of the crude venom resulted in production of the purified polypeptide (ancrod, Arvin), which has now been available for therapeutic use for almost 20 years. A similar thrombin-like enzyme (batroxobin, Defibrase) is extracted from the venom of *Bothrops atrox*.

The mechanism of action of these enzymes is to split fibrinopeptide A (FPA), but not FPB, from fibrinogen. This results in an abnormal fibrin monomer which polymerizes end-to-end only to produce a friable, unstable fibrin which is not cross-linked and which has an increased susceptibility to digestion by plasmin. Following injection of either ancrod or batroxobin into the circulation, there is a rapid fall in the level of thrombin-clottable fibrinogen and evidence of stimulation of fibrinolysis—a fall in the level of plasminogen and the appearance of fibrin fragments X, Y, D and E. How fibrinolysis is stimulated is not understood. The abnormal fibrin, and its degradation products (FDP), are rapidly removed from the circulation by either reticuloendothelial phagocytosis or fibrinolysis, or both. Other coagulation factors and platelet numbers are not affected, but abnormalities of platelet function have been reported, probably due to the high concentrations of FDPs in the blood. The erythrocyte sedimentation rate commonly falls to zero and blood viscosity is reduced. Injections every 12 hours will maintain a fairly constant level of hypofibrinogenaemia.

Like anticoagulant drugs, ancrod and batroxobin are not thrombolytic and their effect would therefore be expected to be limited to prevention of thrombus formation, or thrombus propagation. Despite many clinical studies, however, their role in therapeutics remains uncertain. Probably, they have a similar efficacy to heparin in the prevention and treatment of venous thrombotic disease. They have the disadvantage of being antigenic, which may result in hypersensitivity reactions, and limit the duration and/or frequency of courses of therapy. Although the relatively benign effect of a state of 'therapeutic defibrination' is undoubted, therapy with these agents is still accompanied by an increased risk of bleeding, particularly if clinical risk factors are present. They are contraindicated in pregnancy. Studies with ancrod using subcutaneous dosing regimens have shown benefit in the prevention of deep venous thrombosis after hip surgery—a situation in which, as noted previously, conventional prophylaxis with heparin is generally less successful.

FIBRINOLYTIC STIMULATION WITH ORALLY ACTIVE AGENTS

Several drugs are known to stimulate fibrinolysis when taken by mouth in the medium to long term and some of these have been clinically evaluated in patients with thromboembolic disease. The most widely studied agents are the biguanide phenformin and the anabolic steroids ethyloestrenol and stanozolol, which probably enhance endogenous fibrinolysis by increasing both the synthesis and release of plasminogen activator in the vessel wall. Benefit has been claimed in a variety of circumstances, which include the post-thrombotic syndrome, recurrent DVT, cutaneous vasculitis, Raynaud's phenomenon and Behçet's disease. The main concern about the long-term use of these agents is the possibility of liver damage, since mildly raised serum transaminases are not uncommon. Amenorrhoea, virilization, acne and fluid retention have also been reported.

PLATELET SUPPRESSIVE THERAPY

A growing awareness of the pathogenetic roles of platelets in thromboembolic disease and atherosclerosis has focused attention on the possibility of using drugs which inhibit platelet reactivity as a means of therapeutic intervention. Very many drugs and chemical agents are capable of inhibiting platelets in vitro; very few of these have been adequately assessed in clinical trials. A major problem of such studies is that proof of therapeutic efficacy, especially in arterial disease, can often only come from trials involving several thousands of patients. Such trials are very expensive and time consuming to carry out, and there is often a problem in defining objective end-points. By the time studies have been completed, hypotheses about the scientific rationale of treatments being tested may have changed. This has been a particular problem with aspirin, which has been used in most clinical trials in a dosage much larger than would now be considered optimal.

The antiplatelet drugs which have been subjected to large-scale clinical trial, which are those used most widely in clinical practice, were not developed or introduced because of their potential antithrombotic properties—their effect on platelets was recognized at a later date. More recently available agents were developed more specifically as antithrombotics. Several of these drugs are designed to alter the balance of physiological prostaglandin metabolism which is held to be of key importance in platelet reactivity, and hence thrombogenesis. The more conventional drugs include aspirin, dipyridamole (Persantin) and sulphinpyrazone (Anturan). By inactivation of cyclo-oxygenase, *aspirin* inhibits synthesis of the two principal metabolites of arachidonic acid, thromboxane A_2 (TxA_2) and prostacyclin (PGI_2, epoprostenol). TxA_2, synthesized predominantly by platelets, is a powerful platelet pro-aggregating substance and vasoconstrictor; PGI_2, synthesized by blood vessels, is anti-aggregatory and a vasodilator. In-vitro studies have shown that vascular endothelial cyclo-oxygenase is less sensitive to aspirin than platelet cyclo-oxygenase. Hence, it has been suggested that low doses of aspirin, of the order of 30–40 mg daily or on alternate days, might be more effective than larger conventional doses in enhancing the $PGI_2 : TxA_2$ ratio, and hence have a greater antithrombotic effect. However, if aspirin has such an effect it is possible that it may not be mediated by this mechanism—it is also known, for example, to be capable of enhancing fibrinolysis and causing a reduction in activity of the prothrombin complex clotting factors. *Dipyridamole*, originally introduced as a coronary vasodilator, is now widely promoted as an antithrombotic agent. It increases inhibitory cyclic adenosine monophosphate (cAMP) levels in platelets by inhibition of phosphodiesterase. Possibly, it potentiates the effect of circulating PGI_2. The mechanism of the antiplatelet effect of *sulphinpyrazone*, a uricosuric agent, has not been fully defined. Drugs in the second category include prostacyclin itself, prostaglandin E_1 (PGE_1), agents which specifically inhibit the synthesis or activity of TxA_2, and drugs such as nafazatrom, which may both stimulate prostacyclin synthesis and retard its degradation. An alternative and attractive possibility for platelet suppressive therapy, based mainly on observations in Greenland eskimos, is to alter the balance in favour of 'antithrombotic' prostaglandin metabolites by increasing the dietary intake of various polyunsaturated fatty acids. Eicosapentaenoic acid, a precursor of PGI_3 which can be extracted from certain fish oils, has received particular attention in this respect.

Despite the large amount of effort which has been expended on clinical trials of platelet suppressive agents, there still remain major uncertainties about their indications and optimum dosage. Even without hard evidence of efficacy, however, such agents have attractive qualities which have led to their widespread use in clinical practice. Compared with conventional anticoagulants, they are much less likely to provoke serious bleeding, and they do not require laboratory control. Since firm data concerning the efficacy of anticoagulant therapy are often also lacking, it seems reasonable to opt for the safer and easier alternative. Probably, the best evidence of efficacy of platelet suppressive agents has been obtained in patients with transient cerebral ischaemic attacks (TIAs), where aspirin in doses of 300–1300 mg daily has been found to be beneficial; 300 mg daily or less is now usually preferred. In the primary and secondary prevention of myocardial infarction, there have usually been only minor differences in outcome between drug- and placebo-treated patients, and other methods of prevention

are probably superior. However, aspirin at a dosage of 324 mg daily has been reported to improve the prognosis of patients with unstable angina significantly, and at a dosage of 160 mg daily to augment the favourable effects of streptokinase after myocardial infarction. Both aspirin and dipyridamole, sometimes together with warfarin, have been reported to be of benefit in patients with prosthetic heart valves and after coronary bypass surgery. It should be noted, however, that the overall evidence supporting dipyridamole as a useful antithrombotic drug has been questioned (*Drug and Therapeutics Bulletin*, 1984). Not surprisingly, a different view is taken by the manufacturers.

The newer platelet-suppressing agents have been found to be helpful in diverse conditions, including thrombotic thrombocytopenic purpura, cardiopulmonary bypass, renal dialysis and charcoal haemoperfusion. It remains to be seen, however, whether these 'tailored' agents, or derivatives of them, will prove to be superior to the more conventional drugs which are now used so widely to treat the common occlusive arterial diseases.

SELECTED BIBLIOGRAPHY

Bell W. R., Meek A. G. (1979). Guidelines for the use of thrombolytic agents. *New England Journal of Medicine*, **301**, 1266–1270.

British Society for Haematology (1984). *Guidelines on oral anticoagulation.*

Clouse L. H., Comp P. C. (1986). The regulation of hemostasis: the protein C system. *New England Journal of Medicine*, **314**, 1298–1304.

Colditz G. A., Tuden R. L., Oster G. (1986). Rates of venous thrombosis after general surgery: combined results of randomised clinical trials. *Lancet*, **ii**, 143–146.

Collins R., Scrimgeour A., Yusut S., Peto R. (1988). Reduction in fatal pulmonary embolism and venous thrombosis by perioperative administration of subcutaneous heparin. *New England Journal of Medicine*, **318**, 1162–1173.

Crandon A. J., Peel K. R., Anderson J. A., Thompson V., McNicol G. P. (1980). Postoperative deep vein thrombosis: identifying high-risk patients. *British Medical Journal*, **281**, 343–344.

Drug and Therapeutics Bulletin (1982). Peri-operative low-dose heparin. *Drug and Therapeutics Bulletin*, **20**, 5–7.

Drug and Therapeutics Bulletin (1983). Long-term oral anti-coagulant therapy. *Drug and Therapeutics Bulletin*, **21**, 33–35.

Drug and Therapeutics Bulletin (1984). Doubts about dipyridamole as an antithrombotic drug. *Drug and Therapeutics Bulletin*, **22**, 25–28.

Glomset J. A. (1985). Fish, fatty acids, and human health. *New England Journal of Medicine*, **312**, 1253–1254.

Hirsh J. (1984). New approaches for deep vein thrombosis occurring after surgery. *Journal of the American Medical Association*, **251**, 2985–2986.

Iturbe-Alessio I., Fonseca M. D. C., Mutchinik O., Santos M. A., Zajarias A., Salazar E. (1986). Risks of anti-coagulant therapy in pregnant women with artificial heart valves. *New England Journal of Medicine*, **315**, 1390–1393.

Julian D. G., Pentecost B. L., Chamberlain D. A. (1988). A milestone for myocardial infarction. *British Medical Journal*, **297**, 497.

Lancet (1985). Treatment of coronary thrombosis (leading article). *Lancet*, **i**, 375–376.

Lancet (1986). Aspirin: what dose? (leading article). *Lancet*, **i**, 592–593.

Lancet (1988). Thrombolytic therapy for acute myocardial infarction—round 2. *Lancet*, **i**, 565–567.

Letsky E. A., de Swiet M. (1984). Thromboembolism in pregnancy and its management. *British Journal of Haematology*, **57**, 543–552.

Leyvraz P. F., Richard J., Bachmann F. *et al.* (1983). Adjusted versus fixed-dose subcutaneous heparin in the prevention of deep-vein thrombosis after total hip replacement. *New England Journal of Medicine*, **309**, 954–958.

Lipkin D. P., Reid C. J. (1988). Myocardial infarction: the first 24 hours. *British Medical Journal*, **296**, 947.

Loscalzo J., Braunwald E. (1988). Tissue plasminogen activator. *New England Journal of Medicine*, **319**, 925–932.

Mannucci P. M., Tripodi A. (1987). Laboratory screening of inherited thrombotic syndromes. *Thrombosis and Haemostasis*, **57**, 247–251.

Marder V. J., Sherry, S. (1988). Thrombolytic therapy: current status. *New England Journal of Medicine*, **318**, 925–931, 1512–1520.

Mitchell J. R. A. (1986). Back to the future: so what *will* fibrinolytic therapy offer your patients with myocardial infarction? *British Medical Journal*, **292**, 973–978.

Nilsson I. M., Ljungner H., Tengborn L. (1985). Two different mechanisms in patients with venous thrombosis and defective fibrinolysis: low concentration of plasminogen activator or increased concentration of plasminogen activator inhibitor. *British Medical Journal*, **290**, 1453–1456.

Orme M. (1988). Aspirin all round? *British Medical Journal*, **296**, 307–308.

Preston F. E., Greaves M. (1985). Platelet suppressive therapy in clinical medicine. *British Journal of Haematology*, **60**, 589–597.

Salzman E. W. (1986). Venous thrombosis made easy. *New England Journal of Medicine*, **314**, 847–848.

Salzman E. W. (1986). Low-molecular-weight heparin. Is small beautiful? *New England Journal of Medicine*, **315**, 957–959.

Sandler D. A., Martin J. F. (1985). Liquid crystal thermography as a screening test for deep-vein thrombosis. *Lancet*, **i**, 665–668.

Sherry S. (1985). Tissue plasminogen activator (t-PA). Will it fulfill its promise? *New England Journal of Medicine*, **313**, 1014–1017.

Stehbens W. E. (1985). Relationship of coronary-artery thrombosis to myocardial infarction. *Lancet*, **ii**, 639–642.

Sue-Ling H., Hughes L. E. (1988). Should the pill be stopped preoperatively? *British Medical Journal*, **296**, 447–448.

Thomas D. P. (1985). Venous thrombogenesis. *Annual Review of Medicine*, **36**, 39–50.

Topol E. J. (1987). Advances in thrombolytic therapy. *Journal of Clinical Pharmacology*, **317**, 735–745.

Verstraete M., Collen D. (1986). Thrombolytic therapy in the eighties. *Blood*, **67**, 1529–1541.

INDEX